ACE Advanced Health & Fitness Specialist Manual

The Ultimate Resource for Advanced Fitness Professionals

American Council on Exercise®

Editors
Cedric X. Bryant, Ph.D.
Daniel J. Green

ACE
AMERICAN COUNCIL ON EXERCISE

Library of Congress Catalog Card Number: 2008933559

ISBN 9781890720278

Printed in the United States of America

A B C D

Distributed by:
American Council on Exercise
P.O. Box 910449
San Diego, CA 92191-0449
(858) 279-8227
(858) 279-8064 FAX
www.acefitness.org

Project Editor: Daniel J. Green
Technical Editor: Cedric X. Bryant, Ph.D.
Cover Design & Art Direction: Karen McGuire
Associate Editor: Marion Webb
Special Contributor & Proofreader: Sabrena Merrill
Production: Nancy Garcia
Photography: Dennis Dal Covey
Anatomical Illustrations: James Staunton
Index: Kathi Unger
Chapter Models: Tricia Baglio, Doug Balzarini, Paul Chiappetta, Fabio Comana, Maria Farron, Brian Greenlee, Justis Kao, Kim Lehman, Stephanie Moody, Tracy Neff, Beckie Page, Julia Valentour, Marion Webb

Acknowledgments:
Thanks to the entire American Council on Exercise staff for their support and guidance through the process of creating this manual.

NOTICE

The fitness industry is ever-changing. As new research and clinical experience broaden our knowledge, changes in programming and standards are required. The authors and the publisher of this work have checked with sources believed to be reliable in their efforts to provide information that is complete and generally in accord with the standards accepted at the time of publication. However, in view of the possibility of human error or changes in industry standards, neither the authors nor the publisher nor any other party who has been involved in the preparation or publication of this work warrants that the information contained herein is in every respect accurate or complete, and they are not responsible for any errors or omissions or the results obtained from the use of such information. Readers are encouraged to confirm the information contained herein with other sources.

P08-007

Table of Contents

Reviewers

Lenita Anthony, M.S., is a clinical exercise physiologist and exercise specialist with more than 20 years of experience in group exercise and personal training. She is program coordinator at University of California, San Diego Extension, in the exercise science & fitness instruction certification program and an ACE-approved continuing education provider.

Liz Applegate, Ph.D., FACSM, a nationally renowned expert on nutrition and fitness, is a faculty member in the nutrition department and the director of sports nutrition at the University of California at Davis. Dr. Applegate is on the editorial board of the *International Journal of Sports Nutrition and Exercise Metabolism.* She is a member of the Sports and Cardiovascular Nutritionists, a practice group of the American Dietetics Association. She frequently serves as a keynote speaker at industry, athletic, and scientific meetings, and consults frequently for U.S. Olympic athletes and is the team nutritionist for the Oakland Raiders.

Anthony Carey, M.S., holds a master's degree in biomechanics and athletic training, the Advanced Health & Fitness Specialist certification through ACE, and is a Certified Strength and Conditioning Specialist through the NSCA. Carey is an internationally recognized expert on corrective exercise and working with clients with musculoskeletal challenges. He has authored two best-selling books, four DVDs, and is an international presenter for the health and fitness industry.

Daniel Cipriani, Ph.D., P.T., is a licensed physical therapist and a professor in the School of Exercise and Nutritional Sciences at San Diego State University. Prior to his appointment at SDSU, Dr. Cipriani served as a faculty member at the Medical University of Ohio, teaching in the Physical Therapy curriculum. His areas of teaching and research focus on musculoskeletal/orthopedic intervention and outcome measures. He has more than 20 years of clinical experience as a physical therapist in the orthopedic setting.

James G. Garrick, M.D., is an orthopedic surgeon and the founder and director of the Center for Sports Medicine in San Francisco, California. He also founded the Sports Medicine Division at the University of Washington. Dr. Garrick is a founding member and former board member of the American Orthopaedic Society for Sports Medicine and is also a clinical professor in the Department of Pediatrics at the University of California, San Francisco. Dr. Garrick serves on the editorial boards of *The Physician and Sportsmedicine, The American Journal of Sports Medicine, Medical Problems of Performing Artists,* and *The Journal of Orthopaedic & Sports Physical Therapy*, and is the editor-in-chief of *The Journal of Dance Medicine.*

Reed Humphrey, Ph.D., P.T., is professor and chair, School of Physical Therapy & Rehabilitation Science at The University of Montana in Missoula. He has served as associate editor and contributing author for numerous exercise guidelines published by the American College of Sports Medicine and the American Association of Cardiovascular & Pulmonary Rehabilitation.

Mark Jackman, Ph.D., owns Life Signs[SM], where for 12 years he has specialized in fitness programming for weight management and clients with health conditions. He obtained his doctorate at Duke University, where he did research on occupational stress and health, and has been an upper-level strategic planning manager in the health insurance industry. He is ACE-certified as an Advanced Health & Fitness Specialist, Personal Trainer, and Lifestyle & Weight Management Consultant, and by the American Academy of Health, Fitness, & Rehabilitation as a Medical Exercise Specialist. Dr. Jackman has served on ACE item writing and role delineation panels.

Mary Jayne Johnson, Ph.D., is a 30-year veteran of the health and wellness industry, and was the southwest regional health & fitness manger for the Wellbridge Company. Dr. Johnson is an associate professor at the University of New Mexico, and a faculty member for ACE, Balanced Body University, and Anatomy in Clay. She also participates as a subject-matter expert on the ACE exam-development committee.

Michael E. Rogers, Ph.D., CSCS, FACSM, is the chairperson of the Department of Human Performance Studies at Wichita State University. He is also an associate professor of exercise science and research director for the Center for Physical Activity and Aging at Wichita State University.

Brad A. Roy, Ph.D., FACHE, FACSM, is the administrator of The Summit Medical Fitness Center and part of the administrative team at Kalispell Regional Medical Center in Kalispell, Montana. Dr. Roy has more than 35 years of healthcare and medical fitness experience and facilitated the development of the Facility Standards and Guidelines for the Medical Fitness Association. He is also an active member of the American College of Sports Medicine and the American College of Healthcare Executives.

Kelly Spivey, N.D., is a continuing education provider for health and fitness professionals. As a member of the American Alternative Medical Society, her main focus is on disease prevention and complementary medicine. She is an adjunct professor at the University of Tampa, working in the Exercise Science Department. She also participates as a subject-matter expert on the ACE exam-development committee.

Gregory Welch, M.S., is an exercise physiologist and president of SpeciFit, *An Agency of Wellness,* located in Seal Beach, California. Welch is recognized nationally as an author and lecturer focusing on "real life" functional issues of the special needs population.

Wayne Westcott, Ph.D., is fitness research director at the South Shore YMCA in Quincy, Massachusetts, and adjunct professor of exercise science at Quincy College. Dr. Westcott was a member of the original ACE Personal Trainer Certification Committee.

Patience White, M.D., is the chief public health officer of the Arthritis Foundation. In addition to her work at the national office of the Arthritis Foundation, she is a professor of medicine and pediatrics at the George Washington University School of Medicine and Health Sciences and teaches a Health Policy seminar for Stanford University at the Stanford in Washington campus in Washington, D.C. She has been a practicing rheumatologist caring for both adults and children with rheumatic diseases for more than 25 years.

Foreword

The *ACE Advanced Health & Fitness Specialist Manual* and its accompanying certification represent the latest step in the evolution of the American Council on Exercise—and of the fitness industry itself. Fitness professionals, including those certified by ACE as personal trainers, have traditionally been limited to working with "apparently healthy" adults. Unfortunately, the number of individuals who fall outside that population continues to grow. This is the result of numerous factors, ranging from the obesity epidemic to longer life expectancies. People are now living for decades with one or more substantial health conditions, yet still want to live full, rewarding lives well into their older adult years. It is up to the fitness professional—and the fitness industry—to grow with this trend and acquire the expertise needed to excel in this ever-changing environment and build a bridge to the medical field.

One of the great challenges for the modern fitness professional is the development of the communication and networking skills needed to work as a true member of each client's healthcare team. Gone are the days when a personal trainer demonstrated some simple exercise techniques, developed a program, and then stood back and watched a client work out for an hour or so. One societal change that has had a tremendous impact on the fitness industry is the rising cost of healthcare and the associated limitations of the insurance industry. The combination of these two elements means that individuals who are sick or injured are often released to exercise on their own far earlier than their doctors might prefer. This enables the ACE-certified Advanced Health & Fitness Specialist (ACE-AHFS) to step in as valued team member and help these individuals work toward optimal health and fitness levels while maintaining ongoing communication with the client's physician and other healthcare team members—essentially keeping the individual in the team's care longer than would otherwise be possible.

The ACE-AHFS certification allows fitness professionals to work with a more varied clientele who often are facing multiple health challenges. By focusing exclusively on those conditions that fitness professionals reported encountering in their daily practice, ACE was able to bring an astounding level of detail to each chapter in this new manual. So whether your professional focus is on older adults managing various age-related disorders, obese clients coping with multiple comorbidities, or young athletes recovering from a variety of orthopedic injuries, this manual has everything that you—and your clients—will need to achieve long-lasting success.

Scott Goudeseune
President and CEO

Introduction

It has been a decade since ACE introduced its first advanced certification, the Clinical Exercise Specialist, which addressed the various special populations that fitness professionals might encounter during their careers in the fitness industry. This new manual and certification offer a more focused approach that targets the types of clients that go to health and fitness facilities on a daily basis. The Advanced Health & Fitness Specialist (ACE-AHFS) certification, as stated in Chapter 1, "was developed to enable fitness professionals to collaborate with the healthcare community to support their clients' health and fitness goals."

The exam content outline, which appears as Appendix B in this manual, was created by a team of top experts who represent each branch of required knowledge and also actively work in the health and fitness industry. The creation of this document is not an academic exercise, but rather an attempt to precisely define the roles and responsibilities of an ACE-AHFS, as well as delineate the knowledge and skills needed to meet those responsibilities on a day-to-day basis.

This text is divided into five Parts, the first of which serves as an introduction to this unique certification program. The five chapters in Part One define the scope of practice for an ACE-AHFS and provide broad-stroke guidelines for working with individuals with health challenges. These chapters also offer advice on networking with members of the healthcare community and building a successful and respected business. Finally, the chapter on nutritional considerations for an active lifestyle explains how to stay within the defined scope of practice when giving nutrition advice to clients and encountering supplement use and eating disorders among your clientele.

The next three Parts cover the disorders, diseases, and injuries that fitness professionals most frequently encounter in their daily practices, ranging from blood lipid disorders and diabetes to low-back pain and specific injuries of the upper and lower extremities. Each chapter begins with an overview of its subject, details its etiology, provides specific exercise and programming guidelines, and offers case studies that give practical meaning to the chapter's content. Part Five provides advice and guidelines for working with older adults, youth, and pre- and postnatal exercisers.

The goal of each chapter author—and of this project as a whole—was to enable the certified professional to become an integral and respected part of each client's healthcare team and join in the overall effort to help the client reach his or her optimal health and fitness level. We wish you good luck in your efforts and sincerely hope that this manual serves you well as you prepare to become an ACE-certified Advanced Health & Fitness Specialist and remains a trusted resource throughout your career.

Cedric X. Bryant, Ph.D.
Chief Science Officer

Daniel J. Green
Project Editor

Part One

Introduction

In This Chapter

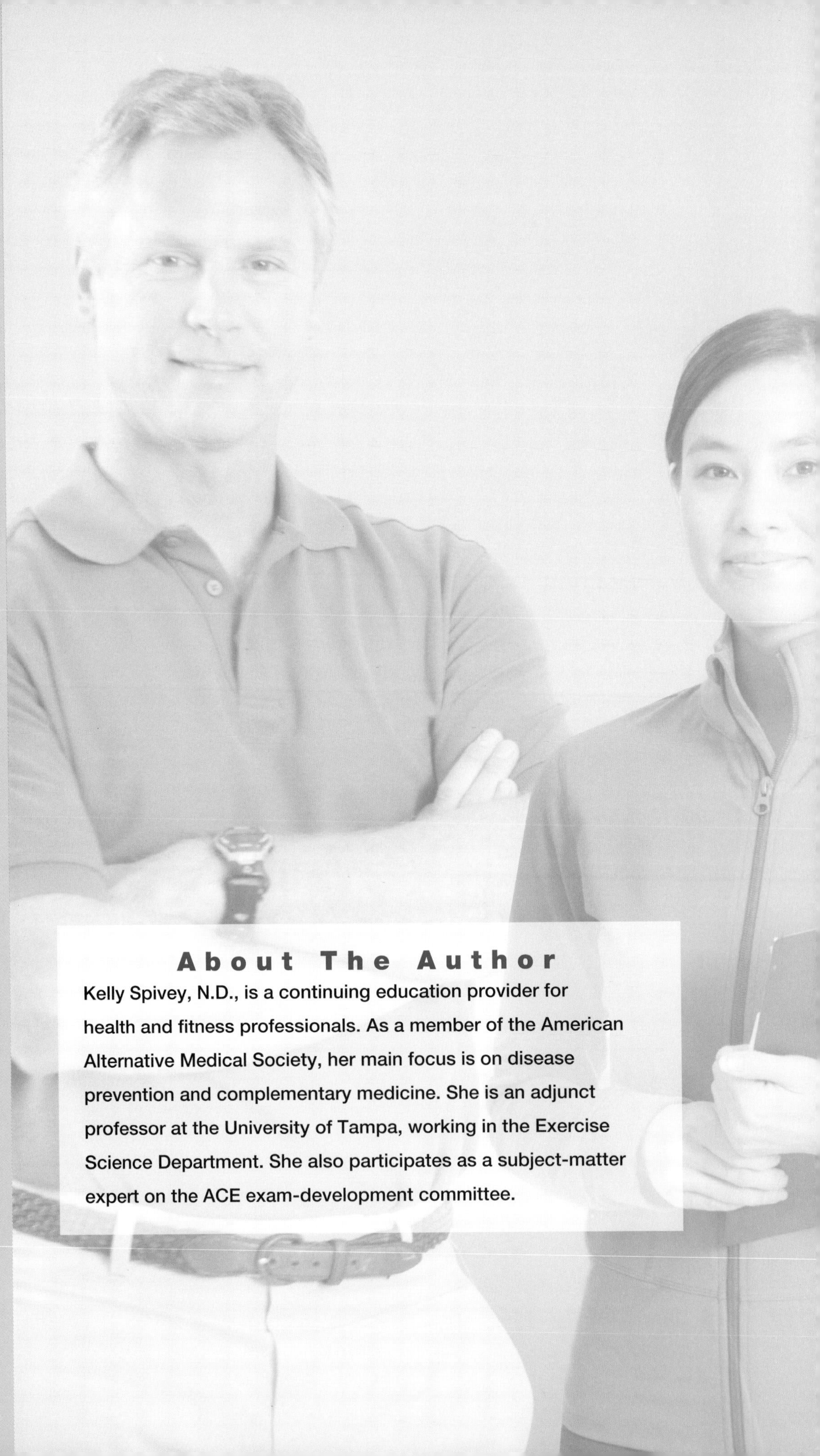

About The Author

Kelly Spivey, N.D., is a continuing education provider for health and fitness professionals. As a member of the American Alternative Medical Society, her main focus is on disease prevention and complementary medicine. She is an adjunct professor at the University of Tampa, working in the Exercise Science Department. She also participates as a subject-matter expert on the ACE exam-development committee.

CHAPTER 1

Role and Scope of Practice for the Advanced Health & Fitness Specialist

Kelly Spivey

The ACE Advanced Health & Fitness Specialist (ACE-AHFS) certification was developed to enable fitness professionals to collaborate with the healthcare community to support their clients' health and fitness goals. In the past, the primary role of an advanced trainer was to bridge the gap between the clinical setting and the traditional fitness center. That role is now changing. Due to the current state of the healthcare system, the majority of healthcare dollars are spent in treating disease and dysfunction. The United States spends more on healthcare than any other nation in the world, largely due to the resources given to treat well-established diseases and dysfunctions, as opposed to preventing the diseased state. Despite the logic associated with disease-prevention practices, the current healthcare system has not made the paradigm shift necessary to modify personal behaviors that affect overall health and well-being. As a result of this void, the role of the ACE-AHFS has evolved into one of health promotion and disease prevention, using a variety of lifestyle interventions (i.e., exercise, nutrition, stress management) and behavior-modification techniques.

An ACE-AHFS has the knowledge, training, and experience to work with clients who currently have, or are at risk for developing, one or more health conditions. The ACE-AHFS must develop a keen understanding of each client's current disease state and then design a safe and effective program that will enable the client to resume optimal function. The ACE-AHFS is not acting as an independent entity, but as a viable part of the healthcare community.

The ACE-AHFS can position him- or herself as an integral component in the healthcare continuum, working with allied health professionals in facilitating lifestyle-modification and disease-prevention strategies. Furthermore, the ACE-AHFS can offer programs that support the existing services provided by licensed healthcare professionals (e.g., supervised exercise to promote weight loss for a client currently working with a certified diabetes educator). There is also a need in the healthcare industry to provide a continuation of care for those who have not reached maximum rehabilitation potential. The many components of a balanced health and fitness program are best facilitated by a certified health and fitness professional, like the ACE-AHFS.

The populations served by the ACE-AHFS include, but are not limited to:

- Those who are at risk for chronic disease or dysfunction
- Those who have borderline health conditions that can be reversed or managed with a progressive health and fitness program
- Those with newly diagnosed cardiovascular, metabolic, or orthopedic conditions and who are in need of professional health and fitness guidance
- Those with chronic cardiovascular, metabolic, or orthopedic conditions and in need of continued health and fitness guidance
- Post-rehabilitation patients following discharge from an outpatient rehabilitation program

The benefits of exercise are well-established, but the majority of allied health professionals have no formal education or practical experience in exercise design and implementation. An individual may be advised to "begin a regular exercise program," but is unlikely to receive much direction from his or her healthcare provider. Clearly, the proper application of exercise is a key to a successful health and fitness program. Because of his or her knowledge and experience in exercise science, an ACE-AHFS can be positioned as a tremendous asset in the healthcare continuum, filling the gap between advice and application.

A client may be referred by a physician or rehabilitation specialist, or walk in on his or her own. To establish a working relationship with other allied healthcare professionals and develop the most appropriate treatment plan, the ACE-AHFS should seek communication with the client's primary healthcare provider and develop strong ties with members of the healthcare team. This book defines an acceptable **scope of practice** for the ACE-AHFS, offers guidelines for developing safe and effective health and fitness programs for special populations, and provides useful strategies that allow the ACE-AHFS to position him- or herself as a vital member of the healthcare team.

The Healthcare Continuum

The ACE-AHFS has a unique place within the healthcare continuum. Any given client may have one or more physicians, depending on the disease or dysfunction. He or she may have worked with a rehabilitation specialist, such as a physical therapist or cardiac rehabilitation nurse, or be seeing a registered dietician (R.D.) or psychiatrist. The role of the ACE-AHFS is to work in conjunction with the current healthcare team to establish the most effective health and fitness plan. This healthcare team takes direction from the client's personal physician. In essence, the physician acts as a "gatekeeper" (Figure 1-1).

Figure 1-1
Who is the ACE-AHFS?

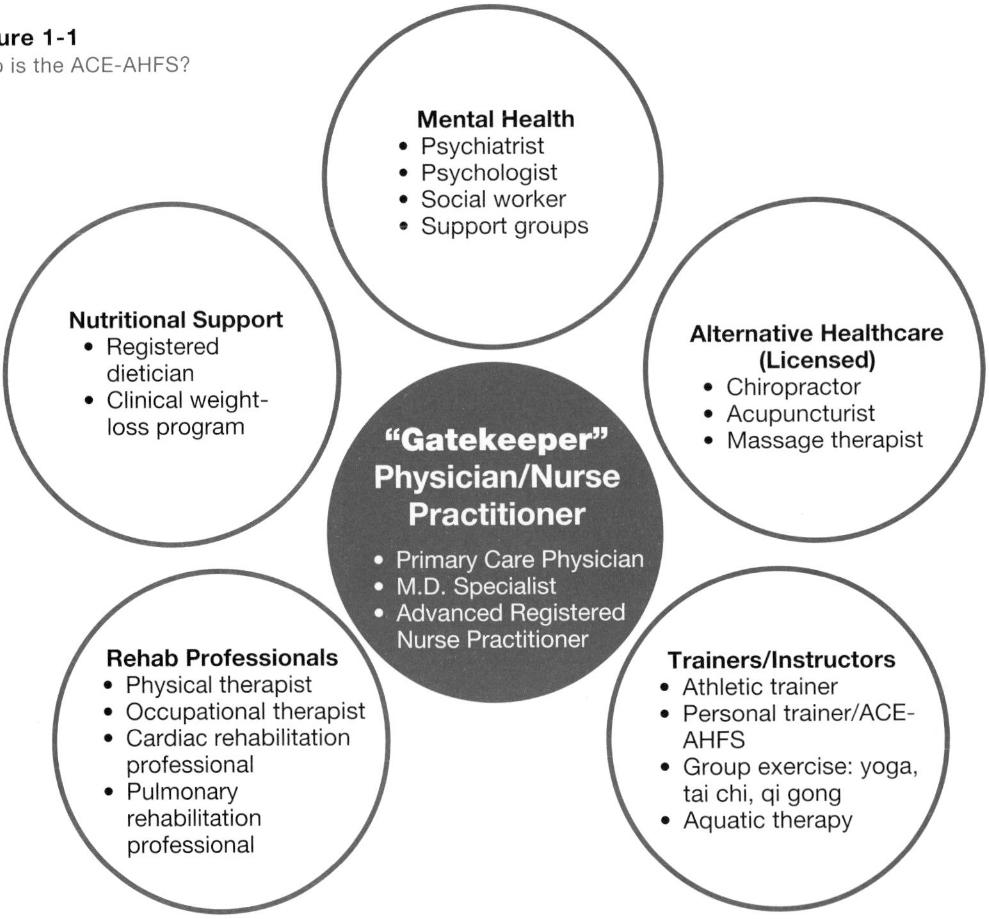

When working with special populations, it is expected that the ACE-AHFS will have the following knowledge and skills as they relate to the populations being served:

- Knowledge of disease **pathophysiology**
- Knowledge of the physician-critical pathway (Figure 1-2) as it relates to treatment of disease and dysfunction, and skill in establishing him- or herself as an integral part of this pathway
- Knowledge of common medications used in the treatment of diseases and dysfunctions, along with the side effects, and skill in applying this information to exercise design and programming (Appendix C)
- Knowledge of common diagnostic tests and skill in designing exercise programs based on the results and/or physician-recommended parameters
- Knowledge and skill in performing an appropriate fitness assessment, including the selection of appropriate methods, measures, endpoints, and special considerations as they relate to the client's disease state and medications, as well as any environmental conditions
- Knowledge of expected exercise progression, from hospital to rehabilitation to mainstream fitness settings and skill in developing a safe and effective exercise program based on these parameters: frequency, intensity, time, and type of exercise, as well as appropriate goals and the customary time needed to achieve predetermined goals
- Knowledge of exercise contraindications as they relate to a variety of accepted values (e.g., blood pressure, blood glucose, **neuropathy**)
- Knowledge and skill in modifying exercise programs to accommodate clients facing health challenges
- Knowledge of current dietary guidelines and skill in educating clients on making appropriate food choices based on solid scientific evidence and sound nutritional practices
- Knowledge of psychological implications related to disease and disability and an ability to empathize with clients who are struggling with their personal health challenges
- Knowledge of recognizable signs and symptoms of improperly managed stress and skill in developing effective coping strategies to eliminate or manage daily stressors
- Knowledge of signs or symptoms that require medical interventions beyond the capability of the ACE-AHFS
- Knowledge of, and ability to perform, first aid, **cardiopulmonary resuscitation (CPR),** and automated external defibrillation (AED) when necessary
- Knowledge of appropriate communication tools and skill in interviewing and communicating effectively with the client and/or healthcare team
- Detailed knowledge of appropriate health and fitness goals (e.g., blood glucose level, joint functioning and **range of motion**, appropriate **body composition**) and the knowledge and skills to help clients progress toward them

Note: Please refer to the AHFS Exam Content Outline in Appendix B for a comprehensive list of the knowledge and skills that an ACE-AHFS should possess.

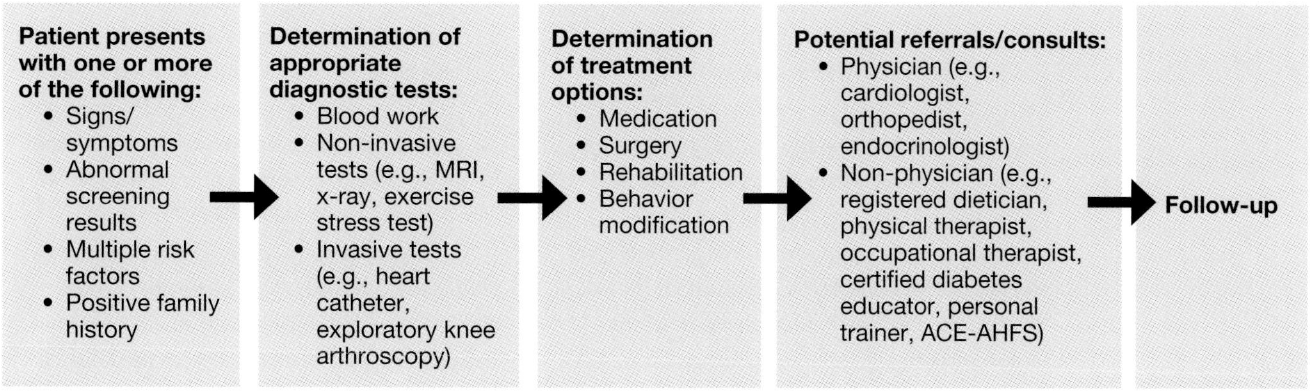
Patient presents with one or more of the following:
• Signs/ symptoms
• Abnormal screening results
• Multiple risk factors
• Positive family history
Determination of appropriate diagnostic tests:
• Blood work
• Non-invasive tests (e.g., MRI, x-ray, exercise stress test)
• Invasive tests (e.g., heart catheter, exploratory knee arthroscopy)
Determination of treatment options:
• Medication
• Surgery
• Rehabilitation
• Behavior modification
Potential referrals/consults:
• Physician (e.g., cardiologist, orthopedist, endocrinologist)
• Non-physician (e.g., registered dietician, physical therapist, occupational therapist, certified diabetes educator, personal trainer, ACE-AHFS)
Follow-up

Figure 1-2
Physician-critical pathway

The Role of the ACE-AHFS Within Allied Healthcare

Physician-critical Pathway

It is important for an ACE-AHFS working within the healthcare system to understand the role of the fitness professional as it relates to the other members of the healthcare team. In many cases, the client has a primary care physician who is responsible for his or her general medical care. If the primary care physician's patient is exhibiting signs or symptoms of disease or is at risk for contracting a particular disease or dysfunction, the doctor will perform a number of diagnostic tests to confirm or deny this suspicion. Once the disease or dysfunction is confirmed, the treatment options will be considered. If the doctor feels that the patient requires medical intervention outside his or her scope of care, the doctor will make a referral. This referral might be to a specialized physician (e.g., cardiologist, orthopedist) or to a registered dietician, a mental health specialist, a rehabilitation professional, or an ACE-AHFS. The referring physician is kept abreast of the patient's progress via regularly written reports. The primary physician will also make decisions on appropriate follow-up (e.g., subsequent office visits, further diagnostic tests). The physician-critical pathway is a decision-making tool to help the physician with the patient's case management (see Figure 1-2).

On average, a personal physician spends approximately 20 minutes with a patient (Mechanic, McAlpine, & Rosenthal, 2001); an R.D. may meet with a patient or client for a one-hour block of time and perhaps one follow-up visit; and a physical therapist or cardiac rehabilitation nurse may see the patient on a regular basis, but often juggles multiple patients at once. The ACE-AHFS is one of the few healthcare professionals who have the opportunity to spend a considerable amount of one-on-one time with a client, which allows for a great deal of information sharing. The ACE-AHFS is likely to know the client on a more personal level and discover detailed information about his or her daily lifestyle habits and behaviors. More importantly, regular appointments give the ACE-AHFS an opportunity to share copious amounts of health information and facilitate the behavior-change process, allowing for permanent adoption of new behaviors. Other allied healthcare professionals will share information and initiate the path to wellness, but the ACE-AHFS will help hold the client accountable and provide regular feedback, enabling the client to reach his or her maximum potential.

Working Within the Healthcare Community

Members of the healthcare community will not always appreciate the value of having an ACE-AHFS on their team. Fortunately, exercise continues to gain recognition and endorsement from the healthcare community as a preventive technique. Challenges for the ACE-AHFS to establish him- or herself as an integral part of the healthcare team may include the following:

- *The ACE-AHFS must demonstrate his or her value to the healthcare team.* The ACE-AHFS will have the benefit of regular meetings with the client, which aids in exercise compliance and enhanced behavior modification. The physician will have peace of mind knowing that his or her patient will be continuously monitored and referred back to the healthcare practitioner if complications arise.
- *The ACE-AHFS must not exceed his or her professional boundaries or go outside the scope of practice.* Providing a sample program design will give the healthcare professional a clearer understanding of the program components.
- *The ACE-AHFS must communicate on a regular basis with either the referring physician or the healthcare team.* An accepted reporting structure includes the following: pre-exercise assessment report; monthly progress reports using a summary of daily **SOAP notes;** post-exercise program summary of progress; and written and/or verbal communication on complications or emergency situations.

Referral sources are certainly not limited to physicians. An ACE-AHFS can also market him- or herself to nurse practitioners, physician assistants, registered dieticians, certified diabetes educators, physical or occupational therapists, cardiac rehabilitation providers, massage therapists, prenatal educators, chiropractors, social workers, clinical psychologists, support groups, weight-loss clinics, and personal trainers.

Scope of Practice

To maintain support from the healthcare community, it is paramount that the ACE-AHFS stay within his or her professional scope of practice. The ACE-AHFS *must* preclude him- or herself from activities that are limited to licensed healthcare professionals. For example, an ACE-AHFS may have seen dozens of clients with **sciatica.** Therefore, he or she is familiar with the symptoms related to sciatica and knows the appropriate treatment plan. But remember, an ACE-AHFS must not diagnose any disease, dysfunction, or condition. Additionally, an ACE-AHFS cannot prescribe specific meal plans or give specific recommendations on supplements or trendy diet plans. An ACE-AHFS cannot provide massage therapy unless he or she is licensed to do so. Also, he or she cannot make recommendations that contradict those of the client's healthcare provider. Table 1-1 lists some examples of practices that fall outside, or within, the ACE-AHFS scope of practice.

The ACE-AHFS should never go against the recommendations of the healthcare team. He or she may recommend certain progressions to the referring physician, based on subjective and objective assessments, but it is essential that no changes be instituted without prior written approval from the licensed healthcare professional.

Each jurisdiction has specific laws and parameters of professional responsibility within any given field. It is the responsibility of the ACE-AHFS to know the laws in his or her geographical area and conform to the professional scope of practice and the laws of the state, province, or country.

Focus on Disease Prevention

Many clients served by an ACE-AHFS may be concerned with one or more health challenges. Their entry into

Table 1-1
Actions That Fall Outside, and Within, the ACE-AHFS Scope of Practice

Outside Scope of Practice	Within the Appropriate Scope of Practice
Diagnose or label an unknown condition	Refer to the appropriate healthcare practitioner for diagnostic tests or additional screening
Design a specific meal plan with daily menus and exact portion sizes	Design a daily eating plan based on the MyPyramid Food Guidance System
Recommend a diet consisting of mostly protein for weight loss and/or muscle gain	Recommend carbohydrate, protein, and fat intake based on the U.S. Recommended Dietary Allowances (RDA) and scientific parameters
Recommend specific supplements and dosages	Refer to a licensed healthcare practitioner for specific guidelines on supplement usage, dosage, and contraindications
Hands-on therapeutic massage for muscle tension	Recommend/demonstrate the use of neuromuscular devices to release muscle tension
Recommend use of over-the-counter medications for a post-exercise strain	Discuss the proper technique for icing a chronic or acute injury
Add the use of the rowing machine to emphasize cross-training, even though the physician stated "treadmill only"	Contact the referring healthcare provider to discuss equipment alternatives and appropriate exercise progression

supervised health and fitness programs may be motivated by a number of factors:

- Financial (e.g., trying to lower their blood pressure so they will not be denied health insurance)
- Quality of life (e.g., trying to restore normal function so they can return to leisure activities like golfing or bowling)
- Morbidity/mortality (e.g., trying to control their diabetes so they do not suffer from complications like neuropathy or vision disturbances; starting an exercise program following a **gastric bypass** procedure to make a serious health change)
- Psychological (e.g., trying to get off medications to regain a sense of health and control)

These clients are not looking for guidance to fit into their "skinny jeans." Rather, they are looking for guidance in quality-of-life issues and disease prevention.

Prevention Defined

Primary Prevention

The U.S. Preventive Services Task Force (1996) defines **primary prevention** measures as "those provided to individuals to prevent the onset of a targeted condition." Primary prevention measures include activities that help avoid a particular disease or dysfunction. Examples include immunization against disease and health education programs promoting the benefits of exercise. Primary prevention is typically considered the most cost-effective form of healthcare because it helps reduce the costs and burdens associated with disease and dysfunction.

Secondary Prevention

Secondary prevention means to "identify and treat asymptomatic persons who have already developed risk factors or preclinical disease but in whom the condition is not clinically apparent" (U.S. Preventive Services Task Force, 1996). The healthcare community focuses on screening for and detecting common asymptomatic diseases that, if left untreated, pose a significant risk for negative outcome. With early detection, the natural course of a disease or dysfunction can often be slowed down or even reversed. This can maximize well-being and minimize suffering.

An example of secondary prevention is a physician determining that his or her patient has developed stage 1 **hypertension.** The physician will implement an appropriate treatment program aimed at reducing the blood pressure values. This plan may include medications, smoking cessation, weight loss, and a supervised exercise program.

Tertiary Prevention

Tertiary prevention focuses on the care of established disease, with attempts made to minimize the negative effects of disease, restore optimal function, and prevent disease-related complications. Since the disease is established, primary and secondary prevention activities may have been unsuccessful or simply ignored. Most likely, involvement in these primary and secondary activities would have minimized the impact of the disease. It is not likely that the ACE-AHFS will work with clients until their disease/dysfunction and associated health risks are deemed manageable or under control. The physician may recommend clinically based therapy programs prior to referral to an ACE-AHFS. The healthcare team needs to keep the individual's primary, secondary, and tertiary prevention needs in mind when prioritizing and guiding care.

Some clients may be trying to prevent disease, while others may be trying to keep their current diseases or dysfunctions at bay, or even reverse the disease process. Some may even be trying to prevent future events from occurring. Whatever the client's motive, the primary task of an ACE-AHFS is to work with the healthcare team to design and implement a comprehensive program aimed at preventing disease and optimizing health outcomes.

Standards of Care

The ACE-AHFS should be familiar with health risks associated with a client's specific disease or dysfunction. Before challenging a client's cardiovascular or musculoskeletal system, a number of safety

Chemoprophylaxis

A relatively new concept in primary disease prevention is **chemoprophylaxis,** which involves the use of drugs, nutritional supplements, or other natural substances to prevent future disease. For example, a client may take it upon him- or herself to take a daily aspirin prophylactically to prevent heart disease. Because aspirin is a drug with potentially serious side effects, the client should consult with his or her personal healthcare provider to discuss the risks and benefits of daily aspirin use.

This example brings up another important point. If a client informs the ACE-AHFS of self-prescribing supplements in megadoses, the ACE-AHFS should recommend that the client consult with his or her doctor or personal pharmacist. Many Americans turn to supplements and herbal remedies because they tend to be less expensive than prescription medications, are often easier to obtain, and the side effects may be negligible when compared to prescription medication. There is a widening gap between the consumer demand and the professional expertise on herbs, vitamins, minerals, and the like. Sales of vitamin, mineral, and herbal supplements exceed 30 million dollars annually. According to the NIH's Institute of Medicine (IOM), an estimated 42% of Americans use herbal products or dietary supplements (IOM, 2005). With so much information available on the Internet, many people will self-treat their conditions using potentially harmful combinations of prescription drugs, over-the-counter medications, and supplements, which may cause serious side effects.

An ACE-AHFS is likely to encounter clients who use over-the-counter medications and/or supplements to prevent disease or dysfunction or to self-medicate. A client may even substitute an herbal supplement for medication prescribed by his or her personal physician. None of these practices should be condoned and the ACE-AHFS should recommend that clients consult with a licensed healthcare professional who specializes in the field of supplementation.

Note that a drug is defined as a substance other than food that is intended to affect the structure or function of the body. This definition includes prescription medications, supplements (e.g., vitamins, minerals, herbs), over-the-counter medications (e.g., aspirin, acetaminophen, ibuprofen), and regularly used chemicals (e.g., caffeine, alcohol, nicotine). All drugs have the potential for side effects and negative interaction with other drugs.

Consider the following examples of harmful combinations of supplements.

A client is taking the following substances, all of which have blood-thinning properties that can cause excessive bleeding:

- Prescription Motrin™ for chronic knee pain
- Self-prescribed aspirin for heart-disease prevention
- Self-prescribed vitamin E as an antioxidant
- Self-prescribed ginkgo biloba as a memory booster

Another example involves a client who is taking the following substances, all of which have stimulant properties and can cause anything from jitteriness to heart palpitations—or worse:

- Self-prescribed diet pills containing Siberian ginseng
- Self-prescribed guarana for energy enhancement
- Daily consumption of caffeinated beverages
- Self-administered over-the-counter allergy medication
- Cigarette usage

concerns and contraindications for exercise testing and programming must be considered. Subsequent chapters provide detailed information on risks and contraindications as related to exercise programming, progression, and appropriate modifications for each specific disease or dysfunction. This section provides information on the following:

- **Physical Activity Readiness Questionnaire (PAR-Q)** and other health-history forms
- Informed consent and release of liability
- Fitness testing guidelines
- Components of program design
- Safety concerns related to program implementation
- Risk management
- Lifelong learning
- Consultation and privacy issues

PAR-Q and Exercise Readiness

As the ACE-AHFS establishes him- or herself as a member of the healthcare team, medical referrals will be customary. Often, a client may enlist the service of an ACE-AHFS without a referral. In this case, the ACE-AHFS must perform due diligence by obtaining some sort of medical clearance or referral form from the healthcare provider who is specifically treating the client (or potential client). It is up to the ACE-AHFS to establish an open line of communication with the client's personal healthcare professional and/or healthcare team, especially if this is a new working relationship. Strategies for successful communication with allied healthcare professionals are detailed in Chapter 3.

Even the "apparently healthy" client may have multiple risk factors for heart disease, which would necessitate a referral from a physician. Refer to Table 1-2 for a list of these major cardiac risks. If a client presents with two or more risk factors, clearance from his or her personal physician is strongly recommended.

To ensure a client's safety, the ACE-AHFS must determine a client's readiness for exercise. The PAR-Q (Figure 1-3) is useful as an initial screening tool, but the information obtained may be insufficient for designing a comprehensive health and fitness program for clients with one or more health concerns. The **Physical Activity Readiness Medical Exam Form (PARmed-X)** (Figure 1-4) is an example of a screening tool used with special populations, as is the Health Status Questionnaire (Figure 1-5).

The PARmed-X has a physical activity–specific checklist to be used by a physician with patients who have had positive responses to the PAR-Q.

Table 1-2
Coronary Heart Disease Risk Factors

Positive Risk Factors

- Family history (premature disease or heart attack in an immediate relative: male <55 yrs; female <65 yrs)
- Hypertension (SBP ≥140 mmHg and or DBP ≥90 mmHg) Confirmed on at least two separate occasions or on antihypertensive medication
- High cholesterol (LDL >130 mg/dL; HDL <40 mg/dL; if LDL is not available, then cholesterol >200 mg/dL), or on lipid-lowering medications
- Physical inactivity (Does not meet the recommended minimum of 30 minutes of physical activity on most days)
- Impaired fasting glucose (fasting blood glucose >100 mg/dL) Confirmed on two separate occasions or on blood glucose–lowering medication
- Current smoker (or quit within the last six months)
- Obesity (BMI >30, or waist girth ≥40 inches (102 cm) for men and ≥35 inches (89 cm) for women, or waist-to-hip ratio ≥0.95 for men and ≥0.86 for women)

Negative Risk Factor

- HDL >60 mg/dL

Note: GXT = Graded exercise test; SBP = Systolic blood pressure; DBP = Diastolic blood pressure; LDL = Low-density lipoprotein; HDL = High-density lipoprotein; BMI = Body mass index

Source: American College of Sports Medicine (2006). *ACSM's Guidelines for Exercise Testing and Prescription* (7th ed.). Philadelphia: Lippincott Williams & Wilkins.

Figure 1-3
The Physical Activity Readiness Questionnaire — PAR-Q

The Physical Activity Readiness Questionnaire — PAR-Q *(revised 2002)*

PAR-Q & YOU (A Questionnaire for People Aged 15 to 69)

Regular physical activity is fun and healthy, and increasingly more people are starting to become more active every day. Being more active is very safe for most people. However, some people should check with their doctor before they start becoming much more physically active.

If you are planning to become much more physically active than you are now, start by answering the seven questions below. If you are between the ages of 15 and 69, the PAR-Q will tell you if you should check with your doctor before you start. If you are over 69 years of age, and you are not used to being very active, check with your doctor.

Common sense is your best guide when you answer these questions. Please read the questions carefully and answer each one honestly: check YES or NO.

YES	NO	
☐	☐	1. Has your doctor ever said that you have a heart condition and that you should only do physical activity recommended by a doctor?
☐	☐	2. Do you feel pain in your chest when you do physical activity?
☐	☐	3. In the past month, have you had chest pain when you were not doing physical activity?
☐	☐	4. Do you lose your balance because of dizziness or do you ever lose consciousness?
☐	☐	5. Do you have a bone or joint problem (for example, back, knee, or hip) that could be made worse by a change in your physical activity?
☐	☐	6. Is your doctor currently prescribing drugs (for example, water pills) for your blood pressure or heart condition?
☐	☐	7. Do you know of any other reason why you should not do physical activity?

If you answered

YES to one or more questions:

Talk with your doctor by phone or in person BEFORE you start becoming much more physically active or BEFORE you have a fitness appraisal. Tell your doctor about the PAR-Q and which questions you answered YES.

- You may be able to do any activity you want—as long as you start slowly and build up gradually. Or, you may need to restrict your activities to those that are safe for you. Talk with your doctor about the kinds of activities you wish to participate in and follow his/her advice.
- Find out which community programs are safe and helpful for you.

NO to all questions

If you answered NO honestly to all PAR-Q questions, you can be reasonably sure that you can:

- Start becoming much more physically active—begin slowly and build up gradually. This is the safest and easiest way to go.
- Take part in a fitness appraisal—this is an excellent way to determine your basic fitness so that you can plan the best way for you to live actively. It is also highly recommended that you have your blood pressure evaluated. If your reading is over 144/94, talk with your doctor before you start becoming much more physically active.

DELAY BECOMING MUCH MORE ACTIVE:

- If you are not feeling well because of a temporary illness such as a cold or a fever—wait until you feel better; or
- If you are or may be pregnant—talk to your doctor before you start becoming more active.

PLEASE NOTE: If your health changes so that you then answer YES to any of the above questions, tell your fitness or health professional. Ask whether you should change your physical activity plan.

Informed Use of the PAR-Q: The Canadian Society for Exercise Physiology, Health Canada, and their agents assume no liability for persons who undertake physical activity, and if in doubt after completing this questionnaire, consult your doctor prior to physical activity.

No changes permitted. You are encouraged to copy the PAR-Q but only if you use the entire form.

Note: If the PAR-Q is being given to a person before he or she participates in a physical activity program or a fitness appraisal, this section may be used for legal or administrative purposes.

I have read, understood, and completed this questionnaire. Any questions I had were answered to my full satisfaction.

NAME ______________________________

SIGNATURE ______________________________ DATE ______________________________

SIGNATURE OF PARENT ______________________________ WITNESS ______________________________
OR GUARDIAN (FOR PARTICIPANTS UNDER THE AGE OF MAJORITY)

Note: This physical activity clearance is valid for a maximum of 12 months from the date it is completed and becomes invalid if your condition changes so that you would answer YES to any of the seven questions.

Source: The Physical Activity Readiness Questionnaire — PAR-Q (revised 2002). Reprinted with permission from the Canadian Society for Exercise Physiology. www.csep.ca/forms.asp

Figure 1-4
PARmed-X

Physical Activity Readiness
Medical Examination
(revised 2002)

PARmed-X PHYSICAL ACTIVITY READINESS MEDICAL EXAMINATION

The PARmed-X is a physical activity-specific checklist to be used by a physician with patients who have had positive responses to the Physical Activity Readiness Questionnaire (PAR-Q). In addition, the Conveyance/Referral Form in the PARmed-X can be used to convey clearance for physical activity participation, or to make a referral to a medically-supervised exercise program.

Regular physical activity is fun and healthy, and increasingly more people are starting to become more active every day. Being more active is very safe for most people. The PAR-Q by itself provides adequate screening for the majority of people. However, some individuals may require a medical evaluation and specific advice (exercise prescription) due to one or more positive responses to the PAR-Q.

Following the participant's evaluation by a physician, a physical activity plan should be devised in consultation with a physical activity professional (CSEP-Professional Fitness & Lifestyle Consultant or CSEP-Exercise Therapist™). To assist in this, the following instructions are provided:

PAGE 1: • Sections A, B, C, and D should be completed by the participant BEFORE the examination by the physician. The bottom section is to be completed by the examining physician.

PAGES 2 & 3: • A checklist of medical conditions requiring special consideration and management.

PAGE 4: • Physical Activity & Lifestyle Advice for people who do not require specific instructions or prescribed exercise.

• Physical Activity Readiness Conveyance/Referral Form - an optional tear-off tab for the physician to convey clearance for physical activity participation, or to make a referral to a medically-supervised exercise program.

This section to be completed by the participant

A PERSONAL INFORMATION:

NAME ____________________

ADDRESS ____________________

____

TELEPHONE ____________________

BIRTHDATE ____________________ GENDER ________

MEDICAL No. ____________________

B PAR-Q: Please indicate the PAR-Q questions to which you answered YES

- ❑ Q 1 Heart condition
- ❑ Q 2 Chest pain during activity
- ❑ Q 3 Chest pain at rest
- ❑ Q 4 Loss of balance, dizziness
- ❑ Q 5 Bone or joint problem
- ❑ Q 6 Blood pressure or heart drugs
- ❑ Q 7 Other reason: ____________________

C RISK FACTORS FOR CARDIOVASCULAR DISEASE:

Check all that apply

- ❑ Less than 30 minutes of moderate physical activity most days of the week.
- ❑ Currently smoker (tobacco smoking 1 or more times per week).
- ❑ High blood pressure reported by physician after repeated measurements.
- ❑ High cholesterol level reported by physician.
- ❑ Excessive accumulation of fat around waist.
- ❑ Family history of heart disease.

Please note: *Many of these risk factors are modifiable. Please refer to page 4 and discuss with your physician.*

D PHYSICAL ACTIVITY INTENTIONS:

What physical activity do you intend to do?

____

____

____

This section to be completed by the examining physician

Physical Exam:

Ht	Wt	BP i) /
		BP ii) /

Conditions limiting physical activity:

- ❑ Cardiovascular
- ❑ Respiratory
- ❑ Other
- ❑ Musculoskeletal
- ❑ Abdominal

Tests required:

- ❑ ECG
- ❑ Exercise Test
- ❑ X-Ray
- ❑ Blood
- ❑ Urinalysis
- ❑ Other

Physical Activity Readiness Conveyance/Referral:

Based upon a current review of health status, I recommend:

Further Information:
❑ Attached
❑ To be forwarded
❑ Available on request

- ❑ No physical activity
- ❑ Only a medically supervised exercise program until further medical clearance
- ❑ Progressive physical activity:
  - ❑ with avoidance of: ____________________
  - ❑ with inclusion of: ____________________
  - ❑ under the supervision of a CSEP-Professional Fitness & Lifestyle Consultant or CSEP-Exercise Therapist™
- ❑ Unrestricted physical activity–start slowly and build up gradually

Supported by: Health Canada Santé Canada

1

Figure 1-4
PARmed-X (continued)

Physical Activity Readiness
Medical Examination
(revised 2002)

PARmed-X PHYSICAL ACTIVITY READINESS MEDICAL EXAMINATION

Following is a checklist of medical conditions for which a degree of precaution and/or special advice should be considered for those who answered "YES" to one or more questions on the PAR-Q, and people over the age of 69. Conditions are grouped by system. Three categories of precautions are provided. Comments under Advice are general, since details and alternatives require clinical judgement in each individual instance.

	Absolute Contraindications	Relative Contraindications	Special Prescriptive Conditions	ADVICE
	Permanent restriction or temporary restriction until condition is treated, stable, and/or past acute phase.	Highly variable. Value of exercise testing and/or program may exceed risk. Activity may be restricted. Desirable to maximize control of condition. Direct or indirect medical supervision of exercise program may be desirable.	Individualized prescriptive advice generally appropriate: · limitations imposed; and/or · special exercises prescribed. May require medical monitoring and/or initial supervision in exercise program.	
Cardiovascular	❑ aortic aneurysm (dissecting) ❑ aortic stenosis (severe) ❑ congestive heart failure ❑ crescendo angina ❑ myocardial infarction (acute) ❑ myocarditis (active or recent) ❑ pulmonary or systemic embolism—acute ❑ thrombophlebitis ❑ ventricular tachycardia and other dangerous dysrhythmias (e.g., multi-focal ventricular activity)	❑ aortic stenosis (moderate) ❑ subaortic stenosis (severe) ❑ marked cardiac enlargement ❑ supraventricular dysrhythmias (uncontrolled or high rate) ❑ ventricular ectopic activity (repetitive or frequent) ❑ ventricular aneurysm ❑ hypertension—untreated or uncontrolled severe (systemic or pulmonary) ❑ hypertrophic cardiomyopathy ❑ compensated congestive heart failure	❑ aortic (or pulmonary) stenosis—mild angina pectoris and other manifestations of coronary insufficiency (e.g., post-acute infarct) ❑ cyanotic heart disease ❑ shunts (intermittent or fixed) ❑ conduction disturbances · complete AV block · left BBB · Wolff-Parkinson-White syndrome ❑ dysrhythmias—controlled ❑ fixed rate pacemakers	· clinical exercise test may be warranted in selected cases, for specific determination of functional capacity and limitations and precautions (if any). · slow progression of exercise to levels based on test performance and individual tolerance. · consider individual need for initial conditioning program under medical supervision (indirect or direct).
			❑ intermittent claudication	progressive exercise to tolerance
			❑ hypertension: systolic 160-180; diastolic 105+	progressive exercise; care with medications (serum electrolytes, post-exercise syncope, etc.)
Infections	❑ acute infectious disease (regardless of etiology)	❑ subacute/chronic/recurrent infectious diseases (e.g., malaria, others)	❑ chronic infections ❑ HIV	variable as to condition
Metabolic		❑ uncontrolled metabolic disorders (diabetes mellitus, thyrotoxicosis, myxedema)	❑ renal, hepatic & other metabolic insufficiency	variable as to status
			❑ obesity ❑ single kidney	dietary moderation, and initial light exercises with slow progression (walking, swimming, cycling)
Pregnancy		❑ complicated pregnancy (e.g., toxemia, hemorrhage, incompetent cervix, etc.)	❑ advanced pregnancy (late 3rd trimester)	refer to the "PARmed-X for PREGNANCY"

References:

Arraix, G.A., Wigle, D.T., Mao, Y. (1992). Risk Assessment of Physical Activity and Physical Fitness in the Canada Health Survey Follow-Up Study. **J. Clin. Epidemiol.** 45:4 419-428.

Mottola, M., Wolfe, L.A. (1994). Active Living and Pregnancy, In: A. Quinney, L. Gauvin, T. Wall (eds.), **Toward Active Living: Proceedings of the International Conference on Physical Activity, Fitness and Health**. Champaign, IL: Human Kinetics.

PAR-Q Validation Report, British Columbia Ministry of Health, 1978.

Thomas, S., Reading, J., Shephard, R.J. (1992). Revision of the Physical Activity Readiness Questionnaire (PAR-Q). **Can. J. Spt. Sci.** 17: 4 338-345.

The PAR-Q and PARmed-X were developed by the British Columbia Ministry of Health. They have been revised by an Expert Advisory Committee of the Canadian Society for Exercise Physiology chaired by Dr. N. Gledhill (2002).

Disponible en français sous le titre «Évaluation médicale de l'aptitude à l'activité physique (X-AAP)»

Continued on page 3...

Figure 1-4
PARmed-X (continued)

Physical Activity Readiness
Medical Examination
(revised 2002)

	Special Prescriptive Conditions	ADVICE
Lung	❑ chronic pulmonary disorders	special relaxation and breathing exercises
	❑ obstructive lung disease ❑ asthma	breath control during endurance exercises to tolerance; avoid polluted air
	❑ exercise-induced bronchospasm	avoid hyperventilation during exercise; avoid extremely cold conditions; warm up adequately; utilize appropriate medication.
Musculoskeletal	❑ low-back conditions (pathological, functional)	avoid or minimize exercise that precipitates or exasperates e.g., forced extreme flexion, extension, and violent twisting; correct posture, proper back exercises
	❑ arthritis—acute (infective, rheumatoid; gout)	treatment, plus judicious blend of rest, splinting and gentle movement
	❑ arthritis—subacute	progressive increase of active exercise therapy
	❑ arthritis—chronic (osteoarthritis and above conditions)	maintenance of mobility and strength; non-weightbearing exercises to minimize joint trauma (e.g., cycling, aquatic activity)
	❑ orthopaedic	highly variable and individualized
	❑ hernia	minimize straining and isometrics; stregthen abdominal muscles
	❑ osteoporosis or low bone density	avoid exercise with high risk for fracture such as push-ups, curl-ups, vertical jump and trunk forward flexion; engage in low-impact weight-bearing activities and resistance training
CNS	❑ convulsive disorder not completely controlled by medication	minimize or avoid exercise in hazardous environments and/or exercising alone (e.g., swimming, mountainclimbing)
	❑ recent concussion	thorough examination if history of two concussions; review for discontinuation of contact sport if three concussions, depending on duration of unconsciousness, retrograde amnesia, persistent headaches, and other objective evidence of cerebral damage
Blood	❑ anemia—severe (< 10 Gm/dl) ❑ electrolyte disturbances	control preferred; exercise as tolerated
Medications	❑ antianginal ❑ antiarrhythmic ❑ antihypertensive ❑ anticonvulsant ❑ beta-blockers ❑ digitalis preparations ❑ diuretics ❑ ganglionic blockers ❑ others	NOTE: consider underlying condition. Potential for: exertional syncope, electrolyte imbalance, bradycardia, dysrhythmias, impaired coordination and reaction time, heat intolerance. May alter resting and exercise ECG's and exercise test performance.
Other	❑ post-exercise syncope	moderate program
	❑ heat intolerance	prolong cool-down with light activities; avoid exercise in extreme heat
	❑ temporary minor illness	postpone until recovered
	❑ cancer	if potential metastases, test by cycle ergometry, consider non-weightbearing exercises; exercise at lower end of prescriptive range (40-65% of heart-rate reserve), depending on condition and recent treatment (radiation, chemotherapy); monitor hemoglobin and lymphocyte counts; add dynamic lifting exercise to strengthen muscles, using machines rather than weights.

*Refer to special publications for elaboration as required

The following companion forms are available online: http://www.csep.ca/forms.asp

The **Physical Activity Readiness Questionnaire (PAR-Q)** - a questionnaire for people aged 15-69 to complete before becoming much more physically active.

The **Physical Activity Readiness Medical Examination for Pregnancy (PARmed-X for PREGNANCY)** - to be used by physicians with pregnant patients who wish to become more physically active.

For more information, please contact the:

Canadian Society for Exercise Physiology
202 - 185 Somerset St. West
Ottawa, ON K2P 0J2
Tel. 1-877-651-3755 • FAX (613) 234-3565 • Online: www.csep.ca

Note to physical activity professionals...
It is a prudent practice to retain the completed Physical Activity Readiness Conveyance/Referral Form in the participant's file.

Supported by: Health Canada Santé Canada

Continued on page 4...

3

Figure 1-4
PARmed-X (continued)

Physical Activity Readiness
Medical Examination
(revised 2002)

PARmed-X PHYSICAL ACTIVITY READINESS MEDICAL EXAMINATION

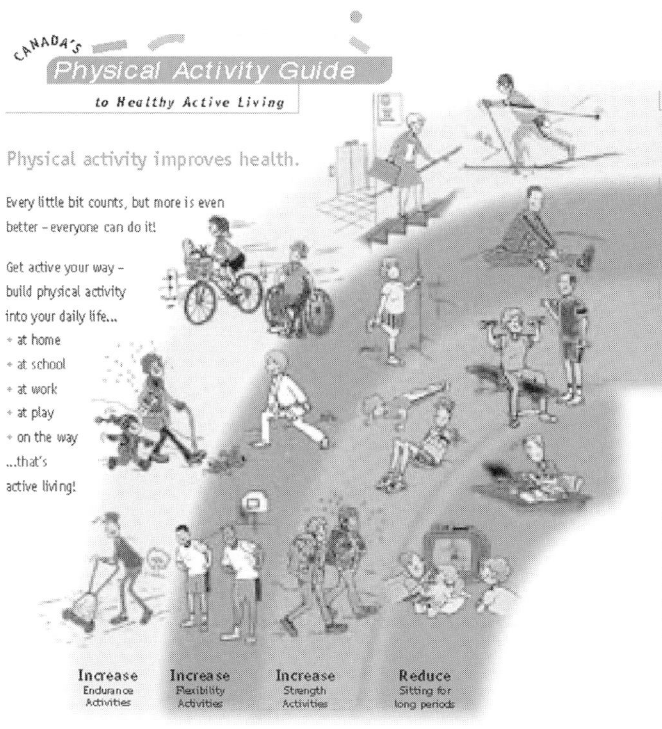

CANADA'S Physical Activity Guide to Healthy Active Living

Physical activity improves health.

Every little bit counts, but more is even better – everyone can do it!

Get active your way – build physical activity into your daily life...
- at home
- at school
- at work
- at play
- on the way

...that's active living!

Choose a variety of activities from these three groups:

Endurance
4-7 days a week
Continuous activities for your heart, lungs and circulatory system.

Flexibility
4-7 days a week
Gentle reaching, bending and stretching activities to keep your muscles relaxed and joints mobile.

Strength
2-4 days a week
Activities against resistance to strengthen muscles and bones and improve posture.

Starting slowly is very safe for most people. Not sure? Consult your health professional.

For a copy of the *Guide Handbook* and more information: **1-888-334-9769**, or **www.paguide.com**

Eating well is also important. Follow *Canada's Food Guide to Healthy Eating* to make wise food choices.

Get Active Your Way, Every Day – For Life!

Scientists say accumulate 60 minutes of physical activity every day to stay healthy or improve your health. As you progress to moderate activities you can cut down to 30 minutes, 4 days a week. Add-up your activities in periods of at least 10 minutes each. Start slowly... and build up.

Time needed depends on effort

Very Light Effort	Light Effort *60 minutes*	Moderate Effort *30-60 minutes*	Vigorous Effort *20-30 minutes*	Maximum Effort
• Strolling • Dusting	• Light walking • Volleyball • Easy gardening • Stretching	• Brisk walking • Biking • Raking leaves • Swimming • Dancing • Water aerobics	• Aerobics • Jogging • Hockey • Basketball • Fast swimming • Fast dancing	• Sprinting • Racing

Range needed to stay healthy

You Can Do It – Getting started is easier than you think

Physical activity doesn t have to be very hard. Build physical activities into your daily routine.

- Walk whenever you can – get off the bus early, use the stairs instead of the elevator.
- Reduce inactivity for long periods, like watching TV.
- Get up from the couch and stretch and bend for a few minutes every hour.
- Play actively with your kids.
- Choose to walk, wheel or cycle for short trips.
- Start with a 10 minute walk – gradually increase the time.
- Find out about walking and cycling paths nearby and use them.
- Observe a physical activity class to see if you want to try it.
- Try one class to start – you don t have to make a long-term commitment.
- Do the activities you are doing now, more often.

Benefits of regular activity:	Health risks of inactivity:
• better health • improved fitness • better posture and balance • better self-esteem • weight control • stronger muscles and bones • feeling more energetic • relaxation and reduced stress • continued independent living in later life	• premature death • heart disease • obesity • high blood pressure • adult-onset diabetes • osteoporosis • stroke • depression • colon cancer

Health Canada Santé Canada   Canadian Society for Exercise Physiology

PARmed-X Physical Activity Readiness Conveyance/Referral Form

Based upon a current review of the health status of ______________________________, I recommend:

❑ No physical activity

❑ Only a medically-supervised exercise program until further medical clearance

❑ Progressive physical activity

  ❑ with avoidance of: ______________________________

  ❑ with inclusion of: ______________________________

  ❑ under the supervision of a CSEP-Professional Fitness & Lifestyle Consultant or CSEP-Exercise Therapist™

❑ Unrestricted physical activity — start slowly and build up gradually

Further Information:
❑ Attached
❑ To be forwarded
❑ Available on request

Physician/clinic stamp:

______________________________ M.D.

______________________________ 20______
(date)

NOTE: This physical activity clearance is valid for a maximum of six months from the date it is completed and becomes invalid if your medical condition becomes worse.

4

Figure 1-5
Health status questionnaire

Source: Bryant, C.X., Franklin, B.A., & Newton-Merrill, S. (2007). *ACE's Guide to Exercise Testing & Program Design* (2nd ed.). Monterey, Calif.: Healthy Learning.

Health Status Questionnaire

Name:____________________ Phone (H):____________________

Address:______________________________________

City:____________________ ZIP: ____________________

Emergency Contact:____________________ Emergency Phone:____________________

Personal Physician: ______________________________________

DOB:__________ Age:__________ Sex: ❑ M ❑ F Physician's Phone:____________________

Section I. Medical History

1. Mark any of the following for which you have been diagnosed or treated:

____ Kidney problem ____ Heart problem ____ Phlebitis ____ Concussion
____ Mononucleosis ____ Cirrhosis, liver ____ Stroke ____ Asthma

2. Mark any medications taken in the last 6 months:

____ Blood thinner ____ Epilepsy medicine ____ Nitroglycerin ____ Cholesterol medicine
____ Diabetes medicine ____ Heart rhythm medicine ____ Insulin ____ Other
____ Blood pressure medicine ____ Diuretic (water pill) ____ Digitalis

3. List any surgeries you have had in the past (e.g., knee, heart, back):

____
____
____

4. Have you ever had back problems, any problems with joints (knee, hip, shoulder, elbow, neck), or been diagnosed with arthritis? __________ If yes, describe:

____
____
____

5. Do you have any other medical conditions or health problems that may affect your exercise plan or safety in any way? __________ If yes, describe:

____
____
____

Section II. Cardiopulmonary and Metabolic Symptoms

Y	N	Do you ever get unusually short of breath with very light exertion?
Y	N	Do you ever have pain, pressure, heaviness, or tightness in the chest area?
Y	N	Do you regularly have unexplained pain in the abdomen, shoulder, or arm?
Y	N	Do you ever have dizzy spells or episodes of fainting?
Y	N	Do you ever feel "skips," palpitations, or runs of fast or slow heart beats in your chest?
Y	N	Has a physician ever told you that you have a heart murmur?
Y	N	Do you regularly get lower -eg pain during walking that is relieved with rest?
Y	N	Do you have any joints that often become swollen and painful? Where:____________________

Figure 1-5
Health status questionnaire (continued)

Section III. Cardiopulmonary/Metabolic Disease

Y N Have you ever had a heart attack, bypass surgery, angioplasty, or been diagnosed with coronary artery disease or other heart disease? _____ If yes, describe:

____

____

____

Y N Do you have emphysema, asthma, or any other chronic lung condition or disease?

____

____

Y N Are you an insulin-dependent diabetic?

____

____

Section IV. Coronary Risk Factor Profile

Y N Have you had high blood pressure ($\geq$140 mmHg systolic or $\geq$90 mmHg diastolic) on more than one occasion?

____

Please list any medications you take for high blood pressure:

____

____

Y N Have you ever been told that your blood cholesterol was high (200 mg/dL or higher)? _________
Cholesterol level___________________________

Y N Do you currently smoke 10 or more cigarettes per day?_________
cigarettes/day___________________________ years smoked___________________________

Y N Have you ever been told that you have high blood sugar or diabetes? ________ If yes, describe:

____

____

Y N Has anyone in your immediate family (parents, siblings) had any heart problems or coronary disease before age 55? ______________ Describe:

____

____

Y N Do you feel you are more than 20 lb overweight? __________________
What do you feel is your realistic ideal weight? ___________________

Section V. Fitness

Circle the average number of times per week you participate in planned moderate-to-strenuous exercise of at least 20 minutes duration (brisk walking, jogging, cycling, swimming, stair climbing, weightlifting, active sports such as tennis, aerobic classes, etc.).

0 1 2 3 4 5 6 7 8 9 10

Y N Can you briskly walk 1 mile without fatigue?
Y N Can you jog 2 miles continuously at a moderate pace without discomfort?
Y N Can you do 20 push-ups?

Please list your body weight:
Now: ________lb/kg 1 year ago: _______lb/kg Age 21:_________lb/kg

Figure 1-5
Health status questionnaire (continued)

Section VI. Lifestyle and Behavioral

1. Describe any aerobic exercise you have done in the past (what, when, how often, for how long).

____
____
____

2. Describe any muscular strength/weight training you have done in the past (what, when, how often, for how long).

____
____
____

3. List any major obstacles that you feel you will have to overcome to stick with your exercise plan long-term (e.g., what has stopped you in the past).

____
____
____

4. Have you ever participated in aerobic or aerobic step classes? _____Yes _____No

5. Please list any recreational physical activities (tennis, golf, etc.) in which you regularly participate and how often.

____
____
____

6. List any favorite activities you would like to include in your exercise plan.

____
____
____

7. List any activities that you definitely do not like and do not want to include.

____
____
____

8. Which do you prefer? ________ Group exercise ________Exercising on your own

9. List the two most important goals or reasons why you want to exercise regularly.

____
____
____

10. Your occupation: ____

11. Do you spend more than 25% of work time doing the following (mark all that apply)?
______Sitting at a desk ______Lifting/carrying loads ______Standing
______Driving ______Walking

12. Number of hours worked per week: ______Hours Any flexible hours? _____Yes _______No

Figure 1-5
Health status questionnaire (continued)

13. Write in the best exercise times for you during a typical week.

	M	Tu	W	Th	F	Sa	Su
AM							
PM							

14. Where do you plan to exercise? ______Club ______Home ______Outside

Other____

15. If at home, list all available equipment.

____

____

____

First, there is a brief self-reporting section to be completed by the client, followed by a comprehensive section to be completed by the examining physician. The physician can also define specific parameters for exercise based on the client's current health condition.

For clients who are pregnant, there is also a PARmed-X for Pregnancy (Figure 1-6). Just as in the standard PARmed-X, this form includes a separate section for the healthcare provider to complete. Note that all three of these forms—PAR-Q, PARmed-X, and PARmed-X for Pregnancy—are available for free download at the Canadian Society for Exercise Physiology's (CSEP) website: www.csep.ca. To preserve the integrity of the content, the CSEP stipulates that their forms are not to be altered in any way.

There are a number of **absolute contraindications** to exercise. As stated in the PARmed-X, the absolute contraindications for exercise include, "dissecting **aortic aneurysm,** severe aortic **stenosis, congestive heart failure (CHF), crescendo angina,** acute **myocardial infarction (MI),** active or recent **myocarditis,** acute pulmonary or systemic **embolism, thrombophlebitis, ventricular tachycardia** and other dangerous **dysrhythmias,** or acute infectious disease." The **relative contraindications** for exercise include moderate aortic stenosis, severe subaortic stenosis, marked cardiac enlargement, uncontrolled or frequent **supraventricular dysrhythmias,** repetitive or frequent ventricular ectopic activity, ventricular aneurysm, untreated or uncontrolled severe hypertension (systemic or pulmonary), **hypertrophic cardiomyopathy,** compensated CHF, subacute/chronic/recurrent infectious disease, uncontrolled metabolic disorder (e.g., diabetes), or complicated pregnancy. Patients with these conditions will either be precluded from exercise or will be referred to a clinical exercise program.

Once the physician or medical professional has completed the appropriate screening and referral forms, it is prudent for the ACE-AHFS to obtain additional diagnostic reports. The client should sign a "release of medical information" form to enable the physician's office to release other pertinent medical information. A client may also be able to provide copies of reports and lab results, saving time for all parties. The following diagnostic test results will be valuable when developing a comprehensive health and fitness program:

- Diagnostic reports
- Lab work, including blood tests
- Progress reports and/or discharge notes from other allied healthcare professionals (e.g., physical therapist, occupational therapist, registered dietitian)
- Medication list

Figure 1-6
PARmed-X for Pregnancy

Physical Activity Readiness
Medical Examination for
Pregnancy (2002)

PARmed-X for PREGNANCY PHYSICAL ACTIVITY READINESS MEDICAL EXAMINATION

PARmed-X for PREGNANCY is a guideline for health screening prior to participation in a prenatal fitness class or other exercise.

Healthy women with uncomplicated pregnancies can integrate physical activity into their daily living and can participate without significant risks either to themselves or to their unborn child. Postulated benefits of such programs include improved aerobic and muscular fitness, promotion of appropriate weight gain, and facilitation of labour. Regular exercise may also help to prevent gestational glucose intolerance and pregnancy-induced hypertension.

The safety of prenatal exercise programs depends on an adequate level of maternal-fetal physiological reserve. PARmed-X for PREGNANCY is a convenient checklist and prescription for use by health care providers to evaluate pregnant patients who want to enter a prenatal fitness program and for ongoing medical surveillance of exercising pregnant patients.

Instructions for use of the 4-page PARmed-X for PREGNANCY are the following:

1. The patient should fill out the section on PATIENT INFORMATION and the PRE-EXERCISE HEALTH CHECKLIST (PART 1, 2, 3, and 4 on p. 1) and give the form to the health care provider monitoring her pregnancy.
2. The health care provider should check the information provided by the patient for accuracy and fill out SECTION C on CONTRAINDICATIONS (p. 2) based on current medical information.
3. If no exercise contraindications exist, the HEALTH EVALUATION FORM (p. 3) should be completed, signed by the health care provider, and given by the patient to her prenatal fitness professional.

In addition to prudent medical care, participation in appropriate types, intensities and amounts of exercise is recommended to increase the likelihood of a beneficial pregnancy outcome. PARmed-X for PREGNANCY provides recommendations for individualized exercise prescription (p. 3) and program safety (p. 4).

NOTE: Sections A and B should be completed by the patient before the appointment with the health care provider.

A PATIENT INFORMATION

NAME ______________________________

ADDRESS ______________________________

TELEPHONE ____________ BIRTHDATE ____________ HEALTH INSURANCE No. ____________

NAME OF PRENATAL FITNESS PROFESSIONAL ____________ PRENATAL FITNESS PROFESSIONAL'S PHONE NUMBER ____________

B PRE-EXERCISE HEALTH CHECKLIST

PART 1: GENERAL HEALTH STATUS

In the past, have you experienced (check YES or NO):

	YES	NO
1. Miscarriage in an earlier pregnacy?	❑	❑
2. Other pregnancy complications?	❑	❑
3. I have completed a PAR-Q within the last 30 days.	❑	❑

If you answered YES to question 1 or 2, please explain:

____

Number of previous pregnancies? _______

PART 2: STATUS OF CURRENT PREGNANCY

Due Date: ______________________________

During this pregnancy, have you experienced:

	YES	NO
1. Marked fatigue?	❑	❑
2. Bleeding from the vagina ("spotting")?	❑	❑
3. Unexplained faintness or dizziness?	❑	❑
4. Unexplained abdominal pain?	❑	❑
5. Sudden swelling of ankles, hands or face?	❑	❑
6. Persistent headaches or problems with headaches?	❑	❑
7. Swelling, pain or redness in the calf of one leg?	❑	❑
8. Absence of fetal movement after 6th month?	❑	❑
9. Failure to gain weight after 5th month?	❑	❑

If you answered YES to any of the above questions, please explain:

____

PART 3: ACTIVITY HABITS DURING THE PAST MONTH

1. List only regular fitness/recreational activities:

____

____

INTENSITY	FREQUENCY (times/week) 1-2	2-4	4+	TIME (minutes/day) <20	20-40	40+
Heavy	___	___	___	___	___	___
Medium	___	___	___	___	___	___
Light	___	___	___	___	___	___

2. Does your regular occupation (job/home) activity involve:

	YES	NO
Heavy Lifting?	❑	❑
Frequent walking/stair climbing?	❑	❑
Occasional walking (>once/hr)?	❑	❑
Prolonged standing?	❑	❑
Mainly sitting?	❑	❑
Normal daily activity?	❑	❑
3. Do you currently smoke tobacco?*	❑	❑
4. Do you consume alcohol?*	❑	❑

PART 4: PHYSICAL ACTIVITY INTENTIONS

What physical activity do you intend to do?

____

Is this a change from what you currently do? ❑ YES ❑ NO

*NOTE: PREGNANT WOMEN ARE STRONGLY ADVISED NOT TO SMOKE OR CONSUME ALCOHOL DURING PREGNANCY AND DURING LACTATION.

1

Figure 1-6
PARmed-X for Pregnancy (continued)

Physical Activity Readiness
Medical Examination for
Pregnancy (2002)

PARmed-X for PREGNANCY PHYSICAL ACTIVITY READINESS MEDICAL EXAMINATION

C CONTRAINDICATIONS TO EXERCISE: to be completed by your health care provider

Absolute Contraindications

Does the patient have:

	YES	NO
1. Ruptured membranes, premature labour?	❑	❑
2. Persistent second or third trimester bleeding/placenta previa?	❑	❑
3. Pregnancy-induced hypertension or pre-eclampsia?	❑	❑
4. Incompetent cervix?	❑	❑
5. Evidence of intrauterine growth restriction?	❑	❑
6. High-order pregnancy (e.g., triplets)?	❑	❑
7. Uncontrolled Type I diabetes, hypertension or thyroid disease, other serious cardiovascular, respiratory or systemic disorder?	❑	❑

Relative Contraindications

Does the patient have:

	YES	NO
1. History of spontaneous abortion or premature labour in previous pregnancies?	❑	❑
2. Mild/moderate cardiovascular or respiratory disease (e.g., chronic hypertension, asthma)?	❑	❑
3. Anemia or iron deficiency? (Hb < 100 g/L)?	❑	❑
4. Malnutrition or eating disorder (anorexia, bulimia)?	❑	❑
5. Twin pregnancy after 28th week?	❑	❑
6. Other significant medical condition?	❑	❑

Please specify: ______________________

NOTE: Risk may exceed benefits of regular physical activity. The decision to be physically active or not should be made with qualified medical advice.

PHYSICAL ACTIVITY RECOMMENDATION: ❑ Recommended/Approved ❑ Contraindicated

Prescription for Aerobic Activity

RATE OF PROGRESSION: The best time to progress is during the second trimester since risks and discomforts of pregnancy are lowest at that time. Aerobic exercise should be increased gradually during the second trimester from a minimum of 15 minutes per session, 3 times per week (at the appropriate target heart rate or RPE to a maximum of approximately 30 minutes per session, 4 times per week (at the appropriate target heart rate or RPE).

WARM-UP/COOL-DOWN: Aerobic activity should be preceded by a brief (10-15 min.) warm-up and followed by a short (10-15 min.) cool-down. Low intensity calesthenics, stretching and relaxation exercises should be included in the warm-up/cool-down.

F	I	T	T
FREQUENCY	**INTENSITY**	**TIME**	**TYPE**
Begin at 3 times per week and progress to four times per week	Exercise within an appropriate RPE range and/or target heart rate zone	Attempt 15 minutes, even if it means reducing the intensity. Rest intervals may be helpful	Non weight-bearing or low-impact endurance exercise using large muscle groups (e.g., walking, stationary cycling, swimming, aquatic exercises, low impact aerobics)

"TALK TEST" - A final check to avoid overexertion is to use the "talk test". The exercise intensity is excessive if you cannot carry on a verbal conversation while exercising.

PRESCRIPTION/MONITORING OF INTENSITY: The best way to prescribe and monitor exercise is by combining the heart rate and rating of perceived exertion (RPE) methods.

TARGET HEART RATE ZONES

The heart rate zones shown below are appropriate for most pregnant women. Work during the lower end of the HR range at the start of a new exercise program and in late pregnancy.

Age	Heart Rate Range
< 20	140-155
20-29	135-150
30-39	130-145

RATING OF PERCEIVED EXERTION (RPE)

Check the accuracy of your heart rate target zone by comparing it to the scale below. A range of about 12-14 (somewhat hard) is appropriate for most pregnant women.

6	
7	Very, very light
8	
9	Somewhat light
10	
11	Fairly light
12	
13	Somewhat hard
14	
15	Hard
16	
17	Very hard
18	
19	Very, very hard
20	

The original PARmed-X for PREGNANCY was developed by L.A. Wolfe, Ph.D., Queen's University. The muscular conditioning component was developed by M.F. Mottola, Ph.D., University of Western Ontario. The document has been revised based on advice from an Expert Advisory Committee of the Canadian Society for Exercise Physiology chaired by Dr. N. Gledhill, with additonal input from Drs. Wolfe and Mottola, and Gregory A.L. Davies, M.D.,FRCS(C) Department of Obstetrics and Gynaecology, Queen's University, 2002.

No changes permitted. Translation and reproduction in its entirety is encouraged.

Disponible en français sous le titre «Examination medicale sur l'aptitude à l'activité physique pour les femmes enceintes (X-AAP pour les femmes enceintes)»

Additional copies of the PARmed-X for PREGNANCY, the PARmed-X and/or the PAR-Q can be downloaded from: http://www.csep.ca/forms.asp.
For more information contact the:

Canadian Society for Exercise Physiology
185 Somerset St. West, Suite 202, Ottawa, Ontario CANADA K2P 0J2
tel.: 1-877-651-3755 FAX (613) 234-3565 www.csep.ca

2

Figure 1-6
PARmed-X for Pregnancy (continued)

Physical Activity Readiness
Medical Examination for
Pregnancy (2002)

PARmed-X for PREGNANCY PHYSICAL ACTIVITY READINESS MEDICAL EXAMINATION

Prescription for Muscular Conditioning

It is important to condition all major muscle groups during both prenatal and postnatal periods.

WARM-UPS & COOL DOWN:
Range of Motion: neck, shoulder girdle, back, arms, hips, knees, ankles, etc.

Static Stretching: all major muscle groups

(DO NOT OVER STRETCH!)

EXAMPLES OF MUSCULAR STRENGTHENING EXERCISES

CATEGORY	PURPOSE	EXAMPLE
Upper back	Promotion of good posture	Shoulder shrugs, shoulder blade pinch
Lower back	Promotion of good posture	Modified standing opposite leg & arm lifts
Abdomen	Promotion of good posture, prevent low-back pain, prevent diastasis recti, strengthen muscles of labour	Abdominal tightening, abdominal curl-ups, head raises lying on side or standing position
Pelvic floor ("Kegels")	Promotion of good bladder control, prevention of urinary incontinence	"Wave", "elevator"
Upper body	Improve muscular support for breasts	Shoulder rotations, modified push-ups against a wall
Buttocks, lower limbs	Facilitation of weight-bearing, prevention of varicose veins	Buttocks squeeze, standing leg lifts, heel raises

PRECAUTIONS FOR MUSCULAR CONDITIONING DURING PREGNANCY

VARIABLE	EFFECTS OF PREGNANCY	EXERCISE MODIFICATIONS
Body Position	• in the supine position (lying on the back), the enlarged uterus may either decrease the flow of blood returning from the lower half of the body as it presses on a major vein (inferior vena cava) or it may decrease flow to a major artery (abdominal aorta)	• past 4 months of gestation, exercises normally done in the supine position should be altered • such exercises should be done side lying or standing
Joint Laxity	• ligaments become relaxed due to increasing hormone levels • joints may be prone to injury	• avoid rapid changes in direction and bouncing during exercises • stretching should be performed with controlled movements
Abdominal Muscles	• presence of a rippling (bulging) of connective tissue along the midline of the pregnant abdomen (diastasis recti) may be seen during abdominal exercise	• abdominal exercises are not recommended if diastasis recti develops
Posture	• increasing weight of enlarged breasts and uterus may cause a forward shift in the centre of gravity and may increase the arch in the lower back • this may also cause shoulders to slump forward	• emphasis on correct posture and neutral pelvic alignment. Neutral pelvic alignment is found by bending the knees, feet shoulder width apart, and aligning the pelvis between accentuated lordosis and the posterior pelvic tilt position.
Precautions for Resistance Exercise	• emphasis must be placed on continuous breathing throughout exercise • exhale on exertion, inhale on relaxation using high repetitions and low weights • Valsalva Manoevre (holding breath while working against a resistance) causes a change in blood pressure and therefore should be avoided • avoid exercise in supine position past 4 months gestation	

PARmed-X for Pregnancy - Health Evaluation Form

(to be completed by patient and given to the prenatal fitness professional after obtaining medical clearance to exercise)

I, ______________________ PLEASE PRINT (patient's name), have discussed my plans to participate in physical activity during my current pregnancy with my health care provider and I have obtained his/her approval to begin participation.

Signed: ______________________ (patient's signature)

Date: ______________________

HEALTH CARE PROVIDER'S COMMENTS:

Name of health care provider: ______________________

Address: ______________________

____

Telephone: ______________________

______________________ (health care provider's signature)

3

Figure 1-6
PARmed-X for Pregnancy (continued)

Physical Activity Readiness
Medical Examination for
Pregnancy (2002)

Advice for Active Living During Pregnancy

Pregnancy is a time when women can make beneficial changes in their health habits to protect and promote the healthy development of their unborn babies. These changes include adopting improved eating habits, abstinence from smoking and alcohol intake, and participating in regular moderate physical activity. Since all of these changes can be carried over into the postnatal period and beyond, pregnancy is a very good time to adopt healthy lifestyle habits that are permanent by integrating physical activity with enjoyable healthy eating and a positive self and body image.

Active Living:

- see your doctor before increasing your activity level during pregnancy
- exercise regularly but don't overexert
- exercise with a pregnant friend or join a prenatal exercise program
- follow FITT principles modified for pregnant women
- know safety considerations for exercise in pregnancy

Healthy Eating:

- the need for calories is higher (about 300 more per day) than before pregnancy
- follow Canada's Food Guide to Healthy Eating and choose healthy foods from the following groups: whole grain or enriched bread or cereal, fruits and vegetables, milk and milk products, meat, fish, poultry and alternatives
- drink 6-8 glasses of fluid, including water, each day
- salt intake should not be restricted
- limit caffeine intake i.e., coffee, tea, chocolate, and cola drinks
- dieting to lose weight is not recommended during pregnancy

Positive Self and Body Image:

- remember that it is normal to gain weight during pregnancy
- accept that your body shape will change during pregnancy
- enjoy your pregnancy as a unique and meaningful experience

For more detailed information and advice about pre- and postnatal exercise, you may wish to obtain a copy of a booklet entitled *Active Living During Pregnancy: Physical Activity Guidelines for Mother and Baby* © 1999. Available from the Canadian Society for Exercise Physiology, 185 Somerset St. West, Suite 202, Ottawa, Ontario Canada K2P 0J2 Tel. 1-877-651-3755 Fax: (613) 234-3565 Email: info@csep.ca (online: www.csep.ca). Cost: $11.95

For more detailed information about the safety of exercise in pregnancy you may wish to obtain a copy of the Clinical Practice Guidelines of the Society of Obstetricians and Gynaecologists of Canada and Canadian Society for Exercise Physiology entitled *Exercise in Pregnancy and Postpartum* © 2003. Available from the Society of Obstetricians and Gynaecologists of Canada online at www.sogc.org

For more detailed information about pregnancy and childbirth you may wish to obtain a copy of *Healthy Beginnings: Your Handbook for Pregnancy and Birth* © 1998. Available from the Society of Obstetricians and Gynaecologists of Canada at 1-877-519-7999 (also available online at www.sogc.org) Cost $12.95.

For more detailed information on healthy eating during pregnancy, you may wish to obtain a copy of *Nutrition for a Healthy Pregnancy: National Guidelines for the Childbearing Years* © 1999. Available from Health Canada, Minister of Public Works and Government Services, Ottawa, Ontario Canada (also available online at www.hc-sc.gc.ca).

SAFETY CONSIDERATIONS

- Avoid exercise in warm/humid environments, especially during the 1st trimester
- Avoid isometric exercise or straining while holding your breath
- Maintain adequate nutrition and hydration — drink liquids before and after exercise
- Avoid exercise while lying on your back past the 4th month of pregnancy
- Avoid activities which involve physical contact or danger of falling
- Know your limits — pregnancy is not a good time to train for athletic competition
- Know the reasons to stop exercise and consult a qualified health care provider immediately if they occur

REASONS TO STOP EXERCISE AND CONSULT YOUR HEALTH CARE PROVIDER

- Excessive shortness of breath
- Chest pain
- Painful uterine contractions (more than 6-8 per hour)
- Vaginal bleeding
- Any "gush" of fluid from vagina (suggesting premature rupture of the membranes)
- Dizziness or faintness

4

Informed Consent and Liability Waivers

The informed consent and liability waiver is an important document designed to protect both the client and the ACE-AHFS. This form serves as an educational tool, informing the client about the assessment process and the potential risks associated with fitness testing and exercise programming. A well-prepared document can also protect the ACE-AHFS from undue legal actions. An informed consent will likely include the following sections:

- The purpose and description of the assessment tests
- An explanation of risks associated with exercise testing and programming
- A listing of the client's rights, including refraining from or terminating any testing procedure or exercise activity at will
- A listing of the client's responsibilities. For example, it is the client's responsibility to communicate openly and honestly with the ACE-AHFS about any health concerns that arise throughout the course of the exercise testing or training program. He or she should also feel free to ask questions about any aspect of the exercise testing or training program.
- A confidentiality clause stating that the ACE-AHFS will maintain strict confidentiality on all client information

The client should of course read the form, but the ACE-AHFS should also verbally review all content areas with the client before the client signs it. For more information on informed consent and liability waivers, refer to the *ACE Personal Trainer Manual* or the *ACE Fitness and Business Forms Handbook*. It is strongly recommended that the ACE-AHFS consult an attorney who specializes in waivers and consent forms in the specific state or jurisdiction where he or she works.

Fitness Assessment

It is expected that the ACE-AHFS is fully trained in the area of fitness assessment. This section simply serves as a synopsis of the initial assessment as it relates to working with special populations.

The ACE-AHFS should take great care in deciding on an appropriate battery of tests. The client may have discharge summaries and diagnostic reports that will eliminate the need for some fitness testing. For example, if the client recently underwent a maximal stress test, there may be no need to complete a submaximal aerobic fitness test. The ACE-AHFS must also consider the client's current health condition and ability to tolerate certain fitness tests.

In general, testing should be conducted to measure:

- Resting heart rate and blood pressure
- Submaximal aerobic fitness
- Body composition
- Muscular fitness
- Joint range of motion
- Neuromuscular function
- Postural alignment

Table 1-3 presents information on assessing clients with health challenges. The ACE-AHFS can find information in the "Special Considerations" column of this table when interpreting the assessment results.

Another necessary piece of background information will come from the client's Health Status Questionnaire (see Figure 1-5). This form will give the ACE-AHFS insight into the client's current and past lifestyle habits. The questionnaire addresses behaviors such as dietary habits, physical-activity patterns, sleep and stress-management activities, as well as family history of early disease or dysfunction.

The initial assessment should conclude by interpreting the results of the client's fitness assessment along with discussing the details of the Health Status Questionnaire. This part of the session should be optimistic, yet realistic and honest, with viable solutions offered for areas in need of improvement. This face-to-face meeting is a great way to build **rapport** and open up lines of communication. Developing an initial plan of action that offers sensible solutions to common behavior-change

Table 1-3
Assessment of Clients With a Health Challenge

PARAMETER	ASSESSMENT	SPECIAL CONSIDERATIONS
RESTING CARDIOVASCULAR FUNCTION		
• Heart rate • Systolic/diastolic blood pressure	Two 30- to 60-second measurements 3–5 min apart	Abnormal: HR >100 bpm Abnormal: SBP ≥140 mmHg and/or DBP ≥90 mmHg
BODY COMPOSITION		
• Height and weight	Record: in/lb or cm/kg	
• BMI	Determined via: weight (kg)/height (m^2)	When BMI ≥30, initiate weight-management strategies: indicates obesity
• Circumference measures	Waist, hip, upper arm, upper thigh WHR	Good measures to confirm loss of inches Abnormal: men >0.95; women >0.86
• Skinfold measures	Recommended: waist, iliac, thigh, subscapular, chest, mid-calf, midaxillary	Requires accurate anatomic location of skinfold sites to determine body fat
• Other techniques	Bioelectrical impedance, hydrostatic weighing, and near-infrared interactance	Requires sophisticated, often costly, equipment
SUBMAXIMAL AEROBIC FITNESS ASSESSMENT		
• Aerobic capacity	In lab setting, use various ergometers: upright bicycle, recumbent bicycle, treadmill, and arm. In field, use walking test.	Use of standard protocol may require modification for some health challenges
	DATA: HR and RPE	Both are good indicators of effort, though HR response may be blunted on certain cardiac medications, including beta blockers
• Endurance performance	Functional assessment must focus on mode of activity familiar to the client DATA: Time to complete known distance	Good means to assess progress for clients who are limited (e.g., cardiac, pulmonary, arthritic, disabled)
MUSCULAR FITNESS MEASURES		
• Muscle strength	Repetition-max test; repetition number specific to client's health status and level of muscular strength	Not appropriate for all persons: Handgrip dynamometer Caution in using these tests Prior strength training and proper cueing important for performing correctly
• Muscle endurance	Number of repetitions before fatigue using: curl-ups, pull-ups, YMCA bench press, or any muscle group	Tests are available with norms, but not all persons can perform such tests. Address specific ability of client to perform repeated movements of any muscle group. Use RPE as a guide to fatigue.
• Joint range of motion (Flexibility)	Upper extremities with goniometer or standardized instrument and lower extremities with goniometer or standardized instrument	Shoulder flexion/extension/abduction and adduction/internal/external rotation. Focus on functional ADL outcomes: sit and reach (low back); hip flexor/extensor; hip adduction and abduction; gastoc-soleus complex; ankle flexibility. Focus on functional ADL outcomes related to balance, coordination, and muscular imbalances.
NEUROMUSCULAR ASSESSMENTS		
	Hand-eye coordination, reaction time, gait analysis, balance	Focus on functional ADL outcomes related to balance, coordination, and muscular imbalances.

Note: HR = Heart rate; SBP = Systolic blood pressure; DBP = Diastolic blood pressure; BMI = Body mass index; WHR = Waist-to-hip ratio; RPE = Rating of perceived exertion; ADL = Activities of daily living obstacles will enhance the client's trust and confidence in the ACE-AHFS. Chapter 3 of this book is devoted to communication strategies and behavior change.

Components of Program Design

The ACE-AHFS is responsible for designing and implementing a progressive health and fitness program. The client should be well-advised of the exercise plan, including short- and long-term goals. To enhance the health and well-being of a client, a comprehensive program should include most, if not all, of the following components:

- Cardiorespiratory endurance
- Muscular strength
- Muscular endurance
- Flexibility
- Body composition
- Balance
- Posture
- Breathing techniques
- Stress management
- Nutrition
- Daily physical-activity plan

The ACE-AHFS should know how to safely and effectively improve the basic components of physical fitness: **cardiorespiratory endurance, muscular strength** and **endurance, flexibility,** and body composition. The remaining components are just as important, but likely will be included as a supplement to the basic fitness components. As an advanced fitness professional, the ACE-AHFS should also know how to make appropriate programming adjustments for specific health conditions, ranging from rotator cuff impingement to obesity. Application of these key elements as they relate to program design and implementation for specific diseases and dysfunctions is discussed in detail in subsequent chapters.

A thorough understanding of the client's condition will enable the ACE-AHFS to design a safe and effective fitness program. Though each program will vary depending on the specific goals and objectives of the client, the basic framework for exercise progression is based on the FITT principle: frequency, intensity, time, and type of exercise.

- F: 3–5 days per week (daily for some clients)
- I: 60–90% of predicted maximum heart rate (MHR)
- T: 20–60 minutes of continuous or accumulated activity
- T: Specific modes of exercise to improve muscular strength and endurance, cardiorespiratory endurance, flexibility, and body composition

When determining the appropriate plan for exercise progression, the ACE-AHFS must assess the objective data (e.g., heart rate and blood pressure, treadmill speeds, sets and repetitions), as well as the subjective data (e.g., **ratings of perceived exertion**, leg pain, difficulty in breathing, excess fatigue). The client-reported information may be more valuable when determining the appropriate modifications in the fitness plan.

Home Exercise Program

One program component that is often overlooked is the home exercise program. The time spent with a client may only total two to three hours per week. To optimize health and wellness, it is important to establish a fitness plan for the remaining time away from the live training sessions. Might the client benefit from a yoga class or a post-rehabilitation support group? Would a weekly aquatic exercise class be an appropriate supplement to land-based training program? The ACE-AHFS will do well to consider a variety of options when designing a comprehensive health and wellness program.

The fact that the ACE-AHFS meets with the client on a regular basis creates a favorable position within the healthcare continuum for optimizing behavioral change and disease management. Using information-gathering techniques, the ACE-AHFS will be able to modify the client's program and enable the successful completion of the agreed-upon goals and objectives. If a problem arises, the ACE-AHFS can discuss his or her concerns with the referring physician before symptoms deteriorate. The ACE-AHFS should hold the client accountable for behavioral modification and provide the necessary tools and support to facilitate positive change. This responsibility starts with the initial evaluation and continues with each and every session.

Developing a Referral Network

It is important to develop a network of referral sources to supplement the program provided by the existing healthcare team. These complementary programs should be directed by health professionals who are reputable and aspire to the same professional standards as an ACE-AHFS. Potential referral sources include the following:

- Mind/body instructors (e.g., yoga, tai chi, qi gong)
- Smoking cessation programs
- Aquatic exercise programs
- Support groups (e.g., cardiac rehab, cancer survivors, Overeaters Anonymous)
- Acupuncturist
- Massage therapist

As the ACE-AHFS develops a referral network, it is important to research the instructors, programs, or organizations before recommending any programs or services to a client. Do they have the proper licensure or certification? Can they provide a list of references? How many years of experience do they have? The ACE-AHFS does not want to jeopardize his or her reputation by referring clients to substandard health and fitness "professionals." With proper networking, the ACE-AHFS may also gain referrals from the other health and fitness professionals within the network.

Safety Concerns Related to Program Implementation

It is the responsibility of the ACE-AHFS to ensure the safety of his or her clients. Prior to each exercise session, it is necessary to conduct a brief pre-exercise assessment. When appropriate, vital signs should be checked and recorded. The client should be asked about any recent symptoms and any problems related to the exercise program itself. The ACE-AHFS should also make observations on the client's current condition. This information should be documented in the client's chart. Based on the client's subjective and objective data, the exercise program may need to be modified from the intended plan.

In addition to the absolute and relative contraindications for exercise testing and programming noted in the "PAR-Q and Exercise Readiness" section of this chapter, there are also some pre-exercise concerns related to exercise. The American College of Sports Medicine (ACSM, 2006) has outlined specific contraindications to exercise-program involvement, including the following:

- *Blood glucose:* If pre-exercise blood glucose (BG) is greater than 250 mg/dL, exercise is not recommended. If BG is less than 80 to 100 mg/dL, the client should ingest carbohydrates to increase BG prior to starting or resuming exercise.
- *Blood pressure:* If resting **systolic blood pressure (SBP)** is greater than 200 mmHg, if exercise SBP rises above 260 mmHg, or if resting or exercise **diastolic blood pressure (DBP)** is greater than 115 mmHg, the exercise session should be terminated. Exercise should also be discontinued if there is a drop in SBP with exercise.

When working with special populations, it is not uncommon for clients to see themselves as their disease. A client may label herself as a "diabetic" as opposed to a 59-year-old woman with diabetes. Clients tend to focus on what they cannot do instead of what they can do and may feel powerless against their conditions. The ACE-AHFS should create a positive atmosphere that is focused on managing or reversing the negative effects of disease. Walking into a health and fitness setting is often a positive first step in achieving a sense of "normalcy."

The role of an ACE-AHFS is to help the client make progress throughout the fitness program. It is gratifying to see a client who is suddenly able to enjoy his or her daily activities because back pain has become tolerable or diabetes has become more manageable.

The client needs to take an active part in establishing viable goals and objectives. It is important that the client accept the program goals and components. The ACE-AHFS needs to establish open, two-way communication and build rapport, ultimately gaining the trust of the client. If a client understands the rationale behind many of the program components, he or she will have a vested interest and feel a sense of accomplishment upon reaching each established milestone. Gaining a sense of control over the condition is empowering.

If a client is limiting activity based on his or her disease/dysfunction, it is important to create a comprehensive program that will enable the client to resume normal activities. For example, if he or she has not been able to golf due to severe sciatica, the ACE-AHFS can provide activities that will help stabilize the spine, strengthen the core, and increase range of motion. It would then be appropriate to create activities in the fitness setting that simulate a golf swing. The client can then progress to putting and chipping, and finally end up at the driving range. This process may take several weeks or even months, but it is important that the client has something meaningful to work toward. (The ACE-AHFS must make sure the client has been cleared by his or her physician to resume such activities.)

There are certain conditions that preclude a client from returning to optimal function. The client may have a hard time coming to terms with this fact. In this case, the ACE-AHFS should look for signs of depression or other negative psychological signs, and be prepared to refer back to the client's physician. Refer to the National Institute of Mental Health's booklet entitled *Depression* for more information on the signs and symptoms of depression (www.nimh.nih.gov).

On occasion, a client's condition may deteriorate. This process may be ever so gradual, but it can often be detected by astute observation. It is up to the ACE-AHFS to recognize warning signs of deterioration and communicate the changes to the appropriate healthcare professional (Table 1-4). In some cases, it may be appropriate to refer the client to his or personal physician for further examination.

A number of contributing factors may prompt a client's turn for the worse. Some may be related to the training program itself. Therefore, a thorough assessment of the client's program is necessary to determine if any activities may have contributed to the client's declining condition. Some symptoms may not be related to the program itself, but result from lifestyle issues, such as improper stress management.

The ACE-AHFS may determine that the signs and symptoms are related to something more serious, which may require a referral back to the primary physician. Some signs and symptoms may result from a worsening disease process, the onset of a new condition, or side effects

Table 1-4
Warning Signs of Deterioration

Physiological Changes	Performance Changes	Psychosocial Changes
• Increase in frequency or severity of symptoms • Increase or decrease in blood sugar • Frequent dizziness • Increase or decrease in blood pressure • Change in posture • Change in gait • Dramatic weight loss or weight gain • Skin discoloration • Change in the amount of sweat	• Higher heart rate at same workload • More frequent difficulty in breathing • Leg cramping • Chest pain with exertion • Increased painful sensations with exercise; tingling numbness; or localized or radiating pain • Decrease in muscular strength or endurance • Decline in pain-free range of motion	• Missed sessions • Failure to achieve agreed-upon behavioral changes • Personality or mood changes

of medications. It will be up to the personal physician to examine his or her patient and then determine the proper course of action.

The 10-step Approach

This manual provides detailed information for designing safe and effective health and fitness programs for addressing the most common diseases and dysfunctions encountered by fitness professionals. It is the responsibility of the ACE-AHFS to apply this information to individual clients. Most chapters provide one or more case studies, but it is simply impossible to cover every situation that may arise when working with special populations. The "10-Step Decision-Making Approach," which is detailed in Appendix D, is a model of reasoning to guide the ACE-AHFS through the critical decision-making steps of client risk assessment, goal-setting, and exercise design and implementation.

Risk Management

The ACE-AHFS must be familiar with the common exercise-induced risks associated with each client's disease or dysfunction. **Risk management** involves being proactive about potential threats to the health and safety of clients, staff, and visitors. There are numerous industry-accepted standards (the minimal performance expectations each facility must meet) and guidelines (recommendations to help each facility achieve higher than minimal expectations) for staffing, programming, equipment, facility layout, and emergency preparedness.

The ACE-AHFS may be working within a facility, from a home studio, or entering a client's home. Each location poses its own risk-management challenges. A written policy will help make certain that all variables have been assessed and addressed, ultimately ensuring the safety and security of the clients. This policy should include sections on risk management and emergency planning, pre-activity screening, client orientation, education, supervision, staff qualifications, facility design, fitness equipment, and operational practices.

The ACE-AHFS may need guidance on federal laws, including the Occupational Safety and Health Administration (OSHA) Blood-borne Pathogen Standard, employment laws, and the Federal Privacy Act. It is important to evaluate state laws and industry standards as they relate to **automated external defibrillator (AED)** availability and cardiopulmonary resuscitation (CPR) certification. Ultimately, being proactive helps fitness professionals protect their clients as well as their own business interests.

Lifelong Learning

The field of health education and disease prevention is constantly changing and evolving. As a responsible ACE-AHFS, it is important to stay abreast of the current research associated with health and fitness, especially as it relates to disease prevention. Knowing where to go for valid health and fitness information is paramount. There are abundant educational sources filled with medical quackery, which makes it challenging to differentiate between what is valid and what is hype. It is important to stay with well-established organizations and industry-accepted publications when searching for information. The information written in consumer magazines should be scrutinized for its content and integrity. Is the author trying to sell something? Is the study size appropriate? Are research findings statistically significant? Who conducted the study? For example, consider the biased findings of a pharmaceutical company's self-funded study of its own supplement. Has the same study been replicated by independent companies with the same or similar results?

The ACE-AHFS should take much care in deciding which reference materials and Internet sources to integrate into his or her collection of educational resources. There is a comprehensive list of references and suggested readings provided at the end of each chapter in this manual.

Additionally, it is recommended that every ACE-AHFS have the following personal references for quick and easy access to pertinent medical information:

- *Physician's Desk Reference* (PDR) and Medline Plus® (www.medlineplus.gov), among other comprehensive guides to prescription drugs

- PDR or other comprehensive guides to supplements
- Medical terminology reference (e.g., *Tabor's Cyclopedic Medical Dictionary*)
- Reputable reference guide to integrative medicine (*The American Pharmaceutical Association Practical Guide to Natural Medicines*)
- Reputable disease-specific medical textbooks, journal subscriptions, or Internet sites

When a client brings his or her list of medications and supplements, the ACE-AHFS should consider the significant side effects of these drugs, especially as they relate to exercise program design and implementation. If a client brings the written results from his or her **magnetic resonance imaging (MRI),** there may be some medical terminology in the report that is unfamiliar. It is important to understand test results, as such interpretation can have an impact on the development of the exercise plan. The ACE-AHFS is likely to encounter a client who is trying one or more alternative medical practices.

The ACE-AHFS should develop and implement a comprehensive exercise and lifestyle-modification plan, and most importantly, include an educational component. Unfortunately, many fitness professionals want their clients to become dependent on their presence. This may temporarily help the trainer's bottom line, but he or she is doing the client a disservice. One of the roles of the ACE-AHFS is to educate clients and help them establish reasonable expectations and develop their own lifelong health and fitness plan.

Consultations/Privacy Issues

During the training sessions, information can be shared with the client to enhance his or her personal knowledge base. The client will likely have many questions about his or her disease or dysfunction, especially if he or she is newly diagnosed with a disease. Due to the vast amount of information that is available on disease prevention and management, there may be a need for further educational support from other health and fitness professionals. The ACE-AHFS should develop a strong network of licensed healthcare professionals who can be consulted with specific questions that may be outside the ACE-AHFS's area of expertise. Refer to Table 1-5 for a viable list of licensed professionals.

Table 1-5
Possible Network of Licensed Professionals

- M.D./D.O.: General practitioner or internist
- M.D. specialist: Cardiologist, orthopedist, neurologist
- Clinical psychologist or psychiatrist
- Chiropractor
- Physical therapist
- Occupational therapist
- Cardiac rehabilitation specialist
- Registered dietician
- Pharmacist
- Massage therapist

As part of the ACE-AHFS's professional responsibility, all client information should remain confidential when consulting with another professional. Pertinent information can be shared, but names and recognizable traits must remain anonymous. If the consulting healthcare professional recommends a referral to a licensed professional, it may be necessary to terminate the training program until the client has received professional help and is referred back to the ACE-AHFS.

An essential aspect of the **standard of care** is knowing one's limitations. The depth of essential knowledge outlined in the performance domains included in the Exam Content Outline (see Appendix B) ranges from basic to advanced. When working with a client with health challenges, it is essential that the ACE-AHFS has more than a familiarity with the disease or dysfunction. Before venturing into unfamiliar territory, it is best to refer the client to another trainer who specializes in the specific condition in question. Trial and error is not an option when dealing with special populations.

That said, an ACE-AHFS need not limit him- or herself to well-known populations. Another important characteristic of the ACE-AHFS is the ability to acquire additional knowledge and training and learn how to safely and effectively apply this knowledge to any future clientele. Experience can be acquired from continuing education courses or through working in conjunction with another trainer who has the sought-after experience. Most hospitals have volunteer opportunities that enable further applied training with the target population. The likely place to volunteer would be in the outpatient physical therapy department or in a cardiac or pulmonary rehabilitation center.

The American Council on Exercise has created a Code of Ethics that governs the professional conduct of its certified health and fitness professionals. As an ACE-certified fitness professional, it is imperative to abide by these professional principles (see Appendix A).

Business Relationships

Medical Referrals

There are many business opportunities available for an ACE-AHFS who specializes in working with special populations. This type of certification brings with it a certain level of expertise in the field of health and fitness, as well as higher expectations from those working in the medical community.

It is unlikely that licensed healthcare providers will refer their patients to someone they do not trust or acknowledge as a competent professional. There are many ways to establish rapport with the medical community. Handing out a flyer is typically not enough to develop a strong referral network. Chapter 4 outlines ways to generate referrals from the medical community.

Self-promotion

Not every physician will be diligent in recommending a supervised health and fitness program. A business-savvy ACE-AHFS will therefore either generate referrals from the surrounding community or market him- or herself effectively to attract new clients.

Create a Written Promotional Piece

An ACE-AHFS should include information on formal education and certifications, as well as applicable career experience and training. It is also a good idea to describe risk management and established safety measures. It is important to define the specific populations being served, and possibly include documented progress achieved with individual clients—while adhering to confidentiality guidelines. Recent research on the importance of exercise in disease prevention is also helpful. Information on the referral process is paramount. The ACE-AHFS may even generate a promotional piece for healthcare professionals and a separate piece of literature for potential clients. Many medical offices welcome marketing flyers in their waiting rooms and patient treatment rooms.

Market Trainer to Trainer

One important referral source that is often overlooked is local personal trainers. Individuals with health challenges may solicit the services of a personal trainer who does not have the appropriate qualifications to work with a specific health condition. Referrals may come from personal trainers whose clients are outside their scope of practice (e.g., a new client who has been screened as inappropriate or a current client who has developed a new disease or dysfunction).

Offer Free Educational Seminars

There are a variety of opportunities for providing health and fitness education. Meeting venues include local fitness centers, YMCAs, churches, community centers, apartment clubhouses, or the local chamber of commerce. Many of these meeting spaces can be accessed at no charge and may even promote the educational seminar within their community. Press releases can greatly enhance public awareness, provided they result in media coverage.

Support groups and civic organizations are always in need of guest speakers. The community events section in local newspapers typically lists meeting schedules and contact information.

Write

For optimal recognition, the ACE-AHFS needs to establish him- or herself as the area's "expert in the field." Writing articles for the local newspaper or community magazine is a great way to develop a recognizable trademark.

Volunteer

Countless nonprofit organizations rely on volunteers for support. The people who are involved with these organizations are often other health and fitness professionals with a passion for the group's specific cause. Working side by side with other like-minded professionals is a great networking opportunity and a very rewarding way to help those in need. The following is a sample list of national organizations, though local hospitals and charities will also have volunteer opportunities:

- American Diabetes Foundation: www.diabetes.org
- American Heart Association: www.americanheart.org
- Arthritis Foundation: www.arthritis.org
- National Osteoporosis Foundation: www.nof.org

Create Packages

Partnering with other health and fitness professionals can generate more business, and also be a great opportunity for an ACE-AHFS to make him- or herself known to other professionals in the geographical area. These packages can even be offered to local charities for silent auctions or other fundraising strategies. A popular package might include:

- Three personal training sessions, complete with risk assessment
- One session with a licensed massage therapist
- One session with a health-conscious personal chef

Utilize ACE Resources

Consumers often do their own research when looking to hire a personal trainer or ACE-AHFS. ACE-certified professionals can market themselves via the ACE website (www.acefitness.org). There are other services available through ACE that can be pursued as a way to promote the programs and services of the ACE-AHFS.

Summary

The current healthcare system spends 80% of its resources treating chronic illness and disease. Resources would be much better spent educating the general population and implementing programs to prevent or manage disease and dysfunction. The ACE-certified Advanced Health & Fitness Specialist is in a perfect position to facilitate this paradigm shift.

It is the responsibility of the ACE-AHFS to stay within his or her scope of practice; educate both the healthcare community as well as the general public on the benefits of supervised, progressive fitness programs; and advocate high standards of professionalism within the field.

There are very few professions that have the opportunity to significantly impact the health and well-being of the clientele they serve. With the necessary knowledge and skills to focus on disease prevention and management, plus the dedication to make a difference in the lives of others, an ACE-AHFS can become an integral part of the healthcare continuum.

References

Institute of Medicine of the National Academies, Committee on the Use of Complementary and Alternative Medicine by the American Public (2005). *Complementary and Alternative Medicine Use in the United States.* Washington, D.C.: National Academies Press.

U.S. Preventive Services Task Force (1996). *Guide to Clinical Preventative Services* (2nd ed.). Baltimore: Williams & Wilkins.

Suggested Reading

American College of Sports Medicine (2007). *ACSM's Health/Fitness Facility Standards and Guidelines* (3rd ed.). Champaign, Ill.: Human Kinetics.

American College of Sports Medicine (2006). *ACSM's Guidelines for Exercise Testing and Prescription* (7th ed.). Philadelphia: Lippincott Williams & Wilkins.

American College of Sports Medicine (2003). *ACSM's Exercise Management for Persons with Chronic Disease and Disabilities* (2nd ed.). Champaign, Ill.: Human Kinetics.

American College of Sports Medicine (1998). AHA/ACSM joint statement: Recommendations for cardiovascular screening, staffing, and emergency policies at health/fitness facilities. *Medicine & Science in Sports & Exercise*, 30, 6, 7–8.

American Council on Exercise (2008). *ACE Lifestyle & Weight Management Consultant Manual* (2nd ed.). San Diego: American Council on Exercise.

American Council on Exercise (2007). *ACE Clinical Exercise Specialist Manual.* San Diego: American Council on Exercise.

American Council on Exercise (2006). *The ACE Fitness and Business Forms Handbook.* Monterey, Calif.: Healthy Learning

American Council on Exercise (2003). *ACE Personal Trainer Manual* (2nd ed.). San Diego: American Council on Exercise.

Medline Plus Reference on Drugs and Supplements (A service of the National Library of Medicine and National Institutes of Health) www.medlineplus.gov.

Physician's Desk Reference (57th ed.) (2003). Montvale, N.J.: PDR.

Pierce, A. (1999). *The American Pharmaceutical Association Practical Guide to Natural Medicines*. New York: Stonesong Press.

Pressman, A. & Shelley, D. (2000). *Integrative Medicine.* New York: St. Martin's Press.

Riegelman, R.K. (2004). *Studying a Study and Testing a Test: How to Read the Medical Evidence.* Philadelphia: Lippincott Williams & Wilkins.

Tabor's Cyclopedic Medical Dictionary (2001). Philadelphia: F.A. Davis Co.

Woolf, S. H., Jonas, S., & Lawrence, R. (1996). *Health Promotion and Disease Prevention in Clinical Practice.* Baltimore: Williams & Wilkins.

In This Chapter

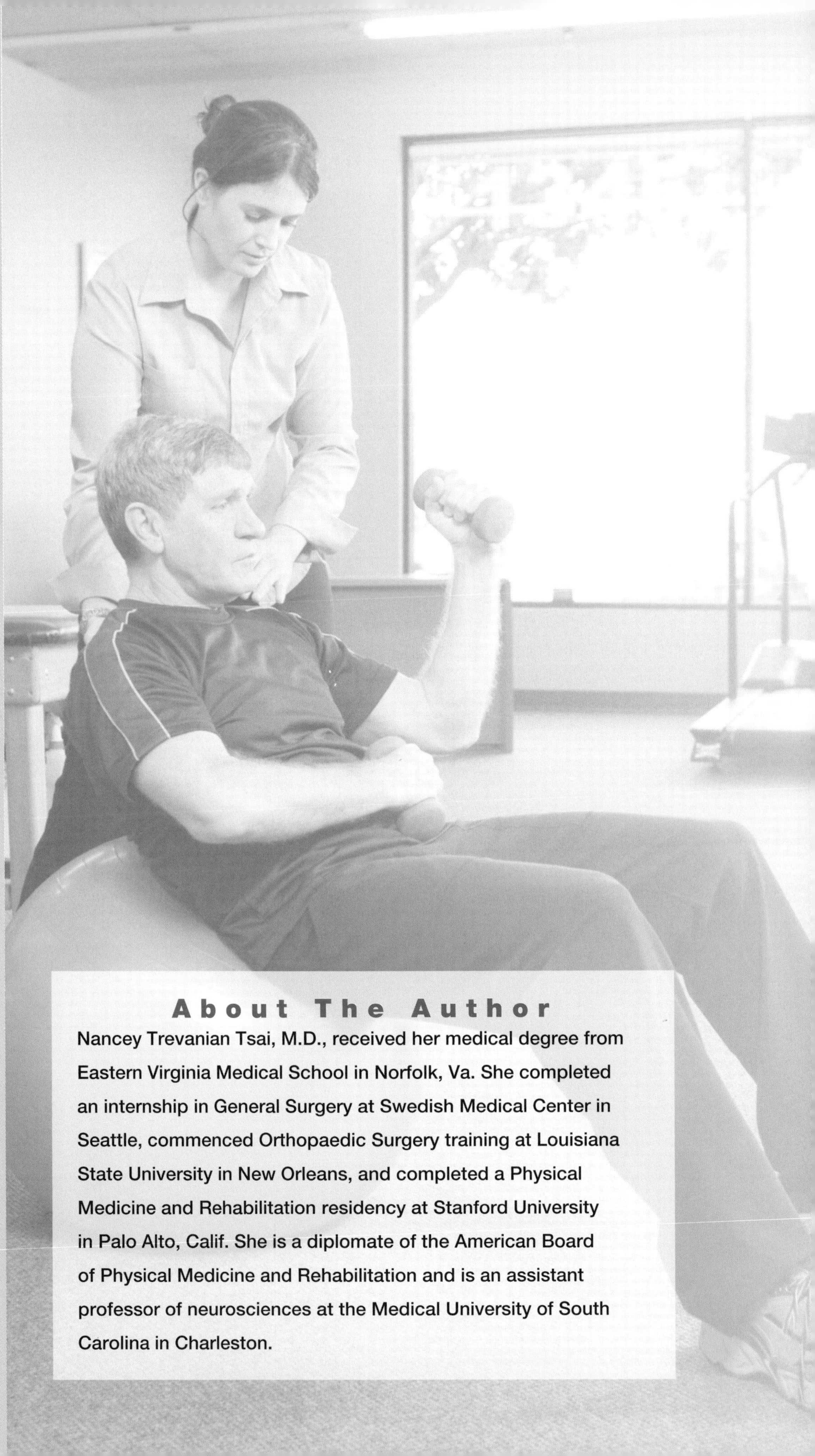

About The Author

Nancey Trevanian Tsai, M.D., received her medical degree from Eastern Virginia Medical School in Norfolk, Va. She completed an internship in General Surgery at Swedish Medical Center in Seattle, commenced Orthopaedic Surgery training at Louisiana State University in New Orleans, and completed a Physical Medicine and Rehabilitation residency at Stanford University in Palo Alto, Calif. She is a diplomate of the American Board of Physical Medicine and Rehabilitation and is an assistant professor of neurosciences at the Medical University of South Carolina in Charleston.

CHAPTER 2

Working With Clients With Health Challenges

Nancey Trevanian Tsai

Mr. James is a 32-year-old man who had been an athlete in high school, but has not been active over the past decade. During that time, he started law school and recently became a junior partner at his firm, which involves working long hours on most days and reviewing documentation frequently on weekends. He is married and likes to go out to eat with his wife several times a week, since they do not spend as much time together as he would like. Upon further questioning, it is revealed that his typical daily diet includes a large coffee drink, a good-sized lunch, and a full restaurant dinner with a glass of wine. He drinks soft drinks or sweet tea throughout the day, occasionally getting a carbohydrate snack, such as pretzels or a bagel. He confesses that he does not exercise, and his hectic study and work schedule are a ready excuse. His weight has steadily increased, as he has added 50 pounds (22.5 kg) to his average-height, medium-build frame. At his last checkup, his blood pressure and blood sugars were mildly elevated, and his cholesterol was high but not requiring of medication. He complains of feeling fatigued all the time and not sleeping well, even when he has time. His wife complains that he is starting to snore more loudly. He is concerned because his father had a heart attack when he was in his late 40s and a stroke shortly after he retired. Between those events, his father developed osteoarthritis of the knees, for which he had joint replacement surgeries. Mr. James' physician has cleared him and recommended regular exercise at least three times a week. He would like fitness and diet recommendations to help him lose weight and manage the early symptoms of the metabolic syndrome.

People are living longer than they have ever lived in history. For the most part, their health is sustained for the duration of their longer lives. However, for many Americans and people in other post-industrial nations, poor lifestyle choices have led to multiple health challenges. For example, **type 2 diabetes** far exceeds the incidence of **type 1 diabetes** in the United States. Researchers have found that the majority (64%) of Americans can now be classified as **overweight,** 15% of children are obese, and an increasing number are considered morbidly obese (Hedley et al., 2004). **Obesity** is associated with other musculoskeletal problems, such as **osteoarthritis** of the spine and extremities, sometimes requiring joint replacement or back surgery. A constellation of symptoms that are often seen together—including borderline **hypertension, hyperglycemia,** and elevated **lipids**—is now termed the **metabolic syndrome.** Fortunately, improving lifestyle choices nearly always improves health status.

It is not uncommon to see clients such as Mr. James who have relatively **sedentary** lifestyles combined with less than optimal nutrition choices. The pattern starts insidiously, typically with a relative decrease in activity due to time constraints. However, to make up for the physical and mental fatigue that accompanies the sedentary lifestyle, food choices that give short bursts of energy are chosen over better balanced meals in the client's effort to "keep going." These habits are developed over years, although it is not unusual for clients to be surprised at their fitness decline. Adding to this constellation of lifestyle choices are the genetic predispositions toward particular diseases. The cause of most health problems is often multifactorial. The solution, however, typically is not overly complex.

Mr. James states that he does not have any significant past medical history, except strep throat and chicken pox as a child and some minor sprains from when he played baseball in high school. He has no significant past surgical history other than wisdom teeth extraction. He does not take any medications at this time and thinks he might be allergic to penicillin. He does not smoke currently, but has chewed tobacco in the past. He does say, "Sometimes, I'll smoke after having a couple beers with my buddies." He denies any illicit drug use. He is also concerned that both of his hands are getting numb, especially at the end of a long day's work on the computer. He asks, "Am I having early signs of heart disease?"

Most lifestyle-related diseases can be addressed successfully by a combination of a sensible diet and a regular exercise program. The major diseases that plague modern productivity include **cardiovascular disease,** hyperglycemia, **diabetes,** and overuse- and obesity-related musculoskeletal disorders such as osteoarthritis and low-back pain. While genetic predisposition can lead to increased risk of developing these diseases, it is obvious that lifestyle remains the single most influential factor in the incidence of these diseases. When working with clients with multiple health challenges, it is important to offer understanding regarding the effects of their disease processes, encourage transparency into their habits, and establish accountability for their choices.

During the ***intake assessment,*** *Mr. James was found to have posterior pelvic tilt and limited flexibility in his hamstrings and hip flexors. His posture was notable for protracted shoulders with a rounded upper back. He was able to comfortably walk on a treadmill, but was having difficulty carrying a normal conversation after three minutes at 4 mph. He continues for 20 minutes and reports feeling spent. The ACE-certified Advanced Health & Fitness Specialist (ACE-AHFS) instructs him to drink several ounces of water and proceed to the cool-down area for stretching. The ACE-AHFS then asks him to list the times when he feels comfortable committing to fitness activities and to keep a journal of his food and drink intake over the next week for review.*

Psychological Impact of Health Challenges

Impact of Disease

The diagnosis of a disease can impact a person's sense of self and wellness. For some, the diagnosis comes after a catastrophic event, such as a heart attack or a **stroke.** For others, it is an insidious process that may only be noticed by loved ones. The reactions to the diagnosis of a disease can be as diverse as abject denial to a clear lifestyle alteration, and is related to the person's coping mechanisms. Furthermore, there is a growing body of evidence that indicates a strong correlation between physical and emotional health. Stress affects wellness physically and emotionally. It is appropriate to ask how a client is coping with the disease and how it impacts his or her life. This is a helpful step in establishing **rapport** and may alter the way a program is designed and progressed. Some clients will experience a crisis and separate themselves from toxic life situations and/or experience a new appreciation for their friends and families. Others may feel helpless, even paralyzed and unable to move toward better choices and better lifestyle decisions. Health challenges bring attention to the need to change bad habits as the person's physiology and life circumstances change.

Although a disease is not necessarily a permanent state, a client can begin to identify him- or herself by a diagnosis. For example, a client may say, "I am diabetic" rather than "I have diabetes." This disease-ridden identity is often one of the barricades that keep a client from seeing him- or herself getting better. With more diagnoses often comes **depression** and chronic pain. Depression often leads to decreased immunity and a greater predisposition to seasonal illnesses. The ACE-AHFS should have frank discussions about a client's disease by identifying the client's knowledge base of the disease, its signs and symptoms, the expectations of its progression or regression with a fitness program, and any concerns the client may have regarding how this disease impacts one's life. If a client is identified as having been traumatized by the sudden onset of the disease process, he or she may need a referral to a psychologist to develop appropriate coping skills. Some clients will use humor as a way to minimize their reaction to their diagnosis, and it is important to offer them a confidential forum to air their feelings. Others will have tremendous **anxiety** and need reassurance that their concerns are heard. It is important to separate the signs and symptoms of the disease from the client's sense of self. A focus on functional gains and separating the person from his or her diseases can dramatically impact a client's outlook in a positive way.

During the initial interview and throughout the program, it is important to ask how the patient feels, preferably as an open-ended question. Depending upon the client's personality, a series of questions may be needed to follow up on the first response. It is helpful to have the client recall a functional gain, a limitation, and a moment when he or she felt good with the circumstances. This verbalization helps to reinforce a positive image of the fitness activity relative to the client's function and helps with program progression. It also extends rapport beyond superficial acquaintance. It is important to affirm clients' feelings, even if the ACE-AHFS does not agree with their beliefs about their state of health. By allowing clients to openly talk about their feelings, the ACE-AHFS offers a way to discharge the negative impact of the health challenge prior to the workout, allowing for more productivity during the exercise session.

There is a growing trend to employ multidisciplinary approaches to treating disease. Integral to this idea is teamwork involving the treating physician, patient/client, physical therapist, fitness professional, and psychologist. Once clearance has been obtained from the physician for an exercise program, the ACE-AHFS has the option of recommending other team members. For some clients, a counselor—a psychologist, social worker, or therapist—may be a valuable team member to assist in functional restoration. This multidisciplinary approach has been demonstrated to be more effective than medication alone or the utilization of any one aspect individually (Schultz et al., 2007; Li et al., 2006; Lillefjell, Krokstad, & Espnes, 2006).

Stress

Dr. Hans Selye (1975) defined stress as "a non-specific response of the body to any demand made upon it." Stress can be good and/or performance-enhancing ("eustress') or bad ("distress"), although most people colloquially associate stress with bad events. A stressor is a particularly difficult concept to define, because it is largely dependent on a person's coping mechanisms. What is stressful for one person may not be stressful at all for another. Furthermore, there are categories of stressors, including positive and negative, and high- and low-impact. The greatest stressors include those events that occur to those closest to the individual, such as the death of a spouse or close family member, a change in marital status, the birth of a child, or a change in employment. The suddenness of these events also changes the impact, depending upon the situation. Some clients will cope with the sudden, unexpected death of a loved one better than others. Others, for example, will have "grieved" for a parent with **Alzheimer's disease** long before he or she passes on. A common theme inherent in stress is the idea of being out of control in one or more situations. As such, the general concept behind coping with stress is to be able to control one's reaction to a stressor, even if one cannot control the context of the stress.

Stressors, or **triggers,** fall into two categories: external and internal. Examples of external stressors include the following:

- *Physical environment:* Noise, lights (bright, direct sunlight, fluorescent lights), temperature (hot or cold), space (confined or open)
- *Social interactions:* With those in a position of power; with rude or angry people
- *Occupational/organizational:* Rules (explicit and implicit), deadlines, power structure, and the expectations of those who are higher ranked
- *Life events:* Death of a spouse or close relative, new job, new child, new home

Examples of internal stressors include the following:

- *Lifestyle choices:* Smoking, excessive alcohol or caffeine intake, poor sleep habits, poor hygiene

- *Negative self-image:* Excessive self-criticism, inherent pessimistic outlook, unrealistic expectations
- *Inability to adapt:* Concrete thinking, taking criticism personally, unwillingness to change or compromise
- *Personality traits:* Type A personalities, perfectionism

In all cases, there are physiological consequences to stress. Cortisol levels are altered in individuals in high-stress environments. Immunity and resistance to disease are lowered during times of stress. Stress can lead to disease states and negatively impact pre-existing diseases by lowering the body's defense mechanisms. The stress reaction consists of a physiological response, including the outpouring of sympathetic **hormones** and alterations of **glucose** and **fatty acids** in the blood to provide energy. **Epinephrine,** also known as adrenaline, causes the "fight-or-flight" response—increasing the **heart rate** and **blood pressure;** increasing mental alertness; and shunting blood flow to the brain, heart, and muscles in preparation for stress. Some people feel euphoric during this time and will continually seek situations that cause these physiological changes. However, others will feel other symptoms more commonly associated with stress, typically some combination of the following categories:

- *Physical:* Headache, chest pains, palpitations, nausea, trembling, diffuse muscle and joint aches and/or stiffness
- *Mental:* Decreased attention, concentration, memory, confusion, indecisiveness
- *Emotional:* Anxiety, depression, irritability, worry, anger, frustration
- *Behavioral:* Tics and other nervous habits such as nail-biting, increased hand-to-mouth activity (eating, smoking, drinking), verbal and/or physical abuse of self or others

Although the triggers can be external or internal, the reaction to stress is almost entirely self-generated. As such, recognizing the stressor and one's reaction to it becomes the first step in coping with stress. If the stress load is overwhelming, it may be important to keep a journal of one's situations and feelings for a week to clearly identify the triggers and their effects. Understanding the stress reaction and altering one's behaviors and thinking are not necessarily easy tasks, because they involve a change in one's outlook on life and general perspective. The development of management and coping skills associated with stress is a multistep process that takes practice. The steps include avoiding stressful situations when possible (boundary creation), altering the situation if it is not avoidable, controlling reactions to stressors, and adaptation.

- *Avoiding stress:* Most people know what situations stress them positively or negatively. When dealing with an avoidable negative stressor, such as a person or a place, limiting interactions with that person or place will decrease the total stress load. People must learn to have healthy boundaries and plan exit strategies ahead of time. Learning to say no is an important part of creating healthy boundaries and maintaining balance. In addition, planning and practicing certain phrases, such as, "I'm sorry to cut this short, but I have a lot to do today and want to get home at a reasonable time," is helpful to maintaining those boundaries. In some cases, it may be necessary to leave the job or relationship that is causing the significant burden in one's life.
- *Altering the context of the stress:* Most stressors are potentially manageable. There are many books and websites devoted to time- and money-management, which are major stressors in many people's lives. Balancing the schedule to reflect positive and negative stress activities is another important step to optimum stress management. The ACE-AHFS can teach clients to schedule in regular exercise, sit down to eat and be conscious of food choices, and plan rewards at regular intervals. These actions will make negative stressors more manageable.
- *Controlling reactions to stressors:* Learning to separate one's feelings and reactions to a stressor is a skill that takes practice. For example, many people are easily angered or upset by criticism from a parent. However, if the emotional reaction is immediately assessed and depersonalized, the stress has

less impact ("I'm not being criticized. He or she is just having a bad day."). It is also helpful to learn phrases, such as, "I can't talk about this right now. I'll get back to you later." It takes effort and practice to stop the immediate emotional reaction that leads to the complex set of behaviors that ensue. However, being able to recognize those internal cues and separate from them will make it easier to practice new behaviors. It is important to remind clients that while a person cannot control the stressors, he or she can control the reaction to them.

- *Adaptation:* This step involves resiliency to challenges. Physical resiliency comes from a well-balanced diet, adequate sleep and relaxation, and regular exercise. Mental resiliency comes from the ability to look at each situation positively and being able to identify opportunities when problems arise. Emotional resiliency is the ability to reject negative thinking and have a sense of humor when situations do not go as well as planned. This is the most creative of all the steps and also the most satisfying.

Impact of Exercise

The 1996 Surgeon General's report states that continuous and consistent physical activity is proven to enhance longevity and the quality of life for people of all ages (U.S. Department of Health and Human Services, 1996). Another study that same year concluded that physical fitness and exercise can reduce the risk of heart disease, non-insulin-dependent **diabetes mellitus,** some cancers, osteoarthritis, **osteoporosis,** and obesity (Paffenbarger, 1996). On the other hand, a sedentary lifestyle prevents the body from utilizing its energy stores and regulating its metabolism effectively. Exercise is crucial to maintaining health, performance capacity, and overall quality of life.

Exercise also improves a person's psychological profile. There are many reasons for this, including the release of **neurotransmitters, endocrine** regulation, and improved sleep. Exercise also discharges the heightened arousal state that results from stress. Satisfaction can also come from the simple act of reaching a goal during each session. Nearly everyone will feel better physically and psychologically after a session of exercise that is appropriate to his or her level of fitness.

Physical activity stimulates the secretion of many "feel-good" hormones. The most obtuse example of this is the reported "runner's high," which is associated with the release of endorphins during a mid- to long-distance run. A person does not need to run several miles or for hours to experience similar effects. Other hormones released during exercise include **growth hormone, norepinephrine,** epinephrine, and **glucagon.** Glucagon is secreted to convert stored **glycogen** into glucose, which improves the efficiency of **insulin** for several hours after each session. Norepinephrine and epinephrine are released in the brain and throughout the body to elevate mood during and immediately after exercise. With regular exercise, the body seeks to continue staying active, sustaining a positive feedback loop.

It has been demonstrated that regular exercise leads to improved sleep quality and duration, which also contributes to the release of nocturnal, reparative neurotransmitters, including growth hormone, **insulin-like growth factors,** and **melatonin.** Although a sleeping person seems inactive, radiography and neurophysiologic studies have demonstrated that the brain is more active during sleep than when a person is performing mundane daily tasks (Prinz et al., 1995; Tannenbaum, Guyda, & Posner, 1983). Sleep-deprivation experiments have demonstrated that pain tolerance is decreased with increased irritability when REM (rapid eye movement) and deep sleep are denied for more than 36 hours. Hallucinations and even death can occur with just 72 hours of complete sleep deprivation. Although there are a number of sleep-induction medications available over-the-counter and by prescription, virtually all of them disrupt the normal sleep patterns. Most of these medications allow a person to fall or stay asleep, but do not allow them to achieve REM or deep sleep. So while a person may feel as if he or she has rested, the cellular repair mechanisms typically taking place during sleep have not occurred. Other clients have no problems falling or staying asleep, but have sleep disturbances, such as **sleep apnea** or nocturnal seizures that require monitoring and interventions with medical devices.

Because sleep is a restorative activity, those who do not sleep well will frequently have other health challenges. Gottlieb et al. (2005) concluded that sleep deprivation affects glucose metabolism, which can lead to the development of type 2 diabetes. Other studies have suggested that sleep deprivation may be linked to obesity, heart disease, and mental illnesses such as bipolar disorder [Institute of Medicine (IOM), 2006]. Many studies suggest that sleep deprivation increases activity on the **hypothalamic-pituitary-adrenal axis** and suppresses growth hormones, leading to poor stress management (IOM, 2006). Animal studies have suggested that sleep deprivation increases stress hormones, reducing new cell production in adult brains (IOM, 2006). Free-radical antioxidation activity is suppressed, leading to poor wound healing and decreased pain tolerance. The great majority of clients will note improved sleep after regular exercise within several weeks of starting their program. They will also experience improved mental clarity and increased creativity with adequate restorative sleep, in addition to improved physical health.

For some clients, the psychological effects of exercise go beyond the hormonal effects of each session. There is the sense of accomplishment in achieving small goals with each session and reaching intermediate goals at set intervals. Some clients may accomplish more during the day due to improved overall function. Some may even complain that they "overdid it" and need to work on setting reasonable limits. The improved sleep resulting from a well-designed exercise program can improve pain thresholds and general life satisfaction. The ACE-AHFS should spend a few minutes with clients to review their subjective feelings since their last session, as doing so may reinforce their perception of progress.

Empathy

During the interview with Mr. James, the ACE-AHFS notices that he looks down at his hands when he talks about his father's medical history and the functional difficulties since the stroke. His voice becomes a little quiet. The ACE-AHFS takes the opportunity to say, "I see that it must be really difficult for you to see him that way. It would be difficult for anyone to see a parent struggle with daily activities. Are you worried that it might happen to you?"

Empathy is the ability to express emotion for another person. It is sometimes described as being able to "walk in another's shoes," or vicariously living through another's experience. As such, empathetic responses typically involve an "I" phrase joining a "you" phrase. For example, "I can see you are very upset by this," or "I understand how exciting this must be for you!" Empathy is slightly different from sympathy, which involves concordance or agreement with the other's feelings. In other words, the ACE-AHFS need not agree with a client's emotional reaction to be empathetic; if the ACE-AHFS did agree with a client's feelings, that would be an example of sympathy. The ability to be empathetic is equivalent to having emotional intelligence. It requires a person to have a large range of emotional experiences from which to draw comparison, awareness of the range of physical expression of those emotions, and the ability to express those emotions with words.

Having empathy requires sensitivity. This can be as simple as acknowledging someone's feelings without dismissal or judgment. It requires a person to be in touch with his or her own feelings so that he or she can recognize another person's emotional reaction. It does not, however, require the person to take on the other's burden. Most clients will be quite subtle in their need for empathy, and it takes practice to acknowledge feelings. During the interview, opportunities to offer empathy will be revealed through active listening, which includes eye contact and cognizance of body language. The keys to effective empathy, as described by Platt (1992) include the following:

- Recognizing the presence of a strong feeling in the interview setting
- Pausing to imagine how the other might be feeling
- Stating the perception of that feeling (e.g., "I can see you are frustrated.")

- Legitimizing the feeling (e.g., "That is understandable.")
- Respecting the effort to cope with the problem
- Offering support and partnership (e.g., "Let's see what we can do to improve...")

Motivational Issues

Mr. James states that his motivation for starting a program is largely driven by a fear that he will not be able to provide for his family if he becomes disabled. He realizes that his disease state is relatively early, but he is afraid that if he does not start now, it might be too hard or too late in the near future.

Motivation has been described as a combination of those factors that determine "why people initiate, choose, or persist in specific actions in specific circumstances" (Mook, 1996). As indicated, motivation is specific and not a generalized term. However, upon closer inspection, it can easily be seen that a person may be motivated to avoid, as opposed to initiate or continue, change. With clients who have health challenges, barriers to change include a self-image that is incongruent with their actual state of health, scheduling and side effects of medication(s), psychological disturbance such as depression or anxiety, and inconvenience.

Persons with new and/or existing health challenges often find themselves despondent. They may feel enslaved by their diseases and treatments. A client may come to the ACE-AHFS by "doctor's orders," and possess no real desire to exercise. Perhaps when this person exercised previously, he or she felt worse afterward. Other barriers include fear of acquiring injuries more easily because of the health challenge. Cultural barriers include the idea that exercise is only for the young and does not benefit older adults. Successful ways to overcome motivational barriers can include frank discussion of fears and worries, as well as strategies employed in the past. It is important to determine a client's **transtheoretical stage of change—precontemplation, contemplation, preparation, action,** or **maintenance**—and use information to assist him or her in moving forward (see Chapter 3). Finally, increasing general function in **activities of daily living (ADL)** is more easily achieved than changing self-perception of health and wellness.

Clients with health challenges who are in the precontemplation stage typically have not considered being in a fitness program. They would benefit from a discussion regarding the costs and benefits of an exercise program with regard to their disease. Many of the common lifestyle diseases will yield more benefit than cost from an exercise program. It is important to stress that diseases are typically not static, but will either worsen or improve based upon the choices made. The ACE-AHFS must have an open discussion about the physical, mental, emotional, and monetary costs of either starting or avoiding a fitness program. The physical costs of starting a program include the discomfort associated with muscle soreness and temporary fatigue with activity; the mental costs include a change of perspective with regards to self-image; the emotional costs include the self-consciousness of being in a fitness facility, working out in front of other people, or having to choose a workout over other social activities; and the monetary costs can include gym membership or equipment, clothing and footwear, and trainer fees. By discussing these costs openly, the ACE-AHFS will be able to customize the program according to the client's preferences once he or she moves on to the next steps. The discussion should also include talk of the benefits of exercise to address all of those cost concerns.

A discussion on the costs of starting a program relatively soon, compared to later on when the disease process has had a chance to progress further, can help clients in the contemplation stage move toward the preparation and action stages. Most people do not equate inaction now with greater costs later, and so it is important to emphasize regular exercise as an investment in each client's overall long-term well-being. The ACE-AHFS can compare this process to a health retirement account: The earlier one commences a program, the longer he or she will be able to draw benefits from that reserve in the future. Having a partnership with clients as they consider positive functional goals will be instrumental in moving them toward action.

For many clients who seek a fitness professional for the first time after a disease diagnosis, the motivation comes from a fear of adverse effects, but that fear tends to subside, which makes it more difficult for the client to stay in the maintenance stage. A return to the contemplation and preparation phases is often needed to reprogram and find positive motivation to stay in a fitness program. For example, rather than stating, "I don't want to have a heart attack," a client can change the motivator to, "I want to be able to enjoy taking longer walks with my spouse (or playing with my children)." Helping the client to identify the activities he or she would like engage in with more freedom will keep the client in the maintenance phase longer and more effectively.

Another barrier to moving toward the action stage and staying in a maintenance stage for those clients with multiple health challenges is the scheduling and side effects of medications. Many medications have peak and trough levels. A blood pressure medication taken one hour before a workout may add to the sensation of fatigue during and at the end of a workout. For those who require insulin, a snack prior to and during a longer session may be necessary to avoid hypoglycemic episodes. Although it initially may be quite tedious to coordinate with a few of these clients and their physicians to optimize medication scheduling and dosing, it is well worth the effort. It is helpful to stay in contact with the physician as a client progresses in the program to adjust dosing as the client's health profile improves. For many of the common health challenges, such as hyperglycemia (early type 2 diabetes) or mild hypertension, staying in a fitness program may eventually obviate the need for medications. Being free of medications and the associated financial and scheduling burden can be effective motivators for many clients.

A client with more complicated health concerns may have restrictions in scheduling appointments or keeping them due to either the diseases or the treatments. It can be challenging to keep the delicate balance between respecting the effect of the diseases and/or treatments while keeping those who may otherwise lack specific positive motivation in check. The ACE-AHFS can work with clients to schedule regular appointments that they are able to keep. Remind them to verbalize their own positive motivators for staying in the program at the beginning and/or end of each session for reinforcement. Maintaining some flexibility while expecting each client to uphold his or her responsibilities will allow all involved to achieve the best results.

The ACE-AHFS directs Mr. James to state positive functional goals in the short-, intermediate-, and long-term. He says that his short-term goals are to increase his exercise stamina, improve his mental clarity at work, and have more restorative sleep. His intermediate goals are to have a normal blood pressure, blood sugar level, and lipid profile, and "finish a 5K with my wife by the end of the year." He chuckles and states that one of his long-term goals is "to out-dance my daughter at her wedding."

Physiological Capacity

Under normal circumstances, physiological capacity increases through childhood and early adulthood and begins to decline in mid- to late-adulthood. As a person ages, **aerobic capacity** can continue to improve at decreased rates, but performance declines. Although aerobic capacity increases in childhood and early adulthood with increases in blood and lung volumes, aerobic capacity declines by about 1% per year and maximal heart rate decreases by one beat per year after reaching maturity. Because muscle cells change in composition, shunting **fast-twitch muscle fibers** toward **intermediate-** and **slow-twitch muscle fibers,** performance of endurance activities tends to improve with age. Strength exercise, although still important, typically produces less actual gains in the elderly than with young adults. However, as the rate of loss is similar between men and women regardless of baseline, it is important to optimize muscle mass and performance during early and mid-adulthood in anticipation of the eventual decline in performance.

Clients with health challenges have altered physiology. For example, those with signs of cardiovascular disease or with known cardiovascular disease have a ceiling to their aerobic capacity. Another example is a client who has smoked for

well known that smokers who do not quit go on to form mal-unions and non-unions more frequently than those who do not smoke. What cannot be described clinically is the persistent pain that interrupts all activities of life, including sleep. Eventually, the pain centralizes and there is no respite, no position that makes it better, and no medication that offers complete relief.

With very rare exception (e.g., in a person diagnosed with paranoid schizophrenia, for whom the psychotic symptoms are known to be attenuated with smoking), there are no health benefits associated with the use of tobacco. For those who choose to quit, most organ systems will reach some level of normalization within one year. Some damage is irreversible, such as the increased alveolar dead space in COPD. Smoking cessation will halt the progression of damage, but cannot reverse the changes. It is always advisable that clients find the motivation and surround themselves with those who will help them to stop smoking.

Food Choices

As mentioned early in this chapter, the majority of Americans are overweight or obese. Although there are a few persons for whom a diagnosis of **hypothyroidism** accounts for a small amount of their weight disparity, it is clearly not the case that more than half of the American population has an endocrine dysfunction that accounts for the prevalence of obesity.

There are some who challenge the traditional Food Guide Pyramid because of its reliance on grain products. When consumed in their least processed form, whole grains are an excellent source of **fiber,** plant **proteins,** and **complex carbohydrates** that offers sustained energy. During the late 1980s and early 1990s, when fat was considered the evil empire, many people found themselves continuing to gain weight and even developing diabetes due to overconsumption of highly refined, highly processed sugary snacks that were "fat-free." Examples of refining processes include the hulling of brown rice, which removes the bran (source of fiber) and the germ (source of protein) from the kernel, leaving only the **carbohydrate** and a minimum of protein inherent in the grain. Many "whole-wheat breads" are made from white flour with a small amount of whole-wheat flour in preparing the dough. A high-quality grain-based diet means choosing whole grain in its natural, unprocessed state.

It is believed that insulin spikes may contribute to the development of the metabolic syndrome. Thus, frequent consumption of highly processed or refined foods may be a cause of the increased incidence of this entity in developed nations. The mildly elevated blood pressure, borderline **hypercholesterolemia,** and persistent hyperglycemia are all symptoms of insulin dysregulation. Some would describe the metabolic syndrome as an early sign of **insulin resistance,** the hallmark of type 2 diabetes (Ford, Giles, & Dietz, 2002). Fortunately, there are also studies that indicate reversal of these early forms of disease with daily activity (Grundy et al., 2004). It is well known that exercise suppresses the release of insulin and improves the cellular uptake of glucose after a meal. Although pharmaceutical companies are developing new drugs to offset this disease of affluence, a 20-minute daily walk can play an important role in helping to normalize blood glucose levels and also increases the release of natural endorphins to improve mood.

Many people have found success with low-carbohydrate diets. These can be expensive, difficult to sustain over long periods of time, and contribute to dehydration if fluids are not consumed in adequate amounts. High-quality proteins should be consumed daily to maintain muscle mass. However, very few individuals need more than 1.0 grams of protein per kilogram of body weight to sustain optimum health. This amount is easily obtained by individuals consuming a normal diet. It is typically recommended to keep total fat below 30% of one's total caloric intake. In addition, no more than 10% of calories should come from saturated fats, and consuming less than 300 mg per day of cholesterol is advised. Fat acts to insulate nerve tissue and internal organs. When not consumed in the diet, it can be converted from an excess of carbohydrate or protein products. However, while skeletal muscle preferentially uses fatty acids as fuel at rest, the brain and other tissues prefer glucose to produce **adenosine triphosphate (ATP).** For those on a diet designed to induce **ketosis,** fatigue and mental sluggishness are side effects that can be counterproductive to an accompanying sensible exercise program.

It is more than vanity that one should be concerned with when working to maintain a healthy weight, as many diseases besides the more common ones like hypertension and diabetes are related to obesity. **Obstructive sleep apnea (OSA)** is increased in those with a **body mass index (BMI)** >30, leading to daytime fatigue, **somnolence,** or **narcolepsy** at its extreme. In women, there is correlation between obesity and polycystic ovaries. Overweight women in their 40s who have not gone through menopause are at risk for gallstones (**cholelithiasis**). Functionally devastating but rare entities such as **pseudotumor cerebri,** in which cerebrospinal fluid outflow is partially obstructed, are 300 to 1000% more common in those who are obese. In men, inguinal hernias requiring surgery present more commonly in the obese than in normal-weight men. Centrally located **adipose tissue** is highly correlated with the incidence of heart attacks. Choosing high quality, nutrient-dense calories to consume in appropriate quantities should be a part of every preventative health plan.

Inactivity

Using bedrest as the extreme example of inactivity, one can infer the relative effects of sedentary lifestyles. For every day a person is immobile, strength decreases by 1 to 1.5%; five weeks of total inactivity will cause a 50% loss of previous muscle strength, with a plateau reached at 25 to 40% of original strength. Simply performing one contraction a day at 50% of maximal strength is enough to prevent this decrease. Most of the muscle fiber diameter loss occurs across type I slow-twitch muscle fibers, which also leads to a decrease in basal metabolism. Lack of gravity resistance causes **osteopenia** and **hypercalcemia.** It is well known that excess calcium in the blood can lead to diffuse abdominal discomfort, depression, pain syndromes, and kidney stones, and calcium is the last mineral to normalize after prolonged inactivity. Osteopenia leads to weakened bones and a higher fracture risk. Blood flow from the lower extremities is attenuated, potentially leading to the development of blood clots. Although it is unlikely that being a "couch potato" will lead to all of these pathologies, lesser manifestations can still be present to some level in a person who chooses to be sedentary.

Alcohol

It is unclear whether moderate alcohol consumption is better for health than teetotaling. There is no doubt that long-term, heavy usage of alcohol, or even occasional binging, leads to altered end-organ function with age. The effects are amplified when the alcohol usage is commenced at an early age.

The most commonly reported disease associated with heavy alcohol use is liver disease. The liver is the first area of processing of most toxins, including alcohol. Some persons are unable to break down alcohol completely and have physiologic reactions, such as flushing and discomfort, and so they will avoid alcohol consumption altogether. Cells that process alcohol also process drugs such as acetaminophen (Tylenol®). If the liver attempts to process more than 4 grams of acetaminophen (about 12 regular or eight extra-strength tablets) or some combination of alcohol and acetaminophen per day, acute liver failure can ensue, leading to increased mortality. More commonly, long-term usage leads to changes in the cyto-histologic features, first as a **fatty liver,** then as a shrunken cirrhotic liver. Because the liver produces nearly all of the non-cellular blood proteins, every tissue in the body becomes more fragile with long-term heavy alcohol consumption.

Alcohol consumption leads to decreased reaction time, decreased motor coordination, and impaired memory at the time of usage.

Caffeine

Caffeine is a substance that is also prevalent in most diets. For many, a morning does not begin until after the first cup of coffee. Others choose sodas or energy drinks. Even some of the effects of chocolate can be attributed to the small amount of caffeine present. Caffeine is a **xanthine** compound, part of a group of **central nervous system (CNS)** stimulants that also includes nicotine.

When consumed in moderation, caffeine can lead to moderate improvements in executive tasks and motor coordination. When consumed in excess, it can lead to nervousness, insomnia, and symptoms that parallel panic and/or heart attacks. It can be an addictive substance for susceptible persons, leading to symptoms of withdrawal if completely and suddenly removed. Because of caffeine's performance-enhancing qualities, many over-the-counter medications containing caffeine have been added to the "banned-substances" list for athletes.

Performance-enhancing Supplements/Drugs

The fine line between supplements and compounds designed to enhance performance continues to be blurred with the advent of genetic technology. A client may have goals that are admirable, but the means of achieving them may not necessarily be acceptable. Over-the-counter supplements designed to increase metabolism, build muscle mass, and/or burn fat are easily accessible. Claims made by manufacturers are not subject to the rigorous testing standards of the Food and Drug Administration (FDA). On the other hand, for the high-performance athlete for whom a few microseconds means the difference between Olympic gold and obscurity, the risk of getting caught is often the basis for making the decision on whether to use supplements, rather than any ethical or health concerns. Unfortunately, this decision is not limited to high-profile athletes, but also affects high school athletes for whom performance can sometimes represent the pathway to a college scholarship or professional sports contract.

The United States Olympic Committee has a published list of banned substances, some of which are sport-specific (such as beta-blockers for archery). Additional information can be obtained at the U.S. Anti-Doping Agency's website (www.usantidoping.org).

Carbonated Beverages

Carbonated beverages are ubiquitous in American life. Soft drinks constitute a multibillion dollar industry that has replaced water for hydration in many people's lives. The refined sugar content in the larger soda sizes has been linked with the increase in the metabolic syndrome and type 2 diabetes. While sugar content is decreased for those who choose diet drinks, the phosphoric acid load still exchanges for calcium, which is then excreted through the kidneys. Although the caffeine content is relatively low in a single serving, those who drink carbonated beverages rarely consume just one serving, which has a cumulative effect.

Illicit Drugs

Occasional use of recreational drugs in the United States is typically done by educated, higher-socioeconomic professionals. The most common drugs used include marijuana, cocaine, and amphetamine-based substances (e.g., ecstasy). Legality issues aside, there are physiological risks that can be harmful. Marijuana leads to decreased reaction time and poor executive function in the immediate phase, with **gynecomastia** (atypical breast tissue development in males) and **microgonadism** (smaller testicles) with long-term use. Cocaine and other CNS stimulants can lead to insomnia in the short-term, and have higher addiction potentials due to their dysphoria-inducing withdrawal symptoms. With long-term amphetamine abuse, irreversible mental states resembling schizophrenia, such as paranoia, poor pain tolerance, and lethargy, can ensue. Users of cocaine are at risk for hypertension and stroke, typically with bleeding into the brain (intracerebral hemorrhage), which has debilitating long-term effects. Ecstasy can lead to symptoms resembling **Parkinson's disease** at a younger age. An ACE-AHFS can reduce professional risk by refusing to work with clients who are known to be using illicit substances.

Sun Exposure

Ultraviolet rays activate vitamin-D precursors at the level of the skin. The amount of exposure this requires is much less than it takes to alter the melanin content of the skin. Most researchers and dermatologists would agree that there is no such thing as "a healthy tan." Contrary to popular belief, getting a "base tan" at a tanning booth does not protect from burns at the beach.

In fact, according to the American Academy of Dermatology, the UVA and UVB exposure from a booth is more detrimental to skin health than typical sunburns. Prolonged sun exposure leads to premature aging and increased risk of skin cancers. It also leads to changes in the eye, including **photokeratitis** and cataract development. Some medications will make the skin more susceptible to burning. When the body is busy repairing its largest organ (the skin) the immune system is rendered more susceptible to viral illnesses and/or reactivations. As such, it is not infrequent that cold sores or herpes will flare up after a session of excess sun exposure. It is important that clients think of tanning as an inflammatory response to an environmental insult. When training clients outdoors, the ACE-AHFS should strongly recommend that sunblock be applied before exposure and reapplied after water exposure or excessive sweating.

Considerations for Clients With Multiple Health Challenges

People with multiple health challenges are some of the most difficult clients to manage. They are often taking numerous medications ("polypharmacy"), and it can be difficult to differentiate the symptoms associated with the diseases from the side effects of their medications. Physical fatigue intermingles with depression and often both are escalated. Furthermore, people with multiple health challenges can place an emotional strain on those who work and live with them, be it their caregivers, physicians, or family members.

The cost of disease is not insignificant. It can be hard for those who are otherwise healthy to imagine the burden imposed on those with chronic and/or multiple disease states. There is the physical burden of the disease itself, which alters function in daily activities, the financial burden of medical bills and medications, the time limitations due to medication dosing and/or side effects, and the emotional burden that comes with a loss of independence in one or more aspect(s) of daily living. Some diseases may have one name, but impact multiple organ systems, such as diabetes. It is worth taking time to ask each client how their disease(s) and treatments have impacted their daily function.

One psychological aspect of having health challenges, especially more than one, is the social isolation the client may feel. Some of this is due to decreased mobility and functional capacity. Some of it can be due to the scheduling of medications and their anticipated side-effects, and some of it can be due to body **dysmorphism** and/or shame. Still others will perseverate on "if only" statements, such as "if only I quit smoking earlier," or "if only I stayed active." Unfortunately, social isolation can be depressing, lead to rumination, and commence a vicious cycle of negative self-talk. The ACE-AHFS may have clients who confess that their calendar revolves around doctors' appointments rather than pleasurable activities. These are some of the most difficult clients to serve, as there is a complex social-emotional pattern that has to be altered. Such clients may have difficulty "finding time" to exercise regularly, but really enjoy it once they attend. It is very important to help them verbalize the positive aspects of exercise on their disease and their overall sense of well-being at the end of each session as positive reinforcement. Remember, behind every great person is a large network of support; in fact, the greatness of the achievement is most frequently proportional to the size of the supporting team. The ACE-AHFS should encourage clients to become part of a network, either through the facility or in their general community outside of the medical concerns. With time, the personal training appointment will become a significant portion of their positive social activity. An ACE-AHFS can be powerfully persuasive in a client's life, not only as a fitness instructor, but also as a coach and encourager. The key is to replace negative self-talk with positive affirmations and explore new social networks.

There are disease processes that are chronic, without definitive cure, and/or with devastating consequences. Some examples include cancer, HIV/AIDS, rheumatoid arthritis, and multiple sclerosis. The diagnosis often becomes a sentinel event, and life is seen as having a "before" and "after" this event. It becomes even more important to foster an environment in which these clients are not defined by their disease through sensitive and effective communication. This process involves acceptance of their feelings, empathy for their hardships, and respect for each of them as an individual. It is also important to maintain reasonable boundaries, especially in terms of time, so that the appointments do not degenerate into solipsism and lose functional exercise as a focus.

Monetary Impact of Multiple Health Challenges

According to the National Coalition on Health Care, the United States spent more than 16% of its gross domestic product on healthcare in 2007. Relatively little of this is actual payment for interaction with physicians. An increasing amount is for prescription pharmaceuticals, "nutriceuticals," and functional assistance in the form of skilled nursing and/or devices. Money spent on preventative measures is comparatively little, despite its potential impact on sustained health. However, as co-pays for medications are increasing—up to $75 for some brand name prescriptions—the session with the ACE-AHFS can seem like a relative bargain when considering the long-term beneficial effects of regular exercise. A person who exercises is less likely to require long-term care or other functional assistance during his or her life. The benefits of exercise range from immediate to lifelong when maintained.

Information and the Internet

Many people now use the Internet as their primary source of information. Unlike professional journals, which are peer-reviewed for accuracy, much of the information available online is anecdotal or merely clever marketing. Clients with multiple health challenges are often susceptible to the barrage of information available to cure their particular ills. Websites can be set up to appear official or professional, but include endorsements of questionable repute. Despite the plethora of evidence that exist for the benefits of daily exercise and good lifestyle choices, many people still fall for "instant cures."

There are many reputable sources on fitness, nutrition, and lifestyle modification. One way to address the potential barrage of web marketing is to keep current on the latest research available in peer-reviewed journals. There are websites and specialty digests, such as the Cochrane Database, that offer abstracts that can be reviewed efficiently in minutes a day. Without discounting the interest a client has demonstrated in his or her own health, an effective ACE-AHFS can guide him or her toward separating sound information from merely good marketing by encouraging interest in the same reputable sources.

Strategies for Successful Communication With Allied Healthcare Professionals

Understanding Allied Healthcare Reporting

Allied healthcare providers communicate very efficiently. The presentation is organized, specific, and concise. In fact, it may sometimes seem direct and impersonal. The ACE-AHFS must understand that this is partly due to the efficiency that must be acquired during the formal education process and continues due to sometimes overwhelming time constraints. An effective ACE-AHFS can develop a very loyal referral base once he or she learns to communicate effectively with other professionals using traditional healthcare language.

Intake History and Physical Exam

The initial visit within the allied health community has specific elements, which have been adapted here for fitness professionals. It is important to note that all documentation must be dated and signed by the ACE-AHFS.

Chief Complaint/Primary Goal

Typically, a patient sees a physician with a primary concern. A question that an ACE-AHFS can ask is, "What is your primary goal in starting an exercise program?" Typically, a client may state that he or she is interested in weight loss, increased flexibility, improved general fitness, or sports-specific improvements. This information sets the tone for fitness programming.

History of Present Illness or Injury

In the medical model, there are usually elements of the chief complaint that require further elucidation. Using pain as an example, a physician will want to know the location of the pain, the onset, duration, whether it is constant or intermittent, how the patient rates the pain (from 0–10), the quality of the pain (e.g., "shooting", "stabbing", "burning", "aching"), and what makes the pain better or worse. For the client starting a fitness program, sometimes there will be a sentinel event, such as a heart attack or recent onset of **sciatica.** To better understand the underlying motive, the ACE-AHFS may consider asking questions about the client's current function and how the recent event has affected him or her, if he or she has any feelings of distress about the sentinel event, and/or what his or her fears may be.

Medical History/Exercise History

An inventory of the other known medical problems is taken to determine how the current problem may be related. An ACE-AHFS who has some training in the basic pathophysiology of diseases may want to take note of these same entities. Perhaps more important to the program development are the client's past exercise habits, his or her interest in those activities, whether the program was successful at achieving the fitness goals, and whether that same type of program or goal is believed to be feasible at this time.

Allergies and Medications

In the medical setting, a patient is asked about allergies and medications. These details are also important information for the ACE-AHFS, as they can be helpful in the event that an accident requires intervention by emergency personnel.

Family and Social History/Support Network

The family history offers a glimpse at a person's genetic predisposition, and the social history provides information about the personal habits, occupation, and environmental modifiers that potentially affect function. It is worth asking about the activity habits of a person's family or social network, as this information helps to identify potential areas of modification needed in the client's fitness goals.

Review of Systems

Most complete medical exams include questions regarding constitution (fever, chills, weight gain or loss), and a systematic review of the different organ systems. For the ACE-AHFS, this may be a good time to allow the client to talk about anything he or she might have otherwise forgotten during the intake.

Physical Exam/Initial Evaluation

A complete medical examination would encompass a general overview of the anatomy and biomechanical function within the scope of the practitioner's practice. For the ACE-AHFS, an initial evaluation will require an assessment of the client's exercise attitudes and physical-activity history prior to starting the first workout. There are some clients who will be easily fatigued and others who will immediately overcome nearly every challenge. It is worthwhile to have progressively more difficult variations of the same exercise to test the client at his or her current level. For example, one set of basic crunches may be too much for a complete novice, while a similar open-chain variation of this exercise using a stability ball and weights in each hand may be necessary to challenge the more advanced athlete. There is a multitude of exercise equipment and training devices offering increasing levels of difficulty for both assessments and programming for any given exercise.

Assessment

This portion of the program requires professional judgment, assimilating the information acquired into a summary of the state of health of a client. For the ACE-AHFS, it may be worth commenting on specific aspects of fitness, such as strength, endurance, balance, and flexibility with respect to the client's stated goals.

Plan

Physicians will typically list elements to be addressed with end goals specified (e.g., "Metoprolol, titrating up from 25 mg twice a day until a target blood pressure of <120/80 mmHg is achieved"). The ACE-AHFS can list short-term and intermediate- to long-term goals based upon measurable results (e.g., "Improve walking speed on treadmill from 3 mph to 3.5 mph, improve duration from 10 minutes to 20 minutes in 15 sessions over four weeks. The client would like to be able to complete a 5K walk with her daughter in six months time.").

SOAP Notes

The standard form of documentation is the **SOAP note**, which stands for subjective, objective, assessment, and plan (see Chapter 4). Wording in each section should be concise and accurately reflect the activities documented. The entire note could be written on an index card, depending on the size of one's writing. It is essential that every SOAP note is dated by the ACE-AHFS.

- *Subjective:* What the client states, often in quotation form. For example: "I feel short of breath walking up two flights of stairs."
- *Objective:* What one observes and can document. For example: Client walked for 10 minutes on the treadmill at a rate of 3 mph. He was able to carry a conversation, speaking six to seven words between breaths.
- *Assessment:* One's professional judgment. For example: Client has improved his exercise tolerance from the initial evaluation one month ago.
- *Plan:* The next steps to achieving mutual goals. For example: Gradual increase of speed on the treadmill to 3.5 mph and duration to 20 minutes, at least three times a week over the next month.

The SOAP note is an elegant and efficient way to communicate both what the client feels and the ACE-AHFS observes in the process of achieving stated functional goals. For allied healthcare professionals, SOAP notes offer a quick and expedient update of the client's progress. Over time, they also document patterns of self-image versus actual performance, and can be useful tools when providing feedback to the client. Again, each section does not need to be elaborate. If necessary, the ACE-AHFS may consider documenting a trend with a narrative, either at the beginning or the end of the SOAP note.

The Role of the ACE-AHFS on the Healthcare Team

It is not uncommon for an ACE-AHFS to have a medical or other healthcare-related background. It is a difficult and necessary task to separate the ACE-AHFS aspects of any client interaction from other knowledge the ACE-AHFS may have, unless he or she is assuming liability as a healthcare professional for that client. It can be the case that an ACE-AHFS will be the first to notice side effects or adverse events that are suspected to be related to a prescription drug or a change in the disease course. The art of communicating this information lies in the diplomacy with which one delivers the information to a healthcare professional who is going to assume risk for changes in treatments.

The assessment portion of the SOAP note is a good place to document one's professional judgment. One way to approach this is to summarize the complaints and effects and state (generically) that it "may be due to" side effects of drugs, change in disease, and/or improvements in physiology due to exercise. Immediately follow this information in the plan portion—"to discuss with client's physician." If an ACE-AHFS suspects the effects are potentially health- or life-threatening, it would behoove him or her to call the attending physician or practitioner sooner rather than later. During the course of the conversation, an effective ACE-AHFS should be able to lead that practitioner to the conclusion without actually stating it. It is not within the scope of practice for an ACE-AHFS to diagnose medical problems or changes in medical conditions, nor is it wise to assume the liability of doing so. It is well within good practice and highly advisable to urge the client to discuss any changes in his or her condition with the attending physician. This empowers the client to be in charge and accountable for his or her own health.

Summary

This chapter serves only as an introduction to the interplay between medical care and exercise science. As with most information, it will not make any difference without a tie-in that makes an emotional impact. Effective fitness professionals, like any effective people, know how to use "feeling" words when conveying important information to induce change in behavior. Every ACE-AHFS should continue learning about all issues that impact functional health and learn to communicate those effects not merely professionally, but also sensitively. However, should there be any doubt with regard to precautions, specific instructions should be obtained from the attending physician.

It is optimistic to state that, at least colloquially, society has moved from "taking medicine" to "receiving healthcare," and that exercise is less about aesthetics and more about fitness. While traditional healthcare professionals are helpful in the reactive phase of disease and disability, the ACE-AHFS can be an effective, lifelong partner in proactive maintenance and/or development of function. The ACE-AHFS has the power to empower, to create a positive vision that will lead each client to a better quality of life.

References

Ford, E.S., Giles, W.H., & Dietz, W.H. (2002). Prevalence of the metabolic syndrome among US adults: Findings from the third national health and nutrition examination survey. *Journal of the American Medical Association,* 287, 356–359.

Fowles, J. et al. (2003). *Chemical Composition of Tobacco and Cigarette Smoke in Two Brands of New Zealand Cigarettes.* New Zealand Ministry of Health Final Report.

Gottlieb, D.J. et al. (2005). Association of sleep time with diabetes mellitus and impaired glucose tolerance. *Archives of Internal Medicine,* 165, 8, 863–867.

Grundy, S.M. et al. (2004). Definition of metabolic syndrome: Report of the National Heart, Lung, and Blood Institute/American Heart Association conference on scientific issues related to definition. *Circulation*, 109, 433–438.

Hedley, A.A. et al. (2004). Prevalence of overweight and obesity among U.S. children, adolescents, and adults, 1999–2002. Journal of the American Medical Association, 291, 2847–2850.

Institute of Medicine (2006). *Sleep Disorders and Sleep Deprivation: An Unmet Public Health Problem.* Washington, D.C.: The National Academy of Sciences.

Li, E.J.Q. et al. (2006) The effect of a "training on work readiness" program for workers with musculoskeletal injuries: A randomized control trial (RCT) study. *Journal of Occupational Rehabilitation,* 16, 4, 529–541.

Lillefjell, M., Krokstad, S., & Espnes, G.A. (2006). Factors predicting work ability following multidisciplinary rehabilitation for chronic musculoskeletal pain. *Journal of Occupational Rehabilitation*, 16, 4, 543–555.

Mook, D.G. (1996). *Motivation: The Organization of Action* (2nd ed.). New York: W.W. Norton.

Paffenbarger, R. (1996). Physical activity and fitness for health and longevity. *Research Quarterly for Exercise and Sports,* 67, 3, 11–30.

Platt, F.W. (1992). Empathy: Can it be taught? *Annals of Internal Medicine,* 117, 8, 700.

Prinz, P.N. et al. (1995). Higher plasma IGF-1 levels are associated with increased delta sleep in healthy older men. *Journal of Gerontology,* 50A, 222–226.

Schultz, I.Z. et al. (2007). Models of return to work for musculoskeletal disorders. *Journal of Occupational Rehabilitation*, 17, 4, 782.

Selye, H. (1975). *Stress Without Distress.* New York: Signet

Tannenbaum, G.S., Guyda, H.J. & Posner, B.I. (1983). Insulin-like growth factors: A role in growth hormone negative feedback and body weight regulation via brain. *Science,* 220, 77–79.

U.S. Department of Health and Human Services (1996). *Physical Activity and Health: A Report of the Surgeon General.* Atlanta: U.S. Department of Health and Human Services, Centers for Disease Control and Prevention, National Center for Chronic Disease Prevention and Health Promotion. S/N 017-023-00196-5.

Suggested Reading

American Council on Exercise (2007). *ACE Clinical Exercise Specialist Manual.* San Diego, Calif.: American Council on Exercise.

American Council on Exercise (2003). *Exercise for Older Adults* (2nd ed.). San Diego, Calif.: American Council on Exercise.

Braddom, R.L. (2006). *Physical Medicine and Rehabilitation* (3rd ed.). Philadelphia: Saunders

Borysenko, J. (2007). *Minding the Body, Mending the Mind.* New York: Da Capo Press.

Haskell, W. (1996). Physical activity, sport, and health: Toward the next century. *Research Quarterly for Exercise and Sport,* 67, 3, 37–51.

Katzmarzyk, P.T. et al. (2003). Targeting the metabolic syndrome with exercise: Evidence from the HERITAGE family study. *Medicine & Science in Sports & Exercise,* 35, 10, 1703–1709.

Malina, R. (1996). Tracking of physical activity and physical fitness across the lifespan. *Research Quarterly for Exercise and Sport*, 67, 3, 48–61.

McNamee, D. (1996). A change in lifestyle may prevent cancer. *Lancet,* 348, 1436.

Additional Resources

American Heart Association: www.americanheart.org

American Cancer Society: www.cancer.org

American Diabetes Association: www.diabetes.org

General medical information: www.WebMD.com; www.medscape.com

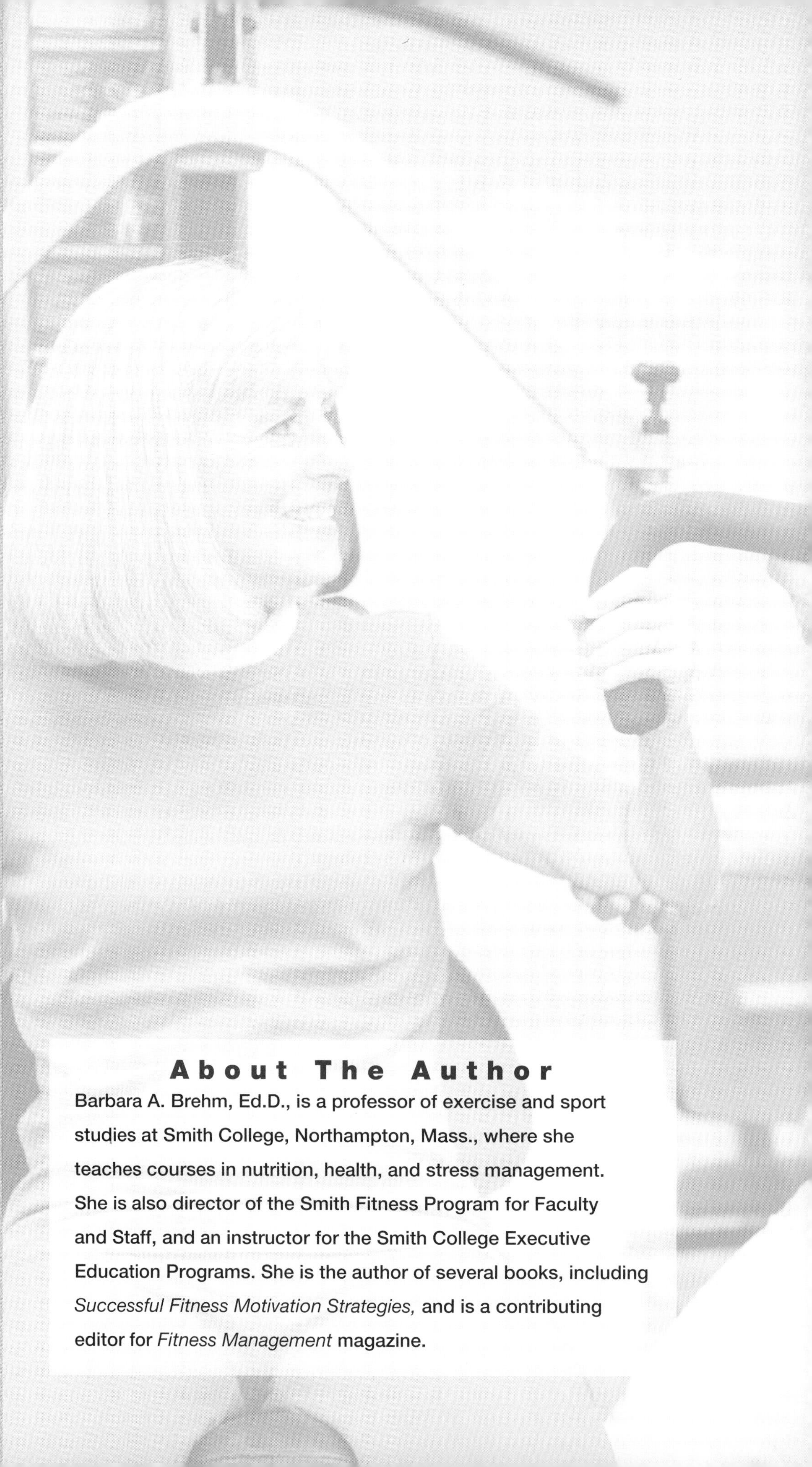

In This Chapter

About The Author

Barbara A. Brehm, Ed.D., is a professor of exercise and sport studies at Smith College, Northampton, Mass., where she teaches courses in nutrition, health, and stress management. She is also director of the Smith Fitness Program for Faculty and Staff, and an instructor for the Smith College Executive Education Programs. She is the author of several books, including *Successful Fitness Motivation Strategies,* and is a contributing editor for *Fitness Management* magazine.

CHAPTER 3

Communication Strategies and Behavior Change

Barbara A. Brehm

Communication and behavior change are integral parts of the fitness profession. Fitness professionals communicate closely with their clients to design effective behavior-change programs, and then support these clients in their efforts. Fitness professionals who are well-versed in exercise science and understand the intricacies of training principles will still lack effectiveness if they do not also have good communication skills, as their knowledge alone will be unlikely to result in positive behavior change. Communication skills are essential when working as part of a group and relating to supervisors and colleagues.

Successful fitness professionals are skilled at working with all kinds of people. They develop **rapport** with their clients in just a few sessions; in fact, the rapport-building process should begin almost immediately, and certainly during the first session. As fitness professionals expand their clientele beyond the healthy, young exercise enthusiasts who walk into the fitness center, they often require more education and training in communication and behavior-change strategies to reach clients who find it difficult to incorporate regular physical activity into their lives. This chapter provides an overview of effective communication skills and presents basic information on how the ACE-certified Advanced Health & Fitness Specialist (ACE-AHFS) can most effectively support clients in their behavior-change efforts.

Developing Rapport

The word "rapport" refers to a relationship marked by mutual understanding and trust. Many factors contribute to the way fitness professionals are perceived. Clients may have preconceived ideas of how an ACE-AHFS should look and behave. Hopefully, clients modify these ideas once they meet the fitness professional and begin a working relationship. This working relationship is built on good communication skills that allow the ACE-AHFS to understand the client's needs, and the client to understand the trainer's recommendations. Rapport and communication help clients develop self-confidence and the motivation to exert the effort required to stick to their exercise programs.

Fitness professionals who have had little difficulty developing rapport with clients of similar age, gender, ethnicity, size, socioeconomic status, educational background, ability, and fitness level may find that it takes a little longer to build trust with people who differ from themselves. Building rapport can take more effort when clients are reluctant to begin exercising, are afraid of getting injured, or are depressed and anxious about their health. Some clients may have had bad experiences that led them to develop prejudices against athletes and physical educators, and thus, may initially be critical of information coming from an ACE-AHFS. Some clients may have less trust in young people, old people, women, people who appear to be overweight, or people of a different ethnicity. Nevertheless, an ACE-AHFS who behaves professionally and employs good communication skills often wins the hearts and trust of even the most reluctant clients.

Knowledge Is Power

An ACE-AHFS can improve his or her rapport-building ability by learning more about each client (Gordon, 2006). An ACE-AHFS should learn about clients' beliefs, attitudes, and lifestyles by talking to others who work with similar groups and reading any information he or she can find about the demographic. For example, some older people and some cultural groups may believe that asking questions is rude and indicates that the speaker has been unclear. Many people pretend they agree and understand a health professional because they want to please the professional, when in fact they may not agree or understand (Wright, Frey, & Sopory, 2007). Sometimes people say they have been performing their exercise programs when in fact they have not been doing so, simply to appear in a good light. As rapport develops between the ACE-AHFS and his or her clients, a working partnership develops as well, and the two parties begin communicating and working more effectively together.

First Impressions

Positive first impressions provide a great start for the rapport-building process. Clients' first impressions are based on many controllable factors, including the appearance and behavior of the ACE-AHFS, who should always wear professional attire, be well groomed, and behave in a friendly and professional manner.

During the first meeting with a new client, the ACE-AHFS should be sure that the client knows about the ACE-AHFS's education, training, certifications, and qualifications. In the allied health professions, these credentials are extremely important for building trust with new clients. During the meeting, the ACE-AHFS should communicate carefully and attentively with the new client, listening with an open mind and conveying a respectful, positive, and supportive attitude.

The work environment contributes to clients' first impressions. The facility should be very clean, neat, and well organized. Offices and staff should have a welcoming and organized appearance. Clients should not have to wait long for appointments, and interactions with the staff should be positive, respectful, and professional.

Communication Skills Build Positive Working Relationships

The work of an ACE-AHFS is built upon effective communication. In the healthcare arena, interpersonal communication skills are strongly related to patient health outcomes (Ambady et al., 2002). Thus, curriculums in many healthcare provider training programs, including those taking place at medical schools, have been expanded to include more training in effective communication skills (Rider & Keefer, 2006).

Verbal and Nonverbal Communication

People's verbal communications are only a small part of the messages they send. People pay attention to much more than words in their effort to decipher messages and understand social situations. While people hear each other's words, they seek to verify verbal content by evaluating the speaker's appearance, facial expressions, body language, and tone of voice. If someone's words ("I am glad to meet you") and body language (lack of eye contact, disinterested facial expression, body turned away, low energy) do not match, people generally trust body language over verbal content (Ambady et al., 2002).

When speaking with clients, it is important to speak clearly and use language that is easily understood by clients. Visual information (e.g., pictures, diagrams, charts) can help illustrate concepts. Exercise demonstrations are sometimes more effective than verbal descriptions, depending on a client's learning preferences. The ACE-AHFS should pause occasionally while speaking to give clients time to ask questions to clarify what's been communicated or show understanding.

The fitness professional's facial expressions and body language should convey sincere interest and a positive regard for the client. Interest is shown via eye contact, appropriate smiling, a body posture directly facing the client, and attention focused solely on the client, not by trying to do two things at once. Most clients can sense when a smile is genuine. Nonverbal communication comes from within; the ACE-AHFS must cultivate an ability to be in the moment with clients, truly paying attention to their work together.

Effective Listening

Some fitness professionals tend to believe that because they get paid to give advice, the more they say, the better. They love to talk about exercise and health, and equate information delivery with performance. Unfortunately, this focus on talking can interfere with communication.

Anyone who works with people needs to be a good listener. The ACE-AHFS must listen carefully to clients to understand their goals and concerns. Listening carefully allows the ACE-AHFS not only to receive information from the client, but also to interpret client reactions to instructions and suggestions.

Effective listening means more than being quiet and giving others some time to speak. It also means actively paying attention to the speaker's verbal and nonverbal communication, being fully engaged, and keeping an open mind while trying to put oneself in the speaker's shoes. Listening carefully allows the ACE-AHFS to gather information to design appropriate exercise programs, and to give clients the impression that their active participation in the ACE-AHFS–client relationship is important.

Effective listening is a difficult habit to develop. People often do not pay attention to what others are saying. Some of the time they pretend to listen, but actually do not hear what the speaker is saying, as their minds may be elsewhere. Or people may hear part of what the speaker is saying, but tune out parts they find offensive or boring. They may tune out parts they do not understand, not bothering to ask for clarification. While the other person is speaking, people might formulate arguments, form judgments about the speaker, or think about what the speaker will say next. They may even daydream about something else entirely or be preoccupied or distracted by their own problems. Even when they try to listen, people may not hear what the speaker is trying to say. People often reconstruct messages to reflect their own beliefs and needs. They may have prejudices about the speaker and look for confirmation of these beliefs in the speaker's words. They may hear only what they expect to hear.

When interacting with clients, the ACE-AHFS should allow clients to speak without interruption. When clients pause, the ACE-AHFS can ask questions for clarification, paraphrase what he or she has heard, and make sure he or she understood correctly. Taking notes on what clients are saying is fine, but the ACE-AHFS should look up repeatedly, make good eye contact with clients, and really listen to what clients are saying.

Barriers to Effective Communication

Even when the ACE-AHFS listens carefully and practices good communication skills, he or she may still find communication difficult. Sometimes the client is reluctant to participate fully, while other times the consultation environment is not conducive to productive conversation.

With effort, most barriers to effective communication can be addressed. Some of the most common barriers encountered by the ACE-AHFS include the following:

- *Cultural differences:* When the ACE-AHFS and the client have significantly different backgrounds, the ACE-AHFS must spend extra time and energy learning about the client. As he or she gains experience with a given population, the ACE-AHFS will become more adept at establishing rapport with clients from that group. It is important to note that while it is important to understand a client's cultural background, the ACE-AHFS must never generalize or stereotype.
- *Emotional health problems:* Clients grappling with **depression** or **anxiety** may tend to focus on negative information, and not hear the positive. Research suggests that people look for information to justify their current mood and beliefs (Ambady & Gray, 2002), which means that when working with clients with mood disorders, the ACE-AHFS must be sure to phrase information in a positive, supportive way. Remember, an ACE-AHFS cannot diagnose these disorders.

- *Too little/too much explanation:* The ACE-AHFS should use language clients can understand and try to meet clients' need for information without "talking down" to them by using technical jargon or providing too much information.
- *Stress/feeling rushed:* By far the largest barrier to quality communication is a lack of effective listening, which is likely to occur when either party feels rushed and distracted, and does not pay attention to what the other person is saying. Cultivating the ability to focus one's attention mindfully is a good antidote to stress and improves communication.
- *Fitness center environment:* Initial meetings between the ACE-AHFS and clients should occur in a comfortable, quiet, private space. Such space is not always readily available in fitness centers. In this case, fitness-center personnel should create a quiet space where clients do not feel like they will be overheard.

Behavior-change Models and Stages of Behavior Change

Fitness professionals may have heard clients say, "I know what to do, but I just can't seem to do it."

Unless people perceive a very good reason for changing, change goes against human nature (Vohs & Heatherton, 2000). People strive for stability to grow and thrive. Psychologists have studied many factors of how people form the intention to change, initiate changes in behavior, and then sustain these changes over the years. An ACE-AHFS must understand these factors if he or she is to help clients negotiate the behavior-change process as they attempt to incorporate regular physical activity into their lives.

Comprehensive coverage of all of the theoretical models that have been proposed to explain behavior change is beyond the scope of this chapter. Instead, this section provides a brief overview of several models that present the most helpful perspective for the ACE-AHFS who is designing exercise programs for clients facing health challenges and choosing to exercise to improve their overall health and fitness. More detailed information on various behavior-change models can be found in the *ACE Lifestyle & Weight Management Consultant Manual* (Second Edition).

The Health Belief Model and the Protection Motivation Theory

The **health belief model** suggests that a person's health beliefs influence decisions about behavior change. Addressing health beliefs is especially important for clients in the early stages of behavior change. The ACE-AHFS should discuss with clients their beliefs about health concerns and physical activity, and correct misperceptions by providing accurate information from quality sources, such as handouts, pamphlets, and websites. The right information will help clients weigh the pros and cons of behavior change and form intentions to modify their lifestyles.

The **protection motivation theory** expands upon the health belief model's assumptions and includes additional factors that influence the relationship between health beliefs and behavior change. Research with adults diagnosed with **coronary artery disease (CAD)** has found that a diagnosis is more likely to lead to behavior change if clients do the following (Reid et al., 2007):

- Perceive CAD to be a serious problem
- Perceive themselves to be susceptible to CAD
- Perceive exercise as an effective way to prevent CAD
- Feel confident in their ability to exercise regularly and safely

According to the protection motivation theory model, the ACE-AHFS should help clients understand personally relevant health concerns and perceive these health concerns as serious, so that they become motivated to take action. However, the ACE-AHFS should remember that people who feel threatened and anxious, and feel like they are unable to deal with the health threat, may avoid, rather than address, a problem (Witte & Allen, 2000). The ACE-AHFS should present health concerns in an informative manner, reassuring the client that taking proper action, such as engaging in regular physical activity, will help reduce the threat posed by the health concern.

When applicable, the ACE-AHFS must help clients conclude that an exercise program is an important means of addressing their health problems and an effective means of reducing the impact of a health problem on the client's daily life, risk of illness, or premature death. In addition, the ACE-AHFS must help clients come to believe that they have the ability to exercise regularly and safely, so that the exercise recommendations seem feasible.

The Transtheoretical Model of Behavior Change

The **transtheoretical model of behavior change (TTM)** emphasizes the importance of viewing behavior change as a process that occurs over time. One aspect of the TTM is called the stages-of-change model, because behavior change is seen to proceed through certain stages. The TTM also describes factors that affect a person's decision to change.

The TTM emphasizes the importance of determining a client's readiness to make a change (Prochaska & Marcus, 1994). According to this model, people who change their behavior go through several stages, from **precontemplation** (not thinking about changing), to **contemplation** (weighing the pros and cons of changing), to **preparation** (getting ready to make a change), to **action** (practicing the new behavior), and finally to **maintenance** (incorporating the new behavior into one's lifestyle) (Table 3-1).

Table 3-1
Stages of Change of Physical Activity

Precontemplation	Not currently active, with no intention of becoming more active
Contemplation	Not currently active, but intending to become more active some day
Preparation	Planning to increase physical activity level soon; taking steps to get ready to increase activity level, or may already be exercising occasionally
Action	Performing regular physical activity for fewer than six months
Maintenance	Performing regular physical activity for longer than six months

Source: Brehm, B.A. (2004). *Successful Fitness Motivation Strategies.* Champaign, Ill.: Human Kinetics. Adapted with permission from Marcus, B.H. et al. (1992). Self-efficacy and the stage of exercise behavior change. *Research Quarterly for Exercise and Sport,* 63, 60–66.

The stages-of-change model from the TTM has been used extensively by fitness professionals (Marcus & Forsyth, 2003). It makes sense that fitness professionals should approach clients already convinced of the benefits of exercise differently from the way they would talk to someone who does not recognize the value of regular exercise and has no intention of becoming more active. Too often, fitness professionals assume that clients have made the decision to become more active, and jump right into exercise program design. While this is often the case, sometimes clients have not yet mentally committed to exerting the effort required to stick to an exercise program. Tailoring actions and recommendations to a client's stage of readiness to change is believed to result in more effective communication and improved adherence.

Precontemplation

People in the precontemplation stage have no intention of becoming more active. They do not exercise and they do not plan to start. They may be unaware that a **sedentary** lifestyle is risky, or, if they are aware of the risk, feel powerless to begin exercising. They may deny the extent or seriousness of the problem and use defensive strategies when others suggest that a sedentary lifestyle is dangerous.

Researchers have further categorized precontemplators into nonbelievers and believers (Reed, 2001). Precontemplation nonbelievers do not believe in the value of physical activity or in their ability to become more active. They may lack information regarding the health benefits of exercise, or they may harbor erroneous beliefs about physical activity. Many people are unaware that a sedentary lifestyle is a serious independent risk factor for chronic illness. Some believe that people only need to exercise if they are overweight. It is commonly believed that exercise makes a person tired, and that if a person is feeling stressed and fatigued, physical activity may make him or her feel worse.

Precontemplation believers, on the other hand, accept to some extent that physical activity is a valuable habit, but the idea of becoming more active is just not a consideration. They may have heard or read about exercise benefits, but have not made the decision to start exercising. Ideas and habits that reinforce their sedentary lifestyle are stronger than beliefs about exercise benefits. They may believe that it takes great quantities and intensities of exercise to achieve beneficial results. Exercise may not be valued by their culture, or they may view it as dangerous.

If the ACE-AHFS finds him- or herself working with a precontemplator, effective strategies include uncovering misinformation, providing education regarding exercise benefits and the dangers of inactivity, and discussing barriers to exercise. The client must make the decision to become active, and the ACE-AHFS can help to facilitate this decision by listening carefully to clients and addressing their concerns.

Contemplation

People in the contemplation stage are sedentary, but are thinking about becoming more active in the near future. They are still weighing the pros and cons of becoming active, and are thinking about whether to exercise regularly. They may be wondering how to begin.

The ACE-AHFS can help contemplators strengthen the pros and weaken the cons of exercise by providing additional information on exercise benefits and addressing the client's concerns about adopting a program of regular physical activity. A contemplator may be more likely to sign on to an exercise program that is perceived to be simple and convenient.

Preparation

People in the preparation stage have decided to become more active, and are preparing to begin. They may have signed up for a class, made an appointment to work with a personal trainer, bought some exercise clothes, or joined a fitness center. People in preparation believe in the benefits of regular physical activity, but may have unrealistic expectations for the changes they hope to achieve by exercising. Their plans may be overly ambitious. They may underestimate the time and energy their exercise plans will take, as well as potential exercise barriers.

The ACE-AHFS can help people in the preparation stage become successful by working with them to set realistic goals and designing convenient exercise programs tailored to clients' abilities and lifestyles. Exercise history can provide insight to what has worked and what has not worked in the past for a specific client.

Action

People in the action stage have begun exercising regularly, but have not yet maintained their exercise behavior for six months. Researchers believe that the first six months of an exercise program are the most difficult (Prochaska & Marcus, 1994), and that people in the action stage may struggle quite a bit to stick to their plans.

Some researchers (Reed, 2001) believe it is helpful to break this group into two subgroups: action/ambivalent and action. People in these groups differ in their confidence in their ability to become regular exercisers. People in the action/ambivalent group exercise regularly, but resemble those in the preparation group in several ways: Their new behavior is fragile, their likelihood of dropout is high, and plans to exercise may be easily disrupted by day-to-day problems.

People in the action group, by contrast, are more confident and are well on their way to dealing with exercise barriers. They believe in physical activity and in their ability to exercise regularly.

Because exercise is a difficult habit to maintain, people in the action/ambivalent and action groups continue to benefit from sustained support from and contact with the ACE-AHFS. Clients in the action group continue to appreciate information on exercise benefits, strategies to best achieve their health and fitness goals, and help with making regular physical activity a lifelong habit.

Maintenance

People in the maintenance stage have been exercising regularly for at least six months.

These clients may seek professional advice on changing their exercise programs to better address their health and fitness goals or to add variety to their exercise programs. For example, committed runners may wish to add strength training or other aeobic activities to their workout routines.

Adherence and Motivation

Sustained behavior change moves a client into the maintenance stage. Exercise **adherence** is the extent to which people follow, or stick to, an exercise program. One of the most important factors that encourage adherence is the client's level of **motivation.** The word motivation refers to the psychological drive that gives purpose and direction to behavior. It is derived from the Latin root *movere,* which means to move. Motivation causes a person to move, do something, or behave in a certain way.

Assessing Self-motivation

A client's level of motivation to exercise regularly is very difficult to measure. For one thing, motivation may change minute to minute, and a client who appears very motivated at a meeting with the ACE-AHFS may still drop out early in the program. Clients may express the idea that they are motivated to increase the amount of exercise they are doing, perhaps wanting to say the right things, but then fail to follow through when challenges arise.

Assessing a client's stage of change will tell the ACE-AHFS something about how far the client has come in making a decision to change. Stage of change may be assessed with a short questionnaire (Figure 3-1) or by asking clients verbally about their exercise habits and intentions.

Even more telling than clients' assessments of their current level of motivation are their previous experiences with exercise programs. A person's exercise history tells the ACE-AHFS a great deal about his or her ability to stick to an exercise program, including the factors thought to be responsible for success, and those responsible for failure. The ACE-AHFS should encourage clients to incorporate factors that have previously enhanced success into their exercise plans, and to plan ways to effectively cope with challenges that have derailed them in the past. Clients who have been successful in the past tend to be more likely to be successful again.

Locus of Control and Learned Helplessness

Research suggests that people who have a stronger sense of control over their lives are more likely to exhibit positive health-related behaviors, such as exercising regularly (Norman et al., 1998). People who tend to attribute events and outcomes to internal factors, such as effort and

Readiness for Exercise Questionnaire

Check the description that best fits you:

❑ 1. I do not exercise and I do not plan to begin exercising in the next six months.

❑ 2. I am not currently exercising, but I am thinking about starting to exercise in the next six months.

❑ 3. I am currently not exercising, or am exercising only occasionally, but I am planning to begin exercising regularly in the next month.

❑ 4. I have been exercising regularly for fewer than six months.

❑ 5. I have been exercising regularly for six months or more.

1 = precontemplation, 2 = contemplation, 3 = preparation, 4 = action, 5 = maintenance

Notes: Regular exercise means three or more times a week, 20 minutes or more each time. Fitness professionals may wish to change the definition of regular exercise to fit their practices.

Figure 3-1
Readiness for exercise questionnaire

Source: Brehm, B.A. (2004). *Successful Fitness Motivation Strategies.* Champaign, Ill.: Human Kinetics. Adapted with permission from Marcus, B.H. et al. (1992). Self-efficacy and the stage of exercise behavior change. *Research Quarterly for Exercise and Sport,* 63, 60–66.

ability, are said to have an internal **locus of control,** while those who generally attribute outcomes to external factors, such as luck or the actions of others, are said to have an external locus of control (Rotter, 1990). People with a stronger internal locus of control in terms of their exercise histories may have more success with sticking to their exercise programs (Kloek et al., 2006).

Clients who seem to fail over and over again are often a special challenge to fitness specialists. **Learned helplessness** refers to a psychological state in which people have come to believe that they are helpless in, or have no power or control over, certain situations (Petersen, Maier, & Seligman, 1995). People who feel like they have little power or control over whether they are able to stick to an exercise program will need extra support to be successful.

People with learned helplessness tend to see failure as inevitable and have learned to attribute their failures to internal, uncontrollable, and stable causes (Petersen, Maier, & Seligman, 1995). This means that they believe failure occurs because of unchangeable and uncontrollable personal qualities in themselves. A client with learned helplessness might think, "I have never had enough energy or organization to stick to an exercise program. I am unable to take care of myself." Contrast this with successful exercisers who view failures as caused by external, controllable, and changeable causes. "The last exercise program didn't work out because I moved to a new town, but I will try to find a new fitness center here."

In conversations with clients who seem to exhibit learned helplessness, the ACE-AHFS should try to help clients view the exercise program as being achievable and under the client's control. When a client starts explaining why the program will not work, the ACE-AHFS can listen carefully, and try to design a program that is as simple and convenient as possible. In addition, the ACE-AHFS should help clients view challenges that arise as a function of controllable and changeable factors, rather than personal failings.

Intrinsic and Extrinsic Motivation

Sports psychology researchers have categorized motivation for exercise in a variety of ways (Duda & Treasure, 2006). One interesting perspective contrasts **intrinsic motivation** and **extrinsic motivation.** People who exercise to achieve an external reward, such as a free T-shirt or the praise of a friend, are said to be extrinsically motivated. People who exercise because they enjoy competition or because exercising feels good are said to be intrinsically motivated. Many clients have both intrinsic and extrinsic motivations for exercise. It is common for people to begin exercising for extrinsic reasons (e.g., a physician told them to or a friend urged them to try a class). People who exercise regularly for extended periods of time, however, often do so because of intrinsic motivations. They have found that exercise makes them feel better or is an enjoyable way to spend time.

Researchers Ryan and Deci (2000) have explored factors related to intrinsic motivation and have formed a theoretical framework known as **self-determination theory.** According to this theory, people need to feel competent, autonomous (i.e., like they are acting on their own accord), and connected to others in many domains of life. When an exercise experience satisfies these needs, clients are more likely to exercise because of intrinsic motivation.

What does this mean for an ACE-AHFS? Exercise will be a more satisfying experience if clients feel competent in their exercise skills and environment, provided they have truly "signed on" to the exercise program and made the decision to adopt an exercise habit. To the greatest extent possible, the ACE-AHFS should incorporate client preferences and input into the exercise program design to satisfy the need for autonomy. And lastly, an exercise program that satisfies the need for connecting with others provides great positive reinforcement for exercise participation. The client may enjoy the connection with fitness professionals, other participants in an exercise group, or other people in the exercise activity and/or environment.

Psychological Benefits of Exercise

People begin exercising for a variety of reasons, but those who continue exercising month after month and year after year often do so because they have found that regular exercise helps them feel good. While they may appreciate the long-term health benefits of regular physical activity, they are especially motivated by the immediate benefits they receive on a daily basis, which strengthens their intrinsic motivation to stick to their exercise programs. These immediate benefits tend to be psychological in nature (Brehm, 2000). People commonly report feeling less anxious, irritable, depressed, and fatigued after an exercise session. They also report positive changes in mood, including feelings of happiness, satisfaction, and vigor. Feelings of energy and vigor have been found to correlate strongly with general feelings of psychological well-being (Park, Peterson, & Seligman, 2004). It should also be noted that regular physical activity (participation for several weeks or more) has been associated with reductions in anxiety, depression, and feelings of stress, and improvements in body image and a sense of well-being (Brehm, 2000). The ACE-AHFS can encourage clients to find immediate and long-term psychological benefits from their participation in regular physical activity in several ways, including the following.

Educate clients about the importance of psychological health. Clients commonly seek the advice of fitness professionals for physical concerns, such as obesity or diabetes. Many do not realize that physical activity may improve psychological well-being. Engaging in regular self-care, including physical activity, helps people maintain or improve emotional balance. And, of course, psychological and physical health go together; poor psychological health is associated with many physical health risks, such as heart disease and hypertension. Similarly, clients with physical health problems often experience psychological problems as well.

Include psychological benefits in health and fitness goals. Many people are concerned about feelings of excess stress, anxiety, and depression, but do not commonly list these issues when asked about their health and fitness goals. Once clients understand that regular physical activity can help reduce feelings of stress and improve mood, they can be encouraged to include these psychological benefits in their health and fitness goals. When clients are consciously aware of the psychological benefits that may result from their exercise programs, they are more likely to experience them, and to figure out what kinds of exercise work best for them.

Recommend effective activities. Some clients may already understand what types of activities give them the greatest stress-reduction benefits. In general, moderately vigorous activities tend to be well-received. The ACE-AHFS should remember, however, that beginners may become too fatigued by overly vigorous options. Therefore, the ACE-AHFS should ask clients about activities they enjoy and then incorporate these into program design whenever possible, as personal preferences have an important influence on intrinsic motivation. Some clients enjoy outdoor options. Some find that exercising with a friend is fun, while others use exercise to get away from people. Activities requiring concentration, such as sports or classes with complicated choreography, can help people change their mental channel and get their minds off their problems. Competitive activities serve a similar function. Healthy, fit clients may experience more stress reduction with very vigorous and relatively higher volumes of exercise.

Measure mood changes with exercise. Some fitness professionals measure mood before and after exercise sessions using a questionnaire such as the exercise-induced feeling inventory (Figure 3-2). Responses can also be compared before and after several weeks of participation in an exercise program.

Principles of Behavior Change

Health-psychology research has studied the behavior-change process extensively. This section presents some of the most useful principles to help guide the ACE-AHFS in designing effective exercise programs that are effective both in terms of meeting a client's health and fitness goals and in encouraging adherence.

Operant Conditioning

Operant conditioning models consider a behavior such as exercise participation as being influenced by many factors. Using this model, the ACE-AHFS can determine the variables that promote or discourage exercise, and then increase the

Figure 3-2
Exercise-induced feeling inventory (EFI) survey

Source: Gauvin, L. & Rejesk, W.J., (1993). The exercise-induced feeling inventory: Development and initial validation. *Journal of Sport & Exercise Psychology,* 15, 4, 409.

Instructions: Please use the following scale to indicate the extent to which each word describes how you feel at this moment in time. Record your responses by checking the appropriate box next to each word.

0 = Do not feel
1 = Feel slightly
2 = Feel moderately
3 = Feel strongly
4 = Feel very strongly

	0	1	2	3	4		0	1	2	3	4
1. Refreshed	☐	☐	☐	☐	☐	**7. Happy**	☐	☐	☐	☐	☐
2. Calm	☐	☐	☐	☐	☐	**8. Tired**	☐	☐	☐	☐	☐
3. Fatigued	☐	☐	☐	☐	☐	**9. Revived**	☐	☐	☐	☐	☐
4. Enthusiastic	☐	☐	☐	☐	☐	**10. Peaceful**	☐	☐	☐	☐	☐
5. Relaxed	☐	☐	☐	☐	☐	**11. Worn out**	☐	☐	☐	☐	☐
6. Energetic	☐	☐	☐	☐	☐	**12. Upbeat**	☐	☐	☐	☐	☐

likelihood that a client will exercise by manipulating these variables.

Variables or factors that precede and influence a client's exercise participation are called **antecedents** or **triggers.** Variables that occur following exercise participation are called **consequences.** With operant conditioning, exercise participation, or a lack of participation, is viewed as part of a **behavior chain,** both preceded and followed by factors that influence whether or not a client participates in physical activity.

Consider a client who has worked with an ACE-AHFS to design an exercise program to improve blood sugar regulation. The client has agreed to begin walking every day around his neighborhood after work for 30 minutes. The client is successful for two days after his meeting with the ACE-AHFS, but on the third day arrives home later than usual from work, feeling hungry and tired, and decides to skip walking. Unfortunately, the next few days are also late days, and the client returns to the ACE-AHFS discouraged and frustrated.

The ACE-AHFS would examine the behavior chain with the client, and find ways to solve the problem by addressing the antecedents and consequences that led to the client's decision to not exercise. Would the client be more successful exercising before work if fatigue at the end of the day is the problem? Would stopping at a fitness center on his way home be an option to avoid the temptations of dinner and rest, which would then be unavailable to reinforce a decision to skip the walk? As the ACE-AHFS and client "take apart" the links in the behavior chain, they can come up with a plan to reinforce the new desired behavior (exercising). This process is called **shaping,** since the ACE-AHFS and client are attempting to shape a new, more productive behavior chain.

Self-efficacy

Self-efficacy refers to a person's confidence that he or she can perform a given task (Bandura, 1997). While self-efficacy is similar to self-confidence, self-efficacy differs in that it is always situation- or behavior-specific. For example, a client may be very confident in his or her ability to use the treadmill, but lack confidence in sticking to a strength-training program. Self-efficacy predicts how much effort clients will exert in sticking to their exercise programs when faced with difficulties. The ACE-AHFS should work to increase client self-efficacy whenever possible, primarily by helping clients become successful. More suggestions for increasing client self-efficacy are given in the "Strategies for Behavior Change" section that follows.

Stress and Negative Emotions

The ACE-AHFS may notice that stress and negative emotions such as anger and worry are common components of behavior chains associated with decisions to skip exercise sessions. Stress and negative emotions make people feel tired and preoccupied with problems and reduce feelings of self-efficacy. Stress and negative emotions "feel bad" and stimulate people to search for ways to feel better.

The drive to cope with negative emotions is stronger for most people than the need to exercise (Tice, Bratslavsky, & Baumeister, 2001). Of course, if the ACE-AHFS can help clients see that exercise will help reduce stress and manage negative emotions, clients may eventually turn to exercise when feeling down. In the meantime, if clients manage stress with harmful actions such as overeating, substance abuse, or sedentary behaviors, these unhealthy behaviors will likely increase when clients are under stress—at the expense of the exercise program.

Exercise Programs Must Be Sustainable

An ACE-AHFS should understand that clients cannot "bank" exercise participation and that **deconditioning** begins within days of resuming a sedentary lifestyle. The ACE-AHFS must help prepare clients for lifelong success by working with them to devise programs that optimize adherence. Exercise programs can and should change over time, as long as regular physical activity continues as a lifelong constant.

Strategies for Behavior Change

Successful behavior change evolves from an understanding and application of the behavior-change theories and principles described in this chapter. The following strategies may be helpful to an ACE-AHFS as he or she works with individuals and groups to promote regular physical activity.

Tailor Exercise Recommendations to Each Client's Stage of Change

Clients in precontemplation and contemplation need help forming an intention to add regular physical activity to their lives. The ACE-AHFS should listen carefully to these clients and provide information to strengthen their perceptions of exercise benefits and address their reservations. Rather than rushing into designing a complicated exercise program, the ACE-AHFS should lead educational discussions to help these clients make the decision to change (Armitage, 2006). Clients should be at least in the preparation stage before starting an exercise program.

Clients who are ready to start exercising will still need a great deal of support and encouragement to sustain their behavior-change efforts. The ACE-AHFS should set clients up for success to build self-efficacy, starting slowly and building gradually to prevent injury.

Help Clients Set Achievable Goals

Many people tend to be overly ambitious when they first decide to begin an exercise program. It is human nature to plan more than can realistically be accomplished with one's given resources, in terms of time, money, and/or energy (Polivy & Herman, 2000). People feel great as they resolve to lose weight, start exercising, or make other lifestyle changes. Just forming a resolution reduces stress. Clients quickly become disillusioned, however, when progress is slower than expected or when life gets busy and finding time to exercise becomes more difficult (Polivy & Herman, 2000).

Lofty goals and promises of success often lure clients into the fitness center, but the ACE-AHFS must avoid the temptation to downplay the time and effort a regular exercise program entails. While the ACE-AHFS should be positive and express confidence in a client's ability to stick to an exercise program, the goals set by the client and ACE-AHFS should be realistic. Fitness goals should include **product goals** as well as **process goals.** A product goal is something measurable, such as increases in strength scores, reductions in resting heart rate, or weight loss. A process goal is something the client does, such as completing an exercise session or attending a talk on stress management. Process goals are great because simply attending the exercise session or event means reaching a goal. More suggestions for helping clients set achievable goals are listed in Table 3-2.

Table 3-2
Tips for Setting Health and Fitness Goals That Motivate Clients for Long-term Adherence

- Listen carefully to understand what clients hope to accomplish with an exercise program.
- Help them define measurable goals.
- Suggest additional goals that clients may not have thought of, such as feeling more energetic and less stressed.
- Break large goals (reachable in six months or more) into small goals (reachable in about eight to 10 weeks) and even weekly goals (e.g., completing a certain number of exercise sessions).
- Include many process goals, such as the completion of exercise sessions. That way, simply completing workouts accomplishes a goal.
- Record goals and set up a record-keeping system to record workouts and track progress toward goals.
- Be sure that clients understand what types of exercise will help them reach their health and fitness goals.
- Reevaluate and revise goals and exercise recommendations periodically to prevent discouragement if large goals are not being met.

Source: Brehm, B.A. (2004). *Successful Fitness Motivation Strategies.* Champaign, Ill.: Human Kinetics.

Incorporate Strategies to Increase Self-efficacy

Self-efficacy helps clients stick to their lifestyle-modification programs. Research suggests that self-efficacy can be increased in many ways (McAuley & Blissmer, 2000).

Set achievable goals. Setting achievable goals is a good start. As the old adage says, success breeds success. Clients will build self-efficacy as they achieve goals and stick to their exercise programs.

Expose clients to role models similar to themselves. People also report increased exercise self-efficacy when they observe people similar to themselves being successful. People of similar age, health status, and other identifying characteristics may help the client think, "If they can do it, so can I."

People with whom the client can interact in real life are best, but people from news reports and other media can provide helpful modeling as well.

Encourage social support. Social support improves exercise adherence (Fraser & Spink, 2002). Social support refers to help from others, including family members, friends, coworkers, and acquaintances. It might mean a spouse who offers extra help with childcare to provide an opportunity for the client to squeeze an exercise session into the day, or a friend who works out with the client. An exercise partner can be an especially effective form of social support that enhances self-efficacy. The exercise partner not only improves the client's adherence, but the exercise sessions also become a more visible and salient component of the client's life. Exercise partners talk about their exercise programs, schedule exercise sessions, and refer to their exercise time together in conversation with others.

Discuss strategies for managing stress and negative moods. Many clients already have stress-management strategies in place, although they may not define them as such. They may also have ways in which they cope with negative moods. The ACE-AHFS should encourage clients to think about ways in which they can cope with negative moods, and strategize about which coping methods are most productive and effective for them. The goal is to help clients see that some strategies (skipping an exercise session or eating a bag of cookies) may make stress worse in the long run, while helpful measures (talking to a friend, watching a funny movie) are more helpful.

The ACE-AHFS can also encourage clients to come up with a list of "healthy pleasures" that can be used more frequently for coping with stress. Clients should be encouraged to mention simple and accessible things like listening to music, watching birds, reading a good book, taking a hot shower, or enjoying hobbies.

The ACE-AHFS should also take the opportunity to reinforce the pleasures and psychological benefits of physical activity, such as reducing feelings of stress, anxiety, depression, and fatigue, and improving mood and energy levels. If clients can learn to turn to exercise to reduce stress and change the channel on negative moods, then clients can shape productive new behavior patterns.

Some clients may find relaxation techniques such as meditation and breathing exercises helpful. Many techniques are very simple to teach and learn (Brehm, 1998). Relaxation techniques can help clients to be more mindfully aware of maladaptive and unnecessary stress response patterns.

Create systems for self-monitoring and problem-solving. Research has shown that self-monitoring is one of the most effective ways to support behavior change, including exercise program adherence (Berkel et al., 2005). Self-monitoring systems, such as an exercise log where clients record their workouts, help in several ways. First, they increase clients' self-awareness. A log with nothing recorded for several days testifies to the fact that clients are neglecting their exercise programs. Self-monitoring acts as a mirror to give clients a more objective view of their behavior.

Second, self-monitoring systems forge an important link between the ACE-AHFS and the client. Clients come to expect careful surveillance of their records, which they present at each session with the ACE-AHFS. Knowing that someone will be checking on their adherence may prod clients into action.

Third, self-monitoring systems can serve as important tools for evaluating behavior-change problems. Clients may note factors that helped or interfered with plans to exercise, as well as their mood before and after exercise sessions. The ACE-AHFS can analyze this information with clients and brainstorm solutions to problems that arise, analyzing links in the behavior chains that influence exercise participation and suggesting changes that will enhance the likelihood of success.

Lastly, self-monitoring records serve as a form of positive reinforcement and help to increase self-efficacy. A completed exercise log shows clients they are being successful in their exercise programs.

Learning Models

Fitness professionals often find themselves in the role of teacher. An ACE-AHFS teaches motor skills such as correct lifting techniques for strength training, how to use exercise machines, and how to perform flexibility exercises. They may also teach clients about information in the **cognitive** domain, explain health problems, and teach how physical activity interacts with physiological variables. The ACE-AHFS may explain the physiology of training effects and injury prevention. Understanding how people learn most effectively can help the ACE-AHFS provide sound instruction to diverse groups of clients.

Motor Learning

Motor learning is the process of acquiring and improving motor skills. Many adult clients are quite self-conscious in the motor skill domain, especially if they have had little experience with sports and physical activity. Fitness professionals with a strong background in physical education and sports are often surprised at the lack of motor ability they see in many adult clients. Motor skills will be taught most effectively if the following points are kept in mind.

Remind beginners that it takes time and practice to improve motor skills. Physical education specialists have noted that many people tend to believe that good coordination and athletic ability are things that a person is born with (Rink, 2004). While ability in the motor-skills domain certainly varies from person to person, motor skills are more strongly related to practice and experience than to natural ability alone. It is important for people new to physical activity to understand that motor-skill improvement takes a great deal of practice; the people they see in exercise classes have often been performing similar movement patterns and choreography for years. The same holds true for athletes in every sport.

Many clients new to exercise feel self-conscious attending a new exercise class or participating in a personal-training situation. They may feel out of place, awkward, and clumsy. The ACE-AHFS must help new clients feel at home in the exercise environment and help new learners understand that most of the people they see working out have been performing these types of activities for months, years, and often, decades.

It is also important to note that even clients with athletic experience may feel awkward when learning new motor skills. Such clients may believe that they should pick up new motor skills quickly, remembering how good they were at sports when they were younger. They may be frustrated if motor learning does not come quickly and easily (Rink, 2004). The ACE-AHFS should reassure new clients that it is okay to be a beginner, and that with practice they will eventually look like a fitness center regular.

If clients appear to be self-conscious and nervous, the ACE-AHFS should encourage them to relax and focus on the task at hand. If the ACE-AHFS is demonstrating a skill, such as using a piece of exercise equipment, and a client does not appear to be watching, the ACE-AHFS should draw the client's attention back to the demonstration and direct the client to focus on details of the motor skill.

Introduce a new skill slowly and clearly. When introducing a new skill, the ACE-AHFS should begin with a very short explanation of what he or she is going to do and why. Explanations should be short and clear. Safety information should be emphasized, along with guidelines for preventing injury. A skill should be explained in terms of what it is accomplishing or why it is important.

When describing certain movements, the ACE-AHFS should focus on the goal of the movement rather than giving distracting details about limb position (Marchant, Clough, & Cramshaw, 2005). For example, the ACE-AHFS would not teach someone how to use an elliptical trainer by describing when to bend and straighten the knees. Instead, the ACE-AHFS would emphasize moving the pedals around in a smooth, steady motion. The ACE-AHFS should demonstrate the skill accurately and allow clients time to watch.

Teaching strength-training exercises or exercise positions does require some explanation of limb position for safety and efficacy. For example, when teaching squats, the ACE-AHFS might ask the client to focus on keeping the knees aligned with the ankles throughout the exercise movement. Descriptions should be brief and simple.

Adapt teaching methods to each client's learning style when possible. Variations in the way people process and retain new information have been called learning style differences. Some clients like a lot of explanation and ask many questions (verbal learning style). Others learn by watching and appreciate longer demonstrations with less talking (visual learning style), while others learn by doing, needing to feel the movement before catching on (kinesthetic learning style). Once the ACE-AHFS has been working with a particular client for a period of time, learning styles may become apparent. Clients may also be able to let the ACE-AHFS know how they learn best, asking for longer demonstrations or explanations. The teaching pace should be comfortable for clients, allowing them to learn one skill before moving on to another.

Allow clients the opportunity for focused practice. People learn more quickly when they focus on performing the motor skill without being distracted by talking or listening. The ACE-AHFS should not talk for a few minutes while the client is trying a new skill, and should encourage the client to give the skill a few tries without talking (except to interrupt the client to prevent an accident or injury) (Coker, Fischman, & Oxendine, 2006).

Give helpful feedback. Once clients have tried the skill, the ACE-AHFS should give the following helpful feedback:

- Provide reinforcement for what was done well
- Correct errors
- Motivate clients to continue practicing and improving

Correcting errors, which may be seen as the more "negative" point, should be sandwiched between reinforcement and motivation (Coker, Fischman, & Oxendine, 2006). An example might be, "Your breathing and timing were just right on the first four lifts. Remember to keep breathing, even as the exercise starts to feel harder. You'll find the work easier now that you are learning how to breathe correctly."

The ACE-AHFS should limit feedback to a few simple points, and decide which errors are the most important to correct first. Most important errors typically include those that involve safety, occur earliest in the movement sequence, or are fundamental in some other way. Feedback should be phrased positively, pointing out what clients should do: "Remember to breathe," rather than "Don't hold your breath."

Cognitive Learning

The ACE-AHFS should also be able to provide effective instruction to clients about health- and exercise-related topics. Clients often ask fitness professionals to explain things like why exercise improves blood sugar regulation, what is meant by **overtraining,** or what is indicated by a pain in a certain area of the body. It is often enough to simply answer the question, giving clients the information they desire without launching into a detailed discussion from an **exercise physiology** class. At other times, the ACE-AHFS may need to teach clients information in a classroom or discussion setting on a particular topic. Guidelines for effective teaching in the cognitive domain include the following:

Clarify instructional goals. Fitness professionals may find themselves teaching material to clients for many reasons. Clarifying instructional goals can help the ACE-AHFS decide on the most effective approach for a given situation.

In many cases, the ACE-AHFS may need to give clients specific directions that should be followed as part of an exercise plan. In such cases, instructions should always be written as well as delivered verbally. Whenever material has an important bearing on the client's behavior, written explanations tailored to the client's educational level and language skills are essential.

Sometimes the ACE-AHFS may wish to stimulate a client to make a change in his or her behavior, perhaps by convincing him or her of the importance of exercise. Many clients appreciate evidence that backs up the points the ACE-AHFS is trying to make. Clients might like a list of helpful websites or well-written articles from respected experts.

Engage learners. Readers who have spent time in classrooms know the sad truth: Dry factual information does not stick and the audience's attention will begin to wander after a very short period of lecturing. Only a very motivated audience learns much from a lecture composed solely of one person talking (Ennis, 2007).

To engage learners, the ACE-AHFS must somehow make the material interesting, meaningful, and relevant to the learner. Pictures promote engagement with the material, as do worksheets that get clients writing. The ACE-AHFS can get clients involved by passing out a questionnaire that enables them to rate themselves on the topic of discussion, such as stress level or diet quality. Clients might interview each other about the topic and report results back to the larger group.

Use instructional media wisely. Audiovisual aids enhance a presentation when used well. Many clients learn more effectively if visual images accompany a speaker's words. Music enhances learners' experiences, but only if learners find the music appealing.

Invite motivational guest speakers. People love personal success stories. The ACE-AHFS can invite role models of the behavior under discussion, such as a former client with diabetes who lost weight via a well-balanced diet and exercise program. Such speakers build client self-efficacy, and thus, enhance exercise adherence.

Entertain the audience. Entertainment should be at the heart of many instructional sessions, since people can be entertained and learn at the same time. It can also be a motivator to return for more fun. Instructional material can be transmitted through personal stories and appropriately funny remarks.

Psychological Issues Related to Illness and Injury

People tend to discuss illness and injury as something that happens to a part of the body, as a physical occurrence with physical causes and physical symptoms. But the physical aspect of illness and injury is only part of the story, just as a person's body is just one part of the person. Thoughts, feelings, and spirit are also important components of the client who is looking to the ACE-AHFS for guidance. While the illness or injury is a guiding consideration when designing safe and effective exercise programs, it is important to consider the whole person when working with clients experiencing illness or injury.

Psychological Response to Illness and Injury

A client's psychological response to a diagnosis of an illness or serious injury is often similar to the process of grieving in response to a significant loss, such as the loss of a loved one. In general, grieving tends to begin with feelings of distress and shock, then move into feelings such as denial, anger, and sadness, and then eventually into resignation, acceptance, and hopefully some form of resolution (Maciejewski et al., 2007). People vary enormously in their responses to illness and injury, depending upon a number of factors.

Severity of the Illness or Injury and Impact on Quality of Life

The more serious the illness or injury, and the more it impacts daily activities, the more adjustment and coping are required from the client. Most medical treatments include therapies such as physical therapy and occupational therapy to help clients improve their ability to perform daily activities while coping with illness or injury. It is important to note that the client's *perception* of the illness or injury is more important than the actual physical nature of the illness or injury—and often is quite different (Brown, 2005).

An illness or injury will obviously have different impacts depending on a client's personal situation. Disruptions in family life, work, school, the ability to produce income, and the ability to participate in fulfilling activities are associated with significant emotional distress.

Expected Outcome

If illness or disease outcome is expected to eventually be positive, clients will feel more positive and less stressed than when coping with an illness or injury that is not expected to significantly improve. Some clients will be living with an illness that may be expected to worsen and lead to significant disability and even premature death. Feeling uncertain about potential outcomes is obviously stressful.

The Client's Personal Resources

Illness and injury can produce not only physical stress, but also financial and social stress. Medical care is expensive on many levels and places significant stress on the patient's partner, family, and friends. Clients with strong financial and social resources may be able to weather these stresses more easily than those with fewer resources.

Personal resources also include individual capacities to adapt and cope with stress. Some people are more resilient than others and find hope in situations when others would give up.

Working With Clients in Distress

An ACE-AHFS is likely to work with clients with significant amounts of emotional distress because of illness and injury. Clients may or may not want to discuss their distress and personal situations. The ACE-AHFS should respect the client's need for privacy and not ask for details irrelevant to exercise program design. When clients share with the ACE-AHFS that times are challenging, the ACE-AHFS can listen with sympathy and acknowledge that life is really hard sometimes. The ACE-AHFS need not try to "fix" everything, but, if appropriate, may recommend helpful resources available to the client. The following strategies may be useful in some situations.

Education

Clients need to understand the health issues and injuries they are coping with and be knowledgeable about rehabilitation and treatment recommendations. However, clients should not be overwhelmed with negative information. Education should focus on answering clients' questions and explaining the most productive ways of coping with the illness or injury. An ACE-AHFS must encourage clients to hope for the best and to view regular physical activity as one of the ways to achieve the best possible outcome for rehabilitation and treatment, and for improving quality of life. Clients must believe in the efficacy of their exercise programs.

Goal-setting and Positive Outlook

Goal-setting improves rehabilitation and treatment adherence. Small, achievable goals help clients feel they are making progress and taking control of their lives (Johnson, Haskvitz, & Brehm, 2009). The ACE-AHFS should encourage clients to have as positive an outlook as possible. While not discounting fear and other negative emotions, the ACE-AHFS should help the client see positive progress. The power of belief will help clients facing illness and injury better cope with the challenges they face.

Social Support

Support from family, friends, and medical staff enhance adherence and help clients feel better. When possible, the ACE-AHFS should welcome a family member or friend to participate with the client. Social support can be especially welcome, and even essential, for clients facing significant difficulties.

Barriers to Exercise

The ACE-AHFS must recognize that clients coping with illness or injury face extra barriers to exercise participation that can interfere with motivation and adherence. These must be taken into consideration as the ACE-AHFS designs exercise programs (Brehm, 2004).

Access to Exercise

Access to exercise opportunities is often limited for many people with health problems. Facilities, classes, and instructors may be inaccessible because of limitations in the physical environment, lack of qualified fitness specialists, or transportation difficulties.

Depression

Depression is more prevalent in people with severe chronic medical conditions than in those without. Some studies estimate that depression affects approximately 10% of individuals receiving medical treatment (Nease & Malouin, 2003). The special challenge of depression is that it often leads to feelings of lethargy and a lack of motivation to be active.

If clients tell the ACE-AHFS that they are coping with depression, the ACE-AHFS should express sympathy and acknowledge that dealing with depression can be very hard. The ACE-AHFS can also remind depressed clients that regular physical activity can help relieve depression symptoms. The ACE-AHFS should also encourage clients to continue current depression treatments, however, and consult their healthcare providers regarding recommendations in this area.

Sometimes the ACE-AHFS may suspect a client is experiencing depression because of persistent negative mood or low energy. If the ACE-AHFS has been working with a client for at least four to six weeks, the ACE-AHFS might ask the client if he or she has considered consulting his or her healthcare provider about the symptoms.

Multiple Health Problems and Medication Side Effects

In addition to a client's primary medical focus, other illnesses and limitations may exist simultaneously. They may be related to the original problem, as when a person with coronary artery disease also has **type 2 diabetes,** or unrelated, as when the same person also has **osteoarthritis.** Medication side effects, such as dizziness, can also interfere with motivation to exercise.

Pain

Pain is associated with many medical problems. Pain is usually a warning to rest the afflicted area. Unfortunately, pain may be continuous in some medical conditions, such as many forms of arthritis, and people with such conditions may need to exercise with some level of pain. Rest and inactivity make some types of pain worse. The ACE-AHFS will need to work closely with such clients and their medical teams to effectively address pain and to help clients understand their exercise limits.

Fear of Harm

People coping with health problems and injury, especially those new to exercise, may feel fragile and vulnerable. Their bodies are already experiencing limitations, and they do not want to compromise their abilities further. For example, clients may fear falling or suffering another heart attack.

Of course, the ACE-AHFS must do everything possible to ensure that clients' exercise programs are safe. When people voice concerns about the safety of their exercise programs, the ACE-AHFS should address these concerns. The ACE-AHFS might remind clients that their physicians recommended these exercises (when that is the case), and that exercise is an important part of the treatment program, emphasizing the substantial benefits that will be gained with regular exercise. Fearful clients should initially be given low levels of exercise to slowly strengthen confidence and improve exercise-specific self-efficacy.

Summary

The ACE-AHFS will be most effective when he or she is able to communicate effectively and build good rapport with clients. An understanding of behavior change models and principles helps the ACE-AHFS plan exercise recommendations and strategies that are most likely to motivate clients to adhere to their exercise programs. As the ACE-AHFS works with clients in the realms of both motor and cognitive learning, good teaching practices facilitate learning.

The ACE-AHFS is likely to work with clients who have significant health challenges, and who may be experiencing psychological distress because of illness or injury. The ACE-AHFS should understand the range of emotional responses people have to illness and injury, and be familiar with the many factors that affect clients' abilities to exercise and their adherence to programs of regular physical activity.

References

Ambady, N. & Gray, H.M. (2002). On being sad and mistaken: Mood effects on the accuracy of thin-slice judgments. *Journal of Personality and Social Psychology*, 83, 4, 947–961.

Ambady, N. et al. (2002). Physical therapists' nonverbal communication predicts geriatric patients' health outcomes. *Psychology and Aging,* 17, 3, 443–452.

Armitage, C.J. (2006). Evidence that implementation intentions promote transitions between the stages of change. *Journal of Consulting and Clinical Psychology,* 74, 1, 141–151.

Bandura, A. (1997). *Self-efficacy: The Exercise of Control.* New York: Freeman.

Berkel, L.A. et al. (2005). Behavioral interventions for obesity. *Journal of the American Dietetic Association,* 105, 5 (Suppl. 1), 35–43.

Brehm, B.A. (2004). *Successful Fitness Motivation Strategies*. Champaign, Ill.: Human Kinetics.

Brehm, B.A. (2000). Maximizing the psychological benefits of physical activity. *ACSM's Health & Fitness Journal,* 4, 6, 7–11, 26.

Brehm, B.A. (1998). *Stress Management: Increasing Your Stress Resistance.* New York: Addison, Wesley, Longman.

Brown, C. (2005). Injuries: The psychology of recovery and rehab. In: Murphy, S. (Ed.) *The Sport Psych Handbook.* Champaign, Ill.: Human Kinetics.

Coker, C.A., Fischman, M.G., & Oxendine, J.B. (2006). Motor skill learning for effective coaching and performance. In: Williams, J.M. (Ed.) *Applied Sport Psychology.* New York: McGraw-Hill.

Duda, J.L. & Treasure, D.C. (2006). Motivational processes and the facilitation of performance, persistence, and well-being in sport. In: Williams, J.M. (Ed.) *Applied Sport Psychology.* New York: McGraw-Hill.

Ennis, C.D. (2007). Defining learning as conceptual change in physical education and physical activity settings. *Research Quarterly for Exercise and Sport,* 78, 3, 138–151.

Fraser, S.N. & Spink, K.S. (2002). Examining the role of social support and group cohesion in exercise compliance. *Journal of Behavioral Medicine,* 25, 3, 233–240.

Gordon, P.M. (2006). Thoughts on communication. *Annals of Family Medicine,* 4, 263–264.

Johnson, J.H., Haskvitz, E.M., & Brehm, B.A. (2009). *Applied Sports Medicine for Coaches*. Philadelphia: Lippincott, Williams, & Wilkins.

Kloek, G.C. et al. (2006). Stages of change for moderate-intensity physical activity in deprived neighborhoods. *Preventive Medicine,* 43, 4, 325–331.

Maciejewski, P.K. et al. (2007). An empirical examination of the stage theory of grief. *Journal of the American Medical Association*, 297, 7, 716–724.

Marchant, D., Clough, P., & Cramshaw, M. (2005). Influence of attentional focusing strategies during practice and performance of a motor skill. *Journal of Sports Sciences,* 23, 11–12, 1258–1259.

Marcus, B.H., & Forsyth, L. (2003). *Motivating People to be Physically Active.* Champaign, Ill.: Human Kinetics.

Marcus, B.H. et al. (1992). Self-efficacy and the stage of exercise behavior change. *Research Quarterly for Exercise and Sport*, 63, 60–66.

McAuley, E. & Blissmer, B. (2000). Self-efficacy determinants and consequences of physical activity. *Exercise and Sport Sciences Reviews,* 28, 2, 85–88.

Nease, D.E. & Malouin, J.M. (2003). Depression screening: A practical strategy. *Journal of Family Practice,* 52, 2, 118–124.

Norman, P. et al. (1998). Health locus of control and behavior. *Journal of Health Psychology* 3, 2, 171–180.

Park, N., Peterson, C., & Seligman, M.E.P. (2004). Strengths of character and well-being. *Journal of Social and Clinical Psychology*, 23, 5, 603–619.

Petersen, C., Maier, S.F., & Seligman, M.E.P. (1995). *Learned Helplessness: A Theory for the Age of Personal Control*. New York: Oxford University Press.

Polivy, J. & Herman, C.P. (2000). The false-hope syndrome: Unfulfilled expectations of self-change. *Current Directions in Psychological Science,* 9, 4, 128–131.

Prochaska, J.O. & Marcus, B.H. (1994). The transtheoretical model: Applications to exercise. In: Dishman, R.K. (Ed.) *Advances in Exercise Adherence*. Champaign, Ill.: Human Kinetics.

Reed, G.R. (2001). Adherence to exercise and the transtheoretical model of behavior change. In: Bull, S. J. (Ed.) *Adherence Issues in Sport and Exercise.* Chichester, West Sussex, England: John Wiley & Sons.

Reid, R.D. et al. (2007). Who will be active? Predicting exercise stage transitions after hospitalization for coronary artery disease. *Canadian Journal of Physiological Pharmacology,* 85, 17–23.

Rider, E.A. & Keefer, C.H. (2006). Communication skills competencies: Definitions and a teaching toolbox. *Medical Education,* 40, 624–629.

Rink, J.E. (2004). It's okay to be a beginner: Teach a motor skill, and the skill may be learned. *Journal of Physical Education, Recreation, and Dance,* 75, 6, 31–35.

Rotter, J.B. (1990). Internal versus external control of reinforcement: A case history of a variable. *American Psychologist,* 45, 4, 489–493.

Ryan, R.M. & Deci, E.L. (2000). Self-determination theory and the facilitation of intrinsic motivation, social development, and well being. *American Psychologist,* 55, 68–68.

Tice, D.M., Bratslavsky, E., & Baumeister, R.F. (2001). Emotional distress regulation takes precedence over impulse control: If you feel bad, do it! *Journal of Personality and Social Psychology,* 80, 1, 53–67.

Vohs, K.D. & Heatherton, T.F. (2000). Self-regulatory failure: A resource-depletion approach. *Psychological Science,* 11, 3, 249–254.

Witte, K. & Allen, M. (2000). A meta-analysis of fear appeals: Implications for effective public health campaigns. *Health Education & Behavior,* 27, 5, 591–615.

Wright, K.B., Frey, L., & Sopory, P. (2007). Willingness to communicate about health as an underlying trait of patient self-advocacy: The development of the willingness to communicate about health (WTCH) measure. *Communication Studies,* 58, 1, 35–52.

Suggested Reading

American Council on Exercise (2008). *ACE Lifestyle & Weight Management Consultant Manual* (2nd ed.). San Diego: American Council on Exercise.

Annesi, J.J. (2002).The exercise support process: Facilitating members' self-management skills. *Fitness Management,* 18, 10 (Suppl.), 24–25.

Brehm, B.A. (2004). *Successful Fitness Motivation Strategies*. Champaign, Ill.: Human Kinetics.

Brehm, B.A. (2000). Maximizing the psychological benefits of physical activity. *ACSM's Health & Fitness Journal,* 4, 6, 7–11, 26.

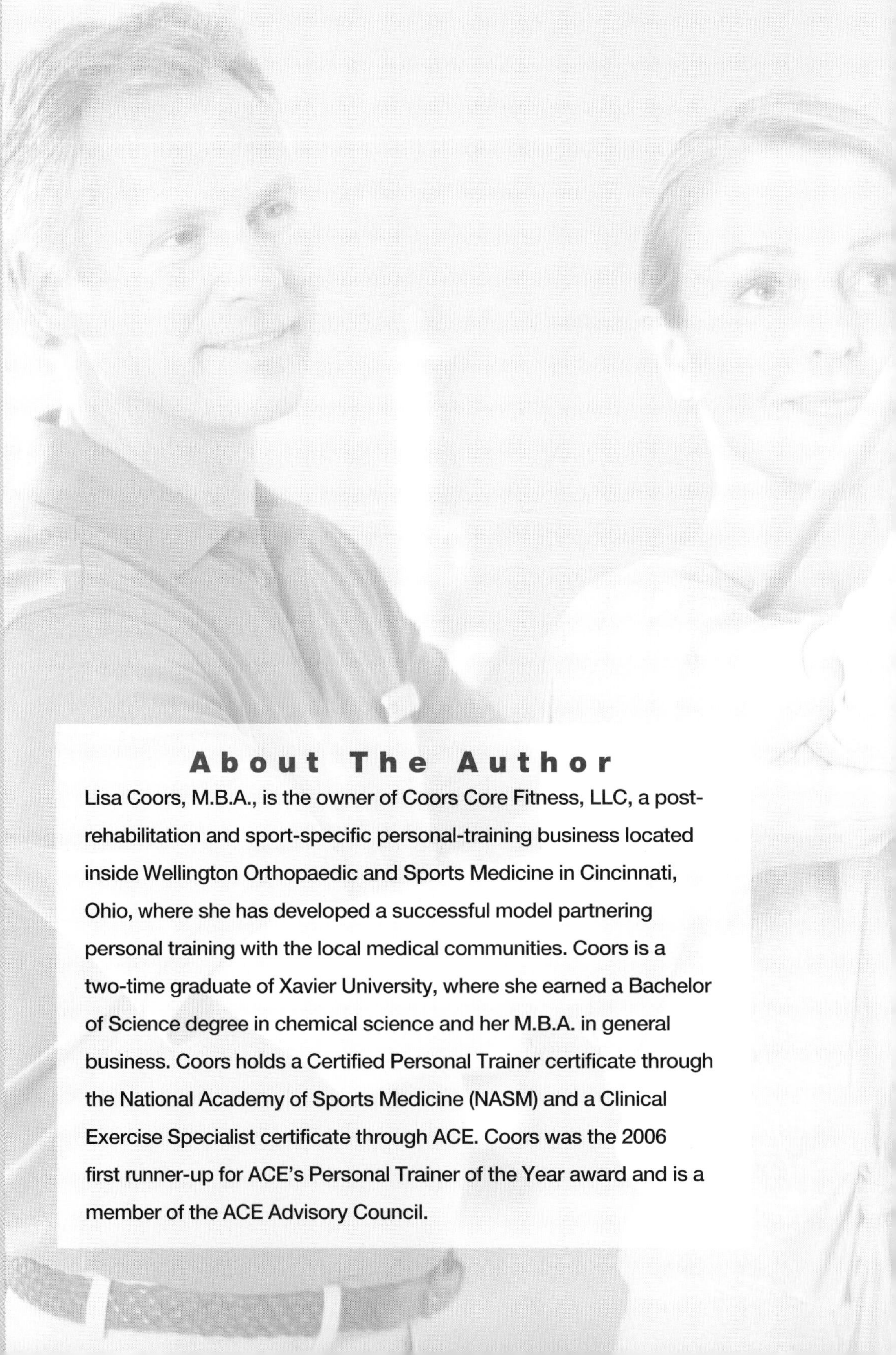

In This Chapter

About The Author

Lisa Coors, M.B.A., is the owner of Coors Core Fitness, LLC, a post-rehabilitation and sport-specific personal-training business located inside Wellington Orthopaedic and Sports Medicine in Cincinnati, Ohio, where she has developed a successful model partnering personal training with the local medical communities. Coors is a two-time graduate of Xavier University, where she earned a Bachelor of Science degree in chemical science and her M.B.A. in general business. Coors holds a Certified Personal Trainer certificate through the National Academy of Sports Medicine (NASM) and a Clinical Exercise Specialist certificate through ACE. Coors was the 2006 first runner-up for ACE's Personal Trainer of the Year award and is a member of the ACE Advisory Council.

CHAPTER 4

Professional Relationships and Business Strategies

Lisa Coors

Communication and Networking With Allied Healthcare Professionals

One of the most important roles of an ACE-certified Advanced Health & Fitness Specialist (ACE-AHFS) is bridging the gap between the fitness industry and the allied healthcare professional field (e.g., physicians, physical therapists, occupational therapists, athletic trainers). Networking is used to facilitate communication between the two parties.

The establishment of this line of communication brings a win-win situation to both parties. By communicating with the ACE-AHFS, allied healthcare professionals can get a better sense of the training progressions a trainer may use while working with one of their patients. Allied healthcare professionals also gain a sense of how an experienced and certified fitness professional can be an important next step for a patient. The ACE-AHFS, meanwhile, can gain a referral base for new clients while learning more about the condition a particular client may have. The allied healthcare professional is an excellent resource for the ACE-AHFS.

Effective communication with a client's physician should be based on the following objectives:

- Determining the physical limitations of a client
- Obtaining medical clearance for a client
- Obtaining recommendations regarding exercise program design
- Introducing the ACE-AHFS and his or her services
- Clarifying questions on the client's health/medical status
- Obtaining special considerations related to the client's health (e.g., a chronic disease such as **diabetes** or **hypertension**)
- Providing progress reports on the exercise program, or receiving health status updates
- Establishing **rapport** with a potential referral source

The best tool for building this "bridge" between the ACE-AHFS and allied healthcare professionals is the medical release. The medical release, once signed by the allied healthcare professional, client, and ACE-AHFS, allows all parties to communicate with one another. It is advised that the ACE-AHFS send a medical release to all allied healthcare professionals that a particular patient/client may be seeing. An example would be a client who has **Parkinson's disease (PD)**, had a hip replacement within the last year, and is obese. An ACE-AHFS should send a medical release to the neurologist (PD), orthopedic physician (hip replacement), physical therapist (hip replacement), and internal medicine doctor (general health and **obesity**). In this scenario, the ACE-AHFS would gain four new contacts with allied healthcare professionals. The ACE-AHFS should maintain a list of all allied healthcare professionals to whom he or she has referred clients for future reference.

There are many options for networking with allied healthcare professionals. However, an ACE-AHFS cannot communicate with any of a client's allied healthcare professionals until the client, the ACE-AHFS, and that particular allied healthcare professional sign the medical release form, which allows the ACE-AHFS to communicate with a particular allied healthcare professional. Any communication without the signing of the medical release form on the part of the client and the ACE-AHFS is a confidentiality breech, a major violation of the ACE Code of Ethics that can lead to revocation of the professional's certification and legal action (see Appendix A).

There are five main options that can be used as means of communicating with a client's allied healthcare professionals: the medical release, progress notes, general communications (e.g., fax, email, phone), visits, and promotional materials and events. The medical release is the first and most important tool in initiating allied healthcare professional communications. Once reviewed by an attorney, the medical release should abide by the Health Insurance Portability and Accountability Act (HIPAA). The medical release should include an area for the ACE-AHFS to write in the conditions that are specific to that client (Figure 4-1). Line item examples could include **osteoporosis,** obesity, and breast cancer. Next, a place is provided where the allied

Figure 4-1
Sample medical release form

Date __________________

Dear Doctor:

Your patient, ____, wishes to start a personalized exercise training program. However, your patient must first obtain a medical clearance prior to initiating exercise due to the following risk factors or conditions:

The activities will involve the following:

(type, frequency, duration, and intensity of activities)

If your patient is taking medications that will affect his or her heart-rate response to exercise, please indicate the manner of the effect (raises, lowers, or has no effect on heart-rate response):

Type of medication____

Effect ____

Please identify any recommendations or restrictions that are appropriate for your patient in this exercise program:

____

____

____

Thank you.
Sincerely,

Fred Fitness
ACE-certified Advanced Health & Fitness Specialist
Address
Phone

____ has my approval to begin an exercise program with the recommendations or restrictions stated above.

Signed____ Date______________ Phone______________ healthcare professional signs his or her name and dates the document. The most important component is the area where the allied healthcare professional is asked to write contraindications and/or restrictions to training this client/patient. Not all allied healthcare professionals will write in this area. It is up to the ACE-AHFS to call the allied healthcare professionals and ask for more clarification, if necessary. An ACE-AHFS, though trained to understand contraindications, should make no assumptions before talking to that particular allied healthcare professional.

An introductory letter or fax cover sheet should accompany the medical release and be used to introduce the ACE-AHFS, present data or **SOAP notes** on that particular client, and present a possible training progression (Figure 4-2). The ACE-AHFS may also wish to include a question regarding client contraindications or restrictions in the introductory letter to emphasize that this information is needed to appropriately train the client.

The introductory letter or fax cover sheet should also include a fax and phone number where the ACE-AHFS can be reached so that the allied healthcare professional can send the signed release back. This is an effective way for an allied healthcare professional to learn what the ACE-AHFS is doing with the patient. It is also a great networking piece for the ACE-AHFS and the fitness industry.

Figure 4-2
Sample introductory letter to a physician

Dear Dr. Cox:

Sedentary lifestyle is considered to be a major health risk factor. Despite the proven benefits of physical activity, more than 50% of U.S. adults do not get enough physical activity to provide health benefits and 25% are not active at all in their leisure time. Additionally, nearly 50% of those who begin exercising stop within the first six months. Exercise has been shown to improve medical outcomes in chronic diseases such as diabetes, hypertension, and coronary artery disease. However, few individuals know how to begin a safe, effective exercise program. I can help.

My name is John Smith and I am a certified Advanced Health & Fitness Specialist at The Health and Fitness Institute in Baltimore. My certification is from the American Council on Exercise (ACE). As an ACE-AHFS, I have a background in evaluating individuals referred to me by their physicians for design and supervision of a safe and effective exercise program. My evaluation includes:

Exercise history
Exercise likes and dislikes
Aerobic capacity (METs)
Body-composition analysis with impedance, anthropometric measurements, and BMI calculations
Muscular fitness assessment
Range-of-motion evaluation

Once I have evaluated the client, with your specific instructions, I tailor an exercise program that usually includes both aerobic and resistance training. I monitor the client's progress and frequently provide you with progress reports and follow-up information.

Our facility provides a wide range of aerobic and resistance-training equipment, a pool for water aerobics, and professionally instructed and supervised aerobic classes.

I would like to offer my services to you and your patients. Enclosed is some material explaining the role of an ACE-AHFS, as well as an article on exercise for special populations. Please feel free to use me as a resource for this type of information, as well as a referral source for your patients.

I would be happy to further discuss referrals at your convenience. My telephone number is 999-999-9999.

I look forward to working with you to help improve your patients' health.

Sincerely,

John Smith
ACE-certified Advanced Health & Fitness Specialist

The second channel in networking is the progress note, which should be typed and sent to each allied healthcare professional from whom the ACE-AHFS has a medical release for a particular client. These progress notes are sent at the discretion of the ACE-AHFS, but it is a good idea to send one every other month or right before a doctor's visit. Information presented may include details on the client's progress (e.g., weight loss, increased flexibility, decreased pain, decreased blood pressure). Information regarding a progression in exercise selection is also an effective means of showing how well a client is performing. Progress notes are essentially any written account of sessions with clients, and these notes can come in the form of SOAP notes, which are covered in subsequent sections of this chapter.

General communications like faxes, emails, and phone calls are great for fine-tuning the communication channels with allied healthcare professionals. An ACE-AHFS should have all physicians' contact information on the initial medical release and health-history forms. When working with physicians who are difficult to get in touch with, finding out who their nurses are can help. Sometimes it is much easier to speak with a physician's nurse or assistant to communicate information about a client. It is important that the ACE-AHFS is respectful and mindful of how busy most physicians are.

A surefire way to network with allied healthcare professionals is to make office visits. The easiest way to do this is to attend a visit with the client. Doing so gives the ACE-AHFS higher credibility in that it shows that he or she truly cares about the client. An ACE-AHFS should also compile a list of all allied healthcare professionals from all clients. He or she should set goals of having one-on-one meetings with each of those professionals over the course of the year. Giving an allied healthcare professional a face to go with the name is a great way for the ACE-AHFS to brand him- or herself and the business.

The last channel of networking is through promotional events. Attending or speaking at a promotional event is a great opportunity for the ACE-AHFS to meet other individuals who are also interested in health and fitness information. Furthermore, many clients with health challenges are aware of events pertaining to their particular condition, such as a "Race for the Cure" for Breast Cancer Awareness Month. Local events, including symposiums, conferences, athletic events/races, and continuing education classes, are great places to meet local allied healthcare professionals.

Promotion within a health facility setting is another great idea for networking. An ACE-AHFS and his or her fitness department can have "open houses" or "networking events" for allied healthcare professionals. This technique works well in that it brings allied healthcare professionals into the fitness facility to see first-hand where their patients will be trained. It also allows them to network with the actual trainers.

Networking with allied healthcare professionals is a great way to expand the awareness of the benefits that an ACE-AHFS can provide to clients. Until recently, allied healthcare professionals and fitness professionals were not working as a team to help patients/clients, but the walls between the two groups are breaking down and important relationships are being formed.

SOAP Notes and Other Documentation

The client folder is the most important item for the ACE-AHFS to maintain. Client folders should include the following:

- Health history
- Medical releases
- Informed consent
- Liability waiver
- Training contracts
- Correspondence sheets
- Initial assessments
- Additional assessments
- Training progressions
- SOAP notes

A good way to start a professionally maintained client folder is to begin with the original documentation, which includes a health history form (Figure 4-3). The health history form is the initial document used in each client's folder. The informed consent and training contract should be drawn up by a lawyer if the ACE-AHFS is

Name____________________ Date__________

Age____________________ Sex ☐ M ☐ F

Physician's Name____________________

Physician's Phone (______) ____________________

Person to contact in case of emergency:

Name____________________ Phone __________

Are you taking any medications or drugs? If so, please list medication, dose, and reason.

____

____

Does your physician know you are participating in this exercise program?

____

____

Describe any physical activity you do somewhat regularly.

____

____

Do you now have, or have you had in the past:	Yes	No
1. History of heart problems, chest pain, or stroke	☐	☐
2. Increased blood pressure	☐	☐
3. Any chronic illness or condition	☐	☐
4. Difficulty with physical exercise	☐	☐
5. Advice from physician not to exercise	☐	☐
6. Recent surgery (last 12 months)	☐	☐
7. Pregnancy (now or within last 3 months)	☐	☐
8. History of breathing or lung problems	☐	☐
9. Muscle, joint, or back disorder, or any previous injury still affecting you	☐	☐
10. Diabetes or thyroid condition	☐	☐
11. Cigarette smoking habit	☐	☐
12. Obesity (more than 20% over ideal body weight)	☐	☐
13. Increased blood cholesterol	☐	☐
14. History of heart problems in immediate family	☐	☐
15. Hernia, or any condition that may be aggravated by lifting weights	☐	☐

Please explain any "yes" answers on the back.

Figure 4-3
Sample health history form

self-employed, or by the fitness facility's attorney. Once an ACE-AHFS starts networking with his or her clients' allied healthcare professionals, all phone notes, emails, and faxes, as well as copies of any progress notes or other correspondence, should be included in the clients' folders.

Other elements of the client folder are the initial assessment data, additional assessments, and the training progression sheet.

SOAP Notes

SOAP is an acronym for subjective, objective, assessment, and plan. A SOAP note is intended to improve communication among all those caring for a given client, communicate pertinent characteristics, and provide the assessment, problems, and plans in an organized format to facilitate the care of the client. Depending on the facility, SOAP notes may also be used for record review and quality control. Documentation of a client's characteristics, program concerns, and related plans must be consistent, concise, and comprehensive. As such, SOAP notes are commonly written by physicians and other licensed healthcare providers, such as a physician's assistant, physical therapist, or licensed nurse practitioner. Many medical offices use the SOAP note format to standardize medical evaluation entries made in clinical records. Given this standard, SOAP notes provide an excellent method for the ACE-AHFS to gather information and communicate client status during the referral process.

The Components of a SOAP Note

Subjective: The initial portion of the SOAP note consists of subjective observations. These are symptoms verbalized by the client or by a significant other. These subjective observations include the client's descriptions of pain or discomfort, the presence of shortness of breath or dizziness on exertion, or a multitude of other descriptions of any dysfunction, discomfort, or illness.

Objective: The next part of the format is the objective observation, which includes symptoms that can actually be measured, seen, heard, touched, or felt. Objective observations include vital signs such as resting heart rate, blood pressure, body weight, percent body fat, waist circumference, and the results of any other related tests or evaluations.

Assessment: The assessment follows the objective observations and is a statement of the client's condition. In some cases, this statement may be clear, such as "moderately obese." In other instances, an assessment may not be as clear and can include several possibilities. *Note:* The word "statement" is used quite intentionally in this description. In the medical field, the assessment is usually a "diagnosis," but the **scope of practice** of an ACE-AHFS does not include making medical diagnoses. Therefore, any reference to a diagnosis should be avoided.

Plan: The last part of the SOAP note is the plan. The plan may include further fitness testing or other diagnostic testing (e.g., **DEXA scan**). This is where a referral to another healthcare professional would be noted. This is also the section where an ACE-AHFS would record his or her appropriate plan in terms of exercise, nutrition, and adherence strategies.

Remember, the SOAP note is not supposed to be as detailed as a progress report. Complete sentences are not necessary and abbreviations are appropriate. However, the ACE-AHFS should avoid using abbreviations until he or she has a thorough knowledge of how they are used. Abbreviations differ for each specialty and should be consistent within the facility in which the ACE-AHFS works. The length of the note will differ depending on the use. SOAP notes that follow each client session will likely be shorter than ones that accompany a referral letter. SOAP notes can be flexible. Many fitness professionals often develop their own styles as they accommodate varied preferences.

SOAP Note Case Example

Peggy is a 55-year-old accountant who just completed her first month of exercise with a trainer. She sits at her desk all day and had not worked out for more than 10 years until one month ago. She was diagnosed with hypertension and is obese. After initial assessment, it is noted that her height is 5'6" (1.7 m), her weight is 180 pounds (81 kg), and her body fat percentage is 40%. Her fitness goals are to lose weight while increasing flexibility and endurance. She was extremely intimidated to start a fitness program because of a fear of overexertion and having a heart attack. After the first month of training, she is experiencing sharp pain in her left hip that she feels while sitting or sleeping at night. She does not feel the pain during exercise.

Associated SOAP Note

Patient Name: Peggy Jones
DOB: 09/17/ 53
Date: 04/27/08

S: Obese accountant with hypertension. Needs to lose significant weight, both lbs and body fat, while increasing flexibility and endurance. Was very intimidated to start exercising. Currently experiencing left hip pain while at rest.

O: 55 years old, height 5'6", weight 180 lb, and body fat 40%.

A: 55-year-old sedentary woman needs a weight-loss program that will also help her manage her hypertension. She complains of left hip pain when she sits in a chair or while sleeping. She needs to see her physician prior to coming back for training.

P: Trainer suggests that the client seek medical attention for left hip. Trainer will not train client until she receives medical clearance.

Approach to Referring Peggy

The ACE-AHFS explains to Peggy that she needs to contact her physician to investigate her left hip pain. The ACE-AHFS should also contact the physician with details on Peggy's training sessions to allow the physician to have additional information for diagnosis.

The ACE-AHFS may also want to ask Peggy for permission to contact her primary care provider before proceeding any further. Permission must be in writing and kept in the client's file. When speaking with or writing to Peggy's physician, the ACE-AHFS must outline his or her concerns, including the intensity of Peggy's program, her current response to exercise, and her stated goals. The ACE-AHFS must ask Peggy's physician to send a letter providing medical clearance to continue exercise, along with any modifications related to the exercise program.

Barriers to Effective Communication

Awareness of communication barriers can greatly facilitate the working relationship with healthcare providers and can lead to better coordinated client care. The ACE-AHFS should use common courtesy, clarify expectations, and communicate clearly to avoid the following barriers to effective communication:

Timeliness of the communication: Does the physician receive the referral letter within days, or within six weeks, of the initial session? Was the ACE-AHFS able to call or send a letter before the physician had a follow-up visit with the client? Does the physician prefer calls or letters? Tardy communication places the physician in a position in which he or she is uninformed of what other team members are doing. This decreases the chance that the physician will send the ACE-AHFS another referral. If the ACE-AHFS knows the client has scheduled an appointment with the physician that will take place before he or she can send a letter, the ACE-AHFS should consider calling the physician's office to give a brief report on any findings and recommendations. It is important to keep written notes in the client's file that detail any phone conversations with the client or physician. The ACE-AHFS should always be prompt with all replies and type them in a professional manner.

Lack of understanding of team member roles: Physicians generally are unfamiliar with the role that the ACE-AHFS can play in the healthcare team. Therefore, the ACE-AHFS is in a position to educate physicians on what he or she has to offer. The method of doing so may include a phone call to let the physician know that he or she can use the ACE-AHFS as a resource for any fitness-related questions. Other means that the ACE-AHFS can use to introduce him- or herself to the physician include explaining his or her areas of expertise in all referral letters, personally visiting the physician's office, and sending pertinent articles on different aspects of personal training and exercise. As the ACE-AHFS develops rapport with physicians, he or she will better understand their information needs.

Unclear expectations: The root problem in many interpersonal and professional relationships is ambiguous or conflicting expectations (Covey, 2004). The ACE-AHFS must be sure to understand what a physician expects, and then strive to deliver it. The ACE-AHFS must be clear about what he or she has to offer the healthcare team and how to apply that expertise. It is important to let the physician know what kind of results clients can expect so that they may provide reinforcement when they see the client.

Reaching beyond the scope of practice: If the ACE-AHFS does not know an answer or cannot help an individual, he or she must be willing to admit it and refer the client to the appropriate member of the healthcare team. See the "Scope of Practice" section later in this chapter for more information.

Confidentiality Issues

Because the ACE-AHFS will keep track of confidential information on each client, it is absolutely essential that this information is kept in a locked file cabinet or be under password protection on a computer. The ACE-AHFS should be the only one able to access these files. Clients expect that their trainers, once they sign a medical release form, keep all information private, which includes abstaining from sharing information with anyone but the client or any medical professionals from whom a medical release has been obtained (see Appendix A for the ACE Code of Ethics). Adherence to confidentiality policies is not only an ethical issue, but may also be a legal issue in some states or municipalities.

If any private information is communicated to someone other than the client or appropriate allied healthcare professional, the ACE-AHFS and/or the facility can face legal action. To prevent a confidentiality breech, the ACE-AHFS should adhere to the following guidelines:

- Client files should be stamped with "confidential" or "private."
- Client files should be kept in a locked file cabinet not accessible to the general public or other facility **employees.**
- Clients' folders should have all documentation papers clipped or stapled in so that papers are not lost.
- Fax machines should be in private areas not accessible to the general public. The ACE-AHFS should be aware of when confidential fax transmittals are arriving so that the information stays private.
- All computer-based client information should be password protected. Firewalls should be used to ensure that no one steals client information.
- All employees working where confidential information is discussed with either another allied healthcare professional or the client should be made to sign a confidentiality policy developed by the company attorney. The policy should specify what legal consequences will occur if the policy is broken.
- All verbal discussion of client information should be done in private. This includes all phone calls and one-on-one client discussions.
- All transmittals such as faxes, email printouts, and written documentation should be put in client files. All other information should be shredded.

The ACE-AHFS must obtain a medical release for each allied healthcare professional he or she wishes to communicate with regarding a client. The client, physician, and ACE-AHFS must sign these documents. This release gives the ACE-AHFS permission to talk to the client's allied healthcare professionals.

Trainers should not talk to their friends, family, employees, or coworkers about client information.

Marketing the Business for Medical Referrals

Marketing is one of the most important business skills for the ACE-AHFS. Marketing is defined as a group of activities designed to expedite transactions by creating, distributing, pricing, and promoting goods, services, and ideas (Ferrell, 2003).

Marketing fitness training services to the medical community does not have to be an expensive endeavor for the ACE-AHFS. Marketing will allow the ACE-AHFS to better bridge exercise for special populations with the allied healthcare field. There are many different marketing channels that are effective means of educating allied healthcare professionals regarding the benefits of using the services of an ACE-AHFS. Before marketing tactics can be discussed, the ACE-AHFS needs to understand what it is that he or she is marketing. What is the competitive advantage? Competitive advantage refers to the way a business and/or individual tries to get consumers to purchase products and services over those offered by the competition (Bearden, Ingram, & LaForge, 2005). In other words, competitive advantage is what a business and/or individual does better than the competitors. Determining the competitive advantage allows the ACE-AHFS to have selling points when communicating with the medical community. An example of a good selling point includes an ACE-AHFS with a specialty in low-back post-rehabilitation.

Once a competitive advantage is determined, the ACE-AHFS can start researching the numerous marketing channels that provide links to the medical community. Some of the most popular channels include:

- Word of mouth from clients, employees, and physician offices
- Local schools and universities
- Orthopedic centers that employ physical therapists, athletic trainers, and occupational therapists
- Local businesses

Word of mouth is the most inexpensive, and often the most beneficial, form of marketing. The easiest place for an ACE-AHFS to start is with current clients. Providing clients with the highest quality and most professional experience can go a long way when it comes to marketing. Continuous quality checks in the form of verbal or written evaluations can also help an ACE-AHFS to improve his or her service. Because every client is different, a trainer has to be able to adapt to all personalities and all medical conditions. This is truly an art, and for most fitness professionals, feedback and evaluations from clients can allow them to make changes that benefit their clients. Satisfied clients will make referrals to friends and family. Of course, word of mouth can be negative as well. If an ACE-AHFS performs poorly, clients will quit and communicate their dissatisfaction to their friends, family, and coworkers. LeBoeuf (1987) noted that "a typical dissatisfied customer will tell eight to 10 people about his problem. One in five will tell 20. It takes 12 positive service incidents to make up for one negative incident."

Word of mouth can also come from non-clients. Employees that work at a fitness center can make referrals, as can a client's allied healthcare professional. An ACE-AHFS can begin networking with fitness center employees by offering a free session to anyone interested. From the person working the front desk to the facility director, it is important to demonstrate the service provided. A client's allied healthcare professionals may become impressed with the communication skills and professionalism of a particular ACE-AHFS. If the allied healthcare professional has good rapport with an ACE-AHFS and/or sees results, he or she will want to promote that ACE-AHFS. It is absolutely essential for an ACE-AHFS to constantly work on cultivating these relationships. Of course, word-of-mouth marketing is not limited to these options.

It may also be productive for an ACE-AHFS to network with local schools and universities. An example of a simple way to network would be to offer a free fitness class or workout session to a local preschool or grade school. To do this, an ACE-AHFS can call schools in his or her area and offer a simple one-time session or a series of programs. One benefit of working with young children is that the ACE-AHFS can give them brochures to take home to their parents, who may then become clients. High schools and universities are great places to find post-rehabilitation athletes. Athletes coming out of physical therapy and transitioning back to their sports may need to learn skills like proper stretching, core training, balance training, and strength training to decrease the chance of re-injury. The options for marketing to local schools are limitless and can allow the ACE-AHFS to build his or her clientele while educating students on the importance of fitness.

Orthopedic centers are in a category of their own due to the high potential for clientele for an

ACE-AHFS. Physical therapists, athletic trainers, and occupational therapists rehabilitate patients after surgery or as a treatment for a particular condition. Once patients have completed their prescribed treatments, they are asked to continue exercising on their own. However, some patients are not educated on what to do aside from the exercises they performed in therapy. They may have a set of exercises that they performed with their therapist, but do not have any progressions for when they work out on their own. Post-rehabilitation personal training is the logical next step for these patients. By building rapport with therapists, an ACE-AHFS may become a referral source. The best way to market the services of an ACE-AHFS is to start with the orthopedic centers used by existing clients. Remember, the ACE-AHFS must have a medical release from a client's physical therapist, occupational therapist, or athletic trainer before initiating a training program. The ACE-AHFS can use these individuals as contacts. Doing a small presentation or meeting with a group of therapists can be extremely beneficial to an ACE-AHFS. Not only can the ACE-AHFS help to decrease the chance of re-injury for a client, but he or she can also increase a client's quality of life, while simultaneously gaining new clientele.

An ACE-AHFS can also market his or her services to local businesses. Athletic shoe stores, athletic apparel shops, and nutrition stores are just some of the places for an ACE-AHFS to promote his or her services. Talking with the owner and/or manager about becoming a referral source is a good start. Offering employees a free session or doing a demonstration of a training session is a great way for an ACE-AHFS to promote his or her services. An ACE-AHFS must be professional in his or her approach and only leave brochures and business cards if permission is granted.

Another way to market to local businesses is for a fitness department or studio to offer an open house event for these vendors. At the open house, an ACE-AHFS can network and demonstrate his or her training services.

Marketing is a critical business skill for any ACE-AHFS. Countless marketing channels can be used to gain new clients. An ACE-AHFS should always have marketing materials prepared, including business cards, portfolios, and/or personal brochures so that all networking opportunities can be maximized.

Billing and Payment Policies

The following factors should be considered when determining the billing and payment procedures:

Pricing: Pricing can be a little more challenging for an ACE-AHFS who is self-employed or an **independent contractor** than for someone is as an employee for a facility. Facilities usually set a particular price per session for the ACE-AHFS. Some facilities offer tiered systems that allow the ACE-AHFS to increase prices and payouts as he or she graduates through the system. Self-employed individuals and independent contractors need to coordinate several factors in their pricing, including insurance, travel, certifications, experience, local market comparisons, and taxes.

Cash, check, or credit card: For an employee, this issue is simple in that the facility takes care of this process. Independent contractors and self-employed individuals who collect their own payments need to be able to track payments for tax purposes. Credit card machines include a charge that needs to be agreed on by the ACE-AHFS and the credit card machine company. An ACE-AHFS who takes credit card payments provides convenience for clients, but has to weigh the costs of the processing fees. An ACE-AHFS who takes cash for payment needs to record this income for tax purposes. Fitness professionals who do not claim cash payments place themselves at risk for tax-related legal issues should they be audited by the Internal Revenue Service (IRS).

Personal-training contract: Employees of fitness facilities normally have a personal-training contract that is designed by the company's attorneys. These forms are handed to each client to sign and cover the following: liability, payment procedures, cancellation procedures, penalties, and late fees. Independent contractors and self-employed individuals need to get their own personal-training contracts designed by an attorney. These signed contracts legally bind clients to the ACE-AHFS in case of missed payments, cancellations, and bounced checks.

Discounts and package plans: Package plans are common incentives to get clients to sign up for training. A discount is often given per session in a package plan. Some facilities offer package plans that include five, 10, or even 20 or more sessions. For independent contractors and self-employed individuals, package plans offer the benefit of up-front payments. Most employees who sell packages get paid only when a session is actually used, whether or not it was part of a package. Sessions used from a package can be tracked using electronic or manual techniques.

In summary, the billing and payment procedures may be already set for the ACE-AHFS if he or she is an employee of a fitness facility. Independent contractors and self-employed individuals have to design a system that is agreeable to their clients. Cancellation policies and late fees are critical factors in receiving on-time payment for services. As noted earlier, an ACE-AHFS should always get legal assistance when drafting his or her billing and payment policies. Having legally reviewed documentation can give clients incentive to make timely payments and adhere to all billing policies.

Legal Issues, Liabilities, and Professional Responsibilities

Ethics Policy

The ethics policy is the umbrella that encompasses legal issues, liability, and professional responsibilities. Adhering to the ACE Code of Ethics will decrease the incidence of these types of issues (see Appendix A). Every business, from a small studio to a large fitness facility, needs to incorporate some type of ethics policy. In facilities where employees are hired, there needs to be a disciplinary policy for individuals that do not abide by the policy. All employees need to sign a contract agreeing that they will follow the ethics policy and that they understand the disciplinary policy for those that breech the contract. Breaking or disregarding these ethics policies can lead to anything from a loss of clients to career-destroying legal allegations.

Legal Issues and Liabilities

There are several legal issues and liabilities that can be avoided if fitness professionals understand the appropriate standard of care. Training high-risk clients can bring about other issues not necessarily considered by trainers who ordinarily work with the "apparently-healthy" population. The three primary areas of concern are scope of practice, qualifications, and appropriate exercise selection.

Scope of Practice

In conjunction with other healthcare professionals, an ACE-AHFS will design, implement, and manage exercise, physical activity, and lifestyle programs for individuals following treatment or rehabilitation for clinically documented chronic disease, musculoskeletal injury, and/or disability. The ACE-AHFS is *not* in the practice of providing the services of his or her profession to the immediate, primary, post-surgical, or post-trauma rehabilitation patient. Rather, the ACE-AHFS provides a safe and effective bridge for the patient to cross from the structured clinical treatment and/or rehabilitation environment to mainstream community or home-based exercise.

Qualifications

Because the ACE-AHFS will be receiving referrals from physicians, it is important for him or her to stay abreast of advancements in the health and fitness industry and complete all continuing education requirements. Times will arise when a client's needs will fall outside an ACE-AHFS's scope of practice and area of expertise, in which case he or she should not hesitate to refer the client back to the allied healthcare professional. For example, just because an ACE-AHFS knows about a particular topic (e.g., post-rehabilitation after a knee injury), this does not mean that he or she is qualified to fill the role of a physical therapist.

Appropriate Exercise Selection

It is recommended that an ACE-AHFS training high-risk clients base exercise selection on the client's health-history data and the healthcare provider's recommendations, when available.

The ACE-AHFS should obtain a medical release from each of the physicians that a particular client is seeing. For example, a client who just finished chemotherapy from breast cancer should have two medical releases, one from the oncologist and one from the internal medicine physician. Along with these releases, an ACE-AHFS can inform the physicians of the exercise progressions that will be used. Having those physicians sign the release allows for suitable exercises to be performed and creates a lower injury risk for the client.

Avoiding Legal Risks

The following are ways that trainers can protect themselves from legal disaster (Riley, 2006):

- Have legal professionals review all documentation used with clients.
- Allow clients to have appropriate time to read and sign all training documentation. Verbally answer questions when necessary.
- Store all documents securely for as long as is required by the state's statute of limitations.
- Be sure to carry sufficient liability insurance for ultimate protection against liability.
- Use a legally reviewed, standardized waiver form with all clients.

Employment Options

Employees

A fitness facility that hires an ACE-AHFS as an employee can control when and how he or she trains clients. Employees are required to sign an employment contract prior to working for the facility. They also receive a salary. Deductions such as withholding tax, social security, and payroll taxes are taken out for the employee by the company. Employees are also protected from discrimination and unfair hiring practices. Some employees are even offered benefits (medical, dental, vision), 401K plans, paid vacation, and paid holidays. In the majority of facilities, the ACE-AHFS would be covered under that facility's **liability insurance.** The ACE-AHFS should ask at the time of employment if additional coverage is required, as determined by the scope of the facility's insurance.

If an ACE-AHFS works for a facility as an employee, in most cases the client will pay the facility, and the ACE-AHFS will receive a paycheck based on how many sessions were produced during a particular pay period. Usually, an ACE-AHFS will take a previously determined percentage of each session's revenue. Keep in mind that an ACE-AHFS may be salaried and make the same amount of money no matter how many clients are seen in a particular pay period.

Independent Contractors

Many fitness facilities hire independent contractors, non-employees who pay their own taxes and insurance. The fitness facility sends a federal 1099 form for tax purposes if an ACE-AHFS has earned $600 or more in a year. Fitness facilities do not have to pay benefits or taxes for the independent contractor, which saves the company money.

In many cases, independent contractors receive direct payment from their clients and then pay the facility certain set fees to rent the use of the facility. Some facilities require clients of independent contractors to pay the facility. In turn, the facility pays the independent contractor a fee that was previously agreed on by both parties.

Self-employed

An ACE-AHFS may also choose to be self-employed by owning a facility, performing in-home training, or training in a facility. When choosing this option, an ACE-AHFS must choose a business entity to file. An ACE-AHFS should get legal advice before forming any business entity. There are three major options to choose from: **sole proprietorship, partnership,** and **corporation,** each of which has several subsets. No matter the business entity, clients will pay either the ACE-AHFS or the business entity. In turn, the ACE-AHFS pays taxes based on the type of business entity chosen. It is essential that the ACE-AHFS consults with his or her tax professional for guidance in determining the best option.

- *Sole proprietorship:* This type of business is owned and operated by one individual. Such owners have total control over business activities, and forming a sole proprietorship is easy and inexpensive. Profits are considered personal income, which makes tax preparation simple. The disadvantage of a sole proprietorship is that the personal liability of the proprietor is not protected. If the business cannot pay its creditors, the ACE-AHFS may be forced to use his or her own money to cover the debts. Personal and business funds are one account, not two different accounts. There is also a limited source of funds and individuals pay a higher marginal tax rate.

- *Partnership:* In a partnership, two or more people agree to operate a business and share profits and losses. A partnership is taxed like a sole proprietorship. There are two main types of partnerships: **general partnerships** and **limited partnerships.**
  - ✔ *General partnership:* Each partner assumes management responsibility and unlimited liability and must have at least a 1% interest in profit and loss.
  - ✔ *Limited partnership:* This is a hybrid organizational form, with both limited and general partners. A limited partner has no voice in management and is legally liable only for the amount of his or her capital contributions, plus any other debt obligations specifically accepted (Harvard Business Essentials, 2001).
- *Corporation:* A corporation is a legal entity recognized by the state, the assets and liabilities of which are separate from its owners. The advantages of a corporation are the limited liability, the ease of transfer of ownership, and the external sources of funds. Disadvantages of a corporation include double taxation, which means that both income and dividends are taxed. Other disadvantages are the costliness of formation and the disclosure of information. There are two subgroups of the corporation: the **S-Corp** and the **limited liability corporation (LLC).**
  - ✔ *S-Corp:* An S-Corp is a form of business ownership taxed as though it were a partnership. It provides limited liability and is restricted to 75 shareholders and one class of stock. All shareholders must be U.S. citizens and cannot be corporations or partnerships.
  - ✔ *LLC:* An LLC is a form of business ownership that provides limited liability but is taxed liked a partnership. It is not limited to a certain number of shareholders and owners do not have to be U.S. citizens.

The Business Plan

A successful ACE-AHFS will not only implement safe and effective programs and services, but will also generate income. Starting a business requires research, advanced preparation, and a sound business strategy. Minimally, it is recommended that the ACE-AHFS consult a lawyer, accountant, and insurance agent. There may also be a small-business development council in the area to assist with the many facets of starting and running a small business. Another excellent resource is the Small Business Administration's website (www.sba.gov).

Before developing a business plan, the ACE-AHFS must determine the purpose of the plan. Possible purposes for the business plan include the following:

- Application for financial assistance (loans, grants, etc.)
- Investor acquisitions
- Overall strategic planning tool

A successful business plan includes, but is not limited to, the following items:

- Mission and vision statements
- Listing of company objectives (how the ACE-AHFS plans to reach the vision)
- Short- and long-term financial and strategic plans
- Detailed budget
- Listing of owners and/or officers of the business and their credentials/bios
- Marketing and public relations plan
- Billing and accounting practices
- Facility safety and security standards
- Equipment maintenance checklists
- Detailed policies and procedures

Another important step is the development of a procedural manual. The procedural manual should be so detailed that another staff person could make important decisions in the absence of the owner or manager by using it as a resource. If the business plan calls for bringing on support staff, it is important to understand the difference between hiring an employee versus hiring an independent contractor. Information can be obtained from the IRS website (www.irs.gov) or by consulting with an accountant or lawyer. For employees or independent contractors, the following items will also be needed:

- Employee forms (i.e., W-4, I-9, and other governmental reporting documents that are in accordance with state and federal requirements)
- Independent contractor agreement and 1099 form
- Employee handbook and personnel manual

Summary

The role of the ACE-AHFS is not only to train clients, but also to exemplify professional business skills in his or her everyday business practices. By working together with allied healthcare professionals, the ACE-AHFS allows the client to receive the safest and most effective training programs. In terms of business development, networking provides a channel for the ACE-AHFS to broaden his or her clientele and areas of expertise.

References

Bearden, W.O., Ingram, T.N., & LaForge, R.W. (2005). *Marketing Principles and Perspectives* (5th ed.). New York: McGraw Hill/Irwin.

Covey, S.R. (2004). *The 7 Habits of Highly Effective People.* New York: Free Press.

Ferrell, O.C. (2003). *Business in a Changing World.* New York: McGraw Hill/Irwin.

Harvard Business Essentials (2001). *Finance for Managers.* Boston: Harvard Business School Publishing.

LeBoeuf, M. (1987). *How To Win Customers & Keep Them For Life.* New York: Berkley Publishing Group.

Riley, S. (2006). The Importance of Protective Legal Documentation. *IDEA Trainer Success,* 3, 1, 10–12.

Suggested Reading

American Council on Exercise (2007). *ACE Clinical Exercise Specialist Manual*. San Diego, Calif.: American Council on Exercise.

American Council on Exercise (2003). *ACE Personal Training Manual* (3rd ed.). San Diego, Calif.: American Council on Exercise.

Ferrell, O.C., Hirt, G., & Ferrell, L. (2007). *Business: A Changing World* (6th ed.). New York: McGraw-Hill.

Harvard Business Essentials (2002). *Finance for Managers.* Boston: Harvard Business School Publishing.

Koeberle, B.E. (1994) *Legal Aspects of Personal Training* (2nd ed.). Canton, Ohio: PRC Publishing.

LeBoeuf, M. (2000). *How To Win Customers & Keep Them For Life*. New York: Berkley Publishing Group.

Longenecker, J. P. et al. (2006). *Small Business Management* (13th ed.). Florence, Ky.: South-Western College Publishing.

Price, R. (2005). *Entrepreneurship* (5th ed.). New York: McGraw-Hill.

Tharrett, S. & Peterson, J.A. (2008). *Fitness Management* (2nd ed.). Monterey, Calif.: Healthy Learning.

In This Chapter

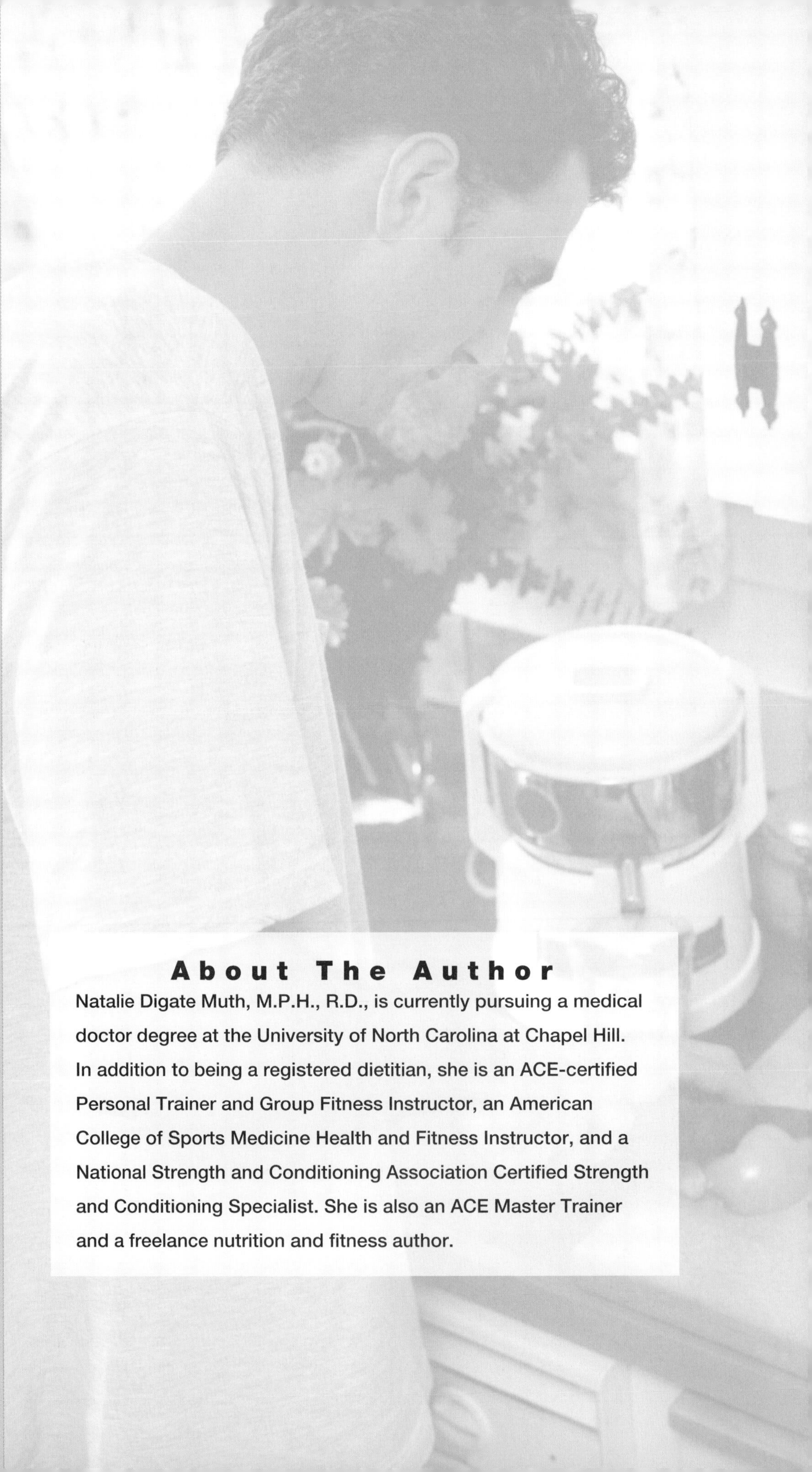

About The Author

Natalie Digate Muth, M.P.H., R.D., is currently pursuing a medical doctor degree at the University of North Carolina at Chapel Hill. In addition to being a registered dietitian, she is an ACE-certified Personal Trainer and Group Fitness Instructor, an American College of Sports Medicine Health and Fitness Instructor, and a National Strength and Conditioning Association Certified Strength and Conditioning Specialist. She is also an ACE Master Trainer and a freelance nutrition and fitness author.

CHAPTER 5

Nutritional Considerations for an Active Lifestyle

Natalie Digate Muth

Personal trainers often seek to broaden their expertise beyond working with "apparently healthy" clientele to a more complex group of individuals who face cardiovascular, pulmonary, metabolic, and musculoskeletal challenges such as heart disease, **asthma, diabetes,** and **arthritis.** Depending on a client's individual goals and challenges, his or her nutritional needs may vary considerably. While a registered dietitian (R.D.) may be best equipped to offer clients a specific and individualized nutrition plan, an ACE-certified Advanced Health & Fitness Specialist (ACE-AHFS) can be a ready source of general nutrition information and education. Furthermore, a grasp of basic nutrition principles will help the ACE-AHFS to better understand the interplay between diet and exercise so that he or she can design the most effective exercise programs for clients. From basic science to applications in sports nutrition, this chapter provides a foundation of knowledge in nutritional sciences, an exciting scientific field that encompasses biology, chemistry, biochemistry, physiology, and psychology. This chapter will help prepare an ACE-AHFS to offer scientifically sound, practical nutrition recommendations for clients, while working within the appropriate **scope of practice.**

Scope of Practice

While only an R.D. is adequately trained to provide specific and individualized nutrition eating plans, an ACE-AHFS can use well-established guidelines to help clients adopt healthful and appropriate nutrition habits. Many clients may have medical diagnoses that require special nutrition recommendations beyond those discussed in the government guidelines. In these cases, it is advisable that the client work closely with his or her physician and a registered dietitian to develop an individualized eating plan. The role of the ACE-AHFS will often be to provide support and encouragement for the client in his or her attempts to follow the recommended plan. This is especially important when working with individuals with complex medical histories and special nutritional requirements.

The role of fitness professional versus registered dietitian has been further delineated in the exercise science and fitness literature (Sass et al., 2007). The authors note that while the certified fitness professional's competencies include *knowledge of* basic nutrition and weight-management information, fitness professionals are not expected to—and should not—*calculate, outline, counsel,* or *prescribe* individual nutrition or weight-management plans. As several lawsuits have demonstrated, fitness professionals tread especially treacherous waters if they recommend supplements or other risky substances (Sass et al., 2007).

Ohio legislators passed a statute in 2006 titled the "Unauthorized Practice of Dietetics" that may serve as a useful example to help clarify scope of practice for "non-licensed individuals"—that is, individuals with occasion to discuss nutrition but without the registered dietitian credential and state license, where necessary (31 states require licensing). Non-licensed individuals can only provide "general nonmedical nutrition information" such as a cooking demonstration; endorsement of government recommendations such as the Dietary Guidelines and **MyPyramid Food Guidance System;** discussion of **macronutrients** and **micronutrients** and how requirements vary by life stage; information about statistics relating to nutrition and **chronic disease;** and education about nutrients contained in particular foods or substances (Sass et al., 2007). This chapter helps equip the ACE-AHFS to provide up-to-date and scientifically sound general nonmedical nutrition information to clients.

Federal Dietary Recommendations

Dietary Guidelines

This chapter explains the role of various nutrients that are essential for optimal functioning. While everyone needs these nutrients, people require varying amounts depending on gender, age, activity level, health status, and other factors. The federal government has taken these differences into consideration when developing recommended intakes. The 2005 Dietary Guidelines [United States Department of Agriculture (USDA), 2005] and MyPyramid Food Guidance System provide individualized nutrition recommendations for a healthy diet.

Published every five years, the Dietary Guidelines are the government's best advice to Americans on how to eat to promote health and prevent chronic diseases such as **cardiovascular disease, stroke, hypertension,** diabetes, **osteoporosis** and some cancers. The 2005 guidelines also emphasize engaging in regular physical activity and decreasing caloric consumption for weight control. The following are the major points in each of the key focus areas:

- *Adequate nutrients within calorie needs:* The Guidelines encourage Americans to choose a variety of nutrient-dense foods such as fruits, vegetables, and whole grains and limit foods high in **saturated** and **trans fats, cholesterol,** added sugars, salt, and alcohol. The food choices should be distributed within a balanced eating plan such as MyPyramid. This strategy allows Americans to get all of the nutrients the body needs without exceeding caloric requirements.
- *Weight management:* The key to weight control is to balance caloric intake from food and beverages with caloric expenditure. Most adults tend to gradually gain weight with age. For adults to prevent weight gain, the guidelines suggest a 50- to 100-calorie decrease in intake each day, combined with 60 minutes of accumulated physical activity per day. Those individuals who are trying to lose weight should aim for a 500-calorie deficit per day achieved through decreased caloric intake and/or increased physical activity. For optimal long-term success and overall health, gradual weight loss is best. And to keep the weight off, clients may need to engage in physical activity for 60 to 90 minutes per day. (Refer to "Nutrition, Exercise, and Weight Control" later in this chapter for more information on weight management.)
- *Physical activity:* All Americans are encouraged to be active and reduce **sedentary** behaviors. To prevent disease, clients should engage in at least 30 minutes of moderate-intensity physical activity most days of the week. More or higher-intensity activity will lead to even greater health benefits and help to prevent weight gain. A balanced physical-activity program includes cardiovascular, resistance, and **flexibility** training.
- *Food groups to encourage*: Fiber-dense fruits, vegetables, and whole grains are the staples of a healthy diet. Americans should aim to consume nine total servings of fruits (2 cups, or four servings) and vegetables (2.5 cups, or five servings) each day for a standard 2000-calorie diet. A colorful variety of fruits and vegetables will optimize **vitamin, mineral,** and **phytochemical** intake. Also, the guidelines encourage Americans to consume three or more servings of whole grains daily to meet **fiber** requirements and three or more cups per day of low-fat milk (or equivalent) products to assure adequate calcium intake.
- *Fats:* The Guidelines advise Americans to eat less than 10% of calories from artery-clogging saturated fat and less than 300 mg per day

of cholesterol. Trans fat, now included on the nutrition label, should be avoided since, like saturated fat, it causes **atherosclerosis.** Ideally, fat intake should contribute 20 to 35% of daily caloric intake, with the majority of fat from **polyunsaturated** or **monounsaturated fat** (fish, nuts, vegetable oils). To minimize unhealthy fat intake, an ACE-AHFS should encourage clients to choose lean, low-fat, or fat-free meat, poultry, dry beans, and milk products.

- *Carbohydrates:* Fiber-rich fruits, vegetables, and whole grains are optimal sources of **carbohydrate.** The Guidelines encourage all Americans to limit added sugars and caloric sweeteners, which contain little nutritional value; practice good oral hygiene; and eat sugar-laden foods less often to prevent dental caries.
- *Sodium and potassium:* To prevent hypertension, people should consume less than 2300 mg of sodium per day (1 tsp salt). In general, fast food, canned food, and frozen dinners contain an abundance of salt and should be avoided in favor of foods with little salt.
- *Alcoholic beverages:* Drink in moderation (one drink per day for women; two drinks per day for men). While a moderate intake of alcohol helps prevent cardiovascular disease, people who do not drink are not encouraged to begin in an effort to realize these benefits. The Guidelines emphasize that people who cannot control intake, pregnant women, children, and those on medications that interact with alcohol should avoid alcoholic beverages.
- *Food safety:* Nearly 76 million people in the United States become ill each year from foodborne illnesses (USDA, 2005). Special populations most at risk include pregnant women, infants and young children, older adults, and people who are **immunocompromised.** The majority of foodborne illnesses are preventable with a few simple precautions, such as washing hands frequently; maintaining clean kitchen counters; separating raw, cooked, and ready-to-eat foods while shopping; cooking foods to a safe temperature to kill microorganisms; refrigerating leftovers within two hours and defrosting foods properly; and avoiding unpasteurized milk products, raw eggs, and raw or undercooked meat. Refer to www.fightbac.org or www.foodsafety.gov for more information.

MyPyramid

MyPyramid is an interactive online tool (www.MyPyramid.gov) designed to replace the well-known but poorly adopted 1992 Food Guide Pyramid. The significance of each component of the MyPyramid symbol is described in Figure 5-1. The goal of MyPyramid is to provide updated guidelines based on the latest scientific research and to offer consumers an online feature to personalize dietary guidelines in accordance with their individual needs and lifestyle.

MyPyramid tailors nutrition advice to individual caloric needs. For example, consumers can go to www.MyPyramid.gov to calculate their estimated energy expenditure based on their age, gender, and their typical amount of physical activity. Within seconds, users will be categorized into one of 12 different energy levels (anywhere from 1000 to 3200 calories) and will be given the recommended number of servings—measured in cups and ounces—to eat from each of the seven food groups. A set number of discretionary calories (i.e., the leftover calories available for sugar or additional fats or an extra serving from any of the food groups) will also be allocated for that individual. By following these recommendations, users will have the optimal diet for disease prevention and weight maintenance based on their personalized needs.

In general, MyPyramid encourages people to consume:

- Mostly whole grains, as opposed to refined sugars
- Ample nutrient-dense dark green and orange vegetables such as broccoli and carrots, rather than disproportionate amounts of starchy vegetables like white potatoes and corn, which contain fewer vitamins and minerals
- A variety of fruits, preferably from whole-food sources, as opposed to fruit juices

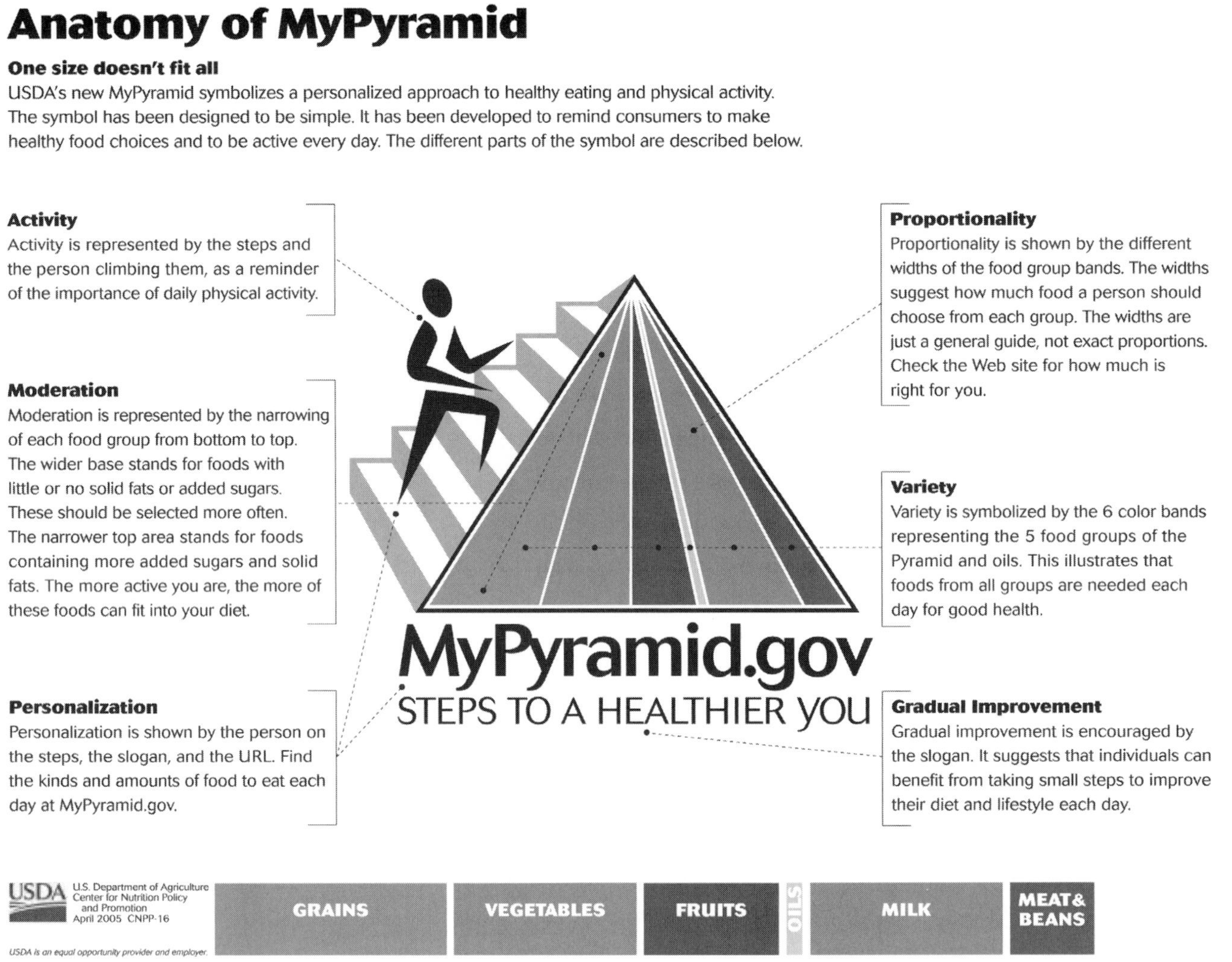
Anatomy of MyPyramid
One size doesn't fit all
USDA's new MyPyramid symbolizes a personalized approach to healthy eating and physical activity. The symbol has been designed to be simple. It has been developed to remind consumers to make healthy food choices and to be active every day. The different parts of the symbol are described below.
Activity
Activity is represented by the steps and the person climbing them, as a reminder of the importance of daily physical activity.
Moderation
Moderation is represented by the narrowing of each food group from bottom to top. The wider base stands for foods with little or no solid fats or added sugars. These should be selected more often. The narrower top area stands for foods containing more added sugars and solid fats. The more active you are, the more of these foods can fit into your diet.
Personalization
Personalization is shown by the person on the steps, the slogan, and the URL. Find the kinds and amounts of food to eat each day at MyPyramid.gov.
Proportionality
Proportionality is shown by the different widths of the food group bands. The widths suggest how much food a person should choose from each group. The widths are just a general guide, not exact proportions. Check the Web site for how much is right for you.
Variety
Variety is symbolized by the 6 color bands representing the 5 food groups of the Pyramid and oils. This illustrates that foods from all groups are needed each day for good health.
Gradual Improvement
Gradual improvement is encouraged by the slogan. It suggests that individuals can benefit from taking small steps to improve their diet and lifestyle each day.
MyPyramid.gov
STEPS TO A HEALTHIER YOU
USDA U.S. Department of Agriculture Center for Nutrition Policy and Promotion April 2005 CNPP-16
USDA is an equal opportunity provider and employer.
GRAINS
VEGETABLES
FRUITS
OILS
MILK
MEAT & BEANS

Figure 5-1
Anatomy of MyPyramid

- Oils in moderation, with an emphasis on mono- or polyunsaturated fats instead of trans or saturated fats
- Low- or nonfat milk products, as opposed to regular whole-milk products
- Lean meat and bean products, instead of higher fat meats such as regular (75 to 80% lean) ground beef or chicken with the skin

The website also has a variety of online tools, including the following:

- *MyPyramid Plan:* Provides an estimate of what and how much food to eat, based on the user's age, gender, and activity level
- *MyPyramid Tracker:* Cites detailed information on the quality of an individual's diet and his or her physical-activity status
- *Inside MyPyramid:* Provides in-depth data for every food group, including recommended daily amounts
- *Tips and Resources:* Offers a variety of suggestions to eat healthier and be more active

MyPyramid also emphasizes the importance of staying active and provides a resource page filled with tips to on how to incorporate more physical activity into a health-conscious lifestyle.

Despite its improvements from the 1992 Food Guide Pyramid, MyPyramid is not perfect. Transferring 85 pages of nutrition information contained in the 2005 Dietary Guidelines Executive Summary into a simple symbol is no easy task. Add the lobbying pressures from the food industry and the relative inaccessibility to seniors and low-income individuals who often do not have access to a computer, and it becomes easy to understand why MyPyramid contains some biases and flaws. Nonetheless, MyPyramid is a valuable tool that the ACE-AHFS can use to help clients improve their nutrition and activity habits.

Dietary Reference Intakes

The description of reference values for optimal intake of various nutrients also has been revamped. In the past, **Recommended Dietary Allowances (RDAs)** were published for the different nutrients based on age and gender. The RDA was defined as "the levels of intake of essential nutrients that, on the basis of scientific knowledge, are judged by the Food and Nutrition Board to be adequate to meet the known needs of practically all healthy persons." Newer reference values, known as **Dietary Reference Intakes (DRIs)** are more descriptive. DRI is a generic term used to refer to three types of reference values: Recommended Dietary Allowance (RDA); **Estimated Average Requirement (EAR),** an adequate intake in 50% of an age- and gender-specific group; and **Tolerable Upper Intake Level (UL),** the maximum intake that is unlikely to pose risk of adverse health effects to almost all individuals in an age- and gender-specific group. **Adequate Intake (AI)**—which is used when a RDA cannot be based on an EAR—is a recommended nutrient intake level that, based on research, appears to be sufficient for good health.

DRIs have been established for calcium, vitamin D, phosphorus, magnesium, and fluoride; **folate** and other B vitamins; **antioxidants** (vitamins C and E, selenium); macronutrients (protein, carbohydrate, and fat); **trace elements** (vitamin A and K, iron, zinc); **electrolytes;** and water. The complete set of DRIs is available at www.iom.edu.

Micronutrient Requirements and Recommendations

Called micronutrients because they are only needed in small amounts, certain nutrients have been identified by the World Health Organization (WHO) as the "'magic wands' that enable the body to produce enzymes, hormones, and other substances essential for proper growth and development" (WHO, 2007). When the body is deprived of micronutrients, the consequences are severe. But when consumed in just the right amounts, they contribute to optimal health and function.

Vitamins

Vitamins are **organic,** non-caloric micronutrients that are essential for normal physiologic function. Vitamins must be consumed through food with only three exceptions: vitamin K and biotin can also be produced by normal intestinal flora (bacteria that live in the intestines and are critical for normal gastrointestinal function) and vitamin D can be self-produced with sun exposure. No "perfect" food contains all the vitamins in just the right amount; rather, a variety of nutrient-dense foods must be consumed to ensure adequate vitamin intakes. Many foods (such as breads and cereals) have been fortified with some nutrients to decrease the risk of vitamin deficiency. Some foods also contain inactive vitamins—called **provitamins.** Fortunately, the human body contains enzymes to convert these inactive vitamins into active vitamins.

Humans need 13 different vitamins, which are divided into two categories: **water-soluble vitamins** and **fat-soluble vitamins.** Thiamin, riboflavin, niacin, pantothenic acid, folate, vitamin B6, vitamin B12, biotin, and vitamin C are the water-soluble vitamins. Their solubility in water (which gives them similar **absorption** and distribution in the body) and their role as **cofactors** of enzymes involved in metabolism (i.e., without them the enzyme will not work) are common traits. With the exception of vitamins B6 and B12, water-soluble vitamins cannot be stored in the body and are readily excreted in urine. This decreases the risk of toxicity from overconsumption, but also makes their regular intake a necessity.

Folate (also known as "folic acid" in its supplement form)—named for its abundance in plant foliage (like green leafy vegetables)—deserves special mention due to its crucial role during pregnancy. Folate is essential for DNA production, red and white blood cell formation, **neurotransmitter** formation, and **amino acid** metabolism. Deficiency is relatively common, as folate is easily lost during food preparation and cooking and because most people do not eat enough green leafy vegetables. Folate deficiency preconception and early in pregnancy can be devastating for a developing fetus, leading to neural tube defects such as spina bifida. Women can be sure to meet their daily folate requirements by taking a vitamin with folic acid every day or by consuming enough folate-rich foods, such as fortified cereal, which provides 100% of the daily value in a single serving. Deficiency also causes a megaloblastic anemia, skins lesions, and poor growth. Notably, excessive consumption of folate can mask a vitamin B12 deficiency.

Vitamins A, D, E, and K are the fat-soluble vitamins. Often found in fat-containing foods and stored in the liver or adipose tissue until needed, fat-soluble vitamins closely associate with fat. If fat absorption is impaired, so is fat-soluble vitamin absorption. Unlike water-soluble vitamins, fat-soluble vitamins can be stored in the body for extended periods of time. This storage capacity increases risk of toxicity from overconsumption, but also decreases risk of deficiency.

Choline, called a "quasi-vitamin" because it can be produced in the body but also provides additional benefits through consumption from food, is also important because it plays a crucial role in neurotransmitter and **platelet** function and may help to prevent **Alzheimer's disease** (McDaniel, Maier, & Einstein, 2003). Table 5-1 lists the vitamin DRIs, common food sources, and functions in the human body.

Minerals

Serving roles that range from regulating enzyme activity and maintaining acid–base balance to assisting with strength and growth, minerals are critical for human life. Unlike vitamins, many minerals are found in the body as well as in food. The body's ability to use the minerals is dependent upon their **bioavailability.** Nearly all minerals, with the exception of iron, are absorbed in their free form—that is, in their ionic state unbound to organic molecules and complexes. When bound to a complex, the mineral is said to not be bioavailable and will be excreted in feces. Typically, minerals with high bioavailability include sodium, potassium, chloride, iodide, and fluoride. Minerals with low bioavailability include iron, chromium, and manganese. All other minerals, including calcium and magnesium, are of medium bioavailability.

An important consideration when consuming minerals, and particularly when taking mineral supplements, is the possibility of mineral-to-mineral interactions. Minerals can interfere with the absorption of other minerals. For example, zinc absorption may be decreased through iron supplementation. Zinc excesses can decrease copper absorption. Too much calcium limits the absorption of manganese, zinc, and iron. When a mineral is not absorbed properly, a deficiency may develop.

Serving a variety of functions in the body, minerals are typically categorized as macrominerals (bulk elements) and microminerals (trace elements). Macrominerals include calcium, phosphorus, magnesium, sulfur, sodium, chloride, and potassium. Microminerals include iron, iodine, selenium, zinc, and various other minerals that do not have an established DRI and will not be discussed here. Table 5-2 presents mineral DRIs, common food sources, and function in the human body.

Macronutrient Requirements and Recommendations

Food is composed of some combination of three macronutrients: carbohydrate, protein, and fat. The term macronutrient simply means that the nutrient is needed in large quantities for normal growth and development. Macronutrients are the body's source of **calories,** or energy to fuel life processes.

Carbohydrates

Carbohydrates contain about four calories per gram and are the body's preferred energy source. The EAR for carbohydrates is 100 grams (about seven servings) for non-pregnant, non-lactating adults and children; 135 grams (about nine servings) for pregnant women; and 160 grams

Table 5-1
Vitamin Facts

Vitamin	RDA/AI* Men†	RDA/AI* Women†	Best Sources	Functions
A (carotene)	**900 µg**	**700 µg**	Yellow or orange fruits and vegetables, green leafy vegetables, fortified oatmeal, liver, dairy products	Formation and maintenance of skin, hair, and mucous membranes; helps people see in dim light; bone and tooth growth
B1 (thiamine)	**1.2 mg**	**1.1 mg**	Fortified cereals and oatmeals, meats, rice and pasta, whole grains, liver	Helps the body release energy from carbohydrates during metabolism; growth and muscle tone
B2 (riboflavin)	**1.3 mg**	**1.1 mg**	Whole grains, green leafy vegetables, organ meats, milk, eggs	Helps the body release energy from protein, fat, and carbohydrates during metabolism
B6 (pyridoxine)	**1.3 mg**	**1.3 mg**	Fish, poultry, lean meats, bananas, prunes, dried beans, whole grains, avocados	Helps build body tissue and aids in metabolism of protein
B12 (cobalamin)	**2.4 µg**	**2.4 µg**	Meats, milk products, seafood	Aids cell development, functioning of the nervous system, and the metabolism of protein and fat
Biotin	30 µg	30 µg	Cereal/grain products, yeast, legumes, liver	Involved in metabolism of protein, fats, and carbohydrates
Choline	550 mg	425 mg	Milk, liver, eggs, peanuts	A precursor of acetylcholine; essential for liver function
Folate (folacin, folic acid)	**400 µg**	**400 µg**‡	Green leafy vegetables, organ meats, dried peas, beans, lentils	Aids in genetic material development; involved in red blood cell production
Niacin	**16 mg**	**14 mg**	Meat, poultry, fish, enriched cereals, peanuts, potatoes, dairy products, eggs	Involved in carbohydrate, protein, and fat metabolism
Pantothenic acid	5 mg	5 mg	Lean meats, whole grains, legumes	Helps release energy from fats and vegetables
C (ascorbic acid)	**90 mg**	**75 mg**	Citrus fruits, berries, and vegetables—especially peppers	Essential for structure of bones, cartilage, muscle, and blood vessels; helps maintain capillaries and gums and aids in absorption of iron
D	5 µg	5 µg	Fortified milk, sunlight, fish, eggs, butter, fortified margarine	Aids in bone and tooth formation; helps maintain heart action and nervous system function
E	**15 mg**	**15 mg**	Fortified and multigrain cereals, nuts, wheat germ, vegetable oils, green leafy vegetables	Protects blood cells, body tissue, and essential fatty acids from harmful destruction in the body
K	120 µg	90 µg	Green leafy vegetables, fruit, dairy, grain products	Essential for blood-clotting functions

* Recommended Dietary Allowances are presented in bold type; Adequate Intakes are presented in non-bolded type.

† RDAs and AIs given are for men aged 31–50 and nonpregnant, nonbreastfeeding women aged 31–50; mg = milligrams; µg = micrograms

‡ This is the amount women of childbearing age should obtain from supplements or fortified foods.

Table 5-2
Mineral Facts

Mineral	RDA/AI* Men[†]	RDA/AI* Women[†]	Best Sources	Functions
Calcium	1,000 mg	1,000 mg	Milk and milk products	Strong bones, teeth, muscle tissue; regulates heart beat, muscle action, and nerve function; blood clotting
Chromium	35 µg	25 µg	Corn oil, clams, whole-grain cereals, brewer's yeast	Glucose metabolism (energy); increases effectiveness of insulin
Copper	900 µg	900 µg	Oysters, nuts, organ meats, legumes	Formation of red blood cells; bone growth and health; works with vitamin C to form elastin
Fluoride	4 mg	3 mg	Fluorinated water, teas, marine fish	Stimulates bone formation; inhibits or even reverses dental caries
Iodine	150 µg	150 µg	Seafood, iodized salt	Component of hormone thyroxine, which controls metabolism
Iron	8 mg	18 mg	Meats, especially organ meats, legumes	Hemoglobin formation; improves blood quality; increases resistance to stress and disease
Magnesium	420 mg	320 mg	Nuts, green vegetables, whole grains	Acid/alkaline balance; important in metabolism of carbohydrates, minerals, and sugar (glucose)
Manganese	2.3 mg	1.8 mg	Nuts, whole grains, vegetables, fruits	Enzyme activation; carbohydrate and fat production; sex hormone production; skeletal development
Molybdenum	45 µg	45 µg	Legumes, grain products, nuts	Functions as a cofactor for a limited number of enzymes in humans
Phosphorus	700 mg	700 mg	Fish, meat, poultry, eggs, grains	Bone development; important in protein, fat, and carbohydrate utilization
Potassium	4700 mg	4700 mg	Lean meat, vegetables, fruits	Fluid balance; controls activity of heart muscle, nervous system, and kidneys
Selenium	55 µg	55 µg	Seafood, organ meats, lean meats, grains	Protects body tissues against oxidative damage from radiation, pollution, and normal metabolic processing
Zinc	11 mg	8 mg	Lean meats, liver, eggs, seafood, whole grains	Involved in digestion and metabolism; important in development of reproductive system; aids in healing

* Recommended Dietary Allowances are presented in bold type; Adequate Intakes are presented in non-bolded type.

† RDAs and AIs given are for men aged 31–50 and nonpregnant, nonbreastfeeding women aged 31–50; mg = milligrams; µg = micrograms

Reprinted with permission from *Dietary Reference Intakes* (various volumes). Copyright 1997, 1998, 2000, 2001 by the National Academy of Sciences. Courtesy of the National Academies Press, Washington, D.C.

(about 11 servings) for lactating women. The American Dietetic Association (ADA) recommends that athletes consume between 6 and10 grams of carbohydrates per kilogram of body weight (3 to 5 g/lb) per day to maintain blood **glucose** levels during exercise and to replace muscle **glycogen** (ADA, 2000).

Carbohydrates are made of sugar chains. A **monosaccharide** is the simplest form of sugar. Monosaccharides are usually found joined together as di-, oligo-, or **polysaccharides.** Three monosaccharides found in nature can be absorbed and utilized by humans—glucose, **galactose,** and **fructose.** Glucose is the predominant sugar in nature and the basic building block of most other carbohydrates. Fructose, or fruit sugar, is the sweetest of the monosaccharides and is found in varying levels in different types of fruits. Galactose joins with glucose to form the disaccharide **lactose,** the principal sugar found in milk. (**Lactose intolerance** results from a deficiency in the enzyme **lactase,** which is necessary to break the bond between the glucose and galactose molecules so that they can be absorbed.) Other disaccharides include **maltose,** which is two glucose molecules bound together, and **sucrose** (table sugar), which is formed by glucose and fructose linked together. Most caloric sweeteners, including raw sugar, granulated sugar, powdered sugar, and honey, are disaccharides. Noncaloric sweeteners—calorie-free because the body cannot metabolize them—also are processed compounds used to add sweet taste to foods and beverages. Aspartame, also known as Equal® in packaged sweetener and NutraSweet® in foods and beverages, acesulfame K (called Sunett® in cooking products and SweetOne® as tabletop sweetener), saccharin, sucralose (Splenda®), and neotame all are approved for use in the United States. While early studies in laboratory rats found that certain sweeteners may cause bladder cancer, subsequent studies of humans have not found an association.

An **oligosaccharide** is a chain of about three to 10 or fewer simple sugars. **Fructooligosaccharides,** a category of oligosaccharides that are mostly indigestible, may help to relieve constipation, improve **triglyceride** levels, and decrease the production of foul-smelling digestive by-products. A long chain of sugar molecules is referred to as a polysaccharide. Glycogen and **starch** are the only polysaccharides that humans can fully digest. Both are long chains of glucose and are referred to as **complex carbohydrates** (versus **simple carbohydrates,** which are short chains of sugar).

Animals store excess carbohydrates as glycogen. Although glycogen can be found in animal products, most glycogen stores are depleted before the meat enters the food supply. Excess carbohydrates from starch or other sugars are stored in the human liver and muscle as glycogen. Because glycogen contains many water molecules, it is large and bulky and therefore unsuitable for long-term energy storage. About 90 grams of glycogen is stored in the liver. At least 150 grams of glycogen is stored in muscle at baseline; this amount can be more than tripled with physical training so that most people have about 200 to 500 grams of glycogen stored in muscle (Mahan & Escott-Stump, 2000). Similar to exercise, carbohydrate loading increases glycogen stores.

Plants store carbohydrates as starch granules. Edible plants make two types of starch: amylase—a small, linear molecule—and the more prevalent amylopectin—a larger, highly branched molecule. Because starches are longer than disaccharides and oligosaccharides, they take longer to digest. Still, humans are able to easily break down and digest starches with specific self-produced **enzymes.** However, the rest of the plant, which is formed largely of the carbohydrate **cellulose** and other fibers such as **hemicellulose, lignin,** gums, and **pectin,** is indigestible because humans do not produce the enzymes necessary to break the sugar bonds. Because no chemical bonds are broken, no energy is released, and therefore fiber does not contain calories.

Fiber is classified as either soluble or insoluble. **Soluble fiber** forms a gel in water. It helps prevent heart disease and stroke by binding bile and cholesterol; diabetes by slowing glucose absorption; and constipation by holding moisture in stools and softening them. Gums found in foods such as oats, legumes, guar, and barley, and pectin found in foods like apples, citrus fruits, strawberries, and carrots are soluble fibers. **Insoluble fiber** comprises the structural part of the plant. It reduces constipation and lowers the risk of hemorrhoids and **diverticulosis** by adding bulk to the feces and reducing transit time in the colon. Insoluble fibers include the cellulose found in whole-wheat flour, bran, and vegetables; hemicellulose found in whole grains and bran; and lignin found in mature vegetables, wheat, and fruits with edible seeds (like strawberries). Increased consumption of soluble and insoluble fiber helps to increase **satiety,** the feeling of fullness, and may lead to decreased caloric intake. As a result, a diet high in fiber may help promote weight loss (ADA, 2002).

Glycemic Index

Historically, much debate has centered on whether the consumption of simple or complex carbohydrates is better for athletic performance. The role of a particular carbohydrate in athletic performance may be better determined by its **glycemic index (GI)** than its structure. GI ranks carbohydrates based on their blood glucose response: high-GI foods break down rapidly, causing a large glucose spike, while low-GI foods are digested more slowly and cause a smaller glucose increase (Table 5-3). **Glycemic load (GL)** accounts for GI as well as portion size:

$$GL = GI \times \text{grams of carbohydrate}$$

Research suggests that a diet based on the consumption of high-GI carbohydrates promotes greater glycogen storage following strenuous exercise (Jentjens & Jeukendrup, 2003). On the other hand, a low-GI eating plan may be better for weight loss (Thomas, Elliott, & Baur, 2007) and for people with diabetes (Brand-Miller et al., 2003). A low-GL diet creates a more favorable glucose and **insulin** response than a high-GL diet, and also leads to a decrease in total cholesterol and the unhealthy **low-density lipoprotein (LDL)** cholesterol (Thomas, Elliott, & Baur, 2007). In general, foods high in soluble fiber, such as whole-grain barley, rye, oats, pasta, and less starchy vegetables, have a low GI. Thus, without having to make drastic dietary changes, individuals may benefit from replacing high-GI grains with low-GI grains and starchy vegetables with less starchy ones, and by cutting down on soft drinks (Liu, 2006).

Table 5-3
Glycemic Index (GI) of Various Foods

High GI ≥70	**Medium GI** 56–69	**Low GI** ≤55
White bread	Rye bread	Pumpernickel bread
Corn Flakes®	Shredded Wheat®	All Bran®
Graham crackers	Ice cream	Plain yogurt
Dried fruit	Blueberries	Strawberries
Instant white rice	Refined pasta	Oatmeal

Fats and Lipids

The most energy-dense of the macronutrients, fat provides nine calories per gram. Ounce for ounce, this is 2.25 times more calories than both carbohydrate and protein. Because of this high caloric value, foods that are high in fat should be consumed in moderation for weight control. The ADA recommends that fats be limited to 20 to 35% of total caloric intake (ADA, 2007). Research suggests that certain types of fat, namely mono- and polyunsaturated fats, are heart-healthy (though still calorie-dense) (Hu & Willett, 2002; Zarraga & Schwarz, 2006). In addition, fats serve many critical functions in the human body, including insulation, support of the cell structure, nerve transmission, vitamin absorption, and hormone production. The compound triglyceride is the principal storage form of fat in the body.

The ADA recommends that fat intake be mostly unsaturated with an emphasis on increasing omega-3 polyunsaturated fat. **Unsaturated fatty acids** contain one or more double bonds between carbon atoms, are typically liquid at room temperature, and are fairly unstable, making them susceptible to oxidative damage and a shortened shelf life. Monounsaturated fat contains one double bond between two carbons. Common sources include olive, canola, and peanut oils. Polyunsaturated fat contains a double bond between two or more sets of carbons. Sources include corn, safflower, and soybean oils and cold-water fish.

Essential fatty acids are a type of polyunsaturated fat that must be obtained from the diet. Unlike other fats, the body cannot produce

omega-3 or **omega-6 fatty acids,** also called **linolenic** and **linoleic acid,** respectively. Omega-3 is an essential fatty acid found in egg yolk, crab, shrimp, oyster, and cold-water fish, such as tuna, salmon, mackerel, and cod. These fatty acids promote a healthy immune system and help protect against heart disease and other diseases. Americans tend not to get enough omega-3 fatty acids. Omega-6, generally consumed in abundance, is an essential fatty acid found in sunflower, safflower, soybean, and corn oils. Polyunsaturated fats decrease total cholesterol, LDL cholesterol, and HDL cholesterol. The ACE-AHFS can help clients consume the appropriate amounts of omega-3 and omega-6 fatty acids by encouraging a dietary pattern containing fruits and vegetables, whole grains, legumes, nuts and seeds, lean protein, fish, and non-hydrogenated margarines and oils (ADA, 2007). Both types of essential fatty acids are used to make **eicosanoids,** which are oxygenated fatty acids that the body uses to signal cellular responses. Those eicosanoids made from omega-6 tend to cause inflammation and increase blood pressure and blood clotting. Eicosanoids made from omega-3 have the opposite effects, as they reduce blood clotting, dilate blood vessels, and reduce inflammation. This balancing act between omega-6 and omega-3 is essential for maintaining normal circulation and other essential processes. Reducing consumption of omega-6 fatty acids and increasing consumption of omega-3 fatty acids may lower chronic disease risk (Simopoulos, 1999), though the research is inconclusive.

Some fats—notably saturated fats and trans fats—lead to a clogging of the arteries, an increased risk for heart disease, and myriad other problems. **Saturated fatty acids** contain no double bonds between carbon atoms, are typically solid at room temperature, and are very stable. Foods high in saturated fat include red meat, full-fat dairy products, and tropical oils like coconut and palm. Saturated fat increases levels of LDL cholesterol. Trans fat, listed as "partially-hydrogenated" oil on a food ingredient list, results from a man-made process used to make unsaturated fat solid at room temperature in an effort to prolong its shelf life. The process involves breaking the double bond of the unsaturated fat. The product is a heart-damaging fat that increases LDL cholesterol even more than saturated fat. Due to legislation requiring food manufacturers to include the amount of trans fat on the nutrition label if it is more than 0.5 grams per serving, many processed foods that used to be high in trans fat, such as chips, crackers, cakes, peanut butter, and margarine, are now "trans-fat free." The ACE-AHFS should encourage clients to check the label and look on the ingredients list for "partially hydrogenated" oil to determine if a food still contains small amounts of trans fat. If so, they should avoid that food.

Cholesterol, a fat-like, waxy, rigid four-ring steroid structure, plays an important role in cell-membrane function. It also helps to make bile acids (which are important for fat absorption), metabolize fat-soluble vitamins (A, D, E, and K), and make vitamin D and some steroid hormones such as estrogen and testosterone. Saturated fat, converted to cholesterol in the liver, is the main dietary cause of **hypercholesterolemia** (high blood levels of cholesterol), though high levels of cholesterol itself are also found in animal products such as egg yolks, meat, poultry, fish, and dairy products. Cholesterol causes problems when there is too much of it in the bloodstream. For cholesterol to get from the liver to the body's cells (in the case of endogenously produced cholesterol), or from the small intestine to the liver and adipose tissue (in the case of exogenously consumed cholesterol), it must be transported through the bloodstream. Because it is fat-soluble, it needs a water-soluble carrier protein to transport it. When the cholesterol combines with this protein en route to the body's cells, it is a low-density lipoprotein, which means that it is susceptible to getting stuck in the bloodstream and clogging the arteries, thus forming a plaque and ultimately causing atherosclerosis. **High-density lipoprotein (HDL)** removes excess cholesterol from the arteries and carries it back to the liver, where it is excreted.

Proteins

Proteins contain four calories per gram and are the building blocks of human and animal structure. The average person requires 0.8 to 1.0 g/kg of body weight per day (0.4 to 0.5 g/lb). Whether active adults have increased protein needs compared to their sedentary counterparts is a source of controversy. Because resistance training and cardiovascular exercise induce beneficial muscular and structural damage and protein helps the muscles and tissues to repair and rebuild themselves, the American Dietetic Association, Dietitians of Canada, and the American College of Sports Medicine recommend that endurance athletes consume about 1.2 to 1.4 g/kg of bodyweight (0.5 to 0.6 g/lb), whereas strength-trained athletes consume up to 1.6 to 1.7 g/kg (0.7 to 0.8 g/lb) (ADA, 2000). However, in a 2002 report, the Institute of Medicine (IOM) concluded that the evidence for increased requirements for active individuals was not compelling, and suggested that 0.8 g/kg of bodyweight (0.3 g/lb) per day was appropriate for athletes (IOM, 2002). Regardless of the amount consumed, the ADA suggests that protein intakes are best met through diet alone without the use of protein or amino-acid supplements (ADA, 2000).

Proteins serve innumerable functions in the human body, including the formation of the brain, nervous system, blood, muscle, skin, and hair, as well as the transport of iron, vitamins, minerals, fats, and oxygen. Proteins are also the key to acid–base and fluid balance. Proteins form enzymes, which speed up chemical reactions to milliseconds that might otherwise take years. Antibodies that the body makes to fight infection are made from proteins. In situations of energy deprivation, the body can break down proteins for energy.

Proteins are built from amino acids, which are nitrogen-containing compounds. Proteins form when amino acids are joined together through **peptide bonds.** The completed protein is a linear chain of amino acids. Attractions between different amino acids then create what are known as helices and pleated structures. These structures fold, creating a unique three-dimensional **polypeptide.** Individual polypeptides may remain free-standing or may bind together to form a larger complex.

Many of the 20 amino acids that bind together to form proteins can be made in the body. These are termed **nonessential amino acids.** Eight to 10 **essential amino acids** have carbon skeletons that humans cannot make and so must be consumed in the diet. Generally, animal products contain all of the essential amino acids in amounts proportional to need and are called **complete proteins.** Usually, proteins in plant foods do not contain all of the essential amino acids in amounts proportional to need and are called **incomplete proteins.** One notable exception is soy, which is a plant-based complete protein. When combined, incomplete plant proteins (such as rice and beans) can together provide all of the essential amino acids; this is called **protein complementarity** (Figure 5-2).

Figure 5-2
Protein complementarity chart

Source: Adapted with permission from Lappé, F.M. (1992). *Diet for a Small Planet.* New York: Ballantine Books.

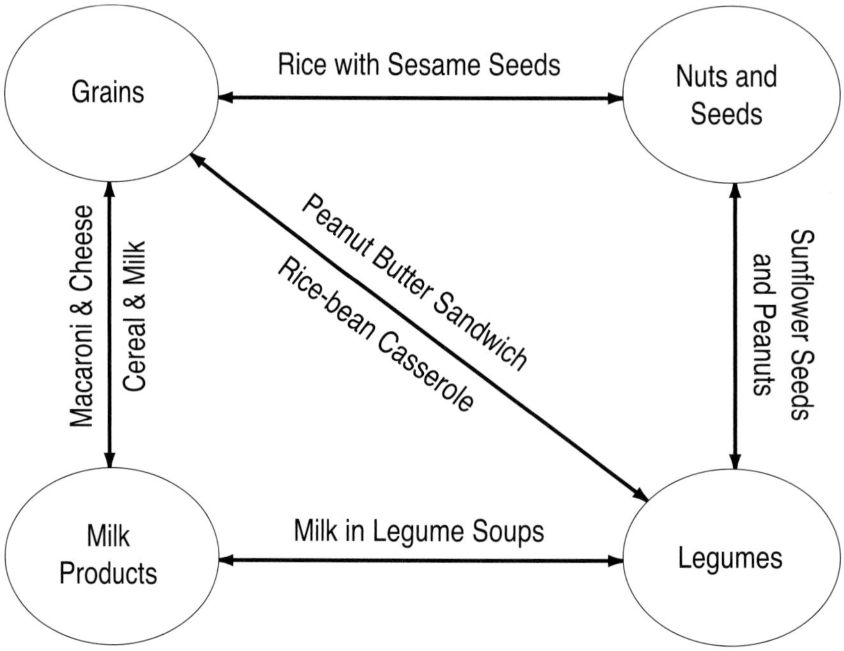

Protein Quality

Adequate protein intake clearly is critical for active individuals to optimize athletic performance and increase muscle mass. Beyond the amount of protein consumed, protein quality is equally important. A specific food's protein quality is determined by assessing its essential amino-acid composition, digestibility, and bioavailability, or the degree to which the amino acids can be absorbed by the body (Food and Agriculture Organization/World Health Organization, 1990). Several scales are used to evaluate protein quality, including the following:

- **Protein efficiency ratio (PER),** a measure based on experiments with lab animals and not discussed in detail here
- **Biological value (BV)**
- **Protein digestibility corrected amino acid score (PDCAAS)**

BV is determined as follows:

BV = Nitrogen used for tissue formation/ Nitrogen absorbed from food x 100

The result of this equation is the percentage of consumed nitrogen utilized by the body, though it is often reported relative to the BV of egg, which is equal to 100. A protein with a high BV is optimal to build tissue and muscle. Whey (104), egg (100), and milk (91) proteins have the highest BV, whereas beef (80), casein (77), soy (74), and wheat gluten (64) proteins have lower BV. Three factors affect a specific protein source's biological value: amino-acid composition (proteins containing all essential amino acids in amounts proportional to need have a higher BV), cooking and preparation (cooking methods that destroy essential amino acids decrease BV), and vitamin and mineral content (foods missing certain critical nutrients have drastically decreased BV). Because the scale does not take these factors into consideration, BV is difficult to apply in practice (Hoffman & Falvo, 2004).

PDCAAS, the preferred method for measuring protein quality, is a somewhat complex mathematical formulation that gives each protein food a score as determined by its chemical score (i.e., essential-amino-acid content in a protein food divided by the amino-acid content in a reference protein food and then multiplied by its digestibility). While an ACE-AHFS will not be calculating PDCAAS scores, he or she can use the published scores to help determine the highest quality proteins. The proteins with highest PDCAAS score—and thus, those considered to be the highest quality—are casein, egg, milk, soy, and whey proteins (all 1.0). Beef comes in next (0.92), followed by black beans (0.75), peanuts (0.52) and wheat gluten (0.25) (Hoffman & Falvo, 2004).

Macronutrient Digestion and Absorption

To fully understand the basics of nutrition, an ACE-AHFS not only needs to know what the macronutrients do in the body, but also how they are converted from a molecule contained within a piece of food or pill into a usable form. These are the processes of **digestion** and absorption.

Digestion

The **gastrointestinal tract** forms a long hollow tube from mouth to anus where digestion and absorption occur (Figure 5-3). Digestion takes two forms: **mechanical digestion**—the process of chewing, swallowing, and propelling food through the gastrointestinal tract—and **chemical digestion**—the addition of enzymes that break down nutrients. At the mere sight or smell of a potential meal, the digestive system prepares to break down the food into nutrients and usable energy by forming enzyme-rich **saliva.** With the first bite, the saliva begins to digest and moisten the food, forming a **bolus.** As a person swallows, the food passes through the pharynx to enter the esophagus (the **epiglottis** prevents food from entering the trachea). Muscles in the esophagus push food to the stomach through a wave-like motion called **peristalsis.** The stomach mixes the food and liquids with its own digestive juices to break down food into absorbable nutrients and energy. Finally, the stomach empties its contents into the small intestine. (The **esophageal sphincter,** also known as the **cardiac sphincter,** prevents food and stomach acid from splashing back into the esophagus from the stomach, while the **pyloric sphincter** separates the stomach from the small intestine). The amount of time it takes for the **gastric emptying** depends on the type of food (carbohydrates are emptied the fastest, followed by protein and then fat), the amount of muscle action of the stomach and small intestine, and several other factors. See "Hydration, Water Balance, and Gastric Emptying" later in this chapter for additional information on gastric emptying.

The gallbladder and pancreas play key roles in digestion, but are not part of the long gastrointestinal tube. With some help from pancreatic digestive juices and bile produced in the liver and stored in the gallbladder, the 22-foot long (6.7 m) small intestine spends about one to four hours further digesting the food, now called **chyme,** and finally absorbing the nutrients and energy into the blood. This blood gets fast-tracked directly to the liver for the processing and distribution of nutrients to the rest of the body. All of the waste and indigestible items left over in the small intestine

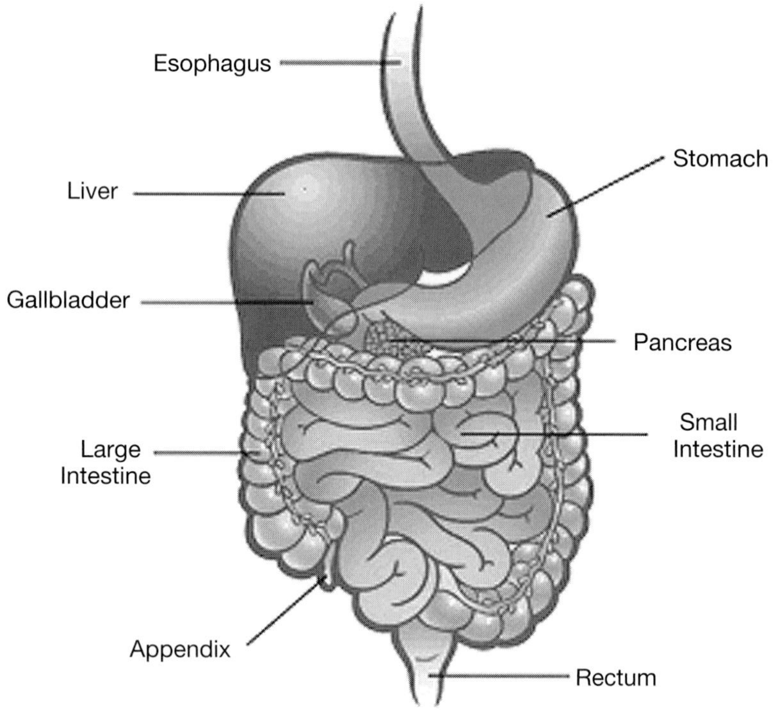

Figure 5-3
The gastrointestinal (GI) tract

Source: This image was provided by KidsHealth, one of the largest resources online for medically reviewed health information written for parents, kids, and teens. www.KidsHealth.org; www.TeensHealth.org.

(such as fiber) are passed through the ileocecal valve to the 5-foot long (1.5 m) large intestine, where a few minerals and a large amount of water are reabsorbed into blood. As more water gets reabsorbed, the waste passing through the colon portion of the large intestine gets harder until it is finally excreted as solid waste from the rectum and anus. Food can stay in the large intestine from hours to days. Total transit time from mouth to anus usually takes anywhere from 18 to 72 hours. Therefore, what's considered to be a "normal" frequency of bowel movements varies among individuals and can range from three times daily to once every three days or more. Of course, a sudden change in the frequency of bowel movements may be a sign of constipation and may warrant further investigation.

Absorption

Carbohydrates, proteins, lipids, vitamins, and minerals are all absorbed through the walls of the small intestine. To maximize surface area, and thus absorptive capacity, the walls of the small intestine contain many folds and hair-like projections called **villi** and **microvilli.** These villous structures form a **brush border** where nutrient absorption occurs.

Nutrients are absorbed by different mechanisms depending on their solubility, size, and relative concentration. Some nutrients, such as water, can readily diffuse across the membrane through **simple diffusion.** Other nutrients, such as water-soluble vitamins, require a carrier; this is known as facilitated diffusion. Amino acids and glucose require **active transport** in which energy is needed to move nutrients across a concentration gradient. Products of lipid digestion and fat-soluble vitamins are carried by micelles to the absorptive surface of the intestinal cells. There they diffuse across the luminal membrane, are converted back into triglycerides, cholesterol, and phospholipids, and join an **apoprotein** to form a **chylomicron.** Other substances, such as vitamin B12, calcium, and iron, have special requirements for absorption. Vitamin B12 must bind with **intrinsic factor,** a glycoprotein—or sugar-protein complex—produced in the stomach that allows vitamin B12 to pass to the **portal circulation** for absorption. Calcium relies on adequate amounts of active vitamin D (1,25-dihydroxycholecalciferol) for absorption. Iron is absorbed in its free form or bound to **hemoglobin** or **myoglobin.** In the intestinal cells, all of the iron is converted into its free form and bound to **transferrin,** its carrier protein, in the blood.

Once across the mucosal membrane, sugar, amino acids, water-soluble vitamins, and minerals enter portal circulation. This system takes nutrients through the bloodstream to the liver. The liver acts to detoxify any harmful substances prior to sending them to the brain or heart. Because chylomicrons are too large to enter the capillaries, fats and fat-soluble vitamins are transferred into the **lymphatic system** and added to the bloodstream through the thoracic duct, a large lymphatic vein that drains into the heart. Ultimately, the nutrients are distributed to muscles, organs, and other tissues.

Impact on Performance and Well-being

The rate and capacity of macronutrient digestion and absorption, in particular that of carbohydrates, influences athletic performance and overall well-being during exercise.

The rate-limiting factor in the process of transferring glucose contained in a sports drink or gel to usable energy to fuel exercise is the rate of absorption of carbohydrate from the small intestine into the bloodstream. Consumption of carbohydrates that contain two or three different saccharides—for example, glucose, fructose, and sucrose—may increase carbohydrate absorption because they each use different transport mechanisms from the small intestine to the bloodstream and so decrease competition for transport. For example, glucose uses a transporter called sodium dependent glucose transporter 1 (SGLT-1), whereas fructose is transported by glucose transporter 5 (GLUT-5). Increased carbohydrate absorption may lead to increased athletic performance by making more fuel available for exercise more quickly (Jeukendrup, 2004).

Not only can consuming foods and drinks that contain more than one kind of carbohydrate enhance athletic performance, but it might also decrease gastrointestinal distress during exercise. By using different transporters for absorption, less carbohydrate remains in the gastrointestinal tract. Less carbohydrate sloshing around the gut means decreased bloating, nausea, and discomfort (Jeukendrup, 2004).

Macronutrient Utilization During Exercise

Anyone who has ever participated in a strenuous athletic endeavor without appropriate fueling and hydration knows that performance can suffer immensely. Careful planning and an understanding of macronutrient utilization during exercise provide the foundation for a successful athletic effort. A basic understanding of nutritional biochemistry will serve an ACE-AHFS well as he or she prepares clients to achieve their personal best.

The basic principle is simple: food provides energy for muscular work. Specifically, energy from food gets converted in the body's cells into usable energy, known as **adenosine triphosphate (ATP).** The energy produced from the breakdown of ATP fuels metabolism, muscle contraction, heart pumping, and the myriad other demands required to maintain exercise performance. Fortunately, people do not have to eat 24 hours a day to supply the body with a constant source of fuel. While ATP is stored in the body in very limited amounts—providing only enough energy for several seconds of exercise—ATP is constantly regenerated through the breakdown of other molecules. For example, as stored ATP breaks down to provide energy, its by-product, **adenosine diphosphate (ADP),** combines with a high-energy phosphate from **creatine phosphate** to produce more ATP. The concentration of high-energy creatine phosphate stored in the muscle is five times that of ATP. Energy from stored ATP and stored creatine phosphate is enough to fuel about five to 10 seconds of an all-out athletic effort. After that, or if moderate exercise proceeds for longer periods, the body must rely on energy-providing nutrients such as carbohydrates, fat, and, in much smaller quantities, protein.

Macronutrient Storage Within the Body

Carbohydrate and fat are stored in the body so that they can be readily available when needed. All protein in the body serves some important purpose; when consumed in excess it gets converted to, and stored as, fat. Liver and muscle store glucose as glycogen. When metabolic demands increase, glucose-releasing enzymes free up the stored glucose, primarily from muscle. When necessary, stored triglycerides (**triacylglycerol**) in adipose tissue are released as energy-rich fatty acids. Intramuscular triglycerides—fat stored in the muscle tissue—also serve as a potential energy source during exercise. While the understanding of how intramuscular triglycerides are utilized during exercise is evolving, the literature to date suggests it is used primarily at the onset of moderate-intensity exercise, and that women use more than men (Roepstorff, Vistisen, & Kiens, 2005). While protein that is not immediately used by the body is converted to, and stored as, fat, the carbon skeleton of some amino acids—whether in the blood from a recent meal or being used by the body in muscle or other tissue—can be used to produce glucose for energy through **gluconeogenesis**, the production of glucose from non-sugar substrates such as amino acids. Depending on the duration and intensity of exercise, these stored macronutrients are broken down to regenerate ATP.

Exercise Hormones

So how does the body know to rev up metabolism during exercise to break down stored nutrients for energy? During exercise, the **sympathetic nervous system**—the body's "fight or flight" response—is activated. The sympathetic nervous system acts to increase blood and oxygen supply to the working muscles. It does this by increasing heart rate, and by shunting blood away from the gastrointestinal system (by constricting the peripheral arteries) and to the working muscles (by dilating the arteries to muscle and liver). The sympathetic nervous system also triggers the release of several exercise hormones. **Epinephrine** is released from the adrenal medulla. It increases blood glucose by inducing the breakdown of liver and muscle glycogen (**glycogenolysis**). Epinephrine also increases glucose by decreasing the release of insulin from the pancreas. **Glucocorticoids,** which are steroid hormones including **cortisol,** are released from the adrenal cortex. The glucocorticoids stimulate glucose production from amino-acid building blocks (gluconeogenesis). The net result is more glucose in the bloodstream and thus more glucose directed to the muscles for energy released as ATP.

Fuel Utilization During Exercise

Perhaps the easiest way to understand the nutritional biochemistry of exercise is with an example, such as that of a marathon training program that incorporates long runs and sprints. The principles presented here also apply to other sports. The same energy systems that predominate during long runs predominate during prolonged biking, swimming, or hiking. Likewise, the main energy systems used during a sprint are also used for resistance training, speed training, and **plyometrics.**

Bobby is a 27-year-old recreational athlete training for a marathon. He trains mostly with long runs, but twice per week he incorporates sprints into his program. Depending on his workout, his body relies on several pathways to varying degrees. The pathways include the **phosphagen system,** in which creatine is the energy source, **anaerobic glycolysis** and **aerobic glycolysis,** where glucose provides energy, and **fatty acid oxidation,** in which energy comes from the breakdown of fat (Table 5-4). Bobby's sprinting program consists of several repetitions of 400-yard (364-m) sprints twice per week. First, it is important to trace his body's energy use through one of these sprints:

- *Seconds 0–8:* Upon starting an all-out physical effort, stored ATP in the muscle is rapidly broken down, releasing ADP, an inorganic phosphate (Pi), and energy:

$$\text{ATP} \Rightarrow \text{ADP} + \text{Pi} + \text{Energy}$$

ADP combines with a high-energy phosphate from stored creatine phosphate to produce more ATP:

$$\text{ADP} + \text{Creatine phosphate} \Rightarrow \text{ATP} + \text{Creatine}$$

Table 5-4
Energy Systems

Energy System	Substrate	Limitation to Produce ATP	Primary Use
Anaerobic			
Phosphagen	CP and stored ATP	Muscle stores very little CP and ATP	High-intensity, short-duration activities; less than 10 seconds to fatigue
Anaerobic glycolysis	Glucose and glycogen	Lactic acid build-up causes rapid fatigue	High-intensity, short-duration activities; from 1–3 minutes to fatigue
Aerobic			
	Fatty acids, glucose, and glycogen	Depletion of muscle glycogen; insufficient O_2 delivery	Long-duration, sub-anaerobic threshold activities; longer than 3 minutes to fatigue

Note: CP = Creatine phosphate; ATP = Adenosine triphosphate

This rapid energy allows for a high-intensity (>85% of $\dot{V}O_2$**max**) effort. By seconds 8–10, the stored ATP and creatine phosphate are depleted.

- *Seconds 8–120:* Anaerobic glycolysis is at full throttle. The body is working on transporting as much glucose as possible to working muscles. The most readily available glucose is floating around in the bloodstream from recently digested carbohydrate and from glycogen stored in the muscle. Glucose is rapidly broken down to produce two ATP molecules per glucose molecule. **Lactic acid,** a metabolic end product, accumulates, causing muscle burn and decreased blood pH. The lowered blood pH interferes with enzymatic action and leads to rapid fatigue. Bobby's sprint is over.

Anaerobic glycolysis (simplified model):

Glucose → Pyruvate → Lactic acid **2 ATP**

- *Recovery:* Bobby is breathing heavily in an involuntary effort to replenish his **oxygen deficit,** the energy supplied to muscles anaerobically at the beginning of exercise. His heavy breathing and **excess post-exercise oxygen consumption (EPOC),** or recovery oxygen consumption, function to provide adequate oxygen to replenish used-up energy stores.

As Bobby nears the peak of his training program, his long runs get longer. The one used in this example is an 18-mile (29-km) run. Unlike the sprint sessions, at the beginning of this workout he starts at a moderate intensity. Again, his initial fuel sources are stored ATP, creatine phosphate, and glucose formed through anaerobic glycolysis, but these are only primary energy sources for the first one to three minutes, until the aerobic glycolysis system is fully functional. Aerobic glycolysis takes longer to provide ATP because it requires adequate oxygen and multiple chemical reactions before ATP is produced. As Bobby breathes in, the oxygen passes from the nasal passages, to the lungs, to the blood, and finally to the muscle cells. Instead of breaking glucose down all the way to lactic acid, the intermediary **pyruvate** enters aerobic glycolysis. Aerobic glycolysis starts with the oxygen-requiring **Kreb's cycle** (also known as the citric acid cycle and the tricarboxylic acid cycle, or TCA cycle). The Kreb's cycle is a series of chemical reactions that act to break pyruvate down to carbon dioxide, water, and many hydrogen-powered molecules known as NADH and FADH2. The hydrogen molecules enter the **electron transport chain** to produce energy through **oxidative phosphorylation,** which is the process by which energy from electrons passed through the electron transport chain are captured and stored to produce ATP. The Kreb's cycle and oxidative phosphorylation occur in the **mitochondria.** Eventually, one molecule of glucose produces a net total of 36 molecules of ATP—clearly more efficient than anaerobic glycolysis, which only produces two ATP molecules.

Aerobic glycolysis (simplified model):
Glucose → Pyruvate → Acetyl-CoA →
Kreb's cycle → Oxidative phosphorylation
36 ATP

After approximately 20 minutes of moderate-intensity aerobic exercise, fat becomes the primary energy source. Triglycerides are broken down to three fatty acids, each of which is broken down further to **acetyl-CoA,** which enters the Kreb's cycle directly; the hydrogen atom by-products are carried into the electron transport chain to produce more ATP. A single fatty acid produces 147 ATP molecules; therefore, each triglyceride produces 441 ATP molecules from fatty-acid oxidation, plus an additional 22 ATP molecules from the breakdown of the glycerol backbone of the triglyceride, for a total of 463 ATP. The increased ATP comes at a price—a marked increase in the amount of oxygen required per molecule of ATP produced.

Triglyceride → 3 Fatty acids → 3 Acetyl-CoA
Kreb's cycle → Oxidative phosphorylation +
22 ATP from glycerol breakdown
463 ATP

As the endurance run continues, both glucose and fatty acids provide fuel for exercise. The proportion depends on the intensity and duration of exercise and the athlete's fitness level. In general, the lower the intensity, the longer the exercise, and the more fit the athlete, the more reliance on fat for fuel. However, it is important to note that fat cannot be metabolized unless carbohydrate is available.

While exercise intensity and duration determine which energy system predominates, at no time does any single energy system provide 100% of energy (see Table 5-4).

Maintaining Glucose Balance During Exercise

When Bobby runs his marathon, he is at risk of "hitting the wall"—a phenomenon that often occurs around mile 20, when extreme fatigue sets in due to drained glycogen stores. When exercise lasts longer than one hour, blood glucose levels begin to dwindle. After one to three hours of continuous moderate-intensity exercise (65–80% $\dot{V}O_2max$), muscle glycogen stores may become depleted. If no glucose is consumed, the blood glucose levels drop, resulting in further depletion of muscle glycogen. When this happens, regardless of the athlete's internal toughness or desire to maintain intensity, performance falters. Athletes can help maintain a ready supply of glucose during endurance activities by consuming about 25 to 30 grams of carbohydrate for every 30 minutes of prolonged exercise lasting longer than one hour. See "Nutrition and Hydration for Optimal Performance" later in this chapter for additional information.

Hydration, Water Balance, and Gastric Emptying

When people think of nutrition, they often forget to think about water. Although it provides no calories and is **inorganic** in nature, water is as important as the oxygen people breathe. Loss of only 20% of total body water may cause death. A 10% loss causes severe disorders. In general, adults can survive up to 10 days without water, while children can live up to five days (Mahan & Escott-Stump, 2000). Water is the single largest component of the human body, comprising about 50 to 70% of body weight. In other words, approximately 85 to 110 pounds (39 to 50 kg) of a 170-pound (77-kg) man is water weight. Physiologically, water has many important functions, including regulating body temperature, protecting vital organs, providing a driving force for nutrient absorption, serving as a medium for all biochemical reactions, and maintaining a high blood volume for optimal athletic performance.

Water volume is influenced by a variety of factors, including food and drink intake; sweat, urine, and feces excretion; metabolic production of small amounts of water; and respiratory losses of water that occur with breathing. These factors play an especially important role during exercise, when metabolism is increased. The generated body heat is released through sweat, a solution of water and sodium and other electrolytes. If fluid intake is not increased to replenish the fluid lost, the body attempts to compensate by retaining more water and excreting more concentrated urine. In this state, the person is said to be dehydrated. Severe **dehydration** can lead to heat stroke. On the other hand, if someone ingests excessive amounts of fluid to compensate for minimal amounts of water lost in sweat, he or she may become overloaded with fluid, leading to low blood sodium levels, a condition called **hyponatremia.** When the blood's water:sodium ratio is severely elevated, excess water can leak into brain tissue, leading to **encephalopathy,** or brain swelling.

Electrolytes help to maintain water balance. Sodium, potassium, and chloride exist as ions in the body and are extremely important for normal cellular function. Sodium and chloride are an extracellular cation and an extracellular anion, respectively, whereas potassium is an intracellular cation. These electrolytes play at least four essential roles in the body: water balance and distribution, osmotic equilibrium (i.e., assuring that the negative ions balance with positive cations when electrolytes move in and out of cells), acid–base balance, and intracellular/extracellular differentials (i.e., assuring that the sodium and chloride stay mostly outside of the cell, while potassium stays mostly inside the cell). When electrolytes are out of balance, such as in the case of dehydration (high concentration of electrolytes) and hyponatremia (low concentration of electrolytes), serious consequences may occur. Symptoms of dehydration include nausea, vomiting, dizziness, disorientation, weakness, irritability, headache, cramps, chills, and decreased performance. Symptoms of hyponatremia include nausea, vomiting, extreme fatigue, respiratory distress, dizziness, confusion, disorientation, coma, and seizures. When severe, both conditions can result in death.

Common wisdom has always said to drink about 64 ounces (1892 mL; eight glasses) of water per day, and to "stay ahead of thirst" while exercising, but the latest recommendations suggest that people follow individualized hydration regimens and let thirst be their guide—if someone is thirsty, he or she should drink water (von Duvillard et al., 2004; ACSM, 2007). Exceptions include infants, heavily exercising athletes, the sick, the elderly, and hospitalized patients; these individuals have higher water needs and should be carefully monitored or, in many cases, encouraged to drink more. "Nutrition and Hydration for Optimal Performance" later in this chapter describes exercise-related hydration recommendations in more detail.

The Gut and Gastric Emptying

The gastrointestinal (GI) system must rapidly digest and absorb fluids and nutrients that fuel exercise. Many exercise-induced GI complaints, such as cramps, reflux, heartburn, bloating, side-stitch, gas, nausea, vomiting, the urge to defecate, loose stool, bloody stool, and diarrhea, occur in response to reduced gastric emptying, delayed transit time, or decreased blood flow. Balancing the factors that affect the GI system's ability to adapt to exercise-induced stresses can help to prevent GI upset and optimize athletic performance.

Gastric emptying refers to the passage of food and fluid from the stomach to the small intestine for further digestion and absorption. When gastric emptying is reduced, food sloshes around in the stomach longer, leading to various GI disturbances. High-intensity exercise (>70% $\dot{V}O_2$max), dehydration, **hyperthermia,** and the consumption of high-energy (>7% carbohydrate) **hypertonic** drinks slow gastric emptying. On the other hand, low- to moderate-intensity exercise helps to speed digestion by stimulating intestinal muscles to contract and push more food waste through the digestive system. Endurance-trained athletes enjoy faster gastric emptying than untrained individuals. This translates into quicker energy availability and decreased GI discomfort following fueling (Murray, 2006).

Exercise-induced sympathetic stimulation diverts blood flow from the GI system to the heart, lungs, and working muscles. The higher the exercise intensity, the more blood flow and colonic tone decrease, causing waste to accumulate in the colon and rectum. The high amount of waste at the end of the GI tract may signal the stomach to slow down, leading to reduced gastric emptying and prolonged transit time. A bulky high-fiber snack prior to intense exercise may increase intestinal distention and water content, contributing to decreased gastric emptying as well as discomforts such as loose stool and an urge to defecate. Notably, trained subjects experience higher blood flow to the gut at any given exercise intensity compared to untrained subjects (Murray, 2006). See Table 5-5 for practical suggestions on how to prepare the gut for an athletic competition.

Table 5-5
Practical Tips to Prepare the Gut for Competition

- Get fit and acclimatized to heat.
- Stay hydrated.
- Practice drinking during training to improve race-day comfort.
- Avoid over-nutrition before and during exercise.
- Avoid high-energy, hypertonic food and drinks before (within 30–60 minutes) and after exercise. Limit protein and fat intake before exercise.
- Ingest a high-energy, high-carbohydrate diet.
- Avoid high-fiber foods before exercise.
- Limit nonsteroidal anti-inflammatory drugs (NSAIDs), alcohol, caffeine, antibiotics, and nutritional supplements before and during exercise. Experiment during training to identify triggers.
- Urinate and defecate prior to exercise.
- Consult a physician if gastrointestinal problems persist, especially abdominal pain, diarrhea, or bloody stool.

Source: Brouns, F. & Beckers, E. (1993). Is the gut an athletic organ? *Sports Medicine,* 15, 242–257.

Nutrition and Hydration for Optimal Performance

Optimal nutrition and hydration before, during, and after exercise support peak athletic performance.

Nutrition Considerations Before, During, and After Exercise

In general, clients should eat about three hours before exercise to give their systems a chance to move the food out of the stomach and begin digestion and absorption. The food should be something that is relatively high in carbohydrate to maximize blood glucose availability, relatively low in fat and fiber to minimize gastrointestinal distress and facilitate gastric emptying, moderate in protein, and well tolerated by the individual. This might be two pancakes, an egg, and a glass of milk for some or a liquid meal for others. If a client is unable to eat three hours before a workout, a small amount of a rapidly digestible carbohydrate like a slice of bread or a banana about 30 minutes to one hour before exercise should suffice.

During training sessions lasting longer than one hour, the exerciser should aim to replace fluid losses with appropriate hydration (see "Hydration Considerations Before, During, and After Exercise" later in this chapter) and consume 30 to 60 grams of carbohydrate per hour of training to maintain blood glucose levels. This is also important when exercising in extreme heat or cold, at high altitude, and when the athlete did not consume adequate amounts of food or drink prior to the training session (ADA, 2000).

Studies show that the best meals for post-workout refueling include an abundance of carbohydrates accompanied by some protein. The carbohydrates replenish the used-up energy that is normally stored as glycogen in muscle and in the liver. The protein helps to rebuild the muscles that were fatigued with exercise. About 75 to 90 grams of carbohydrate (approximately five or six servings of whole grains, fruit, or vegetables) per hour over the course of five hours after training seems to be ideal for optimal refueling, according to one review (Jentjens &

Juekendrup, 2003). The ADA recommends a carbohydrate intake of 1.5 g/kg of body weight in the first 30 minutes after exercise and then every two hours for four to six hours (ADA, 2000). Certainly, the amount of refueling necessary depends on the intensity and duration of the training session (Figure 5-4).

As far as refueling goes, not all carbohydrates are created equal. Carbohydrates with a high GI, such as pancakes and bananas, are more rapidly absorbed and more quickly release sugar into the bloodstream. Therefore, they are more effective at replenishing energy stores than low-GI carbohydrates, which are broken

Figure 5-4
Performance-enhancing post-workout snacks and meals

The following meal ideas provide ample carbohydrate and protein for refueling after an extended early-morning workout. The serving amounts are approximations based on a typical restaurant breakfast.	**This sample post-workout plan is for late-starters who ate before their workout, but still want the performance benefits of post-workout refueling. The snacks should be spaced approximately one to two hours apart:**
French toast: Two slices of French toast with powdered sugar, strawberries, and light syrup; two turkey links; and a glass of orange juice • Carbohydrates: 80 grams • Protein: 17 grams • Calories: 510	*Snack 1:* In the first several minutes after exercise, consume 16 ounces of a sports drink, a power gel, and a medium banana. This snack quickly begins to replenish muscle carbohydrate stores. • Carbohydrates: 73 grams • Protein: 1 gram • Calories: 288
Egg muffin: One poached egg with toasted whole-grain English muffin and low-fat slice of cheese; a glass of low-fat chocolate milk; and an orange • Carbohydrates: 74 grams • Protein: 25 grams • Calories: 490	*Snack 2:* 12 ounces of orange juice and ¼-cup of raisins • Carbohydrates: 70 grams • Protein: 3 grams • Calories: 295
Oatmeal with fruit: One cup of oatmeal with dried fruit, brown sugar, and skim milk; one egg (sunny side up); and a glass of cranberry juice • Carbohydrates: 80 grams • Protein: 17 grams • Calories: 480	*Small meal appetizer:* Salad with spinach, tomatoes, chick peas, green beans, and tuna and a whole grain baguette • Carbohydrates: 69 grams • Protein: 37 grams • Calories: 489
Elvis bagel sandwich: Whole-grain bagel with peanut butter and banana; a glass of water with lemon • Carbohydrates: 76 grams • Protein: 19 grams • Calories: 510	*Small meal main course:* Whole-grain pasta with diced tomatoes • Carbohydrates: 67 grams • Protein: 2 grams • Calories: 292
Omelet: Egg white omelet with tomatoes, spinach, and feta or mozzarella cheese; two slices of whole-wheat toast with jelly; low-fat yogurt with granola; and a glass of tomato juice • Carbohydrates: 72 grams • Protein: 30 grams • Calories: 490	*Dessert:* One cup of frozen yogurt and berries • Carbohydrates: 61 grams • Protein: 8 grams • Calories: 280

down more slowly and take longer to release sugar into the bloodstream. And glucose, found in non-fruit carbohydrates, is better absorbed than fructose, the sugar in fruit (Jentjens & Jeukendrup, 2003). It is important to note that although high-glycemic glucose-rich foods are good for refueling and athletic performance, low-glycemic foods and fruits are a better choice for heart health (see "Glycemic Index" earlier in this chapter). The goal is to find a balance. The ACE-AHFS should remind clients to eat as soon after exercising as possible, preferably within 30 minutes. This is the time when the muscles are best able to replenish energy stores, enabling the body to prepare for the next workout.

Hydration Considerations Before, During, and After Exercise

Hyperconscious of the detrimental health and performance effects of dehydration, health and fitness experts have long warned recreational exercise enthusiasts and athletes alike to hydrate continuously. But research suggests that hyponatremia—severely reduced blood sodium concentration resulting from overhydration—may be of equal or greater concern than dehydration. In response, ACSM has updated its guidelines and the National Athletic Trainer's Association has developed guidelines for optimal hydration during exercise (Table 5-6) (Casa, Clarkson, & Roberts, 2005; Casa et al., 2000).

During exercise, clients should heed the following guidelines:

- *Use thirst to determine fluid needs.* Advise clients to drink when they are thirsty and stop drinking when they feel hydrated.
- *Aim for a 1:1 ratio of fluid replacement to fluid lost in sweat.* Ideally, people should consume the same amount of fluid as is lost in sweat. Clients can check their hydration status by comparing pre- and post-exercise weight. Perfect hydration occurs when no weight is lost or gained during exercise. Another simple way to determine adequate hydration status is to check urine color. Individuals will know that they are adequately hydrated when their urine is clear or pale yellow. Because people sweat at varying rates, the typical recommendation to consume 3 to 6 ounces of water for every 20 minutes of exercise may not be appropriate for everyone. However, when individual assessment is not possible, this recommendation works for most people. Experts advise small athletes exercising in mild environmental conditions to consume slightly smaller amounts of fluids, and competitive athletes working at higher intensities in warmer environments to consume slightly more (Noakes, 2003).
- *Measure fluid amounts.* When exercisers know how much they are actually drinking, they may be able to better assess if they are consuming appropriate amounts.
- *Drink fluids with sodium during prolonged exercise sessions.* If an exercise session lasts longer than two hours or an athlete is participating in an event that stimulates heavy sodium loss (defined as more than 3 to 4 grams of sodium), experts recommend that the athlete drink a sports drink that contains elevated levels of sodium (Coyle, 2004). [Researchers did not find a benefit from sports drinks that contained only the 18 mmol/L (100 mg/8 oz) of sodium typical of most sports drinks and thus concluded that higher levels would be needed to prevent hyponatremia during prolonged exercise (Almond et al., 2005).] Alternatively, exercisers can consume extra sodium with meals and snacks prior to a lengthy exercise session or a day of extensive physical activity (Casa, 2003).
- *Drink carbohydrate-containing sports drinks to reduce fatigue.* With prolonged exercise, muscle glycogen stores become depleted and

Table 5-6
Fluid-intake Recommendations During Exercise

2 hours prior to exercise, drink 500–600 mL (17–20 oz)
Every 10–20 minutes during exercise, drink 200–300 mL (7–10 oz) or, preferably, drink based on sweat losses
Following exercise, drink 450–675 mL for every 0.5 kg body weight lost (or 16–24 oz for every pound)

Source: Adapted with permission from Casa, D.J. et al. (2000). National Athletic Trainers' Association: Position statement: Fluid replacement for athletes. *Journal of Athletic Training,* 35, 212–224.

blood glucose becomes a primary fuel source. To maintain performance levels and prevent fatigue, clients should consume drinks and snacks that provide about 30 to 60 grams of rapidly absorbed carbohydrate for every hour of training (Coyle, 2004). As long as the carbohydrate concentration is less than about 6 to 8%, it will have little effect on gastric emptying (Coombes & Hamilton, 2000).

Following exercise, the athlete should aim to correct any fluid imbalances that occurred during the exercise session. This includes consuming water to restore hydration, carbohydrates to replenish glycogen stores, and electrolytes to speed rehydration (Casa, 2003). Those at greatest risk of hyponatremia should be careful not to consume too much water following exercise and instead focus on replenishing sodium.

Remember that the human body is well-equipped to withstand dramatic variations in fluid intake during exercise and at rest with little or no detrimental health effects. For this reason, most recreational exercisers will never suffer from serious hyponatremia or dehydration and should not be alarmed. However, environmental conditions can dictate whether an exercise experience is safe. Athletes should be particularly conscientious when exercising in extreme conditions. For example, the risk of heat stroke is increased in conditions of elevated temperature and humidity and still wind due to the diminished ability of the body to dissipate heat into the environment (Noakes, 2003). Record-high heat and humidity at the 2007 Chicago marathon forced mid-race cancellation and led to several hospitalizations. To help avoid a negative experience, athletes should aim to be well acclimatized to the environmental conditions and replenish sweat loss with equal amounts of fluid.

Supplements, Alcohol, and Stimulants

Supplements

From multivitamins and herbal supplements to weight-loss pills and **creatine,** the supplement industry is a multibillion dollar industry playing to people's desire to quickly and easily get or stay healthy, lose weight, gain muscle, improve memory, enhance sexual function, and fulfill various other wishes. While some supplements may in fact provide beneficial effects, consumers should purchase and use these products cautiously, as they are not closely regulated by the Food and Drug Administration (FDA). Importantly, no matter how harmless a supplement seems, an ACE-AHFS should never recommend supplements to clients (see Appendix G for ACE's Position Statement on Nutritional Supplements). Not only is it outside the scope of practice of an ACE-AHFS, but recommending supplements without a full medical history and physical exam is dangerous. For example, in "Capati v. Crunch Fitness" a personal trainer and the health club he worked at were sued for $320 million after the trainer recommended a client take a variety of supplements, some of which contained **ephedra.** The client, who was also taking medication for hypertension, became sick and later died of a brain hemorrhage. Research shows that when combined, ephedra and hypertension can be lethal. The case was settled before going to trial, with the gym and trainer liable for $1.75 million (Sass et al., 2007).

The **Dietary Supplement and Health Education Act (DSHEA)** of 1994 dictates supplement production, marketing, and safety guidelines. Fitness professionals and their clients must be aware that savvy product manufacturers and marketing experts have found ingenious ways to get around some of the rules. The following are the basic highlights of the legislation:

- The Act established that a **dietary supplement** is defined as a product (other than tobacco) that functions to supplement the diet and contains one or more of the following ingredients: a vitamin, mineral, herb or other botanical, amino acid, nutritional substance that increases total dietary intake, metabolite, constituent, extract, or some combination of the above ingredients.
- Safety standards provide that the Secretary of the Department of Health and Human Services may declare that a supplement poses imminent risk or hazard to public safety. A supplement is considered *adulterated* if it or one of its ingredients presents a "significant

or unreasonable risk of illness or injury" when used as directed or under normal conditions. It may also be considered adulterated if too little information is known about the risk of an unstudied ingredient.

- Retailers are allowed to display "third-party" materials that provide information about the health-related benefits of dietary supplements. The Act stipulates the guidelines the literature must follow, including the fact that it must not be false or misleading and cannot promote a specific supplement brand.
- Supplements cannot claim to diagnose, prevent, mitigate, treat, or cure a specific disease. Instead, they may describe the supplement's effects on the "structure or function" of the body or the "well-being" achieved by consuming the substance. Unlike other health claims, these nutritional support statements do not need to be approved by the FDA prior to marketing the supplement.
- Supplements must contain an ingredient label including the name and quantity of each dietary ingredient. It must also identify the product as a "dietary supplement" (FDA, 1995).

Alcohol

Alcohol is a non-nutritive calorie-containing beverage (seven calories per gram). Moderate alcohol consumption provides many health benefits, such as increased HDL cholesterol and reduced risk for cardiovascular disease. However, too much alcohol may contribute to weight gain, regretful behavior, and serious accidents. In addition, alcohol during pregnancy is linked to birth defects, and alcohol in excess can cause **cirrhosis** of the liver. The American Heart Association recommends that non-drinkers remain non-drinkers, men drink no more than two drinks per day, and women drink no more than one drink of alcohol per day (Goldberg et al., 2001). One drink is equivalent to:

- 12-oz bottle of beer
- 5-oz glass of wine
- One shot of liquor

Stimulants

A **stimulant** is a substance that activates the **central nervous system** and sympathetic nervous system. It increases heart rate and **cardiac output,** increases glucose availability, and may even suppress appetite. But sometimes stimulants can also be deadly. The Chinese botanical **ma huang,** also known as ephedra, reduces appetite, but also is associated with significant life-threatening side effects, including dangerously increased blood pressure, heart attacks, seizure, stroke, and serious psychiatric illness.

Caffeine, found in coffee, tea, soft drinks, chocolate, and various other foods and drinks, also acts as a stimulant, increasing alertness, mood, and physical performance. However, too much caffeine causes restlessness, irritability, and anxiety. It can also interfere with sleep and cause headaches and abnormal heart rhythms. As a diuretic, caffeine promotes increased urination and may contribute to dehydration. Once a person has developed a dependence on caffeine, withdrawal symptoms such as headache often develop with discontinued use.

Nutrition, Exercise, and Weight Control

The 2005 Dietary Guidelines highlight that the key to weight control is to balance caloric intake from food and beverages with caloric expenditure (USDA, 2005). When more calories are consumed than expended, an individual is in **positive energy balance,** which is necessary during times of growth such as in infancy, childhood, and pregnancy. Otherwise, positive energy balance results in weight gain. When more calories are expended than consumed, an individual is in **negative energy balance,** which is necessary for weight loss.

An ACE-AHFS can help clients to achieve their weight-loss goals by first determining daily energy needs. The ACE-AHFS can use the energy expenditure calculator at www.MyPyramid.gov or utilize the Mifflin-St. Jeor equation, the most accurate estimation of

resting metabolic rate (RMR) (Frankenfield, Routh-Yousey, & Compher, 2005):

Men: RMR = 9.99 x wt (kg) + 6.25 x ht (cm) – 4.92 x age (years) + 5
Women: RMR = 9.99 x wt (kg) + 6.25 x ht (cm) – 4.92 x age (years) – 161

(*Note:* Convert pounds to kilograms by dividing by 2.2; convert inches to centimeters by multiplying by 2.54)

The RMR represents the number of calories needed to fuel ventilation, blood circulation, and temperature regulation. Calories are also required to digest and absorb consumed food and fuel the **activities of daily living (ADL)**. For weight maintenance, moderately active people are generally advised to consume about 1.5 to 1.7 times their calculated resting metabolic rate (ADA, 2000). For example, a 30-year-old female who is 5'6" (1.7 m), weighs 145 pounds (65 kg), and engages in 40 to 60 minutes of vigorous physical activity most days of the week would maintain her weight with an intake of 2200 calories per day. Resting metabolic rate is influenced by various factors (Table 5-7).

Once the ACE-AHFS determines a client's approximate caloric intake for weight maintenance, it is time to develop an exercise program that creates a sufficient energy deficit to help the client reach his or her goals. The 2005 Dietary Guidelines recommend that individuals trying to lose weight aim for a 500-calorie deficit per day achieved through decreased caloric intake and/or increased physical activity (USDA, 2005). Over the course of a week, the 3500-calorie deficit should lead to loss of 1 pound (0.45 kg). For optimal long-term success and overall health, gradual weight loss of no more than 1 to 2 pounds (0.45 to 0.9 kg) per week is best. An ACE-AHFS should encourage clients to consult www.MyPyramid.gov or visit a registered dietitian (R.D.) if they would like help developing an individualized nutrition plan to complement their fitness program.

Table 5-7
Factors Affecting Resting Metabolic Rate

Factor	RMR	Comments
Age	↓	Likely due to a loss of lean body mass
Body Temperature	↑	Seen with temperature extremes: fever and hypothermia (shivering)
Caffeine and Tobacco	↑	These stimulants increase metabolism
Gender	↑↓	Males tend to have more lean body mass
Nervous System Activity	↑	The "fight or flight" hormone norepinephrine can increase RMR
Nutritional Status	↓	Reduced calorie intake can depress RMR
Pregnancy	↑	Periods of growth require extra energy expenditure
Thyroid Hormones	↑↓	People with too much thyroid hormone (hyperthyroidism) have increased RMR, and those with not enough (hypothyroidism) have decreased RMR

Note: ↑ = Increase; ↓ = Decrease; ↑↓ = Variable

Source: Modified from Wardlaw, G.M., Hampl, J.S., & DiSilvestro, R.A. (2004). *Perspectives in Nutrition* (6th ed.). New York: McGraw-Hill.

Exercise and a Vegetarian Diet

A growing number of Americans are **vegetarians.** Vegetarian diets come in several forms, all of which are healthful, nutritionally adequate, and effective in disease prevention if carefully planned. A **lacto-ovo-vegetarian** does not eat meat, fish, or poultry. A **lacto-vegetarian** does not eat eggs, meat, fish, or poultry. A **vegan** does not consume any animal products, including dairy products such as milk and cheese.

Vegetarian diets provide several health advantages. They are low in saturated fat, cholesterol, and animal protein, and high in fiber, folate, vitamins C and E, **carotenoids,** and some phytochemicals. Compared to non-vegetarians, vegetarians have lower rates of **obesity**, death from cardiovascular disease, hypertension, **type 2 diabetes,** and prostate and colon cancer. However, if poorly planned, vegetarian diets may provide insufficient amounts of protein, iron, vitamin B12, vitamin D, calcium, and other nutrients (ADA, 2003).

Athletes have increased protein and energy needs compared to sedentary individuals. While vegetarian diets are capable of providing sufficient energy, some vegetarian athletes may be challenged to eat enough calories to fuel their exercise. Some suggestions to increase caloric intake include eating more frequent meals and snacks; including meat alternatives; and adding dried fruit, seeds, nuts, and other healthful calorie-dense foods. Though vegetarians do not consume complete proteins unless they eat a lot of soy, they can assure adequate protein intake if they choose a variety of foods throughout the day (ADA, 2003). To date, an insufficient number of well-designed research studies have been conducted to determine whether a vegetarian diet affects athletic performance (Venderley & Campbell, 2006).

Eating Disorders and Exercise Disorders

Eating Disorders

Most fitness professionals will at some point face the challenge of helping someone to overcome the powerful grips of an eating disorder. The most infamous and deadly of the eating disorders is **anorexia nervosa (AN)**, which is formally diagnosed when the following conditions are present:

- Refusal to maintain body weight of at least 85% of expected weight
- Intense fear of gaining weight or becoming fat
- Body-image disturbances, including a disproportionate influence of body weight on self-evaluation
- In women, the absence of at least three consecutive menstrual periods **(amenorrhea)**

The disorder is further classified into the restricting type, in which caloric intake is severely reduced to between 300 and 700 calories per day and caloric expenditure is increased, and the binge-eating/purging type, in which the individual uses vomiting, laxatives, diuretics, and/or enemas to lose weight [American Psychiatric Association (APA), 2000]. While a woman's lifetime risk of developing the disorder is about 0.3% and a man's about one-tenth that rate, "sub-threshold" (i.e., symptoms not quite severe enough for diagnosis) forms of anorexia nervosa are much more common (Hoek & VanHoeken, 2003). The causes of anorexia are multifactorial and include the following:

- Genetics
- Personality traits of perfectionism and compulsiveness
- Anxiety disorders
- Family history of depression and obesity
- Peer, cultural, and familial ideals of beauty

The most severe potential consequences of the disorder include osteoporosis, miscarriage and low infant birth weights, abnormalities in cognitive functioning, suicide, and death from starvation or heart **arrhythmias.** While many people with anorexia nervosa are resistant to change and may need inpatient treatment, full recovery of body weight, growth, menstruation, and normal eating behavior and attitudes regarding food and body shape occurs in 50 to 70% or more of treated adolescents. Only 25 to 50% of adults with anorexia severe enough to require hospitalization fully recover (Yager & Andersen, 2005).

Bulimia nervosa (BN) is more difficult to identify than anorexia. While extremely low weight often makes individuals suspicious of anorexia, people with bulimia nervosa are often normal weight or sometimes overweight. Bulimia nervosa is diagnosed when the following criteria are met:

- Recurrent episodes of uncontrolled binge eating
- Recurrent inappropriate compensatory behavior such as self-induced vomiting
- Misuse of laxatives, diuretics, or enemas (purging type)
- Fasting and/or excessive exercise (non-purging type)
- Episodes of binge eating and compensatory behaviors occurring at least twice per week for three months
- Self-evaluation is heavily influenced by body shape and weight
- Episodes do not occur exclusively with episodes of anorexia
- Approximately 1% of women (usually in their late teens to early twenties) suffer from bulimia (Yager & Andersen, 2005). Importantly, anorexia and bulimia often coexist and are caused by many of the same complex social, familial, and personality factors.

The most common of the eating disorders, **binge eating disorder,** also known as compulsive overeating, is characterized by an overwhelming and repeated compulsion to consume unusually large amounts of food, sometimes up to 10,000 to 20,000 calories in a single binge. Symptoms of binge eating disorder include:

- Eating large amounts of food
- Eating despite feeling full
- Eating rapidly during binge episodes
- Feeling that eating behavior is out of control
- Depression
- Anxiety
- Frequent dieting without weight loss
- Frequently eating alone
- Hoarding food
- Hiding empty food containers
- Feeling depressed, disgusted, or upset about one's eating

People with binge eating disorder may be of normal weight or overweight. Interestingly, most people who are obese do not have binge eating disorder.

Exercise Disorders

While people with anorexia and sometimes bulimia engage in excessive amounts of exercise in an effort to lose weight and achieve an elusive state of thinness, people with **muscle dysmorphic disorder** engage in excessive amounts of resistance training in an effort to be muscular and "big." Muscle dysmorphic disorder is diagnosed when the following criteria are met:

- Obsession with the belief that the body should be more lean and muscular, and thus significant amounts of time devoted to weight lifting and a fixation on diet
- Belief that the body is too small or insufficiently muscular
- Two of the following:
  - ✔An uncontrolled focus on a fitness-training regimen causes the person to miss out on career, social, and other activities
  - ✔Circumstances involving body exposure are avoided
  - ✔Performance at work and in social situations is affected by presumed body deficiencies
  - ✔Potentially detrimental effects of the training program fail to dissuade the individual from pursuing hazardous practices

Approximately 100,000 people, mostly men, meet the formal criteria for muscle dysmorphic disorder (Leone et al., 2005).

While hundreds of thousands of people are diagnosed with eating and exercise (body image) disorders, many more suffer from other disordered eating and exercise habits, some of which are referred to as **eating disorders not otherwise specified (EDNOS)** or a body dysmorphia other than muscular dysmorphic disorder. Individuals with severe dietary restriction, compulsive exercise, and subclinical forms of the mentioned disorders should still trigger concern and be helped similarly to those with a diagnosed disorder.

Preventing Eating Disorders and Exercise Disorders in High-risk Populations

Fitness professionals and coaches who work with young people and others at risk for eating disorders play a critically important role in helping to prevent the onset of an obsession with weight, body image, and exercise. The National Eating Disorders Association (www.nationaleatingdisorders.org) offers the following tips for coaches and fitness professionals to help prevent eating disorders:

- Take warning signs seriously. If an ACE-AHFS believes that someone may have an eating disorder, he or she should share those concerns in an open, direct, and sensitive manner, keeping in mind the following "don'ts" when confronting someone with a suspected eating or exercise disorder: Don't oversimplify, diagnose, become the person's therapist, provide exercise advice without first helping the individual get professional help, or get into a battle of wills if the person denies having a problem.
- Deemphasize weight. An ACE-AHFS should not weigh at-risk clients and should eliminate comments about weight, especially with those individuals believed to be at risk for an eating disorder.
- Do not assume that reducing body fat or weight will improve performance or alter the person's body-image misperceptions.
- Help other fitness professionals recognize the signs of eating disorders and be prepared to address them.
- Provide accurate information about weight, weight loss, **body composition,** nutrition, and sports performance. An ACE-AHFS should have a broad network of referrals (such as physicians and registered dietitians) that may also be able to help educate clients when appropriate.
- Emphasize the health risks of low weight, especially for female athletes with menstrual irregularities (in which case, referral to a physician, preferably one who specializes in eating disorders, is warranted).
- Avoid making any derogatory comments about weight or body composition to, or about, anyone.
- Do not curtail athletic performance and gym privileges for an athlete or client who is found to have eating problems unless it is medically necessary and recommended to do so. An ACE-AHFS must consider the individual's physical and emotional health and self-image when deciding how to modify the exercise participation level. It is important that the ACE-AHFS works with the client's healthcare provider to determine the client's ability to continue with exercise.
- Strive to promote a positive self-image and self-esteem in clients and athletes. An ACE-AHFS should carefully assess his or her own assumptions and beliefs.

Training a Client With an Eating Disorder or Exercise Disorder

In addition to being a source of help and empathy, an ACE-AHFS can play an important role in developing structured exercise programs for people recovering from eating and exercise disorders who have already sought help from a qualified medical professional. An important first step is to develop a partnership with the client's treating physician. An ACE-AHFS should seek medical clearance and general recommendations from the physician regarding the maximal duration and intensity of exercise. Note that individuals with a **body mass index (BMI)** of less than 20 may not receive clearance to exercise until they gain a specified amount of weight. When working with such a client, it is important to emphasize the positive psychological and health benefits of appropriate exercise and minimize the focus on appearances and weight. As with all clients, the ACE-AHFS should strive to develop a balanced and well-rounded program that includes cardiovascular training, resistance training, and flexibility exercises. The goal is to help the client learn how to exercise in moderation.

Exercise, Nutrition, and Immune Function

The immune system provides the body's defense against foreign invaders. A prolonged schedule of vigorous physical training can cause immune system impairment and subsequent infection. The immune dysfunction likely results from the immunosuppressive actions of the exercise hormones **adrenaline** and cortisol. Nutritional deficiencies and excesses (especially omega-3 polyunsaturated fats, iron, zinc, and vitamins A and E) also cause immune impairment. A situation of rigorous athletic training combined with nutritional deficiencies provides a very high susceptibility to infection. The following strategies will help clients maintain optimal immune function (Gleeson, Nieman, & Pederson, 2004):

- Maintain adequate calorie, protein, and micronutrient intake, especially iron, zinc, and vitamins A, E, B6, and B12.
- Periodically refuel during prolonged exercise to avoid greater increases in stress hormones.
- Avoid excess intake of vitamins and minerals, especially iron, zinc, and vitamin E, which can impair immune function.
- Avoid high-fat diets, which can suppress some aspects of immune cell function.
- Supplements and antioxidants probably do not boost the immune system, though more research needs to be done.
- Incorporate adequate recovery time following particularly strenuous workout sessions.

Summary

An individual's health is at least partially determined by his or her nutrition habits. While each nutrient has a specific role in the body's well-being, it is the balance among these different nutrients that allows the body to function optimally. As such, a balanced and varied diet forms the foundation for good health. An ACE-AHFS can arm clients with an understanding and appreciation of sports nutrition, as well as the basics of general nutrition, digestion, absorption, and metabolism. Sharing this knowledge will help each client make choices along the path toward optimal health and well-being.

References

Almond, C.S.D. et al. (2005). Hyponatremia among runners in the Boston Marathon. *New England Journal of Medicine*, 352, 15, 1550–1556.

American College of Sports Medicine (2007). American College of Sports Medicine Position Stand: Exercise and fluid replacements. *Medicine & Science in Sports & Exercise,* 39, 2, 377–390.

American Dietetic Association (2007). Position of the American Dietetic Association and Dietitians of Canada: Dietary fatty acids. *Journal of the American Dietetic Association*, 107, 1599–1611.

American Dietetic Association (2003). Position of the American Dietetic Association and Dietitians of Canada: Vegetarian diets. *Journal of the American Dietetic Association,* 103, 6, 748–765.

American Dietetic Association (2002). Position of the American Dietetic Association: Health implications of dietary fiber. *Journal of the American Dietetic Association,* 102, 7, 993–1000.

American Dietetic Association (2000). Position of the American Dietetic Association, Dietitians of Canada, and the American College of Sports Medicine: Nutrition and athletic performance. *Journal of the American Dietetic Association,* 100, 12, 1543–1556.

American Psychiatric Association (2000). *Diagnostic and Statistical Manual of Mental Disorders* (4th ed.) (DSM-IV-TR). Washington, D.C.: American Psychiatric Association.

Brand-Miller, J. et al. (2003). Low-glycemic index diets in the management of diabetes: A meta-analysis of randomized controlled trials. *Diabetes Care,* 26, 8, 2261–2267.

Casa, D.J. (2003). Proper hydration for distance running—Identifying individual fluid needs: A USA Track & Field advisory. www.usatf.org/groups/Coaches/library/hydration/ProperHydrationForDistanceRunning.pdf.

Casa, D.J. et al. (2000). National Athletic Trainers' Association: Position statement: Fluid replacement for athletes. *Journal of Athletic Training,* 35, 212–224.

Casa D.J., Clarkson P.M., & Roberts, W.O. (2005). American College of Sports Medicine roundtable on hydration and physical activity: Consensus statements. *Current Sports Medicine Reports,* 4, 115–127.

Coombes J.S. & Hamilton K.L. (2000). The effectiveness of commercially available sports drinks. *Sports Medicine,* 29, 3, 181–209.

Coyle, E.F. (2004). Fluid and fuel intake during exercise. *Journal of Sports Sciences,* 22, 1, 39–55.

Food and Agriculture Organization/World Health Organization (1995). Protein quality evaluation: Report of the joint FAO/WHO expert consultation. *FAO Food and Nutrition Paper,* 52.

Food and Drug Administration (1995). Dietary Supplement Health and Education Act of 1994. http://www.cfsan.fda.gov/~dms/dietsupp.html

Frankenfield, D., Routh-Yousey, L., & Compher, C. (2005). Comparison of predictive equations of resting metabolic rates in healthy non-obese and obese adults: A systematic review. *Journal of the American Dietetic Association,* 105, 5, 775–789.

Gleeson, M., Nieman, D.C., & Pederson, B.K. (2004). Exercise, nutrition, and immune function. *Journal of Sports Sciences,* 22, 115–125.

Goldberg, I.J. et al. (2001). AHA Science Advisory: Wine and your heart: A science advisory for healthcare professionals from the Nutrition Committee, Council on Epidemiology and Prevention, and Council on Cardiovascular Nursing of the American Heart Association. *Circulation,* 103, 3, 472–475.

Hoek, H.W. & van Hoeken, D. (2003). Review of the prevalence and incidence of eating disorders. *International Journal of Eating Disorders,* 34, 383–396.

Hoffman, J.R. & Falvo, M.J. (2004). Protein: Which is best? *Journal of Sports Science and Medicine,* 3, 118–130.

Hu, F.B. & Willett, W.C. (2002). Optimal diets for prevention of coronary heart disease. *Journal of the American Medical Association,* 288, 2569–2578.

Institute of Medicine, Food and Energy Board (2002). *Dietary Reference Intakes for Energy, Carbohydrate, Fiber, Fat, Fatty Acids, Cholesterol, Protein, and Amino Acids.* Washington, D.C.: National Academy Press.

Jentjens, R. & Jeukendrup, A.E. (2003). Determinants of post-exercise glycogen synthesis during short-term recovery. *Sports Medicine,* 33, 2, 117–144.

Jeukendrup, A.E. (2004). Carbohydrate intake during exercise and performance. *Nutrition,* 20, 669–677.

Leone, J.E. et al. (2005). Recognition and treatment of muscle dysmorphia and related body image disorders. *Journal of Athletic Training*, 40, 4, 353–359.

Liu, S. (2006). Lowering dietary glycemic load for weight control and cardiovascular health: A matter of quality. *Annals of Internal Medicine,* 166, 1438–1439.

Mahan, L.K. & Escott-Stump, S. (2000). *Krause's Food Nutrition and Diet Therapy* (10th ed.). Philadelphia, Pa.: W.B. Saunders Company.

McDaniel, M.A., Maier, S.F., & Einstein, G.O. (2003). "Brain-specific" nutrients: A memory cure? *Nutrition,* 19, 957–975.

Murray, R. (2006). Training the gut for competition. *Current Sports Medicine Reports,* 5, 161–164.

Noakes, T. (2003). Fluid replacement during marathon running. *Clinical Journal of Sport Medicine,* 13, 309–318.

Roepstorff, C., Vistisen, B., & Kiens, B. (2005). Intramuscular triacylglycerol in energy metabolism during exercise in humans. *Exercise and Sports Sciences Reviews,* 33, 4, 182–188.

Sass, C. et al. (2007). Crossing the line: Understanding the scope of practice between registered dietitians and health/fitness professionals. *ACSM's Health & Fitness Journal,* 11, 3, 12–19.

Simopoulos, A.P. (1999). Essential fatty acids in health and chronic disease. *American Journal of Clinical Nutrition,* 70, 560S–569S.

Thomas, D.E., Elliott, E.J., & Baur, L. (2007). Low glycaemic index or low glycaemic load diets for overweight and obesity. *Cochrane Database of Systematic Reviews,* 3, CD005105.

United States Department of Agriculture (2005). *Dietary Guidelines for Americans 2005.* www.health.gov/dietaryguidelines. Executive summary: www.health.gov/dietaryguidelines/dga2005/document/html/executivesummary.htm.

Venderley, A.M. & Campbell, W.W. (2006). Vegetarian diets: Nutritional considerations for athletes. *Sports Medicine,* 36, 4, 293–305.

von Duvillard, S.P. et al. (2004). Fluid and hydration in prolonged endurance performance. *Nutrition,* 20, 651–656.

Wardlaw, G.M., Hampl, J.S., & DiSilvestro, R.A. (2004). *Perspectives in Nutrition* (6th ed.). New York: McGraw-Hill.

World Health Organization (2007). *Micronutrients.* http://www.who.int/nutrition/topics/micronutrients/en/index.html.

Yager, J. & Andersen, A. (2005). Anorexia nervosa. *New England Journal of Medicine,* 353, 14, 1481–1488.

Zarraga, I.G.E. & Schwarz, E.R. (2006). Impact of Dietary Patterns and Interventions on Cardiovascular Health. *Circulation,* 114, 961–973.

Suggested Reading

Dunford, M. (Ed.) (2006). *Sports Nutrition: A Practice Manual for Professionals* (4th ed.). SCAN Dietetic Practice Group and the American Dietetic Association.

Duyff, R.L. & American Dietetic Association (2006). *Complete Food and Nutrition Guide* (3rd ed.). Hoboken, N.J.: John Wiley and Sons.

Kleiner, S.M. (2007). *Power Eating: Build Muscle, Gain Energy, Lose Weight* (3rd ed.). Champaign, Ill.: Human Kinetics.

National Institutes of Health, Office of Dietary Supplements. *Vitamin and Mineral Supplement Fact Sheets*. http://ods.od.nih.gov/Health_Information/Vitamin_and_Mineral_Supplement_Fact_Sheets.aspx

Willett, W. (2006). *Eat, Drink, and Be Healthy: The Harvard Medical School Guide to Healthy Eating* (2nd ed.). New York: Free Press.

Part Two

Major Cardiovascular and Pulmonary Diseases and Disorders

Chapter 6
Coronary Artery Disease

Chapter 7
Blood Lipid Disorders

Chapter 8
Hypertension

Chapter 9
Asthma

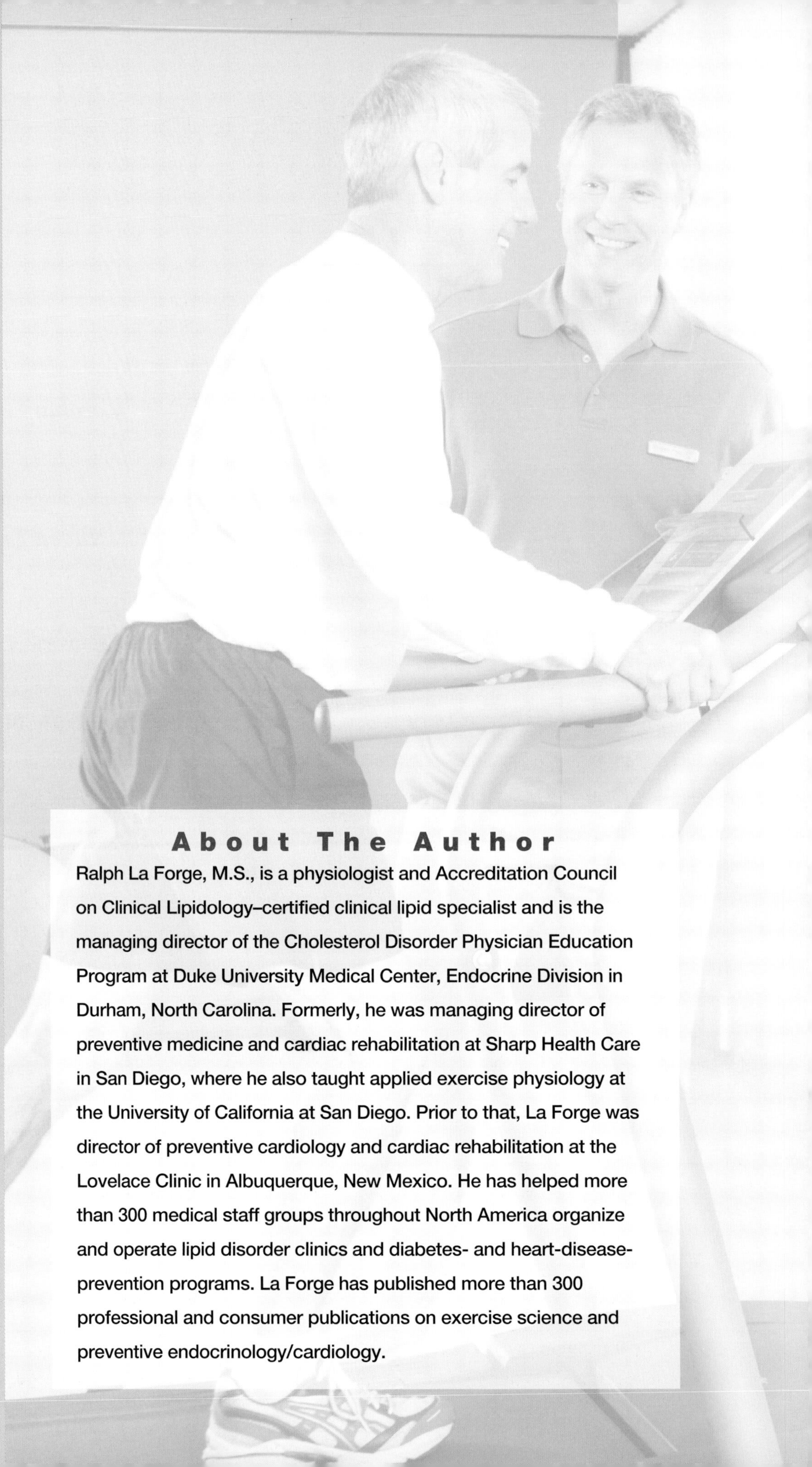

In This Chapter

About The Author

Ralph La Forge, M.S., is a physiologist and Accreditation Council on Clinical Lipidology–certified clinical lipid specialist and is the managing director of the Cholesterol Disorder Physician Education Program at Duke University Medical Center, Endocrine Division in Durham, North Carolina. Formerly, he was managing director of preventive medicine and cardiac rehabilitation at Sharp Health Care in San Diego, where he also taught applied exercise physiology at the University of California at San Diego. Prior to that, La Forge was director of preventive cardiology and cardiac rehabilitation at the Lovelace Clinic in Albuquerque, New Mexico. He has helped more than 300 medical staff groups throughout North America organize and operate lipid disorder clinics and diabetes- and heart-disease-prevention programs. La Forge has published more than 300 professional and consumer publications on exercise science and preventive endocrinology/cardiology.

CHAPTER 6

Coronary Artery Disease

Ralph La Forge

Adults with stable and well-managed **cardiovascular disease (CVD)** represent a key opportunity for competent and experienced personal trainers or ACE-certified Advanced Health & Fitness Specialists (ACE-AHFS). According to the American Heart Association (AHA), an estimated 80.7 million American adults have one or more types of cardiovascular disease. Cardiovascular disease includes the following disease states: **hypertension** (73 million cases in the United States); **coronary artery disease (CAD)**, also known as **coronary heart disease (CHD)** (16 million); heart failure (5.3 million); and stroke (5.8 million) (AHA, 2007).

The purpose of this chapter is to briefly acquaint the ACE-AHFS with the CAD component of CVD, describe its process, and provide appropriate training recommendations. Hypertension, **diabetes, obesity,** and the **metabolic syndrome,** all of which impact the CAD process, are discussed elsewhere in this text. The ACE-AHFS is strongly encouraged to partner the information in this chapter with *ACSM's Guidelines on Exercise Testing and Prescription* (7th edition) [American College of Sports Medicine (ACSM), 2006] and the *ACE Clinical Exercise Specialist Manual* (ACE, 2007), both of which are good resources for the ACE-AHFS who wishes to work with individuals with stable CAD. There is remarkable agreement between these and other guidelines in terms of the recommended quantity and quality of exercise for those with CAD, although there are some minor differences [American Association of Cardiovascular and Pulmonary Rehabilitation (AACVPR), 2003; ACSM, 2006; AHA/American College of Cardiology (ACC), 2006; ACE, 2007]. The ACE-AHFS should see this chapter as somewhat of a synthesis and update of these guidelines.

Fundamentally, the role of the ACE-AHFS who wishes to work with individuals with CAD is to work only with those clients who have stable CAD and are at low risk for exercise-related cardiovascular complications. Furthermore, the principal role of the ACE-AHFS in this context is to design and allocate appropriate and safe levels of physical activity to improve the client's functionality, favorably modify CAD risk factors, and further improve the function of the heart. It is strongly recommended that the clients with whom the ACE-AHFS intends to work have successfully completed phase I and II cardiac rehabilitation by formalized outpatient cardiac rehabilitation programs when these programs are locally available. Phase I cardiac rehabilitation is the in-patient phase that includes teaching and low-level hospital-based ambulatory exercise, while Phase II is the early hospital discharge phase of rehabilitation and includes medically monitored exercise and more concentrated risk-factor education. Fewer than 30% of eligible patients receive phase II care, which would drastically narrow the population of individuals who could work with an ACE-AHFS. Therefore, the ACE-AHFS should target those individuals who have not gone through phase II rehabilitation, as well as those at risk for CAD.

Coronary Artery Disease

Coronary artery disease, also known as ischemic heart disease and atherosclerotic heart disease, is the end result of the accumulation of lipid-rich plaques within the walls of the arteries that supply the **myocardium** (the muscle of the heart). CAD results from the development of atherosclerosis in the coronary arteries. Atherosclerosis is a disease affecting arterial blood vessels. It is a chronic inflammatory response in the walls of arteries, in large part due to the deposition of **lipoproteins** (plasma proteins that carry cholesterol and triglycerides). Atherosclerosis is essentially caused by the formation of multiple plaques within the arteries (Figure 6-1). Today, atherosclerosis is seen not as a disease of the **lumen** of the artery, but a disease of the vessel wall. **Atherogenesis** is the process of the development of these plaques, which involves the infiltration, retention, and oxidation of **low-density lipoprotein (LDL)** cholesterol in the arterial intima, development of fatty streaks, and the calcification of atherosclerotic plaques. Under normal circumstances, the vascular **endothelium** does not bind **leukocytes** (white blood cells) well. However, injury to the endothelium (inner-most layer of the artery wall) causes inflammation that results in the expression of adhesion molecules that facilitate atherosclerosis. It is now understood that an acute coronary event, for example a **myocardial infarction,** is more often caused by rupture of a complicated and vulnerable atherosclerotic plaque than by a gradual closure of the coronary blood vessel.

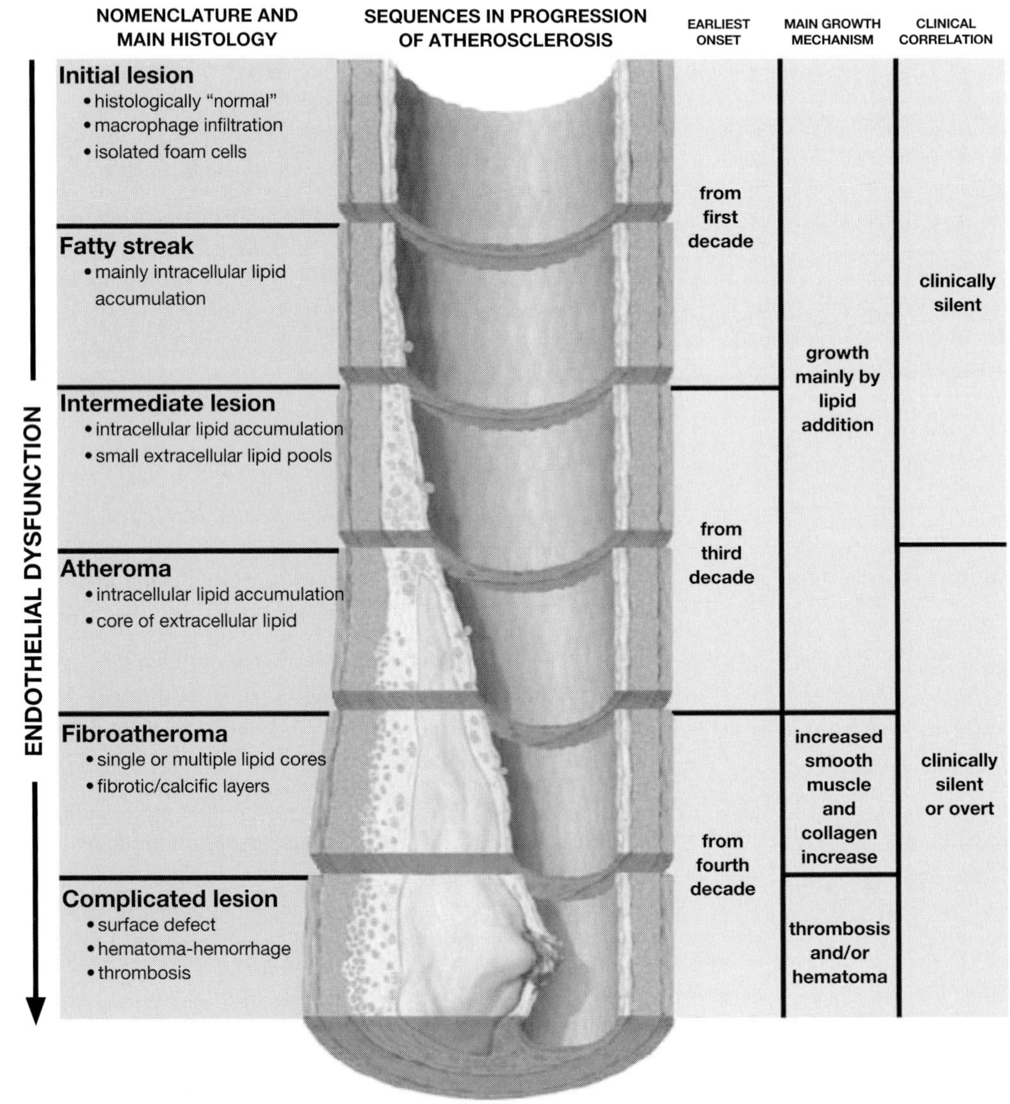

Figure 6-1
The atherosclerotic process: Response to injury

Source: www.en.wikipedia.org/wiki/Atherosclerosis

The vulnerable plaque is essentially characterized by plaques with thin fibrous caps that predispose the plaque to rupture. Rupture of the plaque releases numerous thrombotic substances into the blood that usually stimulate a rapid sequence of events that result in a clot or coronary thrombosis. The formation, progression, and rupture of the vulnerable plaque are viewed as a process related directly to inflammation.

Principal Diagnostic Tests for CAD

There are a number of reasons for a physician to order a battery of diagnostic tests to confirm or rule out cardiovascular disease. In many cases, those with mild to moderate CAD have no major complaints other than fatigue. As the disease progresses, they may develop **angina pectoris** during physical activity. This type of pain typically subsides with rest. It is not uncommon for these symptoms to be ignored. If a patient presents with complaints of periodic chest pain, a physician will likely be aggressive in his or her diagnostics. In some cases, the patient does not have any complaints signifying CAD, but due to his or her multiple risk factors, warrants a closer look (see Table 1-2, page 12). In addition to standard blood work assessing blood **lipids**, glucose, and inflammatory markers, diagnostic tests will be ordered to discover the likelihood of any clinically significant blockage.

Electrocardiogram

An **electrocardiogram (ECG)** is a graphic produced by an electrocardiograph machine, which records the electrical activity of the heart over time. Analysis of the various ECG waveforms and of electrical depolarization and repolarization yields important diagnostic information. Key waveforms of the ECG used for diagnostic purposes include the P wave, P-R interval, QRS complex, S-T segment, and T wave.

ECG Exercise Testing

Essentially, the exercise ECG test is a graded (gradual increase in speed and grade) exercise treadmill test with electrocardiographic recording. The test is considered "positive" if there is a specific standard level of change in the S-T segment component of the ECG. The important diagnostic information that is recorded during a stress ECG is as follows: ECG response (S-T segment, S-T slope, and potential **dysrhythmias**), heart rate (HR) and blood pressure response, symptoms (**angina,** shortness of breath or dyspnea, or dizziness), and the exercise level achieved [e.g., **metabolic equivalent (MET)** capacity]. ECG stress testing can be employed for diagnostic or functional assessment. For functional assessment, the test is used primarily to evaluate the patient's symptomology, MET capacity, and training heart-rate response. The ECG stress test is not as effective as a diagnostic tool as a nuclear stress test.

Radionuclide Stress Test

Radionuclide stress testing involves injecting a radioactive isotope (typically thallium or cardiolyte) into the person's vein, after which an image of the heart becomes visible with a special camera. The radioactive isotopes are absorbed by the normal heart muscle. Nuclear images are obtained in the resting condition and again immediately following exercise. The two sets of images are then compared. During exercise, if a significant blockage in a coronary artery or arteries results in diminished blood flow to a part of the cardiac muscle, this region of the heart will appear as a relative "cold spot" on the nuclear scan, signifying reduced or diminished blood flow. This cold spot may not be visible on the images that are taken while the patient is at rest (when coronary flow is adequate). Radionuclide stress testing, while more time-consuming and expensive than a simple exercise ECG, greatly enhances the accuracy in diagnosing CAD.

Stress Echocardiography

Another supplement to the routine exercise ECG is **stress echocardiography** (cardiac ultrasound). During stress echocardiography, the sound waves of an ultrasound are used to produce images of the heart at rest and at the peak of exercise. In a heart with normal blood supply, all segments of the left ventricle exhibit enhanced contractions of the heart muscle during peak exercise. Conversely, in the setting of CAD, if a segment of the left ventricle does not receive optimal blood flow during exercise, that segment will demonstrate reduced contractions of the heart muscle relative to the rest of the heart on the exercise echocardiogram. Stress echocardiography is very useful in enhancing the interpretation of the exercise ECG, and can be used to exclude the presence of significant CAD in patients suspected of having a "false-positive" stress ECG.

Coronary Angiography (Cardiac Catheterization)

Coronary angiography involves inserting a catheter into the groin area and routing it into the coronary arteries of the heart. This procedure is done for both diagnostic and interventional purposes. A radio contrast agent is passed into the catheter and is visualized on a fluoroscope to evaluate coronary blood flow in the major arteries of the heart. The benefit of this procedure is that while the catheter is inside the heart, the cardiologist can perform a **percutaneous transluminal coronary angioplasty (PTCA).** This technique has several goals:

- To confirm the presence of a suspected blockage in a coronary artery
- To quantify the severity of the disease and its effect on the heart
- To seek the cause of a symptom such as angina, shortness of breath, or other signs of cardiac insufficiency
- To make a patient assessment prior to heart surgery

Vascular Imaging Techniques

Several invasive and noninvasive imaging techniques have been evaluated for use in characterizing atherosclerosis. Invasive coronary angiography has traditionally been the standard clinical tool for visualizing coronary arteries. Since its introduction more than 30 years ago, more than 2 million coronary angiograms have been performed annually in North America. Although coronary angiography is extremely useful in diagnosing obstructive atherosclerosis, it does not effectively define the extent of atherosclerosis in the vessel wall. Intravascular ultrasound is a newer invasive technique that allows for the direct observation of a vessel's plaque volume. The development of noninvasive cardiovascular techniques, such as computed tomography (CT) imaging of coronary artery calcium, CT angiographic imaging, B mode ultrasound of carotid intima-media thickness (CIMT), and cardiovascular magnetic resonance imaging (CMRI), has enabled the more practical non-invasive evaluation of atherosclerosis at a preclinical stage (see page 133).

Appropriate Program Candidates and Stable CAD

The individual in need of a supervised cardiac prevention program may not have diagnosed CAD, but instead merely be interested in preventing heart disease (primary prevention). Candidates for this program may also include those with multiple risk factors for CAD, but may never have had a cardiac event (secondary prevention). Those with documented CAD or unstable CAD are most appropriate for formalized and supervised cardiac rehabilitation. Ideally, the CAD client would have completed phase I and II cardiac rehabilitation programs prior to working with the ACE-AHFS. An experienced ACE-AHFS who wishes to work with CAD clients should work only with those who are under a physician's care and who have stable coronary disease. For purposes of the ACE-AHFS **scope of practice,** stable CAD means that the individual's disease process is well managed (i.e., he or she does not have irregular, unpredictable symptoms, unstable angina, heart failure, or malignant ventricular arrhythmias). Stable also means that the individual is currently under the care of a physician and on appropriate medical therapy for his or her level of CAD. The ACE-AHFS is not expected to discriminate between stable and unstable CAD, but should rely on the client's personal physician's clinical evaluation and judgment—a physician who is currently caring for the client's disease. This physician can be a cardiologist, internist, or, in some cases, a primary care physician such as a family practitioner. One means of confirming stable CAD is periodic exercise electrocardiographic stress testing (exercise ECG) by a physician.

Noninvasive Vascular Imaging Techniques

Coronary CT Angiography

In CT angiography, computed tomography using a contrast material produces detailed pictures. CT imaging uses special x-ray equipment to produce multiple images and a computer to join them together in cross-sectional views. This new test is available to diagnose CAD. In the past, noninvasive functional tests of the heart were used, such as treadmill tests and nuclear studies, to indirectly assess if there were blockages in the coronary arteries. The only way to directly look at the coronary arteries was via a cardiac catheterization and coronary angiogram.

CT scans have been used to look at various anatomic regions, but have not been useful for the heart because the heart is continuously in motion. Today, a new generation of CT scanners that can take 64 pictures a minute is available; with the use of a little medication to slow the heart rate to less than 64, CT images of the coronary arteries are now possible.

High-resolution Magnetic Resonance Imaging

High-resolution cardiovascular magnetic resonance imaging (CMRI) of the arterial wall is emerging as a powerful research technology for characterizing atherosclerotic lesions within carotid arteries and other large vessels. High-resolution magnetic resonance imaging (MRI) is able to noninvasively characterize three important aspects of atherosclerotic lesions: size, composition, and biologic activity. It can quantify not only wall and lumen areas and volumes, but also plaque composition. For example, high-resolution MRI can assess cap thickness and distinguish ruptured plaque caps from thick and stable caps. This technique can also be used to characterize the composition of a plaque by differentiating lipid-free regions from lipid-rich and calcified regions. In addition, high-resolution MRI can identify recent intra-plaque hemorrhages using multi-contrast-weighted studies.

Intravascular Ultrasound

Intravascular ultrasound (IVUS) is a valuable adjunct to coronary angiography. While angiography provides only a two-dimensional assessment of the lumen of the target vessel, IVUS allows the tomographic measurement (the recording of internal body images at a predetermined plane) of artery lumen area, plaque size, plaque distribution, and to some extent, plaque composition. Because the arterial remodeling and plaque deposition that characterize the early stages of atherosclerotic progression occur without decreases in lumen area, IVUS may be able to detect atherosclerotic disease at an earlier state than coronary angiography. In many cases, IVUS may provide the ability to detect some "angiographically silent" **atheromas.**

Coronary Calcium Scoring

Coronary calcification is part of the pathogenesis of atherosclerosis and does not occur in normal vessels. Due to the association between coronary calcification and plaque development, radiographically detected coronary artery calcium (CAC) can provide an estimate of total coronary plaque burden. Studies have reported that CAC scores are independently predictive of CHD outcomes, even after controlling for a variety of risk markers (Greenland et al., 2004). Currently, the primary methods for CAC measurement are electron-beam computed tomography (EBCT) and multi-detector computed tomography (MDCT).

B-mode Ultrasound Assessment

B-mode ultrasound is a noninvasive imaging modality that employs ultrasound to accurately image the walls of arteries and is a useful tool for evaluating carotid intima-media wall thickness (CIMT). The normal arterial wall consists of three layers: the tunica intima, tunica media, and tunica adventitia. The thickness of the two innermost layers in the carotid artery (the intima and media), or the CIMT, is increasingly used as a surrogate marker for early atherosclerosis. Carotid ultrasound measurements correlate well with **histology,** and increased CIMT is associated with the presence of vascular risk factors and more advanced atherosclerosis, including coronary artery disease. Large observational studies have established that CIMT is an independent marker of risk for cardiovascular events. A meta-analysis of eight studies reported that the relative risk per one 0.10-mm difference in common carotid artery CIMT was 1.15 for MI and 1.18 for stroke, adjusted for age and sex (Lorenz, 2007).

Fitness Assessments

Initial Assessment by the ACE-AHFS

Once the ACE-AHFS has received an appropriate referral for training a CAD client, the first step is to review the individual's health history and lifestyle information. Both ACE and ACSM provide comprehensive advice regarding the infrastructure for developing necessary components and formats for this initial assessment (ACE, 2007; ACSM, 2006). The essential components of the pre-training assessment are as follows:

- Medical history
- Current medications
- Existing CAD risk factors (see Table 1-2, page 12)
- Symptoms
- Physical-activity history
- Dietary history

A **Physical Activity Readiness Questionnaire (PAR-Q)** evaluation is also recommended as part of the initial ACE-AHFS evaluation (see Figure 1-3, page 13).

Table 6-1
Overall Recommendations for Training Stable CAD Clients

- Unless otherwise indicated, follow general guidelines for individuals with CAD as put forth by ACSM (2006).
- Ensure that the individual is under appropriate medical care before recommending and/or supervising an exercise program.
- If available, have the individual's physician give a results summary of his or her most recent exercise ECG test (MET level achieved, exercise heart rate, and any relevant exercise-related symptoms).
- Be knowledgeable of the client's current medications and which ones may alter exercise heart rate (ACSM, 2006) (see Appendix C).
- Avoid having the individual exert to muscular contraction "failure."
- Always precede workouts with low-level activity, preferably low-level aerobic activity commensurate with the intensity of the primary conditioning activity.
- Use caution with high- or vigorous-intensity physical activity.
- Avoid sudden strenuous efforts with inadequate warm-up or prior lower-level activity.
- Avoid having the individual perform vigorous exercise when suffering from viral infections, colds, flu, etc.
- Understand and monitor signs and symptoms of cardiac decompensation (excessive shortness of breath, unusual or sudden-onset fatigue, palpitations, lightheadedness or dizziness, chest discomfort) for an extended period of time after cessation of the exercise session.

Fitness Testing

The ACE-AHFS can administer most fitness tests to clients with stable CAD, provided that the client meets the overall considerations in Table 6-1 and has no contraindications to resistance exercise (see Table 6-5, page 140). Appropriate fitness tests include flexibility, muscular endurance, and strength tests in which the client does not exert to muscular contraction "failure." Good cueing will prevent breath-holding (**Valsalva maneuver**). Inappropriate tests are those that push the client to a near-maximal perceived exertion, predicted heart rate, or **$\dot{V}O_2$max.** Submaximum aerobic-endurance tests may be performed, but only when the client has had a recent physician-supervised negative exercise ECG and is free from exercise-related cardiac symptoms (e.g., angina, dysrhythmias). The ACE-AHFS should adhere to the general procedures for submaximal testing of cardiorespiratory fitness as described in the 2006 ACSM guidelines (Table 6-2).

Essential Exercise Recommendations and Manifestations of CAD

The major benefits of exercise training include the following:

- Improved $\dot{V}O_2$max (aerobic capacity)
- Lessening of angina symptoms/raising of the ischemic threshold
- Modest decreases in body fat, blood pressure, total and LDL cholesterol, non–high-density lipoprotein (HDL) cholesterol, and triglycerides
- Increased HDL cholesterol
- Reduction in stress
- Control of diabetes mellitus
- Improved well-being and self-efficacy

Angina Pectoris

Angina pectoris is the discomfort in the chest, arms, shoulders, and even jaw that results from inadequate blood flow, and more specifically oxygen, to the heart. Angina that occurs regularly

Table 6-2
General Procedures for Submaximal Testing of Cardiorespiratory Fitness

- Obtain resting heart rate and blood pressure immediately prior to exercise in the exercise posture.
- The client should be familiarized with the ergometer. If using a cycle ergometer, properly position the client on the ergometer (i.e., upright posture, 5-degree bend in the knee at maximal leg extension, hands in proper position on the handlebars).
- The exercise test should begin with a two- to three-minute warm-up to acquaint the client with the cycle ergometer and prepare him or her for the exercise intensity in the first stage of the test.
- A specific protocol should consist of two- or three-minute stages with appropriate increments in work rate.
- Heart rate should be monitored at least two times during each stage, near the end of the second and third minutes of each stage. If heart rate is >110 beats/minute, steady-state heart rate (i.e., two heart rates within 5 beats/minute) should be reached before the workload is increased.
- Blood pressure should be monitored in the last minute of each stage and repeated (verified) in the event of a hypotensive or hypertensive response.
- Perceived exertion (using either the 6–20 or 0–10 scale) and additional rating scales should be monitored near the end of the last minute of each stage.
- Client appearance and symptoms should be monitored and recorded regularly.
- The test should be terminated when the subject reaches 70% heart-rate reserve (85% of age-predicted maximal heart rate), fails to conform to the exercise test protocol, experiences adverse signs or symptoms, requests to stop, or experiences an emergency situation.
- An appropriate cool-down/recovery period should be initiated consisting of either:
  - ✔ Continued exercise at a work rate equivalent to that of the first stage of the exercise test protocol or lower
  - ✔ A passive cool-down if the subject experiences signs of discomfort or an emergency situation occurs
- All physiologic observations (e.g., heart rate, blood pressures, signs and symptoms) should be continued for at least five minutes of recovery unless abnormal responses occur, which would warrant a longer post-test surveillance period. Continue low-level exercise until heart rate and blood pressure stabilize, but not necessarily until they reach pre-exercise levels.

Source: American College of Sports Medicine (2006). *ACSM's Guidelines for Exercise Testing and Prescription* (7th ed.). Philadelphia: Lippincott Williams & Wilkins.

with activity, upon awakening, or at other *predictable* times is termed **stable angina** and is associated with high-grade narrowings of the coronary arteries. Angina can be easily graded by a simple angina scale (Table 6-3). The angina pain scale is a useful tool for documenting client pain complaints in SOAP notes. The symptoms of angina are often treated with nitrate medicines such as nitroglycerin, which come in short-acting and long-acting forms, and may be self-administered transdermally or sublingually, or orally as needed. **Unstable angina** is angina that changes in intensity, character, or frequency. Unstable angina may precede myocardial infarction and requires urgent medical attention. Individuals who have unstable angina are not appropriate clients for the ACE-AHFS and should always be referred back to their physicians.

Exercise Guidelines for Stable Angina

The ACE-AHFS should ensure that these individuals are medically cleared and are stable. These clients have **myocardial ischemia** (insufficient blood supply to the heart muscle) and are relatively high risk within the category of all CAD patients. Any individual who experiences angina with physical workloads ≤3 METs (i.e., low

Table 6-3
Angina Scale

1 +	Light, barely noticeable
2 ++	Moderate, bothersome
3 +++	Severe, very uncomfortable
4 ++++	Most severe pain ever experienced

physical exertion levels) should not be trained by the ACE-AHFS.

- Progressive aerobic endurance exercise is recommended, as long as it is within the individual's exercise tolerance as indicated by the most recent exercise ECG, or is just below the **anginal threshold** or physician-recommended percent of $\dot{V}O_2$max.
- Intermittent, shorter-duration exercise on a more frequent basis [e.g., three to five sets of five- to 10-minutes of low- to moderate-intensity aerobic exercise bouts (e.g., cycling, treadmill walking)] may be most appropriate in the initial stages of training. Upper-extremity aerobic training (e.g., rowing or arm cranking) may initially exacerbate angina.
- Avoid breath holding, **isometric** exercises, or activities where the individual physically exerts to muscular contraction failure (i.e., very high-resistance exercise).
- Keep close observation of anginal symptoms and ensure that the individual understands when to take angina-resolving medications (e.g., nitroglycerin). Instances when the client uses angina-resolving medications should be documented for the client's physician.

For clients experiencing angina pectoris and who have been prescribed nitroglycerin PRN (as needed), the typical protocol is as follows:

- Discontinue activity and incorporate rest to see if chest discomfort/pain resolves on its own.
- If there is no relief, the client will self-administer one dose of nitroglycerin, either in tablet or spray form. A tablet will be placed sublingually (i.e., under the tongue) or between the cheek and gums. If a spray is used, it would be delivered in the same locations.

The client will then wait five minutes to see if the chest pain is resolved. If not, a second dose will be administered. He or she will then wait five more minutes and then repeat one more time before calling 911. Nitroglycerine is a vasodilator and will dilate vessels, allowing for a greater oxygen delivery to the heart. Side effects of nitroglycerin administration include severe headache and a drop in blood pressure.

Cardiac Dysrhythmias

Cardiac dysrhythmias are cardiac rhythm disturbances that can be of atrial, antrioventricular node (AV node), or ventricular origin. Many patients with CAD and/or who are post-MI or have had heart surgery have ventricular dysrhythmias. Some dysrhythmias are relatively benign, but some represent a high-risk state. For example, some rapid ventricular dysrhythmias can result in cardiac arrest. Cardiologists can prescribe several different classes of medicines or perform specific laboratory procedures (e.g., radio ablation or implantable defibrillators) that can reduce many types of cardiac dysrhythmias.

Cardiac dysrhythmias, especially ventricular arrhythmias, can be heart-rate and physical-effort related, and thus can be elicited by physical exercise. For this reason, the ACE-AHFS should be particularly conscious of symptoms that are induced by exercise-generated ventricular dysrhythmias. Such rhythm disturbances can come on during or after exercise. These symptoms include dizziness, lightheadedness, palpitations, and, in rare occurrences, **syncope** (fainting). Any individual with a history of exercise-induced dysrhythmias should be thoroughly evaluated by a cardiologist. Without physician clearance, these individuals should not be considered stable, although many are or can be well managed by their cardiologist. The two main cautions if such clients are referred to an ACE-AHFS are as follows:

- Always graduate the workload slowly, with no sudden cessation of moderate or vigorous exercise. Always graduate cool-down work.
- Avoid heavy resistance exercise or any exercise in which the client is exerting against

either an isometric load or very high resistance, particularly if the client also holds his or her breath or executes a Valsalva maneuver (expiration against a closed glottis). Inverted hatha yoga poses (head below the level of the heart) or rapid changes in body position are also not advised.

Myocardial Infarction

Acute myocardial infarction (MI), also known as a heart attack, is a medical condition that occurs when the blood supply to the heart muscle is interrupted, most commonly due to the rupture of a lipid-rich, vulnerable, plaque. The resulting oxygen shortage, or **ischemia,** causes damage and potential death of some of the heart muscle cells below the blockage. MI symptoms may include various combinations of pain in the chest, upper extremity, or jaw, or epigastric discomfort with exertion or at rest (i.e., mid-back pain). The discomfort associated with acute MI usually lasts at least 20 minutes. Frequently, the discomfort is diffuse, not localized, not positional, not affected by movement of the region, and may be accompanied by shortness of breath, **diaphoresis**, nausea, or syncope. ECG and cardiac biomarkers (e.g., cardiac troponin taken via blood test at the hospital) also help diagnose an MI. Patients frequently feel suddenly ill. Women often experience different symptoms from men. The most common symptoms of MI in women include shortness of breath, weakness, and fatigue. Approximately one-third of all myocardial infarctions are "silent," without chest pain or other symptoms. Acute MI is a type of **acute coronary syndrome,** which is most frequently (but not always) a manifestation of CAD. In approximately half of all MIs, this is the individual's first indication of CAD. It is very important that the ACE-AHFS be capable of recognizing the signs and symptoms of MI.

Depending on the location of the obstruction in the coronary arteries, different zones of the heart can become injured. Using standard anatomical terms of MI location, one can describe anterior, inferior, lateral, apical, and septal infarctions (and combinations, such as anteroinferior, anterolateral, and so on). For example, an occlusion of the left anterior descending coronary artery will result in an anterior wall MI.

Training the post-MI client requires adherence to precautions very similar to those followed with the angina client. The ACE-AHFS should never be in the position of training a client within four to six weeks of an MI and without direct written authorization and referral from the client's physician. Ideally, the client should have completed at least phase I and II cardiac rehabilitation or equivalent supervised exercise therapy. It is important, however, to note that more than 70% of post-MI patients do not get referred to, or have access to, formal cardiac rehabilitation programs. In such cases, it is imperative that the ACE-AHFS ensures that the individual has an appropriate physician evaluation prior to taking a referral. In all cases, clients should have a physician-supervised exercise ECG prior to working with the ACE-AHFS. All post-MI clients, but especially those with an MI within the preceding three or four months, should begin any and all exercise sessions with very low workloads (e.g., 2 to 3 METs) and progress very gradually. Most post-MI clients who have had symptom-free and negative exercise ECGs can progress to reasonably normal age- and gender-related aerobic and resistance work capacities over six to 12 months.

Congestive Heart Failure

One complication of CAD, particularly MI, is **congestive heart failure (CHF).** An MI may compromise the function of the heart as a pump for the circulatory system, a state called heart failure. There are different types of heart failure. Left- or right-sided heart failure may occur depending on the affected part of the heart, and it is a low-output type of failure. If one of the heart valves is affected, this may cause dysfunction, such as mitral valve regurgitation in the case of left-sided MI. The incidence of heart failure is particularly high in individuals with diabetes and requires special management strategies. These individuals, especially those who have poor **ventricular function** (i.e., the heart has a very poor pumping capacity), are at high risk for exercise-related complications. The ACE-AHFS should not train CHF clients unless otherwise appropriately and specifically authorized by physician referral. There are exceptions among those with New York Heart Association Class I or II CHF (mild CHF with no or slight physical limitations), where low-level progressive exercise is appropriate and helpful. Low-level aerobic activity (2 to 5 METs) and many restorative yoga poses are beneficial when appropriately taught by experienced and qualified yoga teachers.

Post–coronary Artery Bypass Grafting and Percutaneous Transluminal Coronary Angioplasty Intervention

Two interventions most often employed in CAD patients are **coronary artery bypass grafting (CABG)** and percutaneous transluminal coronary angioplasty (PTCA). PTCA will usually include intracoronary stenting (using a wire mesh device to open the artery). The ACE-AHFS can work with all of these clients, as long as they have no complications and are stable from symptom, ventricular function, and ECG perspectives. Most often, these individuals require aggressive risk-factor control, especially blood lipid and blood pressure management. The ACE-AHFS should follow the exercise guidelines and precautions in this chapter for all CAD clients. The most important thing for CABG clients, however, is to avoid traditional resistance-training programs with moderate to heavy weights for the first six weeks post-surgery. This will enable the sternum sufficient time to heal from the CABG sternotomy (surgical opening of the sternum). Graduated upper-extremity range-of-motion exercises and many hatha yoga poses that do not place undue strain on the sternum or upper back are recommended for clients who have had CABG within the previous four to eight weeks. As with the post-MI client, the ACE-AHFS should see these individuals only after physician evaluation and referral.

The success rate for CABG can reach beyond 10 years, but those with multiple risk factors may see coronary blockages in as little as six years post-CABG. Unfortunately, the success rates for angioplasty are not as promising. Up to 30% of post-PTCA clients will experience **restenosis** within the first six months of the procedure. The ACE-AHFS working with clients who are post-PTCA or post-CABG should take notice of any of the following signs and symptoms of restenosis:

- Complaints of general fatigue
- Reduced exercise tolerance or accelerated HR at customary workloads
- Any symptoms of chest discomfort or pain

Since CAD is common among the American population, an astute ACE-AHFS may pick up on these subtle complaints in any of the populations he or she serves.

Essential Recommendations for Exercise Training of the Stable CAD Client

Overall Exercise Energy Expenditure Goals

To optimize the potential for improvement of CAD risk factors and stabilize the disease process, clients should prioritize achieving a total volume of physical activity of 1500 to 2000 kcal or more per week (ACSM, 2006). This volume includes systematic workouts, recreational activities, and **activities of daily living.** The ACE-AHFS must understand how to estimate the energy cost of various physical activities in terms of kcal per session, per day, and per week (Howley, 2006; Ainsworth, Haskell, & Leon, 1993). The ACE-AHFS should adhere to the overall recommendations for exercise in clients with stable CAD as presented in Table 6-1.

Exercise Intensity

Exercise intensity or exercise workload is perhaps the most important, and pliable, component of the exercise program. Work intensity most directly relates to the workload placed on the heart and the coronary arteries. Exercise speed, movement velocity, and resistance load all increase the workload of the heart, primarily through increased heart rate and blood pressure. The two most practical intensity-monitoring strategies for the ACE-AHFS are the client's volitional response to the exercise workload [e.g., **ratings of perceived exertion (RPE)**] and exercise heart rate.

In some cases, HR response may be blunted due to medications (e.g., beta blockers).

ACSM (2006) recommends that the initial stages of aerobic-conditioning programs for low-risk and stable CAD clients have an exercise intensity of 40 to 50% of heart-rate reserve (i.e., approximately 40 to 50% of $\dot{V}O_2max$) or 2 to 4 METs. However, it should be assumed that in most cases the ACE-AHFS will be working with clients who are not in the initial stages of training, but who are in the improvement or maintenance stage of conditioning, in which case an intensity range of 60 to 85% of heart-rate reserve (60 to 85% of $\dot{V}O_2max$) is more appropriate. The majority of CAD clients will do well with 30 to 60 minutes of exercise. For durations of 45 minutes or longer, exercise intensity should be in the moderate range [i.e., 40 to 60% of heart-rate reserve (40 to 60% of $\dot{V}O_2max$)]. It is important to understand that some CAD clients fail to achieve predicted maximal heart rates in the absence of medications that lower heart rate (e.g., beta-blocking agents). This phenomenon is known as **chronotropic incompetence**. These individuals are at higher risk for CVD complications and probably are not within the ACE-AHFS scope of practice.

A good but simple estimate of cardiac workload intensity can be determined using the product of exercise heart rate and **systolic blood pressure (SBP)** divided by 100:

> **The Double Product**
> Myocardial (heart muscle) work = Heart rate (in beats per minute) x Systolic blood pressure (mmHg) / 100
>
> For example:
> 150 beats/minute x 150 mmHg/100 = 225

This expression is known as the **double product,** but is also sometimes referred to as the **rate-pressure product** and corresponds to the anginal threshold (i.e., the point at which angina symptoms occur). Intensive aerobic activities significantly increase heart rate but moderately increase systolic blood pressure, whereas intensive resistance workloads (e.g., resistance training) moderately increase heart rate but cause a more significant rise in systolic blood pressure. Both forms of exercise can dramatically raise the "double product" and therefore raise cardiac workload. Cardiac symptoms and heart-muscle dysfunction are directly related to exertional heart rate and blood pressure. It is not practical for the ACE-AHFS to calculate the double product for each exercise session, but he or she should thoroughly understand the consequences of various aerobic, resistance, and even mindful exercise modalities (e.g., hatha yoga styles, Pilates) and how they influence cardiac work.

It is important for the ACE-AHFS to understand which physical activities and exercises can rapidly increase systolic blood pressure. For example, during heavy resistance exercise where an individual is exerting at ≥80% of maximum voluntary contraction levels, SBP increases quickly along with the **diastolic blood pressure (DBP).** Additionally, when a person exerts to muscular failure during resistance exercise, the ACE-AHFS can assume a peak or near-peak blood pressure response. Even for individuals with relatively stable CAD, this level of arterial pressure (also called "afterload"), which the heart has to pump against, can be dramatic and deserves serious caution.

Exercise Time

Exercise duration for most CAD clients in the maintenance stage of conditioning is usually set between 30 and 60 minutes per day. However, as mentioned previously, many clients will require 60 or more minutes per day to adequately manage body weight, dyslipidemia, and associated risk factors. CAD, diabetes, and metabolic syndrome clients should have exercise programming dosed by daily or weekly energy expenditure rather than separately quantifying only frequency, intensity, and time/duration. The total energy expenditure of the exercise sessions is perhaps the single most important program feature associated with risk-factor reduction.

In most cases, the CAD client will require an activity program that is at least 1500 kcal/week gross energy expenditure. In the case of a CAD client with the metabolic syndrome, **atherogenic**

dyslipidemia, and obesity, the physical-activity program's energy expenditure most often should be ≥2000 kcal per week (gross kcal cost) to meaningfully alter these risk factors. Of course, these energy expenditures are a function of activity mode, frequency, duration, and intensity and therein lies an opportunity for the ACE-AHFS and the client to work together to design a creative and productive activity program. Once again, to constructively do this, the ACE-AHFS will need a good working knowledge of the energy costs of a broad range of physical activities (Ainsworth, Haskell, & Leon, 1993; ACSM, 2006). Refer to Table 7-7, page 159 for a sample program.

Progression to Independent Exercise

For those clients who have been in formal cardiac rehabilitation programs and progress to independent exercise programs in the community, the guidelines in Table 6-4 are appropriate. Note that these guidelines are mostly dependent on recent exercise ECG testing information.

Resistance Training

Resistance-training modalities can clearly improve the client's muscular fitness and functionality. Because there are so many permutations of resistance delivery devices and protocols, certain precautions are important to note. The primary consideration for the ACE-AHFS in this context is the amount and rate of force delivered to the client's muscles relative to his or her capacity and cardiac ventricular function. Table 6-5 denotes criteria for the resistance training of CAD clients. In this instance, resistance training applies to the use of free weights, machines, or other resistive devices that deliver a resistive force ≥40% of the client's maximum voluntary contraction capacity. Table 6-6 describes absolute and relative contraindications to resistance training for individuals

Table 6-5
Criteria for Resistance Training of CAD Clients

- Minimum five weeks after MI or CABG or three weeks after PTCA, including two weeks of supervised cardiorespiratory endurance training
- No evidence of:
    - ✔ Congestive heart failure
    - ✔ Uncontrolled dysrhythmias
    - ✔ Severe cardiac valvular disease
    - ✔ Uncontrolled hypertension
    - ✔ Unstable symptoms

Note: CAD = Coronary artery disease; MI = Myocardial infarction; CABG = Coronary artery bypass grafts ; PTCA = percutaneous transluminal coronary angioplasty

Source: American College of Sports Medicine (2006). *ACSM's Guidelines for Exercise Testing and Prescription* (7th ed.). Philadelphia: Lippincott Williams & Wilkins.

Table 6-4
Guidelines for Progression to Independent Exercise with Minimal or No Supervision

- Estimated functional capacity of ≥7 METs (or measured ≥5 METs) or twice the level of occupational demand
- Appropriate hemodynamic response to exercise (increase in SBP with increasing workload) and recovery
- Appropriate ECG response at peak exercise with normal or unchanged conduction, stable or benign arrhythmias and non-diagnostic ischemic response (i.e., <1 mm ST-segment depression)
- Cardiac symptoms stable or absent
- Stable and/or controlled baseline HR and BP
- Adequate management of risk-factor intervention strategy and safe exercise participation such that the client demonstrates independent and effective management of risk factors with favorable changes in those risk factors
- Demonstrated knowledge of the disease process, abnormal signs and symptoms, medication use and side effects

Note: MET = Metabolic equivalent; SBP = Systolic blood pressure; ECG = Electrocardiogram; HR = Heart rate; BP = Blood pressure

Source: American College of Sports Medicine (2006). *ACSM's Guidelines for Exercise Testing and Prescription* (7th ed.). Philadelphia: Lippincott Williams & Wilkins.

with CAD. These also apply to higher-intensity yoga programs (e.g., Bikram or "hot" yoga and Ashtanga or "power" yoga). The ACE-AHFS should not place him- or herself in the position to recognize these clinical contraindications, but should ensure physician clearance for these contraindications. Table 6-7 lists recommendations for appropriate resistance-training programming and progression. There are no contraindications to Pilates exercises, provided that the same guidelines are adhered to as stated in Tables 6-5, 6-6, and 6-7. As long as the client is not straining to concentrically or eccentrically contract a muscle group or performing breath-holding, Pilates mat or reformer work can be very beneficial to his or her core strength.

Table 6-6
AHA 2007 Contraindications to Resistance Training

Absolute Contraindications
- Unstable CAD
- Decompensated heart failure
- Uncontrolled symptoms
- Severe pulmonary hypertension
- Severe and symptomatic aortic stenosis
- Acute myocarditis, endocarditis, or pericarditis
- Uncontrolled hypertension (>180/110 mmHg)
- Aortic dissection
- Marfan's syndrome
- High-intensity resistance training (80–100% of 1 RM) in clients with active proliferative retinopathy or moderate or worse nonproliferative diabetic retinopathy

Relative Contraindications
- Major risk factors for CHD
- Diabetes at any age
- Uncontrolled hypertension (>160/100 mmHg)
- Low functional capacity (<4 METs)
- Musculoskeletal limitations
- Individuals who have implanted pacemakers or defibrillators

Note: CAD = Coronary artery disease; CHD = Coronary heart disease; MET = Metabolic equivalent 1 RM = One-repetition maximum

Source: American Heart Association (2007). Resistance exercise in individuals with and without cardiovascular disease: 2007 update. A scientific statement from the American Heart Association. *Circulation,* 116, 572–584.

Table 6-7
Recommendations for the Initial Resistance-training Program

Resistance training should be performed:
- In a rhythmical manner at a moderate to slow controlled speed
- Through a full range of motion, avoiding breath-holding and straining (Valsalva maneuver) by exhaling during the contraction or exertion phase of the lift and inhaling during the relaxation phase
- Initially alternating between upper- and lower-body work to allow for adequate rest between exercises

The initial resistance workload should:
- Allow for and be limited to 8–12 repetitions per set for healthy sedentary adults or 10–15 repetitions at a low level of resistance for at-risk adults; for example, <40% of 1 RM for older (>50–60 yrs of age), more frail persons, or cardiac clients
- Be limited to a single set performed two days a week
- Involve the major muscle groups of the upper and lower extremities (e.g., chest, shoulder, triceps, biceps, upper back, lower back, abdominals, quadriceps, hamstrings, and calves)

Note: 1 RM = One-repetition maximum

Source: American Heart Association (2007). Resistance exercise in individuals with and without cardiovascular disease: 2007 update. A scientific statement from the American Heart Association. *Circulation,* 116, 572–584.

Mindful Exercise and the CAD Client

Select forms and styles of mindful exercise modalities are most often appropriate or can be easily adapted for clients with CAD (see Appendix D in the *ACE Personal Trainer Manual*). Table 6-8 lists more suitable forms of mindful exercise that are appropriate for the majority of individuals with CAD.

Mindful exercise programs can range from those requiring very low energy expenditure and deep relaxation qualities to levels that require

Table 6-8
Some Appropriate Forms of Mindful Exercise for Clients With CAD

• Restorative yoga	• Tai chi chuan (moderate pace)
• Kripalu yoga	• Tai chi chih
• Viniyoga	• Yogic breathwork
• Integral yoga	• Pilates mat and reformer work
• Select Iyengar and yoga poses	• NIA at low-to-moderate level

Note: CAD = Coronary artery disease; NIA = Neuromuscular integrative action considerable muscular strength and impose considerable myocardial work. Thus, several considerations are important when choosing particular mindful exercise modalities. Many styles of hatha yoga, for example, involve acute dynamic changes in body position (i.e., the relationship of the head, chest, and lower limbs to each other). It is therefore important to fundamentally understand the **hemodynamic** and cardiac ventricular responses to such exercise and how these may alter cardiac function in individuals with CAD, including clients with hypertension, metabolic syndrome, or diabetes.

Inverted poses where the head is below the heart (e.g., downward facing dog or headstands), or situations in which such a position is alternated with a "head-up" pose, should be avoided. In most cases, those who are initially deconditioned and/or have CAD should minimize acute changes in body position that require the head to be positioned below the level of the heart in early stages of hatha yoga training and use slower transitions from one yoga pose to the next. Because Ashtanga and Iyengar yoga poses and sequences generally require considerable strength, flexibility, and mental concentration, they should be reserved for higher functioning individuals (i.e., clients with >12 MET exercise capacity). Some yoga poses significantly increase blood pressure and may also be inappropriate for older adults with stage II or higher hypertension (i.e., blood pressures ≥160/105 mmHg). One study on intermediate and advanced yoga practitioners showed that some Iyengar poses can rapidly and significantly increase mean and peak systolic blood pressure, particularly with back arch poses (Blank, 2006). This level of blood pressure could impose significant double-product stress on the heart of some CAD clients, particularly if the stress is a sudden increase in systolic blood pressure rather than the gradual workload increase seen with graduated aerobic exercise work levels. It is strongly recommended that the ACE-AHFS start the client with restorative yoga poses prior to engaging in a full complement of Iyengar or equivalent yoga poses.

Perhaps most useful in those with any level of CAD is **yogic breathing.** Although there are many styles of yogic breathing, the breath is generally drawn through the nose during both inhalation and exhalation. Each breath is intentionally slow and deep with an even distribution, or smoothness, of effort. Lengthening exhalations by using the abdominal muscles to expire more air while breathing through the nose will cause a relaxation response. In addition to reduced stress and mental tension, cardiovascular benefits result from yogic breathing. One of the mechanisms responsible for the mental quiescence experienced with yogic breathing is its stimulation of the **parasympathetic nervous system.** When fully stimulated by adequate yogic inspiration and expiration, mechanical receptors in pulmonary tissue (e.g., alveoli) activate parasympathetic nerves, which transiently reduces mental tension and elicits as relaxation response (Pal & Velkumary, 2004). A suitable inhalation/exhalation ratio is to inhale for a 2-count, exhale for a 4-count, and then work up to inhaling for an 8-count and exhaling for a 16-count. To test this relaxation response, the client can feel his or her pulse during this breathing exercise. He or she may notice a reduced pulse rate with prolonged exhalation. This slight slowing of heart rate includes a reciprocal slight increase in heart rate variability—a process that is also called respiratory sinus arrhythmia. Acute reductions in blood pressure also have resulted from yogic breathing training (Murrgesan, Govindarajulu, & Bera, 2000).

Case Study

A 44-year-old mother of three with a history of stage I hypertension, angina, and documented CAD is referred to the ACE-AHFS by an internist. She has a family history of CAD and her father had a myocardial infarction. She has a positive treadmill ECG with mild angina (1 on 4-point scale), achieved a heart rate of 154 bpm, and reached 11 METs. She has been participating in a low-level walking program (five days/week; two-mile walk at 2 to 3 mph).

- Weight: 165 lb (75 kg)
- Height: 5'6" (1.7 m)
- BMI: 36

- Waist circumference: 36 inches (91 cm)
- LDL cholesterol: 115 mg/dL
- HDL cholesterol: 49 mg/dL
- Triglycerides: 195 mg/dL
- Blood pressure: 134/90 mmHg

Medications: Carvedilol (6.25 mg), simvastatin (20 mg), and sublingual nitroglycerin as needed.

Exercise plan: As a supplement to her walking program, the following is added: 1000 kcal/week of a combination of three sessions/week of elliptical trainer exercise (starting with two 10-minute sessions at low-to-moderate level stride rate and progressing to one continuous 30-minute session over a six-week period, keeping exercise heart rate between 120 and 140 bpm). An effort is made to ensure that she is remaining compliant with her medications and low-fat, low-glycemic dietary program. Total weekly physical-activity training energy expenditure is 1900 to 2000 kcal.

Follow-up: At four months, she has lost 11 pounds (5 kg). Her new statistics and labs are as follows:

- Weight: 154 lb (70 kg)
- BMI: 33
- Waist circumference: 34 inches (86 cm)
- LDL cholesterol: 92 mg/dL
- HDL cholesterol: 51 mg/dL
- Triglycerides: 155 mg/dL
- Blood pressure: 130/84 mmHg

One 60-minute variable-terrain walk per week was added, along with two circuit weight-training sessions/week (one or two sets of 10 exercises at 15 RM). Total weekly energy expenditure, including existing walking/elliptical program is 2500 to 2700 kcal.

This client's goals are as follows:

- Weight: <145 lb (66 kg)
- BMI: <30
- Waist circumference: < 30 inches (76 cm)
- LDL cholesterol: <70 mg/dL
- HDL cholesterol: >50 mg/dL
- Triglycerides: <150 mg/dL
- MET capacity: >13 METs

In the absence of significant further reduction in LDL cholesterol, her physician may choose to increase the simvastatin dose to 40 mg. Note that with documented CAD, her ideal therapeutic option LDL cholesterol goal is 70 mg/dL.

Summary

Exercise therapy for the prevention and treatment of CAD works well beyond its moderate lipid-lowering effects by improving functional capacity, antioxidant defenses, arterial endothelial function, insulin sensitization, glucose transport, fibrinolytic capacity, and psychological well-being, and by reducing blood pressure and body fat stores. Ideally, the CAD client would have completed phase I and II cardiac rehabilitation program prior to working with the ACE-AHFS. An experienced ACE-AHFS who wishes to work with CAD clients should work only with those who are under a physician's care and who have stable coronary disease. To optimize the potential for improvement of CAD risk factors and stabilize the disease process, clients should achieve a total volume of physical activity of 1500 to 2000 kcal or more per week. This volume includes systematic workouts (including aerobic, resistance, and select mindful exercise training), recreational activities, and activities of daily living.

References

Ainsworth, B.E., Haskell, W.L., & Leon, A.S. (1993). Compendium of human physical activities: Classification of energy costs of human physical activities. *Medicine & Science in Sports & Exercise,* 25, 71–80.

American Association of Cardiovascular and Pulmonary Rehabilitation (2003). *Guidelines for Cardiac Rehabilitation and Secondary Prevention Programs* (4th ed.). Champaign, Ill.: Human Kinetics.

American College of Sports Medicine (2006). *ACSM's Guidelines for Exercise Testing and Prescription* (7th ed.). Philadelphia: Lippincott Williams & Wilkins.

American Council on Exercise (2007). *ACE Clinical Exercise Specialist Manual*. San Diego, Calif.: American Council on Exercise.

American Council on Exercise (2003). *ACE Personal Trainer Manual* (3rd ed.). San Diego, Calif.: American Council on Exercise.

American Heart Association (2007). Heart disease and stroke statistics—2008 update. A report from the American Heart Association Statistics Committee and Stroke Statistics Subcommittee: 2008 Heart and Stroke Statistical Update. *Circulation,* Dec. 17 online.

American Heart Association/American College of Cardiology (2006). AHA/ACC guidelines for secondary prevention for patients with coronary and other atherosclerotic vascular disease: 2006 update. *Journal of the American College of Cardiology*, 47, 2130–2139.

Blank, S. (2006). Physiological responses to Iyengar yoga poses performed by trained practitioners. *Journal of Exercise Physiology,* 9, 7–23.

Greenland, P. et al. (2004). Coronary artery calcium score combined with Framingham score for risk prediction in asymptomatic individuals. *Journal of the American Medical Association,* 291, 210–215.

Howley, E. (2007). Energy costs of physical activity. In: Howley, E. & Franks, B.D. (Eds.) *Health and Fitness Instructor's Manual* (5th ed.). Champaign, Ill.: Human Kinetics.

Lorenz, M.W. et al. (2007). Prediction of clinical cardiovascular events with carotid intima-media thickness: A systematic review and meta-analysis. *Circulation,* 115, 459–467.

Murrgesan, R., Govindarajulu, N., & Bera, T.K. (2000). Effect of yogic practices on the management of hypertension. *Indian Journal of Physiological Pharmacology,* 44, 207–210.

Pal, G.K., & Velkumary, S. (2004). Effect of short-term practice of breathing exercises on autonomic functions in normal human volunteers. *Indian Journal of Medical Research,* 120, 115–121.

Suggested Reading

American Council on Exercise (2007). ACE *Clinical Exercise Specialist Manual*. San Diego, Calif.: American Council on Exercise.

American Heart Association (2007). Heart disease and stroke statistics—2008 update. A report from the American Heart Association Statistics Committee and Stroke Statistics Subcommittee: 2008 Heart and Stroke Statistical Update. *Circulation,* Dec. 17 online.

American Heart Association (2003). Exercise and physical activity in the prevention and treatment of cardiovascular disease: A statement from the Council of Clinical Cardiology. *Circulation,* 107, 3109–3116.

Schairer, J.R. & Keteyian S.J. (2006). Exercise training in patients with cardiovascular disease. In: Kaminsky, L.A. et al. (Eds.) *ACSM's Resource Manual for Guidelines for Exercise Testing and Prescription* (5th ed.). Philadelphia: Lippincott Williams & Wilkins.

In This Chapter

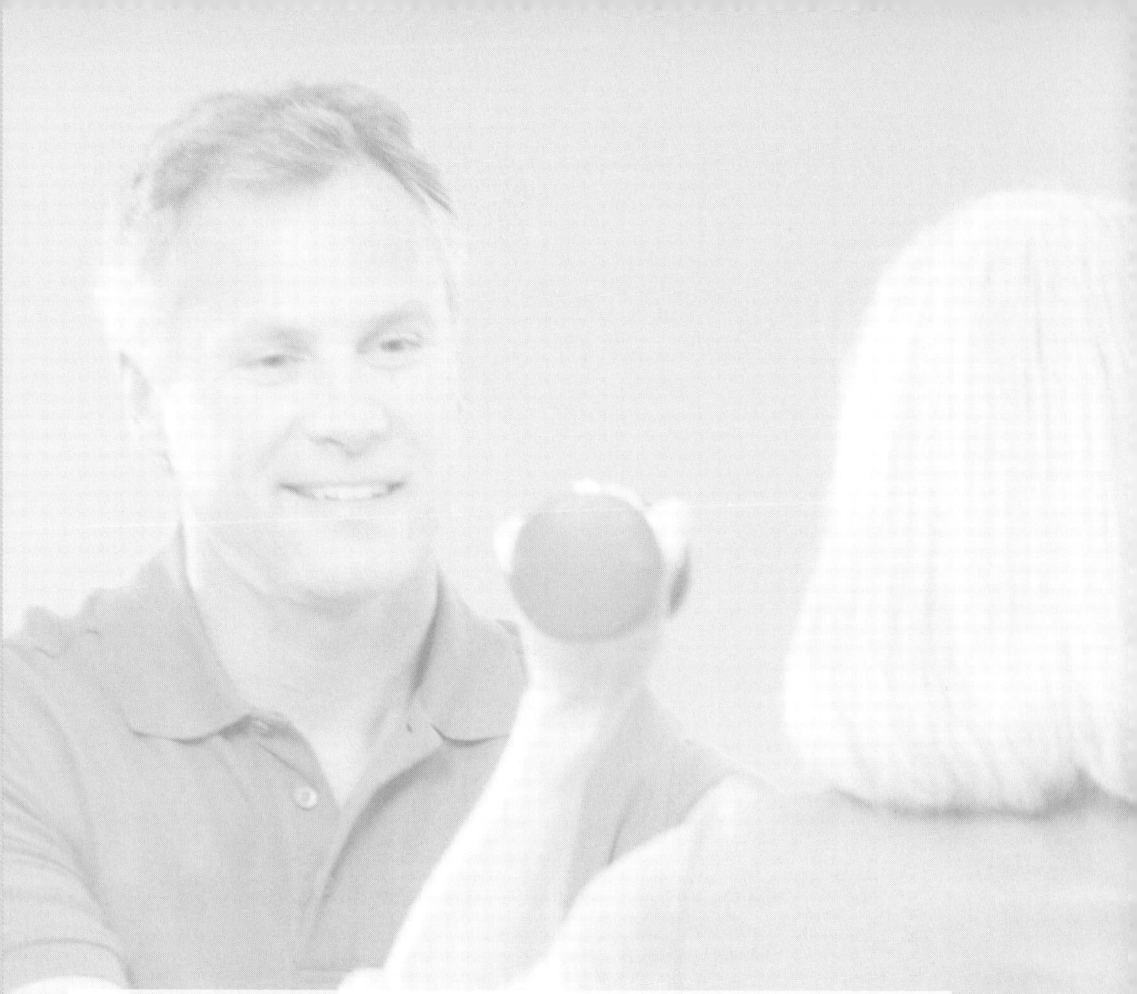

About The Author

Ralph La Forge, M.S., is a physiologist and Accreditation Council on Clinical Lipidology–certified clinical lipid specialist and is the managing director of the Cholesterol Disorder Physician Education Program at Duke University Medical Center, Endocrine Division in Durham, North Carolina. Formerly, he was managing director of preventive medicine and cardiac rehabilitation at Sharp Health Care in San Diego, where he also taught applied exercise physiology at the University of California at San Diego. Prior to that, La Forge was director of preventive cardiology and cardiac rehabilitation at the Lovelace Clinic in Albuquerque, New Mexico. He has helped more than 300 medical staff groups throughout North America organize and operate lipid disorder clinics and diabetes- and heart-disease-prevention programs. La Forge has published more than 300 professional and consumer publications on exercise science and preventive endocrinology/cardiology.

CHAPTER 7

Blood Lipid Disorders

Ralph La Forge

Risk Factors for Coronary Artery Disease

It is imperative that the ACE-certified Advanced Health & Fitness Specialist (ACE-AHFS) understand the principal **coronary artery disease (CAD)** risk factors, as most of these are favorably altered by physical activity. The principal risk factors for CAD include elevated **low-density lipoprotein (LDL)** cholesterol, low **high-density lipoprotein (HDL)** cholesterol, high blood pressure, smoking, and **diabetes.** Of course, **obesity,** age, gender, family history, and stress all play a role, but the central focus of both lifestyle and pharmacologic therapy is on the principal risk factors. Physical activity, weight loss, smoking cessation, dietary behavior changes, and reduction in stress play key behavioral roles in the modification of these principal atherosclerotic risk factors. Other serum and biomarkers of atherosclerotic risk have also been identified, including the following: elevated **triglycerides (TG),** LDL cholesterol particle number, and apolipoprotein B levels; low apolipoprotein A-1 levels; elevated lipoprotein(a); and high C-reactive protein, coronary calcium score, and lipoprotein-associated phospholipase A2. This chapter addresses the importance of blood lipid disorders (**dyslipidemia**) in the prevention and management of CAD. With the exception of smoking, the other principal risk factors are adequately discussed in this text.

Blood Lipid Disorders (Dyslipidemia)

In terms of reducing the risk of CAD progression or a recurrent heart attack, the ACE-AHFS should prioritize a systematic approach to physical activity for the CAD client, while also helping him or her achieve optimal blood lipid control—ideally through therapeutic lifestyle changes. The ACE-AHFS should also understand the role of pharmacotherapy.

A large body of data has established that **serum cholesterol** and associated **lipoproteins** are crucial risk factors for **atherosclerosis.** Blood lipid disorders (also called dyslipidemia or **dyslipoproteinemia**) represent an important modifiable risk factor for the development and progression of **coronary heart disease (CHD).** The 2007 Heart and Stroke Statistical Update, published by the American Heart Association (AHA, 2007), reports that 35.6% of Americans were told that they have high **cholesterol** levels, with the highest percentage in West Virginia at 39.9%. The ACE-AHFS can play a pivotal role in curbing this growing incidence and work directly with physicians in the management of lipid disorders.

Lipids, Lipoproteins, and Atherosclerosis

Cholesterol is a fatty substance that travels in the blood in distinct particles that contain both lipids and proteins. These particles are called lipoproteins. The cholesterol level in the blood is determined partly by genetics and partly by lifestyle factors such as diet, body fat, exercise, and even psychological stress. There are four major classes of lipoproteins found in the blood of a fasting individual:

- Very-low-density lipoprotein (VLDL)
- Low-density lipoprotein (LDL)
- High-density lipoprotein (HDL)
- Non-HDL

VLDL Cholesterol

VLDL is a major carrier of triglycerides in the **plasma.** Triglyceride is a major form of **fat.** A triglyceride consists of three molecules of **fatty acid** combined with a molecule of **glycerol.** Synthesized in the liver, triglyceride-rich VLDL carries endogenously (produced by the body) synthesized triglycerides and cholesterol to their sites of utilization. VLDL also contains 10 to 15% of the body's total serum cholesterol. Increased concentrations of VLDL are associated with a number of lipoprotein disorders, such as familial **hypertriglyceridemia,** obesity, diabetes, and **nephrotic syndrome.** Triglycerides do not accumulate in the vessel wall. Their atherogenicity is based on their association with other substances in the blood. For example, elevated triglycerides tend to be associated with low HDL cholesterol and elevated LDL-particle concentration, especially in individuals with the **metabolic syndrome.** So the risk of having elevated triglycerides is based primarily on its association with other lipoproteins. A very high triglyceride level (>500 mg/dL) is associated with other clinical problems such as **fatty liver** and pancreatitis.

LDL Cholesterol

LDL cholesterol is the major carrier of cholesterol in the circulation. It contains 60 to 70% of the body's total serum cholesterol and is directly correlated with the risk for coronary heart disease. LDL cholesterol and LDL particles play a pivotal role in **atherogenesis,** the early stages of atherosclerosis. This role is illustrated in Figures 7-1 and 7-2, which describe LDL cholesterol infiltration into the arterial endothelium and fatty streak and plaque formation. Although all blood lipids play a role in the development of atherosclerosis, epidemiologic studies suggest that LDL cholesterol is the most significant blood lipid. Without a threshold level of LDL cholesterol and LDL particles, atherosclerosis is rare, despite the presence of other risk factors. LDL cholesterol also is the primary focus of most blood-lipid-lowering therapies. Plasma LDL concentrations are regulated by specialized LDL receptors on the arterial endothelium. When there is a defect in the gene for the synthesis of the LDL receptor, plasma LDL concentrations increase, as seen in individuals with familial **hypercholesterolemia.** Table 7-1 depicts various LDL-cholesterol-lowering strategies and their respective efficacy.

Table 7-1
Generalized Comparative LDL-cholesterol Reduction Strategies

	% LDL Reduction
Dietary modification of fat (e.g., 10–30% dietary fat)	5–35%
Weight loss (e.g., 2–10% fat weight loss)	5–20+%
Exercise training (e.g., 1000–2000 kcal of physical activity/week)	5–15%
Drug therapy (statins, cholesterol transport inhibitors) (e.g., pravastatin 10 mg to rousuvastatin 40 mg)	15–65%

Note: LDL = Low-density lipoprotein

HDL Cholesterol

HDL cholesterol is formed in the intestine and liver. HDL normally contains 20 to 30% of the body's total cholesterol, and HDL levels are inversely correlated with coronary heart disease risk. HDL plays an important role in reverse cholesterol transport (i.e., removal of cholesterol from cells and transporting it back to the liver). By removing excess cholesterol from the circulation, HDL may provide a protective mechanism against the development of atherosclerosis. Research has shown that each mg/dL increase in plasma HDL cholesterol concentration is associated with approximately 3% reduction in CAD risk (Gordon, Probstfield, & Garrison, 1989).

Non-HDL Cholesterol

Non-HDL cholesterol is a very important lipid measure that is strongly associated with the

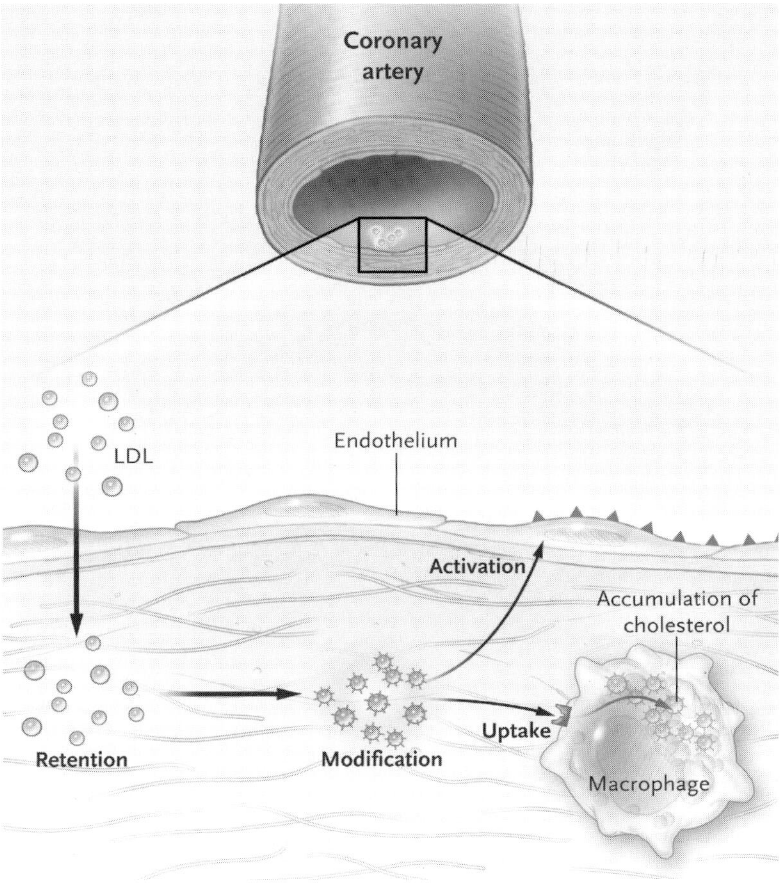

Figure 7-1
Impact of LDL cholesterol infiltration on coronary artery inflammation

Source: Hansson, G.K. (2005). Mechanisms of disease: Inflammation, atherosclerosis, and coronary artery disease. *New England Journal of Medicine*, 352, 1685–1695.

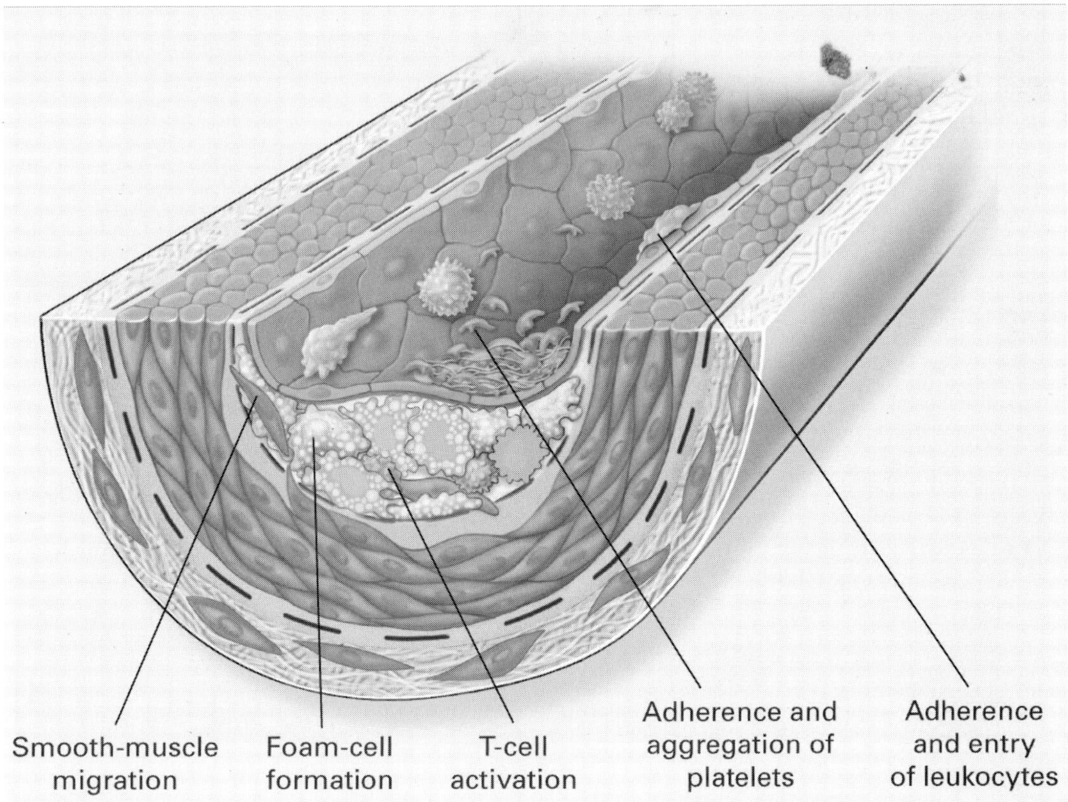

Figure 7-2
Fatty streak formation in atherosclerosis

Source: Ross, R. (1999). Atherosclerosis: An inflammatory disease. *New England Journal of Medicine,* 340, 115–126.

ever-increasing prevalence of obesity, metabolic syndrome, and **type 2 diabetes,** and thus should be of special therapeutic interest to fitness professionals, particularly the ACE-AHFS and lifestyle coaches. Non-HDL should be specifically used as a measure of risk, particularly in those individuals who have fasting triglycerides above 200 mg/dL (e.g., those who have type 2 diabetes, the metabolic syndrome, or who are obese).

Non-HDL cholesterol is calculated as follows:

> Non-HDL cholesterol =
> Total cholesterol – HDL cholesterol

The goal for non-HDL cholesterol is the same number as for LDL-cholesterol for that particular individual, plus 30 mg/dL. For example, someone with diabetes or cardiovascular disease might have an LDL-cholesterol goal of <100 mg/dL. Therefore his or her non-HDL goal would be <130 mg/dL. LDL-cholesterol is still the principal target of therapy for most patients with, or at high risk for, **cardiovascular disease (CVD)** and for all patients with type 2 diabetes, but especially those with both CVD and diabetes. In contrast to LDL cholesterol, non-HDL cholesterol values can be calculated in non-fasting patients without measuring triglycerides.

Why is non-HDL so important? Non-HDL cholesterol level is a more comprehensive measure of atherogenic particles than LDL cholesterol level. Available data suggest that non-HDL cholesterol level is as good as, or better than, LDL cholesterol in predicting cardiovascular risk, especially in individuals who have elevated triglycerides (e.g., those with the metabolic syndrome and/or diabetes) (Cui et al., 2001; Lu et al., 2003; Jiang, 2004; Bittner, 2004).

Non-HDL cholesterol is also a good marker for apoprotein B (also designated as apoB), which is even more atherogenic than the calculated non-HDL. ApoB is a measure of total atherogenic particle load and includes a measure of both triglyceride-rich lipoproteins and LDL cholesterol (i.e., there is one apoB particle attached on the surface of each of these atherogenic lipoproteins). The laboratory assay for apoB has been standardized and is available in most clinical laboratories. Exercise training studies in healthy men and women have demonstrated significant reductions in apo B in comparison to LDL cholesterol (Holme, Hostmark, & Anderssen 2007; Ring-Dimitriou et al., 2007).

In both sexes, non-HDL cholesterol levels correlate closely with obesity and especially **visceral obesity** (Denke, Sempos, & Grundy, 1994). In contrast to total cholesterol and LDL cholesterol, non-HDL cholesterol responds very well to dietary and physical-activity changes, especially in children as demonstrated in the Bogalusa Heart Study (Srinivasan, Myers, & Berenson, 2002). As noted previously, non-HDL cholesterol is a good marker for apoprotein B, which is even more atherogenic than the calculated non-HDL, though apoprotein B is more difficult to measure. An optimal goal for apoprotein B levels would be <80 mg/dL, which would define low-risk.

Other Lipoproteins and Associated Biomarkers of CVD Risk

Besides the major lipoproteins and lipids described earlier, there are other lipoproteins, apoproteins, and lipoprotein fractions such as lipoprotein (a) [also designated as Lp(a)]; apoproteins A, B, C, D, and E; and various subfractions of VLDL, LDL, and HDL [e.g., large- and small-dense LDL cholesterol (also designated as LDL phenotype A and B, respectively)]. These lipoproteins are largely used to more definitively diagnose specific lipid disorders and to provide additional CVD risk prediction. For example, Lp(a) is structurally similar to LDL both in protein and lipid composition and is related to thrombotic (blood coagulation) risk. When significantly elevated (i.e., >30 mg/dL), Lp(a) can also help define coronary heart disease risk, but screening for Lp(a) in the general population is not suggested at this time. Lipoprotein subfractions (e.g., the smaller LDL-particle size) can also help further predict CVD risk, but their measurement requires more advanced laboratory technology [e.g., **nuclear magnetic resonance (NMR)** instrumentation]. The apolipoproteins lie on the surface of the larger lipoproteins and act as **ligands** (points that attach to various receptors) for target receptors and regulate lipoprotein metabolism. Their measurement can help determine the cause, many times genetic, of a particular lipid disorder. For example, in the case of some forms of hypertriglyceridemia, apo CII and apo CIII expression can be the culprit.

Supportive Clinical Trials

Landmark primary and secondary prevention trials involving aggressive cholesterol lowering, especially of LDL cholesterol, have demonstrated significant clinical benefits, including atherosclerotic plaque regression, diminished atherosclerosis progression, increased arterial function, decreased coronary events (e.g., heart attacks), decreased **stroke** incidence, and decreased cardiovascular disease mortality (Sacks et al., 1996; Pederson et al., 1994; Shepard et al., 1995; Gotto, 1997; Downs et al., 1998; Rubins et al., 1999; Collins et al., 2003; Colhoun et al., 2004; Cannon et al., 2004; Petersen et al., 2005; LaRosa et al., 2005). Likewise, trials have shown CAD regression with intensive cholesterol-reduction therapy (Nissen et al., 2006; Ballantyne, 2008). In an older but well-controlled trial, Pitt, Mancini, and Ellis (1995) demonstrated that early aggressive lipid management significantly reduces clinical events such as heart attack, the need for coronary artery bypass surgery, and angioplasty after fewer than six months of therapy. Even in those who were clinically free of coronary heart disease (and had average total cholesterol and LDL), systematic reduction of lipids and lipoproteins has been shown to significantly reduce the incidence of first heart attacks and revascularization procedures (Downs et al., 1998). Evidence also indicates that women benefit from lipid lowering in a way that is similar to men (Pederson et al., 1994; Sacks et al., 1996; Colhoun et al., 2004). Furthermore, adverse changes in plasma lipids and lipoproteins that occur with age in sedentary women are not observed in women who regularly exercise (Stevenson et al., 1995 & 1997; Owens et al., 1992).

The use of a NMR imaging spectroscopy assay to assess lipoproteins has demonstrated that measuring the number of LDL cholesterol particles (i.e., LDL particle concentration or particle number) has shown much promise. There is evidence that the LDL particles themselves, not just LDL cholesterol, are the atherogenic culprits in CAD. Cromwell and others have convincingly shown that in a number of patient populations, but especially in those with the metabolic syndrome, LDL particle number is a better predictor of CVD incidence than LDL cholesterol (Cromwell & Otvos, 2007; Cromwell et al., 2007; Otvos et al., 2006). LDL particle number has a relationship with LDL cholesterol (e.g., 100 mg/dL of LDL cholesterol is equal to ~1100 nm/L of LDL particles).

National Cholesterol Education Program (NCEP) Guidelines

In 2002, the Third Report of the Expert Panel on Detection, Evaluation, and Treatment of High Blood Cholesterol in Adults (Adult Treatment Panel III) was published (abbreviated as ATP III) (NCEP, 2002). It is the most definitive set of guidelines for diagnosing and managing dyslipidemia. The understanding and application of these guidelines is essential for an ACE-AHFS who wishes to work with dyslipidemic individuals.

Two important features in this report are the addition of the metabolic syndrome and multiple risk factors, and the Framingham CHD risk scoring tool (see Appendix E), including several modifications to the lipid and lipoprotein classification. Clinical trial findings have shown that LDL cholesterol target goals are impacted by the presence of multiple CHD risk factors (e.g., smoking and high blood pressure). The other major addition to ATP III is the addition of the diagnosis of the metabolic syndrome. Table 7-2 presents the current classifications of LDL cholesterol, total cholesterol, and HDL-cholesterol, while Table 7-3 presents the classifications for triglycerides.

In 2004, NCEP ATP III was updated (Grundy et al., 2004) and further clarified that more recent research trials have clearly demonstrated that LDL target goals are best determined by global coronary heart disease risk (Table 7-4). This update necessitates the use of the Framingham risk scoring table to classify low, intermediate, high, and very high CHD risk (see Appendix E). These tables estimate the percent probability of a major coronary event (death or a heart attack) over the next 10 years. The following sections present these risk classifications and their relationships with LDL cholesterol goals.

Table 7-2
ATP III Classification of LDL, Total Cholesterol, and HDL Cholesterol (mg/dL)

LDL Cholesterol	
<100	Optimal
100–129	Near optimal/above optimal
130–159	Borderline high
160–189	High
≥190	Very high
Total Cholesterol	
<200	Desirable
200–239	Borderline high
≥240	High
HDL Cholesterol	
<40	Low
≥60	High

Note: LDL = Low-density lipoprotein; HDL = High-density lipoprotien

Table 7-3
Triglycerides (mg/dL)

Normal	<150
Borderline-high	150–199
High	200–499
Very high	≥500

High and Very High Risk

For high-risk individuals, the overall goal remains an LDL level of less than 100 mg/dL. But for people at very high risk, a group that is considered a "subset" of the high-risk category, the update offers a new therapeutic option of reducing LDL to under 70 mg/dL. For very-high-risk people whose LDL levels are already below 100 mg/dL, there is also an option to use drug therapy to reach the <70 mg/dL goal. Note that the very-high-risk category is reserved only for individuals with established cardiovascular disease plus other risk factors.

The NCEP defines high-risk individuals as those who have coronary heart disease or disease of the blood vessels to the brain or extremities, diabetes, or two or more risk factors (e.g., smoking, hypertension) that give them a greater than 20% chance of having a heart attack within 10 years.

Very-high-risk individuals are those who have cardiovascular disease together with either multiple risk factors (especially diabetes), or severe and poorly controlled risk factors (e.g., continued smoking), or the metabolic syndrome (a constellation of risk factors associated with obesity, including high triglycerides and low HDL). Patients hospitalized for acute coronary syndromes such as heart attack are also at very high risk.

Table 7-4
ATP III LDL Cholesterol Goals and Cutpoints for TLC and Drug Therapy in Different Risk Categories and Proposed Modifications Based on Clinical Trial Evidence

Risk Category	LDL Goal	Initiate TLC	Consider Drug Therapy
High risk: CHD or CHD risk equivalents (10-year risk >20%)	<100 mg/dL (optional goal: <70 mg/dL)	≥100 mg/dL	≥100 mg/dL (<100 mg/dL; consider drug options)
Moderately high risk: 2+ risk factors (10-year risk: 10 to 20%)	<130 mg/dL (optional goal: <100 mg/dL)	≥130 mg/dL	≥130 mg/dL (100–129 mg/dL; consider drug options)
Moderate risk: 2+ risk factors (10-year risk: <10%)	<130 mg/dL	≥130 mg/dL	≥160 mg/dL
Low risk: 0–1 risk factor	<160 mg/dL	≥160 mg/dL	≥190 mg/dL (160–189 mg/dL; consider drug options)

Note: LDL = Low-density lipoprotein; TLC = Therapeutic lifestyle changes; CHD = Coronary heart disease

Moderate and Moderately High Risk

For moderately high-risk individuals, the goal remains an LDL <130 mg/dL, but the update provides a therapeutic option to set a lower LDL goal of <100 mg/dL and to use drug therapy at LDL levels of 100 to 129 mg/dL to reach this lower goal. Moderately high-risk individuals are those who have multiple (two or more) risk factors for coronary heart disease together with a 10 to 20% risk of heart attack within 10 years. Moderate-risk individuals also have multiple risk factors, but a less than 10% risk of heart attack within 10 years.

Low Risk

Low-risk individuals have fewer than two risk factors and an LDL-cholesterol goal of <160 mg/dL (see Table 7-4).

The Metabolic Syndrome

The metabolic syndrome, also termed the insulin resistance syndrome—a cluster of factors associated with increased risk for CHD and diabetes—is becoming increasingly common, largely as a result of the increase in the prevalence of obesity (Grundy et al., 2004; Grundy, 2006). The core metabolic risk factors are elevated blood triglycerides, low HDL cholesterol, elevated blood pressure, elevated plasma glucose, a prothrombotic state, and a pro-inflammatory state. The root causes of this syndrome are **overweight**/obesity, physical inactivity, and genetic factors. On the basis of data collected in the 1990s from the National Health and Examination Survey III data, an estimated 47 million U.S. residents have the metabolic syndrome (more likely >50 million today, considering the population growth since the 1990s). The main purpose of identifying individuals with the metabolic syndrome is not to predict CHD or CAD, but to get healthcare providers to pay more attention to the medical aspects of obesity and its complications and to prioritize lifestyle therapy, especially physical activity and healthier dietary behavior.

The term **cardiometabolic risk** has been used to describe a broadened view of the metabolic syndrome. Cardiometabolic risk is essentially defined by a merger of the traditional Framingham CHD risk factors (e.g., smoking, cholesterol, diabetes) and the metabolic syndrome risk factors. Cardiometabolic risk goes beyond the metabolic syndrome. It encompasses a cluster of modifiable risk factors and markers that identify individuals at increased risk of cardiovascular disease (**myocardial infarction,** stroke, **peripheral arterial disease**) and type 2 diabetes. That said, one important utility of the metabolic syndrome itself is that it is a better predictor of persons at high risk for type 2 diabetes than traditional Framingham CHD risk factors (Stern, Williams, & Haffner, 2002). Prospective population studies have shown that the metabolic syndrome confers a twofold relative risk for atherosclerotic cardiovascular events (e.g., heart attack) and a fivefold increase in risk compared with people who do not have the syndrome (Grundy et al., 2005).

Although it is generally agreed that first-line clinical intervention for the metabolic syndrome is lifestyle change, this is insufficient to normalize the risk factors in many patients, and so residual risk could be high enough to justify drug therapy. Elevated triglycerides, low HDL cholesterol, elevated plasma glucose, and excess abdominal fat are among the core metabolic risk factors. A more thorough description and management strategy for the metabolic syndrome is discussed in Chapter 11.

Medications for Dyslipidemia

As indicated in the most recent NCEP guidelines, drug therapy should be considered only after patients have received at least six months of nonpharmacologic therapy, specifically intensive dietary and exercise therapy. Exceptions may include those with overt coronary heart disease, including post–myocardial infarction patients who have lipid disorders. It is important for the ACE-AHFS to recognize these drugs and understand their effects on blood lipids and lipoproteins. The drug classes and drugs most commonly prescribed for patients with lipid disorders include the following.

Bile acid sequestrants (cholestyramine, colestipol, colesevelam): These agents bind bile acids in the small intestine and cause decreased bile acid absorption, in turn lowering total and LDL cholesterol. The agents are available as dry powders in bulk or individual packets, and are usually consumed within one hour of eating and/or are taken with the evening meal. The bile acid sequestrants are quite effective for patients younger than age 55 who have LDL cholesterol between 160 and 220 mg/dL. Side effects are primarily gastrointestinal, with constipation being the most common.

Nicotinic acid (niacin, niaspan, niacor): Niacin is a water-soluble B vitamin that is very effective in lowering LDL cholesterol and triglycerides, but is especially utilized to increase HDL cholesterol when used in relatively high doses (>1,500 mg/day). Nicotinic acid is relatively inexpensive, making it an attractive choice as either single therapy or in combination with other drugs, such as statins. Its chief side effects include significant cutaneous flushing and vasodilatation. Niacin must be used with caution in patients with liver disease, diabetes, or gout and those at risk for peptic ulcer disease. It is important to note that many over-the-counter (OTC) forms of "niacin" consist of inositol hexanicotinate (often termed "no-flush niacin") and are relatively void of sufficient free nicotinic acid, and therefore do very little for LDL, triglycerides, or HDL.

HMG-CoA reductase inhibitors (also known as statins, which include lovastatin, pravastatin, simvastatin, fluvastatin, atorvastatin, rosuvastatin, and pitavastatin in Japan): These drugs effectively lower LDL cholesterol by interfering with cholesterol synthesis. They are competitive inhibitors of HMG-CoA reductase, the enzyme responsible for the rate-limiting step in the cholesterol biosynthetic pathway. They also block the formation of mevalonic acid and decrease intracellular cholesterol synthesis. These drugs are the most effective and expensive class of medications available for lowering LDL cholesterol. Several of the statins have substantial clinical trial support for reducing cardiovascular morbidity and mortality, as well as clinical events and the need for cardiovascular intervention procedures.

Combination nicotinic acid and statin drugs: Advicor® and Simcor® are combination drugs that combine in one pill various combinations of niaspan and lovastatin (Advicor) and niaspan and simvastatin (Simcor).

Fibrates (gemfibrozil, fenofibrate): Gemfibrozil and fenofibrate primarily lower triglycerides and, to a lesser extent, increase HDL cholesterol by reducing VLDL (triglyceride) synthesis and increase VLDL clearance by increasing lipoprotein lipase activity.

Cholesterol transport inhibitors (ezetimibe): These drugs can lower LDL cholesterol by 15 to 20% and are frequently added to statin therapy to further boost LDL-lowering efficacy. Vytorin® (simvastatin + ezetimibe in several formulations) is a potent drug designed to lower LDL cholesterol by 40 to 65%.

Omega-3 fatty acids (select OTC brands or Lovaza®): Marine **omega-3 fatty acid** therapy (fish oil capsules) is prescribed for individuals with high or very high triglycerides. The prescription may be for 1 to 4 grams per day of omega-3 fatty acids in the presence of high or very high triglycerides (200 to 500 mg/dL or higher). It is important to understand that only at the higher intakes of omega-3 fatty acids (≥2 grams/day) are there significant reductions in triglycerides, whereas the lower dosages have other benefits not directly related to triglyceride lowering.

Other agents (non-FDA-approved): A variety of other nutritive and herbal OTC agents are available to consumers. Many of these agents (e.g., "natural cholesterol-lowering products") will be accompanied by ad campaigns claiming the power to lower blood cholesterol. For example, several red yeast rice–based supplements claim on their package inserts that they can lower LDL cholesterol by 13 to 16%. The same holds true for policosanol nutrient products (a sugar-case extract). While not particularly harmful, these products have claims of 15 to 25% reductions in LDL cholesterol. Guggulipid and green tea extract product campaigns also promote lipid lowering and may have some promise in select individuals, but lack controlled clinical trials substantiating their benefit. Consideration must also be given to the potential adverse interaction that these supplements may have when combined with prescription medications. Until better-controlled research is conducted and published, these supplements should not be considered primary modes of therapy in lipid management, and any client considering these supplements should first consult a licensed practitioner.

Overview of Cholesterol and Exercise

Exercise is not generally considered primary therapy for lipid disorders, especially in the current era of lipid-modifying drug therapy. This is unfortunate, because exercise of appropriate quality and quantity can clearly reduce cardiometabolic risk through nonlipid mechanisms, but it can also induce significant favorable changes in the lipid and lipoprotein profile, in part as a result of reductions in adiposity. One meta-analysis of 13 studies representing 613 subjects reported that only triglycerides were significantly altered as a result of exercise training (Kelley, Kelley, & Tran, 2005). However, one must apply caution when attempting to generalize large review studies. Depending on the type of blood lipid disorder and baseline lipids, exercise training of sufficient volume can quite favorably alter blood lipids. Dietary reduction of fat, especially **saturated** and **trans fat**; exercise; and weight loss are still the cornerstones of therapy for individuals who have elevated blood lipids, despite the overwhelming number of lipid-lowering drug trials and LDL-cholesterol-lowering drug promotional campaigns extolling the benefits of statin therapy. With the exception of those who have existing CAD and diabetes, the essential first steps of therapy should be diet and exercise. This recommendation is clearly emphasized in the NCEP ATP III guidelines.

One of the hallmark findings of lipid-lowering drug therapy is improved arterial endothelial function, primarily through enhanced nitric oxide formation and function (nitric oxide is the most potent endogenous arterial vasodilator). Improved endothelial function is thought by many to be one of the primary mechanisms responsible for reduced CVD morbidity and mortality (Bugiardini et al., 2004; Gotto, 1997). Research also has demonstrated similar improvements in endothelial function with sufficient exercise training (Hambrecht et al., 2000; Clarkson et al., 1999; Utriainen et al., 1996).

The Lipid/Lipoprotein Response to Exercise Training

Exercise training of sufficient volume (i.e., kcal energy expenditure per week) generally increases HDL cholesterol and lowers total cholesterol, LDL cholesterol, and triglycerides via a number of mechanisms, including reduced body-fat stores, decreased hepatic lipase activity, and increased lipoprotein lipase activity. Most studies demonstrating exercise-improved lipid profiles have involved subjects with relatively normal blood lipids. There are very few randomized controlled studies appraising the lipid response to exercise training in people with lipid disorders. It is very possible that individuals with lipid disorders may respond differently to a given dose of exercise, depending on the type of dyslipidemia (e.g., those with lipoprotein lipase deficiencies or specific apolipoprotein E genotypes). For most individuals, there appears to be a minimum weekly physical-activity volume required for significant changes in blood lipids. For example, Church and colleagues (2007) reported no significant change in body weight, lipids, or lipoproteins after six months of 400, 800, or 1200 kcal/week exercise training in 464 postmenopausal women. Higher exercise energy expenditure thresholds (e.g., >1,500 kcal/week) are likely required for individuals with elevated total and LDL cholesterol (Crouse et al., 1997; Kraus et al., 2002; ACSM, 2006).

As a general rule, fat weight reduction is required for the most favorable blood lipid response in those who have elevated total and LDL cholesterol. This volume of exercise (150 minutes or more per week, optimally 200 to 300 minutes per week, or ≥2000 kcal per week) is similar to that recommended for obesity (ACSM, 2006). If exercise is of sufficient volume, exercise intensity is not of primary importance in improving the overall blood lipid profile, although most research supports a minimum intensity of at least 40% of peak work capacity (Durstine & Moore, 1997; ACSM, 2006).

Table 7-5 lists factors that play a role in determining serum lipids and the exercise/blood-lipid response. This large number of factors is the reason

Table 7-5
Primary Factors Influencing Blood Lipids and the Exercise Blood Lipid Response

- Frequency, duration, and intensity of exercise (as these increase, total caloric expenditure increases)
- Type of lipid disorder (e.g., variety of genetic hyperlipidemias)
- Total exercise energy expenditure
- Length of training period (e.g., one month, six months, 18 months)
- Coexisting body-fat loss
- Corresponding and compensatory dietary changes
- Concomitant alcohol intake
- Baseline lipid values
- Plasma volume changes
- Gender and menopausal status
- Genetic factors, (e.g., apolipoprotein E isoforms)
- Biologic variation (seasonal and diurnal changes)

the exercise/blood-lipid response is complex and very individualized.

Decreased body fat tends to correlate reasonably well with reduced LDL cholesterol and increased HDL cholesterol, which is why it is important to periodically evaluate body-fat composition in dyslipidemic clients. Most exercise trials support between 700 and nearly 2000 kcal of exercise per week to significantly alter HDL cholesterol and, to a lesser extent, LDL cholesterol (Williams, 1998; Kokkinos et al., 1995; King et al., 1995; Kraus et al., 2002; Shadid et al., 2006).

Prospective Exercise Training Lipid and Lipoprotein Responses

Triglycerides

Compared to other lipids, such as LDL cholesterol, elevated blood triglycerides (TG) are generally more responsive to exercise training. Triglyceride mobilization and utilization appears to be in direct proportion to exercise energy expenditure. Blood triglycerides frequently decrease with exercise training, depending on baseline values and volume of exercise. Unlike total and LDL cholesterol, triglycerides generally decrease immediately after a session of high-volume endurance exercise (e.g., greater than 45 to 50 minutes of sustained effort), and remain lower for up to 48 hours after the session. Trejo-Gutierrez and Fletcher (2007) reported a mean exercise-induced reduction in triglycerides of 24% (range of 4% to 37%).

The exercise program should follow the optimal mode, intensity, duration, and frequency for fat-weight reduction (e.g., 40 to 70% of aerobic capacity for 40 to 60+ minutes, four to six days per week). Four days a week of endurance exercise (e.g., four miles/day of jogging or 400+ kcal of energy expenditure) has been shown in a number of research trials to significantly reduce TG, especially in individuals with elevated baseline triglycerides (Durstine & Haskell, 1994). Overall, a threshold of fat-weight loss may be required for sustained TG reduction. Additionally, a reduction in TG is generally associated with an increase in HDL cholesterol, especially in hypertriglyceridemic subjects.

Subjects who have familial hypertriglyceridemia (e.g., lipoprotein lipase or apo C-II deficiencies) will have fasting triglycerides well above 500 mg/dL and often greater than 1000 mg/dL. While there is very little published research on this population's response to exercise, it is important to note that a relatively high volume of exercise in addition to drug therapy will be the most appropriate combination therapy.

LDL Cholesterol and Total Cholesterol

Most studies evaluating the total cholesterol and/or LDL cholesterol response to exercise training have found zero to only moderate decreases in these lipids and lipoproteins. Many studies used inadequate exercise volumes and/or energy expenditure or failed to control for confounding variables such as training-induced changes in plasma volume, dietary habits, or seasonal variation in cholesterol and lipoproteins (Durstine & Haskell, 1994; Durstine et al., 2002).

The total and LDL cholesterol response to exercise training is quite variable, but tends to positively correlate with associated fat weight loss. LDL cholesterol reduction appears to be slightly more responsive than total cholesterol to endurance exercise training. When LDL cholesterol concentrations are lower (e.g., <130 mg/dL), the reduction has been inversely related to the distance run each week (Wood et al., 1983). Most studies have provided mixed findings for plasma cholesterol concentrations for male runners, female runners, cross-country skiers, and other endurance-trained athletes compared with inactive controls (Superko, 1991; Durstine & Haskell, 1994). More recent results from endurance-training studies have been more encouraging. For example, Halverstadt and colleagues (2007) reported a significant reduction in total cholesterol, LDL cholesterol, and LDL particle concentration in 100 sedentary, healthy 50- to 75-year-olds after 24 weeks of endurance training. Altena and colleagues (2006) compared the effects of four weeks of continuous versus intermittent aerobic exercise on lipoproteins and lipoprotein subfractions and likewise demonstrated significant reductions in total cholesterol, LDL cholesterol, and the total cholesterol:HDL cholesterol ratio. Inactivity also can induce increases in blood lipids. Slentz and colleagues (2007) have shown that 15 days of inactivity can increase LDL cholesterol and LDL particle number and that a modest amount of exercise (approximately 2 miles of walking per week at 40 to 55% of $\dot{V}O_2$**max**) can prevent this increase.

Exercise training that results in weight loss and plasma volume expansion is more likely to result in lower LDL cholesterol and total cholesterol. Most research indicates minimal thresholds of a 1000 kcal of exercise per week (e.g., 12 or more miles of walking per week). Ideally, 2000 kcal or more per week for four to six months is required for significant reductions in LDL cholesterol (ACSM, 2006).

HDL Cholesterol

Overall, there is a modest increase in HDL cholesterol in response to exercise training. When diet is held constant, Leon and Sanchez (2001) reported an average increase in HDL of 4.38% (range –5.8% to +25%) in response to exercise training. There have been mixed findings among studies investigating the relationship between exercise intensity and increases in HDL, with some studies reporting the necessity for more vigorous exercise intensities. Inactive subjects may not increase HDL through energy expenditure as easily as physically active subjects (Durstine & Moore, 1997). Individuals with various genetic forms of very-low-HDL cholesterol (**hypoalphalipoproteinemia**, HDL levels <30 mg/dL) in general will respond minimally to even high levels and volumes of exercise. There are several forms of familial hypoalphalipoproteinemia (genetically related very-low-HDL cholesterol) and the prevalence is approximately one in 50 adults.

Baseline fasting triglycerides also may contribute to the HDL-raising effects of exercise training. Couillard and others (2005) studied 200 men enrolled in the HERITAGE Family Study and demonstrated that regular endurance exercise training may be particularly helpful in men with low HDL cholesterol, elevated triglycerides, and abdominal obesity. Other research suggests that HDL cholesterol may transiently increase after a single bout of endurance exercise in men (Pronk, 1993; Visich et al., 1996). Park and Ransone (2003) observed a 6% increase in 24-hour HDL cholesterol (HDL2 and HDL3 subspecies) after 350 kcal of treadmill exercise at lactate threshold in 18 college-age men. There were no significant changes in HDL cholesterol when these subjects ran at 70% of lactate threshold. Triglycerides also may respond favorably to a single bout of exercise commensurate with an increase in HDL cholesterol. Such acute changes may be realized eight to 12 hours after 300 to 500 kcal of exercise. Sustained increases in HDL cholesterol and HDL-2 appear to require a relatively high exercise-volume threshold. This threshold ranges from running seven miles per week, or approximately 700 kcal (Kokkinos et al., 1995), to running 15 miles per week, or approximately 1500 kcal (Williams, 1996). Hartung (1995) reported that for each six miles run per week, HDL was approximately 3 mg/dL higher in both men and women. In general, for inactive individuals, ≥1,000 kcal per week of exercise above their weekly physical activity baseline may be necessary for significant increases in HDL cholesterol.

There is evidence that HDL cholesterol may be more responsive to a higher daily frequency of exercise (e.g., three 15-minute sessions vs. one 40-minute session). Baseline HDL cholesterol and genetic factors have a significant impact on the capacity to increase HDL via exercise. Research also indicates that exercise-induced HDL cholesterol increases can be independent of exercise intensity, especially in men and women older than 45 to 50 years of age (King et al., 1995; Crouse et al., 1997). Slentz and colleagues (2007) have shown that higher versus moderate volumes of exercise may in some cases be required for significant HDL cholesterol increases. Studies also demonstrate that older adults may take longer to increase HDL cholesterol with exercise training, perhaps as long as two years (King et al., 1995).

Exercise and Postprandial Lipemia

Postprandial lipemia is essentially the blood fat, particularly triglyceride, response to a meal. Depending on how much fat or sugar is consumed in a meal, a person with normal fasting triglycerides will increase their triglycerides by 120 to 300+ mg/dL for two to six hours after the meal. Those with visceral obesity, the metabolic syndrome, or type 2 diabetes can have much larger increases in post-meal triglycerides. The problem of prolonged elevated postprandial triglyceride states is that for the amount of time triglycerides are elevated much above 250 to 300 mg/dL there is diminished arterial function, lower HDL cholesterol, and exposure of the arterial wall to atherogenic lipoprotein particles (e.g., VLDL remnants). Over the past 10 years, there has been abundant research supporting the finding that sufficient exercise timed anywhere from one to 12 hours before a fat-rich meal will reduce postprandial lipemia by 25 to 40% (Zhang et al., 1998; Petitt & Cureton, 2003; Malkova & Gill, 2006). This observation was also found in men with baseline hypertriglyceridemia with a 30 to 39% reduction in postprandial triglycerides with moderate and vigorous exercise, respectively (Zhang, 2006). This somewhat blunted triglyceride response to high-fat or high-glycemic meals is one of the benefits of a daily aerobic exercise program.

Exercise Volume Programming for Overall Lipid Management

Although there will be significant individual variation, it appears that to improve overall lipoprotein status (LDL, HDL, non-HDL, and triglycerides), an exercise volume of at least 1,500+ kcal per week (e.g., running 15 miles or walking 20+ miles per week) may be the minimum necessary based on available research. Optimally, 2000 kcal/week or more is recommended. The ACSM guidelines (2006), based on numerous clinical trials, state that the exercise volume to reduce dyslipidemia should be consistent with the same guidelines for long-term weight control (Table 7-6). Table 7-7 depicts sample exercise protocols with approximate weekly energy expenditures ranging from 600 to 2000+ kcal per week.

Pedometer Stepcounts, Energy Expenditure, and Lipid Dyslipidemia

Systematic use of pedometers (pedometry) or walking stepcounts has been employed as an acceptable estimate of walking energy expenditure. For blood lipid changes or weight loss, the minimal weekly physical-activity goals should be at least 1500 kcal more than entry level physical activity (entry level being evaluated on the first visit). This weekly energy expenditure would be equivalent to about 30,000 or more walking stepcounts *beyond* the client's weekly baseline stepcount. The ACE-AHFS is encouraged to recommend reliable well-engineered pedometers to estimate walking energy expenditure. Perhaps most applicable would be the use of pedometer models that have a step filter, which is incorporated software that minimizes the recording of meaningless spontaneous movements. Optimal goals are ≥2000 kcal/wk, 200+ minutes per week, and/or ≥70,000 total steps per week.

As a general rule, about 2000 steps (+ or – approximately 150 steps) with a step-only pedometer is equivalent to approximately one mile, which is approximately 100 kcal of gross energy expenditure for individuals who are

Table 7-6
Dyslipidemia Physical-activity Guidelines

Based on known therapeutic effects of habitual physical activity, ACSM makes the following recommendations regarding exercise programs for persons with dyslipidemia:

- Primary activity: Aerobic exercise
- Intensity: 40–70% aerobic capacity ($\dot{V}O_2$)
- Frequency: 5 or more days per week
- Duration: 40–60 minutes

Note: This exercise program is consistent with recommendations for long-term weight control: 200–300 minutes/week of moderate physical activity or >2000 kcal/week.

Source: American College of Sports Medicine (2006). *ACSM's Guidelines for Exercise Testing and Prescription* (7th ed.). Philadelphia: Lippincott Williams & Wilkins.

Table 7-7
Sample Graduated Weekly Exercise Energy Expenditures [assumes 160–180 pound (72–81 kg) body weight] (values are expressed in estimated gross energy expenditure costs)

Protocol A (600–800 kcal/wk)
Monday, Wednesday, Friday: Walk 2 miles/day* = 600 kcal
Sunday: 20 minutes of low-level stationary cycling = 100 kcal

Protocol B (1000–1200 kcal/wk)
Monday, Wednesday, Friday: Walk 2 miles/day* = 600 kcal
Tuesday: Walk 3 miles* = 300 kcal
Sunday: Nine holes of golf or 30 minutes of singles tennis = 300 kcal

Protocol C (1500–1800 kcal/wk)
Monday, Wednesday, Friday: Walk 3 miles/day* = 900 kcal
Tuesday, Thursday: 30 min of cycling (50–60% $\dot{V}O_2$max) = 300 kcal
Sunday: 60 min of singles tennis plus 2-mile walk* = 500 kcal

Protocol D (2000+ kcal/wk)
5 days per week, average 300 kcal workout (e.g., 30- to 45-minute aerobic session) = 1500 kcal
1 day per week, perform a long slow-distance workout (e.g., 2-hour moderate- to fast-pace variable-terrain walk) = 600+ kcal

* Walking at moderate pace (2.5–4 mph)

within 10 to 20 pounds of their **ideal body weight.** Of course, for those individuals who have a significantly higher **body mass index (BMI)** (e.g., >35), the gross caloric cost per mile is greater (about 120 to 150 kcal per mile) and in proportion to their body weight.

Resistance Training and Lipid Disorders

As with hypertension management, resistance training is not recommended as the primary form of exercise therapy for individuals with blood lipid disorders. Resistance training certainly may be recommended as a component of a complete exercise program. Research has shown that the blood lipid response to strength training is negligible, with some studies reporting slight-to-moderate reductions in total and LDL cholesterol and others reporting no change (Tucker, Martin, & Harris, 1997; Boyden et al., 1993; Kokkinos et al., 1988). In a study of 8499 men, only those investing more than four hours a week to resistance training maintained this benefit (Tucker, Martin, & Harris, 1997). It is likely, therefore, that the blood lipid response to strength training is related to total net energy expenditure of the session (kcal per workout), as is the case with endurance exercise. One example of a relatively high-energy-expenditure resistance-training session is low-resistance, high-repetition circuit weight training performed for extended periods and approaching 300 kcal or more per session.

Essential Exercise-programming Steps for Individuals With Dyslipidemia

Step 1: Evaluate Health and Lifestyle History

- Relevant comorbidities
- Blood lipid history and current blood lipid profile
- Exercise treadmill test history if at high CVD risk
- Medications, especially lipid-altering medications
- Diet and exercise history

Clients with documented or suspected dyslipidemia frequently have other related clinical conditions (i.e., comorbidities) that also may influence exercise programming. Prolonged elevations in LDL cholesterol, for example, can increase the likelihood of CVD. Other conditions, such as diabetes, especially type 2 diabetes, and obesity, often coexist with lipid disorders and can influence the exercise-lipid response. Although many individuals who have primary lipid disorders do not have associated comorbidities, they should have a thorough health history conducted by the ACE-AHFS for the following conditions or comorbidities:

- Coronary artery disease
- Previous myocardial infarction
- Angina
- Diabetes
- Insulin resistance
- Hypertension
- Obesity
- Metabolic syndrome
- Peripheral vascular disease
- Renal disease
- Chronic obstructive pulmonary disease

Some of these conditions may necessitate a thorough examination by a physician and an exercise electrocardiogram (ECG). It is important in these instances that the ACE-AHFS obtain this medical information and use it to help establish the recommended mode, frequency, duration, intensity, and progression of exercise.

Step 2: Determine the Necessity for Additional Tests or Evaluations

Although the ACE-AHFS will not be in the position to administer or order these tests, he or she can educate the client's physician on ACSM's current recommendations for pre-exercise testing for individuals with lipid disorders. Exercise ECG testing may be required, depending on the client's risk category and planned level of exercise. If the client has existing or suspected diabetes or cardiovascular disease, and has not had an exercise ECG in more than two years, it is recommended that this test be administered by the physician or a qualified exercise laboratory. Please refer to the current ACSM recommendations for exercise testing (ACSM, 2006).

The following evaluations may be appropriate prior to beginning an exercise program for lipid management:

- Baseline lipid/lipoprotein profile
- Exercise ECG
- Physician evaluation
- Clinical dietary assessment and diet prescription
- Evaluation for dyslipidemia medications

Step 3: Perform Anthropometric Measures

Many lipid disorders are sensitive to changes in body-fat stores. For this reason, it is essential that an ACE-AHFS initially and serially assess valid measures of body fat. Body weight, abdominal girth (measured at the level just above the iliac crest, a measure of central visceral fat stores), and/or upper-body skinfolds (e.g., triceps or subscapular) as assessed by Lange or equivalent skinfold calipers should be recorded during the client's initial visit and at four- to six-week intervals throughout the course of exercise training. It is important to focus on the change in waist circumference, BMI, and anthropometric measures rather than their relationship to normative body-fat data. Total cholesterol, LDL cholesterol, non-HDL cholesterol, and triglycerides usually decrease with a diminution in body fat, especially abdominal or visceral fat reduction. HDL cholesterol may or may not directly correlate with fat-weight changes.

Step 4: Set a Realistic Target Lipid Goal for Exercise Therapy

It is important to emphasize that exercise-lipid responses vary among people and that the volume of exercise required for significant changes in blood lipids is generally at a higher weekly energy expenditure threshold than that for reducing blood pressure or improving psychological well-being. For this reason, it may take more time to realize the clinical benefits. The ACE-AHFS must be conservative with short-term lipid-reduction goals, especially with total and LDL cholesterol reductions. A 5 to 15% LDL cholesterol reduction or a 10 to 20% reduction in non-HDL cholesterol is generally a realistic goal for the first 12 to 16 weeks of exercise training, assuming sufficient weekly exercise energy expenditure. Because non-HDL cholesterol includes triglyceride-rich lipoproteins, it may be more responsive and a better target of exercise therapy than LDL cholesterol, depending on baseline LDL cholesterol and triglycerides. Many clients may take six months or longer to show significant decreases in total and LDL cholesterol. This is not unusual, as there are a considerable variety of lipid disorders and blood lipid phenotypes. When possible, the ACE-AHFS should incorporate other co-variants of lipid reduction, such as valid anthropometric measures of obesity and abdominal-visceral fat, to demonstrate progress toward predetermined goals.

Laboratory lipid-assessment values characteristically vary by 8 to 12%, based on biological variation, lab bias, and analytic factors. This is important to consider when interpreting serial blood lipid values. Examples of variation in LDL and HDL cholesterol concentration include hospitalization, **estrogen** replacement therapy, pregnancy, type 2 diabetes, smoking, acute infection, posture, venous occlusion, and seasonal and circadian biological variation. The National Heart, Lung, and Blood Institute (NHLBI) published a comprehensive set of recommendations for laboratories and healthcare providers on ensuring valid lipoprotein measurement and interpretation (NHLBI, 1995).

Step 5: Determine the Exercise Plan From Prior Health History, Level of Fitness, and Current Lipid Profile

The exercise plan should be written clearly and concisely and include exercise mode, frequency, duration, intensity, progression plan, and safety precautions. The client's health history and initial fitness level are integral to formulating the weekly volume. For example, for clients with stable CAD who have had a recent exercise ECG, it will be important to review exercise electrocardiographic and hemodynamic data to appropriately set the exercise intensity and duration range. The individual's exercise capacity in **metabolic equivalents (METs)** or measured $\dot{V}O_2$ will also be helpful in determining initial exercise work levels.

Overall, it may be most straightforward to program exercise by energy expenditure or total weekly caloric expenditure with pedometry (i.e., weekly stepcounts), or simply by duration and intensity. Initial weekly exercise volumes should be set realistically according to the client's initial level of fitness, body composition, and existing comorbidities. See Table 7-7 for a sample set of exercise energy-expenditure protocols. Since many clients may be significantly deconditioned and overweight, it may be most appropriate to start on a progressive walking program. In this case, walking distance, speed, and the difficulty of the terrain should be gradually increased over the course of the program to generate higher energy expenditures. Since overall blood lipid improvement is responsive to weekly exercise volumes (total physical activity energy expenditures) and exercise-generated fat-weight loss, it is imperative that the ACE-AHFS knows how to reliably estimate session, daily, and weekly exercise energy expenditures in kcal. The following are examples of gross energy-expenditure target goals by lipid and lipoprotein:

- Elevated LDL and/or total cholesterol: ≥2000 kcal per week
- Low HDL: ≥1000 kcal per week
- Elevated triglycerides: ≥1000 kcal per week
- Combined dyslipidemia (elevated LDL and triglycerides with low HDL): ≥2000 kcal per week

Step 6: Keep Track of the Client's Lipid-lowering Drugs and Other Medications, if Applicable

If a client is on lipid-lowering drugs, it is wise to know which drug or combination of drugs he or she is taking and any associated dosage changes. The combined use of exercise and lipid-lowering drug therapy can significantly reduce the time needed to achieve the lipid goal. As a group, lipid-lowering drugs have little, if any, effect on exercise **hemodynamics.** Beta-blocking medications, with the exception of the few that have intrinsic **sympathomimetic** activity (e.g., acebutolol and pindolol), will have a tendency to increase triglycerides and decrease HDL cholesterol. Individuals on significant dosages of niacin therapy (e.g., >1500 mg/day) may have a greater tendency to experience a drop in blood pressures after exercise in warm weather. Niacin can also cause flushing and headaches in early stages of this form of pharmacotherapy. As a final note, many lipid-lowering drugs (e.g., statins, fibrates, and niacin) require periodic liver-function tests to assess the possibility of liver toxicity.

Step 7: Track and Document the Client's Musculoskeletal Symptom Status During the Exercise Program

Clients on statins who are exercising at relatively high intensities or volumes are somewhat more susceptible to exercise-associated muscle aches (**myalgia**). One report suggests statin exacerbated exercise-induced skeletal muscle injury, as measured by elevated **creatine kinase (CK)** levels (an index of skeletal muscle injury), in a group of 59 men who took 40 mg of lovastatin per day while embarking on a five-week vigorous endurance-exercise program (Thompson et al., 1997). Although statins are usually well-tolerated, they have occasionally been associated with **myopathy** (myalgia and muscle weakness, with CK elevations) and there is some chance that this situation could be exacerbated with exercise. Myopathy is rapidly reversible if diagnosed early by a physician and treated with discontinuance of drug and hydration. Although the rare occurrence of statin-induced myopathy should not alarm the ACE-AHFS, it does reinforce the need for the ACE-AHFS to keep reasonably close track of any acute and/or recovery musculoskeletal symptoms through at least the early stages of the exercise program and after statin dose changes. The co-administration of approximately 100 mg a day of the antioxidant coenzyme Q_{10} can possibly help reduce statin-related myalgia (Caso et al., 2007) but not all coenzyme Q-statin studies show this benefit, even at higher doses (Young, 2007). The client should discuss adding coenzyme Q_{10} to his or her supplement regimen with a physician.

Step 8: Follow Up

Encourage follow-up blood lipid profile laboratory evaluations in accordance with the referring physician or the lipid clinic's follow-up protocol. Exercise counseling follow-up would ideally be executed in conjunction with the routine lipid clinic follow-up visit, or at six- or eight-week intervals. The exercise plan should be revised as needed, with documentation of weekly energy expenditures and exercise mode(s). Anthropometric measures should be assessed at every clinic evaluation or at the follow-up visit. Dietary and medication compliance should also be routinely assessed at each session.

Step 9: Maintain a Working Knowledge of Other Evidence-based Non-pharmacologic Interventions That Can Help Manage Lipid Disorders

For optimal results, it will often be important to use exercise as a complement to other non-pharmacologic (and pharmacologic) measures. For example, exercise stands the best chance of helping a client reach his or her NCEP lipid goal if it is combined with dietary therapy (NCEP, 2002). Supplemental antioxidant vitamin intake (e.g., vitamin E) may be of value in reducing LDL cholesterol oxidation, although these supplements do not directly affect blood lipid levels (Rimm & Stampfer, 1997). Folic acid, vitamin B6, and vitamin B12 supplementation may also be of help in reducing serum **homocysteine** levels. Homocysteine is an **amino acid** that contributes to the build-up of lipids in **arteries** and increases blood clotting tendency (Wald et al., 1998). The client should discuss adding any of the aforementioned supplements with his or her physician.

Stress- and anger-management interventions, when applicable, should also be included in a comprehensive lipid-management plan. The rationale for such behavioral programs stems from stress-related **catecholamine** production and its putative relationship with LDL oxidation, LDL receptor regulation, and macrophage activation, all of which are integral in the development of atherosclerosis (Williams et al., 1991; Muldoon et al., 1999).

Step 10: Partner With Healthcare Professionals

In some cases, the ACE-AHFS will be collaborating with a physician-directed lipid clinic team in providing therapy. In this sense, the ACE-AHFS is a member of a medical team and may be required to provide progress reports to the lipid clinic's patient record. A helpful description of lipid clinic operations and referral affiliations is available through the National Lipid Association (La Forge, 2006). In other instances, the ACE-AHFS may act independently through self-referral. In this case, it will be necessary to communicate exercise progress to the client's physician and to discuss the relevance of additional tests. Becoming a member of the National Lipid Association (www.lipid.org) is an essential first step.

The Accreditation Council for Clinical Lipidology

The Accreditation Council for Clinical Lipidology (ACCL) (www.lipidspecialist.org) is an independent certifying organization that has developed standards and an examination in the field of clinical lipidology for the growing number of mid- and advanced-level healthcare practitioners who manage individuals with lipid and other related disorders. This organization was developed in association with the National Lipid Association specifically for non-physician advanced-practice clinical professionals, including the ACE-AHFS. An ACE-AHFS can qualify, prepare for, and sit for the ACCL board exam. This is an academically and clinically robust exam that is offered multiple times per year around the U.S. and is very similar to the clinical lipidology board exam offered to physicians. The board credential is "certified clinical lipid specialist." Professional knowledge and skill competencies for this credential include the following:

- Lipoprotein metabolism
- Molecular lipidology
- Epidemiology and clinical trials
- Metabolic syndrome
- Nutrition and nonpharmacologic therapy
- Risk assessment and NCEP guidelines
- Pharmacological therapy
- Safety, behavior, and compliance
- Pharmacodynamics
- Anthropometry

To learn more about this accreditation, visit www.lipidspecialist.org.

Case Study

The client is a 58-year-old male computer programmer with a family history of cardiovascular disease (mother had myocardial infarction at age 51), a 12-year history of obesity, elevated LDL cholesterol (ranging from 168 mg/dL to 185 mg/dL), HDL ranging from 42 to 49 mg/dL, and triglycerides ranging from 170 to 184 mg/dL. He is 5'6" (1.7 m) tall, 175 pounds (79 kg), and has a waist circumference of 35 inches (89 cm). The client's initial level of physical activity was several recreational activities, including participation in a bowling league for two hours a week and a 30- to 40-minute walk twice a week.

Minimal goal: <130 mg/dL LDL cholesterol, <160 non-HDL cholesterol, and <35 inches (89 cm) waist circumference

Optimal lipid goal: <100 mg/dL LDL cholesterol, <130 non-HDL cholesterol

He was put on 10 mg/day of rosuvastatin, but over the last two years failed to consistently take the dose every day. He was also prescribed a NCEP therapeutic lifestyle dietary program (saturated and trans fat reduction). Subsequently, he decreased his LDL cholesterol to 119 mg/dL after complying with 10 mg of rosuvastatin every day, but his body weight remained at 175 pounds (79 kg) and his waist circumference remained at 35 inches (89 cm). Six months ago, the client was encouraged to continue to comply with 10 mg of rosuvastatin once a day, every day, as well as the following exercise program.

Exercise program: 2000+ kcal/week. Variable-terrain walking four times per week at approximately 60% of peak heart rate as determined by his most recent exercise ECG; the walking duration began at 20 minutes per session and progressed to 70 minutes per session after

12 weeks. He also performed two 50-minute aerobic (stationary bike, treadmill, elliptical trainer) exercise sessions a week at a local fitness center, where his average exercise intensity was 65 to 70% of peak heart rate (50 to 65% of heart-rate reserve).

Follow-up: At six months, his initial follow-up (while on the 10 mg rosuvastatin and 2,000 kcal exercise program) showed that he had LDL cholesterol of 102 mg/dL, triglycerides of 111 mg/dL, and HDL cholesterol of 56 mg/dL. His body weight and waist circumference decreased to 164 pounds (74 kg) and 32 inches (81 cm), respectively.

Summary

On average, exercise by itself will reduce LDL cholesterol by 5 to 15% and increase HDL cholesterol by 5 to 15%, depending on exercise volume and the nature of the lipid disorder. Even with a modest 5 to 10% reduction in total and LDL cholesterol, there is a significant decrease in cardiovascular disease risk. Epidemiologic studies have clearly demonstrated that for every 1% reduction in LDL, there is a 2 to 3% reduction in the incidence of CAD (NCEP, 2002).

Lipid management represents a worthwhile opportunity for the ACE-AHFS, given the growth of supportive clinical trials justifying aggressive lipid therapy in dyslipidemic patients and the burgeoning growth of physician-directed lipid and cardiometabolic risk-reduction clinics. Currently, the majority of these programs do not adequately address exercise in any systematic manner. Any ACE-AHFS who is interested in lipid disorders should find this a welcome challenge and seek to forge strong alliances with these outpatient healthcare provider teams.

References

Altena, T.S. et al. (2006). Lipoprotein subfraction changes after continuous or intermittent exercise training. *Medicine & Science in Sports & Exercise,* 38, 367–372.

American College of Sports Medicine (2006). *ACSM's Guidelines for Exercise Testing and Prescription* (7th ed.). Philadelphia: Lippincott Williams & Wilkins.

American Heart Association (2007). Heart Disease and Stroke Statistics—2008 Update. A Report from the American Heart Association Statistics Committee and Stroke Statistics Subcommittee 2008 Heart and Stroke Statistical Update. *Circulation,* Dec. 17 online.

Ballantyne, C.M. et al. (2008). The ASTEROID Investigators: Effect of Rosuvastatin Therapy on Coronary Artery Stenosis Assessed by Quantitative Coronary Angiography in ASTEROID. *Circulation,* doi:10.1161/CIRCULATIONAHA.108.773747.

Bittner, V. (2004). Non-high-density lipoprotein cholesterol: An alternate target for lipid-lowering therapy. *Preventive Cardiology,* 7, 3, 122–126.

Boyden, T.W. et al. (1993). Resistance exercise training is associated with decreases in serum low-density lipoprotein cholesterol levels in premenopausal women. *Archives of Internal Medicine*, 153, 97–100.

Brunzell, J. et al. (2008). Lipoprotein management in patients with cardiometabolic risk: Consensus statement from the American Diabetes Association and the American College of Cardiology Foundation. *Diabetes Care,* 31, 811–822.

Bugiardini, R. et al. (2004). Endothelial function predicts future development of coronary artery disease: A study of women with chest pain and normal coronary angiograms. *Circulation,* 109, 2518–2523.

Cannon, C.P. et al. (2004). Intensive versus moderate lipid lowering with statins after acute coronary syndromes. *New England Journal of Medicine,* 350, 1495–1504.

Caso, G. et al. (2007). Effect of coenzyme-Q10 on myopathic symptoms in patients treated with statins. *American Journal of Cardiology,* 99, 1409–1412.

Church, T.S. et al. (2007). Effects of different doses of physical activity on sedentary or obese post menopausal women with high blood pressure. *Journal of the American Medical Association,* 297, 2081–2091.

Clarkson, P. et al. (1999). Exercise training enhances endothelial function in young men. *Journal of the American College of Cardiology,* 33, 1379–1385.

Colhoun, H.M. et al. (2004). Primary prevention of cardiovascular disease with atorvastatin in type 2 diabetes in the Collaborative Atorvastatin Diabetes Study (CARDS). *Lancet,* 364, 685–696.

Collins, R. et al. (2003). Heart protection study of cholesterol-lowering with simvastatin in 20,536 high risk individuals: A randomized placebo controlled trial. *Lancet,* 360, 7–22.

Couillard, C. et al. (2005). Effects of endurance exercise training on plasma HDL cholesterol levels depend on levels of triglycerides. *Arteriosclerosis, Thrombosis, and Vascular Biology,* 21, 1226–1235.

Cromwell, W. & Otvos, J. (2007). Utilization of lipoprotein subfractions. In: Davidson, M., Toth, P., & Maki, H. (Eds.) *Therapeutic Lipidology*. Totowa, N.J.: Humana Press.

Cromwell, W.C. et al. (2007). LDL particle number and the risk of future cardiovascular disease in the Framingham Offspring study: Implications for LDL-C management. *Journal of Clinical Lipidology,* 1, 583–592.

Crouse, S.F. et al. (1997). Training intensity, blood lipids and apolipoproteins in men with high cholesterol. *Journal of Applied Physiology,* 82, 270–277.

Cui, Y. et al. (2001). Non-high-density lipoprotein cholesterol level as a predictor of cardiovascular disease mortality. *Archives of Internal Medicine,* 161, 1413–1419.

Denke, M.A., Sempos, C.T., & Grundy, S.M. (1994). Excess body weight: An under-recognized contributor to dyslipidemia in white American women. *Archives of Internal Medicine,* 154, 401–410.

Downs, J.R. et al. (1998). Primary prevention of acute coronary events with lovastatin in men and women with average cholesterol levels. *Journal of the American Medical Association,* 279, 1615–1622.

Durstine, J.L. & Haskell, W. (1994). Effects of exercise training on plasma lipids and lipoproteins. *Exercise and Sports Sciences Reviews,* 22, 477–522.

Durstine, J.L. & Moore, G.E. (1997). Hyperlipidemia. In: Durstine, J.L. (Ed.) *ACSM's Exercise Management for Persons with Chronic Diseases and Disabilities.* Champaign, Ill.: Human Kinetics.

Durstine J.L. et al. (2002). Lipids, lipoproteins, and exercise. *Journal of Cardiopulmonary Rehabilitation,* 22, 385–398.

Gordon, D.J., Probstfield, J.L., & Garrison, R.F. (1989). High density lipoprotein cholesterol and cardiovascular disease: Four prospective studies. *Circulation*, 79, 8–15.

Gotto, A.M. (1997). Cholesterol management in theory and practice. *Circulation,* 96, 4424–4430.

Grundy, S.M. (2006). Drug therapy of the metabolic syndrome. *Nature Reviews Drug Discovery,* 5, 295–309.

Grundy, S.M. et al. (2005). Diagnosis and management of the metabolic syndrome: An American Heart Association/National Heart, Lung and

Blood Institute Scientific Statement. *Circulation,* 112, 2735–2752.

Grundy, S.M. et al. (2004). Implications of recent clinical trials for the NCEP ATP III guidelines. *Circulation,* 110, 227–239.

Halverstadt, A. et al. (2007). Endurance exercise training raises high-density lipoprotein cholesterol and lowers small low-density lipoprotein and very low-density lipoprotein independent of body fat phenotypes in older men and women. *Metabolism,* 56, 444–450.

Hambrecht, R. et al. (2000). Effects of exercise on coronary endothelial function in patients with coronary artery disease. *New England Journal of Medicine,* 342, 454.

Hartung, G.H. (1995). Physical activity and high-density lipoprotein cholesterol. *Journal of Sports Medicine and Physical Fitness,* 35, 1–5.

Holme, I., Hostmark, A.T., & Anderssen, S.A. (2007). Apo B but not LDL-cholesterol is reduced by exercise training in overweight healthy men. Results from the 1-year randomized Oslo Diet and Exercise Study. *Journal of Internal Medicine,* 262, 235–243.

Jiang, R. et al. (2004). Non-HDL cholesterol and apolipoprotein B predict cardiovascular disease events among men with type 2 diabetes. *Diabetes Care,* 27, 1991–1997.

Kelley, G.A., Kelley, K.S., & Tran, Z.V. (2005). Aerobic exercise, lipids and lipoproteins in overweight and obese adults: A meta-analysis of randomized controlled trials. *International Journal of Obesity,* 29, 881–893.

King, A. et al. (1995). Long-term effects of varying intensities and formats of physical activity on participation rates, fitness and lipoproteins in men and women aged 50 to 65 years. *Circulation,* 91, 2595–2604.

Kokkinos, P.F. et al. (1995). Miles run per week and high-density lipoprotein cholesterol levels in healthy, middle-aged men. *Archives of Internal Medicine*, 155, 415–420.

Kokkinos, P.F. et al. (1988). Effects of low and high-repetition resistive training on lipoprotein lipid levels. *Medicine & Science in Sports & Exercise,* 20, 50–54.

Kraus, W. et al. (2002). Effects of the amount and intensity of exercise on plasma lipoproteins. *New England Journal of Medicine,* 347, 19, 1522–1524.

La Forge, R. (2006). Key considerations for designing and operating a clinically successful and solvent lipid clinic and other CVD risk reduction programs. *Lipid Spin,* October, 4–11.

LaRosa, J.C. et al. (2005). Intensive lipid lowering with atorvastatin in patients with stable coronary disease. *New England Journal of Medicine,* 352, 1425–1435.

Leon, A. & Sanchez, O.A. (2001). Response of blood lipids to exercise training alone or in combination with dietary intervention. *Medicine & Science in Sports & Exercise,* 33, S502–S515.

Lu, W. et al. (2003). Non-HDL cholesterol as a predictor of cardiovascular disease in type 2 diabetes: The Strong Heart Study. *Diabetes Care,* 26, 16–23.

Malkova, D. & Gill, J. (2006). Effects of exercise on postprandial metabolism. *Future Lipidology,* 1, 743–755.

Muldoon, M.F. et al. (1999). Acute cholesterol responses to mental stress and change in posture. *Archives of Internal Medicine,* 152, 775–780.

National Cholesterol Education Program (2002). Expert Panel on Detection, Evaluation and Treatment of High Blood Cholesterol in Adults. Summary of the 2nd Report of NCEP Expert Panel on Detection, Evaluation and Treatment of High Blood Cholesterol in Adults (Adult Treatment Panel III). NIH Publication 02-5213. Executive summary (2001). *Journal of the American Medical Association,* 285, 2486–2497.

National Heart Lung and Blood Institute (1995). *Recommendations on Lipoprotein Measurement.* NIH Publication # 95-3044.

Nissen, S.E. et al. (2006). Effect of very high-intensity statin therapy on regression of coronary atherosclerosis: The ASTEROID Trial. *Journal of the American Medical Association*. 295, 81–91.

Otvos, J. et al. (2006). LDL and HDL particle subclasses predict coronary events and are changed favorably by gemfibrozil in the Veterans HDL Intervention Trial. *Circulation,* 113, 1556–1563.

Owens, J. et al. (1992). Can physical activity mitigate the effects of aging in middle aged women? *Circulation,* 85, 1265–1270.

Park, D.H. & Ransone, J.W. (2003). Effects of submaximal exercise on high-density lipoprotein cholesterol subfractions. *International Journal of Sports Medicine,* 24, 245–251.

Pederson, T.R. & the Scandinavian Simvastatin Survival Study Group (1994). Randomized trial of cholesterol lowering in 4,444 patients with coronary heart disease. *Lancet,* 344, 1383–1389.

Petersen, T. et. al. (2005). High-dose atorvastatin vs. usual-dose simvastatin for secondary prevention after myocardial infarction: The IDEAL study: A randomized controlled trial. *Journal of the American Medical Association,* 294, 2437–2445.

Petitt, D.S. & Cureton, K.J. (2003). Effects of prior exercise on postprandial lipemia: A quantitative review. *Metabolism,* 52, 418–424.

Pitt, B., Mancini. G.B., & Ellis, S.G. (1995). Pravastatin limitation of atherosclerosis in the coronary arteries (PLAC I). *Journal of the American College of Cardiology,* 26, 133–139.

Pronk, N.P. (1993). Short-term effects of exercise on plasma lipids and lipoproteins in humans. *Sports Medicine,* 16, 431–448.

Rimm, E.B. & Stampfer, M.J. (1997). The role of antioxidants in preventive cardiology. *Current Opinion in Cardiology,* 12, 188–194.

Ring-Dimitriou. S. et al. (2007). Nine months aerobic fitness-induced changes on blood lipids and lipoproteins in untrained subjects versus controls. *European Journal of Applied Physiology,* 99, 291–299.

Rubins, H.B. et al. (1999). Gemfibrozil for the secondary prevention of coronary heart disease in men with low levels of HDL cholesterol: Veterans Affairs HDL-cholesterol Intervention Trial Study Group. *New England Journal of Medicine,* 341, 410–418.

Sacks, F.M. et al. (1996). The effect of pravastatin on coronary events after myocardial infarction in patients with average cholesterol levels. *New England Journal of Medicine,* 225, 1001–1009.

Shadid, S. et al. (2006). Treatment of obesity with diet/exercise versus pioglitazone has distinct effects on lipoprotein size. *Atherosclerosis,*188, 370–376.

Shepard. J. et al. (1995). Prevention of coronary heart disease with Pravastatin in men with hypercholesterolemia. (West of Scotland Coronary Prevention Study). *New England Journal of Medicine,* 333, 1301–1307.

Slentz, C.A. et al. (2007). Inactivity, exercise training and detraining, and plasma lipoproteins. *Journal of Applied Physiology,* 103, 432–442.

Srinivasan, S., Myers, L., & Berenson, G.S. (2002). Distribution and correlates of non-high-density lipoprotein cholesterol in children. The Bogalusa Heart Study. *Pediatrics*, 110, 3, e29.

Stern, M., Williams, K., & Haffner, S.M. (2002). Identification of persons at high risk for type 2 diabetes mellitus: Do we need the glucose tolerance test? *Annals of Internal Medicine,* 136, 575–581.

Stevenson, E.T. et al. (1997). Physically active women demonstrate less adverse age-related changes in plasma lipids and lipoproteins. *American Journal of Cardiology,* 80, 1360–1364.

Stevenson, E.T. et al. (1995). Physical activity is associated with favorable hemostatic and metabolic risk factors for coronary heart disease in healthy non-obese postmenopausal women. *Arteriosclerosis Thrombosis Vascular Biology,* 15, 669–677.

Superko, R. (1991). Exercise training, serum lipids and lipoprotein particles: Is there a change threshold? *Medicine & Science in Sports & Exercise*, 23, 677.

Thompson, P.D. et al. (1997). Lovastatin increases exercise-induced skeletal muscle injury. *Metabolism,* 46, 1206–1210.

Trejo-Gutierrez, J.F. & Fletcher, G. (2007). Impact of exercise on blood lipids and lipoproteins. *Journal of Clinical Lipidology,* 1, 175–181.

Tucker, L.A., Martin, J.R., & Harris K. (1997). Effects of a strength-training program on the blood lipid levels of sedentary adult women. *American Journal of Health Behavior*, 21, 323–332.

Utriainen, T. et al. (1996). Physical fitness and endothelial function (nitric oxide synthesis) are independent determinants of insulin-stimulated blood flow in normal subjects. *Journal of Clinical Endocrinology Metabolism*, 81, 4258–4263.

Visich, P.S. et al. (1996). Effects of exercise with varying energy expenditure on high-density lipoprotein cholesterol. *European Journal of Applied Physiology*, 72, 242–248.

Wald, N. et al. (1998). Homocysteine and ischemic heart disease. *Archives of Internal Medicine,* 158, 862–867.

Williams, P.T. (1998). Relationships of heart disease risk factors to exercise quantity and intensity. *Archives of Internal Medicine,* 158, 3, 237–245.

Williams, P.T. (1996). High-density lipoprotein cholesterol and other risk factors for coronary heart disease in female runners. *New England Journal of Medicine,* 334, 20, 1298–1304.

Williams, R.B. et al. (1991). Biobehavioral basis of coronary-prone behavior in middle-aged men. Part I: Evidence for chronic SNS activation in type A's. *Psychosomatic Medicine*, 53, 517–527.

Wood, P.D. et al. (1983). Increased exercise level and plasma lipoprotein concentrations: A one-year randomized, controlled study in sedentary middle-aged men. *Metabolism*, 32, 31–39.

Young, J.M. (2007). Effect of coenzyme Q10 supplementation on *simvastatin*-induced myalgia. *American Journal of Cardiology,*100, 1400.

Zhang, J.Q. (2006). Effect of exercise on postprandial lipemia in men with hypertriglyceridemia. *European Journal of Applied Physiology,* 98, 575–582.

Zhang, J.Q. et al. (1998). Effect of exercise timing on postprandial lipemia and HDL cholesterol subfractions. *Journal of Applied Physiology,* 85, 1516–1522.

Suggested Reading

American Council on Exercise (2007). *ACE Clinical Exercise Specialist Manual.* San Diego, Calif.: American Council on Exercise.

American Heart Association (2008). *Heart Disease and Stroke Statistics 2008 Update.* www.circulationaha.org

American Heart Association (2003). Exercise and physical activity in the prevention and treatment of cardiovascular disease: A statement from the Council of Clinical Cardiology. *Circulation,* 107, 3109–3116.

Davidson, M.H., Toth, P.P., & Maki, K.C. (2007). *Therapeutic Lipidology,* Totowa, N.J.: Humana Press.

Davignon, J. & Dufour, R. (2007). *Primary Hyperlipidemias: An Atlas of Investigation and Diagnosis*. Oxford: Clinical Publishing.

National Cholesterol Education Program (2002). Expert Panel on Detection, Evaluation and Treatment of High Blood Cholesterol in Adults. Summary of the 2nd Report of NCEP Expert Panel on Detection, Evaluation and Treatment of High Blood Cholesterol in Adults (Adult Treatment Panel III). NIH Publication 02-5213. Executive summary (2001). *Journal of the American Medical Association,* 285, 2486–2497.

National Lipid Association: www.lipid.org.

Schairer, J.R. & Keteyian, S.J. (2006). Exercise training in patients with cardiovascular disease. In: Kaminsky, L.A. (Ed.) *ACSM's Resource Manual for Guidelines for Exercise Testing and Prescription* (5th ed.). Philadelphia: Lippincott Williams & Wilkins.

Stone, N.J. & Blum, C.B. (2006). *Management of Lipids in Clinical Practice* (6th ed.). West Islip, N.Y.: Professional Communications, Inc.

In This Chapter

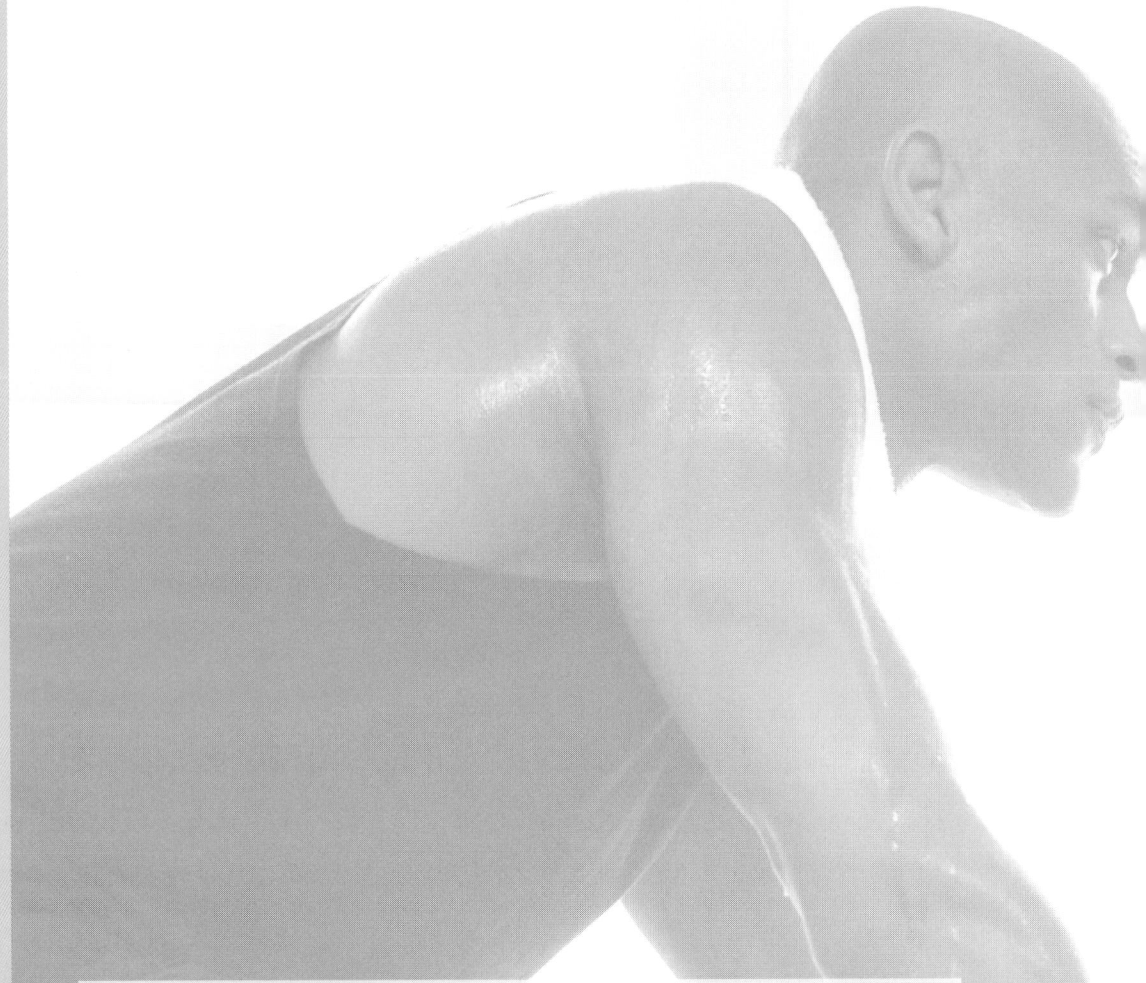

About The Authors

W. Larry Kenney, Ph.D., is a professor of kinesiology and physiology at Pennsylvania State University, and former president of the American College of Sports Medicine. His research focuses on thermal physiology and the biophysics of heat transfer, including the effect of aging and hypertension on human skin blood flow. Dr. Kenney has published more than 150 papers and has been continually funded by that National Institutes of Health since 1985.

Lacy A. Holowatz, Ph.D., is a research associate in kinesiology at Pennsylvania State University. Dr. Holowatz has received awards from the American College of Sports Medicine and the American Physiological Society for her work on impairments in the mechanisms that increase skin blood flow during heat stress in aged and hypertensive populations.

CHAPTER 8

Hypertension

W. Larry Kenney & Lacy A. Holowatz

An independent predictor of mortality, **hypertension** affects more than 70 million adults in the United States [American Heart Association (AHA), 2007]. Exercise is a cornerstone therapy in the prevention and treatment of this disease. It is important for an ACE-certified Advanced Health & Fitness Specialist (ACE-AHFS) to know the role of regular exercise therapy in the management of hypertension and how physical activity produces a decrease in **blood pressure (BP).** Because most hypertensive individuals will take two or more antihypertensive medications to control their BP, it is also important to know the potential effects and interactions of antihypertensive medications on the cardiovascular system during exercise.

Epidemiology

Hypertension is an independent risk factor for **coronary artery disease, stroke,** and **renal failure.** The relationship between BP and adverse cardiovascular events is direct—the higher the BP, the greater the chance of heart attack, heart failure, stoke, and kidney disease (Chobanian et al., 2003). Hypertension is defined as having a **systolic blood pressure (SBP)** ≥140 mmHg, a **diastolic blood pressure (DBP)** ≥90 mmHg, and/or being on antihypertensive medication. According to these criteria, approximately 73 million individuals in the United States and 1 billion individuals worldwide have hypertension (AHA, 2007; Burt et al., 1995; Hajjar & Kotchen, 2003; Rosendorff et al., 2007).

The incidence of hypertension increases with advancing age, with over half of Americans over the age of 65 having some form of hypertension (Rosendorff et al., 2007). The relationship between BP and age is complex. After age 50, SBP steadily increases, whereas DBP plateaus around the sixth decade of life and decreases thereafter. Accordingly, the incidence of isolated systolic hypertension (SBP ≥140 mmHg) or combined systolic-diastolic hypertension (SBP ≥140 mmHg and DBP ≥90 mmHg) increases with age, while the incidence of isolated diastolic hypertension (DBP ≥90 mmHg) decreases with age. The longitudinal Framingham Heart Study has estimated that the 20-year projected risk for developing hypertension is >90% for men and women who are not yet hypertensive by middle age (Vasan et al., 2002).

With the increased mortality risk associated with hypertension, combined with the age-related increase in BP, the early identification and treatment of individuals who will likely become hypertensive has become increasingly important. These individuals are categorized as having "prehypertension"—a SBP of 120 to 139 mmHg or a DBP of 80 to 89 mmHg. For each 20 mmHg rise in SBP or 10 mmHg rise in DBP, the risk of cardiovascular disease doubles (Chobanian et al., 2003). Thus, effective diet, exercise, lifestyle modifications, and pharmacological (drug) therapy to lower BP in prehypertensive and hypertensive individuals is vital to decreasing their total cardiovascular risk. Randomized clinical trials have shown that lowering BP decreases an individual's cardiovascular risk by as much as 50% (Chobanian et al., 2003).

Even though the benefit of reducing and controlling BP in prehypertensive and hypertensive individuals is clear, the control rates for hypertension are undesirable. Approximately 30% of adults in the United States are unaware of their high BP. Of those diagnosed with hypertension, two-thirds are not achieving appropriate BP control (BP <140/90 mmHg) (Chobanian et al., 2003).

Overview of Hypertension (Mechanisms)

Cardiac output is the product of **heart rate** and **stroke volume,** the volume of blood the heart pumps in one beat. BP is the product of cardiac output, the amount of blood the heart pumps out in one minute, and **total peripheral resistance (TPR),** the resistance to blood flow that the blood vessels provide.

Cardiac output = Heart rate x Stroke volume
Blood pressure = Cardiac output x Total peripheral resistance

Stroke volume is altered by the amount of blood filling of the heart (preload), the pressure the heart must pump against (afterload), and the force of cardiac **contractility.** Therefore, alterations in these variables resulting in an increase in either cardiac output or total peripheral resistance can cause hypertension.

Control of Blood Pressure

Short-term Reflex Control of Blood Pressure

Maintaining an adequate BP to ensure sufficient blood flow to the brain is one of the main priorities of the cardiovascular system. Blood pressure is integratively controlled by cardiovascular, neural, renal, and hormonal networks. Like many other controlled variables in physiology, BP is controlled via negative feedback with sensors, a defended set point, and effector responses. The sensors that regulate BP regulation are **baroreceptors** (pressure receptors) and they are located in the aortic arch and the carotid artery walls. Baroreceptors send neural signals to the cardiovascular control centers in the brain regarding the current BP. The cardiovascular control centers in the brain set a predetermined set point and integrate the incoming signals from the baroreceptors regarding the current BP. Depending on what the current BP is and how it compares to this predetermined set point, signals are sent out to the heart, blood vessels, and kidneys via the **autonomic nervous system** to cause a change in BP to bring it closer to the set point. When blood pressure is low or below the set point, there is little stretch on the baroreceptors, resulting in a reduction in the **afferent nervous system** signal going to the brain. The cardiovascular control centers integrate the signal from the baroreceptors and send out signals to the heart and blood vessels in an attempt to increase BP. These efferent signals are carried through the autonomic nervous system (**parasympathetic** and **sympathetic nervous systems**). During a low-BP state, parasympathetic activity to the heart is quickly decreased, which serves to rapidly increase heart rate. In addition, sympathetic nervous system activity increases, which also increases heart rate and cardiac contractility. The actions of the parasympathetic and the sympathetic nervous systems on the heart increase cardiac output. Increased sympathetic activity also causes **vasoconstriction** in the blood vessels, which increases total peripheral resistance (Folkow, 1982).

When blood pressure is high, the baroreceptors are stretched and the afferent signal to the cardiovascular control centers in the brain is increased. The resulting efferent response is to increase parasympathetic activity to the heart to slow heart rate and to inhibit sympathetic activity to cause a passive **vasodilation** of the peripheral blood vessels. This decreases BP, bringing it closer to the set point.

Long-term Neural-hormonal Control of Blood Pressure

In addition to the short-term mechanisms that alter BP, increased sympathetic nervous system activity also has prolonged effects through its action on the kidneys and the release of **hormones** to increase blood volume. During a drop in BP, when there is decreased stretch on the baroreceptors, the hormone **vasopressin** (antidiuretic hormone) is released to help increase blood volume. This hormone causes water to be reabsorbed in the kidneys. In addition to vasopressin release, increased sympathetic nerve activity activates the **beta receptors** in the kidneys, which results in a decrease in blood flow to the kidneys, causing the release of another hormone called **renin.** Renin, in turn, activates a cascade of hormonal events to cause further vasoconstriction in the peripheral blood vessels and an increase in salt and water reabsorption in the kidney to enhance blood volume. Figure 8-1 illustrates the **renin-angiotensin-aldosterone system (RAAS).** Renin is an enzyme released from the kidneys that activates the hormone angiotensinogen by cleaving off part of the protein to form angiotensin I. Angiotensin I is then converted to angiotensin II through another enzyme called angiotensin converting enzyme (ACE). Angiotensin II is a potent vasoconstrictor that binds to receptors on peripheral blood vessels, causing the vascular smooth muscle in the blood vessels to contract. Angiotensin II also causes the mineral corticoid hormone aldosterone to be released from the adrenal cortex. Aldosterone causes sodium and water to be reabsorbed in the kidneys. Overall, the actions of aldosterone serve to increase blood volume. The RAAS system is extremely important for the long-term regulation of BP (Rowell, 1993), and in the pathogenesis of hypertension.

Physiology of Hypertension

Any disturbance in the normal negative feedback control of BP between the cardiovascular, neural, renal, or hormonal systems can result in

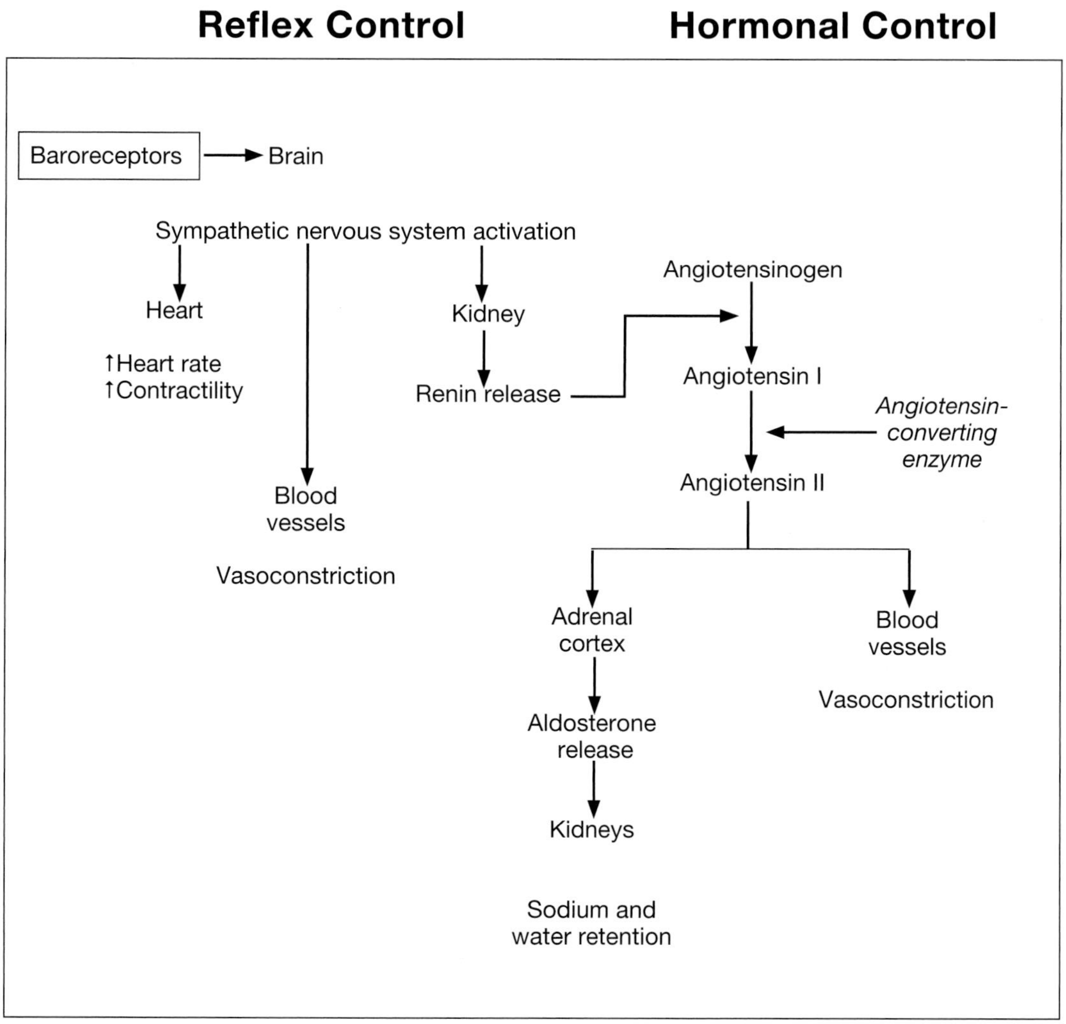

Figure 8-1
The renin-angiotensin-aldosterone system

Source: Kester, M. et al. (2007) *Elsevier's Integrated Pharmacology.* Philadelphia: Elsevier.

hypertension. There are several identifiable causes of hypertension that are summarized in Table 8-1. When there is an identifiable cause of hypertension, this is termed **secondary hypertension,** because it is secondary to a disease state. In these cases, correcting the underlying pathology can sometimes cure the hypertension. However, in greater than 90% of cases of hypertension, there is no single identifiable cause (AHA, 2007a). Hypertension without an identifiable cause is clinically termed **essential** or **primary hypertension.** While the etiology of essential hypertension is unclear, in general, central cardiovascular control centers and the baroreceptors in patients with hypertension acquire a new elevated set point and become less sensitive, meaning that it takes a larger change in BP for the system to respond and correct that change. As a result of the elevated set point, there is a decrease in parasympathetic nerve activity to the heart and an increase in resting sympathetic nerve activity to the heart, vasculature, and kidneys. This situation causes an increase in heart rate and cardiac contractility via stimulation of the beta receptors in the myocardium, as well as an increase in peripheral vasoconstriction via the action of the sympathetic nervous system **neurotransmitters** (e.g., **norepinephrine**) on the blood vessels. Furthermore, in the kidneys, increased sympathetic stimulation causes renin to be released, which activates the RAAS. RAAS activation increases peripheral vasoconstriction through the actions of angiotensin II on the vasculature and increases salt and water reabsorption in the proximal tubules of the kidneys. The resulting increase in total body extracellular volume increases preload on the heart, which serves to further increase cardiac contractility. Thus, feedback regulation in this tightly controlled BP regulatory system is impaired and results in hypertension (Folkow, 1982).

Because the control of BP involves many different organ systems, there can be various mechanisms that ultimately lead to hypertension. There are several common pathophysiological findings associated with high BP. There appears to be a change in the BP set point, an overall increase in sympathetic nervous system activity, and a decrease in the sensitivity of the baroreceptors to a change in BP (Hesse et al., 2007). In addition, there are also alterations in the local control of peripheral blood vessels. To help control blood flow, blood vessels release substances called vasodilators, which cause the blood vessels to open wider, and vasoconstrictors, which cause the blood vessels to narrow. With hypertension, there is a shift from locally released vasodilators to vasoconstrictors. This change is associated with an increase in **free radical** (**oxidant**) stress in the blood vessels. This pro-vasoconstrictor state, along with the elevated pressure on the blood vessels themselves, causes remodeling of the blood vessel walls. This remodeling makes the blood vessel walls **hypertrophy** and become stiff.

Long-term elevations in BP can also induce changes in the heart itself. Just like in the blood vessels, the heart muscle begins to hypertrophy. This is not an advantageous hypertrophy like

Table 8-1
Identifiable Causes of Hypertension

- Sleep apnea
- Drug-induced or related causes (see below)
- Chronic kidney disease
- Primary aldosteronism
- Renovascular disease
- Chronic steroid therapy and Cushing's syndrome
- Pheochromocytoma
- Coarctation of the aorta
- Thyroid or parathyroid disease

Drug-induced or other causes
- Nonadherence
- Inadequate doses
- Inappropriate combinations
- Nonsteroidal anti-inflammatory drugs; cyclooxygenase 2 inhibitors
- Cocaine, amphetamines, other illicit drugs
- Sympathomimetics (decongestants, anorectics)
- Oral contraceptives
- Adrenal steroids
- Cyclosporine and tacrolimus
- Erhythropoietin
- Licorice (including some chewing tobacco)
- Selected over-the-counter dietary supplements and medicines (e.g., ephedra, ma huang, bitter orange)

Associated conditions
- Obesity
- Excess alcohol intake

Source: Chobanian, A.V. et al. (2003). *JNC 7 Express: The Seventh Report of the Joint National Committee on Prevention, Detection, Evaluation, and Treatment of High Blood Pressure.* NIH Publication No. 03-5233. Washington, D.C.: National Institutes of Health & National Heart, Lung, and Blood Institute.

the changes that are induced in the myocardium during endurance-exercise training. Instead, with hypertension, the heart muscle becomes thicker through concentric hypertrophy and less efficient as a pump. This is referred to as left ventricular hypertrophy and can be detected on an **electrocardiogram.**

Prolonged uncontrolled hypertension has many deleterious effects on the cardiovascular system, including remodeling of the myocardium and vascular smooth muscle. This type of remodeling can cause target organ damage in the heart, brain, kidneys, and peripheral blood vessels. Table 8-2 lists the major pathologies caused by hypertension-induced target organ damage.

Table 8-2
Pathologies Cause by Hypertension-induced Target Organ Damage

Heart
- Left ventricular hypertrophy
- Angina or prior myocardial infarction
- Prior coronary revascularization
- Heart failure

Brain
- Stroke or transient ischemic attack

Chronic kidney disease
Peripheral arterial disease
Retinopathy

Source: Chobanian, A.V. et al. (2003). *JNC 7 Express: The Seventh Report of the Joint National Committee on Prevention, Detection, Evaluation, and Treatment of High Blood Pressure.* NIH Publication No. 03-5233. Washington, D.C.: National Institutes of Health & National Heart, Lung, and Blood Institute.

Genetics and Hypertension

The underlying genetic and pathophysiological mechanisms contributing to essential hypertension vary widely and depend on individual characteristics and environmental interactions. Genetic studies in humans to identify the genes that cause essential hypertension are in their infancy. Essential hypertension is genetically encoded on multiple genes and has several phenotypic (outward physical manifestations of disease) and genotypic (genetic code) subtypes. Therefore, each gene that encodes for hypertension only has a small effect on BP (Weder, 2008). However, the genetic predisposition for hypertension is permissive, meaning that environmental influences are necessary for hypertension to ultimately develop.

Considering the genetic and environmental contributing factors in the development of hypertension, it is not surprising that there are many different physiological mechanisms responsible for high BP. The mechanisms that cause hypertension and the individual responses to treatment can differ depending on several variables, including race and age. For example, the incidence of hypertension is greater among African Americans than it is among other ethnic groups. Furthermore, it has also been demonstrated that African Americans respond to certain drug therapies for hypertension better than others (Ferdinand, 2008). Certainly, the data suggest that there are physiological differences in the mechanisms of hypertension depending on genetics, but there are also many environmental and socioeconomic explanations for some of these findings. One additional example to illustrate different causes and physiological mechanisms of hypertension involves individuals who develop high BP at a young age versus those who develop it later in life. In younger individuals, the onset of hypertension is associated with an increase in salt and water retention that results in an increase in cardiac output. In contrast, hypertension in older patients is more commonly associated with an increase in peripheral vascular resistance. These different mechanisms and contributing factors to high BP should be considered, especially when selecting suitable pharmacological and non-pharmacological interventions to treat high BP.

Diagnostic Criteria

Table 8-3 provides the classification of BP for adults 18 and older (Chobanian et al., 2003). These classifications are based on the average of two or more properly measured seated BP readings on two or more occasions.

The auscultatory method of BP measurement with a properly calibrated and validated sphygmomanometer (BP cuff) should be used to measure BP. To obtain a proper resting BP measurement, clients should avoid activities that increase their BP, such as exercise, ingestion of caffeine, and

Table 8-3
Classification of Blood Pressure for Adults Age 18 and Older*

Category	Systolic (mmHg)		Diastolic (mmHg)
Normal†	<120	and	<80
Prehypertension	120–139	or	80–89
Hypertension‡			
Stage 1	140–159	or	90–99
Stage 2	≥160	or	≥100

* Not taking antihypertensive drugs and not acutely ill. When systolic and diastolic blood pressures fall into different categories, the higher category should be selected to classify the individual's blood pressure status. For example, 140/82 mmHg should be classified as stage 1 hypertension, and 154/102 mmHg should be classified as stage 2 hypertension. In addition to classifying stages of hypertension on the basis of average blood pressure levels, clinicians should specify presence or absence of target organ disease and additional risk factors. This specificity is important for risk classification and treatment.

† Normal blood pressure with respect to cardiovascular risk is below 120/80 mmHg. However, unusually low readings should be evaluated for clinical significance.

‡ Based on the average of two or more readings taken at each of two or more visits after an initial screening.

Source: Chobanian, A.V. et al. (2003). *JNC 7 Express: The Seventh Report of the Joint National Committee on Prevention, Detection, Evaluation, and Treatment of High Blood Pressure.* NIH Publication No. 03-5233. Washington, D.C.: National Institutes of Health & National Heart, Lung, and Blood Institute.

smoking, for at least 30 minutes prior to having their BP measured. The client should be seated quietly in a chair with both feet on the floor for at least five minutes prior to obtaining the measurement. BP should be measured with the arm at heart level. The force of gravity will artifactually influence the BP measurement if the arm is not at heart level. In addition, an appropriately sized BP cuff (cuff bladder encircling at least 80% of the arm) should be used to ensure accuracy of the measurement. Most sphygmomanometers have a line on the inside of the cuff (facing the client) that is useful for ensuring that the appropriate size cuff is used. At least two measurements of BP should be made, with five minutes between measurements. The client should continue resting quietly (no talking) in a seated position during the time between BP measurements. When measuring BP, SBP is the pressure at the point where the first of two or more **Korotkoff sounds** is heard. This is the maximum pressure generated when the heart is contracting. DBP is the pressure before the disappearance of the Korotkoff sounds when the heart is relaxed. BP readings should be confirmed by reading BP in the contralateral (i.e., non-dominant) arm. BP can vary by as much as 10 mmHg between arms. However, the higher pressure (usually the lower pressure is in the left arm) more accurately reflects intra-arterial pressure (Grim & Grim, 2008).

It is occasionally necessary to monitor ambulatory BP in individuals to record their BP reading over a period of 24 hours. This is especially necessary in cases of "white coat hypertension," in which BP increases under perceived stressful situations, such as being a patient at a physician's office. In this situation, there is a learned stress response and BP is acutely elevated in the physician's office or under other stressful conditions, but is not chronically elevated. White coat hypertension is suspected when BP is acutely elevated, but there is no history of hypertension or evidence of target organ damage. *Note:* Twenty-four hour ambulatory blood pressure is also more predictive of target organ damage.

NHLBI Guidelines

In 2003, the Seventh Report of the Joint National Committee on Prevention, Detection, Evaluation, and Treatment of High Blood Pressure (JNC-VII) provided guidelines for hypertension prevention and management (Chobanian et al., 2003). These guidelines are based on a systematic evaluation of studies and are meant to increase awareness, prevention, treatment, and control of hypertension.

One of the key elements of the JNC-VII report was the inclusion of a new pre-hypertensive category (see Table 8-3). Those individuals who fall within the prehypertensive category have twice the risk of developing hypertension than those who have a lower BP. The guidelines set forth by the National Heart, Lung, and Blood Institute (NHLBI) emphasize the importance of identification of prehypertensive individuals. Individuals in this category are not candidates for pharmacological treatment of their BP, but instead should adopt lifestyle modifications to control their BP and prevent cardiovascular disease. Importantly, there are a number of causal factors for hypertension, including excess body weight, excess salt intake, inadequate intake of fresh fruits and vegetables, **sedentary** lifestyles, and excess alcohol consumption. Simply modifying these causal factors can treat and prevent hypertension in these individuals. Thus, exercise professionals play a key educational and motivational role in treating individuals with prehypertension and established hypertension.

Figure 8-2 is the algorithm healthcare providers use for the treatment of hypertension. The primary goal of any treatment (non-pharmacological and pharmacological) is to decrease BP to <140/90 mmHg. However, in patients with diabetes or existing chronic kidney disease, the goal of BP treatment is to attain a BP of <130/80 mmHg, as these populations are at an increased risk of further target organ damage and cardiovascular events. The majority of individuals with hypertension will require two or more

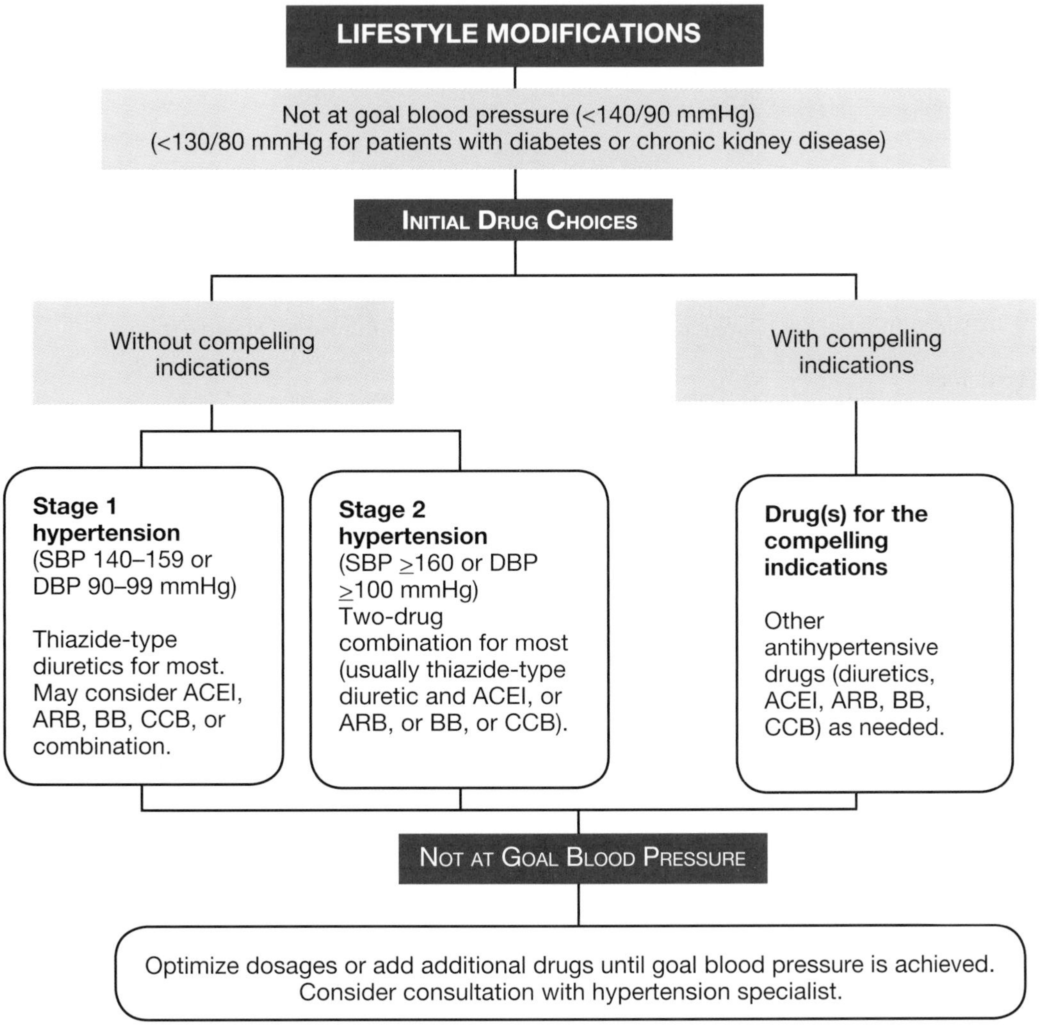

Note: DBP = Diastolic blood pressure; SBP = Systolic blood pressure; ACEI = Angiotensin converting enzyme inhibitor; ARB = Angiotensin receptor blocker; BB = Beta blocker; CCB = Calcium channel blocker

Figure 8-2
Algorithm for treatment of hypertension

Source: Chobanian, A.V. et al. (2003). *JNC 7 Express: The Seventh Report of the Joint National Committee on Prevention, Detection, Evaluation, and Treatment of High Blood Pressure.* NIH Publication No. 03-5233. Washington, D.C.: National Institutes of Health & National Heart, Lung, and Blood Institute.

medications, in addition to lifestyle modifications, to reach their target BP. However, the first line of defense in treating mild hypertension is to adopt a healthy lifestyle that includes regular aerobic exercise. Table 8-4 lists the recommended lifestyle modifications and the resulting average decrease in systolic BP. The most significant decrease in BP with lifestyle modification comes in the form of weight loss. Because exercise is a key component to weight loss and results in a significant decrease in BP, appropriate exercise programs should be incorporated into the treatment plan for clients with hypertension. Lifestyle modifications, including exercise and weight reduction, can prevent a progressive rise in BP and cardiovascular disease, especially in prehypertensive individuals.

If the target BP is not achieved by adopting healthy lifestyle changes, then pharmacotherapy is necessary. Depending on the initial stage of hypertension (see Table 8-3), one to two drugs are initially prescribed to lower BP. For stage I hypertension, the most commonly prescribed drug is a thiazide-type **diuretic.** This type of drug works on the kidneys to decrease salt and water load, thereby decreasing excess extracellular volume. Alternatively, other BP-lowering drugs may be prescribed based on specific individual variables and the primary mechanisms causing the hypertension. With stage II hypertension, a two-drug combination therapy is used to reach the target BP. The therapy regimen typically includes a thiazide-type diuretic and one other antihypertensive drug. If drug therapy is ineffective at reducing BP to the desired level, modification of dosages and the addition of different classes of antihypertensive drugs may be necessary to achieve the goal BP. After antihypertensive therapy is initiated, BP should be routinely monitored to determine the efficacy of treatment and determine if the goal BP has been reached.

Table 8-4
Lifestyle Modifications to Manage Hypertension*†

Modification	Recommendation	Approximate SBP Reduction (Range)
Weight reduction	Maintain normal body weight (body mass index 18.5–24.9 kg/m^2)	5–20 mmHg/10 kg weight loss
Adopt DASH eating plan	Consume a diet rich in fruits, vegetables, and low-fat dairy products with a reduced content of saturated and total fat	8–14 mmHg
Dietary sodium reduction	Reduce dietary sodium intake to no more than 100 mmol per day (2.4 g sodium or 6 g sodium chloride)	2–8 mmHg
Physical activity	Engage in regular aerobic physical activity such as brisk walking (at least 30 minutes per day, most days of the week)	4–9 mmHg
Moderation of alcohol consumption	Limit consumption to no more than two drinks (1 oz or 30 mL ethanol; e.g., 24-oz beer, 10-oz wine, or 3-oz 80-proof whiskey) per day in most men and to no more than one drink per day for women and lighter weight persons	2–4 mmHg

*For overall cardiovascular risk reduction, stop smoking.
†The effects of implementing these modifications are dose- and time-dependent, and could be greater for some individuals.

Note: SBP = Systolic blood pressure; DASH = Dietary Approaches to Stop Hypertension

Source: Chobanian, A.V. et al. (2003). *JNC 7 Express: The Seventh Report of the Joint National Committee on Prevention, Detection, Evaluation, and Treatment of High Blood Pressure.* NIH Publication No. 03-5233. Washington, D.C.: National Institutes of Health & National Heart, Lung, and Blood Institute.

Treatment of Hypertension

The goal of hypertension treatment is to decrease BP to <140/90 mmHg in uncomplicated cases and to <130/80 mmHg in individuals with diabetes or kidney disease. The treatment of hypertension involves adopting a healthy lifestyle, including regular aerobic exercise, and when necessary, pharmacological intervention. In most cases of hypertension, two or more medications will be required to achieve the goal BP. It is important for exercise professionals to work in collaboration with clinicians and nutritionists to optimize the BP-lowering potential of lifestyle modifications with pharmacotherapy. This collaborative relationship creates a support network for clients with hypertension, thereby improving adherence to treatment.

Non-pharmacological Treatment

Non-pharmacological treatments for hypertension include significant lifestyle modifications. These lifestyle modifications, along with the corresponding decrease in systolic BP, are detailed in Table 8-4. Weight reduction of as little as 10 pounds (4.5 kg) in overweight individuals significantly reduces and/or prevents a rise in BP (Hypertension Prevention Research Group, 1997). In addition to weight reduction and incorporating regular aerobic physical activity, it is recommended that hypertensive individuals limit dietary sodium intake to less than 2400 mg per day, which is the equivalent of 1 teaspoon. Most Americans consume at least 75% of their sodium from processed foods (AHA, 2007b). Therefore, adopting a healthy eating plan, including fresh fruits and vegetables, low-fat dairy products, and reduced saturated and total fat content, is vital to reducing dietary sodium intake from prepared foods. There is an additive effect of each of these lifestyle modifications on BP reduction. For example, significantly reducing dietary sodium intake and adopting the **Dietary Approach to Stop Hypertension (DASH) eating plan** has a similar effect on BP as a single pharmacotherapy (Chobanian et al., 2003). Furthermore, the addition of lifestyle modifications to pharmacotherapy results in a greater reduction in BP than pharmacotherapy alone.

The DASH eating plan emphasizes fruits, vegetables, low-fat dairy products, whole grains, poultry, fish, and nuts, and contains only a small amount of red meat, sweets, and sugar-containing beverages (Table 8-5). The DASH eating plan contains a decreased total amount of saturated fat and cholesterol and is lower in total fat. In large clinical trials where total caloric intake was held constant (compared to the pre-diet enrollment), one to two months of dietary modifications with the DASH eating plan reduced SBP by 5 mmHg and DBP by 3 mmHg. Furthermore, reducing the sodium content of the diet had an additive effect on the total reduction in blood pressure combined with the DASH eating plan. Trials that have tested the impact of individual nutrients (e.g., fat, fiber, calcium, or magnesium) on BP have not found an effect large enough to account for the overall DASH-diet response. Thus, the reduction in BP with the DASH eating plan cannot be attributed to any single nutrient, but instead to the total composition of the DASH eating plan.

Pharmacological Treatment

There are many pharmacological options available for the treatment of hypertension. Treatment options depend on other diseases and confounding pathologies that are unique to the individual. Considering that there are many potential contributing mechanisms to the development of hypertension, the optimal pharmacotherapy to treat hypertension will differ for each individual. In general, the following drug classes are used to treat hypertension:

- Diuretics
- Beta blockers
- Angiotensin converting enzyme (ACE) inhibitors
- Angiotensin receptor blockers (ARBs)
- Aldosterone-receptor antagonists
- Alpha 1 blockers
- Ca++ channel blockers
- Centrally acting alpha 2 blockers
- Peripheral vasodilators

Figure 8-3 illustrates where each of the antihypertensive drug classes alters the physiological mechanisms that control BP. The

Table 8-5
The DASH Eating Plan

Food Group	Daily Servings (except as noted)	Serving Sizes	Examples and Notes	Significance of Each Food Group to the DASH Eating Plan
Grains and grain products	7–8	1 slice bread 1 oz dry cereal* ½ cup cooked rice, pasta, or cereal	Whole-wheat bread, English muffin, pita bread, bagel, cereals, grits, oatmeal, crackers, unsalted pretzels, popcorn	Major sources of energy and fiber
Vegetables	4–5	1 cup raw leafy vegetable ½ cup cooked vegetable 6 oz vegetable juice	Tomatoes, potatoes, carrots, green peas, squash, broccoli, turnip greens, collards, kale, spinach, artichokes, green beans, lima beans, sweet potatoes	Rich sources of potassium, magnesium, and fiber
Fruits	4–5	6 oz fruit juice 1 medium fruit ¼ cup dried fruit ½ cup fresh, frozen, or canned fruit	Apricots, bananas, dates, grapes, orange juice, grapefruit, grapefruit juice, mangoes, melons, peaches, pineapples, prunes, raisins, strawberries, tangerines	Important sources of potassium, magnesium, and fiber
Low-fat or fat-free dairy foods	2–3	8 oz milk 1 cup yogurt 1½ oz cheese	Fat-free (skim) or low-fat (1%) milk, fat-free or low-fat buttermilk, fat-free or low-fat regular or frozen yogurt, low-fat and fat-free cheese	Major sources of calcium and protein
Meats, poultry, and fish	2 or less	3 oz cooked meats, poultry, or fish	Select only lean; trim away visible fats; broil, roast, or boil, instead of frying; remove skin from poultry	Rich sources of protein and magnesium
Nuts, seeds, and dry beans	4–5 per week	⅓ cup or 1½ oz nuts 2 Tbsp or ½ oz seeds ½ cup cooked dry beans	Almonds, filberts, mixed nuts, peanuts, walnuts, sunflower seeds, kidney beans, lentils, peas	Rich sources of energy, magnesium, potassium, protein, and fiber
Fats and oils†	2–3	1 tsp soft margarine 1 Tbsp low-fat mayonnaise 2 Tbsp light salad dressing 1 tsp vegetable oil	Soft margarine, low-fat mayonnaise, light salad dressing, vegetable oil (such as olive, corn, canola, or safflower)	DASH has 27% of calories as fat, including fat in or added to foods
Sweets	5 per week	1 Tbsp sugar 1 Tbsp jelly or jam ½ oz jelly beans 8 oz lemonade	Maple syrup, sugar, jelly, jam, fruit-flavored gelatin, jelly beans, hard candy, fruit punch, sorbet, ices	Sweets should be low in fat

* Equals ½–1¼ cups, depending on cereal type. Check the product's Nutrition Facts label.

† Fat content changes serving counts for fats and oils. For example, 1 Tbsp of regular salad dressing equals one serving; 1 Tbsp of a low-fat dressing equals ½ a serving; 1 Tbsp of a fat-free dressing equals 0 servings.

Source: National Heart Lung and Blood Institute of the National Institutes of Health

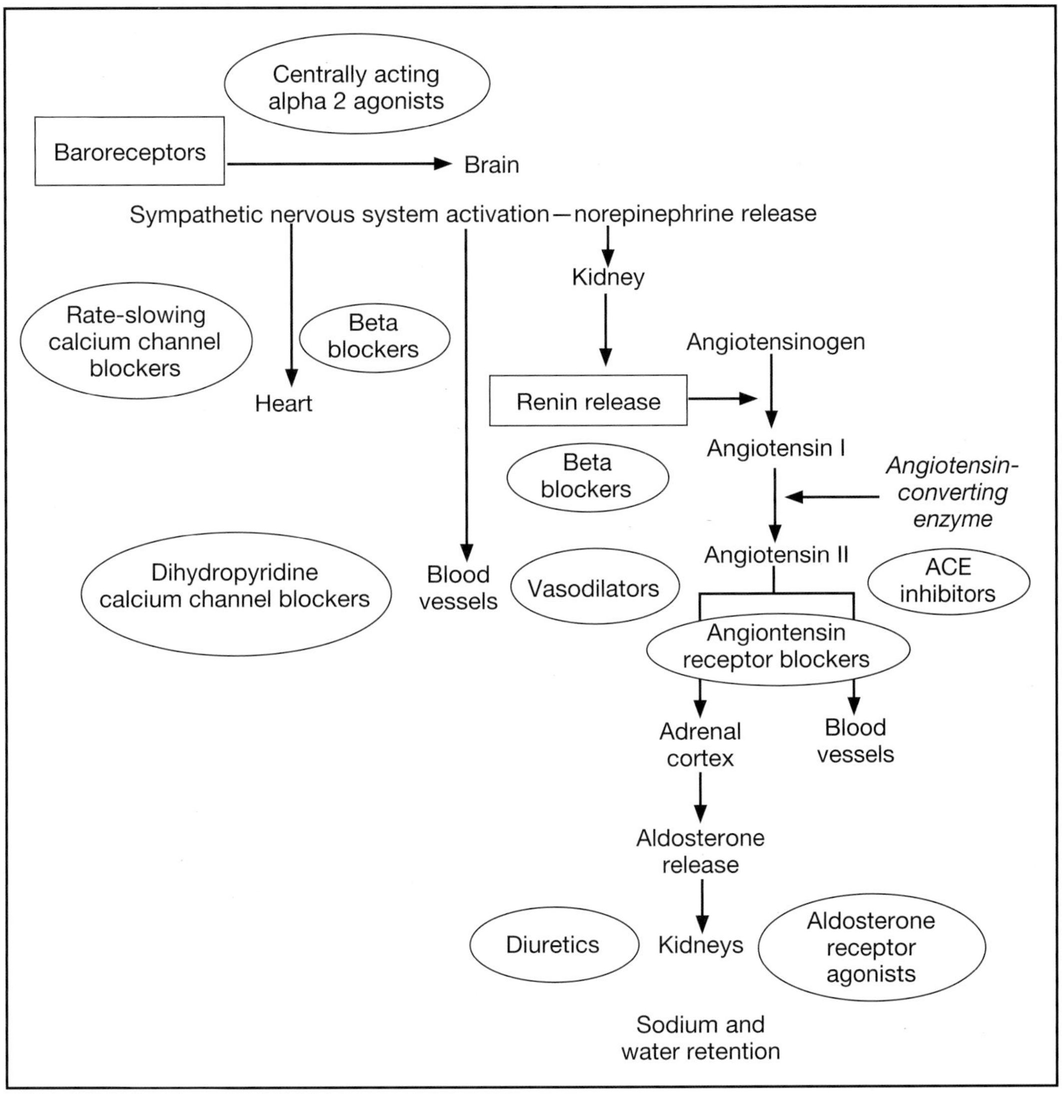

Figure 8-3
The effect of antihypertensive drug classes on the physiological mechanisms that control blood pressure

Source: Kester, M. et al. (2007) *Elsevier's Integrated Pharmacology*. Philadelphia: Elsevier.

different classes of antihypertensive medications exert their effect on one or more of the organ systems that control BP.

Surgical Treatment

There is no surgical treatment option for essential hypertension. In cases of secondary hypertension (see Table 8-1), surgery can be used to correct the underlying cause of hypertension. For example, renal artery stenosis decreases blood flow to the kidney. This condition occurs as a result of congenital defects in the renal artery or as a result of **atherosclerosis.** BP can return to normal if the blockage can be surgically repaired or through removal of the affected kidney.

Another cause of secondary hypertension is an epinephrine-secreting tumor on the adrenal gland called a **pheochromocytoma.** The excess epinephrine caused by the tumor increases heart rate and contractility to increase cardiac output. Treatment for this condition includes surgical removal of the tumor, which normally corrects the hypertension.

Exercise Treatment

For the ACE-AHFS, it is important that clients have appropriate medical clearance from their healthcare providers prior to beginning an exercise program. Incorporation of exercise and a healthy lifestyle is a cornerstone therapy in the treatment of hypertension. However, proper medical clearance is necessary to ensure that exercise is appropriate and will not lead to potential cardiovascular events in unstable hypertensive clients. After a diagnosis of hypertension is made, further medical evaluation is necessary to assess lifestyle, identify other cardiovascular risk factors, and reveal potential identifiable causes of hypertension (see Table 8-1). Medical evaluation is also necessary to assess the presence or absence of target organ damage and cardiovascular disease. In addition to a thorough physical examination, the following routine laboratory tests are recommended:

- An electrocardiogram to assess rate, rhythm, and structural changes in the heart
- Fasting blood glucose measurements to examine the presence or absence of diabetes
- Serum potassium, creatinine, or other measure of glomerular filtration rate to assess kidney function
- A lipid profile that includes the breakdown of high- and low-density lipoprotein concentrations

These laboratory tests help to identify additional risk factors for cardiovascular disease and potential contributing factors to hypertension. If warranted, clinicians may want clients to undergo supervised exercise testing to ensure that it is safe for them to engage in a regular exercise program. Furthermore, these tests are helpful for clinicians to prescribe the appropriate individualized pharmacological and non-pharmacological treatments for hypertension. Table 8-6 lists the major cardiovascular risk factors and associated diseases caused by hypertension-induced target organ damage.

Aerobic exercise training is a cornerstone in the prevention and treatment of hypertension. Exercise training induces many physiological adaptations that lower BP both acutely and chronically. In uncomplicated cases of prehypertension or stage I hypertension, aerobic exercise training along with dietary modification may be sufficient to lower BP to reach the target BP without the addition of pharmacotherapy. In more complicated cases of hypertension, the addition of regular aerobic exercise to pharmacotherapy has an additive effect on BP reduction. Exercise training also modifies other cardiovascular risk factors, including blood lipoprotein profile, insulin sensitivity, and body composition, which combine to decrease cardiovascular risk.

Table 8-6
Cardiovascular Risk Factors

- Hypertension
- Cigarette smoking
- Obesity (body mass index $\geq$30 kg/m^2)
- Physical inactivity
- Dyslipidemia
- Diabetes mellitus
- Microalbuminuria or estimated GFR <60 mL/min
- Age (older than 55 for men, 65 for women)
- Family history of premature cardiovascular disease (men under age 55 or women under age 65)

Note: GFR = Glomerular filtration rate

Source: Chobanian, A.V. et al. (2003). *JNC 7 Express: The Seventh Report of the Joint National Committee on Prevention, Detection, Evaluation, and Treatment of High Blood Pressure.* NIH Publication No. 03-5233. Washington, D.C.: National Institutes of Health & National Heart, Lung, and Blood Institute.

Acute Effects of Exercise

Dynamic exercise induces an acute post-exercise reduction in both SBP and DBP. This response is known as **post-exercise hypotension (PEH).** The PEH cardiovascular response is characterized by a reduction in peripheral vascular resistance that is not compensated for by an increase in cardiac output, resulting in a decrease in BP (Halliwill, 2001). On average, the magnitude of the effect of PEH on BP in hypertensive individuals is approximately 15 and 4 mmHg on SBP and DBP, respectively, and can persist for up to 22 hours following an exercise bout (Pescatello et al., 2004). The PEH response occurs in normotensive and hypertensive men and women of all ages, although the largest reductions in BP occur in hypertensive individuals. This acute exercise-induced reduction in BP is clinically significant. It is unknown whether there is a dose-response effect of exercise duration and intensity on PEH, with longer duration or higher intensity of exercise resulting in a greater reduction in BP. It is known that PEH occurs with relatively short-duration bouts of exercise (as little as three minutes) at low intensities (40% $\dot{V}O_2max$).

Chronic Effects of Exercise

In addition to the acute effects of dynamic exercise on post-exercise BP, there are significant long-term (chronic) effects of exercise on BP. Epidemiological studies show that there is an inverse relationship between physical activity and BP. Analysis of studies examining the effects of exercise on BP show that 150 minutes of exercise weekly reduces systolic BP by 2 to 6 mmHg (Simons-Morton, 2008a). Furthermore, physical activity lowers BP in all populations studied, with the greatest reductions in BP occurring in hypertensive individuals. It is recommended that all prehypertensive and hypertensive individuals engage in regular moderate-intensity physical activity. At a minimum, prehypertensive and hypertensive individuals should participate in 30 minutes of cumulative exercise, such as brisk walking, on most days of the week (Chobanian et al., 2003; Pescatello et al., 2004). As stated previously, exercise alone is sometimes sufficient to reduce blood pressure in prehypertensive individuals and ward off the manifestation of clinically significant hypertension. Furthermore, exercise causes an additional reduction in BP in individuals being treated with antihypertensive medication.

Special Considerations

There are specific safety issues associated with working with hypertensive clients that an ACE-AHFS must consider. First, because dynamic exercise does induce a clinically significant drop in BP through PEH, the ACE-AHFS should remind clients to get up slowly from supine and/or seated positions to avoid a sudden drop in BP (**orthostatic hypotension**). Secondly, many of the drug treatments for hypertension limit peripheral vascular vasoconstriction. Therefore, the hypotensive response upon abruptly ceasing exercise may be greater in clients taking these medications. Clients should extend their cool-down periods. If orthostatic hypotension is a chronic problem, clients should be referred to their healthcare providers to have the dosage or class of antihypertensive medication changed.

Hypertensive Medications and Cardiovascular Response

There are a number of classes of antihypertensive medications. Although lifestyle modification is a cornerstone therapy for treatment of prehypertension and hypertension, most hypertensive individuals will require two or more medications to reach their target BP. It is important that an ACE-AHFS knows the medications his or her clients are taking, how they act on the cardiovascular system to lower BP, and any effects they have on the cardiovascular responses to exercise. Table 8-7 provides a list of different antihypertensive drugs arranged by their class.

Diuretics

Diuretics are the most commonly prescribed BP-lowering drugs and are typically the first-line antihypertensive drugs prescribed for hypertensive patients. This drug class has been used for many years and is very effective at lowering BP, especially in cases in which the hypertension is caused by excess extracellular fluid volume. Diuretics initially work to decrease BP by stimulating the excretion of sodium in the proximal tubule of the nephron (the functional unit of the kidneys). To maintain osmotic balance, water follows the sodium, resulting in a loss of extracellular fluid volume. It is hypothesized that the excess sodium contributes to the peripheral blood vessels' rigidity, thus promoting an increase in peripheral vascular resistance. The long-term BP-lowering capabilities of diuretics may be a result of decreasing sodium and indirectly lowering blood vessel rigidity (Kester et al., 2007).

Clients taking diuretics to manage their hypertension should be instructed to pay particular attention to hydration during exercise, especially when exercising in warm environments. Because diuretics decrease plasma volume, hypertensive clients can easily become dehydrated during exercise. Clients should be instructed to drink fluids throughout exercise to replace the fluid that they are losing through sweat. The volume of sweat lost can be

Table 8-7
Oral Antihypertensive Drugs*

Class	Drug (Trade Name)	Usual Dose Range (mg/day)	Usual Daily Frequency
Thiazide diuretics	Chlorothiazide (Diuril)	125–500	1–2
	Chlorthalidone (generic)	12.5–25	1
	Hydrochlorothiazide (Microzide, HydroDIURIL†)	12.5–50	1
	Polythiazide (Renese)	2–4	1
	Inclapamide (Lozol†)	1.25–2.5	1
	Metolazone (Mykrox)	0.5–1.0	1
	Metolzaone (Zaroxolyn)	2.5–5	1
Loop diuretics	Bumetanide (Bumex†)	0.5–2	2
	Furosemide (Lasix†)	20–80	2
	Torsemide (Demadex†)	2.5–10	1
Potassium-sparing diuretics	Amiloride (Midamore†)	5–10	1–2
	Triamterene (Dyrenium)	50–100	1–2
Aldonsterone receptor blockers	Eplerenone (Inspra)	50–100	1
	Spironolactone (Aldactone†)	25–50	1
Beta blockers	Atenolol (Tenormin†)	25–100	1
	Betaxolol (Kerlone†)	5–20	1
	Bisopropol (Zebeta†)	2.5–10	1
	Metoprolol (Lopressor†)	50–100	1–2
	Metoprolol extended release (Toprol XL)	50–100	1
	Nadolol (Corgard†)	40–120	1
	Propanolol (Inderal†)	40–160	2
	Propanolol long-acting (Inderal LA†)	60–180	1
	Timolol (Blocadren†)	20–40	2
Beta blockers with intrinsic sympathomimetic activity	Acebutolol (Sectral†)	200–800	2
	Penbutolol (Levatol)	10–40	1
	Pindolol (generic)	10–40	2
Combined alpha and beta blockers	Carvedilol (Coreg)	12.5–50	2
	Labetalol (Normodyne, Trandate†)	200–800	2
ACE inhibitors	Benazepril (Lotensin†)	10–40	1
	Captopril (Capoten†)	25–100	2
	Enalapril (Vasotec†)	5–40	1–2
	Fosinopril (Monopril)	10–40	1
	Lisinopril (Prinivil, Zestril†)	10–40	1
	Moexipril (Univasc)	7.5–30	1
	Perindopril (Aceon)	4–8	1
	Quinapril (Accupril)	10–80	1
	Ramipril (Altace)	2.5–20	1
	Trandolapril (Mavik)	1–4	1
Angiotensin II antagonists	Candesartan (Atacand)	8–32	1
	Eprosartan (Teveten)	400–800	1–2
	Irbesartan (Avapro)	150–300	1
	Losartan (Cozaar)	25–100	1–2
	Olmesartan (Benicar)	20–40	1
	Telmisartan (Micardis)	20–80	1
	Valsartan (Diovan)	80–320	1–2

Table 8-7 (continued)

Class	Drug (Trade Name)	Usual Dose Range (mg/day)	Usual Daily Frequency
Calcium channel blockers—non-dihydropyridines	Diltiazem extended release (Cadizem CD, Dilacore XR, Tiazan†)	180–420	1
	Diltiazem extended release (Cardizem LA)	120–540	1
	Verapamil immediate release (Calan, Isoptin†)	80–320	2
	Verapamil long-acting (Calan SR, Isoptin SR†)	120–480	1–2
	Verapamil (Coer, Covera HS, Verelan PM)	120–360	1
Calcium channel blockers—dihydropyridines	Amlodipine (Norasc)	2.5–10	1
	Felodipine (Plendil)	2.5–20	1
	Isradipine (Dynacirc CR)	2.5–10	2
	Nicardipine sustained release (Cardene SR)	60–120	2
	Nifedipine long-acting (Adalat CC, Procardia XL)	30–60	1
	Nisoldipine (Sular)	10–40	1
Alpha 1 blockers	Doxazosin (Cardura)	1–16	1
	Prazosin (Minipress†)	2–20	2–3
	Terazosin (Hytrin)	1–20	1–2
Central alpha 2 agonists and other centrally acting drugs	Clonidine (Catapres†)	0.1–0.8	1
	Clonidine patch (Catpres-TTS)	0.1–0.3	1 weekly
	Methyldopa (Aldomet†)	250–1000	2
	Reserpine (generic)	0.1–0.25	1
	Guanfacine (Tenex†)	0.5–2	1
Direct vasodilators	Hydralazine (Apresoline†)	25–100	2
	Minoxidil (Loniten†)	2.5–80	1–2

*In some patients treated once daily, the antihypertensive effect may diminish toward the end of the dosing interval (trough effect). Blood pressure should be measured just prior to dosing to determine if satisfactory blood pressure control is obtained. Accordingly, an increase in dosage or frequency may need to be considered. These dosages may vary from those listed in the *Physician's Desk Reference,* 57th ed.
†Available now or soon to become available in generic preparations.

Source: Physician's Desk Reference (57th ed.) (2003). Montvale, N.J. PDR.

calculated by taking pre- and post-exercise body weights (accounting for fluid intake or loss via urine). The timing of exercise may also be important, as frequent trips to the restroom can be frustrating to the most avid exercisers.

Beta Blockers

There are many different types of beta blockers with different specificities and mechanisms of action. In general, beta blockers primarily work to lower BP by antagonizing the beta receptors in the heart and the kidneys. In the heart, normal stimulation of beta receptors by epinephrine increases heart rate and increases calcium entry into the myocardial cells, thereby increasing contractility. Stimulation of these receptors causes an increase in cardiac output. Blocking the beta receptors therefore decreases heart rate and contractility, collectively causing a decreased cardiac output. Initially, the antihypertensive effect of beta blockers is due to this decrease in cardiac output.

Beta blockers also inhibit renin release as a result of sympathetic nerve stimulation to the kidney. Recall that the release of renin stimulates a cascade of events that cause peripheral vasoconstriction through angiotensin II, as well as salt and water retention in the kidneys through the RAAS (see Figure 8-1). Thus, blocking the beta receptors in the kidneys inhibits this cascade of events and results in a passive vasodilation of the peripheral vasculature, thereby lowering peripheral vascular resistance.

Beta blockers blunt the normal elevation in heart rate that is observed during exercise. Therefore, gauging exercise intensity via target heart rate when working with hypertensive clients who are taking beta blockers is not appropriate. Instead, **ratings of perceived exertion (RPE)** of "somewhat hard," which equates to a 13 on the Borg scale (6 to 20 scale), should be used to evaluate exercise intensity. This perceived exertion correlates well with exercise intensity in the absence of an appropriate exercise heart-rate response due to the beta-blocker effect.

In addition to the heart-rate response, there are additional precautions that an ACE-AHFS should be aware of with this class of drugs. First, beta blockers can sometimes mask the symptoms of **hypoglycemia** (low blood sugar). Because exercise also decreases blood sugar, significant hypoglycemia during exercise can sometimes occur in clients taking beta blockers. Second, some clients taking beta blockers may complain of exercise intolerance due to the blunted heart-rate response. If this occurs, it is important that the client sees his or her healthcare provider to adjust the dosage of medication. The client must not abruptly stop taking his or her medication, as doing so can result in rebound hypertension. Lastly, beta blockers can cause fatigue, sedation, **depression,** and sexual dysfunction. If a client complains of these symptoms, it is important that he or she sees his or her healthcare provider.

Angiotensin Converting Enzyme (ACE) Inhibitors

ACE inhibitors block the conversion of angiotensin I to angiotensin II in the RAAS (see Figure 8-1), which results in an inhibition of peripheral vasoconstriction mediated by angiotensin II in the vasculature. It also results in an inhibition of aldosterone release from the adrenal cortex, thus preventing sodium and water reabsorption in the kidney. Recall that BP is integratively controlled by many physiological systems working in concert. In some cases, when one component of a body system is altered by pharmacology (such as causing a reduction in peripheral vascular resistance), there is a compensatory response by the other systems (increased cardiac output and sympathetic nerve activity) in an attempt to return to a homeostatic balance. However, in the case of hypertension, the desired effect of the drug treatment is to lower BP, avoiding the compensatory changes that may occur in other systems that regulate BP. One of the advantages of ACE inhibitors is that they cause vasodilation of the peripheral vasculature without inducing a compensatory increase in sympathetic nerve activity.

Angiotensin-receptor Blockers (ARBs)

ARBs are similar to ACE inhibitors in the way that they lower BP. However, instead of inhibiting the production of angiotensin II, they block the receptor on which angiotensin II acts. ARBs cause a decrease in peripheral vasoconstriction, resulting in a decrease in peripheral vascular resistance. Furthermore, ARBs also inhibit the release of aldosterone from the adrenal cortex, which ultimately inhibits sodium and water reabsorption in the kidneys.

Aldosterone-receptor Antagonists

Aldosterone-receptor blockers inhibit the effect of aldosterone on the kidney. Thus, sodium and water are not reabsorbed and plasma volume is decreased.

ACE inhibitors, ARBs, and aldosterone-receptor antagonists can all cause **hyperkalemia** (increase in serum potassium levels). When clients are taking these medications, it is important that the ACE-AHFS monitors them for signs of **electrolyte** imbalances. Signs and symptoms of hyperkalemia can include a general feeling of fatigue, muscle weakness, nausea, tingling sensations, and, most seriously, slow heart beat and a weak pulse.

Alpha Blockers

This class of drugs works by inhibiting the alpha 1 receptors in the peripheral blood vessels, leading to a reduction in vasoconstriction and reduced peripheral vascular resistance. However, when the alpha 1 receptors are blocked, there is a compensatory increase in heart rate in an attempt to increase BP to achieve homeostatic balance. The baroreceptors send signals to the cardiovascular control centers that BP is low and a response ensues through the parasympathetic and sympathetic nervous systems to increase heart rate. However, the effect of the increased sympathetic activity on the peripheral vasculature is blocked by the drug. Alpha 1 blockers are no longer routinely used to manage hypertension.

A common side effect of alpha 1 blockers is orthostatic hypotension. If clients are taking this drug class, they should be reminded to change body positions slowly and to not abruptly stop exercising. In addition, clients should be instructed to do an extended cool-down to limit the potential for a rapid decrease in BP with the cessation of exercise.

Calcium Channel Blockers

Calcium (Ca++) channel blockers prevent calcium from entering the cardiac and vascular smooth muscle cells. This in turn causes a decrease in cardiac contractility, a decrease in conduction of the electrical signal that controls heart rate, and a decrease in peripheral blood vessel vasoconstriction. The BP-lowering action of Ca++ channel blockers is therefore twofold, in that they reduce both cardiac output (decreased stroke volume and heart rate) and peripheral vascular resistance (decreased vasoconstriction). However, some types of Ca++ channel blockers have a greater effect on the heart and others have a greater effect on the peripheral blood vessels.

In relation to exercise training, similar to beta blockers these drugs cause heart rate to be slowed (**bradycardia**) and can cause a substantial drop in BP upon standing. Clients taking these drugs should be advised to use RPE to monitor exercise intensity instead of a target heart rate, prolong the cool-down, and change body positions slowly.

Central Acting Alpha 2 Blockers

Central acting alpha 2 blockers work in the BP control centers in the brain to reset and lower the BP set point, which reduces sympathetic activity to the heart and increases parasympathetic activity, resulting in a slowing of the heart rate. In addition, the reduction in sympathetic activity to the peripheral blood vessels and kidneys decreases vasoconstriction, which decreases renin release and vasoconstriction, resulting in decreased peripheral vascular resistance.

This class of antihypertensive drugs is rarely used in cases of essential hypertension. They have several side effects, including severe sedation. Orthostatic hypotension (low BP upon standing) is also common with central acting alpha 2 blockers, so caution should be used when changing body positions if clients are taking this class of antihypertensive drugs.

Peripheral Vasodilators

These drugs cause vasodilation and reduce BP by relaxing the vascular smooth muscle in the peripheral blood vessels. Typically, peripheral vasodilators are only used in combination with other antihypertensive drugs in cases of resistant hypertension or a hypertensive crisis.

The Role of Exercise in Hypertension Prevention

Unequivocally, regular physical activity and exercise training are associated with a lower incidence of cardiovascular disease. In broad survey-based epidemiological studies, there is a negative association between exercise training and the development of hypertension. Individuals with the highest levels of physical activity or who participate in vigorous sporting activities show the lowest incidence of hypertension. Furthermore, a higher fitness level is also associated with a lower risk for developing hypertension. People with a low fitness level have a higher relative risk of developing hypertension compared with highly fit people (Blair et al., 1984).

Overall, exercise training and greater baseline fitness levels are associated with a lower incidence of hypertension. While exercise training is pivotal for the prevention and treatment of hypertension, hypertension is a multifaceted pathology and is caused by an interaction of genes and environmental factors. There are certain populations with a strong genetic propensity for hypertension, and exercise training may delay the onset of hypertension and/or decrease the severity of the disease.

Exercise-related Treatment and Management of Hypertension

Numerous studies have been conducted to examine the effect of regular aerobic exercise on BP at rest, throughout the day (ambulatory), and during exercise. These studies have examined the effect of dynamic moderate-intensity aerobic exercise such as walking, jogging, running, and cycling. These studies show that resting BP is significantly reduced after aerobic training. The magnitude of the reduction in resting BP is greatest in hypertensive individuals, although people with normal BP still show a reduction in their resting BP after aerobic training. Dynamic exercise training also reduces BP throughout the day and during an acute bout of exercise.

Cardiovascular Responses to Exercise Training

There are many cardiovascular adaptations that cause a reduction in BP as a result of exercise training. Many of these adaptations positively affect BP both at rest and during acute bouts of exercise. An examination of the determinants of mean arterial pressure reveal that for BP to be reduced, a decrease in either cardiac output or total peripheral resistance must occur. With exercise training, there are alterations in the determinants of cardiac output, but the primary mechanism for the decrease in BP is through a decrease in peripheral vascular resistance. The BP-lowering effects of exercise training occur as a result of changes to the systems that integratively control BP.

Changes to the Sympathetic Nervous System

One of the changes that occur as a result of exercise training takes place in the sympathetic nervous system. Essential hypertension is associated with an increase in the nerve traffic from the sympathetic nervous system to the heart and the peripheral blood vessels. In general, there is a decrease in sympathetic nerve traffic with exercise training. Some studies have shown that direct measures of sympathetic nerve traffic at rest decrease after exercise training (Ray & Hume, 1998), though not all studies have been able to consistently replicate this finding (Morlin, Wallin, & Eriksson, 1983).

An additional way to indirectly measure globalized systemic changes in sympathetic nerve activity is to measure the concentration of **norepinephrine** (the sympathetic adrenergic neurotransmitter) in the blood. Recall that the sympathetic nerves release norepinephrine that binds to receptors on blood vessels and causes the peripheral blood vessels to vasoconstrict. Measuring the amount of norepinephrine in the blood is an indirect assessment of sympathetic nerve activity, because the absolute concentration is influenced by how much norepinephrine is released and how well it is cleared. In individuals with hypertension, norepinephrine concentration in the blood has been shown to decrease after exercise training (Meredith, 1990).

Changes to the Renin-Angiotensin-Aldosterone System

The renin-angiotensin-aldosterone system (RAAS) is involved in the long-term regulation of BP. It would be expected that changes to this system would contribute to the reduction in BP observed with exercise training. Decreased renin and angiotensin II are observed in normotensive individuals after exercise training and contribute to the reduction in BP. However, this response is not observed in hypertensive subjects after exercise training (Pescatello et al., 2004).

Changes to the Peripheral Blood Vessels

One prominent change induced by exercise training in hypertensive individuals takes place in the peripheral blood vessels. Exercise training reduces the amount of vasoconstriction that occurs when norepinephrine binds to the receptors on the blood vessels. In addition, there are changes in the locally produced vasoconstrictors and vasodilators in the blood vessels. The two most prominent changes are to a vasoconstrictor called endothelin 1 and the vasodilator nitric oxide. After exercise training, endothelin 1 is reduced and nitric oxide is increased (Pescatello et al., 2004). Long-term exercise training can also cause beneficial adaptations of the structure of the blood vessels themselves, increasing their elasticity. Together, reduced responsiveness to norepinephrine, decreased endothelin 1, increased nitric oxide, and structural adaptations in the blood vessels result in decreased vascular resistance and contribute to the reduction in BP.

Finally, just as there is a complex interaction among genetic and environmental factors in the development of hypertension, there is significant variation in the response to exercise training. Certain genetic profiles may respond more favorably to exercise training. It has been suggested that genetic factors can explain some of the reduction in systolic BP after exercise training (Pescatello et al., 2004).

Thermoregulation

Individuals with hypertension have a diminished ability to dissipate body heat to the environment during heat stress (Kenney, 1985). Thermal heat stress occurs during exercise, passive exposure to hot and humid environments, or the combination that comes with exercising in the heat. The normal physiological response to rising body core temperature during heat stress includes activation of the sympathetic nervous system, which causes an integrated cardiovascular response in an effort to increase blood flow to the skin for **thermoregulation.** Increased skin blood flow allows warm blood from the body core to flow through the cooler skin circulation, where heat is lost through convection. In addition, the evaporation of sweat from the skin cools the skin and serves as a major avenue of heat loss. The integrated cardiovascular response to heat stress includes an increase in heart rate and cardiac contractility, which together increase cardiac output and vasoconstriction in the renal and the splanchnic circulations, thereby allowing the redistribution of blood flow to the skin (Rowell, 1974).

Heat stress significantly challenges the cardiovascular system, especially in individuals with cardiovascular pathologies like hypertension. Most heat-related injuries and deaths occur in individuals with cardiovascular pathology (McGeehin & Mirabelli, 2001). There are several underlying factors contributing to this increased risk, including impairments in the cardiovascular response to heat stress directly caused by the hypertensive disease as well as the inability for the cardiovascular system to respond appropriately during heat stress caused by the pharmacology used to treat hypertension.

Hypertensive individuals have a reduction in skin blood flow during heat stress, which results in a decreased ability to transfer body heat to the environment (Kenney, 1985). The decrease in heat transfer results in a significant increase in body core temperature. There is also a significant reduction in skin blood flow in hypertensive individuals, which is related to structural alteration in the skin blood vessels and to changes in the locally produced signaling molecules in the skin that allow the skin blood vessels to vasodilate during heat stress (Holowatz & Kenney, 2007). In hypertensive individuals, the increase in cardiac work during heat stress is especially dangerous in individuals with cardiac or other end organ damage (left ventricular hypertrophy or coronary artery disease).

In addition to the hypertension-induced physiological changes that occur with heat stress, many of the pharmacological treatments for hypertension also blunt the integrated cardiovascular response to heat stress. Specifically, diuretics decrease plasma volume. Individuals taking diuretics can easily become dehydrated during heat stress, and dehydration alone decreases blood flow to the skin and impairs thermoregulation. Other drugs that adversely affect the cardiovascular response to heat stress include beta blockers, Ca++ channel blockers, and alpha blockers. These drugs impair the central cardiovascular and peripheral blood flow responses that occur during heat stress.

Exercise training has beneficial thermoregulatory effects in hypertensive individuals. Exercise training sufficient to increase $\dot{V}O_2$max strengthens the central cardiovascular system. The amount of cardiac work during exercise at the same absolute workload will be less after exercise training. In addition, peripheral sweating and blood vessel changes allow individuals to start sweating and vasodilating their skin blood vessels at lower body core temperatures. Together, these adaptations confer positive benefits on thermoregulation.

Training Guidelines

Programming and Progression Guidelines and Considerations

Prior to beginning a new exercise program with a hypertensive client, several important safety issues should be addressed. In normal healthy individuals, the initiation of exercise acutely increases SBP. This acute increase in SBP is normal and necessary to increase blood flow to the exercising muscle to deliver oxygen and clear metabolic by-products. However, some hypertensive individuals experience an exaggerated increase in SBP and/or DBP during dynamic exercise, which is predictive of future morbidity from cardiovascular disease. Depending on the initial resting BP and whether the client has target organ damage or additional cardiovascular risk factors, a medically supervised exercise-tolerance test should be conducted. Table 8-8 presents the recommendations for exercise testing prior to engaging in a regular exercise program (Simons-Morton, 2008b). Furthermore, these high-risk clients may benefit from a medically supervised cardiac rehabilitation program. Clients may be unaware that they may qualify for such programs.

Table 8-9 lists the general indications set forth by American College of Sports Medicine (ACSM) for the termination of exercise. An absolute contraindication to exercise is if resting SBP is greater than 200 mmHg or if DBP is greater than 115 mmHg.

Cardiovascular Training

Exercise programming guidelines following the FITT principle (frequency, intensity, time, and type) are suitable for individuals with hypertension. The Centers for Disease Control and Prevention (CDC) and ACSM have endorsed the recommendation that, "Every U.S. adult should accumulate 30 minutes or more of moderate-intensity physical activity on most, preferably all, days of the week" (Pescatello et al., 2004).

The optimal cardiovascular training guidelines necessary to see a reduction in BP are unclear. To a certain extent, the dose of exercise needed to observe a reduction in BP is related to initial fitness level. In sedentary individuals, clinically significant reductions in BP can be observed with relatively modest increases in physical activity. Researchers have found that significant reductions in resting systolic and diastolic BP can occur with as little as 60 minutes of exercise at an intensity

Table 8-8
Recommendations for Exercise Testing Before Exercise Participation

		No known TOD or CVD; 1 or more CVD risk factor		
Exercise intensity	**No TOD or CVD, no risk factors, no symptoms, BP <180/110 mmHg**	**No symptoms; BP <180/110 mmHg**	**Symptoms or BP >180/110 mmHg**	**Known TOD or CVD**
Moderate	Not necessary	Not necessary	Recommended	Recommended
Vigorous	Not necessary	May be beneficial	Recommended	Recommended

Notes: TOD and CVD include ischemic heart disease, heart failure, stroke, renal disease, neuropathy, or retinopathy; also includes diabetes as a "CVD equivalent"
CVD risk factors include hypertension, smoking, dyslipidemia, age older than 60 years, male gender or postmenopausal woman, family history of cardiovascular disease (in women <65 years or in men <55 years).
BP = Blood pressure; TOD = Target organ damage; CVD = Cardiovascular disease

Source: Adapted from American College of Sports Medicine (2004). Position stand: Exercise and hypertension. *Medicine & Science in Sports & Exercise,* 36, 6, 533–553.

Table 8-9
General Indications for Stopping Exercise

- Onset of angina or angina-like symptoms
- Significant drop (20 mmHg) in SBP or a failure of the SBP to rise with an increase in exercise intensity
- Excessive rise in blood pressure: SBP >250 mmHg or DBP >115 mmHg
- Signs of poor perfusion: lightheadedness, confusion, ataxia, pallor, cyanosis, nausea, or cold and clammy skin
- Failure of heart rate to increase with increased exercise intensity
- Noticeable change in heart rhythm
- Subject requests to stop
- Physical or verbal manifestations of severe fatigue
- Failure of the exercise equipment

Note: SPB = Systolic blood pressure; DBP = Diastolic blood pressure

Source: Adapted from American College of Sports Medicine (2006). *ACSM's Guidelines for Exercise Testing and Prescription* (7th ed.). Philadelphia: Lippincott Williams & Wilkins.

of approximately 50% of $\dot{V}O_2$max per week (Ishikawa-Takata, Ohta, & Tanaka, 2003). There is an even greater reduction when the exercise duration was increased to 90 minutes.

Frequency

Studies have consistently shown that training frequencies between three and five days a week will cause a significant reduction in BP. However, increasing the frequency of exercise training to most days of the week may confer additional BP-lowering benefits for hypertensive individuals. These additional benefits are likely due to the acute BP-lowering effects of exercise (i.e., post-exercise hypotension).

Intensity

The intensity of aerobic exercise for hypertensive clients should be moderate. Significant reductions in BP are observed with exercise intensities between 40 and 70% of $\dot{V}O_2$max. Exercise intensities higher than 70% of $\dot{V}O_2$max do not cause greater reductions in BP and may in fact blunt the BP-lowering effect of exercise (Hagberg, Park, & Brown, 2000). Thus, hypertensive clients experience the beneficial effects of exercise at an intensity of 40 to 60% of $\dot{V}O_2$max. This exercise intensity corresponds to approximately a 12 to 13 on the Borg RPE scale (6 to 20 scale). Using the RPE scale to gauge exercise intensity is beneficial, especially when clients are taking antihypertensive medications that alter the cardiovascular responses to exercise (e.g., beta blockers).

Time

The duration of exercise should be at least 30 minutes to have a beneficial effect on cardiovascular health. This 30-minute duration can be continuous or intermittent, but if intermittent exercise is conducted, the bouts should be at least 10 minutes in length and total 30 to 60 minutes of exercise each day. This can also be expressed in terms of calories burned (700 kcal/week is a good initial goal, progressing to 2000 kcal/week).

Type

Aerobic, endurance-type exercise such as walking, jogging, running, swimming, and cycling is recommended. Walking is one of the easiest exercise modalities to start with, especially in previously sedentary clients. Any physical activity that engages the large muscle groups and is rhythmic and aerobic will be beneficial. The type of exercise performed should be individualized so that clients are more likely to adhere to their programs. Thus, the exercises should be relatively simple and offer some variety.

Table 8-10 summarizes the cardiovascular exercise recommendations for hypertensive clients.

Progression

The progression of exercise training in hypertensive clients should follow the basic principles

Table 8-10
Cardiovascular Training Recommendations for Hypertensive Clients

Frequency: On most, preferably all, days of the week

Intensity: Moderate (40–60% $\dot{V}O_2$max or 12–13 RPE)

Time: 30–60 minutes of continuous or accumulated physical activity

Type: Rhythmic aerobic exercise that targets large muscle groups; should be individualized of an initial conditioning stage, an improvement stage, and a maintenance stage that is tailored to the client's initial fitness level and attains the client's specific fitness goals. In general, hypertensive clients should progress to exercising three to seven days per week, for 30 to 60 minutes, at an intensity of 40 to 60% of $\dot{V}O_2max$. The initial conditioning stage should include a moderate level of aerobic exercise that causes minimal muscle soreness or discomfort. For a hypertensive client, this may include walking for two 10-minute bouts twice a week (Simons-Morton, 2008b). This stage may last up to four weeks depending on the adaptation of the individual to the training program. The duration of an exercise session during this initial stage may begin at 15 to 20 minutes and progress to 30 minutes three to four days per week. During the improvement stage, the intensity of exercise is progressively increased every two to three weeks until the client is able to exercise at a moderate intensity for 20 to 30 minutes. During the maintenance stage, the exercise frequency, intensity, and time are maintained while program goals are reviewed and new goals are set.

Resistance Training

There has been significant controversy surrounding the safety of resistance training for hypertensive clients. During **isometric** exercise (resistance), both SBP and DBP increase. The magnitude of the increase in BP with resistance exercise is related to the intensity of exercise and the amount of muscle mass involved in the exercise. This increase in BP is potentially dangerous for hypertensive clients because heavy resistance training can cause large increases in both SPB and DBP. In general, moderate resistance training is beneficial and safe for this population, as long as the hypertension is controlled. According to the guidelines from the AHA, resistance training is contraindicated in individuals with unstable **angina** (chest pain), uncontrolled hypertension (systolic BP $\geq$160 mmHg and/or diastolic BP $\geq$100 mmHg), uncontrolled cardiac arrhythmias, a recent history of congestive heart failure, significant heart valve disease, or pathological enlargement of the heart (**hypertrophic cardiomyopathy**) (Braith & Stewart, 2006). While aerobic exercise is the mainstay in the treatment of hypertension, it can be safely supplemented with resistance training.

Resistance training offers several beneficial physiological effects. It increases muscular strength, endurance, and mass. The increase in muscle mass causes an increased **basal metabolic rate (BMR).** Perhaps one of the most beneficial effects of resistance training on BP results from the positive effects on **insulin** sensitivity. There is a significant link between decreased insulin sensitivity and hypertension. Because consistent and long-term resistance training increases insulin sensitivity, this may be one of the mechanisms mediating the reduction in BP. Resistance training also attenuates the **rate-pressure product** (an index of cardiac work) when lifting any given load, which decreases the demand on the heart when performing **activities of daily living** (ADL) and various work- and recreation-related tasks:

Rate-pressure product = Heart rate (HR) x Systolic blood pressure (SBP)

In addition, resistance training is beneficial for the prevention and management of other chronic conditions, such as low back pain, **osteoporosis, obesity, sarcopenia** (the loss of skeletal muscle mass that may accompany aging), **diabetes,** and the susceptibility to falls. Resistance training of the major muscle groups decreases resting systolic and diastolic BP in hypertensive individuals by approximately 3 mmHg (Braith & Stewart, 2006). In studies examining different types of resistance training (circuit training vs. conventional), no difference in BP reduction was found among modalities. However, because circuit training uses lighter weights with limited rest periods between exercises, thereby introducing an aerobic component, it is the type of resistance training recommended for hypertensive clients.

A preliminary orientation with clients should establish appropriate weight loads, and the ACE-AHFS should instruct the client on proper lifting techniques and correct breathing patterns to avoid straining or performing the

Valsalva maneuver. Straining during resistance training causes significant and dangerous increases in BP. At minimum, one exercise per major muscle group should be performed. For example, a resistance-training program for a hypertensive client might include eight to 12 repetitions of the following exercises performed two to three days per week:

- Chest press
- Seated row
- Shoulder press
- Lower-back extension
- Triceps extension
- Biceps curl
- Abdominal crunch/curl-up
- Quadriceps extension or leg press
- Leg curls (hamstrings)
- Heel raises

Older or frailer clients should initially perform 10 to 15 repetitions at a lower relative resistance to prevent injury. The ACE-AHFS can slowly increase the number of sets until clients are performing three sets two to three days per week.

Mind-body Exercise

Mind-body exercises such as yoga and tai chi are increasingly being incorporated into exercise training programs to promote flexibility, strength, and relaxation. There are few randomized controlled studies examining the effects of these alternative exercise programs specifically on high BP. The few studies that have been conducted suggest a beneficial reduction in BP attributable to both physical activity and relaxation (Santaella et al., 2006; La Forge, 2003).

Randomized clinical studies on the effects of hatha yoga on blood pressure demonstrate a large reduction in SBP with regular yoga therapy. These studies showed a 33 mmHg and 26 mmHg reduction in SBP after practicing yoga and biofeedback for six hours a week for 11 weeks (Patel & North, 1975; Murugesan, Govindarajulu, & Bera, 2000). The combined effects on BP of physical activity and relaxation, as practiced through mind-body exercise, appear to be synergistic, meaning that the combined effect is greater than the individual BP-lowering capabilities of either physical activity or relaxation alone (Cohen & Townsend, 2007).

Mind-body exercise practiced regularly (three times per week for 60 minutes) also improves balance and upper- and lower-body muscular strength and endurance (Taylor-Piliae et al., 2006). Further, these mind-body exercises also improve proprioceptive awareness. Several general precautions should be used when recommending mind-body exercise to hypertensive clients. First, many styles of hatha yoga involve isometric muscle contractions combined with dynamic movement of the body into different positions. This work should be done with caution, because isometric muscle contractions cause significant increases in BP. In addition, hypertensive clients taking certain antihypertensive medications may experience dramatic decreases in BP when changing body position. Specifically, diuretics, alpha blockers, calcium channel blockers, and beta blockers can cause orthostatic hypotension. Hypertensive clients should avoid holding strenuous poses, avoid inverted poses (e.g., downward-facing dog and shoulder stands), and be encouraged to transition slowly between poses. Caution should be used when practicing yoga with stage I and II hypertensive clients. Bikram yoga (rapidly paced yoga in very hot environments) should be avoided altogether because of the impaired thermoregulatory mechanisms seen in hypertensive clients.

Case Studies

Case Study 1

Edith is a 45-year-old woman who would like to start an exercise program to lose weight. She is 5'4" tall (1.6 m) and weighs 150 pounds (68 kg). Her physician has also told her that she has high total cholesterol, with a HDL cholesterol of 68 mg/dL and an LDL cholesterol of 140 mg/dL. She has been diagnosed with hypertension in the past, but admits that she gets very nervous when she visits her doctor's office. She is currently not involved in a regular exercise program but is motivated to start an exercise program to lose weight. Edith's diet is high in total calories, saturated fat, cholesterol, and sodium and low in fruits, vegetables, and fiber. After being seated in a quiet consulting room with both feet on the floor for five minutes, her resting BP is 138/86 mmHg. After an additional five minutes of sitting quietly, her BP drops to 130/82 mmHg.

What is Edith's body mass index? 68 kg ÷ $(1.6 \text{ m})^2 = 26.6$

According to the JNC VII guidelines, is Edith hypertensive? If so what stage of hypertension does she have? Edith has been diagnosed with hypertension in the past. However, her current BP measurements indicate that she is prehypertensive, as her readings fall within the 120/80 to 139/89 mmHg range.

What types of exercise should Edith incorporate into her new training program? How should an ACE-AHFS progress her training program? Edith should begin with an aerobic endurance-training program following the basic principles of an initial conditioning stage, an improvement stage, and a maintenance stage. In general, she should progress to exercising three to seven days per week, for 30 to 60 minutes, at an intensity of 40 to 70% of $\dot{V}O_2$max. The initial conditioning stage should include a moderate level of aerobic exercise that causes minimal muscle soreness or discomfort. This stage may last up to four weeks, depending on her adaptation to the training program. The duration of an exercise session during this initial stage may begin at 15 to 20 minutes and progress to 30 minutes three to four days per week. During the improvement stage, the intensity of exercise is progressively increased every two to three weeks until Edith is able to exercise at a moderate-to-vigorous intensity for 20 to 30 minutes. During the maintenance stage, the exercise frequency, intensity, and time are maintained while program goals are reviewed and new goals are set.

In general, moderate resistance training should be safe for Edith, as long as her hypertension is controlled. While aerobic exercise is the mainstay in the treatment of hypertension, it can be safely supplemented with resistance training. Because circuit training uses lighter weights with limited rest periods between exercises, thereby introducing an aerobic component, it is a good choice for Edith. However, she should be instructed on proper lifting techniques and correct breathing patterns to avoid straining or performing the Valsalva maneuver. Additionally, mind-body exercises such as yoga and tai chi may be incorporated into Edith's exercise training program to promote flexibility, strength, and relaxation.

What other lifestyle modifications should Edith incorporate into her life? Edith can make the following lifestyle modifications (in addition to her exercise program) to help control her BP:

- Weight reduction of as little as 10 pounds (4.5 kg)
- Limiting dietary sodium intake to less than 2400 mg per day
- Adopting a healthy eating plan that includes fresh fruits and vegetables, low-fat dairy products, and reduced saturated and total fat content (DASH eating plan)
- Avoiding or limiting alcohol consumption to no more than one drink per day

Case Study 2

Harry is a 60-year-old man who takes a diuretic and a beta blocker to control his blood pressure. His resting blood pressure with his medication is not very well controlled and today his blood pressure reading is 144/88 mmHg. Harry is relatively healthy, with the exception of his blood pressure, but he does have a strong family history of heart disease (his father died at age 44 from a heart attack). Harry has recently retired from his job and has found that his level of regular physical activity has decreased substantially. Because Harry had a physically demanding job, he has never engaged in a regular exercise program. Harry's age, high blood pressure, family history of heart disease, and current sedentary lifestyle give him four cardiovascular risk factors.

Is Harry's blood pressure adequately controlled with his medication? No, Harry's BP appears unstable.

Should Harry have a supervised exercise test prior to engaging in a new exercise program? Since Harry's BP is less than 180/110 mmHg and he has four cardiovascular disease risk factors, it is not necessary that he have a clinically supervised exercise test prior to participating in a new low-to-moderate intensity (40 to 60% of $\dot{V}O_2max$) exercise program. It may, however, be beneficial to conduct an exercise test if he plans to engage in vigorous-intensity exercise (>60% $\dot{V}O_2max$).

What exercise program should an ACE-AHFS recommend to Harry? In general, an exercise program for Harry should follow the FITT principle and take place on most, preferably all, days of the week, at a moderate intensity (40 to 60% $\dot{V}O_2max$), and be primarily endurance-type activity. Low-resistance, high-repetition resistance training and mind/body activity such as yoga or Pilates can supplement Harry's regular endurance training. The ACE-AHFS should be prepared to assess Harry's BP before, during, and after exercise or as recommended by his physician.

Summary

Exercise is a cornerstone therapy for the treatment and prevention of hypertension. Exercise therapy combined with dietary modification can prevent the development of hypertension in prehypertensive clients, and can have an additive effect with antihypertensive drugs in reducing blood pressure. Exercise therapy for all hypertensive clients should follow the FITT principle and take place on most, preferably all, days of the week, at a moderate intensity (40 to 60% $\dot{V}O_2max$), and be primarily endurance-type activity. Low-resistance, high-repe tition resistance training and mind/body exercise activities can also supplement regular endurance exercise in hypertensive clients.

References

American College of Sports Medicine (2006). *ACSM's Guidelines for Exercise Testing and Prescription* (7th ed.). Philadelphia: Lippincott Williams & Wilkins.

American College of Sports Medicine (2004). Position stand: Exercise and hypertension. *Medicine & Science in Sports & Exercise,* 36, 6, 533–553.

American Heart Association (2007a). Heart disease and stroke statistics—2008 update. A report from the American Heart Association Statistics Committee and Stroke Statistics Subcommittee: 2008 Heart and Stroke Statistical Update. *Circulation,* Dec. 17 online.

American Heart Association (2007b). *Hypertension Statistics*. Dallas: American Heart Association.

Blair, S.N. et al. (1984). Physical fitness and incidence of hypertension in healthy normotensive men and women. *Journal of the American Medical Association,* 252, 487–490.

Braith, R.W. & Stewart, K.J. (2006). Resistance exercise training: Its role in the prevention of cardiovascular disease. *Circulation,* 113, 2642–2650.

Burt, V.L. et al. (1995). Prevalence of hypertension in the U.S. adult population: Results from the Third National Health and Nutrition Examination Survey, 1988–1991. *Hypertension,* 25, 305–313.

Chobanian, A.V. et al. (2003). *JNC 7 Express: The Seventh Report of the Joint National Committee on Prevention, Detection, Evaluation, and Treatment of High Blood Pressure.* NIH Publication No. 03-5233. Washington, D.C.: National Institutes of Health & National Heart, Lung, and Blood Institute.

Cohen, D. & Townsend, R.R. (2007). Yoga and hypertension. *Journal of Clinical Hypertension,* 9, 800–801.

Ferdinand, K.C. (2008). Hypertension in blacks. In: Izzo, J.L. et al. (Eds.) *Hypertension Primer: The Essentials of High Blood Pressure: Basic Science, Population Science, and Clinical Management* (4th ed.). Philadelphia: Lippincott Williams & Williams.

Folkow, B. (1982). Physiological aspects of primary hypertension. *Physiological Reviews,* 62, 347–504.

Grim, C.M. & Grim, C.M. (2008). Blood pressure measurement. In: Izzo, J.L. et al. (Eds.) *Hypertension Primer: The Essentials of High Blood Pressure: Basic Science, Population Science, and Clinical Management*. (4th ed.). Philadelphia: Lippincott Williams & Williams.

Hagberg, J.M., Park, J.J., & Brown, M.D. (2000). The role of exercise training in the treatment of hypertension: An update. *Sports Medicine,* 30, 193–206.

Hajjar, I. & Kotchen, T.A. (2003). Trends in prevalence, awareness, treatment, and control of hypertension in the United States, 1988–2000. *Journal of the American Medical Association,* 290, 199–206.

Halliwill, J.R. (2001). Mechanisms and clinical implications of post-exercise hypotension in humans. *Exercise and Sport Sciences Reviews,* 29, 65–70.

Hesse, C. et al. (2007). Baroreflex sensitivity inversely correlates with ambulatory blood pressure in healthy normotensive humans. *Hypertension,* 50, 41–46.

Holowatz, L.A. & Kenney, W.L. (2007). Up-regulation of arginase activity contributes to attenuated reflex cutaneous vasodilatation in hypertensive humans. *The Journal of Physiology,* 581, 863–872.

Hypertension Prevention Research Group (1997). Effects of weight loss and sodium reduction intervention on blood pressure and hypertension incidence in overweight people with high-normal blood pressure: The Trials of Hypertension Prevention, phase II. *Archives of Internal Medicine,* 157, 657–667.

Ishikawa-Takata, K., Ohta, T., & Tanaka, H. (2003). How much exercise is required to reduce blood pressure in essential hypertensives: A dose-response study. *American Journal of Hypertension,* 16, 629–633.

Kenney, W.L. (1985). Decreased core-to-skin heat transfer in mild essential hypertensives exercising in the heat. *Clinical and Experimental Hypertension,* 7, 1165–1172.

Kester, M.V. et al. (2007). *Elsevier's Integrated Pharmacology.* Philadelphia: Mosby, Inc.

La Forge, R. (2003). Mindful exercise overview for personal trainers. In: American Council on Exercise. *ACE Personal Trainer Manual* (3rd ed.). San Diego: American Council on Exercise.

McGeehin, M.A. & Mirabelli, M. (2001). The potential impacts of climate variability and change on temperature-related morbidity and mortality in the United States. *Environmental Health Perspectives*, 109, Suppl. 2, 185–189.

Meredith, I.T. (1990). Time-course of the antihypertensive and autonomic effects of regular endurance exercise in human subjects. *Journal of Hypertension,* 8, 859–866.

Morlin, C., Wallin, B.G., & Eriksson, B.M. (1983). Muscle sympathetic activity and plasma noradrenaline in normotensive and hypertensive man. *Acta Physiologica Scandinavica,* 119, 117–121.

Murugesan, R., Govindarajulu, N., & Bera, T.K. (2000). Effect of selected yogic practices on the management of hypertension. *Indian Journal of Physiology and Pharmacology*, 44, 207–210.

Patel, C. & North, W.R. (1975). Randomised controlled trial of yoga and bio-feedback in management of hypertension. *Lancet,* 2, 93–95.

Pescatello, L.S. et al. (2004). American College of Sports Medicine position stand: Exercise and hypertension. *Medicine & Science in Sports & Exercise,* 36, 533–553.

Physician's Desk Reference (57th ed.) (2003). Montvale, N.J.: PDR.

Ray, C.A. & Hume, K.M. (1998). Sympathetic neural adaptations to exercise training in humans: Insights from microneurography. *Medicine & Science in Sports & Exercise,* 30, 387–391.

Rosendorff, C. et al. (2007). Treatment of hypertension in the prevention and management of ischemic heart disease: A scientific statement from the American Heart Association Council for High Blood Pressure Research and the Councils on Clinical Cardiology and Epidemiology and Prevention. *Circulation,* 115, 2761–2788.

Rowell, L.B. (1993). *Human Cardiovascular Control.* New York: Oxford University Press.

Rowell, L.B. (1974). Human cardiovascular adjustments to exercise and thermal stress. *Physiological Review*, 54, 75–159.

Santaella, D.F. et al. (2006). Aftereffects of exercise and relaxation on blood pressure. *Clinical Journal of Sports Medicine*, 16, 341–347.

Simons-Morton, D.G. (2008a). Physical activity and blood pressure. In: Izzo, J.L. et al. (Eds.) *Hypertension Primer: The Essentials of High Blood Pressure: Basic Science, Population Science, and Clinical Management* (4th ed.). Philadelphia: Lippincott Williams & Williams.

Simons-Morton, D.G. (2008b). Exercise therapy. In: Izzo, J.L. et al. (Eds.) *Hypertension Primer: The Essentials of High Blood Pressure: Basic Science, Population Science, and Clinical Management* (4th ed.). Philadelphia: Lippincott Williams & Williams.

Taylor-Piliae, R.E. et al. (2006). Improvement in balance, strength, and flexibility after 12 weeks of tai chi exercise in ethnic Chinese adults with cardiovascular disease risk factors. *Alternative Therapies in Health and Medicine,* 12, 50–58.

Vasan, R.S. et al. (2002). Residual lifetime risk for developing hypertension in middle-aged women and men: The Framingham Heart Study. *Journal of the American Medical Association,* 287, 1003–1010.

Weder, A.B. (2008). Genetics of hypertension. In: Izzo, J.L. et al. (Eds.) *Hypertension Primer: The Essentials of High Blood Pressure: Basic Science, Population Science, and Clinical Management* (4th ed.). Philadelphia: Lippincott Williams & Williams.

Suggested Reading

American College of Sports Medicine (2006). *ACSM's Guidelines for Exercise Testing and Prescription* (7th ed.). Philadelphia: Lippincott Williams & Wilkins.

Braith, R.W. & Stewart, K.J. (2006). Resistance exercise training: Its role in the prevention of cardiovascular disease. *Circulation,* 113, 2642–2650.

Chobanian, A.V. et al. (2003). Seventh report of the Joint National Committee on Prevention, Detection, Evaluation, and Treatment of High Blood Pressure. *Hypertension*, 42, 1206–1252.

Cohen, D. & Townsend, R.R. (2007). Yoga and hypertension. *Journal of Clinical Hypertension,* 9, 800–801.

Grim, C.M. & Grim, C.M. (2008). Blood pressure measurement. In: Izzo, J.L. et al. (Eds.) *Hypertension Primer: The Essentials of High Blood Pressure: Basic Science, Population Science, and Clinical Management*. (4th ed.). Philadelphia: Lippincott Williams & Williams.

Pescatello, L.S. et al. (2004). American College of Sports Medicine position stand: Exercise and hypertension. *Medicine & Science in Sports & Exercise*, 36, 533–553.

Simons-Morton, D.G. (2008). Physical activity and blood pressure. In: Izzo, J.L. et al. (Eds.) *Hypertension Primer: The Essentials of High Blood Pressure: Basic Science, Population Science, and Clinical Management* (4th ed.). Philadelphia: Lippincott Williams & Williams.

Simons-Morton, D.G. (2008). Exercise therapy. In: Izzo, J.L. et al. (Eds.) *Hypertension Primer: The Essentials of High Blood Pressure: Basic Science, Population Science, and Clinical Management* (4th ed.). Philadelphia: Lippincott Williams & Williams.

Tipton, C.M. (1991). Exercise, training and hypertension: An update. *Exercise and Sport Sciences Reviews,* 19, 447–505.

Zanesco, A. & Antunes, E. (2007). Effects of exercise training on the cardiovascular system: Pharmacological approaches. *Pharmacology & Therapeutics,* 114, 307–317.

In This Chapter

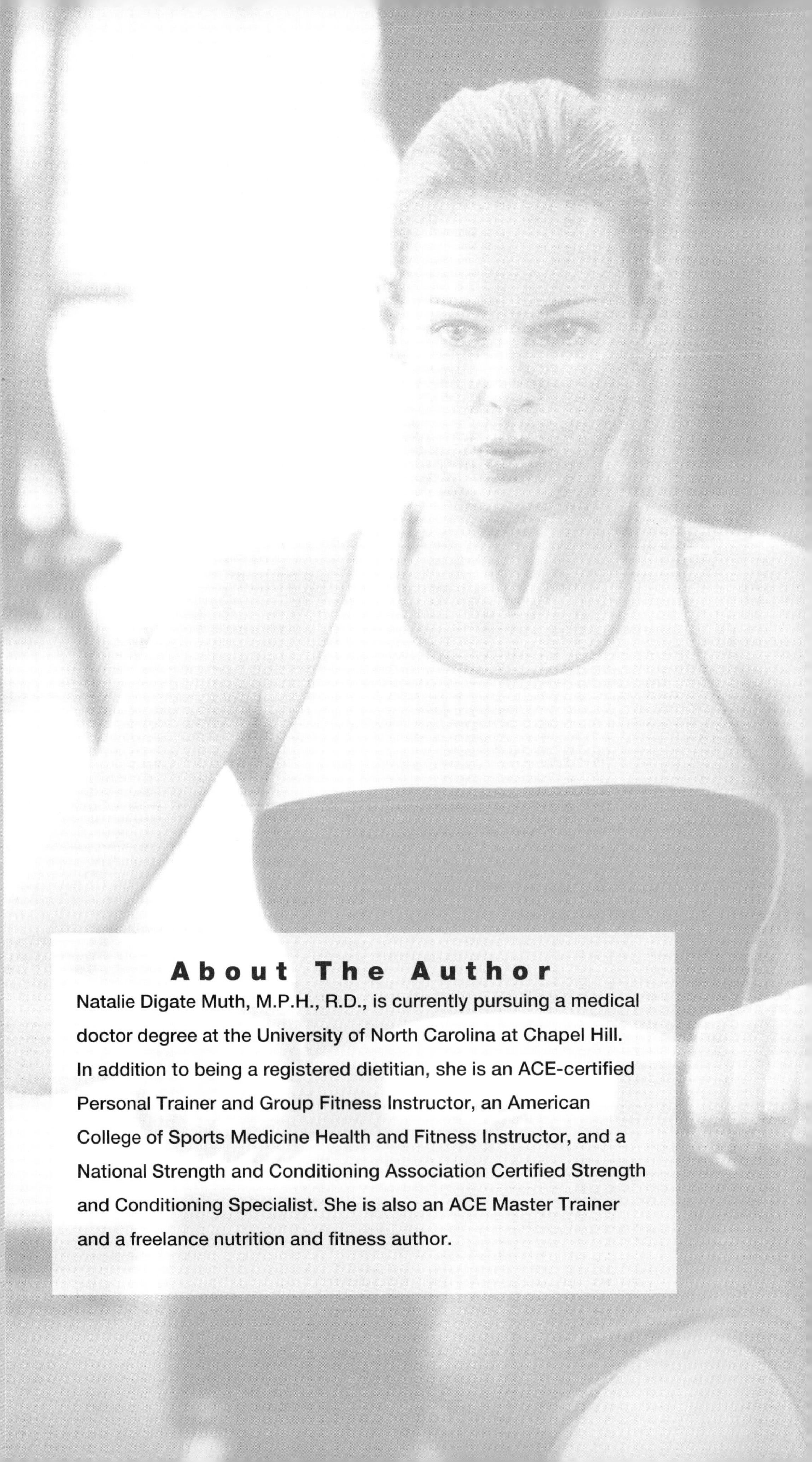

About The Author

Natalie Digate Muth, M.P.H., R.D., is currently pursuing a medical doctor degree at the University of North Carolina at Chapel Hill. In addition to being a registered dietitian, she is an ACE-certified Personal Trainer and Group Fitness Instructor, an American College of Sports Medicine Health and Fitness Instructor, and a National Strength and Conditioning Association Certified Strength and Conditioning Specialist. She is also an ACE Master Trainer and a freelance nutrition and fitness author.

CHAPTER 9

Asthma

Natalie Digate Muth

Pulmonary disorders, including **asthma,** are among the most prevalent chronic diseases that an ACE-certified Advanced Health & Fitness Specialist (ACE-AHFS) will encounter. Asthma, a chronic inflammatory disorder of the airways that causes varying degrees of difficulty breathing, wheezing, coughing, and chest tightness, affects more than 20 million children and adults in the United States [Moorman et al., 2007; National Asthma Education and Prevention Program (NAEEP), 2007].

The disorder is responsible for nearly 500,000 hospitalizations, 2 million emergency room visits, and 4,000 deaths in the United States each year (Moorman et al., 2007). Asthma affects people differently depending on various genetic and environmental factors, though asthma onset begins in childhood for most people. In some individuals, exercise and physical activity can induce an asthmatic response. However, with appropriate medical management and precautions, most severe exercise-related and non-exercise-related asthma responses can be avoided. Furthermore, in many cases, a well-designed and effectively implemented exercise program can help to minimize asthma symptoms and exacerbations. This chapter arms the ACE-AHFS with the basic knowledge and resources necessary to recommend the highest quality and safest exercise programs for clients with asthma.

Overview of Asthma

Asthma is a chronic inflammatory disorder of the airways that affects genetically susceptible individuals in response to various environmental triggers such as **allergens,** viral infections, exercise, cold, and stress. The inflammation leads to narrowing of the airways and **bronchospasm,** making it more difficult to transfer inhaled oxygen through the respiratory system and to the rest of the body. These inflammation-induced airway changes contribute to the severity and frequency of the attacks and are responsible for symptoms such as shortness of breath, wheezing, coughing, and chest tightness. The flow diagram in Figure 9-1 shows the relationship between airway inflammation, airway hyperresponsiveness, and airway obstruction and asthma symptoms. These symptoms are usually worse at night and in the early morning. For some people, chronic inflammation leads to permanent changes in airway structure. Figure 9-2 compares a normal bronchus to an inflamed bronchus.

Asthma severity is categorized based on the frequency of symptoms and the results from pulmonary function tests (Table 9-1). The disease categorization determines the medical treatment and the individual's susceptibility to a severe attack, though it is important to note that asthma severity changes—both for better and worse—over time and even someone with mild intermittent disease can suffer a severe life-threatening asthma exacerbation.

The reason why some individuals develop airway inflammation and subsequently an asthma diagnosis is uncertain. Research suggests that asthma usually begins in childhood in response to various gene-environment interactions (Busse & Lemanske, 2001). The genetic factors that affect disease susceptibility may include the balance between two types

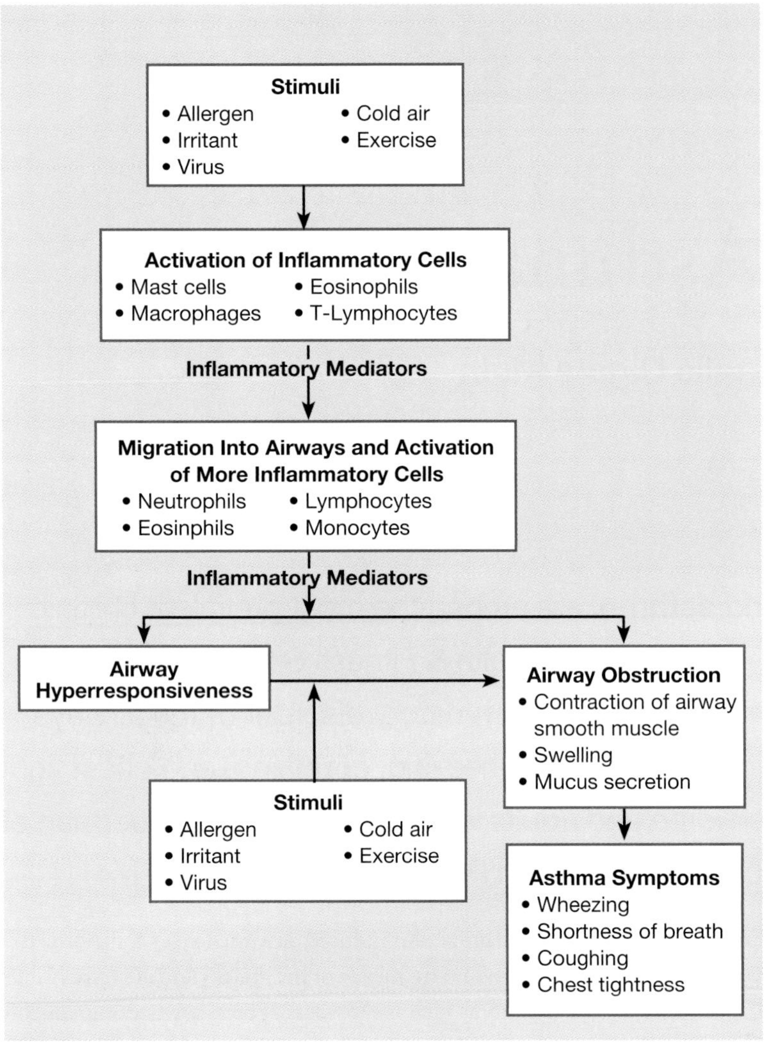

Figure 9-1
Relationships among airway inflammation, airway hyperresponsiveness, airway obstruction, and asthma symptoms

Source: United States Department of Health and Human Services & National Institutes of Health (2003). *Making a Difference in the Management of Asthma: A Guide for Respiratory Therapists.* Pub. No. 02-1064. (http://www.nhlbi.nih.gov/health/prof/lung/asthma/asth_respir.pdf)

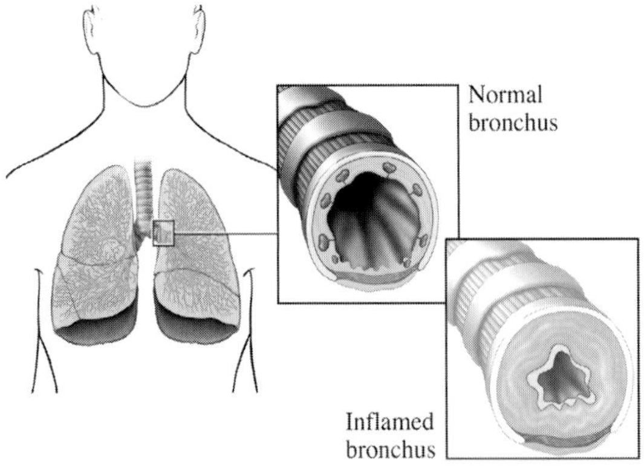

Figure 9-2
A normal versus an inflamed airway

Source: Illustration Copyright © 2008 Nucleus Medical Art, All rights reserved. www.nucleus.com

of Th lymphocytes, which are important in the body's immune response to infection (Figure 9-3); a not yet fully understood complex interaction of certain genes inherited from a susceptible parent; and gender differences (Busse & Lemanske, 2001). Specifically, in childhood, asthma is more prevalent in boys, but at puberty the sex ratio shifts and asthma becomes more common in women (Horwood, Fergusson, & Shannon, 1985). Hormones probably play an important role in this shift, though the precise mechanism is unknown.

Asthma Triggers

Not all genetically susceptible individuals develop asthma. Rather, a gene–environment interaction occurs in some individuals in response to exposure to environmental triggers. The two most important triggers are allergens and viral respiratory infections. Exposure to house-dust mites and cockroaches in early life increases the risk of asthma in susceptible children (Sigurs et al., 2000). Some studies have shown that exposure to dog and cat dander also increases the risk of asthma, but others have found that exposure to dogs and cats in childhood may actually protect against asthma (NAEPP, 2007). Likewise, exposure to **respiratory syncytial virus (RSV)** or parainfluenza virus as an infant seems to increase the risk of asthma in later childhood, with nearly 40% of these infants wheezing or acquiring asthma in later childhood (Sigurs et al., 2000). However, according to the "hygiene hypothesis," exposure to various viral infections, including RSV, in early life decreases the risk of developing asthma by promoting the development of a child's immune system along a "non-allergic" pathway (NAEPP, 2007). Gaining a clearer understanding of the relationship among allergens, viral infections, and the development of asthma is a priority for asthma researchers.

Other environmental factors that may predispose an individual to asthma development include tobacco smoke, certain occupational exposures, possibly a low intake of antioxidants and omega-3 fatty acids, and air pollution (NAEPP, 2007). Notably, a 2002 epidemiologic study found that heavy outdoor exercise (three or more

Table 9-1
Classifying Asthma Severity in Individuals ≥12 Years

COMPONENTS OF SEVERITY	CLASSIFICATION OF ASTHMA SEVERITY			
	INTERMITTENT	PERSISTENT		
		Mild	Moderate	Severe
Symptoms	≤2 days/week	>2 days/week but not daily	Daily	Throughout the day
Nighttime awakenings	≤2x/month	3–4x/month	>1x/week but not nightly	Often 7x/week
Short-acting beta-agonist use for symptom control (not prevention of EIB)	≤2 days/week	>2 days/week but not >1x/day	Daily	Several times/day
Interference with normal activity	None	Minor limitation	Some limitation	Extremely limited
Lung function	Normal FEV1 between exacerbations FEV1>80% predicted	FEV1 >80% predicted	FEV1 >60% but<80% predicted	FEV1 >60% predicted
	FEV1/FVC normal	FEV1/FVC normal	FEV1/FVC reduced 5%	FEV1/FVC reduced 5%
Exacerbations requiring oral systemic corticosteroids	0–1/year	≥2/year	≥2/year	≥2/year

Consider severity and interval since last exacerbation.
Frequency and severity may fluctuate over time for patients in any severity category.
Relative annual risk of exacerbations may be related to FEV1.
Note: EIB = Exercise-induced bronchospasm; FEV1 = Forced expiratory volume in one second; FVC = forced vital capacity

Source: National Asthma Education and Prevention Program (2007). *Expert Panel Report 3: Guidelines for the Diagnosis and Management of Asthma.* Bethesda, Md.: U.S. Department of Health and Human Services, Public Health Service, National Institutes of Health, National Heart, Lung, and Blood Institute. NIH publication number 08-4051. http://www.nhlbi.nih.gov/guidelines/asthma/asthgdln.pdf

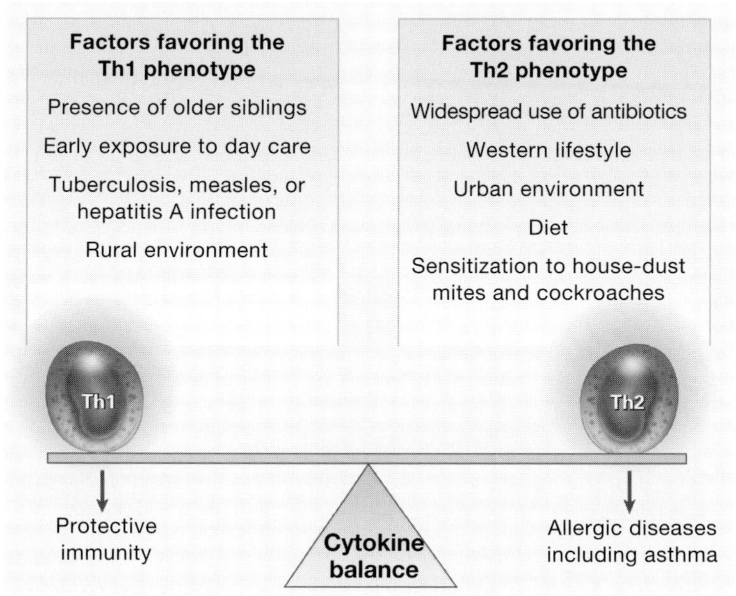

Figure 9-3
Cytokine balance and genetic susceptibility to asthma

Source: Busse, W.W. & Lemanske, R.F. (2001). Advances in immunology. *New England Journal of Medicine,* 344, 350–362.

team sports) in communities with high levels of air pollution was associated with an increased risk of developing asthma in school-age children (McConnell et al., 2002). Individuals with asthma often experience a worsening of symptoms in response to a variety of triggers (Table 9-2). Figure 9-4 provides tips that the ACE-AHFS can share with clients to minimize their exposure to specific triggers.

Table 9-2
Common Asthma Triggers

- Exercise
- Cold air
- Viral infection
- Animals with fur or hair
- House-dust mites (in mattresses, pillows, upholstered furniture, carpets)
- Mold
- Smoke (tobacco, wood)
- Pollen
- Changes in weather
- Strong emotional expressions (intense laughing or crying)
- Airborne chemicals or dusts
- Menstrual cycles
- Stress
- Comorbid conditions such as sinusitis, rhinitis, gastroesophageal reflux disease (GERD), and obstructive sleep apnea (OSA)

Diagnostic Testing and Criteria

A combination of patient history, physical examination, and objective tests is important for physicians to diagnose asthma, as well as assess severity and control of the disease. Patient history often reveals the occurrence of symptoms characteristic of asthma (e.g., shortness of breath, wheezing, coughing, and chest tightness, usually worse in the early morning and at night). Common physical findings in individuals with asthma include the following:

- Use of accessory muscles to breathe
- Appearance of hunched shoulders and/or chest deformity
- Sounds of wheezing during normal breathing or prolonged forced exhalation
- Increased nasal secretion, mucosal swelling, and/or nasal polyp
- Eczema and other signs of an allergic skin condition

Importantly, not all individuals with asthma have these physical findings, and in some people such findings may indicate another medical condition and not asthma (e.g., congestive heart failure, cough secondary to medication). The objective test most often used to diagnose asthma and assess risk of a future asthma event is **spirometry,** a type of **pulmonary function test (PFT).**

Spirometry

Spirometry measures lung function by assessing the amount (volume) and/or speed (flow) of air that can be maximally inhaled and exhaled. Spirometry helps to determine if there is airflow obstruction, its severity, and whether it is reversible. In obstructive lung disease, a narrowing or blockage of the airways causes a decrease in exhaled air flow. In asthma, the narrowing is due to inflammation-induced swelling and sometimes mucous build-up. In spirometric testing, the patient takes a deep breath and blows into a mouthpiece attached to the spirometer. The patient is then instructed to exhale as hard and fast as possible until the lungs feel completely empty. This sequence is repeated until two to three good measurements are recorded. A computerized sensor in the spirometer calculates and graphs the results. The patient is then given a short-acting bronchodilator or nebulizer and the sequence is repeated. A decrease in airflow in people with asthma usually can be partially reversed with short-acting bronchodilators or nebulizers. Spirometry is performed at the time of initial assessment; after treatment is initiated and symptoms and **peak expiratory flow (PEF)** have stabilized; during a period of poorly controlled symptoms; and at least every one to two years to assess maintenance of airway function.

Spirometry Interpretation

A sample spirometry reading in a person with asthma is depicted in Figure 9-5. Note that the person's age, height, and gender are used to determine reference, or predicted, values for

How to Control Things That Make Asthma Worse

This guide suggests things you can do to avoid your asthma triggers. Put a check next to the triggers that you know make your asthma worse and ask your doctor to help you find out if you have other triggers as well. Then decide with your doctor what steps you will take.

Allergens

❑ **Animal Dander**

Some people are allergic to the flakes of skin or dried saliva from animals with fur or feathers.

The best thing to do:

- Keep furred or feathered pets out of your home.

If you can't keep the pet outdoors, then:

- Keep the pet out of the bedroom and other sleeping areas at all times, and keep the door closed.
- Remove carpets and furniture covered with cloth from your home. If that is not possible, keep the pet away from fabric-covered furniture and carpets.

❑ **Dust Mites**

Many people with asthma are allergic to dust mites. Dust mites are tiny bugs that are found in every home—in mattresses, pillows, carpets, upholstered furniture, bedcovers, clothes, stuffed toys, and fabric or other fabric-covered items.

Things that can help:

- Encase your mattress in a special dust-proof cover.
- Encase your pillow in a special dust-proof cover or wash the pillow each week in hot water. Water must be hotter than 130° F (54° C) to kill the mites. Cold or warm water used with detergent and bleach can also be effective.
- Wash the sheets and blankets on your bed each week in hot water.
- Reduce indoor humidity to below 60% (ideally between 30 and 50%). Dehumidifiers or central air conditioners can do this.
- Try not to sleep or lie on cloth-covered cushions.
- Remove carpets from your bedroom and those laid on concrete, if you can.
- Keep stuffed toys out of the bed or wash the toys weekly in hot water or cooler water with detergent and bleach.

❑ **Cockroaches**

Many people with asthma are allergic to the dried droppings and remains of cockroaches.

The best things to do:

- Keep food and garbage in closed containers. Never leave food out.
- Use poison baits, powders, gels, or paste (for example, boric acid). You can also use traps.
- If a spray is used to kill roaches, stay out of the room until the odor goes away.

❑ **Indoor Mold**

- Fix leaky faucets, pipes, or other sources of water that have mold around them.
- Clean moldy surfaces with a cleaner that has bleach in it.

❑ **Pollen and Outdoor Mold**

What to do during your allergy season (when pollen or mold spore counts are high):

- Try to keep your windows closed.
- Stay indoors with windows closed from late morning to afternoon, if you can. Pollen and some mold spore counts are highest at that time.
- Ask your doctor whether you need to take or increase anti-inflammatory medicine before your allergy season starts.

Irritants

❑ **Tobacco Smoke**

- If you smoke, ask your doctor for ways to help you quit. Ask family members to quit smoking, too.
- Do not allow smoking in your home or car.

❑ **Smoke, Strong Odors, and Sprays**

- If possible, do not use a wood-burning stove, kerosene heater, or fireplace.
- Try to stay away from strong odors and sprays, such as perfume, talcum powder, hair spray, and paints.

Other things that bring on asthma symptoms in some people include:

❑ **Vacuum Cleaning**

- Try to get someone else to vacuum for you once or twice a week, if you can. Stay out of rooms while they are being vacuumed and for a short while afterward.
- If you vacuum, use a dust mask (from a hardware store), a double-layered or microfilter vacuum cleaner bag, or a vacuum cleaner with a HEPA filter.

❑ **Other Things That Can Make Asthma Worse**

- Sulfites in foods and beverages: Do not drink beer or wine or eat dried fruit, processed potatoes, or shrimp if they cause asthma symptoms.
- Cold air: Cover your nose and mouth with a scarf on cold and windy days.
- Other medicines: Tell your doctor about all the medicines you take. Include cold medicines, aspirin, vitamins and other supplements, and nonselective beta-blockers (including those in eye drops).

Figure 9-4
How to control things that make asthma worse

Source: National Heart, Lung, and Blood Institute

Figure 9-5
Sample spirometry curves in an individual with asthma

Source: Chobanian, A.V. et al. (2003). *JNC 7 Express: The Seventh Report of the Joint National Committee on Prevention, Detection, Evaluation, and Treatment of High Blood Pressure. NIH Publication No. 03-5233.* Washington, D.C.: National Institutes of Health & National Heart, Lung, and Blood Institute.

SAMPLE SPIROMETRY VOLUME/TIME AND FLOW/VOLUME CURVES

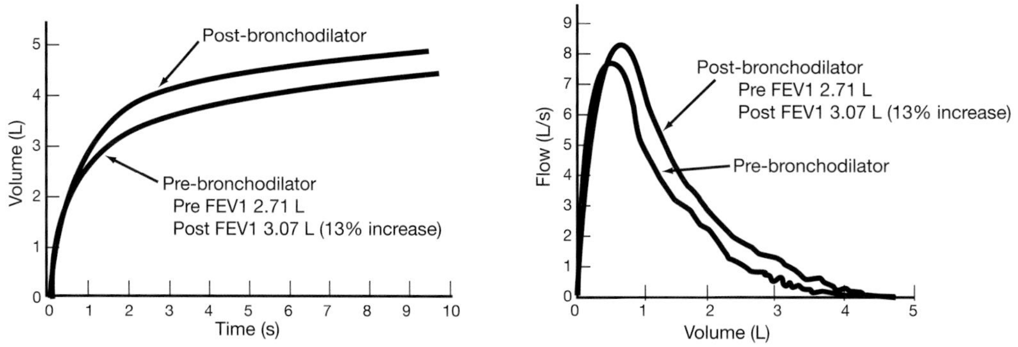

Note: FEV1 = forced expiratory volume in 1 second

REPORT OF SPIROMETRY FINDINGS PRE- AND POST-BRONCHODILATOR

Pre-bronchodilator

Study: bronch Age 59	**ID: Height: 175 cm**	**Test date: 8/7/06 Sex: M**	**Time: 9:38 a.m. System: 7 20 17**
Trial	FVC	FEV1	FEV1/ FVC (%)
1	4.34	2.68	61.8%
2	4.44	2.62	58.9%
3	4.56	2.71	59.4%
Best values	4.56	2.71	59.4%
Predicted values*	4.23	3.40	80.5%
Percent predicted	107.8%	79.7%	73.8%

Interpretations:
FEV1 and FEV1/ FVC are below normal range. The reduced rate at which air is exhaled indicates obstruction to airflow.
*Predicted values from Knudson, R.J. et al. (1983). Changes in the normal maximal expiratory flow-volume curve with growth and aging. *American Review of Respiratory Diseases*, 127, 6, 725–734.

Post-bronchodilator

Study: bronch Age 59	**ID: Height: 175 cm**	**Test date: 8/7/06 Sex: M**	**Time: 9:58 a.m. System: 7 20 17**
Trial	FVC	FEV1	FEV1/ FVC (%)
1	4.73	2.94	62.2%
2	4.76	3.07	64.5%
3	4.78	3.04	63.5%
Best values	4.78	3.07	64.3%
Reference values	4.56	2.71	
Difference (L)	0.22	0.36	
Difference (%)	4.8%	13.4%	

Interpretations:
Significant increases in FEV1 with bronchodilator (≥12% increase after bronchodilator indicates a significant change).

Note: FEV1 = Forced expiratory volume in 1 second; FVC = Forced vital capacity

the individual. The sample patient completed three trials pre-bronchodilator and three trials post-bronchodilator, with the best value used to analyze test results. Refer to the pre-bronchodilator **forced vital capacity (FVC)** and **forced expiratory volume in one second (FEV1)**. FVC is the total amount of air that can be forcibly exhaled after a maximal inhalation, compared to predicted value. Sometimes FEV6 (the amount of air exhaled in the first six seconds of maximal exhalation) is used instead of FVC for older adults who may be unable to complete a maximal expiratory effort to exhale their entire vital capacity. An obstructive lung pattern reveals a reduced FEV1 and a reduced FEV1/FVC ratio. The sample patient in Figure 9-5 has 79.7% of FEV1 and 73.8% of predicted FEV1/FVC. In general, an FEV1 or FEV1/FVC of ≥80% of predicted is normal, while 60 to 79% of predicted indicates mild obstruction; 40 to 59% of predicted indicates moderate obstruction; and <40% indicates severe obstruction, though values vary somewhat with age.

In individuals with an asthma diagnosis, the reduced FEV1 is improved by at least 12% from baseline or 10% of predicted FEV1 after inhalation of a short-acting bronchodilator. For the sample patient in Figure 9-5, the best value from the post-bronchodilator trials showed a 13.4% increase in FEV1 following bronchodilation.

The spirometry volume time and flow volume curves show improved function following bronchodilation, with a greater volume of air expired in the first second of expiration as well as overall (figure on left); and increased maximal flow, area under the curve, and total volume expired (figure on right).

Peak Expiratory Flow

While spirometry is the most useful method for monitoring lung function and asthma control, some individuals and their physicians prefer to also use a peak flow meter to measure how well air moves out of the lungs. Peak flow is used to monitor asthma, not for asthma diagnosis. A peak flow meter is a handheld mechanical or electronic device that provides a simple, reproducible, and quantitative way to measure exhalation capacity. When PEF is used, the individual's personal best peak flow should be used as the reference value. When a patient senses a worsening of symptoms or wants to monitor the response to treatment, he or she compares peak flow to the established reference value. The patient and physician then work together based on the personal best peak flow to set up zones (NAEPP, 2007):

- Green zone (≥80% of personal best) signals good control. No asthma symptoms are present. The individual should take medications as usual.
- Yellow zone (50 to 80% of personal best) signals caution. Measure peak flow several times. If measurements remain in this zone, the individual should take an inhaled short-acting beta agonist. If peak flows continue to be in the yellow zone, this may signal that asthma is not under good control. The client should consult with his or her physician to change or increase daily medications.
- Red zone (<50% of personal best) signals a medical alert. The individual must take a short-acting beta-agonist immediately. The ACE-AHFS should call the client's physician or the emergency room and ask what to do, or take the client directly to the emergency room. If the client is alone, he or she should call 911.

An ACE-AHFS should ask clients with asthma if they use a peak flow meter to monitor symptoms and if they have set up zones to help them decide how to manage PEF results. The ACE-AHFS may find this information beneficial should a client develop symptoms during exercise.

Allergy Testing

A strong relationship exists between asthma and **atopy,** or allergic hypersensitivity. For some individuals with persistent asthma, a thorough evaluation to determine the contributing role of allergens helps to better characterize asthma triggers and aggressively avoid them. After attaining a complete exposure and medical history, a physician may order skin testing or *in vitro* testing to determine the presence of specific **IgE antibodies** to indoor allergens, such as dust mites and animal dander. Importantly, the individual should only be tested for those allergens to which he or she is exposed, as it is impossible to determine whether a specific IgE is responsible for the patient's symptoms.

Asthma Treatment and Education

Treatment

Once an asthma diagnosis has been established, the next step is for the physician to assess the severity of the asthma based on spirometry results and the patient's recall of symptoms over the past two to four weeks. A critically important non-pharmacological treatment is for the patient to aggressively avoid asthma triggers and control comorbid conditions, many of which are listed in Table 9-2.

Medical management consists of a regimen of long-term-control medications and quick-relief medications, depending on asthma classification and severity. Long-term-control medications prevent symptoms, usually by reducing inflammation. These medications must be taken daily and do not typically provide quick relief. Quick-relief medications are short-acting beta-agonists that act to relax muscles around the airway and provide rapid improvement of symptoms. Quick-relief medications should only be used when symptoms occur. The need for these medications on a regular basis may indicate insufficiently controlled asthma and the need to start or increase long-term control medications. Table 9-3 provides a basic overview of the long- and short-term medications used in asthma treatment. Note that the typical response and possible side effects of medication use are included in Table 9-3 as well. Importantly, short-acting beta-agonists, the medications used most often during an exercise-induced asthma exacerbation, also affect the **sympathetic nervous system,** leading to elevated heart rate. Figure 9-6 describes in more detail the evidence-based treatment regimens that physicians use to help an individual best manage asthma symptoms. Some physicians also may recommend sinus surgery for people who have asthma and chronic rhinosinusitis, though results are mixed as to whether surgery improves asthma symptoms.

Table 9-3
Asthma Medications

Long-term-control Medications

- ***Corticosteroids:*** The most potent and effective anti-inflammatory medications currently available. Inhaled corticosteroids are used in the long-term control of asthma. Possible side effects include hoarseness, headache, and mouth infection. A short course of oral corticosteroids is used to gain prompt control of the disease when initiating long-term therapy. Long-term use of systemic steroids is used for severe persistent asthma. Short-term use of oral corticosteroids can cause weight gain, fluid retention, mood changes, and high blood pressure, while long-term use can cause hyperglycemia, osteoporosis, cataracts, muscle weakness, and immune suppression.
- ***Long-acting beta agonists (salmeterol and formoterol):*** Bronchodilators that relax or open airways in the lungs and that work for at least 12 hours. They are used in combination with inhaled corticosteroids for long-term control and prevention of symptoms in moderate or severe persistent asthma, and are the preferred therapy in combination with inhaled corticosteroids for individuals ≥12 years. Possible cardiopulmonary side effects include tremor, rapid heartbeat, elevated blood pressure, and upper airway irritation.
- ***Cromolyn sodium and nedocromil:*** Used as an alternative, not preferred, medication for treatment of mild persistent asthma. They can also be used as preventive treatment prior to exercise or unavoidable exposure to known allergens. Dry cough is a possible side effect.
- ***Immunomodulators (omalizumab):*** Adjunctive therapy for individuals ≥12 years who have allergies and severe persistent asthma. Note that anaphylaxis may occur.
- ***Leukotriene modifiers (montelukast, zafirlukast, 5-lipoxygenase inhibitor):*** Alternative therapy for mild persistent asthma. Note that anaphylaxis may occur.
- ***Methylxanthines (theophylline):*** Mild to moderate bronchodilator used as an alternative adjunctive therapy with inhaled corticosteroids.

Quick-relief Medications

- ***Short-acting beta agonists (albuterol, levalbuterol, pirbuterol):*** Bronchodilators that relax or open airways in the lungs. They are the therapy of choice for relief of acute symptoms and prevention of exercise-induced bronchoconstriction. Bronchodilators activate the sympathetic nervous system and may cause rapid heartbeat, tremors, anxiety, and nausea.
- ***Anticholinergics (ipratropium bromide):*** Reduce vagal tone of the airway leading to dilation. They provide additive benefit to short-acting-bronchodilators in moderate-to-severe asthma exacerbation. Possible side effects include dizziness, nausea, heartburn, and dry mouth.
- ***Oral corticosteroids:*** Though not short-acting, they can be used for moderate and severe exacerbations, in addition to short-acting bronchodilators to speed recovery and prevent recurrence of exacerbations.

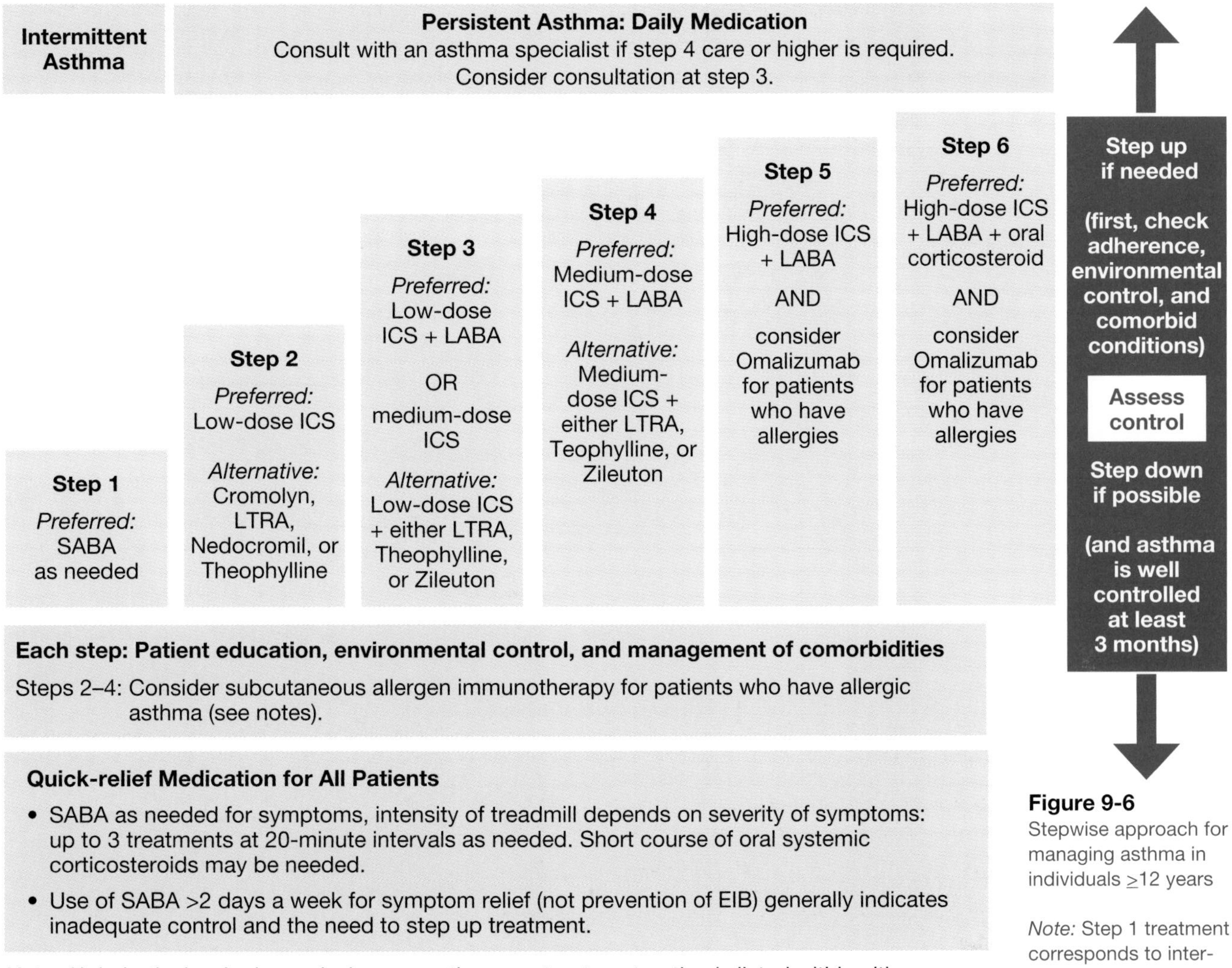
Intermittent Asthma
Persistent Asthma: Daily Medication
Consult with an asthma specialist if step 4 care or higher is required.
Consider consultation at step 3.
Step 1
Preferred:
SABA as needed
Step 2
Preferred:
Low-dose ICS
Alternative:
Cromolyn, LTRA, Nedocromil, or Theophylline
Step 3
Preferred:
Low-dose ICS + LABA
OR
medium-dose ICS
Alternative:
Low-dose ICS + either LTRA, Theophylline, or Zileuton
Step 4
Preferred:
Medium-dose ICS + LABA
Alternative:
Medium-dose ICS + either LTRA, Teophylline, or Zileuton
Step 5
Preferred:
High-dose ICS + LABA
AND
consider Omalizumab for patients who have allergies
Step 6
Preferred:
High-dose ICS + LABA + oral corticosteroid
AND
consider Omalizumab for patients who have allergies
Step up if needed
(first, check adherence, environmental control, and comorbid conditions)
Assess control
Step down if possible
(and asthma is well controlled at least 3 months)
Each step: Patient education, environmental control, and management of comorbidities
Steps 2–4: Consider subcutaneous allergen immunotherapy for patients who have allergic asthma (see notes).
Quick-relief Medication for All Patients
• SABA as needed for symptoms, intensity of treadmill depends on severity of symptoms: up to 3 treatments at 20-minute intervals as needed. Short course of oral systemic corticosteroids may be needed.
• Use of SABA >2 days a week for symptom relief (not prevention of EIB) generally indicates inadequate control and the need to step up treatment.

Note: Alphabetical order is used when more than one treatment option is listed within either preferred or alternative therapy. EIB = Exercise-induced bronchospasm; ICS = Inhaled corticosteroid; LABA = Inhaled long-acting beta-2 agonist; LTRA = Leukotriene antagonist; SABA = Inhaled short-acting beta-2 agonist

Figure 9-6
Stepwise approach for managing asthma in individuals ≥12 years

Note: Step 1 treatment corresponds to intermittent asthma, step 2 treatment corresponds to mild persistent asthma, step 3 and step 4 treatment correspond to moderate persistent asthma, and step 5 and step 6 treatment correspond to severe persistent asthma.

Source: National Asthma Education and Prevention Program (2007). *Expert Panel Report 3: Guidelines for the Diagnosis and Management of Asthma.* Bethesda, Md.: U.S. Department of Health and Human Services, Public Health Service, National Institutes of Health, National Heart, Lung, and Blood Institute. NIH publication number 08-4051. http://www.nhlbi.nih.gov/guidelines/asthma/asthgdln.pdf

Education

While an ACE-AHFS will not prescribe medications or treatment regimens, recognition of the complexity of asthma management will help him or her better understand clients' disease- and asthma-related challenges. Furthermore, the ACE-AHFS can play an important role in helping to reinforce the physician's recommendations, help a client effectively self-monitor, and provide asthma education. Education is a critical component of a successful asthma-management program, as it empowers individuals to effectively carry out complex medication regimens, implement environmental control strategies, detect and self-treat most exacerbations, and communicate effectively with healthcare providers. The ACE-AHFS should ask clients the following questions about their asthma:

- What are your triggers?
- What medications do you take (including those prescribed by a physician and any over-the-counter or alternative therapies)?
- When was your last asthma exacerbation?
- When was the last time you saw your physician?
- Is your physician aware of everything that you have disclosed to me?

The process of answering these questions will force clients to acknowledge and understand

ASTHMA ACTION PLAN

For:______________________ Doctor:______________________ Date:__________

Doctor's Phone Number:__________ Hospital/Emergency Department Phone Number:__________

GREEN ZONE

Doing Well
- No cough, wheeze, chest tightness, or shortness of breath during the day or night
- Can do usual activities

And, if a peak flow meter is used,

Peak flow: more than ________
(80% or more of my best peak flow)

My best peak flow is: ________

Take these long-term control medicines each day (include an anti-inflammatory).

Medicine	How much to take	When to take it

Identify and avoid and control the things that make your asthma worse, like (list here):

Before exercise ❑ __________ ❑ 2 or ❑ 4 puffs __________ 5 to 60 minutes before exercise

YELLOW ZONE

Asthma Is Getting Worse
- Cough, wheeze, chest tightness, or shortness of breath or
- Waking at night due to asthma, or
- Can do some, but not all, usual activities

-Or-

Peak flow: ______ to ______
(50 to 79% of my best peak flow)

First: Add: quick-relief medicine ___ and keep taking your GREEN ZONE medicine.
__________ (short-acting beta-2 agonist) ❑ 2 or ❑ 4 puffs every 20 minutes for up to 1 hour, ❑ Nebulizer, once

Second: **If your symptoms (and peak flow, if used) return to GREEN ZONE after 1 hour of above treatment:**
❑ Continue monitoring to be sure you stay in the green zone.

-Or-

If your symptoms (and peak flow, if used) do not return to GREEN ZONE after 1 hour of above treatment:
❑ Take:__________ (short-acting beta-2 agonist) ❑ 2 or ❑ 4 puffs or ❑ Nebulizer
❑ Add:__________ (oral steroid) mg per day For ______ (3–10) days
❑ Call the doctor ❑ before/ ❑ within ____ hours after taking the oral steroid

RED ZONE

Medical Alert!
- Very short of breath, or
- Quick-relief medicines have not helped, or
- Cannot do usual activities, or
- Symptoms are same or get worse after 24 hours in Yellow Zone

-Or-

Peak flow: ______ to ______
(50% of my best peak flow)

Take this medicine:
❑ __________ (short-acting beta2-agonist) ❑ 4 or ❑ 6 puffs or ❑ Nebulizer
❑ __________ (oral steroid) mg per day

Then call your doctor NOW.
Go to the hospital or call an ambulance if:
- You are still in the red zone after 15 minutes AND
- You have not reached your doctor.

DANGER SIGNS
- Trouble walking and talking due to shortness of breath
- Lips or fingernails are blue

→

- Take 4 or 6 puffs of your quick-relief medicine AND
- Go to the hospital or call for an ambulance ______ (phone) NOW

Figure 9-7
Sample asthma action plan

Source: National Heart, Lung, and Blood Institute

their illness, and perhaps identify discussion points for their next physician visit. The ACE-AHFS can also remind clients to carefully monitor symptoms and adhere to their asthma action plan, which all people with asthma should have developed and discussed with their physicians (Figure 9-7). The asthma action plan will be particularly important should a client develop symptoms during exercise. All people, especially pregnant women and adults with infants and young children (who will be exposed to second-hand smoke), can be encouraged to not smoke or be referred to a smoking cessation program.

Management of Asthma Exacerbation

An **asthma exacerbation,** or asthma attack, is defined as an episode of progressively worsening shortness of breath, cough, wheezing, and/or chest tightness that results in decreases in expiratory airflow. An asthma exacerbation can be triggered by any of the exposures noted in Table 9-2, or by other unknown factors. The intensity of an exacerbation can range from mild to life-threatening. Individuals at highest risk of asthma exacerbation include those who:

- Have had an exacerbation in the past year requiring an emergency room visit, hospitalization, or intensive care unit admission
- Have severe airflow obstruction based on spirometry
- Report feeling in danger or frightened by their asthma
- Have certain demographic and psychosocial characteristics such as female, non-white, non-users of inhaled corticosteroids, current smoking, depression, and stress

People who have had good control of asthma symptoms with inhaled corticosteroid treatment have a decreased risk of an exacerbation. Importantly, individuals who currently may have few symptoms and little impairment of quality of life still are at risk for a potentially life-threatening exacerbation.

Early treatment of an asthma exacerbation is important. Most exacerbations can be managed at home with appropriate advanced planning. Everyone with asthma should have a written asthma action plan to guide self-management. People with asthma should be able to recognize early signs of worsening asthma and promptly take action. Some may find that use of the modified 0 to 10 Borg scale for assessing dyspnea is helpful to characterize the severity of the exacerbation (Table 9-4). When necessary, a person with asthma can intensify therapy by increasing inhaled short-acting beta agonist and, if needed, adding a short course of oral systemic steroids, under his or her physician's guidance. It is also critical to remove the environmental trigger contributing to the exacerbation and promptly communicate with the individual's physician should symptoms not improve (NAEPP, 2007).

In the case of an exacerbation that does not improve with home management, the individual should promptly report to urgent care or the emergency room or call 911. At that time, the individual will receive some combination of oxygen, a short-acting beta agonist plus ipratropium bromide, systemic corticosteroids, serial lung-function measurements, consideration of other adjunct treatment in severe cases, and a discharge plan that includes follow-up in one to four weeks, medication instructions, review of inhaler techniques, and consideration of initiating inhaled corticosteroids. Evidence suggests that methylxanthines, antibiotics (unless necessary for comorbid conditions), aggressive hydration, chest physical therapy, mucolytics, and sedation are not necessary (NAEPP, 2007). Refer to Table 9-5 for a summary of what an

Table 9-4
Modified Borg Dyspnea Scale

0	No breathlessness at all
0.5	Very, very slight (just noticeable)
1	Very slight
2	Slight breathlessness
3	Moderate
4	Somewhat severe
5	Severe breathlessness
6	
7	Very severe breathlessness
8	
9	Very, very severe (almost maximal)
10	Maximal

Table 9-5
What to Do When a Client Has an Asthma Exacerbation During Exercise

- Reduce exercise intensity so that the client can easily administer rescue medication according to his or her asthma action plan. Do not encourage the client to "push through" an attack or stop the exercise abruptly.
- Remove the client from any environmental allergens or irritants, such as cold or polluted air, that may be contributing to the symptoms.
- Provide calm support and coach the client to use diaphragmatic breathing, taking deep breaths in through the nose and extending through the abdomen, and out through the mouth and drawing in the abdomen.
- If symptoms persist, discontinue exercise and seek immediate medical attention.
- Follow the gym or business protocol to document the incident and the actions taken.

ACE-AHFS should do when a client has an asthma exacerbation during exercise.

Exercise and Asthma

For many active individuals of all ages, sports, and levels of competition, exercise can trigger an asthmatic response, known as **exercise-induced bronchospasm (EIB)** or **exercise-induced asthma (EIA),** in which the airways transiently and reversibly narrow, causing symptoms such as cough, shortness of breath, chest pain or tightness, wheezing, or unexpected endurance problems. Up to 80% of people with classic asthma may experience symptoms with exercise (Butcher, 2006). For other individuals, exercise is the only asthma trigger.

EIB results from a loss of heat, water, or both from the lung during exercise due to hyperventilation of air that is cooler and drier than the air of the respiratory tree. Most studies suggest that inflammation plays a role in the cause of EIB, but the precise mechanisms behind EIB are not fully understood.

EIB typically occurs during or shortly after vigorous activity, reaching its peak five to 10 minutes after stopping activity and lasting for 20 to 30 minutes. The individual may also develop a hacking cough two to 12 hours after exercise cessation. The cough may last for one to two days and often is mistaken for an upper respiratory infection. An ACE-AHFS should suspect EIB in a client who experiences asthma symptoms during exercise, especially if this individual has a history of asthma or has been exercising at a vigorous intensity in cold or dry air. The ACE-AHFS should encourage clients to follow their asthma action plan if they have one. Otherwise, the best way to control acute symptoms is usually to markedly decrease or discontinue activity and use a rescue inhaler to open the airways. Clients should seek immediate medical assistance if symptoms persist or worsen. In most cases, symptoms will quickly improve. In those situations, the client can resume exercise as long as the event was not triggered by environmental contaminants such as pollution, cold air, and pollens.

In fact, the client may be least likely to experience asthma symptoms up to one hour following an acute exercise-induced asthma attack. Following the exercise bout, the ACE-AHFS should refer the client to a physician who can then arrange an exercise challenge in which the client engages in sufficiently strenuous activity to increase heart rate to 80% of **maximum heart rate (MHR)** for four to six minutes. A 15% decrease in PEF or FEV1 confirms a diagnosis of EIB.

General Activity Guidelines for Individuals With Asthma

- Avoid asthma triggers during exercise.
- Always have rescue medication nearby for use in the event of an attack.
- Establish a flexible program that can accommodate fluctuations in exercise capacity due to asthma symptoms.
- Utilize an extended warm-up and cool-down.
- Emphasize hydration before, during, and after exercise.
- Have the client practice diaphragmatic breathing.
- Determine exercise intensity according to the client's state of deconditioning, psychological preparedness for exercise, and asthma severity.
- Incorporate intervals for high-intensity training.
- Closely monitor the client for early signs of an asthma attack and respond immediately. Get medical help if symptoms do not subside.
- Use ratings of perceived exertion and the dyspnea scale to communicate with the client regarding symptoms.
- Choose exercise testing methods that accommodate a warm-up period.

Pulmonary Responses to Exercise Training

While the precise mechanisms behind EIB are not fully understood, knowledge of the pulmonary responses to exercise training can help an ACE-AHFS understand why EIB may occur for some people. During physical activity, **minute ventilation**, calculated as the **tidal volume** (the volume of air inspired per breath) multiplied by the **ventilatory rate** (the number of breaths per minute), increases.

Minute ventilation =
Tidal volume x Ventilatory rate

Thus the respiratory system experiences increased demand. The large amounts of relatively cool and dry inspired air must be warmed and humidified by the tracheobronchial mucosa. When the air is warmed and humidified, water evaporates from the epithelial surface of the airway, leading to cooling. One theory is that this process of increased airway cooling provokes bronchoconstriction in individuals with hyperreactive airways. However, research has suggested that perhaps humidity, not air temperature, plays a more important role in causing EIB (Evans et al., 2005), leading to a theory that high minute ventilation in relatively low humidity results in water loss in the airway. The airway drying may then lead to osmotic changes in the epithelium, which causes a release of inflammatory mediators and subsequent bronchospasm (Butcher, 2006).

Because the severity of bronchospasm in EIB is related to the ventilatory rate, the risk of EIB increases with increased exercise intensity. EIB generally occurs at ≥80% of **$\dot{V}O_2$max,** though people who suffer from severe asthma may experience symptoms at much lower intensities. Due to the discomfort that may occur with exercise for people with asthma and other pulmonary diseases, many avoid exercise and become deconditioned. Research suggests that while exercise may not decrease the incidence of EIB or improve pulmonary function, aerobic conditioning decreases risk of an asthma attack in general by reducing the ventilatory requirement for any given activity (NAEPP, 2007). Thus, people with asthma are strongly encouraged to engage in a regular physical-activity program.

While individuals who are susceptible to an exercise-related asthma exacerbation should use caution when lifting heavy weights, as rapid-onset vigorous activity can trigger EIB, they otherwise can follow the standard resistance-training recommendations of the American College of Sports Medicine (ACSM, 2006). Some research suggests that certain relaxation techniques, particularly muscle relaxation, may help to improve lung function (NAEPP, 2007). While some people anticipate that yoga may also provide unique benefits for individuals with asthma, little research is available to confirm or reject this hypothesis (NAEPP, 2007).

Programming and Progression Guidelines and Considerations

Clients with known asthma and/or EIB should receive medical clearance from a physician before beginning an exercise program. The client and his or her physician can discuss what to do in case of an asthmatic episode during exercise and how to best control the underlying asthma to prevent a symptomatic exercise bout. While exercise may be the only asthma trigger for many people, these individuals should still be evaluated by a physician prior to beginning an exercise program.

Individuals with well-controlled asthma who experience few or no symptoms during exercise can follow exercise guidelines for the general population. However, people with poorly controlled asthma or those who experience EIB should follow certain precautions to minimize symptoms and the risk of an exacerbation. First, the client and his or her physician should develop a treatment plan, which may include long-term-control therapy and/or pre-treatment before exercise, if necessary. Long-term-control therapy reduces airway responsiveness and thus decreases the frequency and severity of EIB. Pre-treatment usually includes use of a short-acting bronchodilator (albuterol, pirbuterol) or, less commonly, a long-acting bronchodilator (salmeterol). For mild symptoms, the short-acting bronchodilators are administered as two puffs of an inhaler spaced five to 10 minutes apart, 20 to 40 minutes before exercise. For maximal benefit from the inhaled medications, clients should be sure to consume water after using inhalers to help clear the back of the throat of the medicine. To minimize the risk of EIB, people with asthma should also engage in a prolonged warm-up and cool-down, remain indoors when air pollution or pollen levels are high, exercise with a mask or scarf over the mouth when exercising in cold weather, and avoid dehydration. Avoiding dehydration is especially important because mucous plugging can result from inadequate fluid intake. In practice, the prolonged warm-up and cool-down decrease the risk of EIB, though the mechanisms are speculative. Some believe a prolonged warm-up induces a milder bronchoconstriction, which leads to a refractory period in the hour or so after the warm-up, during which an attack is less likely to occur, and thus the exercise bout can be completed with a lower level of risk. The prolonged cool-down gradually decreases body temperature, which may decrease the risk for EIB that tends to occur immediately following cessation of exercise.

ACSM recommends that people with asthma engage in cardiovascular exercise at least three to four days per week at a comfortable intensity for at least 20 to 45 minutes, either continuously or in bouts intermittent (ACSM, 2006). Clients may use **ratings of perceived exertion (RPE)** to monitor intensity and the Borg dyspnea scale (see Table 9-4) to characterize the extent of breathlessness during exercise and to guide exercise-progression decisions. Swimming is often considered the mode of choice for people with asthma and those with a tendency toward bronchospasm because of its many positive factors: a warm, humid atmosphere; year-round availability; and the way the horizontal position may help mobilize mucus from the bottom of the lungs. Land-based exercise such as walking, leisure biking, and hiking are also good choices, as they are less likely to provoke EIB than other more intense fitness modalities.

Fitness Testing

Fitness-testing protocols may need to be modified to accommodate clients with EIB. Extended stages, smaller increments, and slower progressions in graded exercise tests may be necessary for individuals with functional limitations or early-onset dyspnea. The preferred submaximal testing mode is walking or stationary cycling. Running is not recommended, as it is the exercise most likely to incite EIB. Arm ergometry may be used when appropriate, although it is important to note that upper-extremity cardiovascular exercise can cause increased dyspnea (ACSM, 2006). Exercise testing should be performed in the environment least likely to cause symptoms; therefore, indoor testing is preferred to outdoor testing, as outdoor triggers are more difficult to control. Fitness testing should always be preceded by an extended warm-up and a short-acting medication if the client usually uses medication prior to exercise.

Case Studies

Case Study 1

Sarah is a 55-year-old overweight woman who has struggled with asthma since childhood. She asks the ACE-AHFS to help her begin an exercise program for weight loss. Sarah has never enjoyed exercise, as it caused her some breathing difficulty in the past and she feared that she might have an asthma attack. However, after her physician strongly encouraged her to begin exercising to control her weight and achieve other benefits, she contacted the ACE-AHFS for help. On further questioning, Sarah reveals that she experiences shortness of breath and chest tightness when climbing stairs and playing with her grandchildren (*Note:* Her physician has ruled out any cardiovascular disorder as being responsible for her symptoms.) She is allergic to pollen, mold, dust, and cats. Sarah takes inhaled corticosteroids daily and uses an albuterol inhaler when she experiences symptoms. Her physician ordered spirometry testing, which showed a FEV1 of 75% that was increased to 89% following inhalation of a short-acting bronchodilator.

The ACE-AHFS should begin by reassuring Sarah that he or she will design an exercise program for her that is least likely to cause asthma symptoms and that every effort will be made for her to have a comfortable and enjoyable experience. It is important for the ACE-AHFS to encourage her to discuss any symptoms that she experiences, such as an unusual shortness of breath, chest tightness, coughing, or wheezing. The ACE-AHFS should introduce the RPE and dyspnea scales to provide a communication tool and help Sarah differentiate between exercise-related and asthma-related breathlessness. The ACE-AHFS should also ask Sarah if she has an asthma action plan in place and if she has discussed pre-exercise medication with her physician and what to do should she have an exercise-induced asthma attack. Also, the ACE-AHFS must ask Sarah for permission to contact her physician for medical clearance prior to beginning the exercise program. The ACE-AHFS should perform fitness tests to identify the threshold at which Sarah starts displaying symptoms, and then use this threshold as a baseline. When designing Sarah's exercise program, the ACE-AHFS should start with low-intensity indoor exercise such as treadmill walking, stationary cycling, or indoor aquatic classes, complemented by light resistance training and flexibility exercises. It is important to gradually progress Sarah's program based on her comfort level and her initial response to exercise, with the ultimate goal of safely increasing caloric expenditure for weight loss. It is also a good idea to have Sarah meet with a dietitian.

Case Study 2

Josh is a 19-year-old college student and avid runner who was recently diagnosed with exercise-induced bronchospasm. During the past several months, Josh has noticed increased difficulty breathing during his vigorous training days and his athletic performance has suffered. His physician prescribed a cromolyn sodium inhaler for use three times per day (one time is 20 minutes prior to running) in combination with an albuterol inhaler. While this regimen has helped, he consults the ACE-AHFS to help him maximize his performance for the NYC Marathon in November.

The ACE-AHFS should start by asking Josh more about the symptoms he experiences during his vigorous training days. In addition to difficulty breathing, he may also have chest tightness, wheezing, and cough. The ACE-AHFS should encourage him to pay attention to these symptoms so that he can quickly recognize and respond to them by modifying his training and using his rescue inhaler. Also , the ACE-AHFS should inquire whether other triggers such as pollution, cold air, pollens, or other environmental contaminants cause him to experience symptoms. Josh may consider keeping a workout log, noting the environmental conditions and his symptoms to help him and his physician identify other triggers.

Prior to designing an exercise program or working with Josh to set marathon goals, the ACE-AHFS should arrange for Josh to complete fitness testing to assess his cardiorespiratory fitness level. The ACE-AHFS must remember to choose an indoor test (preferably a running test performed on a treadmill since Josh is preparing for a marathon), incorporate a prolonged warm-up prior to beginning the test, and gradually increase the intensity if a graded exercise test is being utilized. The ACE-AHFS can use these results to program exercise intensities and evaluate Josh's response to a training program. If the data are available, the ACE-AHFS should examine the ventilatory and heart-rate response relationship to determine the heart rate at which Josh's ventilatory response begins to increase disproportionately. With practice, a prolonged warm-up, and medication use, Josh should be able to train at high intensities and progress his training program with few difficulties. However, if Josh experiences repeated asthma exacerbations during his workouts, with exercise performance fluctuating from day to day, he should consult his physician to assess his overall and pre-exercise medication regimen and possible environmental triggers. On the other hand, if Josh consistently cannot tolerate the exercise program, it may be that the program is too difficult, insufficient recovery time has been programmed, or he has reached a training plateau, and the ACE-AHFS should reassess his program and make similar modifications as would be made for a healthy runner.

When preparing Josh for race day, the ACE-AHFS should remind him of the importance of the following:

- Performing a prolonged warm-up
- Covering his mouth with a scarf or mask if the temperature outside is cold
- Taking his medication 20 to 40 minutes before the race and keeping it with him in case he experiences symptoms

- Using a spacer to ensure that the medicine inhaled reaches the lungs and does not simply coat the roof of the mouth or the back of the throat
- Staying well hydrated
- Breathing through the nose as much as possible while running
- Avoiding hyperventilation by using a controlled breathing pattern
- Avoiding any foods known to trigger an attack, as some foods may precipitate an asthma attack in certain individuals (e.g., celery, carrots, peanuts, egg whites, bananas, shrimp)
- Always listening to his body for signs that he should modify his intensity

Summary

Asthma is a common pulmonary disease that can interfere not only with establishing and adhering to a regular exercise program, but also with the individual's quality of life. However, with appropriate precautions and asthma-related education, most people with asthma can effectively control their disease and enjoy a regular and vigorous activity program.

References

American College of Sports Medicine (2006). *ACSM's Guidelines for Exercise Testing and Prescription* (7th ed.). Champaign, Ill.: Lippincott Williams & Wilkins.

Busse, W.W. & Lemanske, R.F. (2001). Advances in immunology: Asthma. *New England Journal of Medicine,* 344, 5, 350–360.

Butcher, J.D. (2006). Exercise-induced asthma in the competitive cold weather athlete. *Current Sports Medicine Reports,* 5, 284–288.

Chobanian, A.V. et al. (2003). *JNC 7 Express: The Seventh Report of the Joint National Committee on Prevention, Detection, Evaluation, and Treatment of High Blood Pressure. NIH Publication No. 03-5233.* Washington, D.C.: National Institutes of Health & National Heart, Lung, and Blood Institute.

Evans, T.M. et al. (2005). Cold air inhalation does not affect the severity of EIB after exercise or eucapnic voluntary hyperventilation. *Medicine & Science in Sports & Exercise,* 37, 544–549.

Horwood, L.J., Fergusson, D.M., & Shannon, F.T. (1985). Social and familial factors in the development of early childhood asthma. *Pediatrics,* 75, 5, 859–868.

McConnell, R. et al. (2002). Asthma in exercising children exposed to ozone: A cohort study. *Lancet,* 359, 9304, 386–391.

Moorman, J.E. et al. (2007). National surveillance for asthma—United States 1980–2004. *Morbidity and Mortality Weekly Report Surveillance Summary,* 56 (SS08), 1–14, 18–54.

National Asthma Education and Prevention Program (2007). *Expert Panel Report 3: Guidelines for the Diagnosis and Management of Asthma.* Bethesda, Md.: U.S. Department of Health and Human Services, Public Health Service, National Institutes of Health, National Heart, Lung, and Blood Institute; NIH publication number 08-4051.

Sigurs, N. et al (2000). Respiratory syncytial virus bronchiolitis in infancy is an important risk factor for asthma and allergy at age 7. *American Journal of Respiratory and Critical Care Medicine,* 161, 5, 1501–1507.

United States Department of Health and Human Services & National Institutes of Health (2003). *Making a Difference in the Management of Asthma: A Guide for Respiratory Therapists.* Pub. No. 02-1064. (http://www.nhlbi.nih.gov/health/prof/lung/asthma/asth_respir.pdf)

Suggested Reading

National Asthma Education and Prevention Program (2007). *Expert Panel Report 3: Guidelines for the Diagnosis and Management of Asthma.* Bethesda, Md.: U.S. Department of Health and Human Services, Public Health Service, National Institutes of Health, National Heart, Lung, and Blood Institute; NIH publication number 08-4051.

Sinha, T. & David, A.K. (2003). Recognition and management of exercise-induced bronchospasm. *American Family Physician,* Vol. 67, No. 4, 769–772.

Part Three

Metabolic Diseases and Disorders

Chapter 10
Overweight and Obesity

Chapter 11
The Metabolic Syndrome

Chapter 12
Diabetes Mellitus

In This Chapter

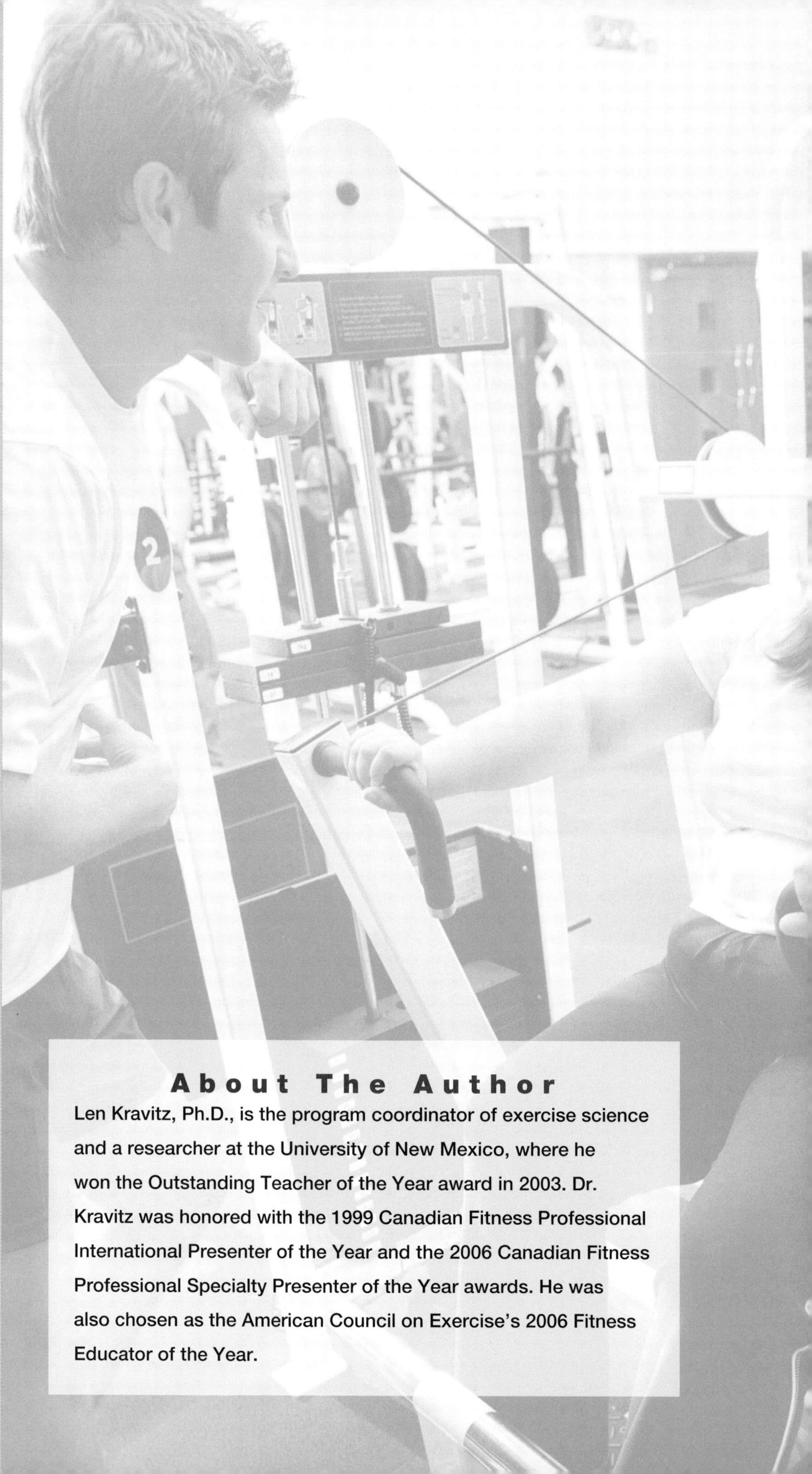

About The Author

Len Kravitz, Ph.D., is the program coordinator of exercise science and a researcher at the University of New Mexico, where he won the Outstanding Teacher of the Year award in 2003. Dr. Kravitz was honored with the 1999 Canadian Fitness Professional International Presenter of the Year and the 2006 Canadian Fitness Professional Specialty Presenter of the Year awards. He was also chosen as the American Council on Exercise's 2006 Fitness Educator of the Year.

CHAPTER 10

Overweight and Obesity

Len Kravitz

Epidemiology of the Epidemic

Worldwide projections by the World Health Organization (WHO) indicate that 1.6 billion people age 15 years or older are **overweight,** with approximately 400 million of them obese (WHO, 2006). Some contributing factors to this epidemic can be credited largely to the progression from a rural lifestyle to a highly technological urban existence, and the tempting capacity of the modern environment to encourage individuals to eat more and move less. Almost all countries are experiencing this dramatic increase in overweight and **obesity.** The WHO further estimates that by 2015, approximately 2.3 billion adults will be overweight and more than 700 million will be obese.

Excess body weight is associated with an increased likelihood to develop heart disease, **hypertension, type 2 diabetes,** gallstones, breathing problems, musculoskeletal disabilities, and certain forms of cancer (endometrial, breast, and colon) [National Institutes of Health (NIH), 2007]. It is also associated with reduced life expectancy and early mortality [American College of Sports Medicine (ACSM), 2006]. In addition, obesity has a deleterious effect on the economy of all countries, as it increases the associated costs for treating the related diseases.

Overview of Overweight and Obesity—The Causes

Ultimately, the primary reason for overweight and obesity is a **positive energy balance,** wherein intake (via calories consumed from food and beverages) is greater than output (energy expenditure from resting metabolism, physical activity, and exercise) (ACSM, 2006). **Energy balance** occurs when energy intake equals energy output, while a **negative energy balance** exists when energy output exceeds energy intake, resulting in weight loss. The human genome has evolved from times when shelter and food were in short supply and famine was a constant threat to life (Loos & Bouchard, 2003). In addition, major amounts of physical exertion were once necessary to obtain food and cope with harsh living environments. Therefore, humans have evolved an outstanding ability to biologically function with great energy efficiency by storing large amounts of excess **fat** as **adipose tissue.** In modern society, many people spend hours every day watching TV, playing video games, using computers, doing schoolwork, and adopting other **sedentary** leisure behaviors. In fact, more than two hours a day of regular TV viewing has been linked to overweight and obesity (NIH, 2007). It is important to also note the existence of obesity disorders such as hypothyroidism, Prader-Willi syndrome, and Cushing's syndrome. With these diseases, metabolic and/or hormonal dysfunctions or impairment contribute to obesity.

An abundance of food may be a by-product of the success of a society, but it clearly creates the conditions for a positive energy balance in the modern lifestyle. Other environmental factors contributing to obesity include not having enough sidewalks, trails, parks, and affordable fitness facilities for all people. Restaurants, fast-food chains, and movie theaters compete for business by offering very large food portions. In addition, healthy food choices are more expensive, making access to these foods less of an option for the financially challenged. And food companies that encourage people of all ages to select high-calorie, high-fat snacks and sugary drinks dominate food advertising.

Overweight and obesity tend to run in families (NIH, 2007). A person's genes may affect the amount of fat he or she stores in the body, as well as where the fat is stored (NIH, 2007). It is well established that fat-site deposition is highly linked to a person's relative health risk. Fat deposited in the hips and thighs, referred to as gluteofemoral or **gynoid** fat (more often observed in females), appears to be quite benign and metabolically inactive. On the other hand, fat found in the trunk area around the internal organs of the abdomen (often observed in men) is referred to as **android** or **visceral** fat. Excess visceral fat is correlated with hypertension, diabetes, high blood **triglycerides** and **coronary heart disease.** It is interesting to observe that with exercise, it is the visceral fat that is often the first to disappear.

Familial factors also contribute to the prevalence of overweight and obesity. For example, families commonly share eating and physical-activity habits. Children tend to adopt the habits of their parents. So, a child with overweight parents who are inactive and eat high-calorie meals may become overweight like the parents. However, if a family adopts healthful food and physical-activity habits, the child's chance of being overweight are reduced (NIH, 2007).

The Biology of Overweight and Obesity

Fat tissue, for the most part, was once understood to be an extra layer of cushioning with few metabolic responsibilities. It was viewed and described like a balloon that inflates when a person eats more food and expends fewer calories, and deflates when there is greater physical activity and less food consumption. More recent research reveals that fat tissue (composed of **adipocyte** cells that specialize in fat storage) functions like other **endocrine** organs (i.e., glands that secretes **hormones**) in the body, sending signals to the brain that affect several intricate physiological mechanisms of energy-expenditure regulation, **insulin** sensitivity, and fat and **carbohydrate** metabolism (Trayhurn, 2005). Two key hormones related to energy metabolism regulation are **leptin** and **adiponectin,** while a host of other hormones are involved in immune reactions in the body.

Leptin

Leptin, which resides in all fat cells, communicates directly with the hypothalamus in the brain, providing information about how much energy is currently stored in the body's fat cells. Leptin functions in what is referred to in biology as a negative feedback loop. For example, when fat cells decrease in size, leptin decreases, sending a message to the hypothalamus to direct the body to eat more. Similarly, when fat cells increase in size, leptin increases and the message sent to the hypothalamus is to instruct the body to eat less. However, it appears that the primary biological role of leptin is to facilitate energy intake when energy storage is low, as opposed to slowing down overconsumption when energy storage is high (Havel, 2002). Leptin production is chiefly regulated by insulin-induced changes in fat-cell metabolism. Havel notes that the consumption of fat (and fructose) actually results in lower circulating leptin levels, which can lead to overeating and weight gain. Thus, diet and, more specifically, intake of foods high in fat and **fructose** may have a direct connection with weight gain. Scientific attempts to take leptin as a pill have not shown any benefit for the overweight, possibly because the digestion process changes the synthetic form of leptin's structure and function.

Adiponectin

Another specialized hormone secreted by fat is adiponectin, which is referred to as "the good-guy" hormone (Liebman, 2004). Adiponectin helps insulin by sending blood **glucose** into the body's cells for storage or use as fuel, thus increasing the cells' insulin sensitivity or glucose metabolism (Havel, 2002). It also helps decrease blood levels of triglycerides by working with insulin to stimulate fat breakdown. If a person has a lot of body fat, then he or she typically will have lower levels of adiponectin, which is predictably low in all overweight individuals and especially low in individuals with **insulin resistance.**

Insulin resistance occurs when the normal amount of insulin secreted by the pancreas is not able to transport glucose into cells. To maintain a normal blood glucose level, the pancreas secretes additional insulin. In some people, when the body cells resist, or do not respond to even high levels of insulin, glucose builds up in the blood, resulting in high blood glucose, which may lead to type 2 diabetes. Even people with diabetes who take medications to control their blood glucose levels can have higher than normal blood insulin levels due to insulin resistance.

Immune Hormones

It is known that fat tissue produces a number of immune-system hormones, such as tumor necrosis factor-alpha, interleukin-6, plasminogen activator inhibitor 1, angiotensin II, and other **cytokines** (Havel, 2002). Cytokines, which are hormone-like **proteins**, function largely as inflammatory proteins, reacting to areas of infection or injury in the body. However, persons with excess fat appear to have an overreaction in terms of the release of these inflammatory proteins. It has been proposed that this is caused by the low oxygen content in the clusters of adipocytes, which are somewhat distant from the tissues' vascular supply (Trayhurn, 2005). The concept of **inflammation** is one of the most critical in obesity biology. Both obesity and diabetes are associated with chronic low-grade inflammation (Trayhurn, 2005). In addition, inflammation is understood to be a key facet in heart disease. The release of these inflammatory proteins may inflame arterial plaque, causing the plaque to rupture and thus lead to a heart attack or **stroke** (Liebman, 2004). Trayhurn (2005) notes that with weight loss there is a corresponding decrease in the circulating levels of these inflammatory proteins. Trayhurn also notes that these fat tissue–derived inflammatory hormones may play a causal role in the development of insulin resistance.

Ghrelin

Another component of the energy reserve regulation in the body involves some of the hormones that control feeding and appetite, which are located in the gastrointestinal tract. Specific hunger signals trigger eating, while satiety messages reduce appetite. These distinctive hormones are often referred to as the "gut hormones," one of which—**ghrelin**—has been proposed to be particularly associated with obesity (Druce, Small, & Bloom, 2005). Ghrelin, secreted by the stomach, plays a chief role in appetite regulation. It is recognized as the "hunger hormone" and has garnered much attention in the research due to its role in the prevalence of obesity.

Working in a positive feedback loop, high levels of ghrelin during a fasted state promote increased food intake, while lower levels of ghrelin are observed after eating a meal. However, when obese individuals lose weight, it often results in an elevation of ghrelin, thereby promoting food intake, which may be a physiological reason why dieters have so much difficulty maintaining their newfound weight. In addition, it appears that food consumption does not suppress ghrelin levels in obese individuals, again contributing to overeating.

Peptide YY

When the body feels that it has eaten enough, the hormone **peptide YY** (and other **satiety** hormones, such as cholecystokin and glucagon-like peptide-1) is released from the intestines. It is particularly stimulated by lipids and carbohydrates (Druce, Small, & Bloom, 2005). This gut hormone is thought to work with the **central nervous system** to regulate the cessation of appetite. Thus, when released, it provides a feeling of satiety (Druce, Small, & Bloom, 2005).

The Sleep–Obesity Connection

It appears that less sleep is highly associated with weight gain (Taheri et al., 2004). People who report regularly sleeping less than seven hours a night, for example, are much more likely to gain weight compared to people who sleep seven to eight hours a night. Those persons who sleep less tend to eat foods that are higher in calories. Hormones, such as leptin, insulin, and ghrelin, are released during sleep to control the body's use of foodstuffs. For example, insulin controls the rise and fall of blood sugar levels during sleep.

People who do not get enough sleep have insulin and blood sugar levels that are similar to those in people who are likely to have diabetes. Taheri and colleagues (2004) note that people who do not get enough sleep on a regular basis seem to have high levels of ghrelin (causing hunger) and low levels of leptin (increasing eating).

Diagnostic Testing of Overweight and Obesity

Body mass index (BMI) is a simple height–weight index that is commonly used for classifying overweight and obesity in adult populations and individuals:

$$\text{BMI} = \text{body weight (kg)}/\text{height}^2\ \text{(m)}$$

However, BMI should only be considered as a useful guide, because it may not correspond to the same degree of fatness in different individuals. For example, BMI does not discriminate between lean mass and fat mass and therefore tends to overestimate body fatness in athletic, heavily muscled individuals. The WHO defines overweight as a BMI ≥25 kg/m^2 and obesity as a BMI ≥30 kg/m^2. These cutoff points provide a benchmark for individual assessment. The WHO is currently developing international growth reference charts for school-age children and adolescents. The Centers for Disease Control and Prevention (CDC) has created BMI charts broken down by age and sex and designed for children and adolescents (www.cdc.gov).

An ACE-certified Advanced Health & Fitness Specialist (ACE-AHFS) can also utilize **waist circumference** to establish health risk. This measurement is made at the narrowest part of the torso between the ribs and iliac crest. The National Cholesterol Education Program (NCEP, 2002) recommends using a waist circumference ≥40 inches (102 cm) for men and ≥35 inches (89 cm) for women as the risk factor threshold for obesity-related metabolic diseases (such as diabetes and insulin resistance) and coronary heart disease.

Another tool for health-risk assessment is the **waist-to-hip ratio,** which is the circumference of the waist divided by the circumference of the hips. This measurement can be taken in inches or centimeters. To determine if a client has a healthy waist-to-hip ratio, the ACE-AHFS can use a measuring tape to determine the smallest part of the waist (usually above the belly button and below the rib cage) and the largest part of the hips (Figures 10-1 and 10-2). The measuring tape must be horizontal all the way around the body when taking a measurement. When measuring the hip circumference, the ACE-AHFS should have the

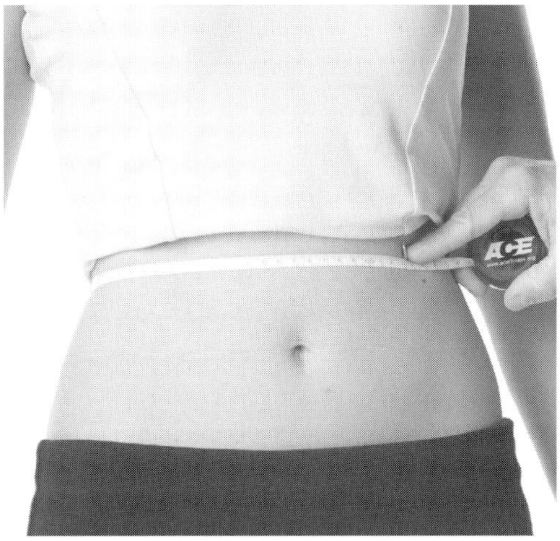

Figure 10-1
Waist circumference

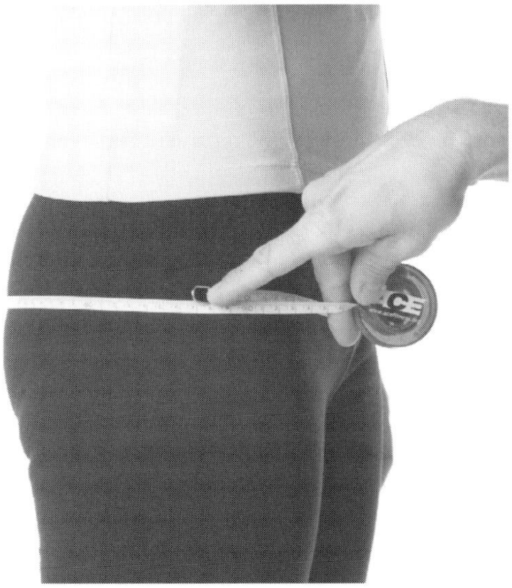

Figure 10-2
Hip circumference

Table 10-1
Waist-to-Hip Ratio—High and Very High Risk Norms for Men and Women

Gender	Age	High Risk	Very High Risk
Men	20–29	0.89–0.94	>0.94
	30–39	0.92–0.96	>0.96
	40–49	0.96–1.00	>1.00
	50–59	0.97–1.02	>1.02
	60–69	0.99–1.03	>1.03
Women	20–29	0.78–0.82	>0.82
	30–39	0.79–0.84	>0.84
	40–49	0.80–0.87	>0.87
	50–59	0.82–0.88	>0.88
	60–69	0.84–0.90	>0.90

Source: Adapted from Heyward, V. (2006). *Advanced Fitness Assessment and Exercise Prescription* (5th ed.). Champaign, Ill.: Human Kinetics.

client stand with his or her feet together. The standards for risk vary with age and sex (Table 10-1).

There are also a variety of assessment methods that can be used to determine a person's body fatness, such as skinfold testing, **hydrostatic weighing, bioelectrical impedance analysis (BIA), infrared interactance, computed tomography, magnetic resonance imaging (MRI),** and **dual-energy x-ray absorptiometry (DEXA).** Women generally have a higher percentage of body fat than men (Table 10-2).

Table 10-2
General Body-fat Percentage Categories

Classification	Women (% fat)	Men (% fat)
Essential fat	10–13%	2–5%
Athletes	14–20%	6–13%
Fitness	21–24%	14–17%
Average	25–31%	18–24%
Obese	32% and higher	25% and higher

The Treatment of Obesity

Losing weight, and then maintaining the weight loss, is often very difficult due to the multifactorial nature of obesity. It is compelling to point out that small changes in body weight result in health benefits. Studies show that a 5 to 10% loss of initial body weight is associated with meaningful improvements in **cholesterol** levels, **hypertension,** and glucose metabolism (Fabricatore & Wadden, 2003). In fact, Fabricatore and Wadden (2003) note that the Diabetes Prevention Program study showed that a four-year lifestyle intervention of physical activity and diet designed to induce a loss of 7% in body weight resulted in experimental subjects having a 58% lowered risk of developing type 2 diabetes as compared to a control group (Diabetes Prevention Program Research Group, 2002). This preventive effect was seen to hold for members of all racial, ethnic, and gender groups in this 3200-subject study. Fabricatore & Wadden (2003) affirm that the guidelines from the NHLBI and the North American Association for the Study of Obesity indicate that the three lifestyle-modification components of a successful obesity treatment program are dietary intervention, behavioral therapy, and physical activity.

Lifestyle Modification

Lifestyle modification refers to changes being made that represent an overall change in the way a person lives his or her life. All too often, individuals view a weight-loss program as an isolated period of time during which a person goes on a diet, takes exercise classes, or employs a personal trainer to get in shape. Others may attempt diet strategies with very unrealistic expectations for weight loss, and then give up when these hopes are not met. It is important to remind clients that they are truly establishing a new way of life, not just a temporary quick fix for some loss of weight. In addition, it is important to emphasize to clients the overall health benefits of increasing physical activity and incorporating a balanced approach to eating and meal planning. These changes can improve the quality of their lives and reduce the risks of developing coronary heart disease, hypertension, colon cancer, and diabetes, while also improving their mental well-being and musculoskeletal function in **activities of daily living (ADL)** (Kravitz, 2007).

Dietary Intervention

Over the past five decades, there has been a remarkable increase in the types of popular diets. Many clients will have tried, with no sustained success, two or more fad diets by the time they begin to work with an ACE-AHFS. The ACE-AHFS may choose to work with nutrition professionals on dietary interventions for some clients. In essence, the goal of the weight-loss dietary intervention is to keep the dietary content nutritionally adequate for health concerns, while introducing simple ways of reducing calorie intake. As acknowledged earlier, modern society has influenced food consumption so dramatically that the attainment of this goal can be easily sabotaged. Evidence suggests that low- and moderate-fat, calorie-restricted diets promote weight loss and are nutritionally sound, and that similar substantiation is lacking for high-protein, high-fat, and low-carbohydrate weight-loss approaches (Boucher, Shafer, & Chaffin, 2001). According to Jakicic and colleagues (2001), absolute dietary energy intake should be adjusted based on body weight to elicit an energy deficit of 500 to 1000 kcal per day. With this deficit, a minimum weight loss of 1 to 2 pounds (0.5 to 1.0 kg) per week is realistic. In addition, ACSM (2006) recommends reducing dietary fat intake to <30% of total energy intake. The NIH (2007) suggests a healthy eating plan that includes the following healthful foods:

- Fruits, which can be canned (in juice or water), fresh, frozen, or dried
- Vegetables, which can be canned (without salt), fresh, frozen, or dried
- Fat-free and low-fat milk and milk products such as low-fat yogurt and cheese
- Lean meat, poultry, fish, lentils, and beans
- Whole-grain foods such as oatmeal, brown rice, bagels, bread, pasta, cereal, tortillas, and crackers
- Canola or olive oils and soft margarines made from these oils in small amounts, because they are high in calories
- Unsalted nuts, like walnuts and almonds, in small amounts due their high caloric value

Behavioral Therapy

The behavioral approaches to weight loss are multifaceted. Costain and Croker (2005) summarize that the behavioral-therapy evidence suggests the following techniques may be successfully incorporated to help clients attain long-term weight control:

- *Properly assess the client's readiness to change.* Weight-loss achievement and maintenance in the long term depends on the individual being ready and able to build new attitudes and behaviors into his or her daily life.
- *Teach accurate self-monitoring of food consumption.* Fabricatore and Wadden (2003) note that obese individuals tend to underestimate how much they eat by approximately 30 to 50%. Therefore, a focus on accurate self-monitoring is vital for long-term success of the weight-management intervention.
- *Set realistic goals.* Unrealistic goal setting may set up a client for failure and cause negative self-talk—"I have no willpower"—when it may actually be the goal that is flawed (Costain & Croker, 2005). The ACE-AHFS should help clients identify modest, achievable goals and the potential barriers that need to be overcome. **SMART goals** are specific, measurable, attainable, relevant, and time-bound. This goal-setting process should be followed with a written and personalized action plan.

For enhanced motivation, the ACE-AHFS and client can together establish rewards along the way for desired outcomes.

- *Incorporate sound dietary change.* Costain and Croker (2005) highlight the following key dietary messages for adults who are seeking to manage body weight:
  - ✔ Include a variety of foods from the main food groups.
  - ✔ Control portion size.
  - ✔ Reduce the proportion of fat, particularly **saturated fat.**
  - ✔ Consume foods rich in **omega-3 fatty acids.**
  - ✔ Increase consumption of fruit and vegetables to at least five portions daily.
  - ✔ Consume low-glycemic, whole-grain, high-fiber, carbohydrate-rich foods in meals.
  - ✔ Reduce sugar intake.
  - ✔ Limit salt intake.
  - ✔ Follow a structured meal pattern, starting with breakfast.
- *Increase physical activity.* See "Physical Activity: Structured Exercise" below.
- *Utilize stimulus control.* **Stimulus control** involves learning how to avoid **triggers** such as the sight of food and dealing with cravings for food. Since food cravings are not fully understood, a few different strategies may need to be attempted. Most importantly, it is essential that clients not adopt a strict diet based on specific food deprivation. In fact, eating craved foods in moderation may quell the craving and prevent overeating. In addition, creating workable diversions to food cravings may be a viable solution.
- *Utilize cognitive restructuring.* **Cognitive restructuring** is a behavioral technique that involves learning how to replace unhealthy or negative thoughts and self-talk regarding weight loss with positive affirmations. Examples of cognitive traps include all-or-nothing thinking (e.g., "I blew my diet last night, so I might as well blow it again today") and discounting the positive (e.g., "I only lost one pound this week instead of two").
- *Utilize relapse management.* Relapse management attempts to makes clients aware that **lapses** and **relapses** are a normal part of behavior change. This strategy helps to relieve the stress of "being a diet failure" that some individuals experience when they miss an exercise session or overindulge in a meal.
- *Establish ongoing support.* Ongoing support involves creatively utilizing communication techniques such as email, phone, and websites that provide maintenance support to clients in an effort to sustain the lifestyle changes that have been made.

Wing and Phelan (2005) have studied and identified the key attributes of successful weight-loss maintainers from the National Weight Control Registry, the largest database in the world of persons sustaining long-term weight loss. Despite using various approaches to lose weight, the chief behavioral characteristics common to these weight-loss maintainers include the following:

- Frequent self-monitoring of body weight and food intake
- Eating a diet low in fat and higher in carbohydrate
- Eating breakfast and regular meals
- Limiting fast food
- Accepting realistic weight goals
- Performing high levels of physical activity (≥1 hour/day)
- Recognizing that weight control is an ongoing process and commitment

Wing and Phelan (2005) further suggest that once successful maintainers have sustained a weight loss for two to five years, the chances of longer-term success greatly improve.

Physical Activity: Structured Exercise

Although there are various evidence-based physical-activity and exercise approaches to weight control, such as the 10,000-steps-a-day model or the >2000 kilocalories per week target goal, the "accumulated time" approach will be highlighted here for designing weight-management programs because of its simplicity and its varied utility for all different forms of exercise (e.g., walking, elliptical training, water exercise, rowing, cycling). The accumulated time approach addresses the fact that energy expenditure is actually a cumulative phenomenon, including both low-intensity activities of daily life, such as walking and recreational dancing, and more vigorous exercise like swimming, elliptical training, and cycling. When pursuing weight-management goals, the evidence suggests that overweight and obese persons should gradually progress to 60 minutes per day of accumulated exercise. There appears to be an optimal dose of maintaining an average of greater than 280 minutes/week (Jakicic & Gallagher, 2003). Jakicic and Gallagher add that these greater weekly volumes of exercise tend to lead to less food consumption in individuals, and the combined exercise and decreased food consumption facilitate weight loss. The ACSM position stand for weight loss and prevention of weight regain recommends progressing to 200 to 300 minutes of accumulated exercise per week (Jakicic et al., 2001).

It is important to note that although resistance exercises are highly recommended for enhanced muscular strength, muscular endurance, physical function, and a host of other health benefits, it is cardiovascular exercise that elicits the needed energy-expenditure deficits for weight loss and the prevention of weight regain (Jakicic et al., 2001). However, research on resistance training and circuit training has shown meaningful changes in **body composition** (Marx et al., 2001). Thus, one of the noteworthy benefits of resistance exercise, as it relates to body composition in overweight populations, is the positive impact of maintaining or increasing fat-free body mass, while encouraging the loss of fat weight via a progressive-overload resistance-training program. Therefore, any resistance-training program designed for overweight and obese persons should be considered very meaningful to the overall health and goals of the client, and an adjunct to the cardiovascular program for weight loss. The data indicate that moderate-intensity exercise is the preferred level of exertion—approximately 60 to 70% of maximal oxygen uptake or a rating of 11 to 13 ("fairly light" to "somewhat hard") on the Borg **ratings of perceived exertion (RPE)** scale (6 to 20 scale) (Jakicic & Gallagher, 2003) (Figure 10-3).

RPE	Category Ratio Scale	
6	0	Nothing at all
7 Very, very light	0.5	Very, very weak
8	1	Very weak
9 Very light	2	Weak
10	3	Moderate
11 Fairly light	4	Somewhat strong
12	5	Strong
13 Somewhat hard	6	
14	7	Very strong
15 Hard	8	
16	9	
17 Very hard	10	Very, very strong
18	*	Maximal
19 Very, very hard		
20		

Figure 10-3
Ratings of perceived exertion

Source: Adapted, with permission, from American College of Sports Medicine (2006). *ACSM's Guidelines for Exercise Testing and Prescription* (7th ed.). Philadelphia: Lippincott Williams & Wilkins.

What Is the Resting Metabolic Rate of Muscle Tissue?

Resting metabolic rate (RMR), which accounts for 60 to 75% of all calorie-burning processes, is the amount of energy required to keep homeostatic processes (the regulation of organ systems and body temperature) performing efficiently. Although muscle is the largest tissue in the body, its estimated RMR is below what has been publicized in the consumer media. In fact, scientific estimation of the metabolic rate of muscle is about 10 to 15 kcal/kg per day, which is approximately 4.5 to 7.0 kcal/lb per day (Elia, 1992).

In an all-inclusive research review, Donnelly and colleagues (2003) note that the majority of peer-reviewed resistance-training studies (lasting from eight to 52 weeks) show increases of 2.2 to 4.5 pounds (1.0 to 2.0 kg) of muscle mass. Therefore, the 4.5 pounds (2.0 kg) of muscle mass would increase the RMR by up to 50 kilocalories per day—far less than what is popularly promoted.

Physical Activity: Unstructured Exercise

In recent years, researchers have been investigating the impact that standing, walking, and fidgeting play on weight gain and obesity. As such, a relatively newly discovered component of energy expenditure is **non-exercise activity thermogenesis (NEAT)** (physiological processes that produce heat). Innovative research in this area has revealed surprising and beneficial information (Levine et al., 2005).

NEAT comprises the energy expenditure of daily activities that are not considered planned physical activity or exercise of a person's daily life. NEAT is measured with sensitive physical-activity monitoring inclinometers and triaxial accelerometers, which are worn on the hips and legs (similar to a pedometer). These devices capture data on body position through all planes of movement 120 times a minute. The combination of this information with other laboratory measurements of energy expenditure leads to a calculation of NEAT. Findings indicate that changes in NEAT accompany changes in energy balance, which are very meaningful in affecting weight loss (Levine et al., 2005).

Levine and colleagues (2005) recruited 20 healthy, sedentary volunteers. As quoted from the article, all subjects were self-proclaimed "couch potatoes." Of the 20 volunteers, five men and five women had BMI measurements of 23±2 kg/m^2 (classifying them as lean) and five men and five women had BMI measurements of 33 ± 2 kg/m^2 (classifying them as mildly obese). A mildly obese population was selected because these individuals were less likely to have medical impediments and orthopedic troubles as compared to a morbidly obese group. With each subject wearing an inclinometer and triaxial accelerometer, the researchers collected data every half-second for 10 days.

The investigators were searching for posture and movement clues of how the 10 lean non-exercisers were different from 10 mildly obese non-exercisers. They found that the obese subjects were seated for 164 minutes longer each day than the lean participants. In addition, the lean participants were upright for 153 minutes longer per day that the obese subjects.

Importantly, sleep times between the groups did not vary at all. The lean subjects had significantly more total-body ambulatory movement, which consisted of standing and walking. In essence, the extra movement by the lean subjects averaged 352±65 calories per day, which is equivalent to 36.5 pounds (16.6 kg) in one year.

In summary, a very important way to help clients achieve their weight-loss goals is to find ways for them to be more active in their daily lives (Table 10-3). Encouraging and educating clients to make small movement changes in their daily lives, in addition to their structured exercise plan, may very well contribute to profound weight-management success.

Table 10-3
Suggestions to Help Clients Be More Active During the Day

- Walk to work.
- Walk during your lunch hour.
- Walk instead of drive whenever you can.
- Take a family walk after dinner.
- Skate to work instead of drive.
- Mow the lawn with a push mower.
- Walk to your place of worship instead of driving.
- Walk your dog.
- Replace the Sunday drive with a Sunday walk.
- Get off the bus or subway a stop early and walk.
- Work and walk around the house.
- Take your dog to the park.
- Wash the car by hand.
- Run or walk fast when doing errands.
- Pace the sidelines at your kids' athletic games.
- Take the wheels off your luggage.
- Walk to a coworker's desk instead of emailing or calling.
- Make time in your day for physical activity.
- Bike to the barbershop or beauty salon instead of driving.
- If you find it difficult to be active after work, try it before work.
- Take a walk break instead of a coffee break.
- Perform gardening and/or home-repair activities.
- Avoid labor-saving devices.
- Take small trips on foot to get your body moving.
- Play with your kids 30 minutes a day.
- Dance to music.
- Walk briskly in the mall.
- Take the long way to the water cooler.
- Take the stairs instead of the escalator.
- Go for a hike.

Source: www.SmallStep.gov.

Obesity Medications and Physiological Responses

Between 2003 and 2007, the U.S. patent office received more than 1700 submissions with the word "obesity" in them (Hickey & Israel, 2007). Hickey and Israel (2007) also note that there are nearly 300 clinical trials currently researching some aspect of obesity. However, there are only two drugs that have been FDA-approved for long-term treatment of obesity: sibutramine (trade name is Meridia™) and orlistat (marketed under the trade name Xenical™ or over-the-counter as Alli™).

Sibutramine prevents the removal of norepinephrine and serotonin in the brain, thus prolonging some of their appetite-suppressing effects. Research on sibutramine showed that individuals who use it average approximately 10 pounds (4.5 kg) greater weight loss, as compared to those who used a placebo over the course of one-year treatments (Li et al., 2005). The research on sibutramine suggests that it is relatively safe, minimally elevating heart rate (4 bpm) and blood pressure (2 to 4 mmHg for both **systolic** and **diastolic blood pressure**). A minor increase of **high-density lipoproteins (HDL)** and a mild reduction in triglycerides have also been observed. No available research exists that has evaluated the use of sibutramine beyond two years.

Orlistat's primary function is preventing the intestinal absorption of fats from the diet, thereby reducing the caloric impact of food consumed. It is intended for use in combination with a physician-supervised reduced-calorie diet. Orlistat is successful at blocking absorption of approximately 30% of dietary fat (Hickey & Israel, 2007). Over the course of a year, the use of orlistat creates approximately 6.5 pounds (2.9 kg) greater weight loss as compared to a placebo (Hickey & Israel, 2007). However, the researchers also note that orlistat has been shown to have considerable gastrointestinal side effects, including abdominal pain, diarrhea, flatulence, bloating, and upset stomach. Long-term research on orlistat has not yet been published.

Clearly, a great deal more needs to be learned about the interplay of food intake and the complex biological, neuroendocrine, and physiological mechanisms of the human body. Although much research is going on in this area of study, simple solutions do not appear to be forthcoming in the near future. In addition, Hickey and Israel (2007) note that the **pathogenesis** (i.e., disease development) of obesity is multifaceted and likely to vary among individuals. This suggests that the idea of one "super pill" for overweight and obesity treatment is unlikely. In addition, it is hoped that any obesity medications will be administered along with lifestyle changes that involve behavior modification, exercise, and healthy food consumption.

In June 2007, Alli became the first over-the-counter diet pill approved by the Food and Drug Administration (FDA). It is a half-strength version of the prescription weight-loss drug Xenical (orlistat). For best results, Alli should be taken before every meal that contains fat. It works by decreasing the amount of fat absorbed by the gastrointestinal tract during the digestive process. Research has shown that when individuals use Alli in combination with diet and exercise, they lose up to 50% more weight on average compared to dieting and exercising alone. As with any drug, Alli has several documented side effects, including excessive flatulence and oily, difficult-to-control bowel movements. Those individuals hailing Alli as the next "magic bullet" for weight loss should bear in mind that most weight-loss experts contend that without the contributory effects of diet and exercise, Alli's beneficial weight-loss effects would be very limited.

Surgical Interventions for Obesity

Bariatrics is the branch of medicine that deals with the causes, prevention, and treatment of obesity. The term bariatrics comes from the Greek root *baro* (weight) and the suffix *iatrics* (a branch of medicine). Surgical treatment of obesity is suggested to be only appropriate for those individuals with a BMI ≥40 kg/m^2 or BMI ≥35 kg/m^2 in the presence of **comorbidities** (one or more disorders or diseases in addition to a primary disease—obesity) (Fabricatore & Wadden, 2003). The two most common surgical procedures for obesity are **gastric bypass** and **vertical banded gastroplasty.** These procedures involve separating a small pouch of stomach with a line of staples to dramatically limit food intake. Bariatric surgery results in a 30% (gastric bypass) and 25% (vertical banded gastroplasty) average reduction of initial weight. Improvements of mood, hypertension, **asthma, sleep apnea,** and diabetes have also been observed (Fabricatore & Wadden, 2003). Clinical trials suggest that gastric bypass surgery is associated with much better weight-loss maintenance than vertical banded gastroplasty, because patients who have undergone gastric bypass surgery and then eat high-fat or high-sugar meals tend to experience stomach cramping and gastrointestinal distress and thus avoid these foods to evade this discomfort. Naturally, before any type of bariatric procedure, individuals need to be rigorously screened to determine if there are any medical or behavioral contraindications to the surgery.

Considerations for Obesity-related Disorders and Diseases

A wide range of diseases and health problems are associated with obesity. The ACE-AHFS should be familiar with the diverse ways that overweight and obesity may be linked with the health and wellness of clients. It is important to note that the research on obesity-related disorders and diseases is very frequently correlational, as opposed to prospective, randomized research. Correlational research explores the statistical association of two or more variables to each other, and this type of study design makes it hard to prove cause and effect. Readers of research results should bear in mind the limitations imposed by the study design. Serious diseases associated with overweight and obesity include coronary heart disease, congestive heart failure, stroke, **emphysema,** chronic **bronchitis,** obstructive pulmonary disease, **deep vein thrombosis,** and some cancers (endometrial, breast, colon) (Patterson et al., 2004; NIH, 2007). The cardiovascular risk factors related to obesity are hypertension, **hypercholesterolemia** (or abnormal cholesterol levels), and type 2 diabetes. Patterson and colleagues (2004) note that the numerous medical conditions linked to obesity include **depression,** migraine headaches, asthma, **gastroesophageal reflux disease,** ulcers, diabetes, bladder infections, **osteoarthritis,** yeast infections, and gallbladder disease. A number of other health concerns associated with obesity include osteoporotic fractures (wrist, hip, forearm), joint pain (neck, back, knee), stress, fatigue, chronic insomnia, **anxiety,** indigestion, heartburn, constipation, skin problems, and allergies (to plants, trees, molds, dust, or animals) (Patterson et al., 2004). This information clearly depicts the health burden of obesity-related disorders and diseases and the challenges faced by fitness, public health, and medical professionals. It is important for an ACE-AHFS to realize that a determination of the absolute risk of morbidity and mortality of an obese client requires a comprehensive evaluation, including a complete medical history, physical examination, and appropriate laboratory tests.

Physiological Responses to Exercise Training

Regular physical activity and exercise has significant benefits in terms of risk reduction for overweight and obesity, insulin resistance, type 2 diabetes, blood lipid and lipoprotein abnormalities, hypertension, **peripheral vascular disease,** cerebrovascular disease, and coronary heart disease. Not everyone who is physically active on a regular basis will remain free from these vascular and metabolic diseases, but the protective effects and the reduction in risk levels are substantial enough to justify the promotion of a physically active lifestyle in all segments of the population, especially the overweight and obese. Continued study of overweight and obese persons is needed to better understand the physiological responses to exercise training for this population. Further epidemiological research (the branch of medicine that deals with the incidence, distribution, and possible control of diseases related to health) may uncover new relationships between obesity and health, and extend the understanding of the health benefits of exercise training. Table 10-4 summarizes the physiological effects of cardiovascular and resistance training.

Table 10-4
Physiological Effects of Cardiovascular and Resistance Training

	Cardiovascular Training	Resistance Training
Bone mineral density	Increase	Increase
Hypertension		
Systolic	Decrease	Possible decrease
Diastolic	Decrease	Possible decrease
Resting heart rate	Decrease	Decrease
Blood lipids		
Triglycerides	Decrease*	Possible decrease
Total cholesterol	Decrease*	Possible decrease
LDL cholesterol	Decrease*	Possible decrease
HDL cholesterol	Increase	Possible increase
Glucose metabolism		
Basal insulin levels	Decrease	Decrease
Insulin sensitivity	Increase	Increase
Cardiovascular endurance	Increase	No change
Body composition		
Fat mass	Decrease	Decrease
Fat-free mass	Increase (mild)	Increase
Resting metabolic rate	No change	Increase (mild)
Musculoskeletal health	Increase (mild)	Increase
Functional capabilities	Increase	Increase
Longevity	Increase	Unknown

*A decrease in triglycerides, total cholesterol, and LDL cholesterol from cardiovascular exercise occurs if there is a concurrent loss of body weight.

Source: Adapted from Kravitz, L. (2007). The 25 most significant health benefits of physical activity and exercise. *IDEA Fitness Journal*, 4, 9, 54–63.

The Role of Exercise in Weight Loss and Weight-gain Prevention

Although it is possible to lose weight with physical activity alone, the combination of exercise with a restricted dietary intake is a more meaningful strategy (Hill & Wyatt, 2005). Hill and Wyatt (2005) also state that exercise positively alters the composition of weight loss so that a greater percentage of weight loss comes from fat, rather than from muscle. In addition, exercise, especially resistance training, helps preserve a person's RMR in weight-loss programs by preserving muscle mass, which has a relatively high metabolic demand. Several investigations (Hill & Wyatt, 2005; Jakicic & Gallagher, 2003) have also demonstrated that persons expending high volumes of weekly exercise (one hour or more each day) have high success rates in long-term weight-loss maintenance. Hill and Wyatt (2005) state that an exertion totaling approximately 2500 to 2800 kcal/week (60 to 90 minutes per day of moderate-intensity physical activity) may be required to maintain substantial weight loss of ≥30 pounds (≥14 kg). The physiological reasons why exercise is so meaningful for long-term weight-loss success are speculative at best. However, Hill and Wyatt (2005) hypothesize that persons who maintain a high level of exercise may be much better at maintaining target food consumption goals as well. In summary, the results of several epidemiological studies consistently reveal that persons who are physically active are much less likely to gain weight over time than those who are not. Although habitual physical activity is an attainable goal, only 48% percent of all American adults currently get ≥30 minutes of moderate-intensity exercise per day on at least five days/week (Morbidity and Mortality Weekly Report, 2003).

Programming and Progressive Exercise Guidelines for Overweight and Obesity

The foundational research for exercise guidelines for overweight and obese persons stems from the ACSM (2006) guidelines for the development and maintenance of cardiorespiratory fitness for endurance exercise (frequency of three to five days per week), using an exercise mode that involves the major muscle groups (in a rhythmic nature) for a prolonged time period. ACSM (2006) recommends an intensity of exercise of 55/65 to 90% of maximum heart rate (or 40/50 to 85% of **oxygen uptake reserve**), with a continuous duration of 20 to 60 minutes per session. Inherent in these guidelines is the concept of individualizing the program for each person's fitness level, health, age, personal goals, risk-factor profile, medications, behavioral characteristics, and individual preferences.

ACSM (2006) has published the following guidelines for overweight and obese clients:

- Establish a long-term reduction in body weight of at least 5 to 10%.
- The primary mode of exercise should be large-muscle-group aerobic activities.
- A combination of weightbearing and non-weightbearing activities is encouraged.
- The initial emphasis of the exercise training should be on duration and frequency (keeping intensity moderate and progressing gradually).
- Frequency of training should be five to seven days per week.
- Accumulate 200 to 300 minutes of aerobic activity per week (which is equivalent to ≥2000 kilocalories of exercise per week); this can be accomplished via exercise bouts lasting as little as 10 minutes.
- Include a reduction in dietary fat intake to <30% of total energy intake.
- Emphasize fruits, vegetables, whole grains, and lean sources of protein.
- Create a negative energy balance of 500 to 1000 kilocalories per day [which is equivalent to a weekly weight loss of 1 to 2 pounds (0.5 to 1.0 kg)].
- Include the use of behavior-management techniques (including relapse prevention).

The concept of periodizing aerobic-training programs is encouraged. **Periodization** training is based on an inverse relationship between intensity and volume of training. With aerobic exercise, intensity can be individualized using percent of heart rate maximum, percent of **$\dot{V}O_2$max (maximal aerobic capacity)**, or RPE, where volume is differentiated by the duration of the session, as well as the frequency of sessions.

The following periodization suggestions can be used to individualize an exercise program to optimize weight loss during aerobic exercise:

- Incorporate frequent cardiorespiratory workouts that are low intensity and longer duration.
- Include some cardiorespiratory workouts that are of higher intensity for a shorter period of time. This objective may best be realized with high-intensity continuous training or with interval training. To avoid physiological and orthopedic stress and injury, it would be prudent to complete only one higher-intensity workout per week.
- Incorporate multi-mode training. The theory of multi-mode training (i.e., employing two or more modes of cardiorespiratory exercise) implies that by doing so the body is protected from getting overly fatigued from overuse of the same muscles in the same movement patterns. This technique helps to thwart the occurrence of musculoskeletal system stress, and aids in the prevention of muscle soreness and injuries. Therefore, theoretically, a person will be able to safely do more work more frequently, which equates to higher total energy expenditure and fat utilization.
- Vary the workout designs regularly. Endeavor to find a satisfactory method for each client by which cardiorespiratory workouts vary within each week, weekly, or bi-weekly using the three ideas just listed. Varying the workouts provides a new stimulus to the body's cardiorespiratory system in an effort to avoid the consequences of overuse exercise fatigue.

Biomechanical Considerations for Obese Clients

Cardiorespiratory Exercise Considerations

The preferred type of cardiorespiratory exercise for overweight and obese is a combination of weightbearing (such as walking and elliptical exercise) and non-weightbearing (such as cycling and swimming) modes. Exercise choices should be based on an individual's preferences and exercise history. Help each client find modes of exercise where he or she has a perceived comfort level with few (if any) negative barriers. The majority of the time spent exercising should be at a low-to-moderate intensity level to avoid joint stress and injury. Therefore, running, jumping, and high-impact movements are not recommended. These physical activities may lead to some musculoskeletal problems associated with body weight and impact forces from the repeated (and forceful) foot strikes on the ground surface. The emphasis of the cardiorespiratory exercise programs should be on performing longer and/or more frequent bouts of exercise. It is important to monitor muscle soreness from the exercise and always ask the client if he or she is experiencing any orthopedic problems or discomfort. Stationary cycling is preferable to road cycling, as it eliminates any balance-related challenges, while also avoiding the hazards of traffic.

Walking is considered a very good initial exercise because it requires no extra skill. When beginning a walking or weightbearing exercise regimen with a client, it is important to keep a few things in mind. Make sure the person has quality fitness shoes with good shock-absorbing qualities. Next, and very importantly, Mattsson, Larsson, and Rossner (1996) presented some very useful data about walking with an obese female population. The most interesting finding of this study was that level walking was much harder work for obese women when compared to normal-weight women. On average, obese women used as much as 56% of $\dot{V}O_2$max during walking, as compared to 36% $\dot{V}O_2$max for normal-weight women. The authors noted that even though obese women do not necessarily walk with a waddle or straddled legs, they do walk with an abnormal gait pattern that increases their relative oxygen cost. The authors conclude that walking may be too exhausting (and sometimes painful) for some obese individuals due to these biomechanical differences in gait and recommend incorporating alternative training modes in the workout design. Swimming and aquatic exercise programs provide total-body exercise with little to no weightbearing due to the buoyancy of water. Buoyancy is also a benefit for overweight and obese people who may have joint problems (such as arthritis of the knee, hip, or ankle, or structural problems of these three joints).

Fitness facilities have a variety of exercise equipment. The ACE-AHFS is encouraged to help clients find exercise devices that are easy to use and that do not cause any back, hip, knee, or ankle discomfort. For example, recumbent bikes are great cycling options for obese individuals, as compared to stationary or road cycling. However, the ACE-AHFS must make sure the bike seat is comfortable for the overweight or obese client. For some obese clients, balance will be an additional challenge with some modes of exercise. If this is the case, the ACE-AHFS should select exercise devices that have handrails to provide balance support and help prevent falling.

Resistance-training Considerations

There are a few biomechanical concerns to note regarding resistance exercise and overweight and obese persons. For some overweight and obese people with mobility and/or balance challenges, seated exercises are good initial options. These types of exercises can be useful in building basic muscle strength. While seated in a chair, individuals are able to do a variety of arm raises, leg lifts, and stretches. Please note that the seats on some exercise machines were not developed for large persons, which may limit the feasibility of using some strength-training equipment. Moreover, weight benches are often quite narrow, which could result in the loss of balance for some clients. In addition, getting into and out of some resistance-training devices may be difficult. It is sometimes preferable not to use exercise devices (such as some abdominal equipment) that are built at floor level, because the overweight person may have great difficulty getting down to, and up from, the floor. Note that some supine exercises may cause breathing difficulty for some obese clients. The ACE-AHFS must always check to make sure that the client's breathing is regular and uninterrupted during all exercises. Prudence should be taken to avoid doing too much lunge and squat work with overweight persons, due to possible knee and back discomfort and injury.

Psychological Issues Associated With Obesity and Related Dietary Patterns

The relationship between obesity and psychological distress is still open for debate. The relationship between obesity and psychological distress is somewhat mixed in the research. Some research does not show statistically significant differences between obese individuals and their non-obese counterparts in psychological health and personality profiles (Huang et al., 2007), while other research shows clear body image, self-esteem, and depression issues (Hill & Williams, 1998; Friedman et al., 2002). Some obese and overweight clients tend to have a higher prevalence of distress then their non-obese counterparts. These clients often experience adverse feelings of body satisfaction and self-esteem. However, there is a growing body of knowledge that substantiates that physical activity improves psychological well-being in most adults (obese and non-obese) (Kravitz, 2000).

It appears that acute exercise bouts (single sessions), as well as sustained exercise training programs (over a period of time), have a positive effect on people with depression (Scully et al., 1998). The research infers that the greatest anti-depressive effects seem to occur after 17 weeks of exercise, although observable effects begin from four weeks onward (Scully et al., 1998). In addition, the effects of exercise on depression seem equivalent in both genders and uninhibited by age or health status. Although no research guidelines exist for actual exercise programming, the evidence suggests following the accepted guidelines for the recommended quantity and quality of exercise for developing and maintaining cardiorespiratory and muscular fitness and flexibility in healthy adults (ACSM, 2006).

Body image is a complex construct that includes feelings, thoughts, and perceptions about one's physique (Scully et al., 1998). Scully and colleagues found that females tend to have a less positive body image than males, and can become very preoccupied with losing weight. When diet and exercise become too dominant in a woman's lifestyle, she is most susceptible to a set of disorders referred to as the **female athlete triad.**

In addition, females tend to focus on their body from an aesthetic viewpoint, whereas males tend to view their bodies in terms of strength, speed, and coordination (Franzoi, 1995). Franzoi (1995) suggests that women are more likely to engage in activities that are non-competitive, such as aerobics, with the goal of keeping fit. Issues such as weight control and attractiveness are bigger concerns for women than men. Misperceptions regarding body image appear to be strongly implicated in the development of eating disorders and clinical depression.

The research suggests that the ACE-AHFS should be very attentive to the design of fitness facilities to make an overweight or obese client feel more comfortable with his or her body image (Scully et al., 1998). For example, having access to private changing facilities is recommended to help reduce feelings of body-image dissatisfaction. In addition, the ACE-AHFS needs to be aware that exercise participation may accentuate a person's body-image dissatisfaction and enhance a person's drive for leanness. Therefore, the suggestion or implication that everyone can attain a "model's body" may perpetuate psychological disorders in some clients. Caution is necessary for all fitness professionals when guiding clients, especially overweight and obese clients, toward healthy physical activity, as opposed to leading them to a path obsessed with thinness and the development of eating disorders.

Exercise has a positive connection to improved self-esteem. This link also appears to be more potent among individuals who have lower self-esteem. At this time, available studies indicate that aerobic exercise may have a more pronounced effect, perhaps only because there is so little research available regarding resistance training and self-esteem. However, self-esteem is quite complex and studies suggest that certain subcomponents contribute to a person's self-esteem, including perceived sport competence, physical condition, an "attractive" body, and strength (Scully et al., 1998). Because of the many variables that influence self-esteem, it is important to note that a person may highly value his or her physical condition and yet have a negative evaluation of his or her body. The meaningful evidence suggests that aerobic exercise seems to have the most consequential influence on individuals who initially have low self-esteem. An optimal exercise design is uncertain at this time based on published research.

Case Studies

Case Study 1

Clare is a 52-year-old client who is 5'6" (1.7 m) and weighs 160 pounds (73 kg). Her blood pressure is 110/70 mmHg, her total cholesterol is 200 mg/dL, and she has 33% body fat. She was very athletic in the past and even competed as a middle-distance runner in high school. Clare takes indoor cycling class lasting 40 minutes three or four times a week and walks leisurely whenever she can. She currently performs no resistance training.

Clare drinks 1.5 liters (0.4 gallons) of water and eats between 2300 and 2500 calories each day, including a small breakfast, light snacking in the morning, a light lunch that sometimes includes protein but usually consists of a salad or just vegetables, an afternoon snack, and a dinner of fish or chicken with vegetables and some fat-free ice cream. She also drinks five cups of decaffeinated coffee during the day and has a glass of wine in the evening five days a week.

Clare reports no health conditions and does not take any medications or vitamins. She has a history of yo-yo dieting and did some fasting in her 20s and 30s. She sleeps 5.5 hours each night and has a high-stress job. Her goals are to lose weight (fat) and "firm up."

The Program

Workout and Lifestyle Plan:

- Cardiovascular exercise (progressed to the following)
  - ✔ 40 minutes of cardiovascular exercise (cycle ergometer or stair stepping) two days a week
  - ✔ Walking for 45 minutes at a self-selected moderate intensity one day a week
  - ✔ Elliptical training for 45 minutes at a self-selected moderate intensity one day a week
  - ✔ Walking moderately for at least 90 minutes (accumulated) during the week
- Resistance training
  - ✔ Circuit resistance-training program three times a week using 10 different exercises (chest, back, biceps, triceps, deltoids, quadriceps, hamstrings, abdominals, buttocks, lower back) (one circuit)

Dietary Pattern:

- Met with a dietician, who gave her a Mediterranean-type diet of approximately 1700 calories a day

Lifestyle:

- Attempted to sleep 7 hours a night when possible
- Did extra stretching exercises on high-stress days

Three-month Outcomes:

- Weight = 148 lb (67 kg)
- Blood pressure = 110/70 mmHg
- Total cholesterol = 184 mg/dL
- Body fat = 28%

Six-month Outcomes:

- Weight = 136 lb (62 kg)
- Blood pressure = 101/70 mmHg
- Total cholesterol = 177 mg/dL
- Body fat = 24%

Case Study 2

Jen is a 19-year-old client who is 5'4" (1.6 m) and weighs 220 pounds (100 kg). Her blood pressure is 124/82 mmHg, her total cholesterol is 210 mg/dL, and she has approximately 60% body fat. Jen walks leisurely twice a week for 45 minutes each time. She currently performs no resistance training.

Jen drinks more than 1.5 liters (0.4 gallons) of water and eats more than 2800 calories of food each day. Her diet is very high in fats (particularly saturated fat) and simple carbohydrates and low in protein. She eats three big meals a day and enjoys a lot of fried and baked foods. She also snacks on sweets (e.g., cookies and cake) during the day. Jen drinks two cups of caffeinated coffee and three or four colas each day. In addition, she drinks three or four alcoholic beverages each weekend.

Jen has prehypertension and hypercholesterolemia and is currently taking no medications or vitamins. She leads what she calls an "inactive lifestyle," sleeps seven hours a night, and has a stress level typical of a college student. Her goal is to lose weight (fat) and get in shape.

The Program

Workout and Lifestyle Plan:

- Cardiovascular exercise (progressed to the following)
  - ✔ 30–60 minutes of cardiovascular exercise (stair stepping, elliptical training, or treadmill walking) four days a week
  - ✔ Walking at a moderate intensity two times a week for 45 minutes each time
- Resistance training
  - ✔ Four days a week using an upper- and lower-body split program; each day she does 5 different exercises, 1 to 5 sets of each (never doing more than 20 sets in a workout).

Dietary Pattern:

- Met with a dietician who gave her a heart-healthy diet as recommended by the American Dietetic Association (lowering the fats and simple sugars and replacing them with healthy fats and more fruits and vegetables and complex carbohydrates)
- Caloric intake gradually decreased to 1500 calories per day

Lifestyle:

- Did meditation 3 or 4 times a week (20 minutes each time) to help manage stress

Three-month Outcomes:

- Weight = 185 lb (84 kg)
- Blood pressure = 110/76 mmHg
- Total cholesterol = 200 mg/dL
- Body fat = 40%

Six-month Outcomes:

- Weight = 150 lb (68 kg)
- Blood pressure = 101/74 mmHg
- Total cholesterol = 185 mg/dL
- Body fat = 32%

Summary

Client education is the framework of successful weight-loss interventions. The ACE-AHFS is encouraged to inform clients of the health risks of overweight and obesity and the benefits that accompany exercise, weight loss, and lifestyle modifications. The ACE-AHFS can help clients establish realistic weight-management goals and strategies, and provide the ongoing support for them to keep up these new behaviors. It is important to regularly remind clients that successful energy balance is a life-long process that starts with a commitment to improve the quality of their lives.

References

American College of Sports Medicine (2006). *ACSM's Guidelines for Exercise Testing and Prescription* (7th ed.). Philadelphia: Lippincott Williams & Wilkins.

Boucher, J.L., Shafer, K.J. & Chafffin, J.A. (2001). Weight loss, diets, and supplements: Does anything work? *Diabetes Spectrum,* 14, 3, 169–175.

Costain, L. & Croker, H. (2005). Helping individuals to help themselves. *Proceedings of the Nutrition Society,* 64, 89–96.

Diabetes Prevention Program Research Group (2002). Reduction in the incidence of type 2 diabetes with lifestyle intervention or metformin. *New England Journal of Medicine,* 346, 393–403.

Donnelly, J.E. et al. (2003). Is resistance training effective for weight management? *Evidence-based Preventive Medicine,* 1, 1, 21–29.

Druce, M.R., Small, C.J., & Bloom, S.R. (2005). Minireview: Gut peptides regulating satiety. *Endocrinology,* 145, 6, 2660–2665.

Elia, M. (1992). Organ and tissue contribution to metabolic weight. In: Kinney, J.M. & Tucker, H.N. (Eds.) *Energy Metabolism: Tissue Determinants and Cellular Corollaries.* pp. 61–79. New York: Raven Press.

Fabricatore, A.N. & Wadden, T.A. (2003). Treatment of obesity. *Clinical Diabetes,* 21, 2, 67–72.

Franzoi, S.L. (1995). The body-as-object versus the body-as-process: Gender differences and gender considerations. *Sex Roles,* 33, 417–433.

Friedman, K. et al. (2002). Body image partially mediates the relationship between obesity and psychological distress. *Obesity Research,* 10, 1, 33–41.

Havel, P.J. (2002). Control of energy homeostasis and insulin action by adipocyte hormones: Leptin, acylation stimulating protein, and adiponectin. *Current Opinion in Lipidology,* 13, 51–59.

Heyward, V. (2006). *Advanced Fitness Assessment and Exercise Prescription* (5th ed.). Champaign, Ill.: Human Kinetics.

Hickey, M.S. & Israel, R.G. (2007). Obesity drugs and drugs in the pipeline. *ACSM's Health & Fitness Journal,* 11, 4, 20–25.

Hill, A.J. & Williams, J. (1998). Psychological health in a non-clinical sample of obese women. *International Journal of Obesity and Related Disorders,* 22, 6, 578–583.

Hill, J.O. & Wyatt, H.R. (2005). Role of physical activity in preventing and treating obesity. *Journal of Applied Physiology,* 99, 765–770.

Huang, J.S. et al. (2007). Body image and self-esteem among adolescents undergoing an intervention targeting dietary and physical activity behaviors. *Journal of Adolescent Health*, 40, 3, 245–251.

Jakicic, J.M. & Gallagher, K.I. (2003). Exercise considerations for the sedentary, overweight adult. *Exercise and Sport Sciences Reviews,* 31, 2, 91–95.

Jakicic, J.M. et al. (2001). ACSM position stand on the appropriate intervention strategies for weight loss and prevention of weight regain for adults. *Medicine & Science in Sports & Exercise,* 33, 2145–2156.

Kravitz, L. (2007). The 25 most significant health benefits of physical activity and exercise. *IDEA Fitness Journal,* 4, 9, 54–63

Kravitz, L. (2000). Exercise and psychological health. *IDEA Personal Trainer,* 11, 10, 19–21.

Levine, J.A. et al. (2005). Interindividual variation in posture allocation: Possible role in human obesity. *Science,* 307, 584–586.

Li, Z. et al. (2005). Meta-analysis: Pharmacologic treatment of obesity. *Annals of Internal Medicine,* 142, 585–589.

Liebman, B. (2004). Fat: More than just a lump of lard. *Nutrition Action Health Letter,* 31, 8, 1, 3–6.

Loos, R.J.F. & Bouchard, C. (2003). Obesity—is it a genetic disorder? *Journal of Internal Medicine,* 254, 401–425.

Marx, J.O. et al. (2001). Low-volume circuit versus high-volume periodized resistance training in women. *Medicine & Science in Sports & Exercise,* 33, 4, 635–643.

Mattsson, E., Larsson, U.E., & Rossner, S. (1996). Is walking for exercise too exhausting for obese women? *International Journal of Obesity and Metabolic Disorders,* 21, 5, 380–386.

Morbidity and Mortality Weekly Report (2003). Prevalence of physical activity, including lifestyle activities among adults—United States, 2000–2001. *Morbidity and Mortality Weekly Report,* 52, 32, 764–769.

National Cholesterol Education Program (2002). Expert Panel on Detection, Evaluation and Treatment of High Blood Cholesterol in Adults. Summary of the 2nd Report of NCEP Expert Panel on Detection, Evaluation and Treatment of High Blood Cholesterol in Adults (Adult Treatment Panel III). NIH Publication 02-5213. Executive summary (2001). *Journal of the American Medical Association,* 285, 2486–2497.

National Institutes of Health (2007). http://www.nhlbi.nih.gov/health/dci/Diseases/obe/obe_whatare.html

Patterson, R.E. et al. (2004). A comprehensive examination of health conditions associated with obesity in older adults. *American Journal of Preventive Medicine,* 97, 5, 385–390.

Scully, D. et al. (1998). Physical exercise and psychological well-being: A critical review. *British Journal of Sports Medicine,* 32, 111–120.

Taheri, S. et al. (2004). Short sleep duration is associated with reduced leptin, elevated ghrelin, and increased body mass index. *PLOS Medicine,* 1, 3, 1–8.

Trayhurn, P. (2005). The biology of obesity. *Proceedings of the Nutrition Society,* 64, 31–38.

Wing, R. R. & Phelan, S. (2005). Long-term weight loss maintenance. *American Journal of Clinical Nutrition,* 82(Suppl.), 222S–225S.

World Health Organization (2006). *Overweight and Obesity.* http://www.who.int/mediacentre/factsheets/fs311/en/

Suggested Reading

Brownell, K.D. (2004). *The LEARN Program for Weight Management* (10th ed.). Dallas: American Health Publishing Co.

Eckel, R.H. (2003). *Obesity: Mechanisms and Clinical Management.* Philadelphia: Lippincott Williams & Wilkins.

Hassink, S.G. (2006). *A Clinical Guide to Pediatric Weight Management and Obesity.* Philadelphia: Lippincott Williams & Wilkins.

U.S. Department of Health and Human Services (1996). *Physical Activity and Health: A Report of the Surgeon General.* Atlanta, Ga.: U.S. Department of Health and Human Services, Centers for Disease Control and Prevention, National Center for Chronic Disease Prevention and Health Promotion. S/N 017-023-00196-5.

Selye, H. (1976). Forty years of stress research: Principal remaining problems and misconceptions. *Canadian Medical Association,* 115, 53–56.

World Health Organization (2006). *Overweight and Obesity.* http://www.who.int/mediacentre/factsheets/fs311/en/

About The Authors

Barry A. Franklin, Ph.D., is director of the Cardiac Rehabilitation and Exercise Laboratories at William Beaumont Hospital in Royal Oak, Michigan, and professor of Physiology at Wayne State University School of Medicine in Detroit, Michigan. Dr. Franklin served as president of the American Association of Cardiovascular and Pulmonary Rehabilitation in 1988 and president of the American College of Sports Medicine in 1999. Currently, he hold editorial positions with numerous scientific and clinical journals, including the *American Journal of Cardiology, Preventive Cardiology, Chest,* and *Medicine & Science in Sports & Exercise.* Dr. Franklin has written or edited more than 500 publications, including 80 book chapters and 23 books.

Wendy M. Miller, M.D., is a graduate of Wayne State University School of Medicine in Detroit, Michigan, and completed her Internal Medicine residency at William Beaumont Hospital in Royal Oak, Michigan. Dr. Miller is Board Certified in Internal Medicine and Bariatric Medicine, and is also certified as a Physician Nutrition Specialist. Currently she serves as medical director of the Beaumont Hospital Weight Control Center in the Division of Nutrition and Preventive Medicine. Dr. Miller is a member of the American College of Physicians and the American College of Preventive Medicine. She has published numerous pieces on obesity and its association with diabetes, inflammation, metabolic syndrome, dyslipidemia, and cardiovascular disease.

Peter A. McCullough, M.D., M.P.H., is the chief of nutrition and preventive medicine at William Beaumont Hospital in Royal Oak, Michigan. After receiving his medical degree from University of Texas Southwestern Medical School, Dr. McCullough went on to complete internal medicine residency at the University of Washington, and cardiology fellowship at William Beaumont Hospital. He holds a master's degree in Public Health from the University of Michigan. Dr. McCullough has more than 200 published scientific communications and is a nationally recognized authority on preventive medicine, chronic kidney disease, obesity, and the primary and secondary prevention of coronary artery disease.

In This Chapter

CHAPTER 11

The Metabolic Syndrome

Barry A. Franklin

Wendy M. Miller

Peter A. McCullough

Complex, mutually reinforcing interactions between **obesity** and **insulin resistance** largely account for the pathogenesis of the **metabolic syndrome** (Figure 11-1). Excess **visceral adiposity** is both necessary and sufficient for the development of this multifaceted disease state (Batsis, Nieto-Martinez, & Lopez-Jimenez, 2007). Genetically predisposed groups, including Hispanics and Asian Indians, have demonstrated a greater intolerance to excess visceral adiposity, and are known to develop the metabolic syndrome at relatively lesser degrees of adiposity (Caballero, 2005; Misra & Vikram, 2004). More than 95% of individuals with the metabolic syndrome have a **body mass index (BMI)** that is ≥ 25 kg/m^2; thus, the BMI as a crude measure identifies the majority of individuals at risk for this medical condition.

Central pathophysiologic features of the metabolic syndrome as a consequence of excess visceral adiposity include the following (Rader, 2007):

- Insulin resistance at the liver and skeletal muscles
- **Atherogenic dyslipidemia,** chiefly manifested as a triad of low **high-density lipoprotein** cholesterol (HDL) together with increases in triglycerides and small, dense **low-density lipoprotein** cholesterol (LDL) particles with fasting and postprandial chylomicrons and glycated LDL particles prone to oxidation
- **Hypertension**
- A proinflammatory state, with increases in acute-phase reactants [e.g., high-sensitivity C-reactive protein (hs-CRP)]
- A prothrombotic state, with increases in plasminogen activator inhibitor (PAI-1) and fibrinogen

Both the proinflammatory and prothrombotic states of the metabolic syndrome derive largely from the secretory activity of intra-abdominal or visceral adipose tissue. Contrary to the traditional concept of **fat** as an inert tissue, **adipocytes** are clearly recognized as secretory cells. **Cytokines** and other inflammatory markers or signaling molecules released by adipocytes (adipokines) include tumor necrosis factor alpha (TNF-alpha), interleukin-6 (IL-6), resistin, and **adiponectin.** Both TNF-alpha and IL-6 are received by the liver through the portal circulation and stimulate hepatocytes to produce inflammatory proteins. Adiponectin is a local paracrine substance produced by adipocytes that is believed to have a favorable physiologic role in maintaining fat mass in **homeostasis.** Accordingly, adiponectin levels are characteristically reduced in the obese and those with the metabolic syndrome, thereby permitting additional growth of adipose tissue (Bodary, Iglay, & Eitzman, 2007).

Hepatic insulin resistance is triggered by resistin, hepatocyte growth factor, and **free fatty acids (FFA),** which are secreted by intraabdominal adipocytes and travel via the portal circulation to the liver. Visceral fat exhibits accelerated lipolytic activity. The subsequent increases in circulating FFA levels result in the development of triglyceride reservoirs in both muscle and

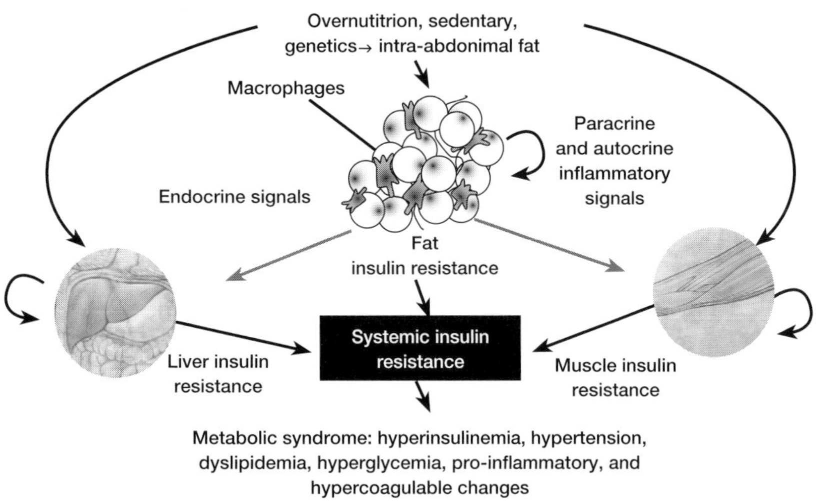

Figure 11-1
Pathogenesis of the metabolic syndrome

liver, depressing **insulin** action and increasing hepatic very-low-density lipoprotein output.

Both the proinflammatory and prothrombotic states resulting from obesity may increase the risk of coronary events. A widely cited report found that increasing BMI was independently associated prothrombotic factors and impaired fibrinolytic activity, including fibrinogen, factor VII, PAI-1, and tissue plasminogen activator in men and women (Rosito et al., 2004). Accordingly, the investigators found greater thrombotic potential in **overweight** and obese subjects. High-sensitivity C-reactive protein is a pivotal acute-phase reactant that is considered an index of inflammation and is associated with increased cardiovascular risk, particularly the provocation of acute coronary syndrome. Values greater than 2 mg/L may serve as a powerful predictor for future cardiovascular events. The American Heart Association/Centers for Disease Control and Prevention (CDC) Scientific Statement on Markers of Intervention and Cardiovascular Disease recommends that in persons with an intermediate Framingham **coronary heart disease (CHD)** 10-year risk (10 to 20%) and an LDL level below the cutoff for pharmacotherapeutic intervention, it may be appropriate to measure hs-CRP to aid in risk stratification (Pearson et al., 2003).

Epidemiology

The epidemiology of the metabolic syndrome directly parallels the obesity pandemic in terms of incidence and prevalence (Ford, Giles, & Dietz, 2002). The many causes for the rise in obesity are complex (see Chapter 10). Follow-up data from the Coronary Artery Risk Development in Young Adults Study

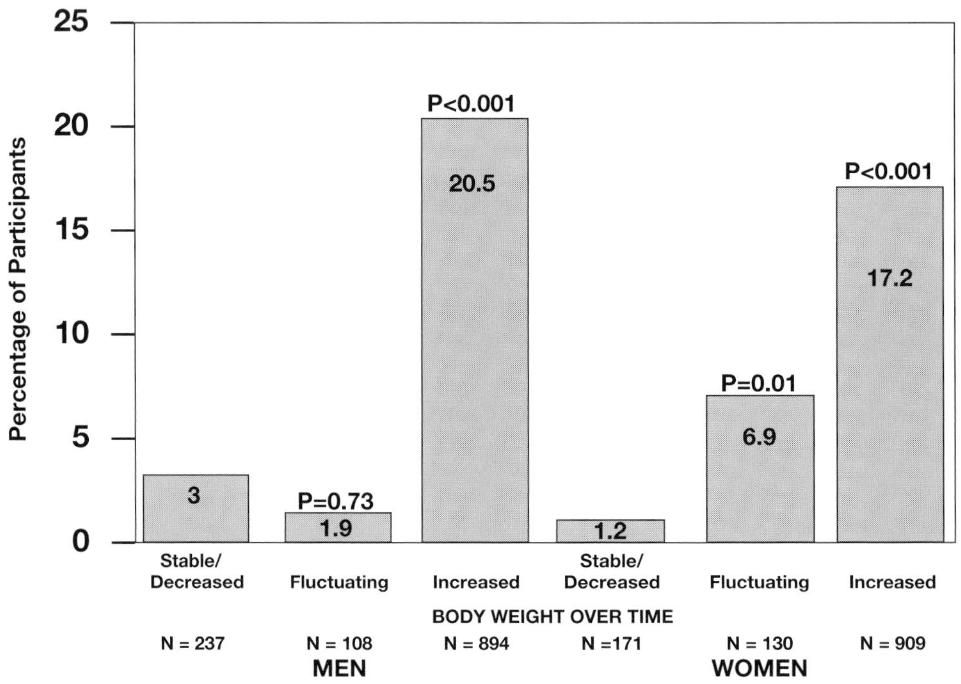

Figure 11-2
Incidence of the metabolic syndrome as reported in the CARDIA study of young adults followed over 15 years

Source: Adapted from Lloyd-Jones D.M. et al. (2007). Consistently stable or decreased body mass index in young adulthood and longitudinal changes in metabolic syndrome components: The Coronary Artery Risk Development in Young Adults Study. *Circulation,* 115, 8, 1004.

(CARDIA) (Figure 11-2) indicate that young adults are at considerable risk for the development of the metabolic syndrome if there has, over time, been a consistent increase in body weight (Lloyd-Jones et al., 2007). Although overall body weight and relative adiposity as reflected in the BMI identify the greater than two-thirds of Western populations at risk for the metabolic syndrome, those with excessive intra-abdominal adiposity are particularly susceptible. This **android** or male pattern of fat deposition in the abdomen is easily recognized and can be accurately quantified. If the abdomen is not **scaphoid**, or concave, on examination, excess visceral adiposity should be considered. Conversely, a predominately **gynoid** pattern of fat deposition in the buttocks and legs with a scaphoid abdomen does not indicate risk for the metabolic syndrome. One practical consideration, however, is that virtually all individuals with a BMI ≥30 kg/m^2 have excess visceral adiposity irrespective of body shape, with the exception of extremely muscular individuals.

Diagnostic Testing and Criteria

The association of visceral obesity and cardiovascular risk stems from the clustering of metabolic conditions, including hypertension, **dyslipidemia,** and **type 2 diabetes mellitus** mediated through insulin resistance leading to the metabolic syndrome. The purpose of this unique designation was to identify those at higher metabolic risk for **cardiovascular disease** and the development of **diabetes** and to respond with more aggressive strategies for prevention. As indicated earlier, the metabolic syndrome should be suspected in all individuals who are overweight or obese with a BMI ≥25 kg/m^2. The National Cholesterol Education Program Adult Treatment Panel III defines the metabolic syndrome as meeting three or more of the following criteria (Grundy et al., 2004):

- Abdominal obesity indicated by a waist circumference ≥40 inches (102 cm) in men and ≥35 inches (88 cm) in women
- Levels of triglyceride ≥150 mg/dL (1.7 mmol/L)
- HDL levels <40 and 50 mg/dL (1.0 and 1.3 mmol/L) in men and women, respectively
- Blood pressure levels ≥130/85 mmHg
- Fasting glucose levels ≥110 mg/dL (6.1 mmol/L)

Additional biomarkers that strongly support the diagnosis of the metabolic syndrome include hsCRP >2 mg/L, **hyperinsulinemia** (fasting C-peptide >4.6 ng/ml), and a urinary albumin:creatinine ratio >30 mg/g, which reflects kidney damage due to the vascular consequences of the disease (Table 11-1).

Table 11-1
Pathophysiologic Processes Associated With the Metabolic Syndrome

- Insulin resistance
- Abnormal fibrinolysis
- Endothelial dysfunction
- Microalbuminuria
- Inflammation
- Procoagulation

Source: Adapted from Grundy S.M. et al. (2004). Implications of recent clinical trials for the National Cholesterol Education Program Adult Treatment Panel III Guidelines. *Circulation,* 110, 2, 227.

The metabolic syndrome is present in 24% of all adults in the United States and in >40% of men and women over the age of 65 (Ford, Giles, & Dietz, 2002). This proportion is expected to grow to approximately two-thirds of the adult population. Each component of the metabolic syndrome is associated with a heightened risk for developing cardiovascular disease and diabetes. Individuals with the metabolic syndrome have a one-and-a-half- to threefold increased risk for developing CHD or **stroke** (Isomaa et al., 2001). In the primary prevention arm of the San Antonio Heart Study, the metabolic syndrome was associated with a twofold higher risk for developing cardiovascular disease over a mean follow-up of 12.7 years (Hunt et al., 2004). This distinguishes the metabolic syndrome as a unique marker for increased cardiovascular risk, highlighting the need for aggressive risk-factor reduction and treatment.

Treatment of the Metabolic Syndrome

The cornerstone treatment of the metabolic syndrome is therapeutic lifestyle modification to reduce body weight and fat stores, increase physical activity, and transition to an anti-atherogenic diet. Reduction of abdominal adiposity, the primary underlying cause of the metabolic syndrome, is the main therapeutic target. Although lifestyle intervention is often overlooked in clinical practice (Grundy, 2006), this non-pharmacologic approach has been shown to reduce cardiovascular risk and prevent or delay progression to diabetes [National Institutes of Health (NIH), 1998; Knowler et al., 2002].

Dietary Treatment

Several dietary approaches have been advocated for cardiovascular risk reduction in overweight and obese individuals. The Third Report of the National Cholesterol Education Program Adult Treatment Panel recommends a therapeutic lifestyle change (TLC) diet. The nutrient composition includes limiting total fat to 25 to 35% of daily calories (approximately 50 to 70 grams for an 1800 kcal/day diet), saturated fat to less than 7% of daily calories (approximately 13 grams for an 1800 kcal/day diet), and total cholesterol to less than 200 mg/day (Expert Panel, 2001). The majority of fat should come from **polyunsaturated** and **monounsaturated fatty acids,** such as fish, nuts, and vegetable oils. These unsaturated fats can help reduce elevated triglycerides and raise the low HDL levels often present in individuals with the metabolic syndrome. **Trans fatty acids,** which can raise LDL levels, should be severely restricted. Sugar and starch (simple carbohydrates) should be eliminated or markedly reduced, since they are major sources of excess calories and promote hyperinsulinemia. Additionally, a daily fiber intake of 20 to 30 grams is recommended. Table 11-2 shows the overall composition of the TLC diet.

Table 11-2
Nutrient Composition of the Therapeutic Lifestyle Changes (TLC) Diet

Nutrient	Recommended Intake
Saturated fat*	<7% of total calories
Polyunsaturated fat	Up to 10% of total calories
Monounsaturated fat	Up to 20% of total calories
Total fat	25–35% of total calories
Carbohydrate†	50–60% of total calories
Fiber	20–30 grams/day
Protein	Approximately 15% of total calories
Cholesterol	<200 mg/day
Total calories	Balance energy intake and expenditure to maintain a desirable body weight/prevent weight gain

*Trans fatty acids are another low-density lipoprotein–raising fat that should be severely restricted.
†Carbohydrates should be derived predominantly from foods rich in complex carbohydrates, including grains, especially whole grains, fruits, and vegetables, with an avoidance of simple carbohydrates, which include sugar and most baked goods and snack foods.

A modified Mediterranean-style diet, which has a similar **macronutrient** composition to the TLC diet, may have particular benefit for individuals with the metabolic syndrome. The diet is high in fruits, vegetables, nuts, whole grains, and olive oil. Limits for daily saturated fat and cholesterol intake of less than 10% and less than 300 mg, respectively, are slightly higher than those recommended in the TLC diet. A two-year randomized, controlled trial of subjects with the metabolic syndrome found superior weight loss with a Mediterranean-style diet as compared with a control prudent diet; moreover, the Mediterranean-style diet group experienced a concomitant reduction in markers of vascular inflammation and insulin (Esposito et al., 2004). Additionally, endothelial function improved in those on the Mediterranean-style diet, but not in the controls.

To achieve weight loss in overweight and obese individuals, a reduction in daily calorie intake of 500 to 1000 kcal is commonly recommended. This degree of caloric deficit should produce a weight loss of 1 pound (0.45 kg) or more per week. Comparisons of popular dietary approaches with unusually high restrictions of various macronutrients, such as very-low-carbohydrate diets, have generally failed to show significant differences in weight loss or cardiovascular risk reduction at one year (Dansinger et al., 2005). Additionally, diets advocating excessive restriction of certain macronutrients are likely to be associated with some nutritional inadequacies and typically are not adhered to over the long term. Therefore, such diet programs should not be recommended. Prevention of weight regain will ultimately depend on the maintenance of substantive lifestyle changes, including healthy dietary modifications and regular physical activity.

Pharmacologic Treatment

Permanent lifestyle changes are generally considered first-line strategies to address the cardiovascular risk factors that characterize the metabolic syndrome. However, pharmacotherapies may be indicated for individuals unable to adopt healthier lifestyle habits or those failing to reach metabolic goals despite lifestyle change. Agents that can modify the cardiovascular risk of the metabolic syndrome may target elevated **blood pressure,** insulin resistance, impaired **glucose** metabolism, dyslipidemia, or combinations thereof.

Elevated blood pressure is often a component of the metabolic syndrome and lowering it reduces the risk for both CHD and stroke. A meta-analysis of several randomized clinical trials indicates that an average reduction of 12 to 13 mmHg in **systolic blood pressure (SBP)** sustained over four years is associated with a 21% reduction in CHD, 37% reduction in stroke, 25% reduction in total cardiovascular mortality, and 13% reduction in all-cause mortality (He & Whelton, 1999).

Although the blood-pressure goal for individuals with the metabolic syndrome is currently unknown, it is reasonable to use the target for diabetes—that is, a value below 130/80 mmHg. There is no consensus on first-line antihypertensive medication in the metabolic syndrome. However, given the relationship between the insulin resistance of the metabolic syndrome and endothelial dysfunction, an agent that blocks the renin-angiotensin system may provide benefits beyond blood pressure reduction. This system plays a central role in endothelial dysfunction and both angiotensin receptor blockers and angiotensin-converting enzyme inhibitors can improve endothelial function (Ruilope, Redón, & Schmieder, 2007).

Insulin resistance places individuals with the metabolic syndrome but without overt type 2 diabetes in a pre-diabetic state. Progression of insulin resistance and a concomitant decline of pancreatic beta cell function ultimately leads to type 2 diabetes. This is a gradual, insidious process and the risk for cardiovascular disease begins to increase 15 years prior to the diagnosis of diabetes (Hu et al., 2002).

The Diabetes Prevention Program study demonstrated that progression to diabetes in individuals with impaired fasting glucose can be prevented or delayed with metformin, a medication that decreases hepatic glucose production, reduces intestinal glucose absorption, and increases insulin sensitivity (Knowler et al., 2002). However, metformin was less effective than intensive lifestyle modification that included a low-calorie, low-fat diet and at least 150 minutes of moderate-intensity exercise per week. Similarly, thiazolidinediones, a medication class that also enhances insulin sensitivity, may be protective against diabetes. In a large randomized, controlled trial, a thiazolidinedione medication reduced the three-year incidence of type 2 diabetes in patients with impaired fasting glucose or impaired glucose tolerance (Gerstein et al., 2006). However, use of metformin for metabolic syndrome prevention may be preferable over thiazolidinediones due to the weight gain associated with the latter.

The two metabolic syndrome criteria most highly correlated with insulin resistance/hyperinsulinemia are **hypertriglyceridemia** and low HDL. On the other hand, the first therapeutic target for cardiovascular risk reduction is LDL (Expert Panel, 2001). For individuals with the metabolic syndrome and cardiovascular disease or diabetes, an LDL of 70 mg/dL or less is recommended (Grundy et al., 2004). LDL targets for others are based on estimation of 10-year CHD risk via Framingham scoring (Expert Panel, 2001). The maximum LDL goal for those without risk factors is less than 160 mg/dL.

First-line pharmacologic treatment for lowering LDL is an HMG-CoA reductase inhibitor (statin), but alternatives include bile acid sequestrants or nicotinic acid. After achieving LDL goals, evaluation of triglyceride and non-HDL levels (HDL = total cholesterol – HDL) should follow. For those with a fasting triglyceride level of 200 mg/dL or greater, non-HDL should be calculated. The goal for non-HDL is 30 mg/dL higher than that of LDL. Non-HDL goals can often be achieved by increasing the dose of the LDL-lowering medication or by adding nicotinic acid or a fibrate.

Surgical Treatment

According to the NIH guidelines, bariatric surgery is indicated for those with a BMI of 40 kg/m^2 or greater, or those with a BMI between 35 and 40 kg/m^2 with at least one comorbid condition such as diabetes, hypertension, obstructive sleep apnea, or CHD (NIH, 1998). Bariatric surgery has shown the highest success rates for obesity management, with an average weight loss of 35 to 38% of initial total body weight (Shah, Simha, & Garg, 2006); moreover, it improves all components of the metabolic syndrome. A meta-analysis of bariatric surgery outcomes found that diabetes improved or resolved in 83%, hypercholesterolemia improved in 95%, and hypertension improved or resolved in 87% of patients who underwent gastric bypass surgery (Buchwald et al., 2004).

Clinical Implications and Associated Disorders of the Metabolic Syndrome

The metabolic syndrome places an individual at high risk for development of type 2 diabetes and cardiovascular disease. Compared to individuals without the metabolic syndrome, those with the diagnostic criteria have about a fivefold increased risk of developing type 2 diabetes and a one-and-a-half- to threefold relative risk of developing cardiovascular disease (Grundy, 2007).

The transition from the metabolic syndrome to overt type 2 diabetes stems from insulin resistance and a decline of pancreatic beta-cell function. Insulin resistance in muscle tissue results in decreased glucose uptake and impaired **glycogen** synthesis. In the liver, insulin resistance results in failure of insulin to suppress hepatic glucose production. Despite these anomalies, individuals are normoglycemic in the early stages of the disease due to a marked increase in pancreatic beta-cell insulin secretion. As the disease progresses, glucotoxicity and lipotoxicity cause beta-cell function to decline, leading to **apoptosis** of pancreatic islet cells (Marchetti et al., 2006). At this point, the lower level of insulin secretion can no longer compensate for the effects of insulin resistance, and serum glucose levels reach the threshold for type 2 diabetes.

A variety of pathophysiologic mechanisms initiated by insulin resistance promote cardiovascular disease. Insulin resistance triggers endothelial dysfunction via glucose intolerance, hyperglycemia, and attenuated vascular production of nitric oxide, a factor involved in vasodilation and endothelial function (Peppa, Uribarri, & Vlassara, 2003; McFarlane, Banerji, & Sowers, 2001). Additionally, insulin resistance is associated with an atherogenic dyslipidemic profile, including hypertriglyceridemia; low HDL; increased proportion of small, dense LDL particles; and increased apolipoprotein B concentrations. Furthermore, insulin resistance contributes to the development of a prothrombotic and proinflammatory state via increased levels of PAI-1 and other inflammatory markers and cytokines, as well as hypertension.

There are other clinical derangements associated with the metabolic syndrome. Fatty liver disease with steatosis can ultimately lead to **fibrosis** and **cirrhosis.** Chronic kidney disease and **microalbuminuria** are more prevalent in those with the metabolic syndrome. There are also relationships between the metabolic syndrome and polycystic ovarian syndrome, obstructive sleep apnea, **hyperuricemia,** and **gout.**

Exercise in the Prevention and Treatment of the Metabolic Syndrome

There is a pathophysiological cascade by which physical inactivity predisposes to a cluster of metabolic diseases, including the metabolic syndrome. With an increasingly hypokinetic lifestyle, skeletal muscle down-regulates its capacity to convert nutritional substrates to energy [**adenosine triphosphate (ATP)**]. Inactive skeletal muscle's impaired ability to oxidize glucose and fatty acids is presumably mediated by several mechanisms, including decreased mitochondrial concentration; a reduced ability to remove glucose from blood due to fewer capillaries and diminished glucose transporter; and an attenuated capacity to hydrolyze blood triglycerides to free fatty acids, secondary to decreased lipoprotein lipase activity (Chakravarthy & Booth, 2003). Collectively, these metabolic perturbations serve to reduce the capacity to burn fuel, resulting in hyperinsulinemia, hypertriglyceridemia, and ultimately increased cardiovascular risk. On the other hand, moderate-to-vigorous leisure-time physical activity diminishes the magnitude of all five risk factors that are associated with the metabolic syndrome (Rennie et al., 2003) (Table 11-3). An increase in physical activity also improves insulin action in obesity, with or without a concomitant reduction in body weight and fat stores (Kelley & Goodpaster, 1999). This is an important (and often overlooked) salutary effect, suggesting that physical activity is as efficacious in preventing insulin resistance as losing body weight.

Researchers in Finland examined the effects of moderate and vigorous physical activity over a four-year period in 612 middle-aged men without evidence of the metabolic syndrome (Laaksonen et al., 2002). Subjects who engaged in more than three hours per week of moderate-intensity leisure-time physical activity (LTPA) were half as likely as sedentary control subjects to develop the metabolic syndrome. Moreover, vigorous LTPA had an even stronger inverse association, particularly in unfit men. Men in the upper third of $\dot{V}O_2max$ were 75% less likely than unfit men to develop the metabolic syndrome. This was the first prospective study to show that low levels of leisure-time physical activity and aerobic fitness predict the development of the metabolic syndrome, even after adjustments for potential confounding variables (age, BMI, smoking habit, alcohol intake, socioeconomic status, and other coronary risk factors).

Table 11-3
Influence of Physical Activity (and Inactivity) on the Characteristics of the Metabolic Syndrome

CHARACTERISTICS OF THE METABOLIC SYNDROME	IMPACT OF PHYSICAL ACTIVITY	IMPACT OF PHYSICAL INACTIVITY
Large abdominal circumference: Women ≥35 inches (88 cm) Men ≥40 inches (102 cm)	Decreases	Increases
Hypertriglyceridemia: ≥150 mg/dL	Decreases	Increases
Low HDL: Women <50 mg/dL Men <40 mg/dL	Increases	Decreases
High blood pressure: ≥130/85 mmHg	Decreases	Increases
High fasting blood glucose: ≥110 mg/dL	Decreases	Increases

Source: Adapted from the Expert Panel on Detection, Evaluation, and Treatment of High Blood Cholesterol in Adults (2001). Executive Summary of the Third Report of the National Cholesterol Education Program (NCEP) Expert Panel on Detection, Evaluation, and Treatment of High Blood Cholesterol in Adults (Adult Treatment Panel III). *Journal of the American Medical Association,* 285, 19, 2486.

Several investigators have also examined the relationships among habitual physical activity, cardiorespiratory fitness, the metabolic syndrome, and all-cause and cardiovascular mortality. Overall, these studies suggest that higher levels of daily physical activity and/or aerobic fitness are associated with a decreased clustering of risk factors that delineate the metabolic syndrome (Carroll, Cooke, & Butterly, 2000; Farrell, Cheng, & Blair, 2004; Kullo, Hensrud, & Allison, 2002; LaMonte et al., 2005). In one widely cited report (Whaley et al., 1999), the age-adjusted cumulative odds ratio for abnormal markers of the metabolic syndrome was 3.0 for the least-fit men compared with moderately fit ones, and 10.1 when compared with the most-fit men (Figure 11-3). Among women, the age-adjusted cumulative odds ratio was 2.7 for the least-fit women when compared with moderately fit ones, and 4.9 when compared with the most-fit women (see Figure 11-3). Others have reported that higher levels of cardiorespiratory fitness are associated with a substantial reduction in health risk for a given level of visceral and subcutaneous fat (Lee et al., 2005),

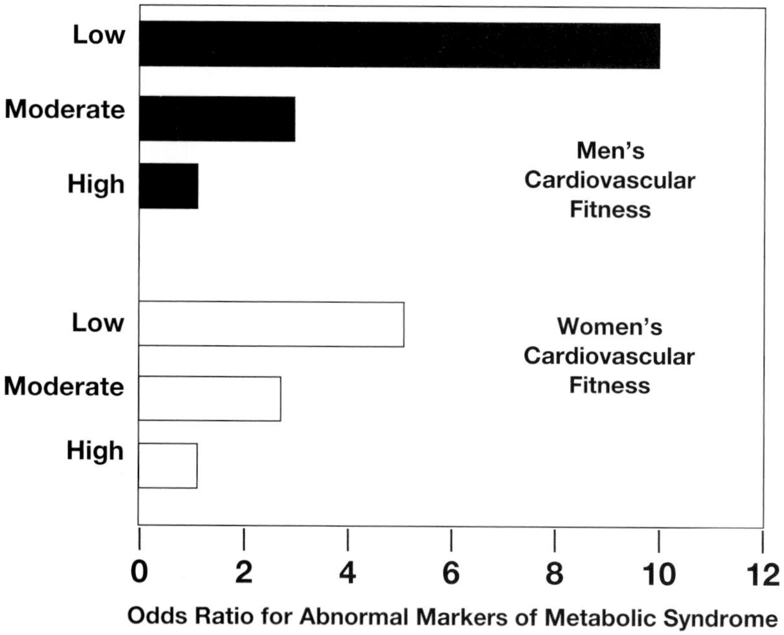

Figure 11-3
Prevalence of metabolic syndrome increases as cardiovascular fitness decreases

Source: Adapted from Whaley, M.H. et al. (1999). Physical fitness and clustering of risk factors associated with the metabolic syndrome. *Medicine & Science in Sports & Exercise*, 31, 2, 287.

and that fitness provides a strong protective effect against all-cause and cardiovascular mortality in men with the metabolic syndrome (Katzmarzyk, Church, & Blair, 2004; Katzmarzyk et al., 2005). Accordingly, these data strongly support the role of structured exercise, regular physical activity, or both, in interventions designed to prevent and treat the metabolic syndrome (Janiszewski, Saunders, & Ross, 2008).

Physiologic Responses to Exercise

There is considerable evidence that the metabolic syndrome is associated with an impaired exercise tolerance, especially among overweight/obese individuals and those destined to develop type 2 diabetes (Alexander, 1964). Most studies have reported a decreased aerobic capacity (approximately 10 to 20% or more), expressed as milliliters of oxygen per kilogram of body weight per minute (mL O_2/kg/min) or as **metabolic equivalents** (METs; 1 MET = 3.5 mL/kg/min), among individuals with insulin resistance syndrome, as compared with age- and activity-matched controls (Shahid & Schneider, 2000). Moreover, there is an inverse graded relationship between BMI and cardiorespiratory fitness (Gallagher et al., 2005). Common characteristics of overweight/obese individuals that may contribute to their reduced functional capacity include heat intolerance; **hyperpnea/dyspnea;** movement restriction; orthopedic pain or discomfort; localized muscular weakness; agility problems; and anxiety about loss of balance during moderate-to-vigorous physical activity.

The metabolic syndrome may also serve as a respiratory stress, especially in individuals with concomitant abdominal obesity (Buskirk, 1971; deJong et al., 2008). As adiposity develops, breathing requires increased effort, owing to the expanded mass of the chest wall, elevation of the diaphragm, and compression of a protruding abdomen. Dyspnea on exertion may result because the depth of breathing (i.e., **tidal volume**) is compromised, and the only way increased ventilation can occur is by increasing the individual's breathing frequency. Varied indices of breathing economy may be adversely affected, such as the minute ventilation/oxygen consumption slope or the minute ventilation/carbon dioxide production slope (Gallagher et al., 2005), as well as associated responses, including **hypoxia, hypercapnia, respiratory acidosis, somnolence,** and **pulmonary hypertension.** Conversely, these pulmonary abnormalities may exacerbate the obesity because the breathlessness on exertion stimulates the afflicted individuals to avoid moderate-to-vigorous physical activity (Buskirk, 1971).

Individuals with the metabolic syndrome may also be susceptible to altered cardiovascular, hemodynamic, and thermoregulatory responses to exercise. During a progressive treadmill walk, obese individuals demonstrate a higher heart rate and SBP at any given work rate as compared with their leaner counterparts (Alexander, 1964). Because subcutaneous fat provides thermal insulation against cold, performance of a given submaximal workload in the cold is accomplished by the obese person with a lower body surface temperature but a higher core temperature than a lean person. On the other hand, performance of a fixed work rate involving transport of body weight in a warm environment causes greater thermal strain on the obese (Buskirk, 1971). The added heat stress results in a higher heart rate and core temperature and a greater sweat rate than in the lean individual.

Exercise Programming and Progression Guidelines

Because obesity is at the core of the metabolic syndrome, the exercise program should generally follow the guidelines published by the American College of Sports Medicine (ACSM) for the treatment of overweight and obese clients (BMI $\geq$25 kg/m^2 and $\geq$30 kg/m^2, respectively) (Jakicic et al., 2001), but other components of the cluster of risk factors associated with the condition (i.e., dyslipidemia, hypertension, and if applicable, diabetes) also should be considered. Overall, individuals with the metabolic syndrome have an increased risk of mortality and morbidity from cardiovascular disease and developing diabetes as compared to their age- and gender-matched counterparts without this syndrome. Accordingly, a careful cardiovascular assessment including peak or symptom-limited exercise testing should be considered before beginning a vigorous ($\geq$60% $\dot{V}O_2$ reserve) exercise training program.

$\dot{V}O_2$reserve formula = percent intensity x ($\dot{V}O_2$peak – $\dot{V}O_2$rest) + $\dot{V}O_2$rest

Both the American College of Cardiology/American Heart Association guidelines on exercise testing and the ACSM guidelines recommend exercise testing before vigorous training can be conducted with clients with **diabetes mellitus** (Thompson et al., 2007).

Type of Exercise

Aerobic (or endurance) exercise has been the most frequently studied mode of exercise, and has consistently resulted in improvements in the components of the metabolic syndrome (Shahid & Schneider, 2000). The most effective exercises for the endurance phase employ large muscle groups, are maintained continuously, and are rhythmic in nature, such as walking, jogging, elliptical training, stationary or outdoor cycling, swimming, rowing, stair climbing, and combined arm-leg ergometry. Clearly it is difficult to achieve an adequate volume of exercising muscle (and caloric expenditure) if the lower extremities are excluded. Other exercise modalities commonly used in physical-conditioning programs for clients with the metabolic syndrome include calisthenics, particularly those involving sustained total-body movement; recreational games; and resistance training. The latter is a particularly important option, since traditional aerobic-conditioning regimens often fail to accommodate participants who have an interest in improving muscular strength and endurance. Moreover, studies have shown that muscular strength is inversely associated with all-cause mortality (FitzGerald et al., 2004) and the prevalence of the metabolic syndrome (Jurca et al., 2005), independent of cardiorespiratory fitness levels.

Walking has several advantages over other forms of exercise during the initial phase of a physical-conditioning program. Brisk walking programs can result in a substantial increase in aerobic capacity and a reduction in body weight and fat stores, particularly when the walking duration exceeds 30 minutes (Pollock et al., 1971). Walking offers an easily tolerable exercise intensity and causes fewer musculoskeletal and orthopedic problems of the legs, knees, and feet than jogging or running. Moreover, it is a "companionable" activity that requires no special equipment other than a pair of well-fitted athletic shoes. Walking in water, with a backpack, or with a weighted vest are additional options for those who seek to lose body weight and fatness and improve cardiorespiratory fitness.

Because most overweight/obese clients prefer to walk at moderate intensities, it is helpful to recognize that walking on level ground at 2 and 3 mph (3.2 and 4.8 km/h) approximates 2 and 3 METs, respectively. For clients who prefer the slower walking pace (2 mph; 3.2 km/h), each 3.5% increase in treadmill grade adds approximately 1 MET to the gross energy cost. For example, if a client desires to walk at a 2 mph (3.2 km/h) pace, but requires a 4-MET workload for training, he or she would be advised to add 7% grade to this speed. For clients who can negotiate the faster walking speed (3 mph; 4.8 km/h), each 2.5% increase in treadmill grade adds an additional MET to the gross energy expenditure. Accordingly, a workload of 3.0 mph (4.8 km/h) at a 5.0% grade would approximate an aerobic requirement of 5 METs. Using this practical rule can be helpful to the ACE-certified Advanced Health & Fitness Specialist (ACE-AHFS) in counseling clients regarding walking workloads for training.

Although resistance exercise has generally been considered to be less effective in treating individuals with the metabolic syndrome, some reviews suggest that high-volume resistance training has independent and additive effects to an aerobic exercise program for virtually the entire cluster of associated cardiovascular risk factors (Braith & Stewart, 2006; Williams et al., 2007). For example, numerous studies show that resistance training improves insulin action, significantly decreases **glycosylated hemoglobin (HbA1c)** and blood pressure in diabetic and hypertensive adults, respectively, and reduces total body-fat mass and visceral adipose tissue in both men and women. In addition, the maintained or enhanced muscle mass resulting from chronic resistance training is associated with a modest increase in **basal metabolic rate (BMR)** which, over time, may facilitate greater success at weight reduction than can be achieved with aerobic exercise alone. Weight training has been shown to attenuate the **rate-pressure product** when any given load is lifted (McCartney et al., 1993), which may reduce cardiac demands during daily activities such as carrying packages or lifting moderate-to-heavy objects. There are also intriguing data to suggest that strength training can increase muscular endurance capacity without an accompanying increase in cardiorespiratory fitness (Hickson, Rosenkoetter, & Brown, 1980).

Despite the widely cited CDC/ACSM exercise guidelines (Pate et al., 1995) and the much-heralded Surgeon General's report (United States Department of Health and Human Services, 1996), the traditional model for getting people to be more physically active (i.e., a regimented or structured exercise program) has been only marginally effective. The skyrocketing prevalence of the metabolic syndrome (approximately 47 million U.S. adults, or nearly 25% of the population) suggests the need for "real world" interventions designed to circumvent and attenuate barriers to achieving an adequate daily energy expenditure. Accordingly, the ACE-AHFS should counsel clients to integrate multiple short bouts of physical activity into their daily lives. The Activity Pyramid (Figure 11-4) has been suggested as a model to combat America's increasingly hypokinetic

Figure 11-4
The Activity Pyramid

Source: Adapted from The Activity Pyramid © ParkNicolletHealthSource,® Minneapolis, U.S.A. Used with permission.

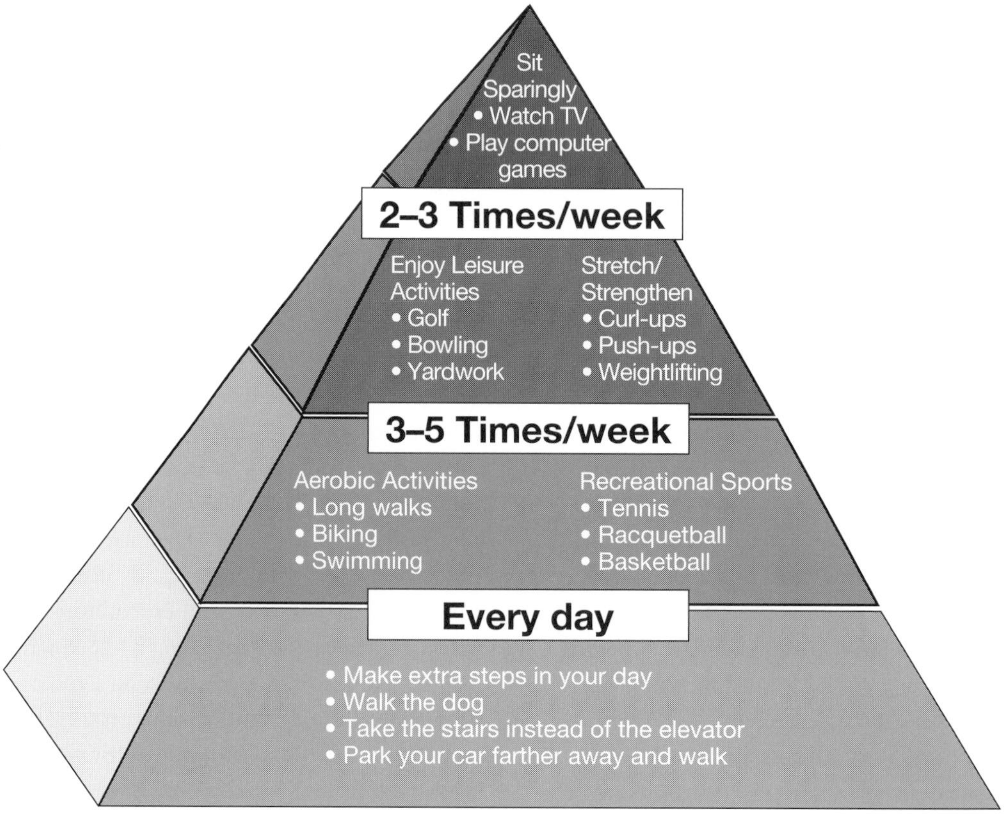

environment (Leon & Norstrom, 1995). This schematic presents a tiered set of weekly goals to promote improved aerobic fitness and health, building on a base that emphasizes the importance of accumulating at least 30 minutes of moderate-intensity activity on five or more days per week (Haskell et al., 2007).

Intensity and Duration

Structured exercise training sessions should include a preliminary aerobic warm-up (approximately 10 minutes) followed by stretching activities, a conditioning phase (30 minutes or more), a cool-down (five to 10 minutes), and ideally, an optional recreational game. The warm-up facilitates the transition from rest to the conditioning phase by stretching postural muscles and increasing blood flow. More important, a gradual warm-up may reduce the potential for exercise-induced ischemic responses, which can occur with sudden strenuous exertion (Barnard et al., 1973). A walking cool-down enhances venous return during recovery, reducing the possibility of post-exercise hypotension and related **sequelae.** In addition, it facilitates more rapid removal of **lactic acid** than stationary recovery and ameliorates the potential deleterious effects of the post-exercise rise in plasma catecholamines (Dimsdale et al., 1984).

There is some controversy regarding the most appropriate exercise intensity and duration that are needed to optimally train individuals with the metabolic syndrome (Shahid & Schneider, 2000). Different risk factors associated with this condition may optimally respond to different exercise dosages. For example, a randomized, controlled trial of sedentary, overweight men and women with mild-to-moderate dyslipidemia compared the effectiveness of three different exercise regimens versus controls: high-amount, high-intensity exercise; low-amount, high-intensity exercise; and low-amount, moderate-intensity exercise (Kraus et al., 2002). Although all exercise groups had better responses on a variety of **lipid** and **lipoprotein** variables than the control group, the most beneficial effect of exercise was seen most clearly with the high amount of high-intensity exercise. Because the metabolic syndrome has been associated with a **sedentary** lifestyle and low cardiorespiratory fitness, the initial exercise program should approximate at least 30% of the $\dot{V}O_2$ reserve or 60% of maximal heart rate (Swain & Franklin, 2002) for a minimum accumulated duration of 30 minutes. Over time, the exercise intensity should be increased to 50 to 75% $\dot{V}O_2$ reserve (or maximal heart-rate reserve) to provide the stimulus to improve cardiorespiratory fitness and facilitate a progressive overload (i.e., attainment of goal energy expenditure).

Frequency

The frequency of exercise is an important consideration when structured exercise and/or increased lifestyle activity are used to treat the abnormalities associated with the metabolic syndrome, especially insulin sensitivity and glucose utilization. Because much of the benefit of exercise is related to the cumulative effects of individual bouts of exercise, exercising five or more times a week is ultimately necessary to maximize benefits.

A summary of the physical-activity recommendations for clients with the metabolic syndrome is shown in Table 11-4, with specific reference to the FITT principle (frequency, intensity, time, and type of exercise) variables required to provide a safe and effective exercise program.

Case Study

James, a 57-year-old asymptomatic male, is interested in starting a weight-reduction program, including exercise. His medical history reveals that he is obese, pre-diabetic, has hypertension and hyperlipidemia, is currently sedentary, does not smoke cigarettes, and has a family history of premature atherosclerotic cardiovascular disease (i.e., his father suffered his first acute myocardial infarction at 53 years of age). James is currently taking Toprol XL® (metoprolol SR) 50 mg once daily for hypertension, Lipitor® (atorvastatin) 40 mg once daily for hyperlipidemia, Niaspan® (niacin extended-release tablets) 500 mg twice daily for a reduced HDL level, and aspirin 81 mg once daily for prophylaxis of acute myocardial infarction. Because he has three or more components of the metabolic syndrome, or takes medications to control them, he is considered to have the metabolic syndrome.

Table 11-4
Physical-activity Recommendations for Clients With the Metabolic Syndrome: The FITT Principle*

Component	Recommendations
Frequency	*Five days per week or daily.* More frequent structured exercise bouts are desirable, but care should be taken to initially establish a regular exercise habit (3–5 days/week); 3–4 sessions per week are required to elicit beneficial metabolic effects, whereas 4–5 sessions per week (or more) may be needed to reduce body weight and fat stores.
Intensity	*30/45–75% $\dot{V}O_2$reserve.*† To avoid musculoskeletal injuries and maximize compliance, start at a light-to-moderate intensity‡ and gradually progress over the course of several weeks or months to vigorous exercise (≥60% $\dot{V}O_2$reserve or heart-rate reserve) (if desired by the client). Initially emphasize increasing duration rather than intensity, with the goal of optimizing caloric expenditure.
Time	*30 to 90 minutes/day, using a gradual progression.* Multiple shorter periods of exercise (10- to 15-minute exercise bouts) accumulated throughout the day may elicit similar (or even greater) reductions in body weight and fat stores as a single long bout of the same total duration.
Type**	*Low-impact activities (walking, low-impact aerobics, cycling).* These activities are convenient, accessible, and perceived as enjoyable by the client, supplemented by adjunctive resistance training to assist in the maintenance of basal metabolic rate and an increase in daily lifestyle activities (walking breaks at work, gardening, household work).

*FITT: frequency, intensity, time, and type of exercise provide a framework of evidence-based recommendations for a safe and effective exercise program.

† $\dot{V}O_2$reserve formula = ($\dot{V}O_2$peak – $\dot{V}O_2$rest) x 30–75% intensity +$\dot{V}O_2$rest, where $\dot{V}O_2$ values are expressed as metabolic equivalents (METs).

‡ A light-to-moderate intensity workout approximates 50–76% of the maximal heart rate or a rating of perceived exertion of 11–13 (“fairly light” to “somewhat hard”) on the 6–20 category exertion scale.

**Aerobic exercise should be preceded by a warm-up (approximately 10 minutes) and followed by a cool-down (5–10 minutes) at a reduced exercise intensity (e.g., slow walking). Stretching (5–10 minutes) may be incorporated before or after the endurance exercise phase.

On physical examination, his height and weight are 5'7" (1.7 m) and 255 pounds (115 kg), corresponding to a body mass index of 40 kg/m². He has a waist circumference of 46 inches (117 cm); seated resting blood pressure of 146/94 mmHg; resting pulse of 64 beats per minute (regular); and a fasting plasma glucose of 122 mg/dL. With the exception of a low HDL (37 mg/dL), his serum lipids and lipoproteins are at the goal level. The remainder of the physical examination was unremarkable from an exercise programming perspective (e.g., no limiting orthopedic or musculoskeletal problems).

James performed a peak or symptom-limited exercise stress test to volitional fatigue using the conventional Bruce treadmill protocol. He intends to exercise at a health club after work and the exercise test was performed in the late afternoon. James typically takes his metoprolol SR after breakfast and was instructed to do so on the morning of the exercise test.

Immediately prior to the exercise test, in the standing position, his heart rate was 76 bpm and blood pressure was 152/94 mmHg. During the exercise test, James demonstrated infrequent unifocal **premature ventricular contractions (PVCs)** and occasional **premature atrial contractions (PACs)** but did not develop chest discomfort, lightheadedness, or significant ST-segment depression. The test was terminated after five minutes because of volitional fatigue [ratings of perceived exertion (RPE) of 18/20, signifying “very hard” work] and increasing dyspnea (3/4, corresponding to “moderately severe” shortness of breath), indicating an estimated functional capacity of 6.6 METs. He achieved a peak heart rate and blood pressure of 136 bpm (83% of his estimated maximal heart rate) and 186/92 mmHg, respectively. His blunted peak heart rate was most likely attributed, at least in part, to his beta-blocker therapy for hypertension.

Based on James' medical history, physical examination, and graded exercise test results, the following exercise program was formulated.

Aerobic exercise program:

- Type: Treadmill walking and combined arm-leg ergometry
- Frequency: Initially three days/week; increase gradually to five to seven days/week
- Duration: Initially 15 to 20 minutes/session, which may be accumulated in two 10-minute exercise bouts; to build up gradually to 45 to 60 or more minutes/session by adding approximately five minutes each week as tolerated
- Intensity: Target heart rate set at 40–75% heart-rate reserve = 100–121 bpm and target RPE (6–20 scale) set at 11–14; target MET range initially set at 40–75% $\dot{V}O_2$reserve = 3.2–5.2 METs). Estimated treadmill workloads at the lower end of this intensity range (approximately 3.2 METs) might be 2.0 mph, 3.5% grade or, for clients who prefer a faster walking pace, 3.0 mph, 0% grade.

James was informed that the time interval between his taking metoprolol SR and exercise training could modify his heart-rate response to exercise, since the effects of beta-blocker therapy are not necessarily uniform over time. Moreover, he was counseled about the importance of warming up and cooling down, as well as the significance of warning signs and symptoms (e.g., heart rhythm irregularities, exertional chest pain or pressure, lightheadedness, unusual shortness of breath) that require the cessation of exercise and immediate medical review.

Resistance exercise program:

James was counseled to complement his aerobic exercise regimen with resistance training. Initially, he was advised to perform one set of 10 to 15 repetitions of eight to 10 different exercises that condition the major muscle groups on two or three days/week. He was advised regarding appropriate lifting and breathing techniques (e.g., avoid the **Valsalva maneuver**), and encouraged to increase the weight/resistance gradually [approximately 2 to 5 pounds/week (0.9 to 2.25 kg/week) for arms and 5 to 10 pounds/week (2.25 to 4.5 kg/week) for legs] as tolerated.

Lifestyle activity:

James was also counseled to integrate multiple short bouts of walking into his daily routine. To this end, he purchased a quality pedometer to enhance his awareness of daily physical activity by progressively increasing step totals. Baseline ambulatory studies conducted over one week revealed that he took approximately 3000 steps/day on average. He was advised to add at least an additional 500 steps/day each week, to ultimately increase his daily step totals to 8000 to 10,000 steps/day. Moreover, he was provided a "log" to document and track his progress in this regard.

Summary

Obesity and insulin resistance largely account for the pathogenesis of the metabolic syndrome. Although overall body weight and relative adiposity as reflected in the BMI identify the greater than two-thirds of Western populations at risk for the metabolic syndrome, those with excessive intra-abdominal adiposity are particularly susceptible.

The cornerstone treatment of the metabolic syndrome is therapeutic lifestyle modification to reduce body weight and fat stores, increase physical activity, and transition to an anti-atherogenic diet. Although lifestyle intervention is often overlooked in clinical practice, this non-pharmacologic approach has been shown to reduce cardiovascular risk and prevent or delay progression to diabetes. The ACE-AHFS can play an important role in providing a safe and effective exercise program that corresponds with the lifestyle-intervention component of metabolic syndrome treatment. Because obesity is at the core of the metabolic syndrome, the ACE-AHFS should generally follow the guidelines published by ACSM for the treatment of overweight and obese clients when designing exercise programs for this population. Aerobic exercise, resistance training, and increased lifestyle activity are recommended for individuals with the metabolic syndrome.

References

Alexander, J.K. (1964). Obesity and cardiac performance. *American Journal Cardiology*, 14, 860.

Barnard, R.J. et al. (1973). Ischemic response to sudden strenuous exercise in healthy men. *Circulation*, 48, 5, 936.

Batsis, J.A., Nieto-Martinez, R.E., & Lopez-Jimenez, F. (2007). Metabolic syndrome: From global epidemiology to individualized medicine. *Clinical Pharmacology & Therapeutics*, 82, 5, 509.

Bodary, P.F., Iglay, H.B., & Eitzman, D.T. (2007). Strategies to reduce vascular risk associated with obesity. *Current Vascular Pharmacology*, 5, 4, 249.

Braith, R.W. & Stewart, K.J. (2006). Resistance exercise training: Its role in the prevention of cardiovascular disease. *Circulation*, 113, 22, 2642.

Buchwald, H. et al. (2004). Bariatric surgery: A systematic review and meta-analysis. *Journal of the American Medical Association*, 292, 14, 1724.

Buskirk, E.R. (1971). Obesity. In: Downey, J.A., & Darling, R.C. (Eds.) *Physiologic Basis of Rehabilitation Medicine*. Philadelphia: W.B. Saunders Co, pp. 229–242.

Caballero, A.E. (2005). Diabetes in the Hispanic or Latino population: Genes, environment, culture, and more. *Current Diabetes Reports*, 5, 3, 217.

Carroll, S., Cooke, C.B. & Butterly, R.J. (2000). Metabolic clustering, physical activity and fitness in nonsmoking, middle-aged men. *Medicine & Science in Sports & Exercise*, 32, 12, 2079.

Chakravarthy, M.V. & Booth, F.W. (2003). *Hot Topics: Exercise*. Philadelphia: Hanley and Belfus (Elsevier).

Dansinger, M.L. et al. (2005). Comparison of the Atkins, Ornish, Weight Watchers, and Zone diets for weight loss and heart disease risk reduction: A randomized trial. *Journal of the American Medical Association*, 293, 1, 43.

deJong, A.T. et al. (2008). Peak oxygen consumption and the minute ventilation/carbon dioxide production relation slope in morbidly obese men and women: Influence of subject effort and body mass index. *Preventive Cardiology,* 11, 2, 100.

Dimsdale, J.E. et al. (1984). Post exercise peril: Plasma catecholamines and exercise. *Journal of the American Medical Association*, 25, 5, 630.

Esposito, K. et al. (2004). Effect of a Mediterranean-style diet on endothelial dysfunction and markers of vascular inflammation in the metabolic syndrome: A randomized trial. *Journal of the American Medical Association*, 292, 12, 1440.

Expert Panel on Detection, Evaluation, and Treatment of High Blood Cholesterol in Adults (2001). Executive summary of the Third Report of the National Cholesterol Education Program (NCEP) Expert Panel on the detection, evaluation, and treatment of high blood cholesterol in adults (Adult Treatment Panel III). *Journal of the American Medical Association*, 285, 19, 2486.

Farrell, S.W., Cheng, Y.J., & Blair, S.N. (2004). Prevalence of the metabolic syndrome across cardiorespiratory fitness levels in women. *Obesity Research*, 12, 5, 824.

FitzGerald, S.J. et al. (2004). Muscular fitness and all-cause mortality: Prospective observations. *Journal of Physical Activity & Health*, 1, 1, 7.

Ford, E.S., Giles, W.H., & Dietz, W.H. (2002). Prevalence of the metabolic syndrome among U.S. adults: Findings from the third National Health and Nutritional Examination Survey. *Journal of the American Medical Association*, 287, 3, 356.

Gallagher, M.J. et al. (2005). Comparative impact of morbid obesity vs. heart failure on cardiorespiratory fitness. *Chest*, 127, 6, 2197.

Gerstein, H.C. et al. of the DREAM (Diabetes Reduction Assessment with ramipril and rosiglitazone Medication) Trial Investigators (2006). Effect of rosiglitazone on the frequency of diabetes in patients with impaired glucose tolerance or impaired fasting glucose: a randomized controlled trial. *Lancet*, 368, 9541, 1096.

Grundy, S.M. (2007). Cardiovascular and metabolic risk factors: How can we improve outcomes in the high-risk patient? *The American Journal of Medicine*, 120, 9, Suppl. 1, S3.

Grundy, S.M. (2006). Metabolic syndrome: Connecting and reconciling cardiovascular and diabetes worlds. *Journal of the American College of Cardiology*, 47, 6, 1093.

Grundy, S.M. et al. (2004). Implications of recent clinical trials for the National Cholesterol Education Program Adult Treatment Panel III guidelines. *Circulation*, 110, 2, 227.

Haskell, W.L. et al. (2007). Physical activity and public health: Updated recommendation for adults from the American College of Sports Medicine and the American Heart Association. *Circulation*, 116, 9, 1081.

He, J. & Whelton, P.K. (1999). Elevated systolic blood pressure and risk of cardiovascular and renal disease: Overview of evidence from observational epidemiologic studies and randomized controlled trials. *American Heart Journal*, 138, 3 Pt 2, 211.

Hickson, R.C., Rosenkoetter, M.A., & Brown, M.M. (1980). Strength training effects on aerobic power and short-term endurance. *Medicine & Science in Sports & Exercise*, 12, 5, 336.

Hu, F.B. et al. (2002). Elevated risk of cardiovascular disease prior to clinical diagnosis of type 2 diabetes. *Diabetes Care*, 25, 7, 1129.

Hunt, K.J. et al. (2004). National Cholesterol Education Program versus World Health Organization metabolic syndrome in relation to all-cause and cardiovascular mortality in the San Antonio Heart Study. *Circulation*, 110, 10, 1251.

Isomaa, B. et al. (2001). Cardiovascular morbidity and mortality associated with the metabolic syndrome. *Diabetes Care*, 24, 4, 683.

Jakicic, J.M. et al. (2001). American College of Sports Medicine position stand: Appropriate intervention strategies for weight loss and prevention of weight regain for adults. *Medicine & Science in Sports & Exercise*, 33, 12, 2145.

Janiszewski, P.M., Saunders, T.J., & Ross, R. (2008). Lifestyle treatment of the metabolic syndrome. *American Journal of Lifestyle Medicine*, 2, 2, 99.

Jurca, R. et al. (2005). Association of muscular strength with incidence of metabolic syndrome in men. *Medicine & Science in Sports & Exercise*, 37, 11, 1849.

Katzmarzyk, P.T., Church, T.S, & Blair, S.N. (2004). Cardiorespiratory fitness attenuates the effects of the metabolic syndrome on all-cause and cardiovascular disease mortality in men. *Archives of Internal Medicine* 164, 10, 1092.

Katzmarzyk, P.T. et al. (2005). Metabolic syndrome, obesity, and mortality. *Diabetes Care*, 28, 2, 391.

Kelley, D.E. & Goodpaster, B.H. (1999). Effects of physical activity on insulin action and glucose tolerance in obesity. *Medicine & Science in Sports & Exercise*, 31, (6 Suppl), S619.

Knowler, W.C. et al. for the Diabetes Prevention Program Research Group (2002). Reduction in the incidence of type 2 diabetes with lifestyle intervention or metformin. *New England Journal of Medicine*, 346, 6, 393.

Kraus, W.E. et al. (2002). Effects of the amount and intensity of exercise on plasma lipoproteins. *New England Journal of Medicine*, 347, 19, 1483.

Kullo, I.J., Hensrud, D.D., & Allison, T.G. (2002). Relation of low cardiorespiratory fitness to the metabolic syndrome in middle-aged men. *American Journal of Cardiology*, 90, 7, 795.

Laaksonen, D.E. et al. (2002). Low levels of leisure-time physical activity and cardiorespiratory fitness predict development of the metabolic syndrome. *Diabetes Care*, 25, 9, 1612.

LaMonte, M.J. et al. (2005). Cardiorespiratory fitness is inversely associated with the incidence of metabolic syndrome: A prospective study of men and women. *Circulation*, 112, 4, 505.

Lee, S. et al. (2005). Cardiorespiratory fitness attenuates metabolic risk independent of abdominal subcutaneous and visceral fat in men. *Diabetes Care*, 28, 4, 895.

Leon, A.S. & Norstrom, J. (1995). Evidence of the role of physical activity and cardiorespiratory fitness in the prevention of coronary heart disease. *Quest*, 47, 3, 311.

Lloyd-Jones, D.M. et al. (2007). Consistently stable or decreased body mass index in young adulthood and longitudinal changes in metabolic syndrome components: The Coronary Artery Risk Development in Young Adults Study. *Circulation*, 115, 8, 1004.

Marchetti, P. et al. (2006). The pancreatic beta-cell in human type 2 diabetes. *Nutrition, Metabolism, and Cardiovascular Diseases*, 16, Suppl. 1, S3.

McCartney, N. et al. (1993). Weight-training-induced attenuation of the circulatory response of older males to weight lifting. *Journal of Applied Physiology*, 74, 3, 1056.

McFarlane, S.I., Banerji, M., & Sowers, J.R. (2001). Insulin resistance and cardiovascular disease. *Journal of Clinical Endocrinology and Metabolism*, 86, 2, 713.

Misra, A. & Vikram, N.K. (2004). Insulin resistance syndrome (metabolic syndrome) and obesity in Asian Indians: Evidence and implications. *Nutrition*, 20, 5, 482.

National Institutes of Health (1998). Clinical guidelines on the identification, evaluation, and treatment of overweight and obesity in adults: The Evidence Report. *Obesity Research*, 6, Suppl. 2, 51S.

Pate, R.R. et al. (1995). Physical activity and public health: A recommendation from the Centers for Disease Control and Prevention and the American College of Sports Medicine. *Journal of the American Medical Association*, 273, 5, 402.

Pearson, T.A. et al. (2003). Markers of inflammation and cardiovascular disease: A statement for healthcare professionals from the Centers for Disease Control and Prevention and the American Heart Association. *Circulation*, 107, 499–511.

Peppa, M., Uribarri, J., & Vlassara, H. (2003). Glucose, advanced glycation end products, and diabetes complications: What is new and what works. *Clinical Diabetes*, 21, 4, 186.

Pollock, M.L. et al. (1971). Effects of walking on body composition and cardiovascular function of middle-aged men. *Journal of Applied Physiology,* 30, 1, 126.

Rader, D.J. (2007). Effect of insulin resistance, dyslipidemia, and intra-abdominal adiposity on the development of cardiovascular disease and diabetes mellitus. *American Journal of Medicine*, 120, 3, Suppl. 1, S12.

Rennie, K.L. et al. (2003). Association of the metabolic syndrome with both vigorous and moderate physical activity. *International Journal of Epidemiology,* 32, 4, 600.

Rosito, G.A. et al. (2004). Association between obesity and a prothrombotic state: The Framingham Offspring Study. *Thrombosis and Haemostasis*, 91, 4, 683.

Ruilope, L.M., Redón, J., & Schmieder, R. (2007). Cardiovascular risk reduction by reversing endothelial dysfunction: ARBs, ACE inhibitors, or both? Expectations from the ONTARGET Trial Programme. *Vascular Health Risk Management*, 3, 1, 1.

Shah, M., Simha, V., & Garg, A. (2006). Review: Long-term impact of bariatric surgery on body weight, comorbidities, and nutritional status. *Journal of Clinical Endocrinology and Metabolism*, 91, 11, 4223.

Shahid, S.K. & Schneider, S.H. (2000). Effects of exercise on insulin resistance syndrome. *Coronary Artery Disease*, 11, 2, 103.

Swain, D.P. & Franklin, B.A. (2002). $\dot{V}O_2$ reserve and the minimal intensity for improving cardiorespiratory fitness. *Medicine & Science in Sports & Exercise*, 34, 1, 152.

Thompson, P.D. et al. (2007). AHA Scientific Statement: Exercise and acute cardiovascular events. Placing the risks into perspective. *Circulation*, 115, 17, 2358.

United States Department of Health and Human Services (1996). *Physical Activity and Health: A Report of the Surgeon General*. Atlanta: U.S. Department of Health and Human Services, Centers for Disease Control and Prevention, National Center for Chronic Disease Prevention and Health Promotion.

Whaley, M.H. et al. (1999). Physical fitness and clustering of risk factors associated with the metabolic syndrome. *Medicine & Science in Sports & Exercise,* 31, 2, 287.

Williams, MA. et al. (2007). AHA Scientific Statement: Resistance exercise in individuals with and without cardiovascular disease: 2007 update. *Circulation*, 116, 5, 572.

Suggested Reading

Chakravarthy, M.V. & Booth, F.W. (2003). *Hot Topics: Exercise.* Philadelphia: Hanley and Belfus (Elsevier).

Durstine, J.L. et al. (Eds.) (2008). *Pollock's Textbook of Cardiovascular Disease and Rehabilitation.* Champaign, Ill.: Human Kinetics.

Franklin, B.A. & Gordon, N.F. (2005). *Contemporary Diagnosis and Management in Cardiovascular Exercise.* Newtown, Penn.: Handbooks in Healthcare Company.

Grundy, S.M. et al. (2005). Diagnosis and management of the metabolic syndrome: An American Heart Association/National Heart, Lung, and Blood Institute Scientific Statement. *Circulation,* 112, 17, 2735.

Janiszewski, P.M., Saunders, T.J., & Ross, R. (2008). Lifestyle treatment of the metabolic syndrome. *American Journal of Lifestyle Medicine*, 2, 2, 99.

Nor Janosz, K.E. et al. (2008). Clinical resolution of type 2 diabetes with reduction of body mass index using meal replacement based weight loss. *Vascular Disease Prevention*, in press.

In This Chapter

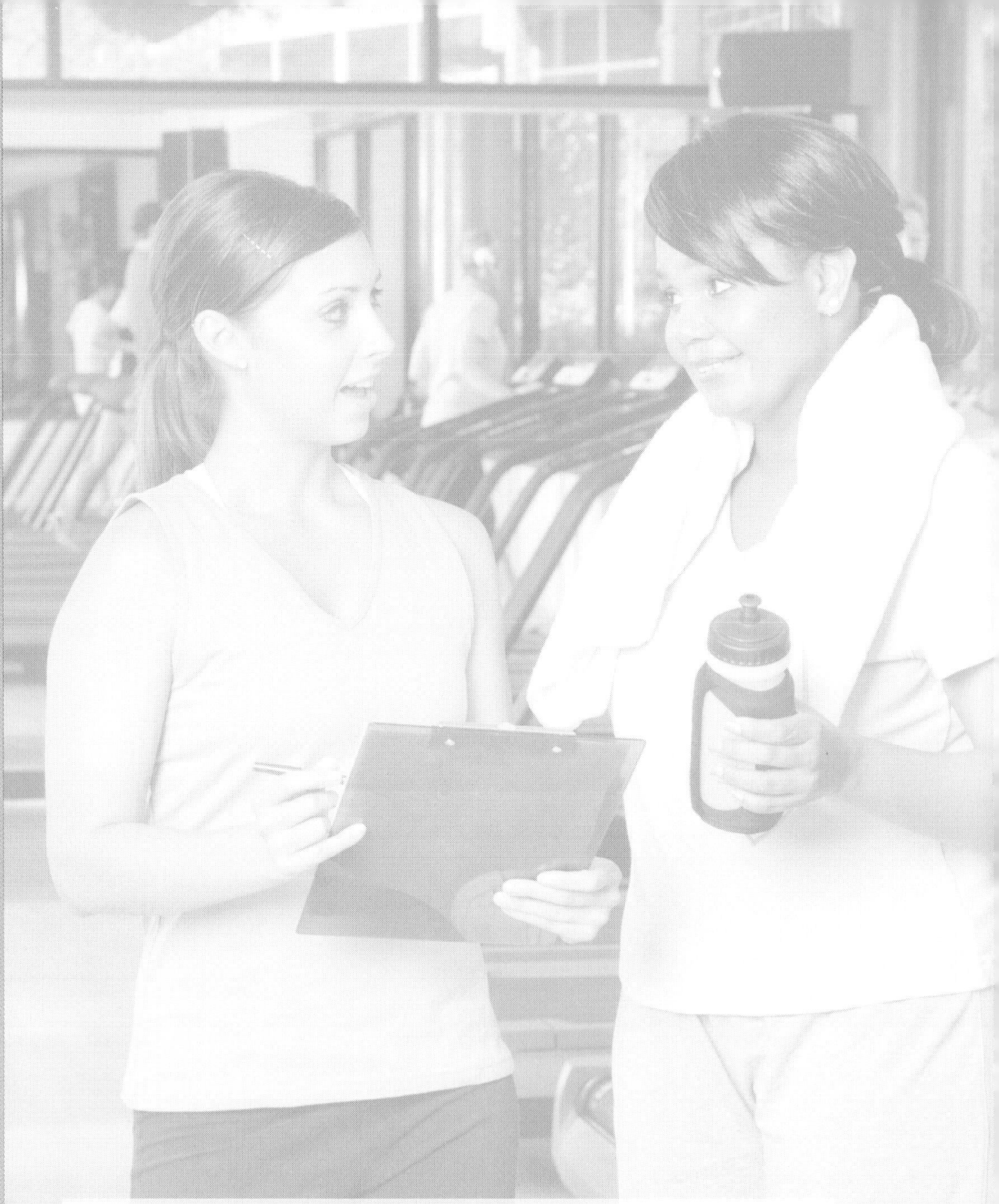

About The Author

Larry S. Verity, Ph.D., FACSM, is a professor of exercise physiology in the School of Exercise and Nutritional Sciences at San Diego State University. He is a fellow of the American College of Sports Medicine (ACSM) and is certified as an Exercise Specialist. Dr. Verity served on ACSM's CCRB Publications Subcommittee and is co-editor of ACSM's *Certified News,* has written manual chapters for the American Council on Exercise, and has published reviews and original manuscripts on diabetes and exercise in many refereed publications. He has managed type 1 diabetes for more than 32 years and is without complications.

CHAPTER 12

Diabetes Mellitus

Larry S. Verity

Only three decades ago, physical exercise for persons with **diabetes**—also called **diabetes mellitus**—was frowned upon. In fact, diabetes was seen as an excuse to avoid exercise. Questions continue to be asked regarding whether a person with diabetes can safely participate in exercise or physical activity. Questions that an ACE-certified Advanced Health & Fitness Specialist (ACE-AHFS) may be asked include the following:

- Does exercise actually help a person with diabetes or does it hamper his or her condition?
- Can exercise actually control diabetes?
- Is it safe for persons with diabetes to exercise at any time?
- Do diabetes complications affect the ability to regularly and safely participate in exercise?

To answer these questions, the ACE-AHFS must have a solid understanding of the different types of diabetes to recommended exercise interventions for individuals with this disease, identify practical aspects of physical activity for diabetics, and design and modify exercise programs to improve disease management and health outcomes. This chapter provides a thorough overview of the different types of diabetes, the benefits and risks of exercise for this disease, and assessments that may be performed by the ACE-AHFS that could aid in the design of a safe and effective exercise program.

Epidemiology

According to the Centers for Disease Control and Prevention (CDC, 2005), an estimated 21 million people in the United States have diabetes, with more than 6 million undiagnosed cases, while prevalence is approximately 7.0% of the population. **Type 2 diabetes mellitus (T2DM)** accounts for 90 to 95% of all cases of diabetes mellitus, and there is a slightly greater prevalence in men (10.5%) versus women (8.8%) (CDC, 2005). The burden of diabetes disproportionately affects minorities. The prevalence rates are about twofold greater in Hispanic Americans, African Americans, Native Americans, Asians, and Pacific Islanders when compared with non-Hispanic whites. **Type 1 diabetes mellitus (T1DM)** accounts for 5 to 10% of all cases of diabetes (CDC, 2005). Although T1DM is one of the most commonly diagnosed chronic diseases in children, diagnosis of T2DM in youth has risen dramatically over the past decade [American Diabetes Association (ADA), 2000].

The ACE-AHFS should realize that diabetes mellitus is a heterogeneous disease composed of three primary categories: T1DM, T2DM, and **gestational diabetes mellitus (GDM)** (ADA, 2004a). Diagnostic and classification criteria of diabetes focus on cause and pathogenesis (ADA, 2007a). The two major etiopathogenetic categories of diabetes are T1DM and T2DM, each of which has distinguishing characteristics (Table 12-1). All persons with diabetes have elevated blood **glucose** levels, or **hyperglycemia**, caused by either an absolute or relative lack of **insulin**, along with abnormal protein and fat metabolism (ADA, 2007b). Low blood glucose, or **hypoglycemia**, occurs most often in T1DM, but persons with T2DM and GDM can also experience episodes of hypoglycemia, although these are infrequent (ADA, 2004b; 2004a; 2007b). Acute complications can occur when hypoglycemia or hyperglycemia are present for relatively short periods of time.

Table 12-1
Distinguishing Characteristics of Type 1 and Type 2 Diabetes Mellitus

	T1DM	T2DM
Synonyms	Insulin requiring (formerly: juvenile onset)	Non-insulin requiring (formerly: adult onset)
Former Abbreviation	IDDM	NIDDM
Age of Onset	<30 years	>30 Years
Cases of Diabetes in U.S.	5–10%	90–95%
Pathological Factor	Auto-immune deficiency	Family history
Insulin Use	100%	~27%
Body Weight History	Recent weight loss	Weight gain
Obese at Diagnosis	Uncommon	Common (~80% obese)
Insulin Production	None	Deficient
Ketoacidodic Episodes	Common	Uncommon
Response to Diet Alone	Absent	In some mild forms
Insulin Resistance	Uncommon; may be present	Common

Diabetes mellitus increases the risk for cardiovascular disease, along with other complications. Most notably, macrovascular, microvascular, and nerve disease complications are commonly linked to hyperglycemia and diabetes. An ACE-AHFS should know whether a client has complications, which reflect the severity and duration of the disease and may contribute to accelerated morbidity and excessive mortality.

Diabetes mellitus afflicts 9.6% of American adults over the age of 20 years (CDC, 2005). Interestingly, 20.9% of people from 60 years and older have diabetes, while one in three people born in the United States in the year 2000 are projected to develop diabetes in their lifetime (Narayan et al., 2003). Overall, diabetes contributes to more than 200,000 deaths in the U.S. each year (CDC, 2005), with heart disease being the leading cause of diabetes-related deaths. The presence of diabetes-related complications (DRCs) exacerbates morbidity and increases the likelihood of physical limitation or disability (ADA, 2007a). Hyperglycemia for extended periods is linked with chronic abnormalities that worsen macrovascular, microvascular, and neural disease processes. As shown in Table 12-2, DRCs can be quite serious. Because of the daily fluctuations in blood glucose that occur in diabetes, therapeutic interventions are focused on the effective management and control of blood glucose and heart disease risk factors, along with prevention of DRCs (ADA, 2007a; Buse et al., 2007; Grundy et al., 1999).

Table 12-2
Diabetes-related Complications

- Coronary heart disease death rates in adults with diabetes are two to four times higher than in adults without diabetes.
- Stroke risk is two to four times higher among adults with diabetes.
- Hypertension is present in approximately 73% of adults with diabetes.
- Retinopathy is the leading cause of new cases of blindness among adults 20 to 74 years old.
- Diabetic nephropathy is a leading cause of end-stage renal disease, accounting for 43% of new cases.
- Neuropathy, mild to severe forms of nervous system damage involving peripheral motor sensory nerves and autonomic nerves, affects approximately 65% of people with T1DM or T2DM.
- Severe forms of diabetic nerve disease are major contributing causes of lower-extremity amputations; more than 60% of non-traumatic lower-limb amputations in the United States occur among people with diabetes.

Sources: American Diabetes Association (2007b). Standards of medical care in diabetes—2007: Position Statement. *Diabetes Care,* 30 (suppl 1), S4–S41; Centers for Disease Control and Prevention (2005). *National Diabetes Fact Sheet: National Estimates and General Information on Diabetes in the United States—2005.* Atlanta, Ga: U.S. Department of Health and Human Services, Centers for Disease Control and Prevention; Joint National Committee on Prevention, Detection, Evaluation, and Treatment of High Blood Pressure (2003). The seventh report of the Joint National Committee on prevention, detection, evaluation, and treatment of high blood pressure (JNC-VII). *Journal of the American Medical Association,* 289, 2560– 2572; Vinik A.I. & Erbas, T. (2002). Neuropathy. In: Ruderman, N. et al. (Eds.) *Handbook of Exercise in Diabetes (2nd ed.).* Alexandria, Va: American Diabetes Association (pp. 463–496).

Etiology of Type 1 Diabetes Mellitus

T1DM usually afflicts persons younger than 30 years old, and is an immune-mediated disease that selectively destroys the pancreatic **beta cells,** leading to a "central defect" in insulin release upon stimulation, or **hypoinsulinemia** (waning of the insulin dose), and resultant hyperglycemia (ADA, 2007a). Serologic markers of pancreatic beta-cell destruction [(e.g., islet cell autoantibodies, insulin autoantibodies, glutamic acid decarboxylase (GAD), and human leukocyte antigens (HLA)] are common at diagnosis and provide evidence for its autoimmune nature (ADA, 2004a).

Onset of T1DM is usually abrupt and accompanied by "classic" signs of diabetes, including frequent urination **(polyuria),** constant hunger **(polyphagia),** excessive thirst **(polydipsia),** and unexplained weight loss (ADA, 2004a). An absolute lack of insulin production in T1DM requires exogenous insulin administration (e.g., injections, pump, or inhalation) to maintain normal glucose levels, minimize complications, and prevent excessive use of **fatty acids** for energy, resulting in **ketoacidosis.**

Ketoacidosis occurs when a high level of **ketones** (beta hydroxybutyrate, acetoacetate) are produced as a by-product of fatty-acid metabolism. In T1DM, the combination of deficient insulin and increased counter-regulatory hormones (e.g., **catecholamines, cortisol, glucagon**) results in excessive ketone production and metabolic acidosis. **Diabetic ketoacidosis (DKA)** can result from an infection, but is more commonly linked to a lack of insulin, dehydration, and failure to manage glucose levels. Signs and symptoms of DKA include confusion, gastrointestinal (GI) upset, extreme thirst, lethargy, and a fruity breath odor (ADA 2004c; 2007a). DKA is a serious health issue for individuals with T1DM and, if left untreated, can result in coma or death.

Etiology of Type 2 Diabetes Mellitus

T2DM usually afflicts persons older than 30 years of age, and is directly related to insulin resistance (ADA, 2007a). In 2007, the American Heart Association put forth an educational program entitled *The Heart of Diabetes:*[SM] *Understanding Insulin Resistance* to help individuals with T2DM reduce their risk for heart disease and **stroke.** For those with T2DM, insulin resistance creates a health burden that worsens the ability to manage blood glucose,and significantly increases morbidity and mortality associated with vascular complications of diabetes (ADA, 2007a; Cerosimo & DeFronzo, 2006). The pathology and natural history of T2DM onset is illustrated in Figure 12-1. Interestingly, onset of T2DM may actually be present approximately 10 years prior to diagnosis.

The role of diabetes and insulin resistance in advancing heart disease and DRCs, or disorders of the eyes, kidneys, heart, blood vessels, and nerves, is well established (ADA, 2007a; AHA, 2007). T2DM is highly linked with typical **cardiovascular disease (CVD)** risk factors, such as **obesity, hypertension,** and **dyslipidemia** (ADA, 2007b). Alarmingly, the incidence of T2DM in children and adolescents has increased in recent years, to the point where approximately 85% of children diagnosed with T2DM are overweight or obese at diagnosis, presumably related to increased levels of obesity secondary to excess caloric intake and too little caloric expenditure (ADA, 2000). To this end, the ACE-AHFS must have a solid understanding of T2DM onset to develop an effective exercise program that can aid in managing T2DM and countering the common coexisting conditions of this disease.

Varying degrees of endogenous insulin production (e.g., normal or elevated) are present in T2DM, which is characterized by insulin resistance or a relative lack of activity in insulin-sensitive tissues to maintain **normoglycemia** (i.e., normal glucose levels) (ADA, 2007a). Insulin resistance is considered a "peripheral defect" because of a decrease in insulin-mediated uptake and storage of glucose in the liver and skeletal muscle. Reduced insulin receptor binding at target tissues and impaired post-receptor activities related to insulin function manifest as insulin resistance. Central to post-receptor deficiencies are abnormal translocation of muscle glucose transporters (GLUT-4) and insulin receptor substrates (IRS) that perform important intermediary phosphorylation processes (ADA, 2004a). Interestingly, these

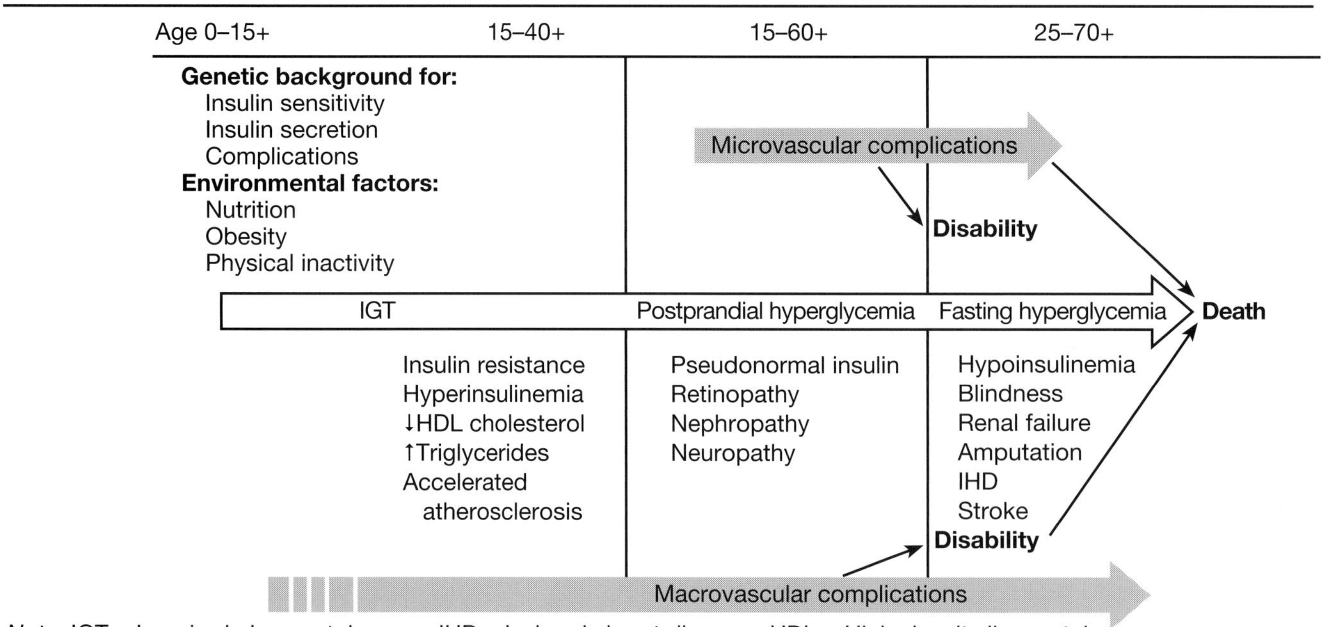

Note: IGT = Impaired glucose tolerance; IHD = Ischemic heart disease ; HDL = High-density lipoprotein

Figure 12-1
Pathology and history of onset of T2DM

Source: Peters, A. (2000). The clinical implications of insulin resistance. *American Journal of Managed Care,* 6, 13 Suppl., S668–S674.

abnormalities are reversible through weight loss, proper diet, and physical activity (Albright et al., 2000; ADA, 2007a). The hyperglycemia present in T2DM suggests that insulin release is inadequate to compensate for the insulin resistance. Over time, the pancreas loses its ability to produce insulin, and the need for exogenous insulin to control blood glucose increases (ADA, 2007a).

Control of glucose levels in T2DM is essential to prevent **hyperosmolar hyperglycemic nonketotic syndrome (HHNS),** an emergency condition in which elevated glucose levels are accompanied by dehydration without ketones in the blood or urine (ADA, 2004c). Usually, HHNS affects individuals with T2DM and, if not treated over several days to weeks, can lead to coma or death.

Onset of T2DM is associated with genetic, environmental, and cultural factors (ADA, 2004a; 2007a). The risk of T2DM rises with family history, age, obesity, and inactivity. About 80% of adults and 85% of adolescents with T2DM are obese and physically inactive, both of which are related to increased insulin resistance (CDC, 2005). Lifestyle interventions focusing on weight loss and physical activity are essential strategies to manage diabetes (ADA, 2007a), lessen the onset of DRCs (Aeillo et al., 2002; Vinik & Erbas, 2002; Waxman & Nesto, 2002), prevent the onset of T2DM [Ruderman, 2002; Diabetes Prevention Program Research Group (DPP), 2005], and prevent the onset of CVD (Buse et al., 2007; Cerosimo & DeFronzo, 2006; Grundy et al., 1999).

Etiology of Gestational Diabetes Mellitus

The ACE-AHFS should have a sound understanding of all types of diabetes, including the type that occurs during pregnancy. In essence, GDM is an inability to maintain normal glucose or any degree of glucose intolerance during pregnancy, despite being treated with either diet or insulin. GDM occurs in about 7% of all pregnancies (ADA, 2004b). High-risk factors for developing GDM include obesity, personal or family history of GDM, and **glycosuria** (an excretion of glucose in the urine) (ADA, 2004a; 2007b; 2007a). GDM is usually diagnosed by an oral glucose tolerance test between 24 and 28 weeks of gestation. If GDM is diagnosed, therapeutic strategies are used to monitor and manage maternal blood glucose to prevent fetal **macrosomia** and maternal complications (ADA, 2004b). GDM resolves postpartum, yet many women who experience GDM eventually develop T2DM. Although not identical in pathophysiology, GDM resembles etiologic features of T2DM, including obesity, insulin resistance, family history, and physical inactivity (ADA, 2004b; 2007a). As in T2DM, GDM onset is related to genetic predisposition, insulin resistance, and subsequent deficient insulin release (ADA, 2004a; 2007b). Management of GDM focuses on interventions similar to those that are commonly recommended in T2DM. However, insulin therapy, not oral agent therapy, is usually initiated when glucose control is not achieved (ADA, 2004a). Referring women with GDM to an exercise setting that can provide heart-rate monitoring of both mother and fetus is the most appropriate action for the ACE-AHFS, as women with GDM typically require close medical supervision during exercise.

Clinical Features of Diabetes Mellitus

The diagnosis of diabetes mellitus is based on established criteria (ADA, 2004a; 2007b) (Table 12-3). After diagnosis, clinical emphasis is placed on frequent blood glucose monitoring (i.e., three to six glucose checks per day) in conjunction with diet and physical activity to control glucose levels and reduce the risk of complications (ADA, 2007a). Glycemic control is assessed using **glycosylated hemoglobin (HbA1c)**, which reflects a time-averaged blood glucose concentration over the previous two to three months. The recommended A1C goal is set at less than 7.0%, which is approximately 1% above the non-diabetic range (A1C <6.0%), and it is recommended that it be assessed every three to four months (ADA, 2007b; 2007a).

Assessment of overall health, especially identification of coexisting CVD risk factors and DRCs, is an essential component of effective diabetes care (ADA, 2007b; 2007a). A relatively new term has been used to address the complex relationship between diabetes and cardiac risk—**cardiometabolic risk.** The existence of multiple risk factors for CVD, along with metabolic- and diabetes-specific factors, creates an unusually increased likelihood for those with diabetes to develop CVD (Figure 12-2). Recommendations focus on aggressive management of CVD risk factors (ADA, 2007a; Buse et al., 2007). Glucose-lowering agents are the primary medications used in diabetes management, supplemented by drugs to prevent CVD, such as antihypertensive drugs, lipid-lowering agents, and antiplatelet medications (ADA, 2007a; CDC, 2005).

Table 12-3
Diagnostic Criteria of Diabetes Mellitus

- Fasting blood glucose ≥126 mg/dL
- Diabetes symptoms, plus casual plasma glucose ≥200 mg/dL (casual glucose is taken without regard for last meal)
- Two-hour glucose ≥200 mg/dL during an oral glucose tolerance test using a 75-gram glucose load

Source: Copyright © 2007 American Diabetes Association. From *Diabetes Care,*® Vol. 30, 2007; S42-S47. Reprinted with permission from The American Diabetes Association.

Whereas body weight is usually normal in T1DM, obesity prevails in T2DM and GDM. **Body mass index (BMI)** often exceeds 30 kg/m^2 and abdominal girth is often large [men ≥40 inches (102 cm); women ≥35 inches (88 cm)] in those with T2DM, placing many patients at high risk for CVD and cancer [ADA, 2007b; National Institutes of Health (NIH) and National Heart, Lung, and Blood Institute (NHLBI), 1998]. Therefore, weight loss is a primary treatment goal to improve insulin action in persons with T2DM (ADA, 2007a).

The Metabolic Syndrome

The **metabolic syndrome (MetS)**, also called **insulin-resistance syndrome** or **syndrome X,** is commonly seen in T2DM (Grundy et al., 1999) and is linked to physical inactivity, diet, and genetic factors [Joint National Committee (JNC) on Prevention, Detection, Evaluation, and Treatment of High Blood Pressure, 2003]. The MetS is characterized by a constellation of disorders, including insulin resistance, obesity, central adiposity, glucose intolerance,

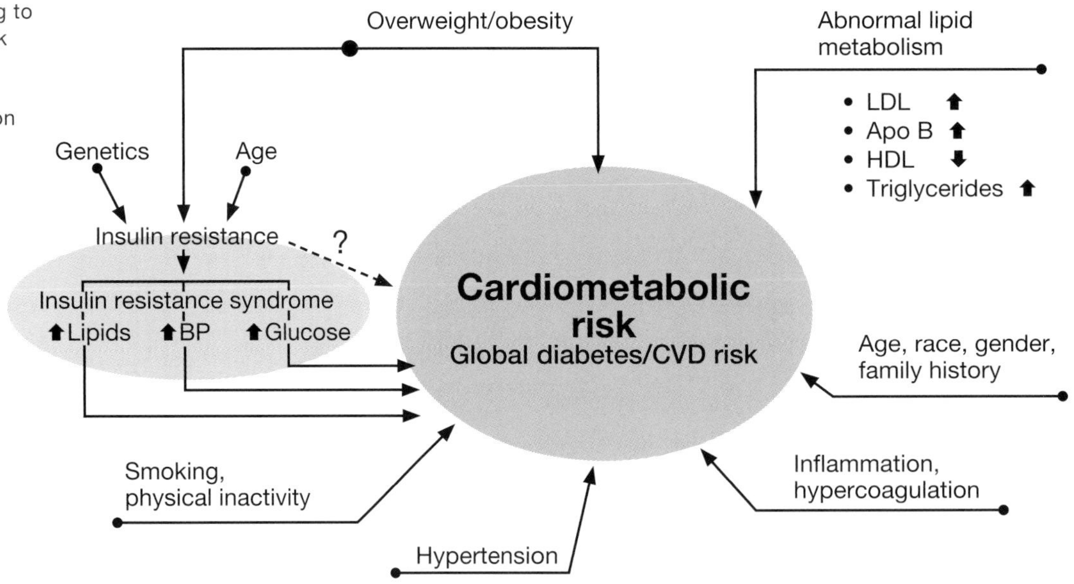

Figure 12-2
Factors contributing to cardiometabolic risk

Source: American Diabetes Association www.diabetes.org

Note: BP = Blood pressure; LDL = Low-density lipoprotein; Apo B = Apolipoprotein B; HDL = High-density lipoprotein; CVD = Cardiovascular disease

dyslipidemia, and hypertension (Table 12-4) (NIH/NHLBI, 1998). The presence of the MetS substantially increases the risk of developing both T2DM and cardiovascular disease. Insulin resistance is a cornerstone in diagnosing MetS and appears to worsen the risk for CVD and hasten the onset of T2DM. Insulin resistance is also commonly present in most individuals with T2DM.

Table 12-4
Criteria for the Diagnosis of the Metabolic Syndrome (MetS)

At least three of the following factors must be present for MetS to be confirmed:

- SBP ≥130 mmHg or DBP ≥85 mmHg
- Fasting glucose ≥110 mg/dL
- HDL cholesterol <40 mg/dL for men and <50 mg/dL for women
- Triglycerides ≥150 mg/dL
- Waist circumference ≥40 inches (102 cm) for men and ≥35 inches (88 cm) for women

Note: SBP = systolic blood pressure; DBP = diastolic blood pressure; HDL = high-density lipoprotein

Source: Joint National Committee on Prevention, Detection, Evaluation, and Treatment of High Blood Pressure (2003). The seventh report of the Joint National Committee on prevention, detection, evaluation, and treatment of high blood pressure (JNC-VII). *Journal of the American Medical Association,* 289, 2560–2572.

Pathological Consequences of Diabetes Mellitus

Diabetes leads to a variety of metabolic, physiologic, vascular, and neural problems. The pathology of this disease results in DRCs that primarily affect the macrovascular (e.g., cardiovascular disease, peripheral vasculature, cerebral vasculature), microvascular (e.g. small vessels of the retina and kidney), and neural (e.g., peripheral motor and sensory nerves, and autonomic nerves) systems. It is important to note that these DRCs are not always present in clients with diabetes. Diabetes self-management principles suggest maintaining near-normal glucose levels and managing CVD risk factors to reduce the risk for complications. In essence, good metabolic control is associated with a significant reduction in vascular and neural diabetes complications.

Macrovascular, microvascular, and nerve disease complications are commonly linked to hyperglycemia and diabetes (ADA, 2007a; AHA, 2007; Buse et al., 2007). DRCs reflect the severity and duration of the disease and contribute to accelerated morbidity and excessive mortality in diabetics. Diabetes increases mortality risk from CVD. Thus, the ACE-AHFS must know the health profile of any client with diabetes to ensure safe and effective exercise participation, while also minimizing risks for untoward outcomes.

Macrovascular Disease

Large-vessel disease, or **macrovascular disease,** is common in persons with diabetes. One type of macrovascular disease, **coronary heart disease,** is accelerated in people with diabetes and leads to premature morbidity and mortality. Additionally, diabetes contributes to an accelerated atherogenic process in other large vessels, including those in the lower extremities (peripheral vasculature) and in the brain (cerebral vasculature). Lower-extremity complications usually limit the weightbearing tolerance of afflicted individuals and contribute to a greater risk of non-traumatic amputations. **Cerebral vascular disease** is another serious complication worsened by high blood pressure that increases the risk of stroke in people with diabetes. Consequently, knowing whether a client with diabetes has macrovascular disease is a crucial part of the pre-activity screening process. If macrovascular disease is present, obtaining physician approval of exercise and modifying the assessment, programming, and leadership accordingly is prudent.

Multiple, coexisting risk factors for macrovascular disease are commonly present in T1DM and T2DM, as indicated by the cardiometabolic risk profile in diabetes (Buse et al., Grundy et al., 1999). As in non-diabetic populations, modification of CVD risk factors (e.g., smoking, elevated lipid levels, high blood pressure, and physical inactivity) aid in minimizing the risk of macrovascular disease (ADA, 2007a). Additionally, T2DM is the most common form of diabetes among individuals of older age or with obesity, visceral fat, **insulin resistance,** hypertension, dyslipidemia, and inactivity, which commonly coexist, and thus, increase the risk for macrovascular disease (ADA, 2007a; AHA, 2007; Buse et al., 2007; Grundy et al., 1999).

Physiological and metabolic abnormalities of diabetes that are believed to exacerbate the macrovascular atherogenic process are glucose intolerance, hyperglycemia, and insulin resistance (Cerosimo & DeFronzo, 2006). Though there may be different mechanisms responsible for the pathogenesis of atherosclerosis in T1DM and T2DM, modification of CVD risk factors (ADA, 2007a; Buse et al., 2007; Grundy et al., 1999) and improvement of glucose control (ADA, 2003a; 2003b) and insulin sensitivity (Cerosimo & DeFronzo, 2006) are keys to lessening the risk of atherosclerotic vascular disease.

Microvascular and Neural Complications

Small-vessel diseases, or microvascular complications, and nerve diseases are common outcomes of long-standing diabetes. Usually, the onset of **microvascular disease** progressively contributes to failure of the target tissue involved. The three different types of microvascular and neural complications are **retinopathy** (eye disease), **nephropathy** (kidney disease), and **neuropathy** (nerve disease). These complications of diabetes are the leading causes of new blindness, end-stage renal disease and kidney failure in adults, and nervous system damage leading to numerous amputations, respectively (see Table 12-2). Moreover, these complications affect work performance and tolerance, as well as the mode and intensity of work performed. The ACE-AHFS must know whether microvascular complications exist to safely and effectively devise an exercise program for a client with diabetes.

Interestingly, near-normalization of blood glucose reduced the risk for onset and/or progression of microvascular disease in T1DM by over 50% (ADA, 2003a), and similar outcomes for T2DM have been published (ADA, 2003b). Compelling data link diabetes complications with poor blood glucose control, and provide diabetes healthcare professionals with persuasive evidence about the importance of vigilant management of metabolic factors through **self–blood glucose monitoring [SBGM]** to prevent or delay the progression of complications. Thus, an ACE-AHFS can help in diabetes management by encouraging clients to maximize glucose control and regulation, while lessening the progression of small-vessel complications in these clients.

Glucose Regulation

Precise hormonal and metabolic events that normally regulate glucose **homeostasis** are disrupted in diabetes because of defects in insulin release, action, or both, and result in an excess release of counter-regulatory hormones. Glucose control requires near-normal balance between hepatic glucose production and peripheral glucose uptake, combined with effective insulin responses. In diabetes, an inability to precisely match glucose production with glucose use results in daily glucose excursions that require regular glucose monitoring and adjustments in the dosage of exogenous insulin dose or oral agent, combined with adjustments in dietary intake, particularly when anticipating exercise or physical activity.

The ACE-AHFS should have a general understanding of common medications that are prescribed for individuals with diabetes mellitus, their action(s), and the impact of exercise with respect to the medication. Classically, there are different diabetes medications that aid in controlling blood glucose. The ACE-AHFS should recognize that medication is taken by injection/infusion or orally.

Insulin Injections or Continuous Subcutaneous Insulin Infusion

Individuals with T1DM require multiple daily insulin injections or must use an insulin pump—also called continuous subcutaneous insulin infusion (CSII)—to facilitate glucose uptake and control glucose levels (ADA, 2007a). An insulin pump can be used by some individuals to manage T2DM and GDM. Insulin administered by syringe is injected into subcutaneous tissue using a rotation of sites, including the abdomen (fastest absorption rate), upper arms, lateral thigh, and buttocks (Berger, 2002). CSII is subcutaneously delivered only in the abdominal area.

Insulin administered by syringe can be rapid-acting (peak action: 30 minutes to one hour) (Humalog®), short-acting (peak action: two to three hours) (Regular), intermediate-acting (peak action: four to 10 hours) (Humulin L or N), or long-acting (peak action: sustained for 20 to 24 hours) (Humulin U). A mixed dose of different types of insulin produces a more normal glucose response and is used most commonly in T1DM. Usually, rapid-acting insulin is used with CSII. Exercise can accelerate the mobilization of insulin if the injection site is in the exercising muscle. Therefore, it is essential that the ACE-AHFS understands the importance of avoiding injection of insulin into working muscle. Also, insulin dosage (pump or injection) can be reduced prior to exercise to avoid hypoglycemia. Frequent adjustments in insulin administration are generally needed to effectively manage diabetes. These insulin adjustments involve a trial-and-error process that requires an understanding of insulin action and the impact of exercise, food intake, and medication on glucose excursions, combined with frequent routine SBGM (Berger, 2002; Toni et al., 2006).

There are also two injectable medications that aid glucose management and are used by individuals with T1DM and/or T2DM: Byetta® (exenatide or extendin-4) and Symlin® (pramlintide), a synthetic form of amylin, which is a hormone co-released from pancreatic beta cells with insulin (Joy, Rogers, & Scates, 2005; Ryan, Jobe, & Martin, 2005). For the ACE-AHFS, the main exercise-related concern with these medications is that they both delay the emptying of food from the gut after a meal and could slow the release of ingested carbohydrates taken to prevent or treat low blood glucose levels during a bout of exercise. Consequently, to err on the side of safety, neither Byettan nor Symlin should be injected within two hours prior to scheduled physical activity.

Oral Hypoglycemic Agents

Oral agents are widely prescribed for individuals with T2DM when onset is recent and little or no insulin is taken (e.g., <20 units) (ADA, 2007a). As with insulin injections, oral agents are prescribed individually or in combination to optimize glucose control in T2DM. Four major groups of oral agents are used to control glucose:

beta-cell stimulants for insulin release, drugs to improve insulin sensitivity, drugs to abate intestinal absorption of carbohydrates, and drugs to extend the action of insulin. Their mechanisms of action and effects on exercise are discussed in the following sections.

Beta-cell Stimulants for Insulin Release

Sulfonylurea and meglitinide drugs are taken at mealtime to stimulate insulin release and manage **postprandial glycemia.** Because of insulin stimulation, these oral agents can lead to hypoglycemia with or without exercise. The prolonged length of action in these oral agents increases the risk for low blood glucose and requires more frequent monitoring during exercise. Sulfonylureas include the following:

- Chlorpropamide (Diabinese®)
- Glipizide (Glucotrol® and Glucotrol XL®)
- Glyburide (Micronase®, Glynase®, and Diabeta®)
- Glimepiride (Amaryl®)

Repaglinide (Prandin®) and nateglinide (Starlix®) are the only meglintinides currently on the market (ACSM, 2006). The ACE-AHFS should recognize that individuals taking these types of longer-lasting oral hypoglycemic medications will need to check their blood glucose levels more often when exercising (and afterward). When exercise becomes a habit, it is a good idea to encourage these clients to check with their health-care providers about lowering their medication doses, particularly if they are experiencing more frequent low glucose readings with exercise.

Drugs to Improve Insulin Sensitivity

The thiazolidinediones [rosiglitazone (Avandia®) and pioglitazone (Actos®)] improve insulin sensitivity at muscle and adipose tissue, and the biguanides [e.g., metformin (Glucophage® and Glucophage XR®)] promote muscle glucose uptake and inhibit hepatic glucose output overnight. Consequently, these types of medications have little effect on exercise responses. Insulin sensitizers mainly improve the action of insulin at rest, not during exercise, so the risk of them causing exercise-associated hypoglycemia is very low (ACSM, 2006).

Drugs to Abate Intestinal Absorption of Carbohydrates

Alpha-glucosidase inhibitors [acarbose (Precose®) and miglitol (Glyset®)] decrease the carbohydrate absorption rate and slow the increase in postprandial blood glucose level. These medications do not directly affect exercise, but can delay effective treatment of hypoglycemia during activities by slowing the absorption of carbohydrates ingested to treat this condition (ACSM, 2006).

Drugs to Extend the Action of Insulin

Dipeptidyl peptidase-4 inhibitors (DDP-4 inhibitors) are the newest class of oral diabetic drugs. The primary action of these drugs is to extend the action of insulin, but they may not increase the risk of exercise-induced hypoglycemia in individuals with type 2 diabetes who are already being treated with metformin (Charbonnel et al., 2006).

Diabetes Management

Exercise intervention for persons with diabetes involves a multidisciplinary team of specialists that includes the diabetes physician, diabetes nurse educator, registered dietician, and exercise specialist to facilitate patient education and necessary lifestyle changes to manage this disease (ADA, 2007a). Intensive SBGM, combined with balancing diet, oral drugs or exogenous insulin (or both), and exercise are the established cornerstones of therapy to facilitate near-normal to normal metabolic function (ADA, 2007a). In general, management of blood glucose level in diabetes involves a planned regimen of insulin or oral medication (or both), frequent SBGM, an individualized medical nutrition therapy (MNT) plan, and participation in a regular physical-activity program. Self-management skills are essential to the successful management of diabetes. The use of diabetes self-management education (DSME) is also an important tool to improve control (ADA, 2007a). The use of a continuous glucose monitoring system (CGMS) has been shown to improve the management of diabetes, but remains a limited therapeutic intervention due to third-party reimbursement issues.

The primary goal of therapy for all diabetics focuses on SBGM to achieve acceptable blood glucose control (A1C <7.0%), thereby limiting the development and progression of DRCs (ADA, 2007a). Both T1DM (ADA, 2003a) and T2DM (ADA, 2003b) show reduced risk for retinopathy, nephropathy, and neuropathy with intensive therapy and the potential for a reduction of cardiovascular disease with improved glycemic control. Glycemic control is best achieved through SBGM combined with nutrition, adjustment of medications, and physical activity.

The ACE-AHFS should address the ABC's of diabetes with respect to clients' health (AHA, 2007):

- *A1C% (glycosylated hemoglobin):* <7%; checked at least twice a year
- *Blood pressure:* <130/80 mmHg; checked at every doctor's visit
- *Cholesterol:* LDL <100 mg/dL; checked at least once a year

Managing the ABC's of diabetes aids in reducing cardiometabolic risk and managing risk for CVD onset. Cardiovascular risk factors, along with symptomatic and asymptomatic CVD, are common in diabetes (ADA, 2007b; Buse et al., 2007; Cerosimo & DeFronzo, 2006). Identification of macrovascular disease and comorbidities of diabetes and aggressive intervention are crucial in minimizing their progression, particularly factors linked with the MetS (Buse et al., 2007; Grundy et al., 1999). CVD morbidity and mortality in diabetes can be favorably affected through lifestyle interventions. Prudent lifestyle interventions in diabetes care focus on minimizing progression of CVD through the management of CVD risk factors. Lifestyle strategies lower CVD risk factors by favorably modifying blood pressure, blood lipids, glucose tolerance, and body weight. Lifestyle strategies for managing CVD risk in diabetes include the following (ADA, 2007a):

- Dietary intervention where calories and fat intake are restricted
- Weight management and/or weight loss
- Regular physical activity
- Smoking cessation
- DSME

The coexistence of multiple CVD risk factors and hyperglycemia requires a vigilant lifestyle intervention to lessen risk and prevent CVD (Buse et al., 2007).

Therapeutic Interventions for Diabetes Mellitus

The cornerstones of diabetes therapy for self-management of this disease include insulin (or oral drugs), diet, and exercise, as well as a focus on blood glucose regulation. The primary goal of treating diabetes is not only to normalize glucose metabolism, but also to delay or prevent disease complications common to diabetes. Therapeutic strategies for diabetes treatment encompass various allied health professionals in conjunction with the physician to enhance self-care management of the disease (Figure 12-3). The ACE-AHFS is part of the diabetes management team and can help in motivating clients to safely and regularly participate in physical activity. Also, proactive communication with other members of the diabetes treatment team (e.g., personal physician, nurse educator) to ensure the safety and effectiveness of a physical-activity program is an essential responsibility of the ACE-AHFS.

The Role of Exercise in Diabetes Management

Regular physical activity and exercise offer multiple well-known health benefits for both T1DM and T2DM (Table 12-5). Mild-to-moderate intensity exercise may assist with daily glucose regulation on a short-term basis for both T1DM and T2DM, which may explain the role of regular exercise to favorably alter metabolic functions related to glucose metabolism. Regular exercise helps lessen CVD and cardiometabolic risk factors, such as mild to moderate hypertension, insulin action and resistance, glucose metabolism, vascular inflammation and altered vascular reactivity, impaired **fibrinolysis,** and abnormal lipid profiles. Also, regular exercise favorably affects not only cardiovascular and metabolic health, but also the psychological and cognitive health of individuals with T1DM and T2DM. Clearly, the ACE-AHFS should understand the benefits of chronic exercise and its adaptations in clients with diabetes.

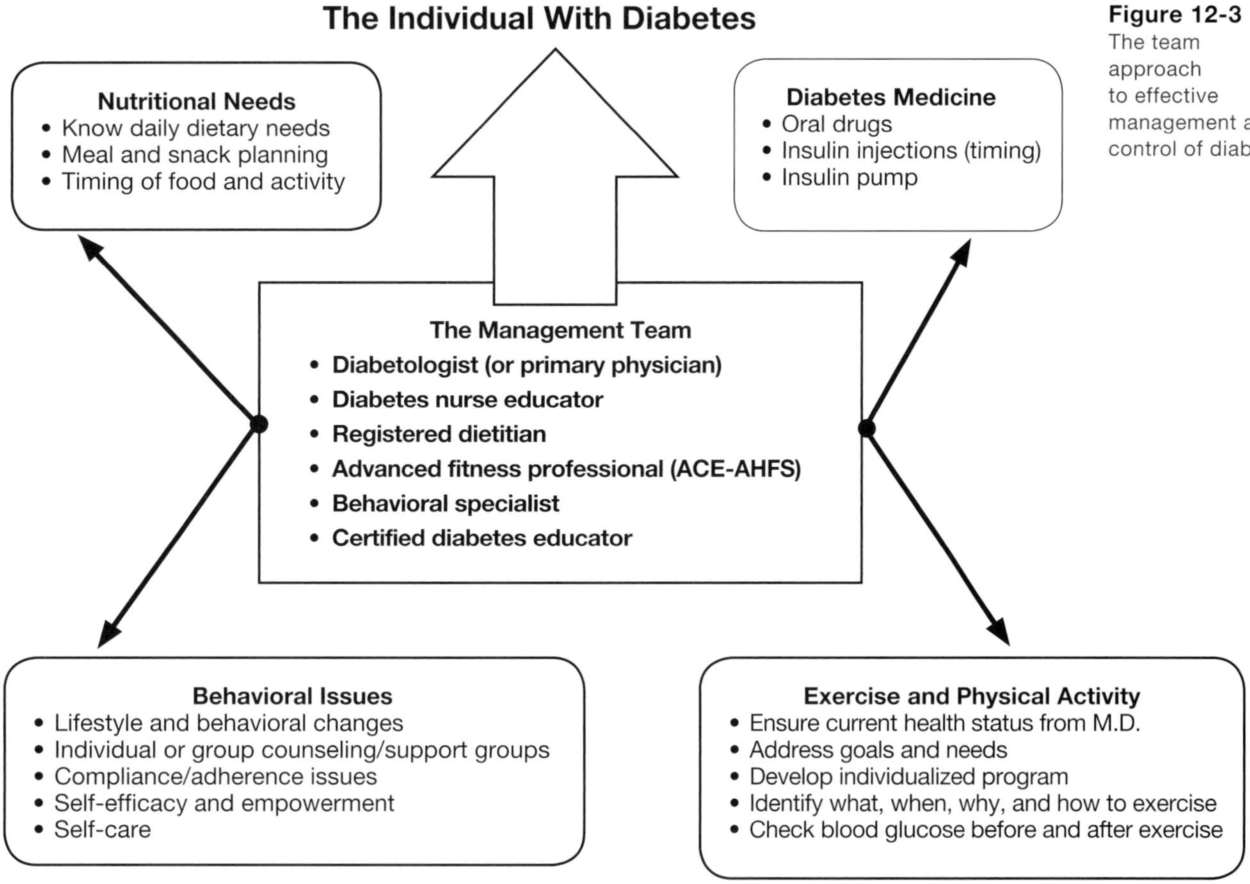

Figure 12-3
The team approach to effective management and control of diabetes

Long-term Benefits of Exercise in T1DM

Current knowledge about the long-term benefits of regular exercise on various health aspects offers a persuasive rationale for persons with T1DM to participate in physical activities. While effective exercise programming is based upon an understanding of short-term benefits, it is the benefits of chronic exercise that help to maximize health and manage risks for CVD and DRCs.

A single session of exercise acutely lowers blood glucose in individuals with T1DM for a variable amount of time, as long as the pre-exercise blood glucose level is approximately 250 mg/dL or less. The synergistic effect of exercise and insulin on lowering blood glucose is well established, and is the typical focus regarding the role of exercise as part of diabetes management. As the pre-exercise blood glucose increases beyond 250 to 300 mg/dL (with or without ketones), exercise causes skeletal muscle to increase blood glucose utilization; however, the relative amount of glucose use is countered with an excessive amount of glucose production from the liver. Thus, the ACE-

Table 12-5
The Benefits of Regular Exercise in T1DM and T2DM

	Relative Change
Cardiovascular Aspects	
• Aerobic capacity, or fitness level	↑
• Resting heart rate	↓
• Blood pressure—chronic outcome	↓
Lipid/Lipoprotein Alterations	
• HDL	↑
• LDL	↔ ↓
• VLDL/triglycerides	↓
• Total cholesterol	↔
• Risk ratio (total cholesterol/HDL)	↓
Body Composition	
• Body fat, especially in obese	↓
• Fat-free mass	↑
• Visceral body fat	↓
Metabolic Aspects	
• Insulin sensitivity	↑
• Glucose metabolism	↑
• Intracellular insulin action—insulin signaling	↑
• Basal and postprandial insulin needs	↓
Psychological Aspects	
• Self-concept/self-esteem	↑
• Depression	↓
• Stressor response to psychologic stimuli	↓

Note: ↑ = increase; ↓ = decrease; ↔ = no change

AHFS should understand that the pre-exercise blood glucose has an effect on the exercise-related blood glucose response. Requiring blood glucose checks for all individuals with T1DM before and after exercise is a safe and effective strategy to minimize untoward outcomes of exercise.

In T1DM, aerobic capacity has been suggested to be lower than that of non-diabetic, healthy individuals (Riddell & Iscoe, 2006). Nonetheless, physical training through aerobic workouts and/or resistance training is commonly recommended for individuals with T1DM who are without complications. Such individuals tend to exhibit chronic exercise benefits similar to those observed in non-diabetics (ADA, 2004d). However, regular exercise is not effective for improving blood glucose control of T1DM and should not be the sole means of controlling blood glucose (ACSM, 2006; ADA, 2004d; Verity, 2006). Adjusting therapeutic medication and nutritional regimens is an important management strategy for individuals with T1DM, along with SBGM (ADA, 2004d). Although regular exercise improves metabolism in individuals with T1DM, it does not facilitate the desired level of metabolic control. The ACE-AHFS should help educate clients on daily use of SBGM, insulin adjustment, and nutritional needs combined with regular exercise to facilitate the management of glucose.

The ACE-AHFS should recommend regular physical exercise for cardiovascular conditioning and modification of cardiovascular risk factors in individuals with T1DM, rather than only as a means for better glucose control. Research suggests that cardiovascular training in T1DM favorably alters common CVD risk factors, including blood lipids, blood pressure, insulin resistance, and glucose control (ADA, 2004d; Giannini, Mohn, & Chiarelli, 2006; Herbst et al., 2005). Therefore, improving aerobic fitness and muscular fitness in individuals with T1DM is central to improving cardiovascular health and lessening CVD risk.

The ACE-AHFS must understand that physical training (e.g., cardiorespiratory or resistance training) enhances the sensitivity of peripheral tissue to insulin action in T1DM, as is commonly reflected by reduced daily insulin dosage (Berger, 2002; Giannini, Mohn, & Chiarelli, 2006; Riddell & Iscoe, 2006). While physical activity augments insulin-mediated glucose disposal into skeletal muscle and improves insulin action, physical inactivity independently improves glucose uptake through important glucose transport activities (e.g., GLUT-4) (Zierath, 2002). Physical activity has a short-term, or transient, effect on glucose transport because insulin sensitivity begins to decline within days after physical activity ceases. To minimize insulin needs and maximize insulin action, regular exercise participation is strongly recommended for individuals with T1DM.

Beyond the physiological and metabolic benefits of chronic exercise, the psychological benefits of regular exercise for those with T1DM are beginning to receive attention. The rigors of diabetes management are emotionally stressful, particularly for young children and adolescents. **Depression** is common in people with T1DM and can adversely influence adherence to diabetes self-management regimens and result in poor glycemic control (Lustman & Clouse, 2005; Lustman, et al., 2000; Van Tillburg et al., 2001). Because of poor glycemic control, T1DM can also increase the risk for diabetes complications (de Groot et al., 2001). Given that regular exercise may help lessen physiological reactivity to mental stressors, it may help reduce stress, thereby enhancing psychological well-being, lessening depressed feelings, and improving the quality of life for individuals with T1DM (Zacker, 2004). Chronic exercise is a powerful tool for those with T1DM to empower themselves to keep control of their lives. The ACE-AHFS must continually promote the mind-body value of exercise for individuals with T1DM.

Long-term Benefits of Exercise in T2DM

Of the many coexisting conditions presented in T2DM, insulin resistance is central to muscle glucose metabolism and numerous health-related problems that only worsen the health profile. Consequently, the strategic focus of therapeutic interventions in waging war against these combined health risks is to manage glucose levels and reverse insulin resistance, or improve insulin sensitivity, which favorably affect glucose metabolism, glucose control, lipid metabolism, inflammatory reactions, and vascular wall functions—all while focusing on the reduction of cardiometabolic risk. Individuals with T2DM may also suffer from abnormal insulin secretion and hepatic and peripheral insulin resistance. Obesity, hyperglycemia, **hyperinsulinemia,** dyslipidemia, and physical inactivity also contribute to insulin resistance. Presently, diabetes management includes strategies to not only control blood glucose levels, but also to lessen morbidity and mortality in T2DM via aggressive lifestyle interventions.

In addition to glucose control through self-management skills, T2DM interventions also include nutritional changes, weight loss, CVD risk-factor management, and physical activity. These strategies are recommended based on results of the Diabetes Prevention Program (2005), where modest lifestyle changes—including dietary changes in line with current recommendations, weight loss between 5 and 7%, and increased physical activity—reduced the risk of T2DM onset by 58% in those with impaired glucose tolerance. Just as these lifestyle strategies are used to prevent the onset of T2DM, the same strategies can be implemented secondarily to lessen the progression of cardiometabolic risks associated with T2DM (Buse et al., 2007).

The favorable effects of regular exercise have been reported for insulin signaling (Zeirath, 2002), insulin resistance (Praet & van Loon, 2007), and T2DM (Albright et al., 2000; Sigal et al., 2004). It can be stated that the more that individuals with T2DM engage in physical activity throughout each week, the lower the insulin levels and the greater the insulin sensitivity or the lower the insulin resistance. To maximize health benefits, regular aerobic and resistance exercise, combined with individualized nutrition therapy, are the key weapons used to combat T2DM and insulin resistance (Buse et al., 2007; Sigal et al., 2007; Stewart, 2002). The combined therapeutic interventions promote myriad beneficial health outcomes, including improved cardiovascular and metabolic functions (Cerosimo & DeFronzo, 2006), reduced risk of cardiac morbidity and mortality (Buse et al., 2007), and favorable changes in lipids and lipoproteins (increased HDL; decreased triglycerides and LDL), blood pressure, body weight, fat-free mass (maintained or decreased), fat mass, body-fat distribution and morphology, insulin sensitivity and insulin concentrations, and glucose metabolism (ADA, 2004d; Albright et al., 2000; Sigal et al., 2004). Also, strength training has been shown to improve muscle function and quality, while increasing insulin sensitivity in individuals with T2DM (Castenada et al., 2002; Cheng et al., 2007; Dunstan et al., 2002; Sigal et al., 2007). Most importantly, the glucose metabolic defects found in previously sedentary individuals with T2DM are reversed with exercise, while both insulin signaling and exercise signaling of glucose transport are markedly improved with moderate-intensity exercise performed consistently over time (Ziereath, 2002). Consequently, regular exercise training improves glucose control (e.g., A1C) in T2DM, primarily through improved insulin signaling and insulin sensitivity. These combined physiological changes can actually lower daily medication dose (e.g., insulin and/or oral agent) for individuals with T2DM.

Interestingly, increased energy expenditure through aerobic exercise and/or strength training is independently linked with reducing insulin resistance, while improving insulin sensitivity. Both physical activity/aerobic exercise and muscle-strengthening activities have been shown to improve insulin-mediated glucose uptake, GLUT-4 transporters, insulin signaling capabilities, and insulin sensitivity—all of which are essential in glucose metabolism and management. In general, exercise training appears to reverse inflammatory markers and postreceptor insulin signaling defects, and encourage intramuscular and abdominal fat use, while simultaneously lowering the metabolic and atherosclerotic risks associated with T2DM (ACSM, 2006; ADA, 2007a; Grundy et al., 1999; Stewart, 2002; Zierath, 2002).

Additionally, regular exercise may favorably alter stress-related psychological factors and cognitive function in diabetes. Depression is common in people with diabetes (de Groot et al., 2001; Engum et al., 2005; Lustman & Clouse, 2005; Lustman et al., 2000). Unfortunately, depression can interfere with the management of diabetes and worsen glucose control in T2DM. Because glucose control plays a pivotal role in minimizing the risk for complications, individuals with T2DM are at increased risk for diabetes complications. Thus, regular exercise may assist in countering depression/**anxiety,** while improving glucose control and lessening the risk for complications. Moreover, non-traditional exercise modalities in which mind-body interventions are the focus have become more popular and have been integrated into the overall programs of clients with diabetes (Rice, 2001). For example, tai chi, yoga, and Pilates are becoming more common as alternative exercises for clients with T2DM. These types of exercise not only improve functional fitness and flexibility, but also aid in glucose management. Because the mind-body interventions aid in self-care and self-knowledge, there is a psychological outcome that has important outcomes for those with T2DM. Furthermore, regular exercise may enhance psychological well-being and quality of life for individuals with T2DM when other therapies fail (Zacker, 2004). The ACE-AHFS must recognize the value of traditional and non-traditional exercise to facilitate improved diabetes management and health outcomes in individuals with T2DM.

Pre-exercise Screening and Client Assessment

The diabetes management team must encourage clients to participate in physical activity. While regular exercise carries significant benefits, the risks are also undeniable. It is best to proceed cautiously. Before initiating exercise with clients who have diabetes, the ACE-AHFS must acquire information about his or her client to ensure safe and effective participation in physical activity. By implementing the pre-activity questionnaires (e.g., PAR-Q and PARmed-X), the ACE-AHFS will have crucial information about the client's current health and risk factors, evidence of any DRCs and physical limitations, and exercise-intensity recommendations from the physician. Thus, the pre-activity questionnaires provide an excellent opportunity for the ACE-AHFS to obtain important health information about a client with diabetes. Assessment of clients with diabetes includes the following key areas related to diabetes:

- Medical information
- Physician approval
- Lifestyle and habits questionnaire
    - ✓ PAR-Q (see Figure 1-3; page 13)
    - ✓ PARmed-X (see Figure 1-4; page 14)
- Pre-test screening
- Health-related fitness assessment

Medical Information and Physician Approval

For most clients with diabetes, physician approval is the first step to safely beginning an exercise program. Due to the high prevalence of asymptomatic coronary heart disease, there may be a need for the client with diabetes to undergo an exercise test before initiating a modest exercise program (Buse et al., 2007). The ACE-AHFS should know the health of his or her client and whether vascular and/or neural complications exist. Therefore, learning about a client's health and clinical status is essential for the ACE-AHFS to effectively engage a client with diabetes in an exercise program. Additionally, identifying questions that reflect the potential needs of the client is encouraged, including the following:

- How long has the client suffered from diabetes?
- How long has he or she taken medication?
- Are other coexisting conditions present (e.g., hypertension, elevated lipids, smoking habits, obesity)?

Because diabetes is a disease that increases the risk for coexisting conditions, the ACE-AHFS should develop a continuing-care plan that requires clients to have periodic medical evaluations (e.g., at least one physician visit per year). These follow-up visits may identify the onset or progression of complications.

Depending on the client's age, duration of diabetes, and presence of additional CVD risk factors or microvascular and/or nerve disease, a stress test may be advisable before the start of an exercise program (ACSM, 2006; Sigal et al., 2004). Stress tests are advisable for all persons with diabetes who are older than 35 years of age, and for people who are older than 25 years of age who have had T1DM for more than 15 years or T2DM for more than 10 years (ADA, 2004d; 2007a). Also, a stress test may be needed to assess cardiorespiratory integrity if a client is to embark on moderate-to-high intensity physical activity and is at high risk for underlying cardiovascular disease (ADA, 2004d). CVD risk is increased with both T1DM and T2DM, and an exercise test may aid in identifying safe exercise heart-rate limits for persons with or without neural complications (e.g., **autonomic neuropathy**), and/or hypertensive response(s) to exercise. From this physician-derived information, the ACE-AHFS may then design a safe program for this type of higher-risk client with diabetes.

The ACE-AHFS must understand the nature of each client's health- and diabetes-management plan. Given this perspective, the ACE-AHFS should ask his or her clients about current medication(s) for diabetes and any other coexisting conditions (e.g., high blood pressure, abnormal lipids). All individuals with T1DM and some with T2DM use insulin to aid in lowering blood glucose, while many, but not all, people with T2DM use oral medications to manage blood glucose levels. Thus, prior to initiating any exercise program, it is important for the ACE-AHFS to pinpoint the daily dose(s) of insulin and the location of the insulin injection. He or she must also keep a ready supply of simple sugar (e.g., candy bar, snacks) to counter the likelihood of low blood glucose, or hypoglycemia. In some clients who require insulin injections, physical activity combined with close monitoring of blood glucose may contribute to a lowering of the daily insulin requirement. However, any adjustment of insulin dosage must be carefully balanced with nutritional needs and close glucose monitoring. Any change must also be thoroughly discussed with the client's physician, diabetes educator, or nurse practitioner. Under no circumstances should an ACE-AHFS recommend an unusual lowering of daily insulin dosage.

Oral medications are commonly prescribed for those with T2DM, while fewer than 20% of individuals with T2DM are prescribed insulin alone or in combination with oral medications (CDC, 2005). The purpose of oral drugs is to lower blood glucose by augmenting insulin release and insulin action or sensitivity. Once again, the ACE-AHFS should ask clients to identify the daily dosage of oral medications. Oral agents to lower blood glucose for T2DM include:

- Glucotrol XL® (glipizide extended release)
- Prandin® (repaglinide)
- Amaryl® (glimepiride)
- Rezulin® (troglitazone)
- Glucophage® (metformin)
- Micronase® (glyburide)

Medication dosage can be reduced following a period of weight loss and/or physical activity. However, only the client's physician should make changes in oral medications. The ACE-AHFS should encourage clients who are taking oral medications to regularly monitor and record their blood glucose and then provide this information to a physician, which may help the physician in determining dosage.

About 73% of all persons with diabetes develop hypertension (CDC, 2005). Hypertensive medications are outlined in Chapter 8. Drugs commonly prescribed to treat high blood pressure can adversely elevate blood glucose. These include **diuretics,** beta blockers, and calcium-channel blockers. Furthermore, beta blockers are known to mask the symptoms related to low blood glucose. Other hypertensive medications may actually lower blood glucose, including ACE inhibitors and alpha-adrenergic antagonists (JNC, 2003). The varying effect of hypertensive medications is further reason to monitor blood glucose.

The ACE-AHFS should follow standard fitness screening procedures (ACSM, 2006; 2008). Using a questionnaire (e.g., PAR-Q and PARmed-X) is appropriate. If the client responds positively to a question, its significance must be ascertained through a follow-up with the client's physician. Also, if any client with diabetes has been diagnosed with CVD, or has suffered a heart attack, he or she requires medical approval to exercise. Whenever a client with diabetes presents a history of heart disease, the ACE-AHFS should refer the client to a clinical setting for supervised exercise.

Lifestyle and Habits Questionnaire

The ACE-AHFS should consider a number of factors before developing an exercise program for clients with diabetes. Based on current health profile, fitness assessment outcomes, and limitations identified by the physician, a safe and effective individualized exercise program can be devised. Central to the safety of an exercise program is ensuring the client with diabetes monitor and manage his or her blood glucose to minimize risks of exercise and onset of diabetes complications. To motivate the client, the ACE-AHFS should devise an exercise program that considers personal interests, past and/or present exercise habits, and short- and long-term goals that are achievable, as doing so is central to the client's successful adherence to the exercise program. Because more than 70% of diabetics do not engage in regular physical activity (Ford & Herman, 1995), developing an activity program that is motivational, develops long-term habits, and addresses each client's personal goals is key to a successful program.

Identifying the personal goals and needs in a physical-activity program is crucial to maintain the interest and focus of a client with T2DM. Additionally, past exercise habits can provide important insight regarding present exercise interests, commitments, and/or habits. Previous habits and interests can also provide information about the client's awareness and knowledge of his or her disease, and about his or her effort in trying to control blood glucose. Glucose control is a life-long habit and helps ensure that exercise is safe and effective.

Education about the role of SBGM before and after each exercise session is usually presented in diabetes education classes. If a client with diabetes has not participated in a series of diabetes education classes, the ACE-AHFS should encourage him or her to do so. These classes will increase the client's understanding of the disease and reemphasize the importance of regular glucose monitoring. Also, the ACE-AHFS may provide the client with a list of diabetes educators and other resources.

Screening

The ACE-AHFS should administer the PAR-Q, PARmed-X, informed consent, and possibly release forms, and then measure resting heart rate and blood pressure. From his or her most recent physician visit, the client with diabetes should know his or her A1C (%) and inform the ACE-AHFS of this value for baseline information. Also, the client with diabetes should bring his or her glucose meter on the day of the health-related fitness assessment and on subsequent exercise days for glucose monitoring before and after each exercise session.

Resting heart rate and blood pressure assessment are commonly used as screening aids for apparently healthy persons who wish to partake in physical activity. About 73% of persons with diabetes have hypertension. Some medications used to treat hypertension may actually lower the resting heart rate; however, resting blood pressure may remain elevated. Consequently, a client with diabetes may have a normal resting heart rate but elevated blood pressure.

A resting heart rate above 120 bpm and resting blood pressure exceeding 180/105 mmHg are contraindications to exercise (Gordon, 2002). Other contraindications to exercise follow previously established guidelines (ACSM, 2006).

Health-related Fitness Assessment

Fitness assessments are integral to effective exercise programming. The ACE-AHFS can chart client progression and set goals to motivate clients. Fitness evaluations may include body morphology and/or composition, cardiorespiratory fitness, and musculoskeletal fitness tests. Although fitness assessments can be administered, the ACE-AHFS may have to adapt the procedure for some clients with diabetes. Whenever testing procedures are changed, the ACE-AHFS should record the modifications of the client's initial test so that subsequent evaluations are consistent.

Body Morphology and/or Composition

Excessive body weight and/or body fat is common in individuals with T2DM, while those with T1DM are commonly normal weight. Most persons with T2DM are overweight or obese (ADA, 2007b), while the distribution of body fat is predominantly in the abdominal region. This type of body morphology, or body-fat distribution, increases the risk for CVD, insulin resistance, and abnormal lipids. The preferred method to determine body composition is by using skinfold thickness measures. The use of circumferential measures aids the ACE-AHFS in understanding the distribution of body fat, or the client's morphology (ACSM, 2008). Normally, it is acceptable to use the same generalized equations that have established norms for age and gender of apparently healthy persons for those with T1DM. When working with individuals with T2DM, the determination of body fat is difficult and may not be very useful, as most of these individuals are obese. However, the ACE-AHFS can measure and record skinfold thickness to observe subtle changes over time. Also, circumference measures (e.g., abdominal, waist, hip) can be obtained and recorded for clients with T2DM to derive a baseline from which program goals may be targeted. Overall, these types of morphologic measures have far greater practical outcomes and can be easily compared with previous assessments.

Cardiorespiratory Fitness

Clients with diabetes tend to participate less frequently in regular physical activity than non-diabetics (Ford & Herman, 1995). Low cardiorespiratory fitness is strongly linked with cardiac mortality in individuals with diabetes (Boulé et al., 2003). Moreover, research suggests that people with T2DM consume a lower amount of oxygen than non-diabetics across different intensity levels of work (Regensteimer et al., 1995). Therefore, improving cardiorespiratory fitness is an extremely important health outcome that can be accomplished through regular participation in exercise (Boulé et al., 2003; Buse et al., 2007; Stewart, 2002). The ACE-AHFS is encouraged to use standard submaximal testing protocols to assess cardiorespiratory fitness in persons with diabetes. Also, heart-rate data and **ratings of perceived exertion (RPE)** should be obtained during cardiorespiratory assessments. However, administering a valid submaximal test can be difficult with diabetics.

Many persons with diabetes are hypertensive and take heart-rate-altering medications, which make a submaximal test to assess cardiorespiratory fitness invalid. In some clients, a bicycle protocol may be appropriate (e.g., YMCA protocol). To ensure the validity of submaximal outcomes, the ACE-AHFS must know whether a client has a neural condition called **cardiac autonomic neuropathy,** because this DRC slows the heart rate and limits the validity of submaximal protocols that assess heart-rate responses to submaximal work.

The ACE-AHFS may find field tests (e.g., 12-minute walk/run test) to be suitable for clients with T1DM, but not for those with T2DM. Performance in this type of test requires motivation to achieve a near-maximal effort and knowledge of pacing oneself. The use of a field test of this type may only be useful for those who have a recent history of regular exercise.

For those clients who undergo a stress test with their physicians, it is always a good idea to obtain a copy of this report through client consent. In cases where the cardiorespiratory fitness assessment cannot be administered, the information from a stress test can be used to aid in developing an aerobic program for a client.

Musculoskeletal Fitness

Administration of tests to assess muscle endurance, muscle strength, and joint flexibility in clients with diabetes is appropriate only in those who are not limited by diagnosed complications, especially microvascular complications (Aiello et al., 2002; Albright et al., 2000). Prior to initiating any portion of the muscular-strength and/or endurance assessments, the ACE-AHFS should ensure an appropriate medical health status, especially the absence of microvascular complications. The ACE-AHFS is encouraged to use standard testing protocols that do not use **one-repetition maximum (1 RM)** to assess musculoskeletal fitness in persons with diabetes (e.g., YMCA).

Guidelines for Exercise Programming

The ACE-AHFS must have a solid understanding of the client with diabetes. Some of the more distinguishing factors to keep in mind when devising an exercise plan for diabetes clients are as follows:

- Diabetics are less active than non-diabetics. Approximately 70% of persons with diabetes are sedentary (Ford & Herman, 1995).
- Diabetics are older, perceive their health more poorly, and identify physical or orthopedic limitations four times more frequently than their non-diabetic counterparts (Ford & Herman, 1995).

Developing an exercise plan by using the FITT acronym is commonplace. Incorporating RPE to identify exercise intensity is prudent, as disease progression and complications (e.g., autonomic and **peripheral neuropathy**) can limit the ability to accurately assess heart rate. Additionally, the FITT program differs for those with T1DM and T2DM (Table 12-6), in that a T1DM program can emphasize exercise at a moderate to high intensity for shorter durations, while a program for individuals with T2DM can emphasize caloric expenditure where lower-intensity and longer-duration exercise is strongly encouraged. In those with T1DM without complications, exercise recommendations are closely aligned with apparently healthy persons (Wasserman & Zinman, 1994), while recommendations for those withT2DM are more closely aligned with obesity and hypertension guidelines (Sigal et al., 2004; Stewart, 2002) due to the prevalence of these comorbidities in T2DM. Also, individuals with T2DM are encouraged to engage in at least 150 minutes of moderate-intensity exercise each week (or 90 minutes of vigorous exercise each week), primarily focusing on caloric expenditure and weight-management issues (ADA, 2004d). The ACE-AHFS must consider the risk for muscular injury whenever he or she recommends higher-intensity exercise, especially for clients with T2DM. For long-term weight-loss maintenance, larger volumes of exercise (seven hours/week of moderate or vigorous activity, with an expenditure of more than 2000 kcals/week) are recommended for clients with T2DM (ADA, 2004d; Sigal et al., 2004). Consideration of personal interests, past and/or present activity habits, and the goals and needs of a physical-activity program is critical for successful participation, especially in those with T2DM (Albright et al., 2000; Praet & van Loon, 2007). Individuals who use insulin may prefer to engage in daily physical activity to improve the balance between insulin dose and caloric needs (Albright et al., 2000; ADA, 2004b; Berger, 2002).

Table 12-6
Recommended FITT Program for Aerobic Training in Individuals With Diabetes

Variable	T1DM	T2DM
Frequency	3–7 days/week	3–7 days/week
Intensity	50–80% HRR RPE = 12–16 (6–20 scale)	50–80% HRR* RPE = 12–16 (6–20 scale)
Time Moderate ~50–70% HRmax Vigorous >70% HRmax	20–60 minutes/session At least 150 minutes/week At least 90 minutes/week	30–60 minutes/session At least 150 minutes/week At least 90 minutes/week
Type*	Walking, cycling, jogging, aquatic exercise	Walking, cycling, aquatic exercise, leisure activities, house- and yardwork

*Some individuals may need to perform non-weightbearing activity or alternate with weightbearing activities due to orthopedic limitations and/or peripheral vascular disease.

Note: HRR = heart-rate reserve; RPE = ratings of perceived exertion; HRmax = maximum heart rate

Sources: American Diabetes Association (2004). Physical activity/exercise and diabetes: Position statement. *Diabetes Care,* 27 (Suppl 1), S58–S64; Sigal, R.J. et al. (2004). Physical activity/exercise and type 2 diabetes: Technical Review. *Diabetes Care,* 27, 10, 2518–2539.

Resistance training is recommended for persons with diabetes who have no contraindications (Albright,et al., 2000; ADA, 2004d) and follows apparently healthy guidelines, with age and experience as prime considerations in program development (Table 12-7). When working with clients who have diabetes complications, the ACE-AHFS must either obtain specific instructions from the physician for safe and effective participation, or refer the client to an appropriately monitored setting. Strength or resistance training appears to offer specific improvements in insulin sensitivity (Cheng et al., 2007) and glucose control in those with T2DM (Castenada et al., 2002; Dunstan et al., 2002; Sigal et al., 2007). Therefore, the ACE-AHFS is strongly encouraged to have all appropriate diabetes clients engage in resistance training to accrue its many potential benefits. Appropriate attention to modifying the intensity of the resistance-training session may lessen the risk for elevations in blood pressure and glucose, and for the onset of musculoskeletal injury (Albright et al., 2000; ADA, 2004d). Research suggests that higher-intensity resistance exercise is safe and effective in lowering A1C (Castenada et al., 2002; Dunstan et al., 2002). Caution should be reserved when recommending higher-intensity resistance exercise for those with diabetes. For safe and effective exercise participation, it is imperative that glucose levels be carefully managed. Moreover, initiation of a resistance-exercise program requires that clients do not have complications that might prevent safe and effective outcomes. To lessen exercise-induced blood pressure elevations, modifications may need to be made, including lowering the intensity of each lift, requiring higher repetitions, foregoing lifting to exhaustion, and limiting isometric contractions.

Flexibility exercises are strongly recommended for those with diabetes (Albright et al., 2000; Gordon, 2002; Verity, 2006) and aid in maintaining normal joint function. Balancing the selection of exercises between the upper and lower body, as well as for the core area, is important. Essentially, the flexibility-exercise recommendations are very similar between T1DM and T2DM (Table 12-8). The ACE-AHFS must ensure that clients do not hold their breath for the entire range of motion of any movement, even when statically holding a given stretch. Proper breathing will limit the **Valsalva maneuver**, which causes elevated SBP and may be detrimental to individuals with CVD or to those who have DRCs (Gordon, 2002).

Exercise Programming in T1DM

Daily aerobic exercise has been recommended for individuals with T1DM to better

Table 12-7
Recommended FITT Program for Resistance Training in Individuals With Diabetes

Variable	T1DM	T2DM
Frequency	2–3 days/week	2–3 days/week*
Intensity	60–80% 1 RM Low-to-moderate intensity RPE ~13–16 (6–20 scale)	60–80% 1 RM Low intensity RPE ~11–15 (6–20 scale)
Time	8–12 reps/exercise 2–3 sets/exercise	8–12 reps/exercise reps (up to 20) 2–3 sets/exercise
Type of exercise	8–10 muscle groups Upper body: 4–5 exercises Lower body: 4–5 exercises	8–10 muscle groups Upper body: 4–5 exercises Lower body: 4–5 exercises

*3 days/week is strongly encouraged
Note: T1DM = Type 1 diabetes mellitus; T2DM = Type 2 diabetes mellitus; 1 RM = One-repetition maximum; RPE = Ratings of perceived exertion

Sources: American Diabetes Association (2004). Physical activity/exercise and diabetes: Position statement. *Diabetes Care,* 27 (Suppl 1), S58–S64; Sigal, R.J. et al. (2004). Physical activity/exercise and type 2 diabetes: Technical Review. *Diabetes Care,* 27, 10, 2518–2539.

Table 12-8
Recommended FITT Program for Flexibility Training in Individuals With Diabetes

Variable	T1DM	T2DM
Frequency	2–3 days/week	2–3 days/week
Intensity	Stretch to ROM tightness	Stretch to ROM tightness
Time	15–30 seconds/stretch 2–4 reps/stretch	15–30 seconds/stretch 2–4 reps/stretch
Type of stretching exercise	Upper body: 4–5 exercises Lower body: 4–5 exercises	Upper body: 4–5 exercises Lower body: 4–5 exercises

Note: ROM = Range of motion

Sources: American Diabetes Association (2004). Physical activity/exercise and diabetes: Position statement. *Diabetes Care,* 27 (Suppl 1), S58–S64; Sigal, R.J. et al. (2004). Physical activity/exercise and type 2 diabetes: Technical Review. *Diabetes Care,* 27, 10, 2518–2539.

regulate insulin dosage and diet needs for glucose control (ADA, 2003a; 2003b). Improving glucose control for individuals with T1DM is best achieved through intensive insulin therapy combined with SBGM (ADA, 2007a). Therefore, clients with T1DM are best served to follow the FITT principle in Table 12-6 and exercise three to five days per week to improve aerobic capacity and accrue other health-related benefits. The ACE-AHFS should know that exercise is not recommended for glucose control in T1DM, and that daily exercise may be unrealistic. Moreover, high-intensity activity can increase the risk of elevating blood glucose and suffering musculoskeletal injuries (Gordon, 2002; Hornsby & Albright, 2003). Clients with T1DM who do not have complications can comfortably exercise between 55 and 75% of functional capacity, or at an RPE of 11 to 14 (using the 6 to 20 scale) or 3 to 5 (using the 0 to 10 scale). Each activity session should last about 30 minutes to spur improved aerobic fitness and health-related benefits.

Finally, strength training for clients with T1DM may increase aerobic capacity , as well as increase muscle mass and improve glucose control, by increasing insulin sensitivity (Riddell & Iscoe, 2006). Clients with T1DM who do not have complications can participate in a moderate-intensity strength-training program that mimics a program non-diabetics would use (see Table 12-7). Clients with a longer history of T1DM should seek physician approval and heed limits on participation.

Exercise Programming in T2DM

Exercise programming for individuals with T2DM follows the FITT principle (see Table 12-6). The focus of such programming is to burn calories and lose weight (ACSM, 2006; ADA, 2004d; Sigal et al., 2004). Physical activity of 40 to 60 minutes in duration at a low intensity of 40 to 60% of functional capacity (or 50 to 70% of HRmax) is appropriate for overweight/obese persons to burn an adequate number of calories. Lower-intensity walking improves aerobic capacity, insulin action, and glucose control (Boulé et al., 2001; 2003) and aids in weight management for individuals with T2DM (Yamanouchi et al., 1995). Overall, the therapeutic effects of regular exercise have enormous health benefits for those with T2DM (Praet & van Loon, 2007; Sigal et al., 2004; Stewart, 2002). Because obesity is a problem for individuals with T2DM, more moderate exercise reduces the likelihood of foot irritation and/or musculoskeletal injury (Gordon, 2002; Verity, 2006).

Exercising five to six days per week maximizes the caloric expenditure necessary for weight management. Although walking is the most convenient activity, persons with **claudication** pain may have to perform low- or non-weightbearing activity (e.g., swimming, aquatic exercise, stationary cycling), or alternate between weightbearing and non-weightbearing activities. Moreover, peripheral neuropathy, which may lead to foot irritation, may preclude weightbearing activities due to the possibility of foot irritation.

Finally, it may also benefit individuals with T2DM to engage in moderate-intensity resistance training (see Table 12-7), which increases muscle mass, lowers basal insulin levels, improves insulin action and sensitivity, and aids in glucose control. Resistance training is a safe, effective, and highly recommended component of a comprehensive exercise program that provides cardiovascular and metabolic benefits for those with T2DM (Hornsby & Albright, 2003). However, it is important for clients with T2DM to participate regularly in an aerobic-training program before the start of a resistance-training program. Most of these clients are severely deconditioned. Dynamic, whole-body activity in the aerobic exercise program will enhance their abilities to accommodate the muscular strength, endurance, and flexibility requirements.

Guidelines for Exercise Leadership

Clients with diabetes should consider numerous factors before starting an exercise program. Safety before, during, and after exercise is of paramount importance. Ensuring that clients learn certain practical information before exercising is central to safe and effective exercise participation, and providing practical exercise advice for clients with diabetes is a strong asset for an ACE-AHFS (Table 12-9).

Documenting each exercise session helps when communicating with a client's physician about cardiovascular adaptations and metabolic changes resulting from regular exercise. A daily log may be a particularly efficient way to record vital information—both quantitative and qualitative.

In fact, a qualitative assessment of the client's ability and performance is essential. Additionally, evaluating the client's self-concept, self-esteem, motivation to exercise regularly, and other quality-of-life issues is important for the ACE-AHFS to understand. Any noticeable dysfunctional changes should immediately be reported to the client's physician. These changes may include:

- An inability to accurately palpate and obtain a heart rate
- A loss of sensation in the feet or toes during weightbearing activities
- Increasing pain in the legs during weightbearing activities
- Difficulty reading the RPE chart
- Unusual forgetfulness or memory problems
- Persistent fatigue

The ACE-AHFS must evaluate the client on a daily basis and report both quantitative and qualitative information regarding the exercise session. Barring more immediate problems, written documentation can be submitted to the client's physician on an annual basis. This documentation may compare various fitness assessments to those from the previous year. They may include the frequency and amount of daily submaximal work and heart rate, medication doses, glucose levels before and after sessions (averaged weekly or monthly), and any qualitative assessments previously described.

Risks of Exercise in Clients With T1DM and Clients With T2DM Who Require Insulin

Although individuals with T1DM and some individuals with T2DM require exogenous insulin derived from an injection site, or through a continuous infusion pump, exogenous insulin absorption does not mimic the normal insulin secretory pattern, especially during physical exercise. Consequently, insulin administration poses a potential problem for these individuals as they work to sustain near-normal glucose levels while exercising (Toni et al., 2006). In nondiabetics, metabolic responses to most exercise are balanced between adequate insulin release and an intricately matched glucose utilization and glucose production (Figure 12-4a). The maintenance of a normal glucose response, or **euglycemia,** during exercise is always achieved in normal clientele. Because of the need for exogenous insulin for diabetics, it is important

Table 12-9
Practical Tips for Clients With T1DM and T2DM When Engaging in Exercise

Check with your physician.
- Clients may need to limit the intensity of physical activity, especially if disease complications are present.
- Clients may need to join a supervised program for guidance and assistance, especially if they have not been physically active for a long period of time.

Utilize self–blood glucose monitoring (SBGM).
- Clients should perform SBGM before and after each physical-activity session. SBGM is excellent cognitive training for diabetics to understand individual glucose response to physical activity. It is important to ensure that blood glucose is in relatively good control before engaging in purposeful exercise. If blood glucose is:
  - ✔ >250 mg/dL with ketones, physical activity should be postponed
  - ✔ <100 mg/dL, the client should eat a snack consisting of carbohydrates and recheck blood glucose before exercising
  - ✔ Between 100 and 250 mg/dL, physical activity can be safely performed

Keep a daily log.
- Clients should record the value and the time of day the SBGM is performed and the amount/timing of any pharmacologic agent (e.g., oral drugs or insulin). Also, they should include approximate time (minutes), intensity (heart rate), and distance (miles or meters) of each activity session. This information will aid the diabetic in understanding the type of response to possibly expect from specific physical-activity bouts.

Plan for an exercise session.
- How much activity is anticipated (e.g., time and intensity)?
- If needed, clients should carry extra carbohydrate feedings (~20–30 g of carbohydrate per 30 minutes of exercise).

Exercise with a partner.
- Exercising with a partner affords a "support system" for the physical-activity habit. Initially, diabetics should exercise with a partner until glucose response is known. Ideally, a partner who accompanies the physically active diabetic will be a source of social support and encourage continued participation in this healthy lifestyle.

Wear a diabetes I.D.
- Never leave home without it. Hypoglycemia or other problems can arise that require an understanding of the condition.

Wear good shoes.
- Proper-fitting and comfortable footwear can minimize foot irritations and sores, and reduce the occurrence of orthopedic injuries to the foot and lower leg.

Practice good hygiene.
- Clients should always take extra care to inspect their feet for any irritation spots to prevent possible infection. They should tend to all sores immediately and report hard-to-heal sores to a physician. Clients can prevent irritations when physically active by using Vaseline™ on the feet and wearing socks inside-out.

Modify caloric intake accordingly.
- Through frequent SBGM, caloric intake can be regulated more carefully on days of, and following, physical activity. For those clients requiring insulin, blood glucose can drop significantly after physical activity and latent post-exercise hypoglycemia can be prevented via SBGM. Also, in consultation with the client's physician, a decrease in insulin dosage may be necessary.

for the ACE-AHFS to identify the risks for individuals with T1DM and T2DM who wish to safely participate in exercise.

Insulin injection therapy for most individuals with T1DM typically consists of multiple-dose insulin injections, while those who use CSII infuse a single type of fast-acting insulin (Toni et al., 2006). In some clients with T2DM, insulin is commonly introduced into an existing treatment regimen of oral medications as a single evening or bedtime dose of basal insulin. Because of this regimen, those with T2DM are less likely to experience the common risks of insulin injections/infusions observed in those with T1DM.

Exogenous insulin absorption is not well regulated and results in varying degrees of insulin excess or deficiency in the peripheral blood. Insulin levels are very important during the increased metabolic demands of physical exercise. In T1DM, several factors influence the blood glucose response to exercise, including the time of the insulin injection; the location of insulin injection (e.g., active vs. non-active muscle); pre-exercise glucose; pre-exercise nutrition; intensity and duration of the exercise session; and the novelty of the exercise performed (Toni et al., 2006).

Given so many factors to regulate, it is not surprising that physical exercise brings about unpredictable blood glucose responses in individuals with T1DM. Because of the dependency on exogenous insulin and an inability to regulate the absorption of insulin, people with T1DM commonly oscillate between insulin excess and insulin deficiency. Hence, the degree of "insulinization" and the level of blood glucose before the start of exercise determine the blood glucose response during and after exercise for those with T1DM. In well-controlled or well-insulinized T1DM clients, a single session of moderate exercise brings about normal metabolic responses. Under certain conditions, blood glucose may increase or decrease, depending on insulin levels (Figure 12-4).

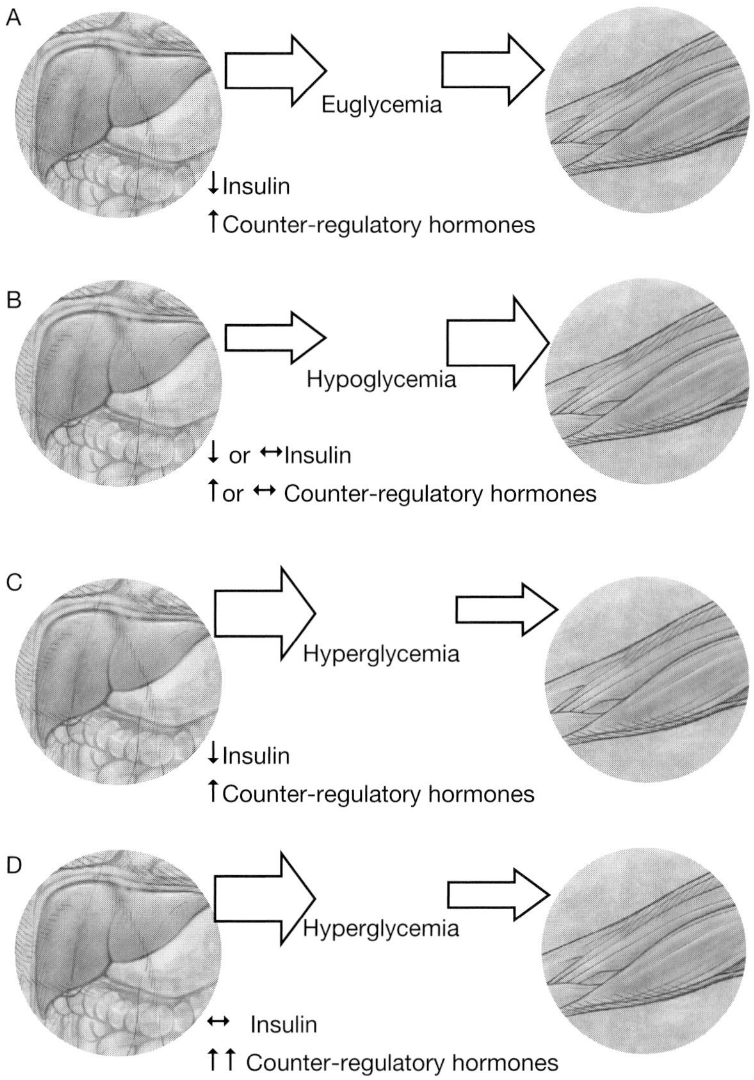

Figure 12-4
Schematic illustration of the blood glucose response to exercise. (A) Non-diabetic response or ideally controlled T1DM where hepatic glucose production matches skeletal muscle glucose utilization and blood glucose does not change. (B) Hyperinsulinemia, or excessive insulin, results in low hepatic glucose production and enhanced skeletal muscle glucose uptake, yielding a low blood glucose, or hypoglycemia.(C) Hypoinsulinemia, or insulin deficiency, results in elevated counter-regulatory hormones, causing an imbalance between excessive hepatic blood glucose production and an inadequate skeletal muscle glucose uptake, thereby yielding an increase in blood glucose. (D) The stress of high-intensity exercise, competition, or heat can dramatically increase counter-regulatory hormones that increase hepatic glucose output with diminished skeletal muscle glucose uptake resulting in hyperglycemia.

Note: ↑= Increase; ↓= Decrease; ↔ = No change; ↑↑= Large increase

Source: Riddell, M.C. & Iscoe, K.E. (2006). Physical activity, sport, and pediatric diabetes. *Pediatric Diabetes,* 7, 60–70.

Hypoinsulinemia

Hypoinsulinemia, or insulin deficiency, results in elevated blood glucose and ketone bodies before exercise (Figure 12-4c). Insulin-deficient diabetics rely heavily upon **free fatty acids (FFA)** as a primary energy source, which leads to elevated ketones in the blood and urine.

What happens when an insulin-deficient client exercises? As work increases, there is an increase in metabolic functions to provide adequate fuel for the body. Unfortunately, a person with inadequate insulin is not able to adequately regulate blood glucose levels, and therefore experiences an increase in blood glucose, along with an increase in FFA use and ketone production. Exercise seems to worsen hyperglycemia in an insulin-deficient state because insulin action does not promote normal metabolic functions. Clients with diabetes should use SBGM before exercise, as this is the safest way to determine whether exercise will help improve insulin action and lower glucose levels.

Exercise-induced Hyperglycemia

During heavy, or high-intensity, exercise in clients with T1DM, glucose levels increase because of stress responses to the intensity of work that result in excessive release of glucose from the liver and limit skeletal muscle glucose use. Typically, the T1DM is in good control prior to exercise and the elevation of blood glucose is singularly due to the stressors of high-intensity exercise. Therefore, the ACE-AHFS should always have his or her T1DM clients check their blood glucose to enhance effective management of their exercise-induced responses.

Hyperinsulinemia

Hyperinsulinemia, or high insulin levels, usually occurs when exogenous insulin is accelerated by increased muscle contraction and blood flow (Figure 12-4b). This situation can cause exercise-induced hypoglycemia. Insulin injection into non-active muscle is recommended on exercising days, although the strict use of non-active muscle as an injection site may not prevent hypoglycemia during exercise in those with T1DM (Toni et al., 2006).

Elevated insulin levels suppress hepatic glucose production, which causes an imbalance between the rate of peripheral glucose use and production, and results in the lowering of blood glucose. Although a decrease in blood glucose is a beneficial short-term effect of exercise, prolonged exercise can bring about hypoglycemia. Consequently, blood glucose lowering is dependent upon such factors as pre-exercise levels of blood glucose and insulin, antecedent nutrition, and exercise duration and intensity. Regular SBGM and modifying food intake and insulin dose on exercise days are useful strategies to prevent hypoglycemia in clients with T1DM.

Post-exercise Hypoglycemia

Although hypoglycemia can occur during exercise, low blood glucose can develop many hours after an acute exercise bout in those with T1DM. Although short-lived, post-exercise metabolic adjustments increase the risk for hypoglycemia in the first few hours following an exercise bout. To prevent acute and late-onset hypoglycemia, strategies should combine aggressive post-exercise SBGM with the adjustment of pre- and post-exercise insulin and caloric intake, as changes in insulin dose and caloric intake are not totally effective.

Postprandial Exercise Responses

The majority of individuals with T1DM exercise after a meal, rather than in a post-absorptive, or fasted, state. Usually, persons with T1DM have glucose fluctuations with each meal, due to the relative timing of insulin injection or infusion and the rate of insulin absorption from the injection/infusion site. Mild exercise after breakfast blunts glucose elevations throughout the course of a day in those with T1DM. Exercise performed after breakfast may also prove valuable because of a reduced risk for hypoglycemia during and following exercise. However, the postprandial (i.e., after-meal) response to exercise in those with T1DM is quite variable, and is dependent upon the pre-exercise glucose level, the timing of the insulin injection and food consumption before activity, and exercise intensity and duration.

Management of Exercise Risks in Clients With Diabetes

As a client with diabetes engages in regular physical activity, are there risks associated with participation? Will he or she develop problems? If so, what are the signs and symptoms of these problems?

The ACE-AHFS should know that the most common problem encountered by exercising clients with T1DM (and some T2DM) is low blood glucose, or hypoglycemia. Hypoglycemia can occur at any time (e.g., before, during, or after exercise) and is defined as blood glucose less than 80 mg/dL. Clients may be experiencing hypoglycemia or an insulin reaction when they:

- Sweat profusely
- Are clammy and look pale
- Get shaky
- Have difficulty answering specific questions

- Slur their speech
- Seem exhausted
- Become lightheaded or pass out

It is important for a client showing any of these symptoms to ingest a simple sugar snack (e.g., candy) or drink (e.g., orange juice) that contains about 20 to 30 grams of carbohydrate. After five minutes, blood glucose should be checked to determine whether more carbohydrates are needed. This cycle should be repeated until a client's blood glucose returns close to 100 mg/dL before engaging in exercise. Following an insulin reaction, the client may not feel comfortable exercising. At this point, the exercise session should be terminated.

Hypoglycemia is not totally preventable. Exercise-induced hypoglycemia most commonly occurs in insulin-requiring diabetics. To minimize the occurrence of low blood glucose, the ACE-AHFS should link each exercise session to the timing and site of insulin injection or the use of CSII, the antecedent and post-exercise nutrition, the time of day, and the pre- and post-exercise blood glucose monitoring.

For those who use insulin injections, the insulin injection should occur at least one hour before exercising, and preferably in a non-exercising area. Some insulin-requiring clients can reduce the dosage of intermediate insulin by 30 to 50%, whether using injections or CSII (Toni et al., 2006). For persons on insulin pumps, a reduction in basal insulin dosage is recommended during and after mild to moderate exercise to minimize the risk of acute and late-onset hypoglycemia (Verity, 2006).

Consumption of carbohydrates is critical for individuals with T1DM to avoid low blood glucose levels. Between 15 and 30 grams of carbohydrates should be consumed for every 30 minutes of moderate exercise (Verity, 2006). A complex carbohydrate snack helps lessen post-exercise reductions in blood glucose and late-onset hypoglycemia.

The timing of exercise for those with T1DM may be a key in avoiding hypoglycemia. Depending on insulin administration and nutrient intake, the best time for some clients with T1DM to exercise is one to two hours after breakfast, or at least in the morning hours. For some with T1DM, postprandial exercise aids in mitigating glucose excursions throughout the day, and leaves them less susceptible to dramatic decrements in blood glucose (Toni et al., 2006). It is also important to individualize an exercise regimen. A program must fit into a client's schedule.

SBGM is essential for clients with T1DM and is strongly recommended for those with T2DM. Glucose monitoring is appropriate before and after exercising. Given the understanding of glucose levels, those with diabetes can minimize severe glucose shifts, especially after exercise.

Elevated blood glucose occurs in clients with diabetes who are not well insulinized because of excessive caloric intake and/or not enough insulin. Exercise will only worsen the hyperglycemia and ketone levels when pre-exercise glucose levels are elevated. Pre-exercise glucose levels exceeding 250 mg/dL with ketones indicate poor control and necessitate postponement of exercise. A log enables a management team to evaluate glucose excursions and prevent a reoccurrence. When blood glucose is high, clients with T1DM need an appropriate dosage of insulin, while those with T2DM may be able to engage in low-intensity physical activity without medication adjustment. For those with T1DM, exercise is not recommended until blood glucose is below 250 mg/dL.

High-intensity exercise has been found to elevate blood glucose from a normal to hyperglycemic level. It is believed that the role of counter-regulatory hormones on glucose production plays a major part in this type of glycemic excursion. Moderate-intensity exercise is recommended to facilitate more normal glucose levels and lessen the likelihood of musculoskeletal injury.

Progression of the Program

The progression of the aerobic and musculoskeletal programs is determined by several factors, including age, functional capacity, medical and disease complications, and personal preferences and goals (Albright et al., 2000; ADA, 2004d; Gordon, 2002). Initial changes in FITT programming for clients with diabetes should focus on the duration of the exercise session rather than the intensity, particularly for those with T2DM. This programming adjustment can prevent blood glucose increases, provide a safe and effective workout that is not unduly taxing, and increase the likelihood that the program will be sustained.

For clients without complications, initial ability levels are quite different between types of diabetes. For example, individuals with T1DM follow a similar FITT program to that of apparently healthy persons. They can initially engage in continuous, moderate-intensity physical activity for 20 minutes, while those with T2DM may only be able to engage in low-intensity physical activity for five to 10 minutes before fatiguing. The initial phase of FITT programming for clients with T2DM requires low-intensity and short-duration (e.g., less than 15 minutes) activity at least three times per week, and preferably five times per week (Albright et al., 2000; ADA, 2004d; Sigal et al., 2004). But individuals with T1DM may not require significant modifications in the initial phase of FITT programming. By closely observing client response to a program and modifying it to prevent fatigue, the ACE-AHFS will enhance the client's enjoyment and commitment to such a lifestyle change.

Progression of the program after the initial phase should be approached with caution, especially when working with clients with T2DM. For both types of diabetes, the duration of an activity should be increased before the intensity. The duration should be gradually increased to accommodate the ability and clinical status of each client. Because clients with T2DM are more likely to be obese and older, they may require a longer period of time to adapt to program changes. Once the client is able to exercise for a desired amount of time, programmatic changes should be small and be approached with caution to lessen the risk of undue fatigue, musculoskeletal injuries, and/or relapse.

Some clients with well-controlled T1DM may set a goal to participate in competitive athletics (e.g., 10Ks, marathons, triathlons, biathlons). A small number of these clients may require higher-intensity, longer-duration workouts. Successful participation in competitive athletics by an individual with T1DM is dependent upon rigorous SBGM, appropriate insulinization, proper nutrient intake, and regular medical visits. Still, most diabetics will not strive to compete in athletics. Instead, they will need to improve functional aspects that relate to quality of life. Because T2DM onset is related to older age, obesity, and dysfunction of physiologic and neurologic processes, the most valuable aspect of any program should relate to functional outcomes specific to each client and his or her abilities and limitations.

Medical Concerns and Disease Complications

Although complications are common in diabetes (ADA, 2007a), their existence does not preclude physical activity. Rather, there are physical-activity precautions and limitations for clients with diabetes who have one or more types of microvascular and/or neural complications. The options for diabetics with disease complications are discussed in the following sections. The ACE-AHFS should familiarize him- or herself with the many diabetic complications. Clients with diabetes-related complications should often be referred to a clinical setting where close supervision and monitoring of exercise can safely occur.

Retinopathy

Although exercise increases systemic and retinal blood pressure, there is no evidence that physical activity acutely worsens the retinopathy present in diabetes (Aiello et al., 2002). Diabetics with proliferative retinopathy who engage in low-intensity exercise can significantly improve cardiovascular function. However, systolic blood pressure should be monitored during each exercise session and limited to 20 to 30 mmHg above resting. Clients with retinopathy may exercise safely when they are properly supervised.

Clients with retinopathy should not engage in activities that require them to raise their arms over their heads, such as with certain strength-training movements. These activities may cause systolic blood pressure to rise dramatically. Under such circumstances, increased blood pressure may increase the likelihood of retinal hemorrhaging when proliferative retinopathy is present (Aiello et al., 2002).

Nephropathy

Approximately one-third of individuals with T1DM develop nephropathy, while some clients with T2DM develop nephropathy (Mogensen, 2002). Increased blood pressure is a common precursor to worsening of this microvascular disease (ADA, 2007a). It is prudent to avoid activities that cause systolic blood pressure to rise to 180 to 200 mmHg (e.g., Valsalva maneuver, high-intensity aerobic or strength exercises), as systemic pressure increases could potentially exacerbate the progression of this disease. Persons with progressive nephropathy or end-stage renal disease may benefit from lower-intensity physical activities. Most clients with nephropathy should be referred to a clinical setting where their fragile metabolic condition may be carefully monitored. In many cases, clients with this disease participate in physical-activity sessions while undergoing renal dialysis.

Neuropathy

Neuropathy is a nerve disorder. The two main nerve diseases related to diabetes are autonomic neuropathy (AN), and peripheral neuropathy (PN). When this disease affects the autonomic nerves to the heart, it is called cardiac autonomic neuropathy (CAN). The heart rate is altered. The maximal heart rate is blunted, while resting heart rate (HRrest) increases (e.g., HRrest >100 bpm). CAN causes hypertension and hypotension and increases the risk for exercise-induced hypotension after strenuous activity (Vinik & Erbas, 2002). Persons with AN have impaired sweating and thermoregulatory abilities and impaired hypoglycemia awareness. Persons with CAN exhibit a lower fitness level and fatigue at relatively low workloads due to the disruption in nerve innervation to the heart (Vinik & Erbas, 2002). Consequently, physical activity for these persons should focus on low-level daily activities, where mild changes in heart rate and blood pressure can be accommodated. Before beginning any exercise program for persons with AN or CAN, the ACE-AHFS should gain physician approval and proceed cautiously.

Peripheral nerve disease affects the extremities, especially the lower legs and feet. Repeated weightbearing activities on insensitive feet can lead to chronic irritation, open sores, and musculoskeletal injuries, especially fractures. Persons with PN are susceptible to overstretching due to loss of sensation, as well as infection, particularly when daily hygiene is lacking. Proper footwear for any weightbearing activity is important to prevent undetectable sores, which may turn into infections. However, people with PN should also participate in non-weightbearing activities (Vinik & Erbas, 2002). Such interventions may include aquatic exercise, recumbent cycling, chair exercises, and upper-extremity exercises. Additionally, activities requiring a full range of joint motion are highly effective in reducing stiffness due to muscle contractures. Some nontraditional exercises (e.g., yoga, Pilates, and tai chi) may be prudent for the client who has PN.

Case Studies

Case Study 1

Jim has T1DM. He is 35 years old and has had diabetes since the age of 13. He is 5'10" (1.8 m) and weighs 165 pounds (75 kg). Jim was highly involved in high school and college sports, but has not been regularly active for about 12 years. He currently uses an insulin pump and monitors his blood glucose once or twice each day. He visits his doctor each year and his self-reported health is good. He reports no diabetes-related complications and believes his A1C was 8.5% when it was measured about eight months ago. Jim's goal is to begin an aerobic program so that he can run a 10K with his son, who is a teenager. He has come to an ACE-AHFS for professional assistance.

As a general rule, an ACE-AHFS must obtain more information about Jim's health before developing an exercise program. According to established guidelines (ACSM, 2006), Jim is considered a higher-risk client. It is prudent for the ACE-AHFS to obtain physician approval before working with Jim, since he has had diabetes for 22 years. Also, it is essential that Jim completes the PAR-Q and PARmed-X questionnaires to ascertain any known cardiovascular disease, with the physician's completion of the PARmed-X to address diabetes-related complications and potential limitations with exercise. Additionally, the ACE-AHFS should assess Jim's exercise history and obtain information about his usual meal times and insulin pump routine before developing an exercise plan.

From this screening, Jim should either plan to visit his diabetes educator or enroll in a diabetes education class to improve his diabetes self-management skills and education. Although Jim uses an insulin pump, his one or two daily blood glucose checks are not adequate to effectively manage his blood glucose levels. He should try to do better. Also, his A1C is high. He should strive to get his A1C below 7.0%. More frequent A1C assessments are strongly encouraged, as A1C is highly linked with risk for cardiovascular disease, as well as onset/progression of DRCs. With more rigorous monitoring and visits with his diabetes educator, Jim may see his A1C gradually decline. SBGM before and after each exercise session is a requirement for him.

To develop an appropriate exercise regimen, the ACE-AHFS should conduct a fitness assessment (ACSM, 2008). Results from the submaximal YMCA bicycle protocol found Jim's aerobic fitness to be average for his age and gender. His percent body fat as determined from skinfold assessment was 17%, while his musculoskeletal fitness was good. Results from the fitness and exercise habits assessments suggest that Jim can immediately participate in aerobic activity. His desire to participate in a 10K does not preclude alternate activities (e.g., recumbent cycle ergometer, upright cycle ergometer, stair stepping). Blood glucose readings should be recorded, and if his pre-exercise blood glucose is above 250 mg/dL, the ACE-AHFS should postpone the session until his glucose is below 250 mg/dL. If Jim's pre-exercise blood glucose is less than 100 mg/dL, he should consume about 15 to 20 grams of carbohydrates for every 30 minutes of anticipated exercise to limit hypoglycemia onset.

When initiating the resistance-training program, the ACE-AHFS should begin at the lower end of the range of each FITT element. It is essential that Jim learns proper lifting techniques and breathing cues (e.g., breath on effort) before starting a resistance program. If Jim does the resistance-training program following the aerobic regimen, he should check his blood glucose after completing his aerobic session and resistance-training session. If there is a long delay (e.g., several hours) between the aerobic and resistance-training programs, then Jim should do the SBGM before and after each respective regimen.

Case Study 2

Jane is 55 years old and was diagnosed with T2DM about three years ago. Jane is 5'3" (1.6 m) and weighs 180 pounds (82 kg). She is currently taking an oral medication (troglitazone) for her diabetes and antihypertensive medications for her high blood pressure (ACE inhibitor: lisinopril, 40 mg; beta blocker: atenolol, 25 mg) and does not regularly monitor her blood glucose. She reports SBGM about twice per week and her A1C is about 9.0%. Jane reports that her health is good. She does not suffer from diabetes complications, but gets easily fatigued doing housework and cleaning. Furthermore, she reports that taking a 15- to 25-minute stroll with her husband at the local mall creates discomfort in her knees and hips. She has not seen her doctor in more than a year; however, her diabetes educator has encouraged her to participate in regular physical activity. She has asked the ACE-AHFS for assistance in the development of an exercise/physical-activity program. Her goals are to improve her endurance and lose about 45 pounds (20 kg).

Jane requires an annual check-up on the clinical status of her diabetes (e.g., the evaluation of the presence/absence/progression of disease complications). She must receive her physician's approval to begin an exercise program with the ACE-AHFS, who should encourage this client to improve management of her diabetes by getting routine physician check-ups and blood work. Also, the ACE-AHFS should recommend that Jane work with a registered dietician who is a certified diabetes educator to determine the most appropriate method of safely and effectively losing the desired weight.

Because Jane is 55 years old and has T2DM, she should complete the PAR-Q and PARmed-X questionnaires to ensure physician approval and identify possible limits in her exercise program. Her discomfort while walking requires further evaluation. The lack of regular blood glucose monitoring must be addressed, along with her elevated A1C%. The use of the questionnaires may aid physician encouragement for more frequent glucose monitoring and A1C checkups. Also, these questionnaires improve the safety and appropriateness of an exercise program for Jane.

Once the ACE-AHFS has gotten physician approval with possible information from a stress test (if needed), and disease status and limitations are obtained, he or she can develop an exercise regimen for Jane. Of greatest importance are the client's personal interests and goals. Because Jane has difficulty with short-term weightbearing activity, the ACE-AHFS can help her choose activities that are less wearing on her joints and identify enjoyable activities that she would more likely engage in on a regular basis. Due to her desire to lose about 45 pounds (20 kg), Jane should be encouraged to seek out weight-management professionals to advise her about that goal.

Jane should exercise wherever the social stigma of obesity and overweight issues is minimized. She must feel comfortable in her exercise surroundings. This is an important issue because the wrong exercise environment could cripple her motivation to maintain her physical-activity program.

What health-related fitness assessments can be administered? One of Jane's blood pressure medications is a heart rate–altering medication (e.g., beta blocker) that eliminates the use of a cardiorespiratory fitness assessment using submaximal protocols that base aerobic capacity on heart rate measurement. A field test requiring a weightbearing exercise (e.g., 1.5 mile walk/run test or a 12-minute walk/run test) is inappropriate, given her excessive weight. Fortunately, a stress test was conducted by her physician and is an excellent starting point for program development. From the stress test, resting and maximum parameters, including heart rate, blood pressure, and RPE can be identified. Jane's physician probably determined the upper limit of exercise intensity on the PARmed-X. Based on this information, she was not to exercise at over 70% of her maximum heart rate. From this information, an individualized FITT program can be devised for Jane that focuses on the lower end of the range for each FITT element. The program must be safe, effective, reasonable, and prudent for this type of client. The FITT should look as follows:

- F = 4–6 days per week
- I = 50–60% of maximal heart rate, or RPE approximately 2–3 (on the 0–10 scale)
- T = 15–30 minutes
- T = alternate between weightbearing (e.g., walking) and non-weightbearing (e.g., aquatic exercise; recumbent ergometer; chair exercises) activities

Body composition assessment is not necessary when someone is already known to be obese, but a morphological assessment can be easily administered. Initial measures should include body weight, selected skinfold site thicknesses, as well as abdominal, hip, and waist circumferences. These measurements provide a good baseline for serial assessments. Jane's measurements were as follows:

- Body weight: 180 lb (82 kg)
- Abdominal skinfold: 36 mm
- Iliac skinfold: 32 mm
- Thigh skinfold: 40 mm
- Triceps skinfold: 34 mm
- Chest skinfold: 28 mm
- Waist circumference: 42 in (107 cm)
- Hip circumference: 48 in (123 cm)
- Upper-arm circumference: 18 in (46 cm)
- Thigh circumference: 22 in (56 cm)

From these measurements, it is obvious that weight loss will have a favorable impact on Jane's anthropometric measurements. The measurements can also be motivating for Jane as she strives to improve her fitness and lose weight.

Musculoskeletal fitness should not be assessed in the initial phase of the program. Jane has enough to do at this point. Incorporating an additional routine into Jane's activity regimen is not appropriate at the outset. As previously indicated, the ACE-AHFS should start with an aerobic program to engage Jane in an exercise routine before initiating the resistance-training program.

The ACE-AHFS must require SBGM before and after each exercise session as a prerequisite to safe exercise programming. Jane may be able to engage in low-intensity exercise (e.g., 40% HRmax) if her pre-exercise blood glucose is above 250 mg/dL. If Jane's pre-exercise blood glucose is below 100 mg/dL, then she should consume about 15 to 20 grams of carbohydrates for every 30 minutes of anticipated exercise. Jane's beta blocker for hypertension can mask hyperglycemia, so the ACE-AHFS should periodically check her blood pressure, especially at the start of a program.

Jane is willing to come to a fitness facility two days each week. For Jane to succeed in her exercise program, she should exercise on two additional days. She should be instructed on the correct use of RPE to ensure a safe and effective exercise environment when she is not supervised.

The ACE-AHFS should always encourage clients to drink adequate amounts of water, especially clients prone to dehydration. The ACE-AHFS should also discourage clients from exercising when the temperature is above 80° F (27° C).

During the first activity session, Jane should be closely supervised and should be comfortable when exercising. The intensity level should be appropriate. She should expend energy. Also, she must accurately monitor her blood glucose. For Jane to exercise for the recommended 30- to 60-minute exercise period, she may need to alternate between a circuit of five-minute aerobic activities with 10-minute rest intervals or initiate a low-intensity aerobic interval program of similar work and rest intervals. Keep in mind that a client with T2DM must be closely monitored and given prompt feedback about accomplishments and progress. Also, the ACE-AHFS must ensure that blood glucose levels are normal when the client leaves the facility to minimize the risk of low glucose or hypoglycemia problems.

Summary

The ACE-AHFS must realize that physical activity and/or exercise is an essential part of the therapeutic regimen in diabetes management and care. Diabetes presents challenges for exercise that requires the ACE-AHFS to perform careful assessment of client status, determine client ability, and individualize the exercise program to meet the needs and goals of those with either T1DM or T2DM. Careful attention to the client and their diabetes-related comorbidities is a must for safe and effective exercise-training administration. The ACE-AHFS should also maintain close communication with each client's physician to update progress or address any issues/concerns of the exercise program and/or responses that may need attention.

References

Aiello L.P. et al. (2002). Retinopathy. In: Ruderman, N. et al. (Eds). *Handbook of Exercise in Diabetes* (2nd ed.) pp. 401–413. Alexandria, Va: American Diabetes Association.

Albright, A. et al. (2000). Exercise and type 2 diabetes: Position stand. *Medicine & Science in Sports & Exercise,* 32, 1345–1360.

American College of Sports Medicine (2008). *ACSM's Health-related Physical Fitness Assessment Manual* (2nd ed.). Philadelphia: Lippincott Williams & Wilkins.

American College of Sports Medicine (2006). *ACSM's Guidelines for Exercise Testing and Prescription* (7th ed.). Philadelphia: Lippincott Williams & Wilkins.

American Diabetes Association (2007a). Standards of medical care in diabetes—2007: Position statement. *Diabetes Care,* 30 (Suppl. 1), S4–S41.

American Diabetes Association (2007b). Diagnosis and classification of diabetes mellitus. *Diabetes Care,* 30 (Suppl. 1), S42–S47.

American Diabetes Association (2004a). Report of the expert committee on the diagnosis and classification of diabetes mellitus. *Diabetes Care,* 27 (Suppl. 1), S5–S35.

American Diabetes Association (2004b). Gestational diabetes mellitus: Position statement. *Diabetes Care,* 27 (Suppl. 1), S88–S93.

American Diabetes Association (2004c). Hyperglycemic crises in patients with diabetes mellitus. *Diabetes Care,* 27 (Suppl.1), S94–S102.

American Diabetes Association (2004d). Physical activity/exercise and diabetes: Position statement. *Diabetes Care,* 27 (Suppl. 1), S58–S64.

American Diabetes Association (2003a). Implications of the diabetes control and complications trial: Position statement. *Diabetes Care,* 26 (Suppl. 1), S25–S27.

American Diabetes Association (2003b). Implications of the United Kingdom prospective diabetes study: Position statement. *Diabetes Care,* 26 (Suppl. 1), S28–S32.

American Diabetes Association (2000). Type 2 diabetes in children and adolescents: Position statement. *Diabetes Care,* 23, 3, 381–389.

American Heart Association (2007). *The Heart of Diabetes:℠ Understanding Insulin Resistance.* http://www.americanheart.org/presenter.jhtml?identifier=11243.

Berger M. (2002). Adjustment of insulin and oral agent therapy. In: Ruderman, N. et al. (Eds.). *Handbook of Exercise in Diabetes* (2nd ed.) pp. 365–381. Alexandria, Va: American Diabetes Association.

Boulé, N.G. et al. (2003). Meta-analysis of the effect of structures exercise training on cardiorespiratory fitness in type 2 diabetes. *Diabetologia,* 46, 1071–1081.

Boulé, N.G. et al. (2001). Effects of exercise on glycemic control and body mass in type 2 diabetes mellitus: A meta-analysis of controlled clinical trials. *Journal of the American Medical Association,* 286, 1218–1227.

Buse, J.B. et al. (2007). Primary prevention of cardiovascular diseases in people with diabetes mellitus: A scientific statement from the American Heart Association and the American Diabetes Association. *Circulation,* 115, 114–126.

Castenada, C. et al. (2002). A randomized controlled trial of resistance exercise training to improve glycemic control in older adults with type 2 diabetes. *Diabetes Care,* 25, 2335–2341.

Centers for Disease Control and Prevention (2005). *National Diabetes Fact Sheet: National Estimates and General Information on Diabetes in the United States—2005.* Atlanta, Ga: U.S. Department of Health and Human Services, Centers for Disease Control and Prevention.

Cerosimo, E. & DeFronzo, R.A. (2006). Insulin resistance and endothelial dysfunction: The road map to cardiovascular diseases. *Diabetes/Metabolism Research and Reviews*, 22, 423–436.

Charbonnel, B. et al. for the Sitagliptin Study 020 Group (2006). Efficacy and safety of the dipeptidyl peptidase-4 inhibitor sitagliptin added to ongoing metformin therapy in patients with type 2 diabetes inadequately controlled with metformin alone. *Diabetes Care,* 29, 12, 2638–2643.

Cheng, Y.J. et al. (2007). Muscle-strengthening activity and its association with insulin sensitivity. *Diabetes Care,* 30, 9, 2264–2270.

de Groot, M. et al. (2001). Association of depression and diabetes complications: A meta-analysis. *Psychosomatic Medicine,* 63, 619–630.

Diabetes Prevention Program Research Group (2005). Impact of intensive lifestyle and metformin therapy on cardiovascular disease risk factors in the diabetes prevention program. *Diabetes Care,* 28, 4, 888–894.

Dunstan, D.W. et al. (2002). High-intensity resistance training improves glycemic control in older patients with type 2 diabetes. *Diabetes Care,* 25, 1729–1736.

Engum, A. et al. (2005). Depression and diabetes. *Diabetes Care,* 28, 1904–1909.

Ford, E.S. & Herman, W.H. (1995). Leisure-time physical activity patterns in the U.S. diabetic population: Findings from the 1990 national health interview survey—health promotion and disease prevention supplement. *Diabetes Care,* 18, 1, 27–33.

Giannini, C., Mohn, A., & Chiarelli, F. (2006). Physical exercise and diabetes during childhood. *ACTA Biomedica,* 77 (Suppl. 1), 18–25.

Gordon N. (2002). The exercise prescription. In: Ruderman, N. et al. (Eds.). *Handbook of Exercise in Diabetes* (2nd ed.) pp. 269–288. Alexandria, Va: American Diabetes Association.

Grundy, S.M. et al. (1999). Diabetes and cardiovascular disease: A statement for healthcare professionals from the American Heart Association. *Circulation,* 100, 1134–1146.

Herbst, A. et al. (2007). Impact of physical activity on cardiovascular risk factors in children with type 1 diabetes. *Diabetes Care,* 30, 2098–2100.

Hornsby W.G. & Albright, A.L. (2003). Diabetes. In: Durstine, L. & Moore, G. (Eds.). *ACSM's Exercise Management for Persons with Chronic Disease and Disabilities* (2nd ed.) pp. 133–141. Champaign, Ill.: Human Kinetics.

Joint National Committee on Prevention, Detection, Evaluation, and Treatment of High Blood Pressure (2003). The seventh report of the Joint National Committee on prevention, detection, evaluation, and treatment of high blood pressure (JNC-VII). *Journal of the American Medical Association,* 289, 2560–2572.

Joy, S., Rodgers, P., & Scates, A. (2005). Incretin mimetics as emerging treatment for type 2 diabetes. *Annals of Pharmacotherapy,* 39, 1, 110–118.

Lustman, P.J. & Clouse, R.E. (2005). Depression in diabetic patients: The relationship between mood and glycemic control. *Journal of Diabetes and Its Complications*, 19, 2, 113–122.

Lustman, P.J. et al. (2000). Depression and poor glycemic control. *Diabetes Care,* 23, 934–942.

Mogensen, C.E. (2002). Nephropathy: Early. In: Ruderman, N. et al. (Eds.). *Handbook of Exercise in Diabetes* (2nd ed.) pp. 433–449. Alexandria, Va: American Diabetes Association.

Narayan, K.M. et al. (2003). Lifetime risk for diabetes mellitus in the United States. *Journal of the American Medical Association,* 290, 1884–1890.

National Institutes of Health and National Heart, Lung, and Blood Institute (1998). *Clinical Guidelines on the Identification, Evaluation, and Treatment of Overweight and Obesity in Adults: Evidence Report.* Bethesda, Md: NIH Publication No. 98-4083.

Praet, S. & van Loon, L. (2007). Optimizing the therapeutic benefits of exercise in type 2 diabetes. *Journal of Applied Physiology,* 103, 1113–1120.

Regensteiner, J. et al. (1995). Effects of non-insulin dependent diabetes on oxygen consumption during treadmill exercise. *Medicine & Science in Sports & Exercise*, 27, 875–881.

Rice, B.I. (2001). Mind-body interventions. *Diabetes Spectrum,* 14, 4, 213–217.

Riddell, M.C. & Iscoe, K.C. (2006). Review article: Physical activity, sport, and pediatric diabetes. *Pediatric Diabetes,* 7, 60–70.

Ruderman, N. (2002). A target population for diabetes prevention: The metabolically obese, normal-weight individual. In: Ruderman, N. et al. (Eds.). *Handbook of Exercise in Diabetes* (2nd ed.) pp. 235–249. Alexandria, Va.: American Diabetes Association.

Ryan, G., Jobe, L., & Martin, R. (2005). Pramlintide in the treatment of type 1 and type 2 diabetes mellitus. *Clinical Therapeutics*, 27, 10, 1500–1512.

Sigal, R.J. et al. (2007). Effect of aerobic training, resistance training, or both on glycemic control in type 2 diabetes: A randomized control. *Annals of Internal Medicine,* 147, 357–369.

Sigal, R.J. et al. (2004). Physical activity/exercise and type 2 diabetes: Technical review. *Diabetes Care,* 27, 10, 2518–2539.

Stewart, K.J. (2002). Exercise training and the cardiovascular consequences of type 2 diabetes and hypertension: Plausible mechanisms for improving cardiovascular health. *Journal of the American Medical Association,* 288, 13, 1622–1631.

Toni, S. et al. (2006). *ACTA Biomedica,* 77 (Suppl. 1), 34–40.

Van Tillburg, M. et al. (2001). Depressed mood is a factor in glycemic control in type 1 diabetes. *Psychosomatic Medicine*, 63, 551–555.

Verity, L.S. (2006). Diabetes mellitus and exercise. In : Kaminsky, L.S. (Ed.). *ACSM's Resource Manual for Guidelines for Exercise Testing and Prescription* (5th ed.) pp. 470–488. Philadelphia: Lippincott Williams & Wilkins.

Vinik A.I. & Erbas, T. (2002). Neuropathy. In: Ruderman, N. (Eds.) *Handbook of Exercise in Diabetes* (2nd ed.) pp. 463–496. Alexandria, Va.: American Diabetes Association.

Wasserman D. & Zinman, B. (1994). Exercise in individuals with IDDM. *Diabetes Care,* 17, 924–937.

Waxman, S. & Nesto, R.W. (2002). Cardiovascular complications. In: Ruderman, N. et al. (Eds.). *Handbook of Exercise in Diabetes* (2nd ed.) pp. 415-432. Alexandria, Va.: American Diabetes Association.

Yamanouchi, K. et al. (1995). Daily walking combined with diet therapy is a useful means for obese NIDDM patients not only to reduce body weight but also to improve insulin sensitivity. *Diabetes Care,* 18, 775–778.

Zacker, R.J. (2004). Exercise: A key component of diabetes management. *Diabetes Spectrum,* 17, 3, 142–144.

Zierath, J.R. (2002). Exercise effects of muscle insulin signaling and action—Invited review: Exercise training-induced changes in insulin signaling in skeletal muscle. *Journal of Applied Physiology,* 93, 773–781.

Suggested Reading

American College of Sports Medicine (2003). *ACSM's Exercise Management for Persons with Chronic Disease and Disabilities* (2nd ed.). Champaign, Ill.: Human Kinetics.

American College of Sports Medicine and American Diabetes Association (1997). Diabetes mellitus and exercise: A joint position statement of the American College of Sports Medicine and the American Diabetes Association. *Medicine & Science in Sports & Exercise*, 29, i–vi.

American Diabetes Association (2007). Clinical practice recommendations. *Diabetes Care,* 30 (Suppl. 1), S1–S103.

American Diabetes Association (2003). Physical activity/exercise and diabetes mellitus: Position statement. *Diabetes Care,* 26 (Suppl.1), S73–S77.

Bernbaum, M. et al. (1989). Cardiovascular conditioning in individuals with diabetic retinopathy. *Diabetes Care,* 12, 740–742.

Riddell M.C. et al. (2002). Exercise physiology and diabetes: From antiquity to the age of the exercise sciences. In: Ruderman, N. et al. (Eds.). *Handbook of Exercise in Diabetes* (2nd ed.) pp. 3–15. Alexandria, Va: American Diabetes Association.

Ruderman N. et al. (Eds.) (2002). *Handbook of Exercise in Diabetes* (2nd ed.). Alexandria, Va.: American Diabetes Association.

Part Four

Musculoskeletal Disorders

Chapter 13
Posture and Movement

Chapter 14
Mobility, Gait, and Balance

Chapter 15
Arthritis

Chapter 16
Osteoporosis and Osteopenia

Chapter 17
Principles of Post-orthopedic Rehabilitation

Chapter 18
Musculoskeletal Injuries of the Lower Extremity

Chapter 19
Musculoskeletal Injuries of the Upper Extremity

Chapter 20
Low-back Pain

In This Chapter

About The Authors

Wendy Williamson, Ph.D., is nationally recognized as a leading educator and fitness professional and is a sought-after speaker in the areas of general personal-training education, medical exercise services, and post-rehabilitation. She was recognized by the American Council on Exercise (ACE) as one of the leading personal trainers in the nation in 2005 and 2006 and holds multiple personal training certificates from ACE and the National Academy of Sports Medicine. Dr. Williamson, who is a faculty member for ACE, recently completed her Ph.D. in exercise science at Oklahoma State University. She consults and continues to provide hands-on post-rehabilitation training in Wichita, Kansas. She also has an extensive track record in corporate and public health with an emphasis on middle school, high school, and college/university health and wellness curricula development.

Fabio Comana, M.A., M.S., is an exercise physiologist and spokesperson for the American Council on Exercise and faculty at San Diego State University and UC San Diego, teaching courses in exercise science and nutrition. He holds two master's degrees, one in Exercise Physiology and one in Nutrition, and certifications through ACE, ACSM, NSCA, and ISSN. Prior to joining ACE, he was a college head coach and the strength and conditioning coach at SDSU. Comana also managed health clubs for Club One. He lectures, conducts workshops, and writes on many topics related to exercise, fitness, and nutrition both nationally and internationally. As an ACE spokesperson and presenter, he is frequently featured in numerous media outlets including television, radio, Internet, and more than 100 nationwide newspaper and print publications. Comana has authored chapters in various textbooks.

CHAPTER 13

Posture and Movement

Wendy Williamson

Fabio Comana

The human body is designed to move and develop in response to the stresses placed upon the joints, bones, muscles, and tissues. Efficient movement often originates from good posture, defined as that state of musculoskeletal alignment and balance that allows muscles, joints, and nerves to function efficiently (Kendall et al., 2005). Correct posture contributes to the well-being of the individual by placing less stress on muscles, bones, and joints (Shultz, Houglum, & Perrin, 2005). Poor posture, on the other hand, is the faulty alignment of various body parts, producing increased stress and strain on supporting structures, ultimately compromising balance and movement efficiency and leading to degenerative changes and pain (Kendall et al., 2005). It is often perpetuated by muscle imbalance (Houglum, 2005).

"Stand tall… stop slouching… pull your shoulders back…" These familiar comments, which most people heard repeatedly throughout childhood and adolescence, are equally important in adulthood to cue better posture. Occupational and lifestyle positions (e.g., driving a car, working at a computer, repetitive movements, wearing high heels, holding static positions for long periods, improper weight-training techniques) and poor movement technique often create postural challenges that, over time, can result in poor posture and muscle imbalance. Muscle imbalance and postural deviations can be attributed to many factors, including the following:

- Repetitive movement (pattern overload)
- Habitual poor posture (positions and movements)
- Side dominance
- Poor joint integrity and stabilization
- Poor neuromuscular efficiency
- Poor or imbalanced muscle training
- Congenital conditions (e.g., scoliosis, polio)
- Pathologies (e.g., rheumatoid arthritis)
- Structural deviations (e.g., tibial or femoral torsion, femoral anteversion)
- Trauma (e.g.., surgery, injury, amputations)

Muscle imbalance generally alters physiological properties and function within muscle by changing the muscle's length-tension curve and force-coupling relationship (Sahrmann, 2002). This often alters movement at the joint (arthokinetics) and beyond the joint of origin (e.g., an anterior pelvic tilt may change the static position, and movement of, the cervical vertebrae) (Whiting & Rugg, 2006). As joints bear weight and move abnormally, the body strives to discover paths of lesser resistance (**law of facilitation**), potentially overloading the musculoskeletal system. This inevitably increases the likelihood of discomfort, injury, and pain. This sequence is illustrated in Figure 13-1. Often, the more advanced the dysfunction, and the more time that lapses, the more difficult the dysfunctions are to address.

Correct body mechanics can certainly assist in alignment and muscle balance and should always be the focus with restorative exercise. When there is associated pain, the ACE-certified Advanced Health & Fitness Specialist (ACE-AHFS) must always consult with a qualified medical professional.

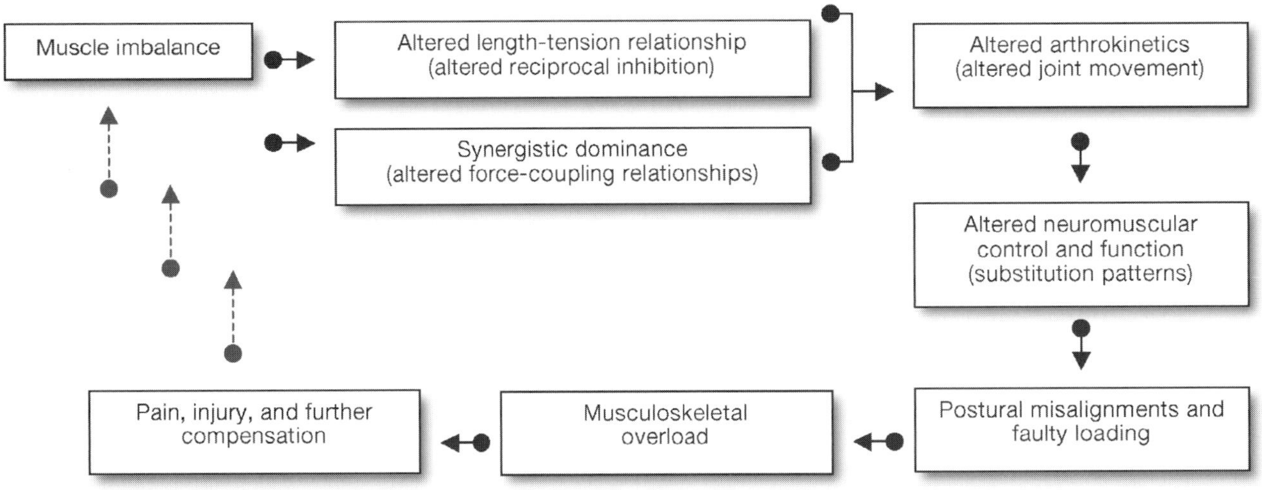

Figure 13-1
Pain-compensation cycle associated with muscle imbalance

Muscle Imbalance—Physiological Properties

The cause of muscle imbalance is often a loss of motion or flexibility within a muscle or muscle group, coupled with lengthening and weakening in the opposing muscle or muscle group. Generally, if an **agonist** shortens, its **antagonist** lengthens (Kendall et al., 2005). When faulty muscle positions are sustained over a period of time, a muscle's force-generating capacity changes in accordance with the length-tension curve.

Length-tension Relationship

The length-tension relationship explains the force-generating capacity of a **sarcomere,** the smallest functional unit of a muscle, and the orientation between the contractile proteins (e.g., **actin** and **myosin**) within a sarcomere. As illustrated in Figure 13-2, a slight stretching of the sarcomere beyond normal resting length increases the spatial arrangement between the muscle's contractile proteins and increases its force-generating capacity (Wilmore, Costill, & Kenney, 2008). Further stretching beyond optimal lengths, however, reduces the potential for contractile protein binding and reduces force-generating capacities. Since muscle is elastic, a sarcomere can generally elongate to 150 to 167% of its resting length, reaching thresholds for tissue failure beyond that point (MacIntosh, Gardiner, & McComas, 2006). In contrast, shortening the sarcomere beyond resting length results in an overlap of contractile proteins and also reduces force-generating potential.

Muscles can shorten in as little as two to four weeks when held in passively shortened positions without any stretching or use through a full or functional **range of motion (ROM).** For example, continuous bouts of sitting without any hip

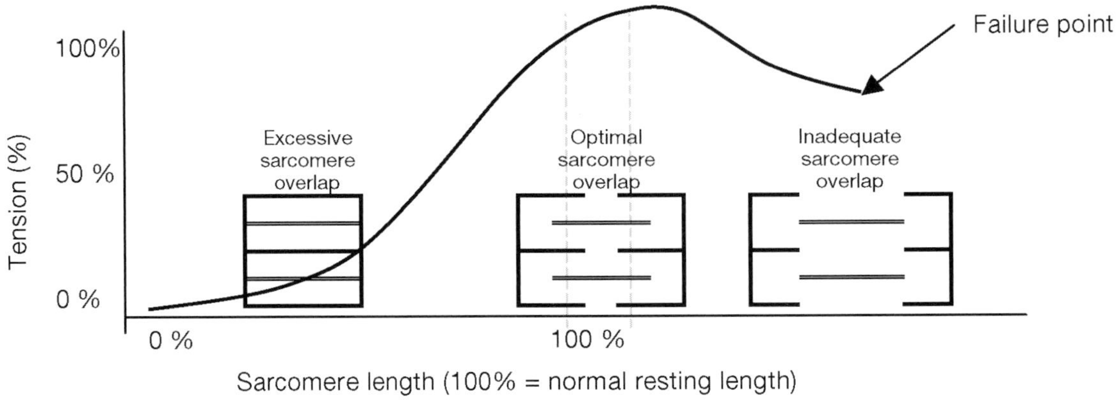

Figure 13-2
Length-tension relationship of a sarcomere

extension activity can shorten the iliopsoas. The adaptive shortening represents a loss of sarcomeres, shifting the length-tension curve to the left as illustrated in Figure 13-3 (MacIntosh, Gardiner, & McComas, 2006). The muscle may demonstrate greater force-generating capacities in shortened positions, but has reduced force-generating capacity in the normal resting-length or lengthened positions. Simply stretching a tight muscle does not restore its force-generating capacity in the normal-resting or stretched positions due to inadequate sarcomere quantity and sarcomere overlap. Following sustained periods of passive elongation of a tightened muscle, additional sarcomeres are added in series that will help restore normal resting-length and length-tension forces.

Muscles will also gradually lengthen when placed in elongated positions for prolonged periods of time. For example, repetitive sleeping on one's side moves the upper leg into **adduction,** potentially lengthening and weakening the gluteus medius. Repetitive sleeping on one's back with the weight of covers over the feet may potentially lengthen and weaken the dorsiflexors of the feet. Muscle lengthening represents the addition of sarcomeres in series, shifting the length-tension curve to the right and creating muscle weakness in normal resting-length positions due to the overlap of contractile proteins (MacIntosh, Gardiner, & McComas, 2006). The muscle may demonstrate greater force-generating capacities in lengthened positions (e.g., increasing the joint angle by 10 to 15 degrees), but has reduced force-generating capacity in the normal resting-length or shortened positions. Restoring normal resting-length and force-generating capacity requires a reverse of the physiological adaptation to lengthening and is best achieved by strengthening a muscle in normal resting-length positions and not in lengthened positions.

A tight agonist experiences a lowered activation threshold, which can be described as becoming overactive or **hypertonic.** Hypertonic muscles decrease neural activity to the lengthened antagonists via reciprocal inhibition and contribute to a progressive weakening (latency) of that muscle (Whittle, 2007). This may also produce another condition called **synergistic dominance**, in which the synergists carry out the primary function of a weakened or inhibited prime mover (Whittle, 2007). For example, a tight hip flexor may inhibit normal gluteus maximus function in hip extension. This forces a compensatory action of the hamstrings in extending the hip. The hamstrings, a synergist in hip extension, then act as a prime mover, potentially overtaxing the muscle and predisposing it to greater risk for injury.

Force-couple Relationship

Muscles rarely work in isolation, but rather function as integrated groups. Many muscles serve to provide opposing, directional, or contralateral pulls to achieve balanced movement, a term called force-coupling. For example, when the abdominal muscles pull upward on the anterior pelvis and the hamstring muscles pull downward on the ischial tuberosity of the pelvis, this creates a **force-couple** to rotate the pelvis posteriorly and flatten the lumbar spine. On the other hand, when the back extensors pull upward on the pelvis and the hip flexors pull downward on the pelvis, these muscles work as a force-couple to

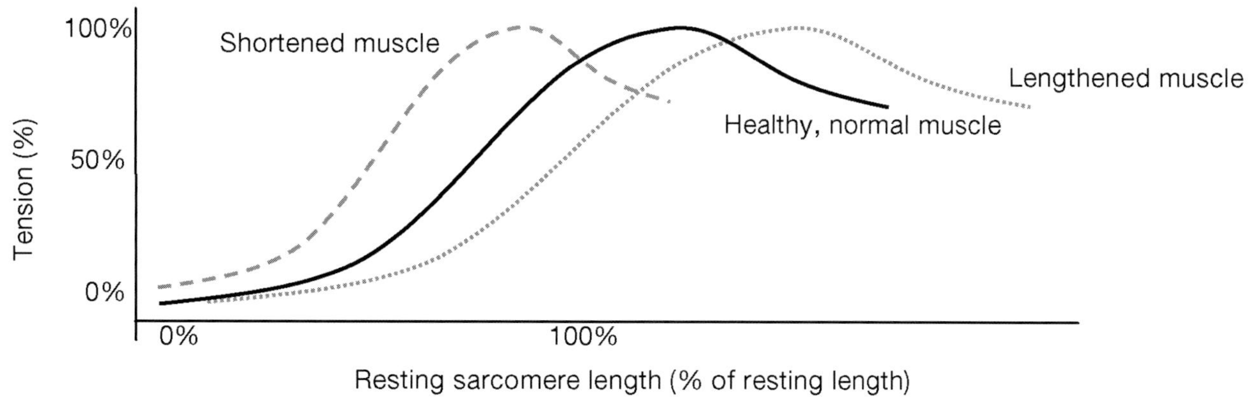

Figure 13-3
Alterations to the length-tension relationship of a sarcomere

rotate the pelvis anteriorly and extend the lumbar spine (Sahrmann, 2002). A neutral pelvis involves combined activation of the four muscles as illustrated in Figure 13-4:

- The rectus abdominis pulling upward on the anterior, inferior pelvis
- The hip flexors pulling downward on the anterior, superior pelvis
- The hamstrings pulling downward on the posterior, inferior pelvis
- The erector spinae group pulling upward on the posterior, superior pelvis

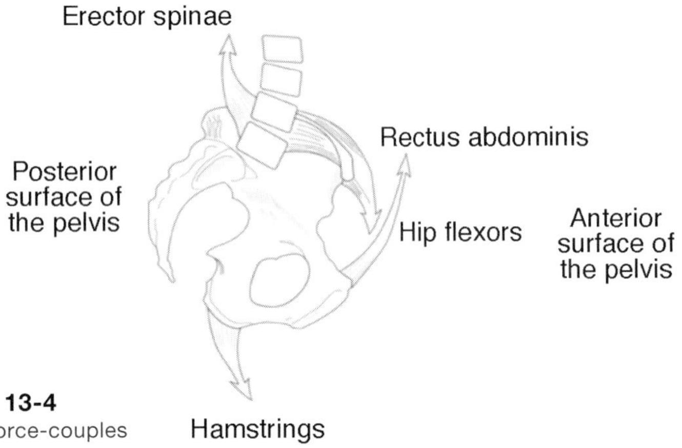

Figure 13-4
Pelvic force-couples

When these muscle groups are in balance, the pelvis achieves neutral position. Muscle imbalance, however, can position the pelvis into an anterior or posterior tilt. Vladimir Janda, a pioneer in postural research, termed this condition **lower cross syndrome** (Sahrmann, 2002). For example, hip flexor tightness pulls the pelvis anteriorly, producing possible shortening and tightening in the erector spinae group while the rectus abdominis and possibly the hamstrings become lengthened and weakened.

The shoulder has several force-couples that function during arm movement. It is important that the muscles within each of these force-couples remain balanced to provide optimal function. In the glenohumeral joint, the infraspinatus and teres minor form a force-couple with the subscapularis to control rotation of the humerus, and the rotator cuff group forms a force-couple with the deltoid to control arm **abduction** (Figure 13-5).

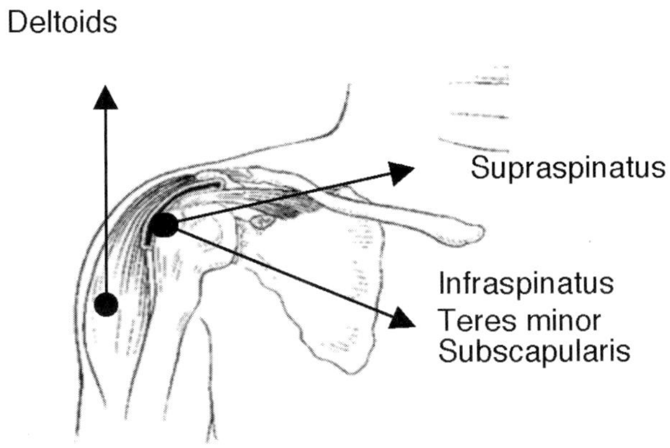

Figure 13-5
Force-couple at the shoulder

Force-couples that control rotation of the scapula include the upper and lower trapezius and the serratus anterior, which act to rotate the scapula upward, and the pectoralis minor, levator scapulae, and rhomboids, which control downward scapular rotation. The muscles within each force-couple must work cooperatively in both timing and level of intensity to produce the desired activity (Houglum, 2005).

The latissimus dorsi and pectoralis major are often overdeveloped in body builders and athletes compared to their posterior deltoids and rotator cuffs (infraspinatus and teres minor). This imbalance internally rotates the humerus, altering the articulation of the humeral head within the glenoid fossa and increasing musculoskeletal overload within the joint (Sahrmann, 2002). Likewise, the deltoids are often overdeveloped in body builders and athletes compared to the rotator cuff muscles. This destabilizes the glenohumeral joint during abduction. If upper trapezius action exceeds that of the lower trapezius and serratus anterior, the scapula may not rotate correctly during abduction and impingement of the rotator cuff may occur. However, the ACE-AHFS must also recognize that the body is an integrated chain and that trunk and lower-extremity stability and strength are important for scapular function. The legs and trunk provide 51 to 55% of the total kinetic energy and total force produced to complete overhead activities, while the shoulder itself only contributes 13% to the total energy production and 21% of the total force produced. For this reason, exercises for hip and trunk should be included in a shoulder strengthening, maintenance, or rehabilitation program (Houglum, 2005).

Forces generated from the legs, hips, trunk, shoulders, and arms are delivered through summation via the body's kinetic chain and ultimately delivered to the distal joint, or driver. These forces must be timed, directed, and applied in a specific sequence if the body is to work efficiently and effectively. This process requires a balance of muscle strength throughout all of the delivery systems involved (Houglum, 2005).

The following classification of muscles may assist in the understanding of how the muscles are applied within force-couples:

- *Agonist:* Prime mover; muscle that causes a desired motion
- *Antagonist:* Muscle that has the potential to oppose the action of the agonist
- *Synergist:* Muscle that assists the agonist in causing a desired action; may act as a joint stabilizer, neutralize rotation, or be activated when the external resistance increases, or when an agonist becomes fatigued or inhibited
- *Co-contraction:* Occurs when the agonist and antagonist contract together and a joint must be stabilized
- *Stabilizer:* A muscle that co-contracts to protect a joint and maintain alignment via strength and endurance

Overview of Postural Assessment

Postural assessments can provide information that guides exercise programming and helps the ACE-AHFS achieve an important objective of "straightening the body before strengthening it." This may potentially avoid exacerbating existing postural and movement compensations and muscle–joint imbalances. It is important to remember, however, that while postural assessments provide valuable information, they are only one piece (a starting point) of the movement efficiency puzzle, and therefore should not be overemphasized. The ACE-AHFS is encouraged to focus on the obvious, gross imbalances, and avoid getting caught up on minor postural asymmetries. Regardless, the ACE-AHFS must always respect the **scope of practice,** particularly in the presence of pain or injury, and understand the need for referral to more qualified professionals.

A static postural assessment may offer valuable insight into the following (Sahrmann, 2002):

- Muscle imbalance at a joint and the working relationships of muscles around a joint (e.g., agonists, antagonists, stabilizers)
- Potentially dysfunctional movement
- Altered neuromuscular coordination and control (sensory input and motor output)

A comprehensive approach to observing posture and its potential impact on movement involves three sequential steps (Figure 13-6):

- Client history (written and verbal)
  - ✔Collecting information on musculoskeletal issues, congenital issues, trauma, injuries, pain and discomfort, site(s) of pain or discomfort, and what aggravates and relieves pain or discomfort
  - ✔Collecting lifestyle information, including occupation, side dominance, and habitual patterns, although this piece of information may take time to gather
- Visual observation
  - ✔Identifying observable postural deviations
- Manual assessment
  - ✔ Verifying of muscle imbalance via muscle-length (and strength) testing
  - ✔ Determining impact on movement using movement screens
  - ✔ Cueing proper posture to distinguish correctible from non-correctible compensations (this may precede movement screens)

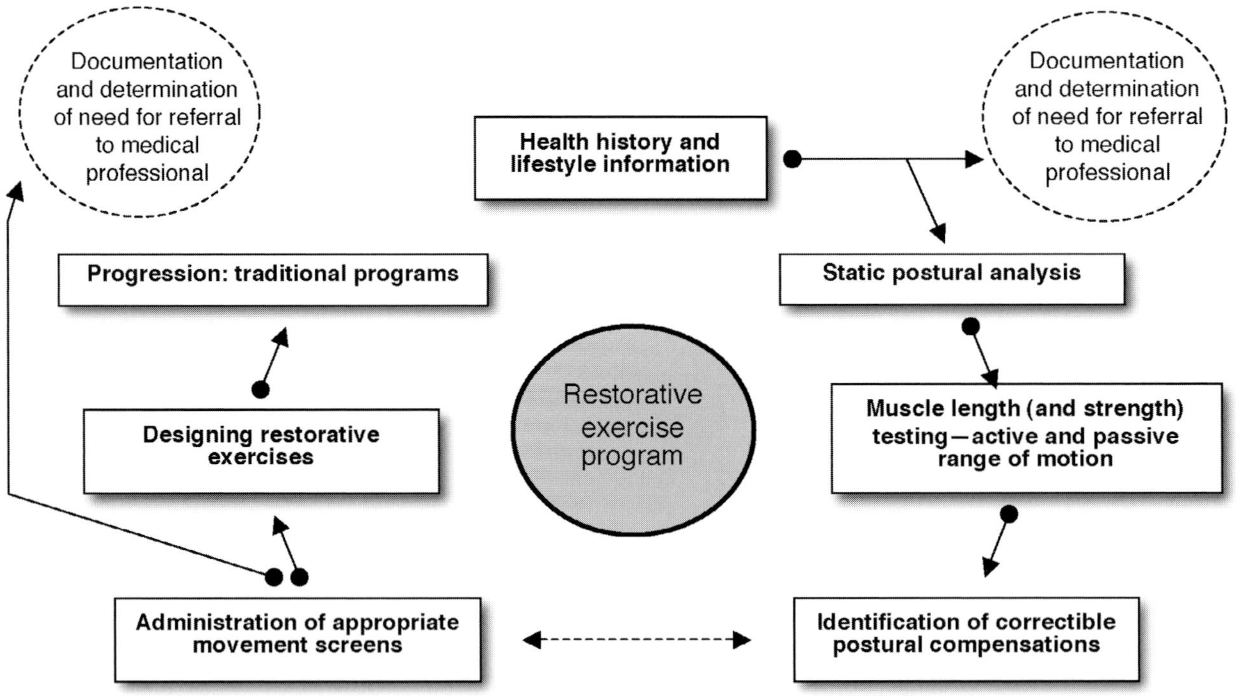

Figure 13-6
A chronological plan for observing posture and its potential impact on movement

The Right Angle Design of the Body

This model demonstrates how the human body represents itself in vertical alignment across four joints: the three main weightbearing joints and the shoulder joint (considered a minimal weightbearing joint). The main weightbearing joints are:

- The ankle (and subtalar) joint
- The knee joint
- The hip joint

This process divides the body into two hemispheres while observing symmetry between the joints in all three planes of motion. This implies a state in the **frontal plane** wherein the two halves appear as mirror images and in the **sagittal plane** where the anterior and posterior surfaces appear in balance, allowing the spine to display its natural curves (Figure 13-7) (Kendall et al., 2005). The body is in neutral position when the body parts are symmetrically balanced around the body's line of gravity, which represents the intersection of the mid-frontal and mid-sagittal planes. The reference of the body's line of gravity is achieved by hanging a plumbline from a fixed point above the client and positioning him or her behind the line in multiple planes to observe triplanar symmetry.

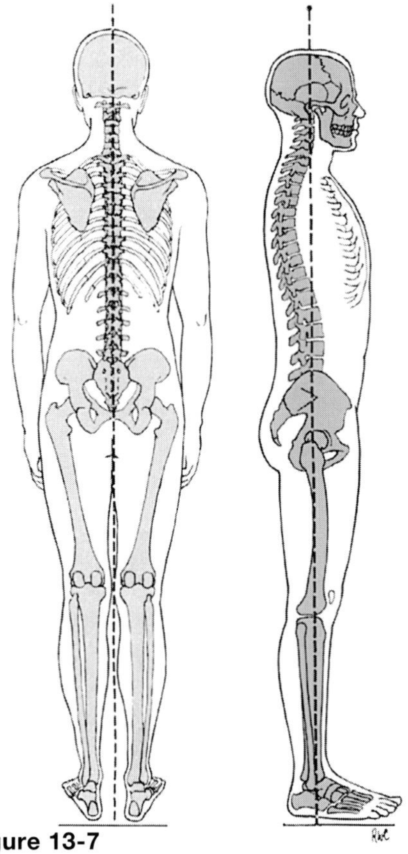

Figure 13-7
The right angle rule (frontal and sagittal views)

Source: LifeART image copyright 2008 Wolters Kluwer Health, Inc., Lippincott Williams & Wilkins.

Plumbline and Client Positioning, and Observation Guidelines

- Suspend a plumbline from the ceiling or a fixed point so that it hangs to approximately 0.5 to 1 inch (1.25 to 2.5 cm) above the floor.
- Use a solid, plain wall or backdrop, or a grid pattern that offers contrast against the client.
- Clients should wear form-fitting athletic-style clothing that exposes joints and bony landmarks. They should also remove their shoes.
- The use of adhesive dots placed on the bony landmarks may assist in identifying postural deviations.
- Focus on gross deviations that differ by ≥0.25 inches (0.6 cm)
- Understand that clients will consciously or subconsciously attempt to correct their posture under observation. Therefore, the ACE-AHFS should encourage them to assume a normal, relaxed position. Getting a person to talk as a distraction may relax his or her posture.
- Anterior view:
  - ✔ Position the individual between the plumbline and wall, facing the plumbline with the feet equidistant from the suspended line (use the medial malleoli as a reference).
  - ✔ The plumbline should ideally pass equidistant between the feet and ankles, intersecting the pubis, umbilicus, sternum, manubrium, mandible (chin), maxilla (face) and frontal bone (forehead) (Kendall et al., 2005; Shultz, Houglum, & Perrin, 2005).
- Posterior view:
  - ✔ Position the individual between the plumbline and wall, facing away from the plumbline with the heels equidistant from the suspended line.
  - ✔ The pumbline should ideally pass equidistant between the heels, intersecting the sacrum and overlapping the spinous processes of the vertebrae (Kendall et al., 2005; Shultz, Houglum, & Perrin, 2005).
- Sagittal view:
  - ✔ Position the individual between the plumbline and wall, facing sideways with the plumbline aligned immediately anterior to the lateral malleolus (i.e., the ankle bone).
  - ✔ The plumbline should ideally pass immediately anterior to the lateral malleolus, the anterior third of the knee, the greater trochanter of the femur, and the acromio-clavicular (A-C) joint, and slightly anterior to the mastoid process of the temporal bone of the skull (in line with the earlobe) or external auditory meatus (ear canal) (Kendall et al., 2005; Shultz, Houglum, & Perrin, 2005).
- Transverse view:
  - ✔ Transverse views involve the client standing in the frontal and sagittal plane positions.

Limitations

The ACE-AHFS must understand that limitations exist in using the right-angle model to identify postural imbalances. These limitations, which may not be correctible, include:

- Postural deviations attributed to congenital issues (e.g., scoliosis, polio, birth defects)
- Postural deviations attributed to pathologies (e.g., rheumatoid arthritis)
- Postural deviations attributed to structural issues (e.g., tibial or femoral torsion, femoral anteversion)
- Postural deviations attributed to trauma-type events (e.g., surgery, injury, amputation)

As the body ages, postural deviations become more pronounced. As muscles naturally weaken with age, structures become increasingly tight and less flexible. Therefore, pathological posture becomes even more apparent with aging, further increasing joint and muscle stresses

(Houglum, 2005). When removing stress or action from a joint, such as when lying supine at rest, it is possible that the body will assume a more neutral position. However, if a joint has remained out of correct anatomical position for a significant amount of time, this neutral return may be unlikely. In this case, while muscle imbalance can be improved or corrected, the structure may not return to neutral position.

Sometimes an individual acquires incorrect postural alignment because genetically determined joint or soft-tissue characteristics cause the deformity over time, or because the deformity present from birth becomes more apparent as the person ages (Kendall et al., 2005; Shultz, Houglum, & Perrin, 2005).

Standard Postural Deviations

Kyphosis represents excessive posterior curvature of the thoracic spine (Figure 13-8). The upper thoracic spine normally has a rounded contour, but this curve can be accentuated secondarily due to congenital factors, compensatory changes, muscular imbalance, joint disease, compression fractures, **osteoporosis** in older adults, and **Scheuermann's disease** in youth (i.e., juvenile kyphosis). Scheuermann's disease is a growth disorder characterized by inflammation and **osteochondritis** of the thoracic vertebrae. This degenerative condition narrows the anterior vertebral body at three or more levels secondary to axial and flexion overload (Shultz, Houglum, & Perrin, 2005).

Kyphosis is typically associated with rounded shoulders and tightness in the pectoralis major and minor and intercostals, counterbalanced by elongation and weakness in the thoracic erector spinae, rhomboids, and trapezius muscles (Kendall et al., 2005; Houglum, 2005). Scapulae abduction or protraction greater than the normal 2 inches (5 cm) from the vertebral spinous process is evident. Forward-head position generally results in tightness in the cervical extensors and lengthening in the cervical flexors.

It is common to see excessive thoracic kyphosis in response to excessive lumbar lordosis. This posture decreases the angle between the pelvis and the thigh anteriorly, resulting in tightness in the hip flexors with possible tightness in the low-back

Figure 13-8
Kyphosis-lordosis posture

Source: LifeART image copyright 2008 Wolters Kluwer Health, Inc., Lippincott Williams & Wilkins.

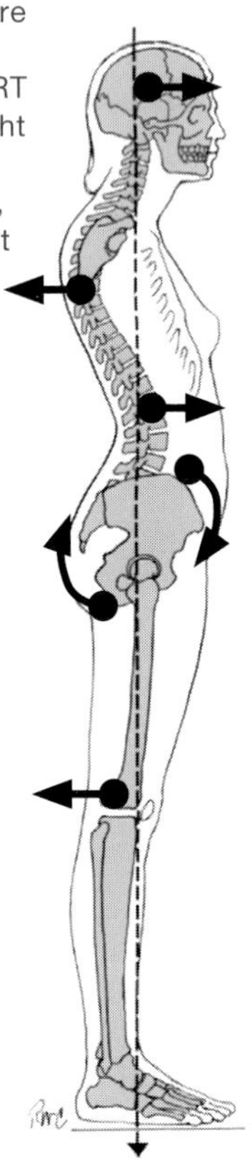

Static Position (sagittal)

Ankle and foot: Slight plantarflexion due to backward leg inclination
Knees: Slightly hyperextended
Hips and pelvis: Anterior tilt, flexed hip joint
Lumbar spine: Increased lordosis
Thoracic spine: Increased kyphosis
Shoulders (scapulae): Abducted (protraction)
Cervical spine: Hyperextended
Head: Forward

General Muscle Compensations

Hypertonic (short, tight, and strong)
- Calves
- Hip flexors
- Possibly lumbar extensors (if back does not flatten with sitting)
- Anterior chest muscles
- Neck extensors

Lengthened (weak and inhibited)
- Hip extensors (including hamstrings unless synergistically dominant)
- External oblique (may exclude rectus abdominis given chest depression with kyphosis)
- Upper-back extensors
- Scapular stabilizers
- Neck flexors

extensors if the back does not flatten with sitting (Kendall et al., 2005). While the external obliques are generally weak and elongated, the rectus abdominis may not be, given the chest depression associated with kyphosis (Kendall et al., 2005; Shultz, Houglum, & Perrin, 2005). The hamstrings are generally slightly elongated, but may not be weak given their increased responsibility in hip extension due to an inhibited gluteus maximus (synergistic dominance).

An individual with excessive lumbar lordosis may experience pain because of the extension in the lumbar spine (Sahrmann, 2002). The cause of lordosis varies; however, several common reasons are tight hip flexors, weak low-back extensors, and weak abdominal muscles, especially lower abdominals. If not addressed, the lordotic curve can eventually cause nerve root compression, **sciatica,** joint inflammation, degenerative disk problems, and vertebral changes as a result of the pressure and possible narrowing of the vertebral disk spaces. Accordingly, this narrowing of disk space may cause a narrowing of the intervertebral foramen and approximation of the vertebral articular facets.

Swayback posture is a long outward curve of the thoracic spine with a backward shift of the trunk starting from the pelvis (Figure 13-9). Swayback posture indicates a posterior tilt at the pelvis with hip extension, forward translation of the pelvis, and a flattening of the natural curve in the low back, although a backward lean is evident (Kendall et al., 2005). The ACE-AHFS must avoid confusion between swayback and excessive lordosis. Because the swayback alignment decreases the demands on the hip extensors, the gluteal muscles appear underdeveloped and usually test weak (Sahrmann, 2002). Clients who stand with a swayback posture will often walk with minimal use of the gluteus maximus muscle during the stance phase of **gait.** Runners with swayback posture who have atrophy and weakness of the gluteus maximus muscles can be predisposed to hamstring muscle strain (Sahrmann, 2002).

In a swayback state, the elongated and weak muscles include the neck flexors, external oblique, upper-back extensors, and one-joint hip joint flexors. The hamstrings and upper fibers of the internal obliques remain strong, but are shortened (Kendall et al., 2005).

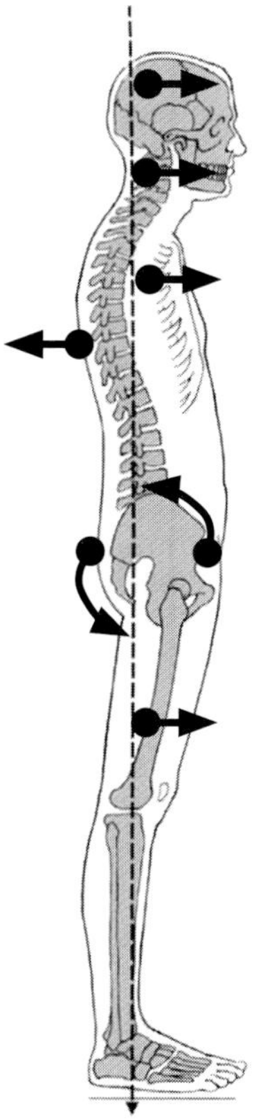

Figure 13-9
Swayback posture

Source: LifeART image copyright 2008 Wolters Kluwer Health, Inc., Lippincott Williams & Wilkins.

Static Position (sagittal)

Ankle and foot: Neutral (anterior displacement usually occurs between the knees and hips)
Knees: Hyperextended
Hips and pelvis: Hyperextended, anterior displacement and posterior tilt
Lumbar spine: Flattened (straight)
Thoracic spine: Increased kyphosis with posterior displacement of the upper trunk
Shoulders (scapulae): Varies
Cervical spine: Slightly extended
Head: Forward

General Muscle Compensations

Hypertonic (short, tight, and strong)
- Hamstrings
- Upper fibers of the internal oblique (posterior tilt), not the lower fibers (anterior displacement)
- Lumbar extensors (may not be short due to the posterior lean)
- Neck extensors

Lengthened (weak and inhibited)
- One-joint hip flexors
- Possibly rectus femoris (if posterior tilt is significant and knee hyperextension is small)
- External oblique (as the pelvis displaces anteriorly)
- Upper-back extensors
- Neck flexors

Similar to the swayback position, in the flat-back position the pelvis tilts backward and translates forward with the hip joint in extension and the low back flattened (Figure 13-10) (Kendall et al., 2005; Sahrmann, 2002). There is a corresponding decrease in the normal lordotic curve of the lower back and kyphotic curve in the upper back. As a result of the flat thoracic spine, the scapula appears to be winged (Sahrmann, 2002).

Lordotic, or military, posture is associated with an anterior tilt of the pelvis, increasing lordosis in the lumbar spine (Figure 13-11)

Figure 13-10
Flat-back posture

Source: LifeART image copyright 2008 Wolters Kluwer Health, Inc., Lippincott Williams & Wilkins. All rights reserved.

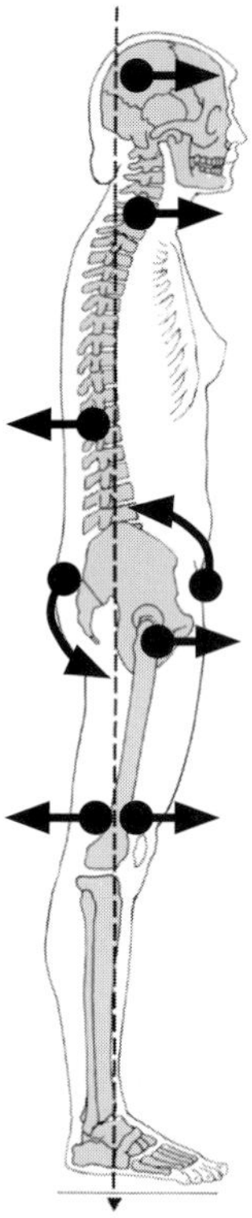

Static Position (sagittal)

Ankle and foot: Slight plantarflexion (slight backward leg inclination and knee extension)
Knees: Hyperextended or possibly in slight flexion
Hips and pelvis: Slight anterior displacement and posterior tilt, extended hips
Lumbar spine: Flattened or flexed (straight)
Thoracic spine: Flattened (straight) with increased flexion in the upper thoracic region
Shoulders (scapulae): Varies
Cervical spine: Slightly extended
Head: Forward

General Muscle Compensations

Hypertonic (short, tight, and strong)
- Hamstrings (especially if knees are in flexion)
- Rectus abdominis
- Possibly upper-back extensors
- Neck extensors
- Possibly ankle plantarflexors (if in plantarflexion)

Lengthened (weak and inhibited)
- One-joint hip flexors
- Possibly internal oblique (if pelvis does not displace anteriorly)
- Lumbar extensors
- Neck flexors

Figure 13-11
Lordotic, or military, posture

Source: LifeART image copyright 2008 Wolters Kluwer Health, Inc., Lippincott Williams & Wilkins. All rights reserved.

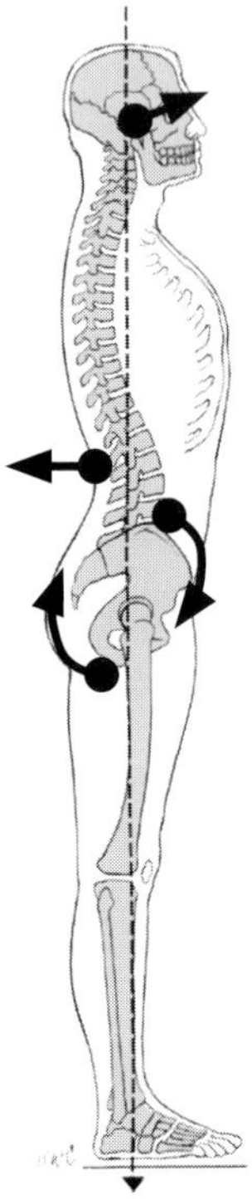

Static Position (sagittal)

Ankle and foot: Slightly plantarflexed
Knees: Slightly hyperextended
Hips and pelvis: Anterior tilt
Lumbar spine: Increased lordosis
Thoracic spine: Normal kyphosis
Shoulders (scapulae): Retracted, possible scapular adduction
Cervical spine: Normal lordosis or possible extension
Head: Neutral or possible upward head tilt

General Muscle Compensations

Hypertonic (short, tight, and strong)
- Hip flexors
- Low-back extensors
- Possibly neck extensors (with upward head tilt)

Lengthened (weak and inhibited)
- Rectus abdominis
- External oblique
- Hamstrings
- Possibly neck flexors (with upward head tilt)

(Kendall et al., 2005). This may create plantarflexion at the ankle and hyperextension in the knees. Additionally, the upper extremity might exhibit scapular adduction and extension in the cervical spine.

Side Dominance

Also called handedness, side dominance often begins at an early age and can result in postural changes due to a general over-reliance on the dominant side (Kendall et al., 2005). A right-handed individual may exhibit a right shoulder that is lower than the left given the frequency of reaching and the tendency to lean toward the right side. Consequently, the right hip appears higher than the left due to the right sideways lean of the body, which involves adducting the right hip and lengthening the right gluteus medius. This sideways lean may cause a slight deviation of the spine toward the left and force the left foot into more excessive pronation than the right foot.

Postural Assessment

The Ankle and Foot

Landmarks—frontal and transverse planes

- The client should remove his or her shoes and socks.
- The feet normally face forward approximately 3 inches (7.5 cm) apart, either in parallel or with an 8- to 10-degree toe-out from the midline. This small amount of toe-out is considered normal due to the ankle joint lying in an oblique plane with the medial malleolus slightly anterior to the lateral malleolus.
- The toes should be aligned neutrally with no abduction or adduction.
- No appearance of pronation or supination should exist at the subtalar joint. To help determine the subtalar position, the ACE-AHFS can palpate the joint by placing the thumb and index finger immediately behind the tendons of the extensor hallucis longus and digitorum longus (immediately anterior to the malleoli). The ACE-AHFS should ask the client to maximally pronate and supinate the foot to determine which movement demonstrates a greater degree of movement. This indicates whether he or she normally stands more in pronation or supination.
- The Achilles tendon orientates at 90 degrees with the floor (posterior view).

Landmarks—sagittal plane

- The plumbline lies slightly anterior of the lateral malleolus of the fibula.
- The longitudinal arch of foot appears neutral with the weight evenly distributed over the heel and ball of the foot.
- There appears to be 5 to 10 degrees of ankle dorsiflexion from vertical alignment.

Common deviations

- Overpronation at the subtalar joint that generally forces foot eversion (Figure 13-12).
- Lack of dorsiflexion at the ankle joint that usually follows overpronation. Pronation abducts the foot and raises the lateral side of the heel, potentially shortening the gastrocnemius and soleus.

Overpronation at the subtalar joint generally internally rotates the tibia, resulting in knee abduction (**valgus** strain). During gait, the knee tries to align itself forward in the sagittal plane to facilitate knee flexion and extension. An everted foot changes the loading at the foot, transferring more to the medial surface of the foot, consequently increasing the likelihood of bunions at the first metatarsal head. Abduction of the big toe and calluses along the medial surface of the big toe may also be present. Adjusting the subtalar and foot position may result in the client demonstrating a toe grip due to the reduced or altered base of support. Tightness and tenderness in the plantar fascia are often experienced

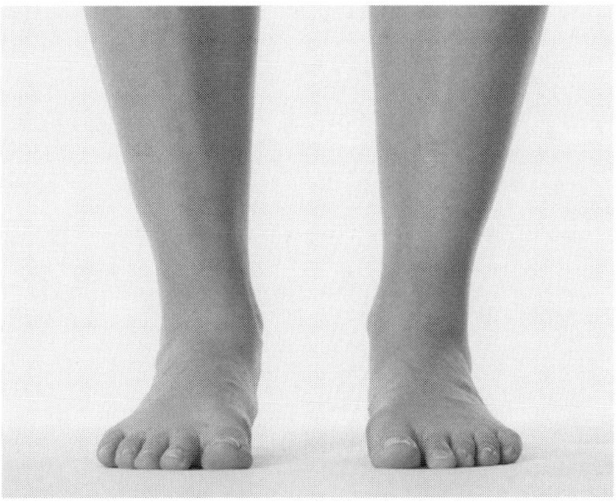

Figure 13-12
Overpronation

with pronation due to lengthening of the fascia. Tables 13-1 and 13-2 list the key deviations of the ankle and foot in various planes of motion.

The Knee

Landmarks—frontal and transverse planes

- Direction of patella (anterior view)—internal or external rotation
- Direction of popliteal groove (posterior view)—internal or external rotation

Landmarks—sagittal plane

- The plumbline should pass through the anterior third of the knee.

Common deviations

- Internal rotation at the knee is generally associated with pronation and may force valgus strain (Figure 13-13). However, the ACE-AHFS must be aware of tibial torsion that creates anomalies. To determine the difference, the ACE-AHFS can have the client establish neutral subtalar position and observe the orientation of the tibia and knee.
- Hyperextension at the knee associated with tight posterior muscles and swayback posture

The design of the knee imparts little support to joint stability, because it sits in the middle of

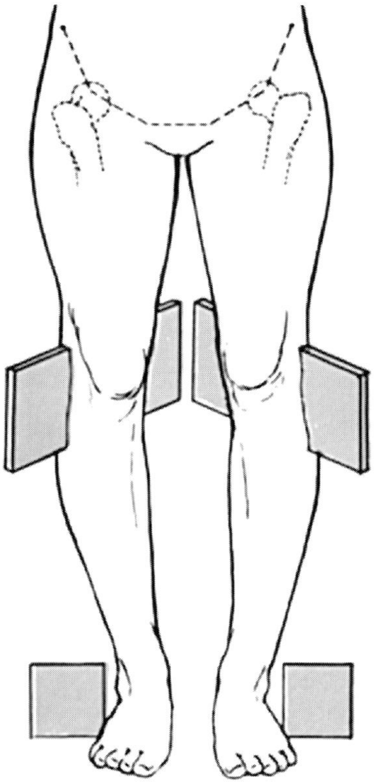

Figure 13-13
Internal rotation of the knees

Source: LifeART image copyright 2008 Wolters Kluwer Health, Inc., Lippincott Williams & Wilkins. All rights reserved.

Table 13-1
Key Deviations of the Ankle and Foot—Frontal and Transverse Planes

Observation	Criteria	Tightness	Lengthening
Pronation	Flattened longitudinal arch in pronation (flat feet)	Peroneal group and toe extensors	Tibialis posterior, toe flexors, and possibly tibialis anterior
Supination	Increased longitudinal arch in supination (high arch)	Tibialis anterior and posterior	Peroneal group and toe flexors

Table 13-2
Key Deviations of the Ankle and Foot—Sagittal Plane

Observation	Criteria	Tightness	Lengthening
Dorsiflexed ankle	Greater than 10 degrees of ankle dorsiflexion from vertical (weight shifted forward)	Anterior muscles (tibialis and peroneal groups)	Gastrocnemius and soleus
Plantarflexed ankle	Less than 5 degrees of ankle dorsiflexion from vertical (weight shifted backward)	Gastrocnemius and soleus	Anterior muscles (tibialis and peroneal groups)

two long lever-arms exposed to large forces. Gray and Tiberio (2007) refer to the knee as a "reactor," as it simply responds to drivers from above and below that act in three dimensions. These drivers constitute ground reaction forces, gravity, loads, and momentum. During loading of the foot, the ankle joint creates a chain reaction from the ground up that influences the knee. The natural tendency is toward calcaneal eversion and pronation, coupled with internal tibial rotation and knee abduction (valgus position), and internal femoral rotation, placing heavier stresses on the anterior cruciate ligament (ACL). The body is designed to resist this internal rotational movement and corresponding stresses by having:

- Big posterior-lateral muscles at the hips to decelerate the internal rotation
- A big medial collateral ligament (MCL) to resist excessive knee abduction
- Stronger deltoid ligaments (medial surface at the ankle) to resist excessive pronation

The ACL is a very important stabilizer of the femur on the tibia and serves to prevent the tibia from sliding forward (anterior translation) and rotating excessively inward during agility, jumping, and deceleration activities. Greater engagement of the gluteus maximus during knee and hip flexion prevents excessive internal tibial rotation and knee abduction, thereby helping unload the ACL (Gray & Tiberio, 2007). Additionally, greater engagement of the gluteus maximus during knee flexion activates the hamstrings that pull backward on the posterior tibia, helping unload the ACL. Tables 13-3 and 13-4 list key deviations of the knee in various planes.

The Lumbo-pelvic Region and Hip

Hip landmarks—frontal and transverse planes

- Alignment of the iliac crest and greater trochanters (anterior view)
- Discrepancies in the level of the gluteal folds and differences in gluteal definition (posterior view)

Table 13-3
Key Deviations of the Knee—Frontal and Transverse Plane

Observation	Criteria	Tightness	Lengthening
Knee position	Asymmetries between knee heights and spacing from plumbline may indicate limb-length discrepancies.		
Genu valgum (valgus)	Knock-knee appearance (hip adduction and knee abduction, ankle pronation)	Medial hip rotators, TFL, and lateral knee joint structures	Medial knee joint structures
Genu varum (varus)	Bow-legged appearance (hip joint medial rotation, knee joint hyperextension, ankle pronation)	Medial hip rotators, quadriceps, foot everters	Hip lateral rotators popliteus, and tibialis posterior

Note: TFL = Tensor fasciae latae

Table 13-4
Key Deviations of the Knee—Sagittal Plane

Observation	Criteria	Tightness	Lengthening
Hyperextended knee*	Associated with plantarflexion at the ankle	Quadriceps and soleus (not gastrocnemius) due to knee hyperextension	Hamstrings
Flexed knee*	Less common, associated with ankle dorsiflexion	Hamstrings and gastrocnemius	Quadriceps and soleus

*Dependent on pelvic position (tilt and translation)

Pelvis landmarks—frontal and transverse planes
- Position of the iliac crests, anterior superior iliac spine (ASIS) and posterior superior iliac spine (PSIS)
- Using a dowel across the hips can help identify a level pelvis (Figure 13-14)
- Relationship of the umbilicus and pubis reflects lumbo-pelvic alignment and possible lumbar deviation or pelvic listing

Hip landmark—sagittal plane
- Plumbline passing through the greater trochanter of the femur

Pelvis landmarks—sagittal plane (Figure 13-15)
- Relative positions of the ASIS and PSIS, although this is not a valid marker for estimating pelvic tilt, given structural variations in the pelvis. Generally, the ASIS lies lower than the PSIS, with the ASIS–PSIS angle deviating approximately 10 to 15 degrees from horizontal in men and between 5 and 10 degrees in women. In addition, the PSIS is difficult to locate, especially in obese individuals.

Alternative methods to determine pelvic tilt include observing the angle of the waistline of pants or observing the alignment of the pubic bone and the ASIS, which lie vertical in a neutral pelvis.

Common deviations
- Anterior pelvic tilt due to tight hip flexors (see Figure 13-15)
- Hip adduction (and lateral pelvic tilt) on the more dominant side due to the sideways lean to the dominant side (Figure 13-16).
- Excessive pronation at the foot and associated internal rotation at the knee normally internally rotates the femur and forces an anterior tilt at the pelvis to accommodate femural rotation, increasing lordosis in the lumbar spine.

Tables 13-5 and 13-6 list key deviations of the lumbo-pelvic region and hip in various planes.

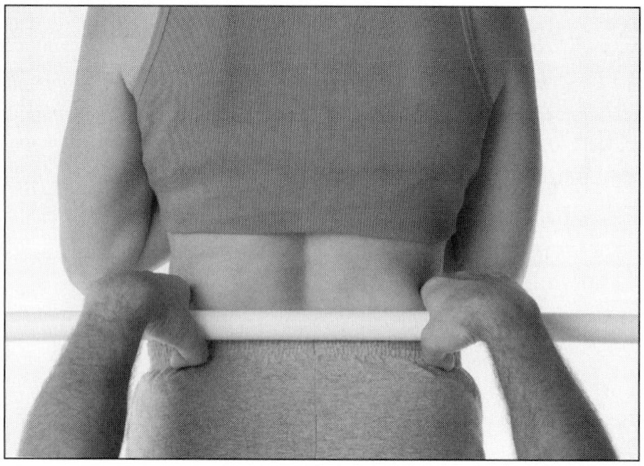

Figure 13-14
Dowel placement to determine level pelvis

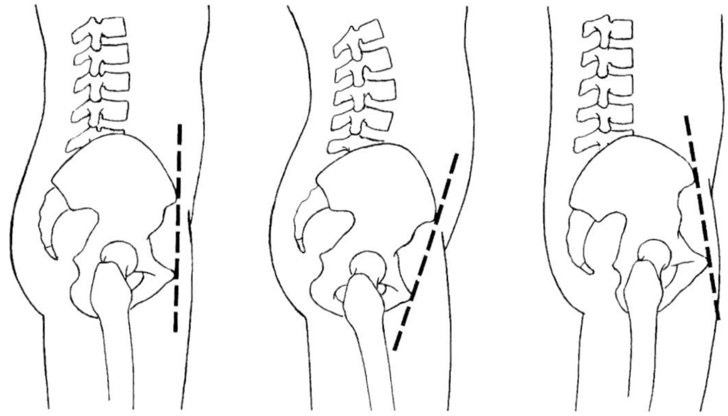

Figure 13-15
Alignment of the ASIS and pubic bone

Source: LifeART image copyright 2008 Wolters Kluwer Health, Inc., Lippincott Williams & Wilkins.

The Thoracic Spine and Shoulders

Spine landmarks—frontal and transverse planes
- Alignment of the umbilicus, sternum, and manubrium with the plumbline (anterior view)
- Even spacing between arms and torso on each side (anterior and posterior view)
- Alignment of the spinous processes of the spine with the plumbline (posterior view)

Shoulder landmarks—frontal and transverse plane
- Acromioclavicular (AC) joint, clavicle, antecubital fossa. and hand position (anterior view)

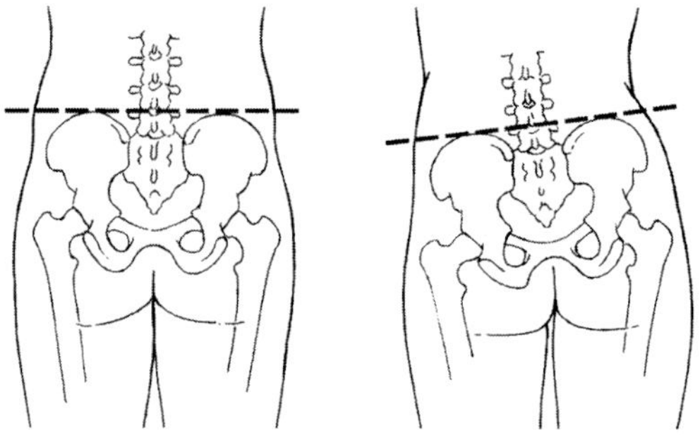

Figure 13-16
Normal hip position versus right hip adduction

Source: LifeART image copyright 2008 Wolters Kluwer Health, Inc., Lippincott Williams & Wilkins.

Table 13-5
Key Deviations of the Lumbo-pelvic Region and Hip—Frontal and Transverse Planes

Observation	Criteria	Tightness	Lengthening
Hip adduction (with possible c-curve in spine)	Hip tilts laterally	High-side adductors, low-side abductors and TFL, high-side lateral trunk muscles	High-side abductors (especially gluteus medius) and TFL, low-side adductors, low-side lateral trunk muscles
Medial (forward) rotation	>0.25-inch (0.6 cm) difference between ASIS positions	TFL, anterior fibers of gluteus medius	Lateral hip rotators
Lateral (backward) rotation	>0.25-inch (0.6 cm) difference between ASIS positions	Lateral hip rotators	TFL, anterior fibers of gluteus medius

Note: TFL = Tensor fasciae latae; ASIS = Anterior superior iliac spine

Table 13-6
Key Deviations of the Lumbo-pelvic Region and Hip—Sagittal Plane

Observation	Criteria	Tightness	Lengthening
Lordosis	Anterior pelvic tilt with excessive lumbar spine extension	Lumbar extensors (if back does not flatten with sitting), upper internal oblique	Rectus abdominis (if chest does not depress), external oblique
Flat back	Posterior pelvic tilt and anterior displacement with lumbar spine flexion	Rectus abdominis, external oblique	Lumbar extensors, internal oblique (if pelvis does not displace anteriorly)
Swayback	Posterior pelvic tilt and anterior displacement with flattened spine and posterior lean	Upper fibers of external oblique (due to posterior tilt—not lower fibers due to anterior displacement), lumbar extensors (short, but strong)	External oblique as pelvis displaces anteriorly

- Use of a dowel placed across the spine of the scapula can help determine if the shoulders are level.
- Spine of the scapula, inferior angle and medial border of scapula, and elbow (posterior view)
- The scapulae should lie flat against the upper back with up to 30 degrees of forward rotation in the frontal plane due to the rounded shape of the ribcage
- Vertebral border approximately 2 to 2.5 inches (5 to 6 cm) from the spine. The ACE-AHFS can look at the width and breadth of the ribcage to make this determination.
- Arm position with hands in neutral position (palms parallel to torso)

Spine landmarks—sagittal plane

- Increases or losses in the natural spinal curves
- Differentiate between kyphosis and scapular protraction, or winging
- Orientation of the top of the manubrium versus the C-7 spinous process. A higher position of C-7 is generally evident with kyphosis.

Shoulder landmarks—sagittal plane

- Acromioclavicular (AC) joint position relative to the plumbline
- Left and right elbow position relative to the plumbline
- Scapulae position (**protraction, retraction,** and anterior tilting)

Common deviations

- Excessive kyphosis and depressed chest
- Winging scapula or protracted scapula
- Internal rotation of humerus due to lifestyle-related factors such as repetitive motion and awkward postures

Tables 13-7 and 13-8 list key deviations of the thoracic spine and shoulders in various planes.

The Neck and Head

Landmarks—frontal and transverse plane

- Alignment of the chin, eyes, and forehead with the plumbline (anterior view)

Table 13-7
Key Deviations of the Thoracic Spine and Shoulders—Frontal and Transverse Planes

Observation	Criteria	Tightness	Lengthening
Spine			
Arm spacing	Differences in arm space may indicate lateral torso deviation		
Lateral flexion	Deviation of spinous processes from plumbline	Lateral trunk flexors (flexed side)	Lateral trunk flexors (extended side)
Paraspinal asymmetry	≥0.5 inch (1.3 cm) difference in muscle hypertrophy (spine rotates toward the hypertrophied side) Tightness in the paraspinal muscles on the rotated side		
Spinal rotation or scoliosis	Identified with a forward bend movement, with ribs possibly more prominent on one side		
Shoulders			
Elevated scapulae	Scapula lying higher than T2 position	Upper trapezius, levator scapula, and rhomboids	Lower trapezius
Abducted (forward) scapulae	Vertebral border >3 inches (7.5 cm) from the spine and rotated in the frontal plane >30 degrees, usually accompanied by elevated shoulders	Serratus anterior, anterior scapulohumeral muscles, upper trapezius	Rhomboids, lower trapezius muscles
Medially rotated humerus	Cubital fossa faces medially, olecranon process faces laterally, hands may be internally rotated	Pectoralis major, latissimus dorsi, and medial rotator cuff muscle	Lateral rotator cuff muscles, posterior deltoid

Table 13-8
Key Deviations of the Thoracic Spine and Shoulders—Sagittal Plane

Observation	Criteria	Tightness	Lengthening
Thoracic Spine			
Kyphosis and depressed chest	Thoracic spine flexion, diminished intercostal space	Shoulder adductors, pectoralis minor, and rectus abdominis; internal obliques with depressed chest	Thoracic paraspinal muscles and middle/lower trapezius
Flat back	Loss of the natural spinal curves	Thoracic paraspinal muscles, external obliques	Lateral hip rotators
Swayback	Position with hips forward in posterior tilt position while shoulders are >2 inches (5 cm) posterior to greater trochanters	Rectus abdominis, internal obliques	Lengthening of the external obliques
Shoulders			
Winging (anterior tilt)	Inferior angle and vertebral border protrude from the thorax (may occur with a flat thorax)	Serratus anterior, pectoralis minor, teres major, anterior scapulohumeral muscles	Lower trapezius muscles
Forward shoulders	Usually abducted and elevated	Serratus anterior, pectoralis minor, upper trapezius	Middle and lower trapezius

- Alignment of the cervical vertebra with the plumbline (posterior view)

Landmarks—sagittal plane

- Alignment of the mastoid process with the plumbline and the level of the chin as landmarks
- Head orientation (tilting)

Most common deviation

- Forward head position (Figure 13-17). The ACE-AHFS can look at the alignment of the cheek bone to collarbone; they should almost be in vertical alignment.

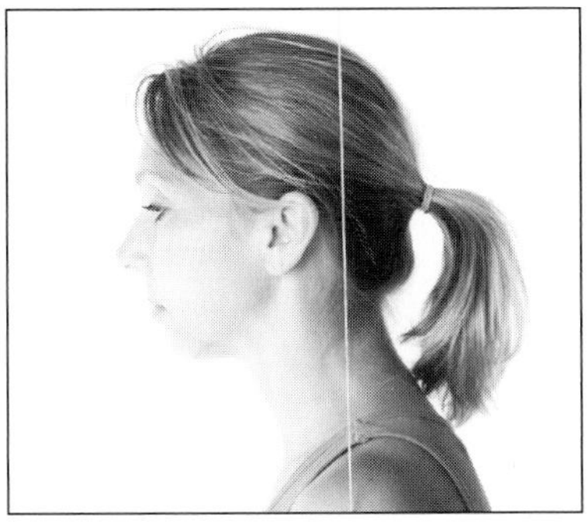

Figure 13-17
Forward head position

Tables 13-9 and 13-10 list key deviations of the neck and head in various planes.

The checklists and worksheets presented in Tables 13-1 through 13-10 and Figures 13-18 through 13-20 may be useful tools to use when performing postural assessments.

Musculoskeletal and Congenital Considerations

Most postural deviations observed in childhood fall into the category of developmental deviations; when patterns become habitual, they may result in postural faults. Developmental deviations are those that appear in many children at approximately the same age and that improve or disappear without any corrective treatment, sometimes even despite unfavorable environmental influences.

Table 13-9
Key Deviations of the Neck and Head—Frontal and Transverse Plane

Observation	Criteria	Tightness	Lengthening
Head rotation	Deviation of landmarks from plumbline in transverse plane; contraction of the SCM rotates the head in the opposite direction	Ipsilateral capitus (spinalis, longissimus, and smaller muscles); contralateral SCM	Contralateral capitus (spinalis, longissimus, and smaller muscles); ipsilateral SCM
Head lateral tilt	Deviation of landmarks from plumbline in frontal plane; contraction of the SCM	Ipsilateral capitus (spinalis, longissimus and smaller muscles); ipsilateral SCM	Contralateral capitus (spinalis, longissimus, and smaller muscles); contralateral SCM

Note: SCM = Sternocleidomastoid

Table 13-10
Key Deviations of the Head and Neck—Sagittal Plane

Observation	Criteria	Tightness	Lengthening
Head forward tilt	Chin should sit higher than the clavicle [>1–2 inches (2.5–5 cm)]	Cervical spine flexors	Cervical spine extensors
Head forward position	Head forward with straight cervical spine	Cervical spine extensors, upper trapezius, levator scapulae	Cervical spine flexors

Figure 13-18
Postural assessment checklist

Frontal View	
☐	Overall body symmetry: symmetrical alignment of the left and right hemispheres
☐	Ankle position: observe for pronation and supination
☐	Foot position: observe for inversion and eversion
☐	Knees: rotation and height discrepancies
☐	Hip adduction and shifting: observe for shifting to a side as witnessed by the position of the pubis in relation to the plumbline
☐	Alignment of the iliac crests
☐	Alignment of the torso: position of the umbilicus and sternum in relation to the plumbline
☐	Alignment of the shoulders
☐	Arm spacing: observe the space to the sides of the torso
☐	Hand position: observe the position relative to the torso
☐	Head position: alignment of the ears, nose, eyes, and chin
Posterior View	
☐	Overall body symmetry: symmetrical alignment of the left and right hemispheres
☐	Achilles alignment: observe for vertical orientation of tendon
☐	Calf development and tone
☐	Alignment of the popliteal line: observe for valgus/varus strain
☐	Alignment of the gluteal folds: observe for muscle tone
☐	Alignments of the iliac crests and PSIS: observe oblique folds immediately above the iliac crest
☐	Alignment of the spine: vertical alignment of the spinous processes (may require forward bending)
☐	Alignment of the scapulae: inferior angle of scapulae and presences of winged scapulae
☐	Alignment of the shoulders
☐	Head position: alignment of the ears
Sagittal View	
☐	Overall body symmetry: symmetrical alignment of load-bearing joint landmarks with the plumbline
☐	Knees: flexion or extension
☐	Hip position: forward (swayback) or back position
☐	Pelvic alignment for tilting: relationship of ASIS to PSIS
☐	Spinal curves: observe for thoracic kyphosis, lumbar lordosis, or flat-back position
☐	Shoulder position: evidence of forward rounding (protraction) of the scapulae
☐	Head position: neutral cervical curvature (forward position) and level (position above the clavicle)
Transverse View	
☐	Overall body symmetry: rotational deviations from all views
☐	Ankles and feet: observe for inversion or eversion
☐	Knees/femurs: observe for internal or external rotation at the knees
☐	Hips: observe for rotation of ASIS and PSIS
☐	Arms: observe for internal or external rotation of the arms by hand position
☐	Chest: observe for rotational deviation of thorax (sternum from the plumbline)
☐	Head position: rotational deviation

Note: PSIS = Posterior superior iliac spine; ASIS = Anterior superior iliac spine

Figure 13-19
Anterior/posterior worksheet

Anterior View:			**Posterior View:**		
L	**R**	**Deviation**	**L**	**R**	**Deviation**
☐	☐	1. ______	☐	☐	1. ______
☐	☐	2. ______	☐	☐	2. ______
☐	☐	3. ______	☐	☐	3. ______
☐	☐	4. ______	☐	☐	4. ______
☐	☐	5. ______	☐	☐	5. ______
☐	☐	6. ______	☐	☐	6. ______
☐	☐	7. ______	☐	☐	7. ______

Circle or mark observed deviations

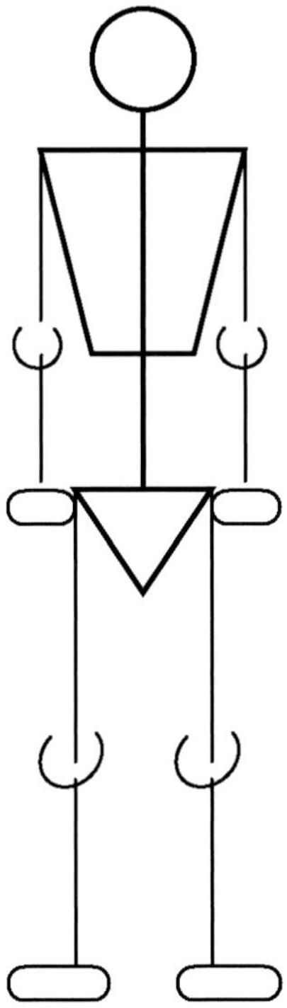

Circle or mark observed deviations

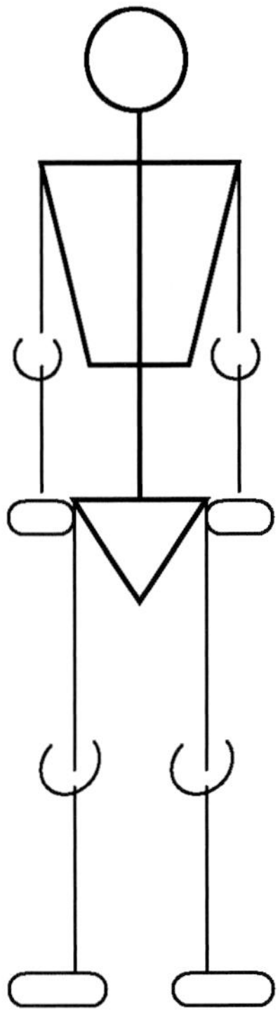

Figure 13-20
Sagittal worksheet

Sagittal: Left Side		**Sagittal: Right Side**	
L	**Deviation**	**R**	**Deviation**
☐	1. ______	☐	1. ______
☐	2. ______	☐	2. ______
☐	3. ______	☐	3. ______
☐	4. ______	☐	4. ______
☐	5. ______	☐	5. ______
☐	6. ______	☐	6. ______
☐	7. ______	☐	7. ______

Circle or mark observed deviations

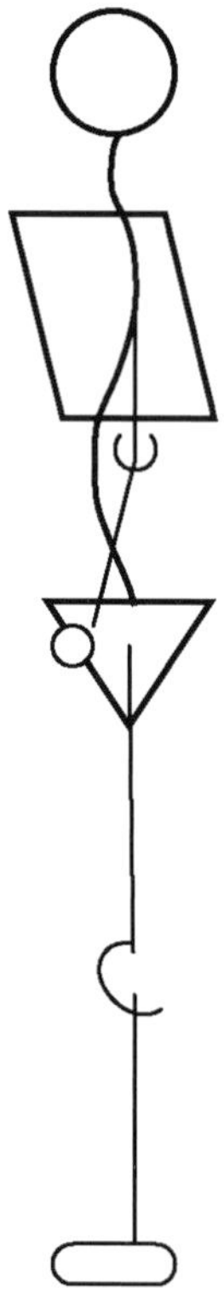

Circle or mark observed deviations

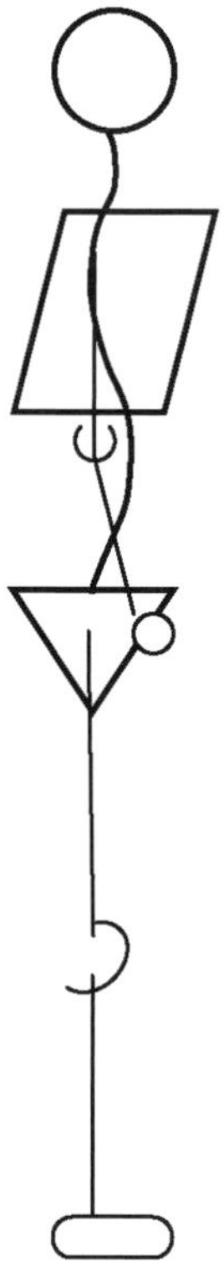

If deviations become static or the deviations increase, corrective measures are indicated. Severe faults need treatment as soon as they are observed, regardless of the age of the individual. A young child is not likely to have habitual faults and can actually be harmed by unnecessary corrective measures.

Incorrect posture can gradually develop with changes in the muscles, tendons, or fascial support. Children under the age of four generally have good posture and mechanics. As young as elementary school, children develop poor sitting and standing habits, and abnormal posture becomes apparent. By the time children reach their teenage or young-adult years, abnormal postural habits are entrenched. Poor posture becomes more exaggerated as people age and develop progressively greater tightness and weakness in already shortened or lengthened soft-tissue structures, resulting in changes in bone alignment and stress distribution (Shultz, Houglum, & Perrin, 2005).

Maintaining good nutrition is particularly significant for the proper structural development of skeletal and muscular tissues. After growth is completed, poor nutrition is less likely to cause structural faults that directly affect posture.

Certain physical defects, diseases, and disabilities have associated postural problems (e.g., visual and auditory impairments, clubfoot, hip dislocation, amputations of a lower extremity) (Kendall et al., 2005).

Children who have postural faults may also experience bowlegs **(varus).** Postural bowing is a deviation associated with knee hyperextension and hip medial rotation. Bowlegs may also be a result of compensation for knock knees **(valgus).** This condition usually disappears when an individual is in a recumbent position (Kendall et al., 2005).

Muscle Length Testing

As illustrated in Figure 13-6, after completing the static postural assessment, the ACE-AHFS may want to validate his or her observations by measuring the length of specific muscles. Table 13-11 provides the average range of motion for healthy adults for movements at each joint.

Determining Correctible Posture

It is imperative to distinguish correctible from non-correctible postural compensations. While a client's health history may provide valuable information to make this determination, the objective is to cue the client to move the joint in question toward neutral and evaluate his or her ability to do so without compromise or pain. Because the body is one continuous kinetic chain, the desired movement of one joint may require undesirable compensation at another (e.g., an individual presenting with kyphosis may increase lordosis when moving into thoracic extension). It is important to differentiate undesirable compensations from desirable compensations (e.g., an undesirable compensation to avoid is increasing lordosis with thoracic extension, while a desirable compensation is to facilitate natural posterior tilting of the pelvis as one moves into supination at the feet).

When cueing clients into neutral posture, effective strategies to increase awareness of muscle imbalance include the use of mirrors and touching so that clients can observe and feel the correction to a desired position. The ACE-AHFS must provide cues to help clients understand the desired joint movement (e.g., when cueing abdominal engagement and a posterior pelvic tilt, the ACE-AHFS can instruct the client to place his or her hands over the iliac crest and ASIS, look down to count the number of visible fingers, then cue a contraction to see more fingers). When cueing a movement toward neutral, the ACE-AHFS should have the client attempt to hold the position for 10 to 15 seconds. Success in achieving this position without pain or undesirable compensation along the kinetic chain gives a good indication that the muscle imbalance is correctible (e.g., while stabilizing the low back firmly against a backrest of a chair, a kyphotic individual is successful in moving into thoracic extension for 10 to 15 seconds). As this may prove difficult with more deconditioned individuals or those suffering from poor posture, the ACE-AHFS

Table 13-11
Average Range of Motion for Healthy Adults

Joint and Movement	ROM (degrees)	Joint and Movement	ROM (degrees)
Shoulder		**Thoraco-lumbar Spine**	
Flexion	150–180	Flexion	60–80
Extension	50–60	Extension	20–30
Abduction	180	Lateral flexion	25–35
Medial rotation	70–80	Rotation	30–45
Lateral rotation	90		
Horizontal abduction	90*	**Hip**	
Horizontal adduction	30–40*	Flexion	100–120
		Extension	30
Elbow		Abduction	40–45
Flexion	145	Adduction	20–30
Extension	0	Medial rotation	35–45
		Lateral rotation	45–50
Radio-ulnar			
Pronation	90	**Knee**	
Supination	90	Flexion	125–145
		Extension	0–10
Wrist			
Flexion	80	**Ankle**	
Extension	70	Dorsiflexion	20
Radial deviation	20	Plantarflexion	45–50
Ulnar deviation	45		
		Subtalar	
Cervical Spine		Inversion	30–35
Flexion	45–50	Eversion	15–20
Extension	45–75		
Lateral flexion	45		
Rotation	65–75		

*Zero point (0 degrees) is with the arm abducted to shoulder height.

Source: Kendall, F.P. et al. (2005). *Muscles: Testing and Function With Posture and Pain* (5th ed.). Philadelphia: Lippincott Williams & Wilkins.

can position them in more supported environments (lying supine, seated in a chair) to avoid or minimize the undesirable compensations along the chain.

The ACE-AHFS must always respect the scope of practice and the need for referral to qualified professionals. It is important to remember that an ACE-AHFS does not diagnose conditions or injuries, but can determine whether a restorative program will be effective at correcting muscle imbalance. If a client experiences any musculoskeletal pain, the ACE-AHFS should refer him or her for medical evaluation.

Movement Screens

When muscle tightness is a primary limitation, it is evident with passive muscle stretching. However, when compensatory movements occur during active muscle contraction or movement, it is usually indicative of faulty neural control. Consequently, active movement is an effective method to determine the influence that muscle imbalance and poor posture have on neural control, and to identify limitations to movement. The active movements selected as screens, however, must be skill- and conditioning-level appropriate, allow practice trials, and be specific to the client's needs. It is important to remember that almost any screen can evaluate functional capacity, as long as it is relevant to a client's needs and challenges and provides useful feedback on movement efficiency.

Gait analysis is arguably the most functional movement screen, given the dependence on walking to complete most daily activities. Gait analysis provides valuable information about the integrated roles and limitations of the lower and upper extremity in all three planes of movement. However, understanding the complexities of gait requires advanced learning. The ACE-AHFS is encouraged to review the fundamentals of gait presented in Chapter 14 and study gait in more detail before attempting to analyze it.

Recognizing the complexities of gait analysis, simplified movement screens have been developed that assess the ability to perform basic movements. Gray Cook created seven functional movement screens (FMS) that mimic primary movements and basic **activities of daily living (ADL)** (Cook, 2003; Esquerre et al., 2000). A big advantage to these movement screens is in their simplicity of scoring, using a simple 0 through 3 scale according to movement efficiency.

3 = movements performed without compensation or deviation from the intended planes of movement

2 = movements performed, but with some compensation, deviation, or assistance

1 = an inability to perform the movements

0 = pain associated with the movement and a need for referral

Many movement screens have not undergone validation studies, but have validity in mimicking functional or primary movement. Primary human movement, a topic addressed in more detail in Chapter 14, involves single-leg stands, bending and lifting, pushes (vertical and horizontal), pulls (vertical and horizontal), and rotations. All movement of the human body is essentially one of, or combinations of, these movements. Hence, movement screens should mimic the primary movements (e.g., the functional movement screens), but more importantly, they should be relevant to the challenges the client faces in performing his or her daily activities. For example, an older client who struggles to get into and out of a bathtub or car should perform a single-leg stand, lifting the opposite leg to clear an obstacle as tall as the tub wall or the car's doorsill. It is important to realize that not only do the screens monitor relative improvement, but they also serve as the exercises.

Several movement screens are presented here as examples, but the ACE-AHFS is encouraged to refer to the references and suggested readings at the end of this chapter for additional screens. The ACE-AHFS must always clear clients for pain before conducting any movement screens, especially when administering screens involving movement of the spine.

Forward Bend and Return

Source: Sahrmann, 2002

Objective: This screen examines bilateral mobility in the hips and lumbar spine during a forward bend and observes neural control and movement efficiency during the return from a forward bend.

Instructions:

- The client stands with feet hip-width apart and hands placed palm down on the front of the thighs.
- The ACE-AHFS should instruct the client to exhale gently, engage the abdominals, and slowly bend forward at the hips and lumber spine, sliding the hands down the front of the thighs as far as possible (Figure 13-21).

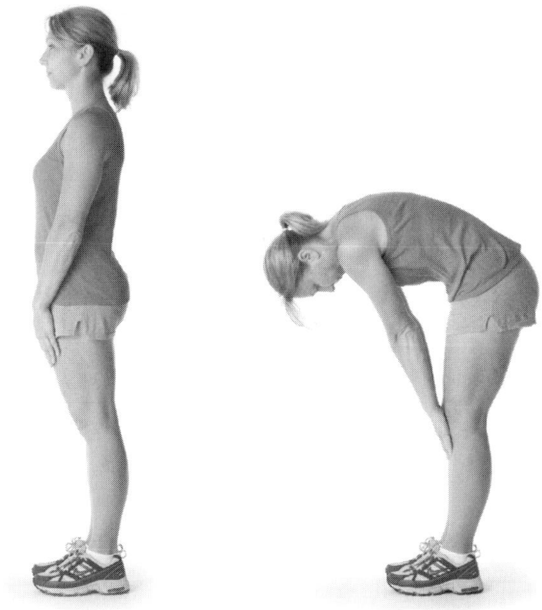

Figure 13-21
The forward bend and return

- The ACE-AHFS should allow sufficient practice trials to accommodate learning before administrating the test screen.

General Interpretations:

- This screen mimics a key primary movement of bending and lifting.
- The ACE-AHFS can identify the origin of the movement limitation or compensation and evaluate its impact on the entire kinetic chain.
- Normal forward bending is initiated at the hips, producing 80 degrees of hip flexion coupled with approximately 20 degrees of lumbar flexion.
- The hips normally flex faster than the spine during the first 50 degrees of motion.
- The return movement is initiated with hip extension.

Table 13-12 lists the movement compensations for the forward bend and return and provides interpretations of each.

Modified Hurdle-step Stand

Source: Adapted from Sahrmann, 2002 and Cook, 2003

Objective: This screen examines simultaneous mobility of one limb and stability of the **contralateral** (opposite) limb, while maintaining both hip and torso stabilization under a balance challenge of standing on one leg.

Equipment:

- Two uprights to anchor the string (chairs or table legs)
- 36-inch (91-cm) long piece of string
- 48-inch (122-cm) wooden or plastic dowel

Instructions:

- This screen is performed wearing shoes.
- The ACE-AHFS fastens a piece of string spanning two points at the height where the raised leg will flex the hip to 70 degrees (i.e., equal to a height where the sole of the raised foot is aligned halfway up the tibia).

Table 13-12
Forward Bend and Return—Movement Compensations and Interpretations

Movement Compensation	Interpretation
Excessive lumbar flexion or lumbar spine flexing faster than the hips during the first 50 degrees of motion	May indicate tightness in the hip extensor muscles and weakness (lengthening) in the lumbar extensor muscles
Inadequate lumbar flexion (flat back)	May indicate tightness in the lumbar extensor muscles
Inadequate hip flexion (men <75 degrees; women <85 degrees)	May indicate tightness in the hip extensor muscles or a potentially long trunk
Excessive hip flexion (>100 degrees)	May indicate lengthening of the hamstrings
Hips shift more than 5 inches (13 cm) posteriorly during flexion	May indicate tightness in the plantarflexor muscles
Return movement initiated with the spine, with hip extension occurring after the first third of the range of motion	May indicate dominance in the lumbar extensor muscles or tightness in the hip flexor muscles
Forward hip sway with lumbar extension and marked dorsiflexion at the feet	May indicate weakness in the hip extensor muscles

- The client stands with the feet together and aligns the front edge of the toes directly beneath the string.
- The dowel is placed across the shoulders in a traditional squat position and parallel to the floor.
- The ACE-AHFS instructs the client to slowly load onto one leg and slowly lift the opposite leg over the string, raising the hip to 70 degrees to clear the string, and gently touching the heel of the raised leg to the floor in front of the string before slowly returning to the starting position (Figure 13-22).
- Repeat with the opposite leg.
- It is important to allow sufficient practice trials to accommodate learning before administrating the test screens.

General Interpretations:

- This screen mimics key movements essential to gait.
- The ACE-AHFS can identify the origin of the movement limitation or compensation and evaluate its impact on the entire kinetic chain.
- If the ACE-AHFS suspects poor mobility (flexibility) as the limitation, he or she may elect to administer a passive flexibility test on the suspected muscle to verify muscle shortening.

Table 13-13 lists the movement compensations for the modified hurdle-step stand and provides interpretations of each.

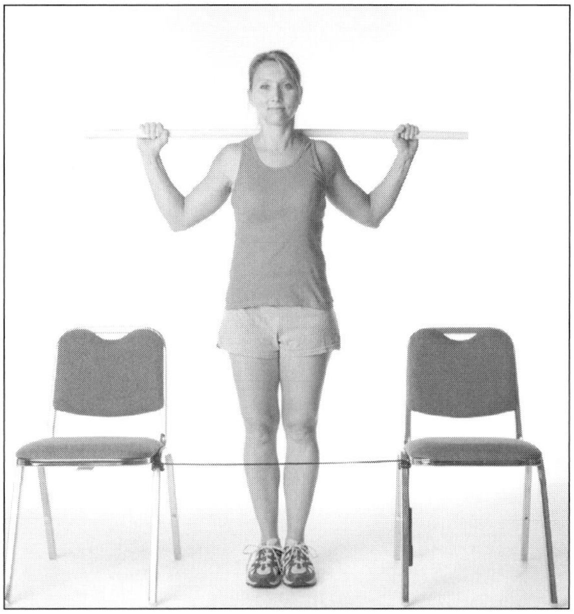

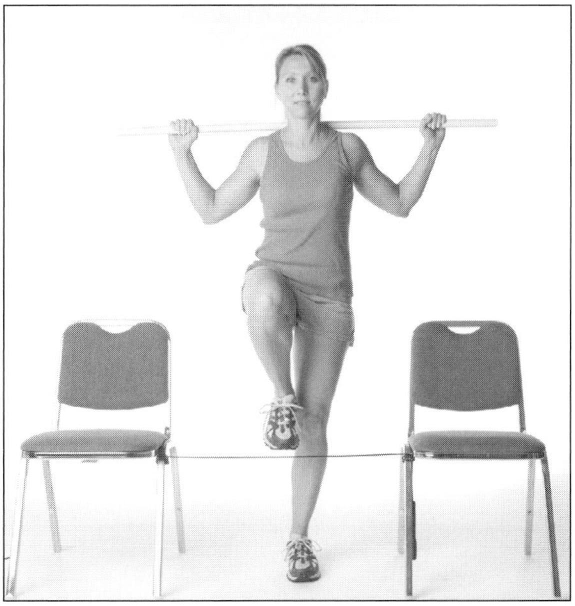

Figure 13-22
The modified hurdle-step stand screen

Active Straight-leg Raise

Source: Cook, 2003

Objective: This screen examines hamstring and contralateral hip-flexor mobility while maintaining simultaneous trunk stability.

Equipment:

- Measuring tape
- 48-inch (123-cm) dowel
- Small riser [e.g., 2 x 4 inches (5 x 10 cm)]

Instructions:

- The client lies supine with legs extended, ankles dorsiflexed (shoes removed), arms at sides with palms facing upward, and a neutral spine.
- If any space exists under the knees or lower thigh, the ACE-AHFS can place the small riser beneath to make light contact with the posterior knee or thigh.
- Using the measuring tape, the ACE-AHFS locates the mid-point of the thigh, midway between the ASIS and the knee joint.
- He or she then positions the dowel vertically at that location.
- The ACE-AHFS instructs the client to actively raise one leg keeping the knee

Table 13-13
Modified Hurdle-step Stand—Movement Compensations and Interpretations

Movement Compensation	Interpretation
Excessive stance-leg adduction or downward tilting of the pelvis toward the opposite side [lateral hip shift >1.5–2 inches (3.8–5 cm)]	May indicate weakness in the stance-leg abductors
Lateral trunk flexion toward the stance leg (dowel movement in the frontal plane)	May indicate weakness in the stance-leg abductors with a compensatory lean of the torso to maintain balance
Pelvic rotation toward the stance leg (medial rotation)	May indicate weakness in the raised-leg lateral rotators, allowing the pelvis to rotate May indicate tightness in the raised-leg internal rotators
Hip rotation (stance leg rotates internally)	May indicate weakness in the stance-leg lateral rotators
Deviation from frontal alignment in the raised leg	May indicate weakness in the hip flexor raising the thigh May indicate tightness in the stance-leg hip flexor preventing posterior hip rotation (when raising toward 90 degrees of flexion) May indicate tightness in the raised-leg hip extensors (when raising toward 90 degrees of flexion)
Anterior tilt in the pelvis or forward lean in the torso (dowel movement in the sagittal plane)	May indicate tightness in the stance-leg hip flexors May indicate weakness in the rectus abdominals and hip extensors of the stance leg
Forward flexion in the torso with the leg raise	May indicate weakness in the raised-leg hip flexors (when raising toward 90 degrees of flexion)
Excessive pronation of the stance foot	May indicate weakness in the gluteus muscle group of the stance leg, forcing medial rotation May indicate weakness in the tibialis posterior and anterior to eccentrically stabilize against pronation
Inability to control torso movements and maintain balance	May indicate poor core stability and balance

extended and foot dorsiflexed while attempting to keep the contralateral (opposite) leg in contact with the riser (Figure 13-23).

- The client should continue to raise the leg until the contralateral leg lifts off the riser.
- The torso, arms, and head should remain motionless throughout the screen.
- It is important to allow sufficient practice trials to accommodate learning before administrating the test screens.

Scoring:

- The ACE-AHFS scores each leg independently, using the lowest score attained on each side (Table 13-14).

Figure 13-23
Active straight-leg raise

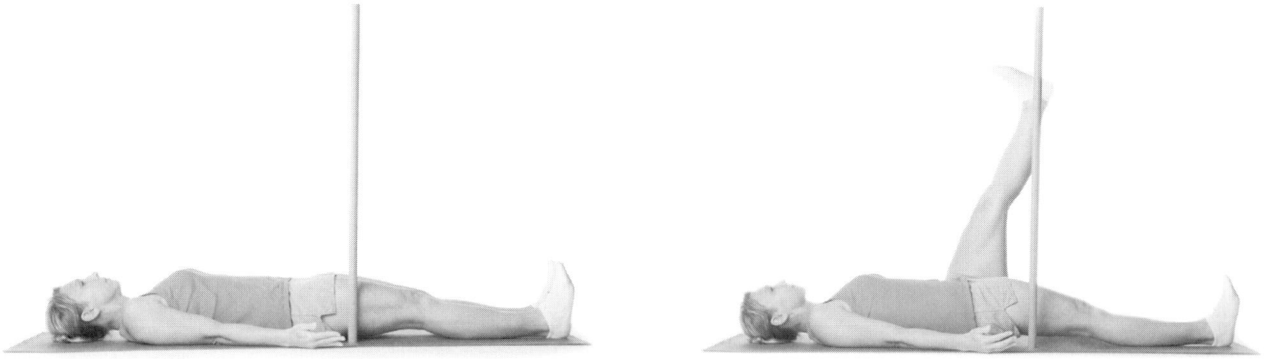

General Interpretations:

- This screen reflects the ability to perform walking and bending movements that require mobility around the hips.
- The ACE-AHFS can identify the origin of the movement limitations or compensations and evaluate their impact on the entire kinetic chain.

Table 13-15 lists the movement compensations for the active straight-leg raise and provides interpretations of each.

Active Lordosis With Active Knee Extension and Ankle Dorsiflexion

Source: Adapted from Sahrmann, 2002

Objective: This movement screen examines active hamstring and lumbar stability, or active hamstring mobility without low-back compensation.

Instructions:

- The client sits toward the front edge of a seat or table top without any contact against a backrest, with the legs hanging freely off the floor.
- The ACE-AHFS instructs the client to extend the lumbar spine into lordosis, aligning the torso at 90 degrees to the hips.
- Next, the ACE-AHFS instructs the client to extend the knee to within 10 degrees of full extension, while maintaining lumbar extension and dorsiflexion at the ankle (Figure 13-24).
- Repeat the movement with a dorsiflexed ankle to 10 degrees.
- Repeat with the opposite leg.

Table 13-16 lists the movement compensations for active lordosis with active knee extension and ankle dorsiflexion and provides interpretations of each.

Active Lordosis With Active Hip Flexion

Source: Adapted from Sahrmann, 2002

Objective: This movement screen examines hip flexor performance and lumbar stability without low-back compensation.

Table 13-14
Scoring the Active Straight-leg Raise Screen

Score	Criteria
3	Actively raising the leg until the malleolus passes the dowel with no contralateral leg or trunk movement. Both legs remain extended with the ankles in dorsiflexion, exhibiting no internal or external rotation.
2	The movement screen is completed, but the raised leg only reaches a position where the dowel is aligned between the knee and malleolus before the trunk or contralateral leg movement occurs.
1	The client is unable to complete the movement screen or the raised leg only reaches a position where the knee does not pass the dowel.
0	Pain is indicated (terminate the movement screen and refer the client to a qualified healthcare professional).

Table 13-15
Active Straight-leg Raise—Movement Compensations and Interpretations

Movement Compensation	Interpretation
Lumbar flexion and limited hip flexion	May indicate tightness in the hamstring muscles
Early lifting of the contralateral leg and lumbar extension	May indicate tightness in the hip flexors
Lateral femoral rotation	May indicate tightness in lateral hip rotators and hip flexors
Medial femoral rotation	May indicate weakness in lateral hip rotators and hip flexors

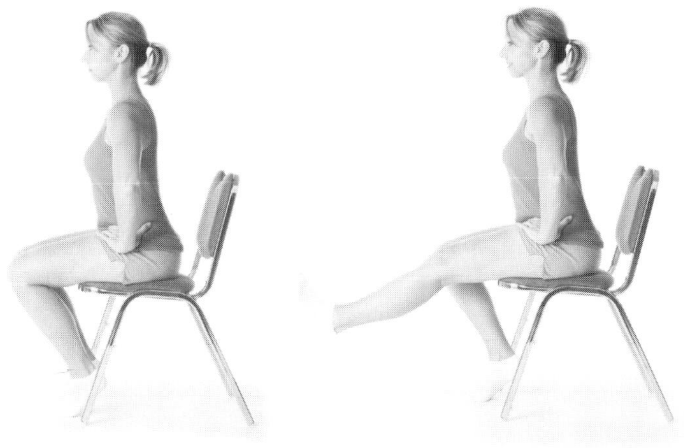

Figure 13-24
Active lordosis with active knee extension and ankle dorsiflexion

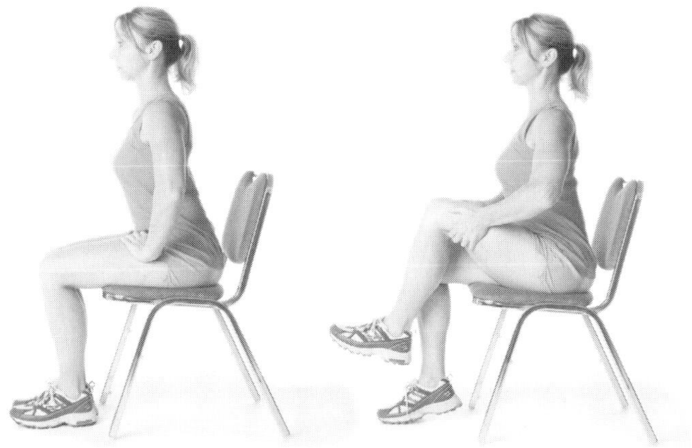

Figure 13-25
Active lordosis with active hip flexion

Instructions:
- The client sits toward the front edge of a seat or table top without any contact against a backrest, with the legs hanging freely off the floor.
- The ACE-AHFS instructs the client to extend the lumbar spine into lordosis, aligning the torso at 90 degrees to the hips.
- Using both hands, the client lifts one thigh as high as possible toward the chest without altering low-back lordosis or tilting the pelvis (Figure 13-25).
- Next, the client releases the leg hold and attempts to maintain the same position for five to 10 seconds using the hip flexors.
- Repeat the procedure, but add isometric resistance for five to 10 seconds by having the client push down with the hand on top of the thigh.
- Repeat with the opposite leg.

Table 13-17 lists the movement compensations for active lordosis with active hip flexion and provides interpretations of each.

Table 13-16
Active Lordosis With Active Knee Extension and Ankle Dorsiflexion—Movement Compensations and Interpretations

Movement/Movement Compensation	Interpretation
Active lumbar lordosis cannot be maintained throughout movement	May indicate weakness in the lumbar back extensor muscles May indicate tightness in the hamstrings
Active lumbar lordosis maintained throughout the movement	May indicate lumbar stability
The knee is extended without any change in pelvic position (plantarflexion at the ankle)	May indicate active flexibility in the hamstrings
The knee is extended without any change in pelvic position (dorsiflexion at the ankle)	May indicate active flexibility in the gastrocnemius
Leg alignment (ASIS, knee, and second toe) is maintained throughout the movement	May indicate potential muscle balance between the medial and lateral hip rotators

Note: ASIS = Anterior superior iliac spine

Table 13-17
Active Lordosis With Active Hip Flexion—Movement Compensations and Interpretations

Movement/Movement Compensation	Interpretation
Active lumbar lordosis cannot be maintained throughout the movement	May indicate weakness in the lumbar back extensor muscles
Active lumbar lordosis maintained throughout the movement	May indicate lumbar stability
The hip flexes to 120 degrees and isometric resistance is tolerated without any change in lordosis or pelvic titling	May indicate appropriate engagement of the hip flexors
The hip flexor is unable to tolerate resistance at 120 degrees, but can between 100 and 120 degrees, or the movement cannot be completed without hiking the pelvis	May indicate lengthening of the hip flexors with mild weakness
The hip flexor is unable to tolerate resistance at any range	May indicate significant weakness in the hip flexors

Standing Wall Screens

Source: Adapted from Sahrmann, 2002

Objective: These movement screens examine bilateral mobility of the shoulder girdle and key upper-extremity muscle groups during overhead movement patterns.

Instructions—First movement:

- The client faces the wall as close as possible with the elbows bent, forearms and little fingers touching the wall, and forearms out to the side (Figure 13-26a).
- The client should engage the abdominals to stiffen and immobilize the trunk prior to any arm movement.
- The ACE-AHFS instructs the client to slide his or her arms up the wall to an overhead, abducted position (135 degrees) where the scapulae have abducted and upwardly rotated.
- The client adducts the scapulae to lift the arms off the wall (Figure 13-26b).

Instructions—Second movement:

- The client faces the wall as close as possible with elbows bent, arms close to the body, and forearms and little fingers touching the wall (Figure 13-26c).
- The client should engage the abdominals to stiffen and immobilize the trunk prior to any arm movement.
- The ACE-AHFS should instruct the client to depress his or her scapulae and hold that position while sliding the arms vertically up the wall to an overhead position (170 degrees) where the scapulae have abducted and upwardly rotated (Figure 13-26d).
- The client returns to the starting position, then proceeds to shrug the shoulders and hold that position while repeating the shoulder flexion movement.
- It is important to allow sufficient practice trials to accommodate learning before administrating the test screens.

Table 13-18 lists the movement compensations for the standing wall screens and provides interpretations of each.

Restorative Exercise for Postural Compensation

The overall goal with programming is to restore muscle balance, enhance muscle's physiological properties, and improve neuromuscular control of movement by re-educating faulty neural pathways. However, unless *awareness* of poor posture, and *intention* to improve are key objectives of the program, individuals are not likely to attain great success. Table 13-19 presents the basic programming principles surrounding:

- Stretching hypertonic (tight and overactive) muscles through passive elongation to increase the number of sarcomeres in series
- Strengthening **latent** (weak and inactive) muscles with isometric or limited range-of-motion exercises in normal resting-length positions

Figure 13-26
Standing wall screens

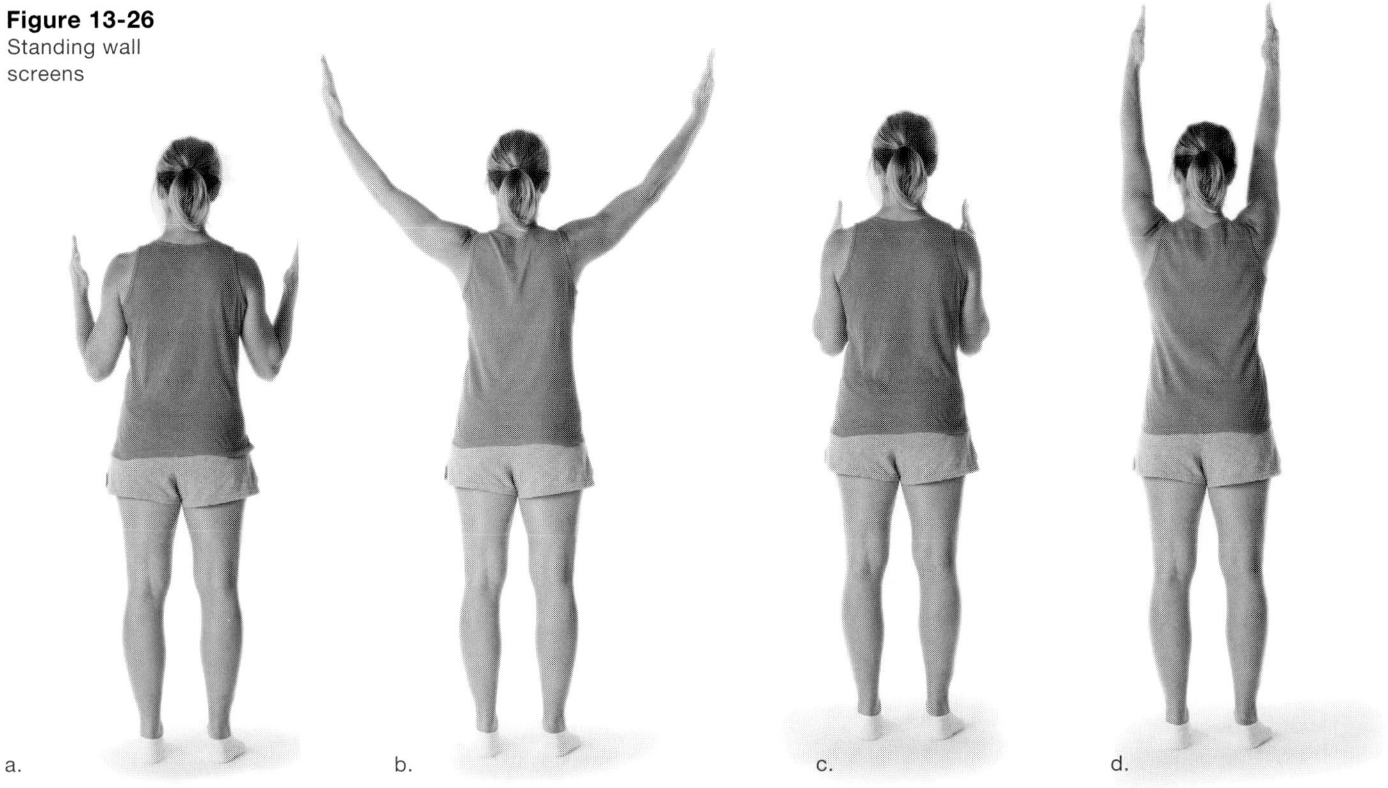

The initial emphasis placed on passive elongation (static stretching) to reduce muscle tightness may not be considered functional by some, but its objective is to reset muscle tone (in the hypertonic muscle), correct side asymmetry, and introduce normal range of motion and muscle length prior to integrating movement patterns. This is especially important if muscle length or tone restricts efficient movement. McGill (2007), however, claims that static stretching deadens the muscle from a neural perspective, diminishing the stretch reflex and reducing peak strength and power. Consequently, the dominance of static-type stretching should be limited to the initial part of the program until the client is capable of integrating movement patterns. As the client progresses through the program, the static-type stretches will be replaced with more dynamic-type movement patterns.

Many fitness professionals implement **myofascial release** as a modality to reduce muscle hypertonicity before stretching and after workouts. The use of foam rollers or "sticks" to apply sweeping strokes to longer muscles or more directed pressure to the sensitive areas in short muscles can certainly improve flexibility via **autogenic inhibition.** However, foam rollers can be difficult to use for some deconditioned and less agile clients.

A common issue of debate is whether hypertonic agonists should first be stretched or the weakened antagonists should first be strengthened. Several approaches exist, but a basic approach of stretch-then-strengthen delivers effective results. This approach involves inhibiting and reducing tension in the hypertonic (tight) muscles, and stretching the tight muscles before strengthening the latent (weakened) muscles to facilitate their full activation. Janda studied EMG activity on hypertonic erector spinae and normotensive rectus abdominis muscles during trunk flexion exercises (Arokoski et al., 2001). Test subjects demonstrated reduced rectus abdominis activity with tight erector spinae during normal trunk flexion, yet when the erector spinae were first stretched, they exhibited increased rectus abdominis activity and reduced erector spinae

Table 13-18
Standing Wall Screens—Movement Compensations and Interpretations

Movement Compensation	Interpretation
First Movement	
Abduction: Unable to abduct arms to 135 degrees with adequate upward scapular rotation	May indicate tightness in the rhomboid muscle group and weakness in the trapezius and serratus anterior muscles
Adduction: Unable to adduct scapulae and lift arms off wall on completion of arm abduction to 135 degrees	May indicate weakness in the lower trapezius and possibly the rhomboid muscle group
Elevation: Scapular elevation occurs very early during the movement	May indicate tightness in the upper trapezius May indicate weakness in the lower trapezius
Second Movement	
Flexion: Unable to achieve 170 degrees of shoulder flexion	May indicate tightness in the pectoralis group, latissimus dorsi, and teres major
Elevation: Unable to prevent scapular elevation	May indicate tightness in the upper trapezius May indicate weakness in the lower trapezius
Adduction: Unable to adduct scapulae on completion of shoulder flexion	May indicate tightness in the pectoralis minor May indicate weakness in the lower trapezius and possibly the rhomboid muscle group
Depression: Unable to maintain a shoulder shrug during the flexion movement	May indicate tightness in the rhomboid muscle group and weakness in the trapezius and serratus anterior
Increased lumbar lordosis during the flexion movement	May indicate tightness in the latissimus dorsi May indicate weakness in the rectus abdominis

Table 13-19
Key Steps of Restorative Exercise Programming

Restorative Progression Steps	Modality
Inhibit hypertonic muscles	Myofascial release, static stretching, PNF, isometric contractions, active isolated stretches
Lengthen hypertonic muscles	Static stretching, PNF
Activation of latent muscles	Isometric contractions, active isolated stretches, muscle activation techniques, dynamic contractions
Integration into functional movement*	Part-to-whole progression of movement patterns

*An example of integrated movement is the progression from a shoulder-bridge knee-tuck to stretch tight hip flexors and activate a weak gluteus maximus to more functional walking lunges with overhead triplanar arm reaches that engage more of the entire body.

Note: PNF = Proprioceptive neuromuscular facilitation

activity. It therefore appears that the neurological principles of autogenic inhibition serve an important role in restorative exercise.

Low-force, longer-duration static stretches evoke low-grade muscle spindle activity and a temporary increase in muscle tension due to muscle lengthening. This low-grade muscle response progressively decreases due to a gradual desensitization of the muscle spindle activity as the duration of the stretch progresses. After approximately seven to 10 seconds of a low-force stretch, the increase in muscle tension activates a **Golgi tendon organ (GTO)** response. Under GTO activation, muscle spindle activity within the stretched muscle is temporarily inhibited, allowing further muscle stretching. This concept defines autogenic inhibition (Whittle, 2007). For example, passively holding a hamstrings stretch to the point of resistance for the appropriate timeframe will elicit this neurological response. After the removal of the stretch stimulus, however, the muscle spindle quickly reestablishes its stretch threshold to approximately 70% of full recovery within the first five seconds (MacIntosh, Gardiner, & McComas, 2006).

Increasing the number of sarcomeres in series is best accomplished through prolonged passive elongation at lower intensities (Sahrmann, 2002). While passively positioning shortened muscles in elongated positions for 10-minute-plus intervals effectively stimulates increases in sarcomere number, these timeframes prove unrealistic and unmanageable for most. Consequently, the ACE-AHFS must encourage clients to follow their stretching programs as frequently as possible, as stretching adaptations are dose-dependent on volume (repetitions x duration x frequency) and the quality of the repetitions completed.

Active agonist contraction and reciprocal inhibition are alternative approaches to restorative exercise. Active agonist contractions involve a series of repeated, low-grade isometric or dynamic contractions of the hypertonic agonist to reduce its irritability threshold via GTO activation (MacIntosh, Gardiner, & McComas, 2006). This facilitates stretching of the agonist, which is followed by strengthening of the antagonist. For example, a sequence at the pelvis would include low-grade concentric or isometric contractions of the hip flexors preceding hip flexor stretching, followed by gluteus maximus strengthening.

Reciprocal inhibition involves first performing isometric or dynamic contraction with the weakened antagonist to reciprocally inhibit the hypertonic agonist, which can then be stretched. Low-grade muscle contractions at approximately 50% of maximum force in the antagonist for a total duration of six to 15 seconds inhibit or reduce muscle spindle activity within the agonist muscle (Whittle, 2007). For example, a low-grade isometric contraction of the gluteus maximus reciprocally inhibits the hip flexors, which can then be stretched, followed again by gluteus maximus strengthening.

Table 13-20 provides general guidelines for the ACE-AHFS to follow when designing a restorative exercise program for a client.

Exercise Considerations

Generally, faulty movement patterns in the **transverse plane,** followed by the frontal plane, are most significant in developing disruptions to normal motion and precipitating injury (Gray & Tiberio, 2007). While textbooks often define muscle function in its most common plane of movement, many muscles play active roles in triplanar movement [(e.g., hip flexors are involved concentrically in hip flexion, external rotation (femur), and hip abduction; the gluteus maximus is involved concentrically in hip extension, external rotation, and hip abduction)] (Gray & Tiberio, 2007). A restorative exercise program must ultimately load muscles in all planes of movement. Initially, however, the ACE-AHFS can emphasize supported exercises and muscle isolation in single planes prior to integration of unsupported multi-joint and multiplanar patterns. Janda divided muscles into functional groups prone to weakness and prone to tightness (Cook, 2003), as depicted in Table 13-21. Programs, including maintenance programs, improve passive and active range of motion in groups prone to tightness, and aim to strengthen or condition muscle groups prone to weakness. For example, the gluteus maximus is traditionally a weak muscle and functions three-dimensionally. Therefore, good activation and conditioning exercises would include the following:

- Forward lunges with simultaneous bilateral arm reaches to the floor, adding light dumbbell resistance as conditioning improves (activates gluteus maximus to decelerate and loads it for hip extension)—1 set x 10 reps
- Side lunges with simultaneous bilateral arm reaches to the opposite side (at hip height), forcing hip adduction (activates gluteus maximus to decelerate and loads it for hip abduction)—1 set x 10 reps
- Crossover lunges (step over and in front with the leading leg), with simultaneous bilateral

Table 13-20
Restorative Exercise Programming Guidelines (F.I.R.S.T.)

Program Modality	Tightened Muscles—Stretching	Lengthened Muscles—Strengthening
Frequency	Best accomplished with prolonged passive elongations (10-minute-plus intervals), but unrealistic/unmanageable for most As adaptations are dose-dependent, aim for 1–2 times/day	Perform 1–2 times/day with the stretching program
Intensity	Static stretching: To the point of tension Always control joint movements in bi-articulate (two-joint) muscles Dynamic patterns: Controlled tempos to the point of resistance Maintain full neuromuscular control of movement—higher intensities may call upon existing faulty strategies	Provide small overload in controlled positions Generally only need around 50% of MVC Focus on strengthening with the joint position near neutral position Use the body's resistance or fixed surfaces (e.g., the floor) Higher intensities may call upon existing faulty strategies Lower intensities also allow faster muscle recovery and more frequent training
Repetitions and sets	Static stretching: 2–4 reps x 30–60 seconds each Dynamic movements: 1–2 sets x 5–10 repetitions progressing to 3 sets x 15–20 repetitions	Isometric contractions: 2–4 reps x 5–10 seconds each Emphasize uniplanar action Dynamic contractions: 1–2 sets x 12–20 repetitions with slow, controlled tempos Progress to 2–3 sets x 10–15 repetitions Introduce triplanar action
Timeframe	Plan sessions between 30–45 minutes (depending on the amount of muscle imbalance noted) Plan for 1–3 months of participation, depending on the degree of imbalance and volume of exercise performed, or until noticeable body alignment and movement efficiency is restored After 2 weeks of overload, small strength gains are evident, but they are 20% morphological and 80% neural 4–6 weeks may be required to demonstrate more significant morphological changes in muscle	

Note: MVC = Maximum voluntary contraction

Table 13-21
Janda's Functional Division of Muscle Groups

Muscles Prone to Weakness	Muscles Prone to Tightness
Peroneal group Tibialis anterior Vastus medialis and lateralis Gluteus group Rectus abdominis Serratus anterior Rhomboids Lower trapezius Cervical flexors Extensors of the arm	Gastrocnemius and soleus Tibialis posterior Hip adductors Hamstrings Rectus femoris Iliopsoas Tensor fasciae latae Piriformis Erector spinae Quadratus lumborum Pectoralis group Upper trapezius Levator scapulae Scalenes Flexors of the arm

arm rotations toward the leading leg (at hip height), forcing internal hip rotation (activates gluteus maximus to decelerate and loads it for hip external rotation)—1 set x 10 reps

Exercise Examples for Stability and Mobility

This section provides basic examples of stretches and exercises to improve mobility and stability of the scapulothoracic and lumbopelvic regions.

Supine overhead reach: This exercise promotes thoracic extension and scapular mobility. The client lies supine in a bent-knee position, engages his or her abdominals to stabilize the spine against the floor, and places the arms at the sides. While holding the abdominal engagement, the client moves the arms overhead into 180 degrees of shoulder flexion with the arms extended. From this position, the client performs shrugs and depressions of the scapulae. This exercise can be progressed to the quadruped position, with the client performing the arm movements unilaterally.

Wipers: Also called snow angels, this exercise promotes scapular adduction and upward and downward rotation (mobility). The client assumes the same starting position as for the supine overhead reaches, and then adducts the scapulae, extends the thoracic spine, and bends the elbows to 90 degrees with the arms positioned at the sides. The client slowly performs a wiper movement, moving the hands to touch overhead, while maintaining contact of the spine, head, and back of the arms with the floor throughout the movement. This exercise can be progressed to the quadruped position, with the client performing the arm movements unilaterally.

Supine letters: This exercise promotes scapular mobility and stability. The client assumes the same starting position as for the supine overhead reaches, and moves his or her arms into letter "Y" and "T" positions. At each position, the client reaches and retracts the arms through scapular movement while maintaining abdominal engagement. This exercise can be progressed to the quadruped position, with the client performing the arm movements unilaterally.

Supine lying on a foam roller: This movement facilitates thoracic extension. The client lies supine with a foam roller positioned directly under the spine, from the head to the coccyx. People with longer torsos may need to have a pillow for the head; however, the spine must be kept on the roller. With knees bent and feet flat on the floor, the client engages the abdominals to flatten the lumbar spine and abducts and externally rotates the arms, allowing gravity to gently pull the arms toward the floor, thereby increasing thoracic extension and stretching of the chest muscles.

Wall crawls: This activity promotes thoracic extension and scapular position. To perform this exercise, the client stands close to a wall. He or she places the heels approximately 3 inches (7.6 cm) from the wall with the hips touching the wall, and engages the abdominals to stabilize the lumbar spine against the wall. The client abducts and externally rotates the arms to a "goal post" position. If possible, the client should place his or her elbows and the backs of the hands against the wall, then slowly slide the arms up the wall to an overhead position without arching the back. This exercise will be difficult for individuals with swayback, kyphosis, or lordosis conditions.

Additional stretches for the scapulothoracic region include the following:

- Pendulum exercises (a.k.a. Codman's exercise) to relax the muscles around the shoulder girdle
- Passive stretches
- Inferior capsule stretch—to improve shoulder elevation
  - ✔Posterior capsule stretch to gain medial rotation and horizontal flexion; to stretch the posterior rotator cuff
  - ✔Anterior capsule stretch to gain horizontal extension and lateral rotation; to stretch the pectoralis major
  - ✔Superior capsule stretch to stretch the superior capsule

✔Medial rotation stretch to increase medial rotation and stretch the capsule

✔Lateral rotation stretch to increase lateral rotation and stretch the capsule

Strengthening exercises for the scapulothoracic area may appear basic to the ACE-AHFS. However, it is critical that the ACE-AHFS understand how to "set" the scapulae to strengthen the necessary muscles in the correct neutral positions. In terms of posture, the scapulae are the "chief engineers" of the scapulothoracic region. The priority must be to facilitate retraction and **depression** of the scapulae using the surrounding musculature to return the posture to its origin.

Additionally, the deltoid is often strengthened with lateral raises and overhead shoulder presses to the point where the muscular imbalances between the rotator muscles and the deltoids are extreme. The rotator cuff muscles secure the humeral head into the glenohumeral joint. The ACE-AHFS will often need to utilize rotator cuff exercises before trying to strengthen a client's deltoids, as the imbalance could lead to injuries, including rotator cuff strains and tears.

Scapular protraction: From a supine position, the client presses upward against manual resistance. The serratus anterior is the primary muscle providing this motion. Alternatives include wall push-ups with an emphasis on the additional push at the end to facilitate the serratus anterior. Once the elbows are extended, the client pushes the body away even further by moving the scapulae forward around the ribcage.

Scapular retraction: The client performs a row exercise, pulling the elbows back and squeezing the scapulae together. This exercise can be performed sitting or standing.

Scapular depression: The client performs lat pull-downs or single-rope depressions, utilizing the lower trapezius and pectoralis minor muscles.

Bouhler exercises: These exercises strengthen the lower trapezius as it functions in upward rotation of the scapula. Performed in shoulder flexion with elbows extended and the back against the wall, this exercise consists of three steps: arms overhead with the palms facing each other; backs of the hands against the wall; and arms further away from the ears in a "V" placement against the wall. An advanced version of this exercise involves lying prone on a stability ball, in which case the arms are in flexion and extend with small weights .

Scapular elevation: Shrugs and exercises that involve pressing upward with straight arms strengthen the upper trapezius and levator scapulae.

Glenohumeral exercise (external rotation): These exercises strengthen the infraspinatus, teres minor, and posterior deltoid.

Glenohumeral exercise (internal rotation): These exercises strengthen the subcapularis.

Glenohumeral exercise (abduction): This motion, which stabilizes the glenohumeral joint during elevation and abduction, is produced by force-couple activity of the deltoid with the supraspinatus.

Exercises and stretches for the lumbopelvic region performed in the supine position should include abdominal engagement to stabilize the lumbar spine against the floor.

Hip flexor stretch: From the supine position, the client starts in the bent-knee position, slowly extending the legs unilaterally while attempting to maintain low-back contact with the floor.

Supine bridge with unilateral knee tucks: This exercise aims to reciprocally inhibit tight hip flexors and simultaneously activate the gluteus maximus. From a supine bent-knee position with both feet on the floor, the client first performs a shoulder bridge by raising the hips off the floor as high as possible. The client then returns to the floor, tucking one knee to the chest and repeating the bridge movement. This position stretches the non-tucked hip flexor under gluteus activation.

Modified supine hamstrings stretch: The hamstrings, a biarticulate muscle, can be effectively targeted via a simple modification to a standard supine hamstrings stretch. The client lies supine inside a door jamb, resting one leg against a wall while the opposite leg lies through the door jamb in a bent-knee position. From a passively elongated position, the client engages the hip flexors to anteriorly tilt the pelvis and increase the stretch on the hamstrings.

Multijoint stretch of the hip flexors and quadriceps: This exercise involves lying supine on a table with the hips aligned to the table edge and legs hanging freely over the edge of the table. The client gently pulls one knee toward the chest while engaging the abdominals to stabilize the lumbar spine. While stretching the hip flexor in the non-tucked knee, the client can also stretch the quadriceps of the same leg by flexing the knee without any internal or external rotation of the leg.

Additional stretches for the lumbopelvic region include the following:

- Child's pose to stretch the lumbar and hip extensors
- Cat-camels (in quadruped position) to stretch the lumbar extensors
- Supine piriformis stretch to stretch the lateral hip rotators
- Supine wall rotations to stretch the hip abductors and adductors
- Kneeling triplanar lunges with arms overhead to stretch the hip flexors

Strengthening exercises for the lumbopelvic area may also appear basic to the ACE-AHFS, but it is important to understand how to "set" the pelvis to strengthen the necessary muscles in the appropriate positions.

- Spine bent-knee pillow squeezes and resisted abductions activate and strengthen the hip abductors and adductors and mobilize the sacroiliac joint.
- Quadruped hip extensions (avoiding hip and torso rotation) activate and strengthen the hip extensors.
- Side-lying hip abduction with elastic ankle cuffs activate and strengthen the hip abductors.
- Single-leg quarter squats with internal rotation activate and strengthen the hip extensors and lateral hip rotators.

Other Considerations

In situations where there are imbalances between the strength of muscles on each side of the body, unilateral machines will reveal the differences in strength. For example, the muscles surrounding the right scapula may be stronger than the muscles surrounding the left scapula. Keep in mind that the exercises may progress from the seated, stationary position to standing, unbalanced positions, and then to multijoint exercises.

Sitting Postures

All sitting postures should provide for good spinal alignment and normal spinal curves. The head should not be forward (anteriorly translated) and the shoulders should not be rounded forward. It is known that prolonged sitting can lead to new injury or the aggravation of an old injury (Houglum, 2005).

Technically, chairs should be firm and fitted to the individual. Individuals will be at risk when they sit on a very soft padded seat, such as a couch or deep-sinking chair. The seat height must allow the individual's feet to rest comfortably on the floor with the knees and hips at 90 degrees. The seat depth should be such that the edge of the seat does not press against the back of the individual's knees. The chair back should support the lumbar and thoracic spine and come to the lower border of the scapulae. In addition, if the chair has arms, they should be at a level that provides for shoulder relaxation and permits the forearms to rest comfortably with the elbows at 90 degrees (Houglum, 2005).

Exercises that strengthen the sitting posture will most likely involve a stability ball. When a client is sitting upright with the shoulders retracted and the chest elevated, the unstable ball will require the abdominals to engage. The ball should be the size that creates 90-degree angles at the hips and knees, and no less (Table 13-22). At less than 90-degree angles, the load on the knees, hips, and low back become increased.

Body Mechanics in the Gym Setting

Many fitness/health facilities have standard resistance equipment that is adaptable to individuals of various sizes. An ACE-AHFS can assist guests or visitors as they "fit" the equipment to their particular needs. Just because one individual is 5'9" (1.8 m), this does not mean that the equipment will be optimally set for another person of the same height, as some individuals have longer legs and others have longer torsos.

Fitness equipment often has joint "cam" markers on the equipment for the knees, shoulders, or

Table 13-22
Stability Ball Selection Criteria

Height	Ball Size
Under 4'6" (137 cm)	30 cm (12 inches)
4'6" to 5'0" (137 to 152 cm)	45 cm (18 inches)
5'1" to 5'7" (155 to 170 cm)	55 cm (22 inches)
5'8" to 6'2" (173 to 188 cm)	65 cm (26 inches)
Over 6'2" (188 cm)	75 cm (30 inches)

hips. These markers should assist with the placement of seat heights, backrests, or leg lengths on the equipment. Individuals new to the fitness facility should begin on the equipment that requires settings and not perform multijoint exercises until they have adequate body awareness and strength.

Once the fixed equipment is mastered and muscle memory is created with correct postural movement, the client can advance to the cable machines. After the cable equipment is mastered, multijoint functional movement patterns can be implemented with resistance bands, stability balls, and unstable surfaces. For an ACE-AHFS, having a varied program design allows for creativity, as long as the joint alignments are correct and not placed in faulty torque positions.

Physiological Considerations

Several issues need to be considered when discussing posture and movement. It is essential to have a physician's authorization when postural compensation has been detected and the client is experiencing sharp pain or pain that has become chronic. A great rule of thumb is to initially decrease the range of motion and progress as muscle memory and strength are accrued. For compensation of the upper scapulothoracic region, it is often necessary to perform three or four rhomboid/scapula-retraction exercises for every chest (pectoralis major) exercise. The corrective exercises can thereby prevail as dominant while still working the opposite muscle group. Keep in mind that when retracting the scapula, the client is also stretching the tight pectoral muscles. It is important not to forget the coupling effect that the agonist and antagonist have on one another.

Case Study

A 59-year-old professional male presents for a fitness assessment. During the standing overhead reach against the wall, the following observations are made:

- As shoulder flexion begins, the lower back arches off of the wall.
- He cannot reach full shoulder flexion.
- He cannot keep the shoulders pressed against the wall.

In addition, when performing the back scratch test, he cannot place either hand at the middle of his back. What can be determined from this information? The inability to keep the shoulders flat against the wall or perform the back scratch could mean that he is kyphotic. In addition, his latissimus dorsi are likely tight if he arches off of the wall when his arms move to shoulder flexion.

The client must be medically screened before the ACE-AHFS can perform assessments or begin a restorative program. The screening should eliminate concern about any spinal injuries or diseases. The ACE-AHFS may feel the need to assess the length of various muscles to determine which movements are limited. The ACE-AHFS should also keep in mind that there are many approaches to resolve this client's issues and various options may need to be considered. To begin, if the scapulae appear to be elevated and protracted, the ACE-AHFS should begin by working on positioning the scapula in depression and retraction. The ACE-AHFS may need to instruct the client how to perform these movements, cueing with mirrors and kinesthetic touch. The scapulae may initially move with difficulty, but once the movement is achieved and he has awareness and feels the muscle action, the stretching and strengthening program can begin. This may include the use of a foam roller along with the stretching and strengthening exercises to promote better posture.

Summary

Efficient movement often originates from good posture. Therefore, an assessment of static posture should be considered a prerequisite screening for all programming. Postural restorative exercises strive to "straighten the body before strengthening it" and potentially avoid exacerbating existing postural and movement compensations, muscle-joint imbalances caused by numerous factors including occupational and lifestyle positions, and poor movement technique. These factors alter key physiological properties and functions within muscle, changing arthokinetics at and beyond the joint of origin.

Postural assessments follow the right angle rule, identifying how the body aligns across four joints. This model divides the body into two hemispheres while observing symmetry between the joints in all three planes of motion. Following a postural assessment, the ACE-AHFS may want to validate his or her observations by measuring the length of specific muscles and conduct movement screens to evaluate the impact of muscle imbalance on movement. When muscle tightness is a primary limitation, limitations are evident with passive muscle stretching. However, when compensatory movements occur during active muscle contraction or movement, it is usually indicative of faulty neural control. Consequently, active movement is an effective method of determining the effect that muscle imbalance and poor posture have on neural control, and to identify limitations to movement. The active movements selected as screens, however, must be skill- and conditioning-level appropriate, allow practice trials, and be specific to the client's needs. It is important to remember that almost any screen can evaluate functional capacity, as long as it is relevant to client needs and challenges and provides useful feedback on movement efficiency. It is also imperative to distinguish correctible from non-correctible postural compensations. While a client's health history may provide valuable information to determine this, the objective is to coach the client to move the joint in question toward neutral and evaluate his or her ability to do so without compromise or pain.

The overall goal with exercise programming is to restore muscle balance and muscle's physiological properties, and improve neuromuscular control of movement by re-educating faulty neural pathways. However, unless awareness of poor posture and intention to improve are key objectives of this program, individuals are not likely to achieve great success. Restorative exercise programs focus upon stretching hypertonic muscles through passive elongation to increase the number of sarcomeres in series and then strengthen latent muscles with isometric or limited range-of-motion exercises in normal resting-length positions.

References

Arokoski, J.P. et al. (2001). Back and abdominal muscle function during stabilization exercises. *Archives Physical Medicine and Rehabilitation,* 82, 1089–1098.

Cook, G. (2003). *Athletic Body in Balance*. Champaign, Ill.: Human Kinetics.

Esquerre, R. et al. (2000). *Beyond Sets and Reps: Reebok Reactive Neuromuscular Training: A Reebok University Programming Option for Personal Trainers,* Toronto: Reebok University.

Gray, G. & Tiberio, D. (2007) *Chain Reaction*. Adrian, Mich.: Wynn Marketing.

Houglum, P.A. (2005). *Therapeutic Exercise for Musculoskeletal Injuries* (2nd ed.). Champaign, Ill.: Human Kinetics.

Kendall, F.P. et al. (2005), *Muscles: Testing and Function With Posture and Pain* (5th ed.). Philadelphia: Lippincott Williams & Wilkins.

MacIntosh, B.R., Gardiner, P., & McComas, A.J. (2006). *Skeletal Muscle* (2nd ed.). Champaign, Ill.: Human Kinetics.

McGill, S.M. (2007). *Low Back Disorders: Evidence-based Prevention and Rehabilitation* (2nd ed.). Champaign, Ill.: Human Kinetics.

Sahrmann, S.A. (2002). *Diagnosis and Treatment of Movement Impairment Syndromes*. St. Louis, Mo.: Mosby.

Shultz, S.J., Houglum, P.A., & Perrin, D.H. (2005). *Examination of Musculoskeletal Injuries* (2nd ed.). Champaign, Ill.: Human Kinetics.

Whiting W.C. & Rugg, S. (2006). *Dynatomy: Dynamic Human Anatomy*. Champaign, Ill.: Human Kinetics.

Whittle, M. W. (2007). *Gait Analysis: An Introduction* (4th ed.). Edinburgh: Butterworth Heineman Elsevier.

Wilmore, J.H., Costill, D.L., & Kenney, W.L (2008). *Physiology of Sport and Exercise* (4th ed.). Champaign, Ill.: Human Kinetics.

Suggested Reading

Cook, G. (2003). *Athletic Body in Balance.* Champaign, Ill.: Human Kinetics.

Kendall, F.P. et al. (2005), *Muscles: Testing and Function With Posture and Pain* (5th ed.). Philadelphia: Lippincott Williams & Wilkins.

Sahrmann, S.A. (2002). *Diagnosis and Treatment of Movement Impairment Syndromes.* St. Louis, Mo.: Mosby.

In This Chapter

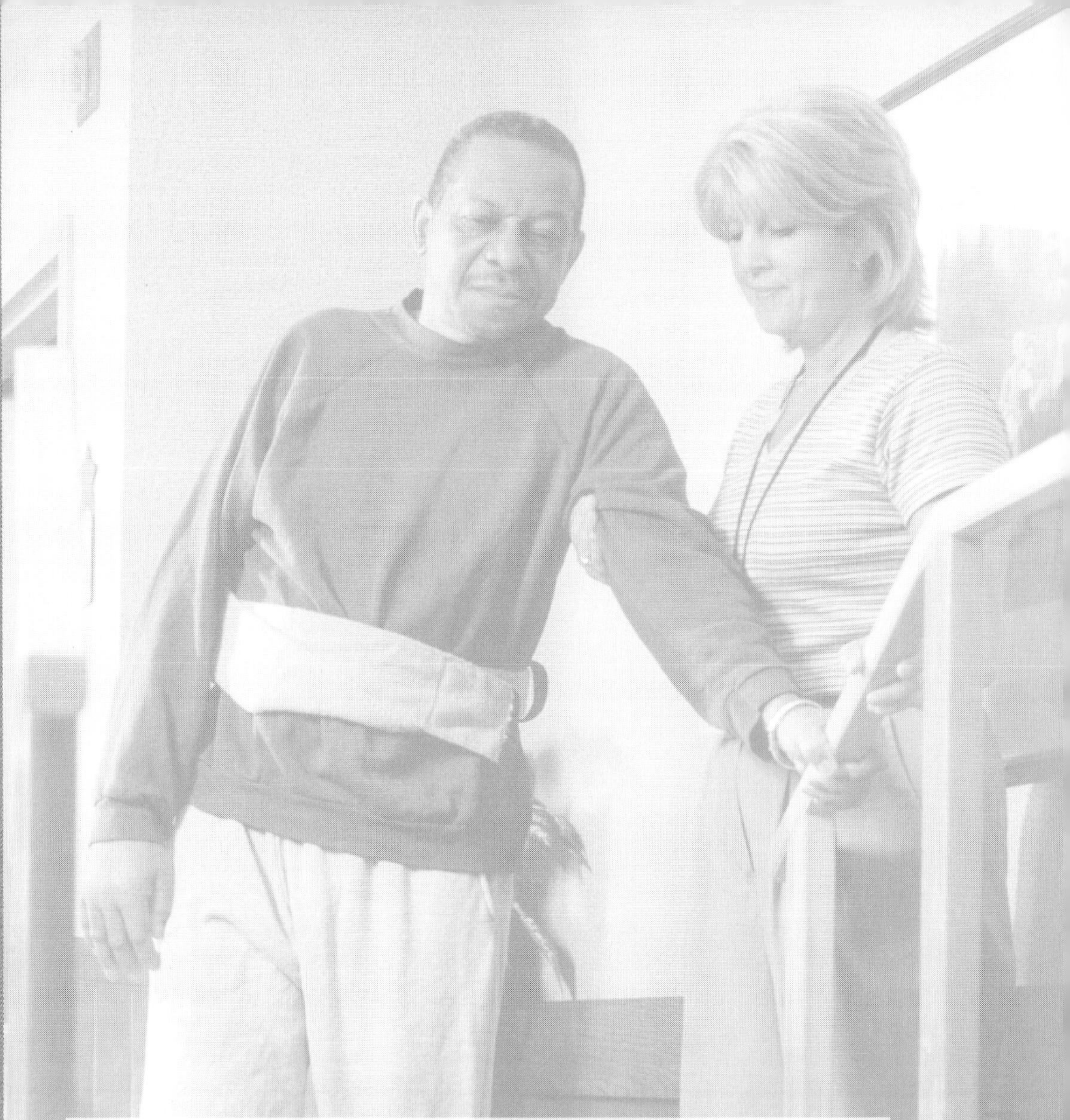

About The Author

Fabio Comana, M.A., M.S., is an exercise physiologist and spokesperson for the American Council on Exercise and faculty at San Diego State University and UC San Diego, teaching courses in exercise science and nutrition. He holds two master's degrees, one in Exercise Physiology and one in Nutrition, and certifications through ACE, ACSM, NSCA, and ISSN. Prior to joining ACE, he was a college head coach and the strength and conditioning coach at SDSU. Comana also managed health clubs for Club One. He lectures, conducts workshops, and writes on many topics related to exercise, fitness, and nutrition both nationally and internationally. As an ACE spokesperson and presenter, he is frequently featured in numerous media outlets including television, radio, Internet, and more than 100 nationwide newspaper and print publications. Comana has authored chapters in various textbooks.

CHAPTER 14

Mobility, Gait, and Balance

Fabio Comana

Movement is essential to complete all **activities of daily living (ADL),** and a person's ability to move efficiently requires control of the body's postural alignment. Control of posture is termed **balance,** which is defined as the maintenance of postural stability. More specifically, balance is subdivided into **static balance**—referring to the ability to maintain the body's **center of mass (COM)** within its **base of support (BOS)**—and **dynamic balance**—referring to the ability to move outside of the body's base of support, yet maintain postural control (Shumway-Cook & Woollacott, 2001; Whiting & Rugg, 2006; Gambetta, 2007).

A body's **center of gravity (COG)**, or COM, is that point around which all weight is evenly distributed. It is generally located 2 inches (5 cm) anterior to the spine in the S2 (second sacral vertebra) location (Figure 14-1), but the location varies by gender, body shape, body size, and even age (Kendall et al., 2005; Rose, 2003). The COG in males tends to be slightly higher than in females because of the greater quantity of upper-body musculature. Additionally, the body's COG continually shifts by changing position, moving, or adding external resistance.

The BOS can be described as the two-dimensional distance between and including a body's **points of contact (POC)** with a surface (Houglum, 2005). For example, when standing with the feet 12 inches (30 cm) apart, the base of support represents the areas that the feet contact and the area between the feet. Moving the feet to 6 inches (15 cm) apart reduces this area and the BOS, thereby reducing balance.

A body is stable when its **line of gravity** falls within its base of support. The line of gravity is a theoretical vertical line passing through the COG, dissecting the body into two hemispheres. When this line of gravity or the COG falls outside of the base of support, or when the body's **limits of stability (LOS)** are challenged, maintaining balance becomes more difficult. The LOS is the degree of allowable sway from the line of gravity without a need to change the base of support. Healthy adults normally tolerate about 12.5 degrees in anterior-posterior sway and about 16 degrees laterally (Rose, 2003; Sherlock, 1996). Muscle weakness, a deconditioned core, reduced **joint mobility,** and neurological and proprioceptive losses reduce LOS.

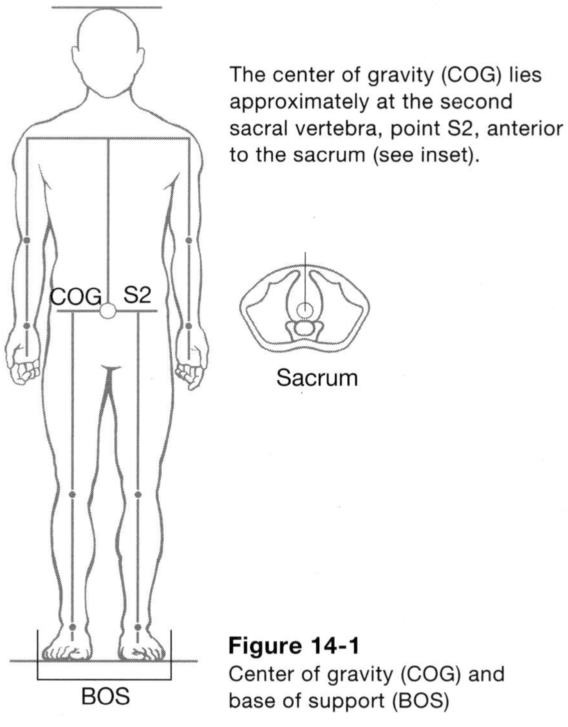

The center of gravity (COG) lies approximately at the second sacral vertebra, point S2, anterior to the sacrum (see inset).
COG
S2
Sacrum
BOS

Figure 14-1
Center of gravity (COG) and base of support (BOS)

Good balance generally exists because multiple systems provide accurate and precise information and commands. Sensory input from the visual, vestibular, and kinesthetic receptors provide important sensory information to the **peripheral** and **central nervous systems,** while motor responses result in reflexive or voluntary muscle action. Voluntary motor commands are relatively slow in comparison to automated or reflexive movements. Therefore, balance efficiency is dependent, in part, on the effectiveness of automated or reflexive systems.

Three measurable dimensions of balance exist and merit consideration when evaluating postural control and designing programs for improving balance and mobility: anticipatory, reactive, and adaptive postural control (Whiting & Rugg, 2006).

Anticipatory postural control involves stabilization of the body in anticipation of voluntary disruptive events that may require postural changes and potential losses in balance.

Reactive postural control occurs in response to unexpected threats to balance that cause the line of gravity to move away from the BOS. This control is necessary to restore balance and prevent a fall. If the disturbance does not exceed the LOS, the righting response may not require a change to the BOS, but if the disturbance is significantly large, it does require a change in BOS (e.g., taking a step or multiple steps to avoid a fall).

Adaptive postural control is the control of posture through the integration of afferent information from all three sensory systems and efferent (neuromuscular) commands. This allows the body to modify the sensory and motor systems in response to the environment and situational changes.

Maintaining balance relies on three distinct strategies utilized consciously or subconsciously. They involve the ankle, knee, and hip (Whiting & Rugg, 2006). These strategies normally function in sequence and along a continuum, depending on the magnitude and speed of the balance disturbance (Figure 14-2). While these strategies are discussed relative to the **sagittal plane,** they also apply to balance disturbances in the **frontal** and **transverse planes** as an individual exceeds the LOS.

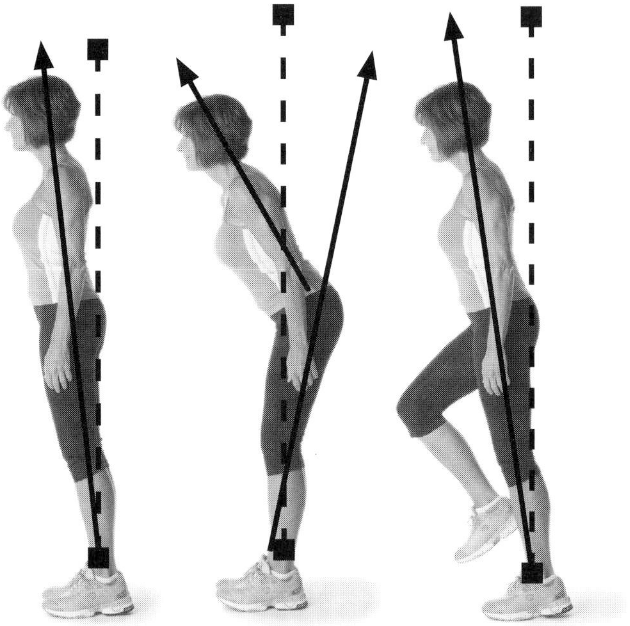

Figure 14-2
Three postural control strategies used to control balance

Ankle strategies occur in response to small disturbances in balance to restore the COG within the BOS by action at the ankle joint. This strategy primarily involves activation of either the plantarflexors or dorsiflexors, resulting in simultaneous sway, or movement of the upper and lower body in the same direction to restore balance. Given the relative weakness of the musculature of the ankle, this strategy generates small amounts of force and responds to minimal balance disturbances, such as normal postural sway.

Hip strategies occur in response to larger and/or faster disturbances in balance necessitating faster restorations of the COG within the BOS. Given the larger magnitude of correction required, the larger hip muscles are recruited to move the lower and upper extremities in opposite directions to restore balance.

Knee or step strategies respond when ankle and hip strategies are ineffective in restoring balance, given that the balance disturbance has exceeded the body's static LOS. Movement is required in the direction of the disturbance by taking a step to restore balance under a new BOS without losing postural control. Knee or hip strategies are vital to maintaining dynamic balance during movement.

These strategies require adequate flexibility at the involved joints, along with strength, power, reactivity, and normal neuromuscular input and responses. Three peripheral systems—visual, somatosensory, and vestibular—provide sensory input:

- The visual system provides visual layouts; spatial location relative to objects; a reference of verticality and head motion; navigation, anticipation, and avoidance; and generally accounts for 75% of human sensory input.
- The somatosensory system provides spatial position and movement relative to support surfaces, position and movement of body segments relative to each other, and assists with balance and navigation in the absence of vision.
- The vestibular system provides internal gravitational, linear, and angular acceleration information in relation to inertial space and head position, and becomes important when visual and somatosensory inputs are absent, distorted, or in conflict (e.g., the sensation of a vehicle rolling at stoplight when another vehicle pulls alongside).

Any change to these intrinsic systems reduces the ability to accurately and rapidly perceive sensory information, compromising balance and mobility.

The Core in Balance

Balance is the foundational skill element to all programming, whether functional or sports-related. Balance not only enhances physical performance, but also contributes to improving the cognitive and affective (emotional) domains and building self-efficacy and confidence. Improvements to balance result from increased postural stability, a key function of the core musculature. Core conditioning therefore involves balance and the use of controlled, yet exaggerated, positions of static and dynamic imbalance to generate effective neural feedback and evoke appropriate levels of neuromuscular responses.

The concept of the core refers to the trunk, or more specifically the lumbo-pelvic region. Although many definitions exist, postural stability is the ability of the core musculature to effectively control the position and motion of the trunk relative to the pelvis and legs (Willardson, 2007). Panjabi (1992a; 1992b) defines core stability as the capacity of the stabilizing systems to maintain the inter-vertebral neutral zones within physiological limits. The stabilizing system consists of three components (McGill et al., 2003):

- The passive joint subsystem (spinal column, fascia, joint shape, joint structure, and ligaments)
- The active muscle subsystem (muscle action)
- The neural subsystem (feedback and control)

As the passive subsystem generally allows the lumbar spine to support a limited load of about 22 pounds (10 kg), it is the active muscle subsystem that must contribute significantly to supporting body mass, plus any additional loads associated with external resistance and dynamic movement. The active muscle subsystem therefore plays a critical role in stabilization of the lumbo-pelvic region (Figure 14-3) (McGill, 2001; McGill et al., 2003).

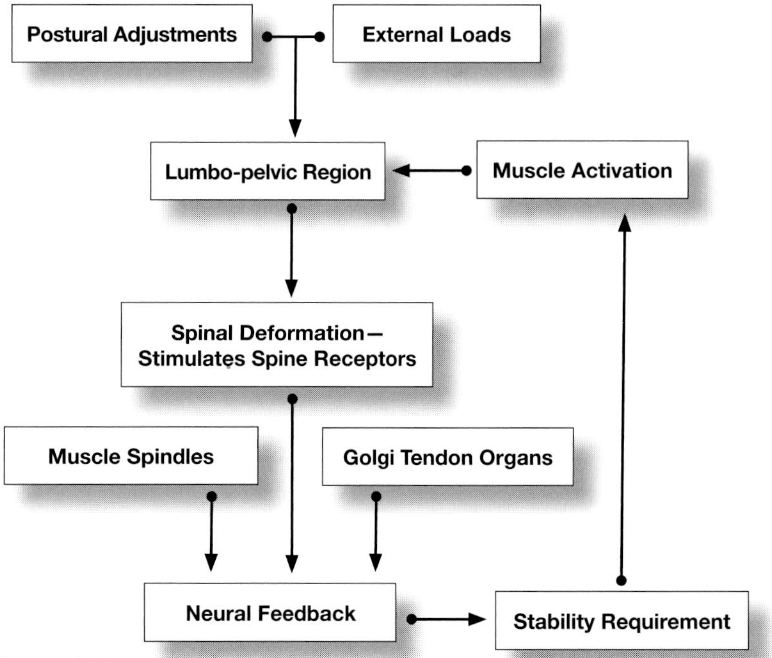

Figure 14-3
Model of core stability

Source: Willardson, J.M. (2007). Core stability training: Applications to sports conditioning programs. *Journal of Strength and Conditioning Research,* 21, 3, 979–985.

Core Anatomy

The different layers of muscles within this region each have specific roles in movement and stabilization. The larger, more superficial muscles are primarily responsible for movement and force transfer between the pelvis and thoracic cage, while the smaller, deeper muscles are more responsible for intersegmental motion and stabilization of the spine.

Cresswell and Thortensson (1994) demonstrated that the key muscle that works with the neural subsystem is the transverse abdominis. It functions primarily to increase intra-abdominal pressure, reducing compressive forces along the spine. In healthy individuals, this muscle fires in anticipation of voluntary or involuntary loading of the spine to reduce compressive forces (Hodges & Richardson, 1996; Hodges et al., 1996)). Given the different roles muscles play within this region, it may be easier to review the muscle anatomy by function and location, rather than exclusively by location.

The deep layer, or inner unit, consists of small muscles (rotatores, interspinali, intertransversarii) that span single vertebrae and are generally too small to offer stabilization of the entire spine. They offer segmental stabilization of each vertebra, especially at end ranges of motion, and are rich in sensory nerve endings that provide feedback information to the brain relating to spinal position.

The middle layer forms a box spanning several vertebrae, from the diaphragm to the pelvic floor, with muscles and fascia enclosing the back, front, and sides (Figure 14-4). The group consists of the transverse abdominis, multifidus, quadratus lumborum, posterior fibers of the internal oblique, the diaphragm, the pelvic floor musculature, and the adjoining fascia (i.e., linea alba, thoracolumbar fascia). This box allows the spine and sacroiliac joint to stiffen in anticipation of loading and movement, and provides a working foundation from which the body can operate (Bergmark, 1989).

The relationship between the vertebrae and core musculature (local layer) can be likened to a segmented flagpole with guy wires controlled by the neural subsystem (Figure 14-5) (Bergmark, 1989). The segmented pole represents the vertebra, while the guy wires represent the core muscles. Balanced tension within the guy wires increases tension to stiffen the flagpole or lumbar vertebrae and enhance spinal stability.

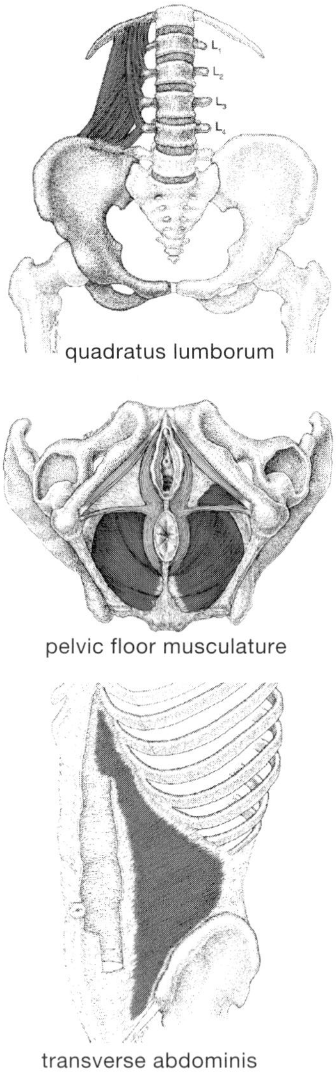

Figure 14-4
Middle layer of core muscles
Source: LifeART image copyright 2008 Wolters Kluwer Health, Inc., Lippincott Williams & Wilkins. All rights reserved.

The outer layer consists of big powerful muscles that span many vertebrae and are involved in gross movement of the trunk (Figure 14-6) (Bergmark, 1989). These muscles include the rectus abdominis, erector spinae group, external and internal oblique, iliopsoas, and latissimus dorsi.

In healthy individuals without low-back pain, the core musculature functions reflexively to stabilize the spine under voluntary or involuntary loading without the need for conscious muscle

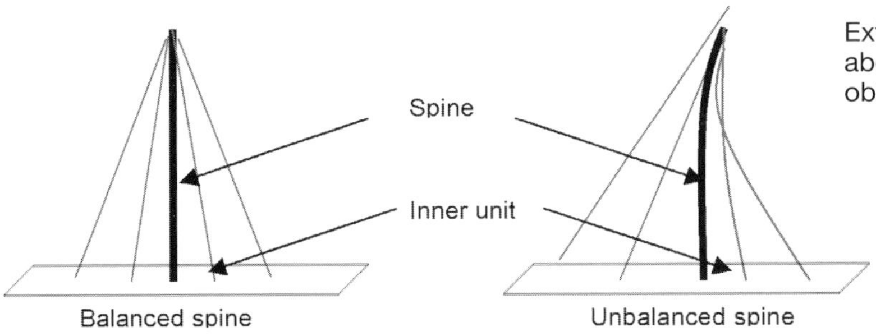

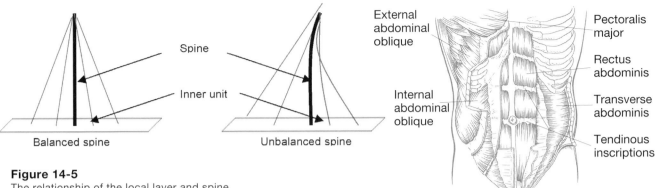

Figure 14-5
The relationship of the local layer and spine

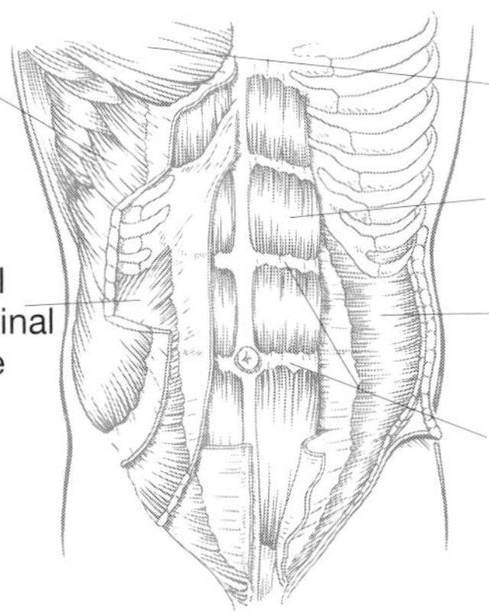

Figure 14-6
Muscles of the abdominal wall

control. This anticipatory muscle action minimizes the equilibrium disturbances provoked by the voluntary action. During voluntary or involuntary multiplanar loading and movement, effective core action optimizes force production and transfer through the trunk to the extremities, thereby enabling more efficient control of integrated movement; improving the ability to tolerate loading forces; protecting the spine from potential injury; and improving balance, coordination, dynamic postural strength, and control.

Hodges and Richardson (1996) discovered that delayed activation or minimal activation of the transverse abdominis muscle and limited co-contraction of core muscles in individuals suffering from low-back pain indicated some neural control deficits. Delayed onset of the transverse abdominis may cause inadequate stabilization of the lumbar spine during movements of the upper extremity (Sahrmann, 2002). Deconditioned individuals who spend much of their time in supported devices (back rests, etc.) may demonstrate similar neural control deficits. Consequently, balance and core training must begin with exercises that emphasize re-education of these faulty motor patterns and is best achieved by activating the core musculature in isolation in stable, supported environments.

McGill (2002) claims that the relative contributions of the core muscles continually change throughout movement to accommodate postural adjustments and spinal loading. Core muscle involvement therefore is dynamic, and effective core training must ultimately simulate the patterns and planes of natural movement. McGill also states that the development of core endurance should take precedence over core strength, as muscular endurance better correlates with spinal stability and a lower risk of injury. Arokoski and colleagues (2001) agree, indicating that the lumbar-stabilizing multifidi muscles are primarily type I fibers, best trained with lighter loads and more repetitions.

McGill (2002) also states that while **abdominal hollowing,** or "centering," the isolated activation of the inner unit that draws the umbilicus inward and upward, serves essential motor re-education purposes, it does not ensure the same degree of stability as "bracing," which involves the co-contraction of both the core and abdominal muscles to create a more rigid and wider BOS for spinal stabilization. Ultimately, clients should implement bracing, as it is a more effective method of stabilizing the spine (Gambetta, 2007).

Intra-abdominal Pressure

Contraction of the inner unit produces a "hoop tension" effect similar to the effect of cinching a belt. This contraction, primarily of the transverse abdominis, pulls on the linea alba, thereby pulling the abdominal wall inward and upward. This contraction compresses the internal organs to push upward against the diaphragm and downward against the pelvic floor musculature. According to Cresswell and Thorstensson (1994) this increases intra-abdominal pressure (IAP), creating a lift pressure against the diaphragm. Since the diaphragm has attachments on the second and third lumbar vertebra, contraction of the inner unit pulls them upward, increasing traction between the lumbar vertebra. The increased traction reduces joint and disk compression on the lumbar discs by as much as 40% and creates a rigid cylinder (spinal stiffening) to stabilize the spine during loading.

Thoracolumbar Fascia Gain

The synergistic contractions of the transverse abdominis and obliques, and increased IAP, generate lateral tension on the thoracolumbar fascia, creating an extension force on the second through fifth lumbar vertebrae (Gracovetsky, Farfar, & Lamy, 1992; Gracovetsky, Farfar, & Helleur, 1985; McGill, 2002). This extension force is termed thoracolumbar fascia gain and is believed to assist with buffering force transfer between the muscular and ligament systems of the spine during trunk flexion and extension movements. Only a small amount of muscle activity in the multifidi and transverse abdominis is required to create this effect.

Movement

Movement involves integrated action along the kinetic chain, where action at one segment affects successive segments within the chain. Efficient movement involves the synergistic contributions of mechanics, and the cohesive actions of the neurological and physiological systems working together to achieve simultaneous stability and mobility at the moving joints. The effective contributions of these systems allows the body to accurately receive and interpret sensory information, anticipate stabilization and movement demands, and allow for the selection and execution of appropriate motor responses to bring about efficient movement (Figure 14-7) (Cook, 2003).

Joint mobility is the range of uninhibited movement around a joint or body segment. **Joint stability** is the ability to maintain or control joint movement or position. Both joint mobility and stability are attained by the interaction of all components surrounding the joints and the neuromuscular system. Joint mobility must never be attained by compromising joint stability.

Flawed movement patterns, poor posture, improper exercise technique, and poorly designed exercise equipment may force unnatural joint movements and muscle action, thereby overtaxing muscles and increasing the potential for muscle imbalance. These types of misalignments and compensated movements due to faulty mechanics ultimately result in injury.

Locomotion is the act of moving from one location to another. **Gait** defines a particular form of locomotion, most commonly used in the context of describing walking and running (Whiting & Rugg, 2006). Although gait differs between people, there are basic similarities. Major differences result from postural variations, muscle weaknesses and imbalances, and structural abnormalities or variances (Houglum, 2005). While walking appears to be a simple movement task, it actually entails a complex set of coordinated neuromuscular and mechanical events. This section provides a comprehensive review of the gait cycle and describes the movements involved.

Although the higher brain centers provide overall control, variation, and adaptability to gait patterns, neuron complexes (central pattern generators) in the spinal cord control rhythmic and subconscious muscle activation and coordination

Figure 14-7
The movement efficiency model

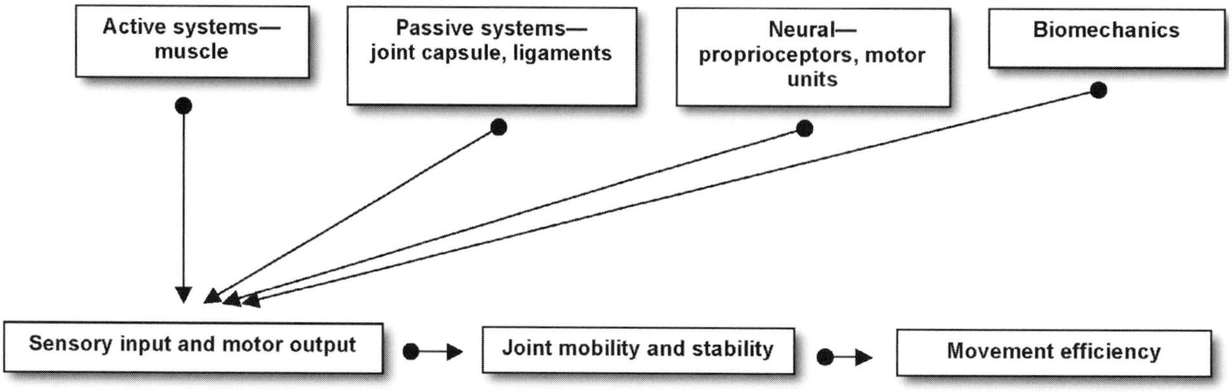

patterns during walking. These patterns integrate sensory information from the three sensory systems (vision, vestibular, and somatosensory) that control and modify gait in anticipation of, or in reaction to, obstacles (Rose, 2003). Proactive visual control involves avoidance strategies, momentary modifications in gait patterns to avoid obstacles, accommodation strategies, and the adaptation of gait patterns in response to changing surfaces. The vestibular system works together with the visual system to stabilize vision during gait while the head is moving via the vestibulo-occular reflex. Somatosensory feedback provides continual information regarding limb orientation during the gait cycle.

The Gait Cycle

The gait cycle is the time between the first contact with the ground by the heel of one foot and the next heel-ground contact with the same foot. This period of **ipsilateral** (i.e., same side) contact is called a stride and is composed of two steps. A step is defined as the period from initial contact of one leg to the initial contact of the **contralateral** (i.e., opposite side) leg (Figure 14-8). Because of their taller stature, men have stride and step lengths that are approximately 14% greater than women (Whiting & Rugg, 2006). Normal stride lengths average 57 to 59 inches (1.45 to 1.50 m) in men and 50 to 52 inches (1.27 to 1.32 m) in women, while normal step lengths average 28.5 to 29.5 inches (0.73 to 0.75 m) in men and 25 to 26 inches (0.64 to 0.66 m) in women (Lehmann & DeLater, 1990). Step width is measured between the medial surfaces of the foot and normally equals 2 to 4 inches (5 to 10 cm) during walking and decreases to 0 inches (0 cm) or even demonstrates some crossover during running (Whiting & Rugg, 2006; Lehmann & DeLater, 1990).

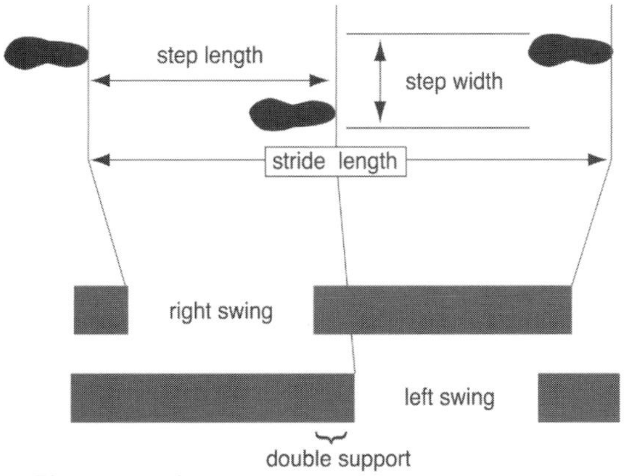

Figure 14-8
Step length, stride length, and step width

Step rate is called cadence and is important in determining speed (velocity). Walking speed is calculated as follows:

Walking speed = Cadence (steps/minute) x Step length (inches) x 0.00095

For example, at a step length of 25.5 inches (0.65 m) and a cadence of 110 steps/minute, an individual's walking speed would be approximately 2.7 mph (4.3 km/h). To determine speed in miles per hour (mph), perform the following calculations:

- Walking speed = cadence (steps/minute) x step length (inches) x 0.00095
- Walking speed = 110 steps/minute x 25.5 (inches) x 0.00095
- Walking speed = 2.7 mph (4.3 km/h)

Normal cadence in adults is between 90 and 120 steps/minute, with women typically demonstrating rates six to nine steps faster/minute than men (Lehmann & DeLater, 1990).

Walking speed differs depending on numerous factors, including age, size (limb length), physical condition, injury, and disability. A significant age-related change is a reduction in gait speed due to reductions in stride and step length, but also decreased step frequency, increased time spent in double-support time, more cautious load acceptance, increased transition times from heel strike to toe-off, reduced limb advancement and swing, reduced knee flexion during the swing phase, and reduced torso rotations.

During gait, each leg alternates between periods when the foot is in contact with the ground (stance phase) and when it is moving forward through the air (swing phase). When only one foot is in contact with the ground and is solely supporting the entire body, it is termed single-support, and when both feet are in contact with the ground, it is termed double-support. During each stride, there are two single-support times, each accounting for 40% of the gait cycle, and two double-support times, each accounting for approximately 10% of the gait cycle (Whiting & Rugg, 2006; Rose, 2003).

The human gait cycle consists of two phases for each foot (Figure 14-9) (Houglum, 2005):

- *Stance phase:* Accounts for 62% of the gait cycle and consists of five instants when the foot is in contact with the floor and the extremity is bearing partial or total weight
  - ✔The initial contact (heel strike) and load response instants are the weight-acceptance periods of the stance phase, when one foot is preparing to accept weight while the other is preparing for toe-off.
  - ✔The midstance instant involves single-leg support and forward movement of the stance-leg tibia over the stationary foot.
  - ✔The terminal stance (heel-off) and pre-swing (toe-off) instants involve weight unloading in preparation for leg swing.
- *Swing phase:* Accounts for 38% of the gait cycle when the foot is in the air and not in contact with the surface.
  - ✔The initial, acceleration, or early-swing instant occurs when the foot is lifted off the floor, with knee flexion and ankle dorsiflexion allowing the limb to accelerate forward.
  - ✔The midswing or swing-through instant occurs when the swing leg moves forward and adjacent to the stance leg (in midstance).
  - ✔The terminal, deceleration, or late-swing instant slows down the swinging limb in preparation for heel strike and loading.

Normal gait requires the ability to execute simultaneous and controlled movements at multiple joints and in multiple planes (Table 14-1). Any disturbances to the sequencing or level of muscle activation may alter gait mechanics and create a need for compensatory muscle action and patterns.

To achieve normal gait patterns, an individual must possess the following (Rose, 2003):

- Adequate ranges of motion in all necessary planes across the involved joints
- Adequate strength levels within each of the involved muscles
- Unimpaired sensory input from the visual, somatosensory, and vestibular systems
- Appropriate magnitude and timing of muscle activation and coordination

During gait, three major tasks must be achieved to ensure normal gait patterns: weight acceptance, single-leg support, and limb advancement (Figure 14-10). Appropriate magnitudes and timing of muscle action in the lower extremity is essential for normal gait function and

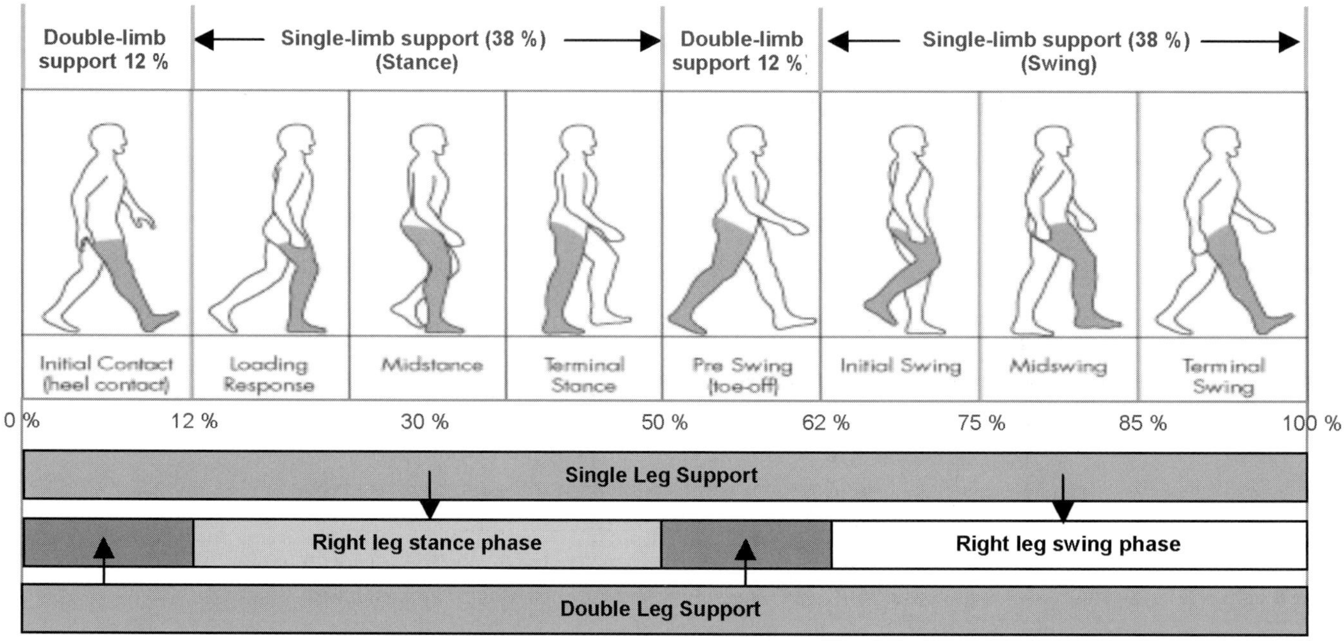

Figure 14-9
The phases and instants of the gait cycle

Source: Adapted from Whiting W.C. & Rugg, S. (2006). *Dynatomy: Dynamic Human Anatomy.* Champaign, Ill.: Human Kinetics.

Table 14-1
Joint Movement During Gait

Reference Limb	Initial Contact (IC)	Load Response (LR)	Midstance (MST)	Terminal Stance (TST)	Pre-swing (PS)	Initial Swing (IS)	Midswing (MSW)	Terminal Swing (TSW)
Opposite Limb	**PS**	**PS**	**IS, MSW**	**MSW, TSW**	**IC, LR**	**MST**	**MST**	**TST**
	Weight Acceptance		Single-leg Support			Limb Advancement		
Trunk	Erect with some rotation	Erect	Erect with some rotation	Erect with some rotation	Erect with some rotation	Erect with some rotation	Erect	Erect with some rotation
Reference Limb	Initial Contact (IC)	Load Response (LR)	Midstance (MST)	Terminal Stance (TST)	Pre-swing (PS)	Initial Swing (IS)	Midswing (MSW)	Terminal Swing (TSW)
Opposite Limb	PS	PS	IS, MSW	MSW, TSW	IC, LR	MST	MST	TST
	Weight Acceptance		Single-leg Support			Limb Advancement		
Pelvis	4–5° anterior tilt 4° medial rotation Lateral elevation, but dropping	Moves into posterior tilt 4° medial rotation	Neutral Rotating laterally Lateral elevation	Posterior tilt 4° lateral rotation Lateral dropping	4–5° posterior tilt 4° lateral rotation	Move into anterior tilt 4° lateral rotation Lateral elevation	Neutral Lateral elevation	4–5° anterior tilt 4° medial rotation
Hip	30° flexion, slight adduction/ medial rotation	30° flexion	Neutral	10–15° extension	Neutral, slight abduction, lateral rotation	15–20° flexion	20–30° flexion	30° flexion
Knee	0° flexion 8–10° lateral rotation	15° flexion	15–0°, medial rotation	0°, moving into lateral rotation	35° flexion	60° flexion, moving into medial rotation	60–30° flexion	0°
Ankle	0° Supinated	10–15° plantarflexion, moves into pronation	0–10° dorsiflexion, pronation	10–0° dorsiflexion, moves into supination	20° plantarflexion, supination	10–0° plantarflexion, pronated	0°	0°, moves into supination

even subtle muscle deficiencies can significantly affect movement efficiency. The key muscles groups involved in gait are the hip and knee extensors, and the plantar- and dorsiflexors that collectively bring about specific control of movements throughout the gait cycle (Rose, 2003). Key muscle-group functions during each instant include (Whiting & Rugg, 2006):

- *Initial contact and load response:* Hip abductors eccentrically prevent excessive lateral pelvic tilting, the knee extensors eccentrically prevent excessive flexion, and the ankle dorsiflexors eccentrically control plantarflexion. This results in weight acceptance, pelvic stabilization, and deceleration.
- *Midstance:* Hip abductors and adductors stabilize hip and knee alignment over the foot, the gastrocnemius helps stabilize the knee, the contralateral quadratus lumborum controls lateral pelvic tilting, and the plantarflexors eccentrically control tibial advancement over the foot.
- *Terminal stance:* The loaded hip extensor and contralateral arm begin to control rotation and ready the body for propulsion.
- *Pre-swing and initial swing:* The loaded hip extensor and contralateral arm provide propulsion and the hip flexors initiate hip flexion.
- *Initial swing and midswing:* Ankle dorsiflexors act concentrically to help clear the foot.
- *Midswing and terminal swing:* Ankle dorsiflexors eccentrically control plantarflexion, the hamstrings act eccentrically to slow knee extension, and the contralateral erector spinae group stabilizes the sacroiliac joint and maintains trunk extension in preparation for initial contact.

Forward pelvic rotation in the transverse plane allows the femur to move further forward and increases step length without requiring a downward pelvic shift. Normal pelvic rotation totals 8 degrees, with a 4-degree forward rotation on the swing leg and a 4-degree backward rotation on the stance leg. This prevents excessive dropping of the center of gravity to achieve desirable step lengths (Houglum, 2005). Research by Bruijn and colleagues (2007) demonstrates that at walking velocities greater than 1.9 mph (3 km/h), the pelvic and thoracic contributions to total body angular momentum was less than 10% of the total, while the contributions from the legs and arms totaled 90%. This finding implies that the counter-rotation of the torso against the pelvis is relatively unimportant to total angular momentum when increasing gait speed.

Vertical pelvic shifting, or "hiking," during the midstance instant also lowers the center of gravity. As the support leg achieves its highest point at midstance, the downward lateral tilt and lowering of the swing leg lowers the center of gravity by almost 5 degrees.

Figure 14-10
Accomplishment of the three major tasks during in the gait cycle

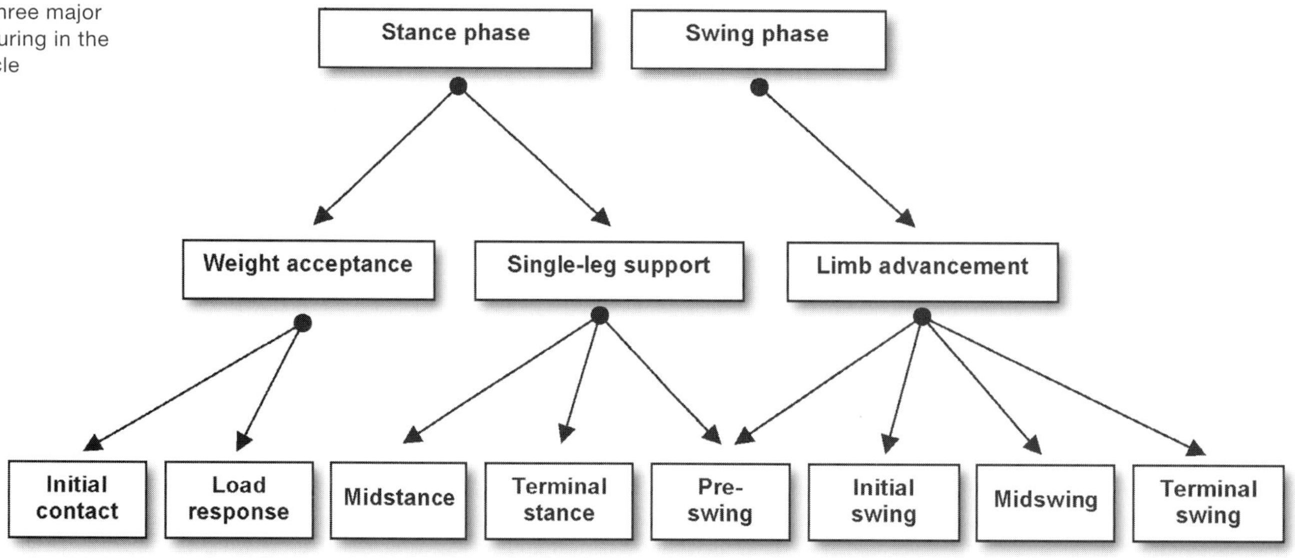

A small lateral pelvic shift, or "list," occurs during the single-leg time to support the body on one leg. If the femur and tibia were aligned in parallel fashion, a shift of up to 6 inches (15 cm) would be needed to support the center of gravity during single-leg support. Given that the femurs are not aligned in parallel fashion (**Q-angle** effect), but angled medially, a shift of only 1 to 2 inches (2.5 to 5 cm) is generally needed to support the center of gravity over one leg, as during the midstance instant.

Following initial contact, the knee moves into flexion to help minimize the center of gravity's vertical excursion at midstance, when the movement of the hips is at its highest position. The center of gravity at the ankle is highest at initial contact (heel strike) and at the pre-swing (toe-off) instants, but lowest during midsta nce, reducing the vertical excursion of the center of gravity.

The combined efforts of pelvic rotation, pelvic tilting, and the knee and ankle motions are responsible for reducing the vertical excursion of the center of gravity by 1 inch (2.5 cm) and improving overall stability during the gait. This downward excursion in the center of gravity reduces the total vertical excursion at midstance to less than 2 inches (5 cm). This smoothens the movement transitions into the midstance instant, thereby reducing the energy expenditure needed to lift the body's center of gravity, and improves movement efficiency (Houglum, 2005).

During running, the duration of the stance phase decreases, although loading forces increase almost threefold, and a float, or double-unsupported, phase occurs while the double-limb support phase disappears. The run cycle contains four phases:

- Stance phase (40%)
- First float phase (15%)
- Swing phase (30%)
- Second float phase (15%)

Myofascial Slings

Newton's third law addresses reactive forces to actions. The body generally distributes these reactive forces over large surface areas to dissipate excessive force build-up on individual muscles or joints. This process reduces the potential for injury. These forces transfer to other muscles, tendons, ligaments, fascia, joint capsules, and bones that lie in series or in parallel to actively moving joints or muscles, creating continuous lines of action called **myofascial slings.** The body contains numerous myofascial slings that act ipsilaterally and contralaterally to integrate movement and dissipate forces between the lower and upper extremities.

There are four systems within the body that provide a dynamic stabilization during movement (Vleeming et al., 1990a; 1990b; 2007). In particular, Vleeming and colleagues (2007) give attention to the ligaments and muscles spanning the sacroiliac joint, given its capacity for movement and the need for stabilization in controlling force transfer between the trunk and lower limbs. Stabilization or force closure relates to the ability of the muscle system, through its attachments into connective tissue, to compress the joint surfaces of the sacrum and iliac bones together. During gait, ground reactive forces transmit superiorly, while the force of gravity transmits forces inferiorly. While these myofascial slings facilitate efficient movement and help stabilize joints, they buffer forces, distributing them throughout the kinetic chain. These slings are defined as the posterior longitudinal, or deep longitudinal, system; the lateral system; the anterior oblique system; and the posterior oblique system (Vleeming et al., 2007; Myers, 2001). The actions of these four slings are effectively illustrated in the Premier Personal Training Solutions DVD collection (Premier Training International, 2005). In addition to the four slings identified by Vleeming and colleagues (2007), other slings have been identified, including the **serape effect**, which describes a sling that facilitates rotational movements of the torso.

The Posterior Longitudinal, or Deep Longitudinal, Sling

This sling provides stabilization to the sacroiliac joint during the swing phase and as the body prepares for heel strike. It includes the peroneus longus, tibialis anterior, biceps femoris, sacrotuberous ligament linking the ischium and sacrum, and the contralateral erector spinae group (Figure 14-11).

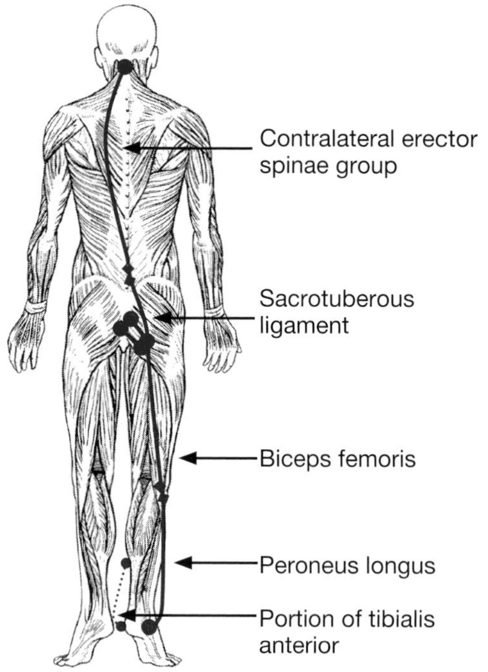

Figure 14-11
The posterior longitudinal, or deep longitudinal, myofascial sling

Source: LifeART image copyright 2008 Wolters Kluwer Health, Inc., Lippincott Williams & Wilkins. All rights reserved.

During the swing phase, as the swing leg moves forward, it produces rotation in the hip and torso, thereby generating tension within the contralateral erector spinae group that pulls superiorly on the sacrotuberous ligament. Conversely, the eccentric deceleration of hip flexion and knee extension by the biceps femoris pulls inferiorly on the sacrotuberous ligament. These opposing forces at the sacrotuberous ligament act to stabilize the sacroiliac joint in extension. Tension placed on the sacrotuberous ligament causes closure of this joint.

In anticipation of initial contact, the tibialis anterior prepares to eccentrically decelerate plantarflexion, while the peroneus longus eccentrically acts to control foot pronation, thereby stabilizing the foot. These muscles act collectively to stabilize and dissipate forces over a larger surface area of the sling and help stabilize the sacroiliac joint in extension through initial contact.

The Lateral System

During load response and through midstance, the lateral system plays an important role in stabilizing the pelvis and maintaining alignment of the hip and knee over the foot. It includes the gluteus medius and minimus, the adductor group, and contralateral quadratus lumborum (Figure 14-12). This sling is very important during single-leg stance positions, especially in individuals with larger Q-angles, given knee instability and consequent potential for hip adduction.

The balanced action of the gluteus and adductor groups stabilize the pelvis with the knee, maintaining alignment over the second toe and preventing excessive pelvic adduction during the stance phase. In normal walking, during the early and midstance instants of a given leg, the pelvis tends to drop toward the contralateral side. The degree of drop is controlled by the eccentric action of the stance-leg abductors (gluteus medius and minimus) and the concentric action of the contralateral quadratus lumborum (see Figure 14-12). Weak hip abductors allow excessive pelvic drop characteristic of **Trendelenburg gait,** which involves a drop of the pelvis on the side opposite of the stance leg, indicating weakness on the side of the stance leg (Houglum, 2005). This hip adduction collapses the knee and ankle inward while hiking that same hip upward, exacerbating the potential for injury.

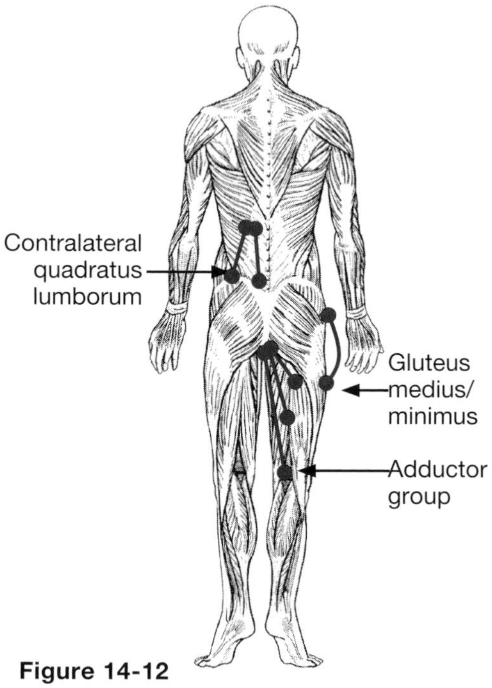

Figure 14-12
The lateral myofascial sling

Source: LifeART image copyright 2008 Wolters Kluwer Health, Inc., Lippincott Williams & Wilkins. All rights reserved.

The contralateral quadratus lumborum is unable to prevent that hip adduction and, in turn, can become weakened. As a compensatory mechanism to this condition, individuals usually demonstrate a lean in their trunks toward the stance leg.

The Anterior Oblique Sling

During the stance phase, the swing leg will advance forward of the stance leg to its new position. While the adductors act to anchor and fix the pelvis, the torso undergoes rotation to facilitate the leg swing. This sling includes the adductor group, ipsilateral internal oblique, contralateral external oblique, and intervening anterior abdominal fascia (Figure 14-13). These structures act to provide anterior stabilization of the sacroiliac joint during forward rotational movements in the stance phase of gait. As the stance-leg assumes load and allows the opposite leg to prepare its forward swing, the stance-leg adductors fire to stabilize the hip. Simultaneous action in the ipsilateral internal oblique and contralateral external oblique rotate the torso forward (see Figure 14-13).

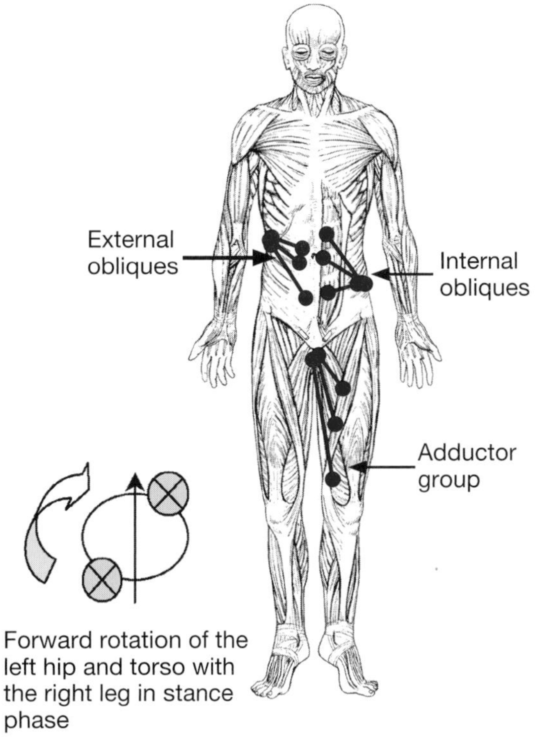

Figure 14-13
The anterior oblique sling

Source: LifeART image copyright 2008 Wolters Kluwer Health, Inc., Lippincott Williams & Wilkins. All rights reserved.

The Posterior Oblique System

During the terminal stance instant, the stance-leg hip moves into extension in preparation for toe-off and swing. Gluteus maximus activation extends the hip and externally rotates the femur, generating a rotational force upon the body. The contralateral latissimus dorsi is activated to oppose this rotational force. This sling, therefore, is composed of the stance-leg gluteus maximus, contralateral latissimus dorsi, and intervening thoracolumbar fascia and provides posterior stabilization of the sacroiliac joint during backward rotational movements during the toe-off instant of gait (Figure 14-14).

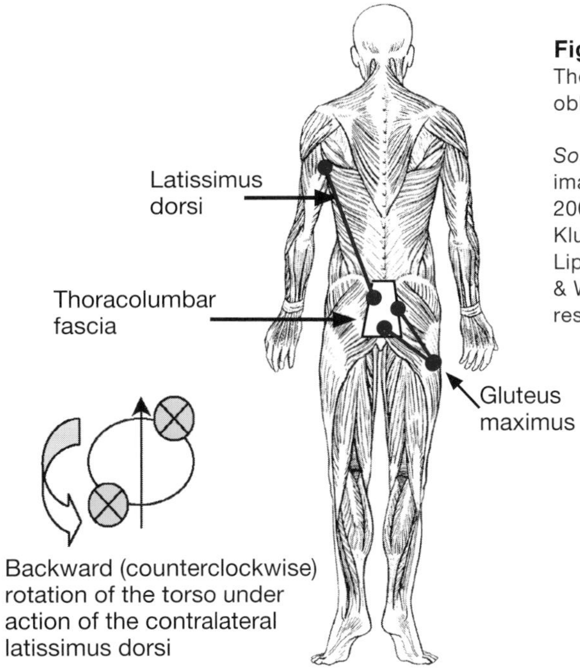

Figure 14-14
The posterior oblique sling

Source: LifeART image copyright 2008 Wolters Kluwer Health, Inc., Lippincott Williams & Wilkins. All rights reserved.

Concentric contraction of the gluteus maximus pulls the hip into extension and slight posterior rotation, pulling inferiorly on the thoracolumbar fascia. Simultaneously, the contralateral latissimus dorsi contracts, extending and posteriorly rotating the shoulder in the opposite direction of the hips and pulling superiorly upon the thoracolumbar fascia.

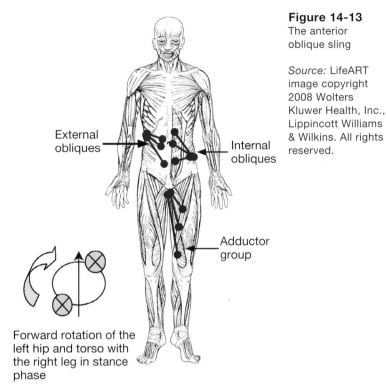

As this sling system runs at right angles to the joint plane of the sacroiliac joint, it causes closure of the joint when these muscles contract. Furthermore, as the gluteus maximus and thoracolumbar fascia have investments into the sacrotuberous ligament, tension placed on this ligament will also cause closure of the sacroiliac joint. This co-activation of opposing forces creates an extensor force on the thoracolumbar fascia and stabilizes the sacroiliac joint in extension during the toe-off instant.

Primary Movements

All human movement can essentially be broken down and described by primary movements:

- Single-leg movements (single-leg stance)
- Squatting movements (bending and lifting)
- Pushing movements (in vertical and horizontal planes)
- Pulling movements (in vertical and horizontal planes)
- Rotational movements

Activities of daily living are essentially the integration of multiple movements. For example, the action of picking up a child and turning to place him or her in a car seat involves a squatting movement, a rotational movement, a possible single-leg movement (if a step in involved), a pushing movement, and finally a pulling movement as the child is lowered into the seat.

Efficiency in executing these primary movements relies in part upon one or several myofascial slings:

- Single-leg movements rely predominantly on the lateral system.
- Squatting movements rely predominantly on the posterior longitudinal or deep longitudinal system.
- Pushing movements rely on the lateral and deep longitudinal systems.
- Pulling movements rely predominantly on the lateral and deep longitudinal systems.
- Any rotational movements rely predominantly on the anterior (push) and posterior oblique (pull) systems.

It makes sense that functional training should include integrated movements that train these sling patterns, perhaps starting with more isolated exercises to correct muscle imbalances (weaknesses) and establish neuromuscular control before progressing to integrated, multiplanar, and multijoint movement patterns. Yet, some fitness professionals teach advanced skills without first evaluating an individual's ability to perform the primary movements.

Single-leg Stance and Stepping

This movement involves weight transference over the stance leg (diminished base of support), while preserving optimal alignment among the hip, knee, and foot. Weight transference generally requires 1 to 2 inches (2.5 to 5 cm) of lateral shift over the stance leg with only a small hip hike (≤4 to 5 degrees of hip abduction). The ability to control hip adduction and the amount of lateral shift is a concern in women given their knee instability and 18-degree Q-angle, compared to the 13-degree Q-angle seen in men (Houglum, 2005). A wider pelvis, coupled with shorter bones, exaggerates the Q-angle, but greater joint laxity, smaller ligaments and surface area for attachment, and weaker muscles all compound the potential for injury. The anatomy of the knee imparts little support to joint stability, as the knee sits in the middle of two long lever-arms exposed to large forces. Gary Gray refers to the knee as a "reactor," as it simply responds to drivers from above and below (Gray, 2007). These drivers can take the form of ground reaction forces, gravity, momentum, loading, the hands and feet, or even the eyes tracking movement. During foot loading, the ankle joint creates a chain reaction from the ground up that influences the knee. The natural tendency on impact is toward calcaneal eversion and foot pronation, coupled with internal tibial rotation and knee abduction (**valgus** position) and internal femoral rotation (Kendall et al., 2005). These place stress upon the anterior cruciate ligament (ACL), increasing its potential for injury. The body is designed to resist these movements and corresponding stresses through the presence of big posterior-lateral muscles at the hips to decelerate internal rotation, a big medial collateral ligament (MCL) to resist excessive knee abduction, and strong deltoid ligaments on the medial surface at the ankle to resist excessive pronation. These elements protect their respective joints and reduce the loading upon the ACL. The ACE-AHFS needs to teach clients how to load into a stance-leg position without placing additional stresses on the knee. The single-leg stand movement screen presented in Chapter 13 serves as a good exercise to control these movements at the ankle, knee, and hip.

Bend and Lift (Squat or Dead Lift)

This lower-extremity primary movement can also place large stresses on the ACL if performed improperly. The ACL is also a very important stabilizer of the femur on the tibia and serves to prevent the tibia from sliding forward (anterior translation) and rotating inward excessively during agility, jumping, and deceleration activities (Houglum, 2005). Gluteus maximus (and posterior fibers of the gluteus medius) engagement during knee and hip flexion prevents excessive internal tibial rotation and knee abduction, helping unload the ACL. Additionally, greater gluteus dominance during knee flexion pulls on the hamstrings, which in turn pull on the posterior tibia and help unload the ACL (Gray, 2007). Individuals who are quadriceps dominant in their bend-and-lift technique will experience diminished strength and power by not engaging the gluteus maximus concentrically and may predispose the knees to greater risk for injury. The gluteus maximus and posterior fibers of the gluteus medius function in three planes and should therefore be trained in all three planes:

- Hip extension (sagittal plane)
- Lateral rotation of the hip (transverse plane)
- Abduction (frontal plane)

When instructing clients to perform a bend-and-lift movement, the ACE-AHFS can follow these guidelines:

Starting, standing position

- Before loading the spine, brace the trunk (co-contraction of the core and abdominal muscles to stabilize the spine).
- Position the feet in neutral to 8 to 10 degrees of eversion.
- Toe-tap to shift weight onto the heels.
- The heads-up position will help shift weight over the heels.
- A slight anterior tilt in the pelvis will help the client balance the barbell.

Downward phase

- Hip disengagement (anterior tilt) will shift the hips backward and initiate the downward movement, creating a pivot-like movement at the knees. This reduces premature anterior translation at the knee and downward sheering forces between the tibia and femur.
- The shoulders and hips drop together.
- As the downward movement continues, strong abdominal engagement generates a slight posterior pelvic tilt to position the spine more neutrally and avoid excessive lumbar lordosis.

Lowered position

- The client should align the ASIS and the knee over the second toe as well as possible (ASIS alignment will vary given differences in body shape).
- Anterior translation of the tibia will assist with balance and help the client avoid excessive hip flexion
- The client should maintain a figure-4 position with the tibia and torso in parallel and the thighs parallel to the floor.
- No visible evidence of lateral weight shifting or torso rotation should be seen over the dominant limb.

Upward phase

- Pushing is initiated through the heels while maintaining the heads-up position.
- The hips and shoulders rise together to avoid the lumbar strain associated with the hips-then-shoulders movement.

Rotational Movement

Rotation is a primary movement required in many sports and daily activities. Many mass movement patterns stored in the brain are spiral and diagonal motions, which match the spiral and rotary characteristics of the bones and joints (Voss, Ionta, & Myers, 1985). Rotation occurs in the transverse plane, where breakdowns occur most frequently due to the increased stresses placed along the spine. Therefore, correct form when performing these movements is critical to ensure safe and effective movement. Two triplanar movements requiring diagonal and spiral movements of the arms, shoulders, trunks, hips, and legs are the wood chop and hay bailer that are discussed in greater detail later in this chapter.

Assessment of Balance and Gait

A thorough medical screening is always a prerequisite to conducting assessments and includes a review of medications and any potential side effects the medications may have on balance (e.g., psychotropic and antihypertensive medications). The ACE-AHFS should also conduct a needs assessment to determine the appropriateness of testing based upon the client's needs, skill level, and functional capacity. The ACE-AHFS must then give consideration to prioritizing the assessments and establish timelines for testing, as many clients may find a battery of tests conducted at the onset overwhelming. To further complicate matters, the scope of practice of the ACE-AHFS includes additional evaluations such as posture and movement. Figure 14-15 provides an overview of how an ACE-AHFS can sequence assessments.

The use of population-specific protocols that are appropriate to functional capacity is recommended when working with older adults, given their propensity for functional limitations and considering the fact that many industry-standardized protocols are not appropriate nor validated for this age group (Nagi, 1991; Ricki & Jones, 2001). Figure 14-16 illustrates the progression of age-related changes in physiological function toward disability.

Several researchers and practitioners have developed and validated population-specific protocols. These protocols generally evaluate a cross-section of the major health- and skill-related fitness components associated with independent living, including balance. Balance tests assess basic static balance (standing or unsupported sitting); static balance challenges (manipulating BOS and

Figure 14-15
Sequencing of assessments

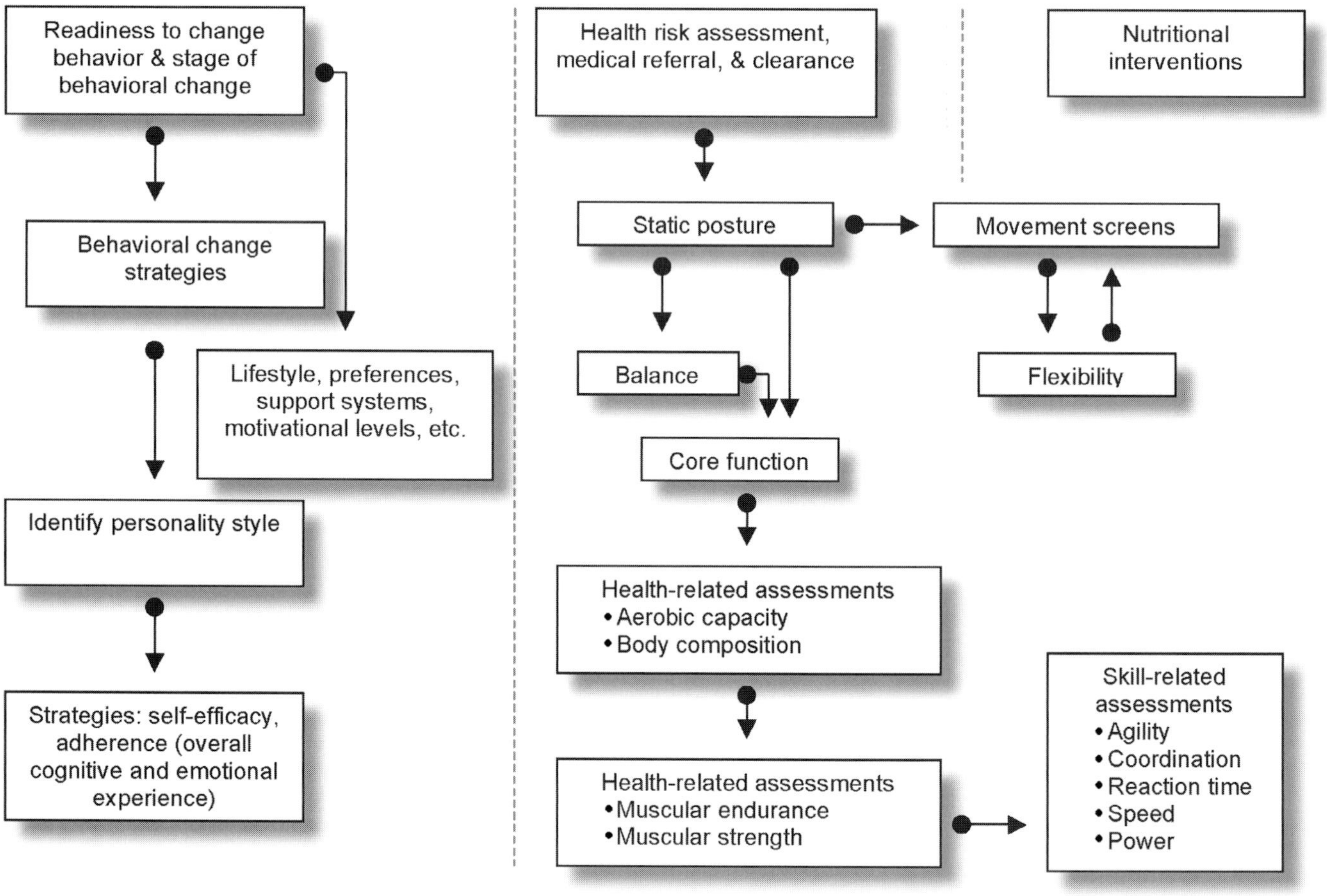

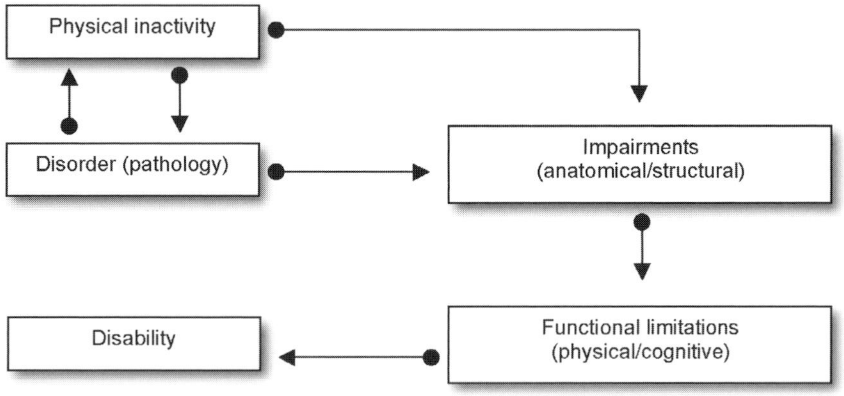

Figure 14-16
The modified disability model

Source: Adapted from Nagi, S.S (1991). Disability concepts revisited: Implication for prevention. In: Pope, A.M. & Tarlov, A.R. (Eds). *Disability in America: Toward a National Agenda for Prevention.* Washington, D.C.: National Academy Press.

COG, challenging LOS, and sensory integration); dynamic balance (rising out of chairs and gait); and anticipatory or adaptive control (movement around and over obstacles). Rose's *Fall Proof* (2003) and Rikli and Jones's *Senior Fitness Tests* (2001) are excellent resources for many of these protocols. Some of these population-specific protocols include:

- Berg Balance Scale (BBS)
- Fullerton Advanced Balance (FAB) Scale
- Fullerton Functional Fitness Tests (FFFT)
- Modified Clinical Test for Sensory Interaction in Balance (M-CTSIB)
- Multidirectional Reach Test (MDRT)
- Romberg and Sharpened Romberg
- Tinetti Balance and Gait Evaluation

For more information on some of these population-specific balance protocols, refer to Chapter 21 and Appendix F.

Older adults are broadly categorized into five functional levels based on their physical ability to perform ADL—physically elite, physically fit, physically independent, physically frail, and physically dependent—before being considered disabled (Spirduso, Francis, & MacRae, 2005). Activities of daily living can be classified as advanced (AADL), which include participation in sports, vacation, travel, and gardening; instrumental (IADL), which include housecleaning, doing laundry, and shopping; or basic (BADL), which include six primary functions:

- Feeding
- Continence
- Transference (e.g., moving about between a bed and chair)
- Toileting
- Dressing
- Bathing

The physically elite participate in physical training on a daily or near-daily basis and compete in age-appropriate events. This category also includes older adults holding physically demanding jobs. They generally possess physical capacities superior to many younger, untrained adults and this elite status is perhaps due to a genetic predisposition or sustained activity levels throughout adulthood. While they certainly could be assessed with the same protocols as younger adults, it is advised they are assessed under physician supervision due to their age.

The physically fit are frequently active or exercise two to seven days per week, primarily for health, recreation, and well-being. They tend to be consistent in maintaining health and exercise habits, and exhibit a significant difference between chronological and physical age. They too could be assessed using standardized protocols, as their functional capacities exceed most population-specific tests for older adults, but should also be assessed under physician supervision.

The physically independent generally do not participate in regular exercise or activity and have no significant desire to maintain their health through exercise and activity. They typically have no debilitating diseases or conditions impairing their functional independence, but may have small functional limitations in that they are no longer able to perform certain tasks or activities. While they remain mobile and independent, they exhibit borderline health (usually on medications) and have meager physical reserves. They live independently, but lack the aerobic capacity and lower-extremity strength and power for standardized protocols. Therefore, they must be thoroughly screened and assessed using population-specific protocols.

The physically frail exhibit multisystem reductions in their reserve capacity. Several physiological systems are close to the threshold for symptomatic, clinical failure. The significant reductions in musculoskeletal function, aerobic capacity, cognitive and neurological function (motor control), and nutritional reserves observed in the physically frail negatively impact overall functional capacity. Individuals in this category must be thoroughly screened and may only be capable of completing the basic population-specific protocols.

The physically dependent rely on others to perform many ADL, as they lack the physical ability to perform physiological assessments. Their functional capacity is primarily assessed with ADL-IADL inventories, questionnaires, and surveys. Figure 14-17 presents an overview of functional capacities.

Figure 14-17
Functional capacity classifications in older adults

Note: ADL = Activities of daily living; AADL = Advanced ADL; IADL = Instrumental ADL; BADL = Basic ADL

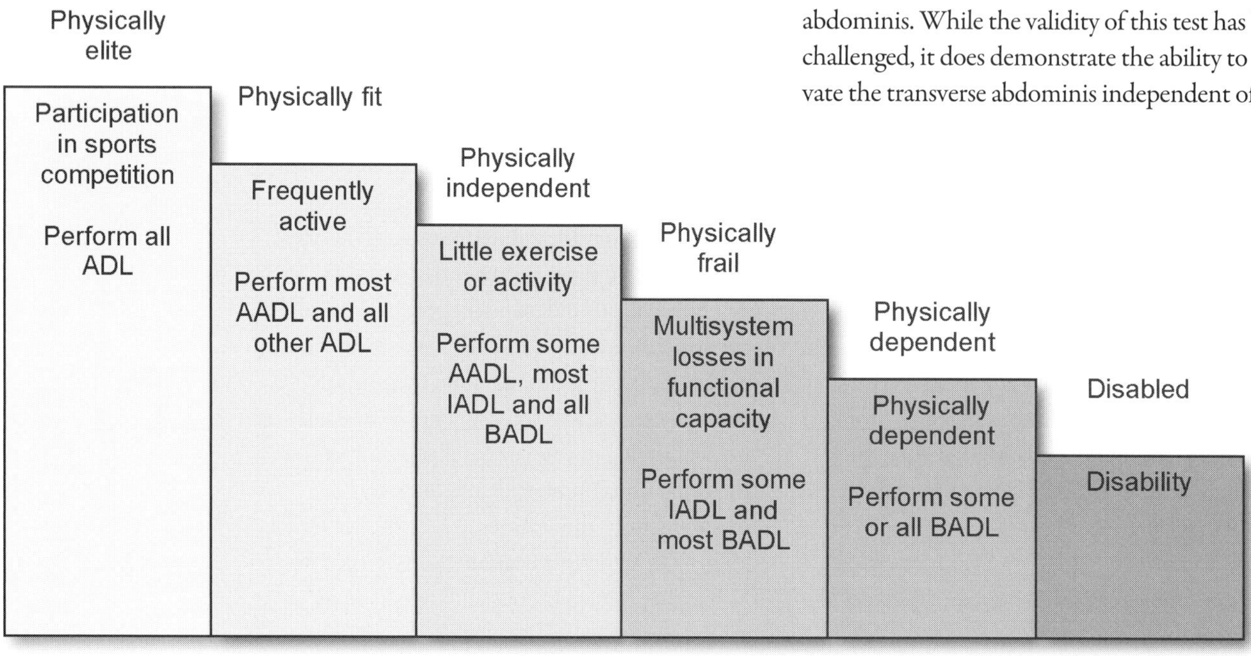

Core Function Assessments

The assessment of core musculature and function is not a simple process. While the transverse abdominis plays a key role in spinal stabilization by drawing the umbilicus toward the spine to increase intra-abdominal pressure, it works collectively with many other muscles to stabilize the spine and reduce the potential for back injury. What McGill et al. (1999) state as more relevant, however, is the evaluation of endurance of the abdominal muscles and their ability to function together, given their involvement in low-back pain. They recommend a small battery of tests that evaluate muscle balance among the torso flexors, extensors, and lateral muscles, given their strong reliability coefficients. The ACE-AHFS must properly screen a client for low-back pain before performing any of the following assessments.

Transverse Abdominis Testing

Simple tests that isolate muscle groups are difficult to find, especially when evaluating the isolated action of the transverse abdominis. Richardson and colleagues (1999) outlined some tests, including one to assess the ability to draw in the abdominal wall through coordination of the transverse abdominis and related inner unit musculature without activation of the rectus abdominis. While the validity of this test has been challenged, it does demonstrate the ability to activate the transverse abdominis independent of the rectus abdominis, an important function in centering or drawing-in. To perform this test:

- Have the client lie prone and place the bladder of the blood pressure cuff directly under his or her umbilicus and pump the bulb to between 40 and 70 mmHg at end-tidal volume (after exhalation) (Figure 14-18). The ACE-AHFS can use any number between 40 and 70 mmHg if 70 mmHg proves to be uncomfortable.

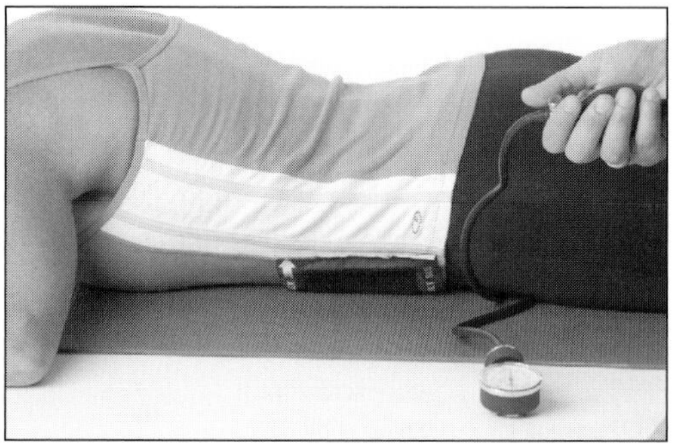

Figure 14-18
Transverse abdominis testing

- Following a few normal breaths, instruct the client to exhale, relax, and attempt to draw his or her umbilicus toward the spine, lifting it off the cuff. The ACE-AHFS should carefully monitor any limb or torso movement, including leverage through the legs and arms, flexing the hips, activating the gluteus maximus, or lifting the ribcage.
- An indicator of normal transverse abdominis activation is a reduction in cuff pressure reading by 10 mmHg.
- Faulty recruitment patterns that rely on the rectus abdominis commonly increase the pressure reading, as the contraction of the muscle pushes downward on the bladder.

Flexor Endurance Test

- The client assumes a seated bent-knee position (knees and hips flexed 90 degrees) with the arms folded across the chest, hands placed on the opposite shoulders, and feet planted firmly on the floor (the toes can be anchored under a strap or held by the test administrator if needed) (Figure 14-19).
- The client leans back to rest the upper extremity against a support at a 60-degree angle.

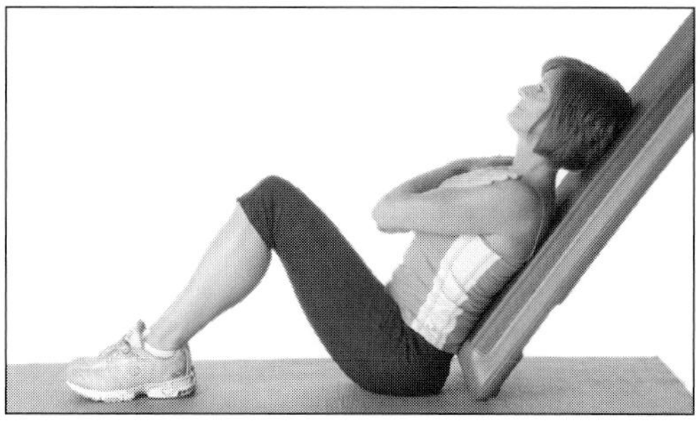

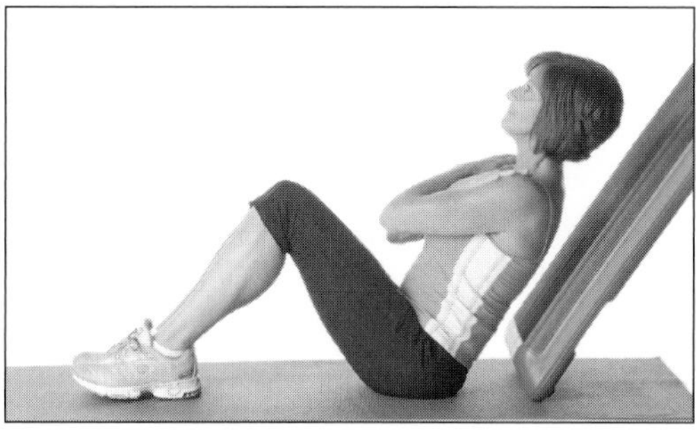

Figure 14-19
The flexor endurance test

- The ACE-AHFS slowly removes the back support by sliding it back 4 inches (10 cm) while the client maintains this isometric position.
- The ACE-AHFS records the time to fatigue when any part of the back touches the back rest.

Back Extensor Endurance Test

- The client assumes a prone position on a table with the iliac crest aligned with the table edge and the upper extremity hanging perpendicular to the floor (Biering-Sorenson position).
- The pelvis, knees, and hips are secured on the table top, with the hands folded across the chest and touching the opposite shoulder.
- The client extends the upper extremity parallel to the floor (Figure 14-20). The ACE-AHFS records the time that this position is held until fatigue—when the parallel position can no longer be maintained.

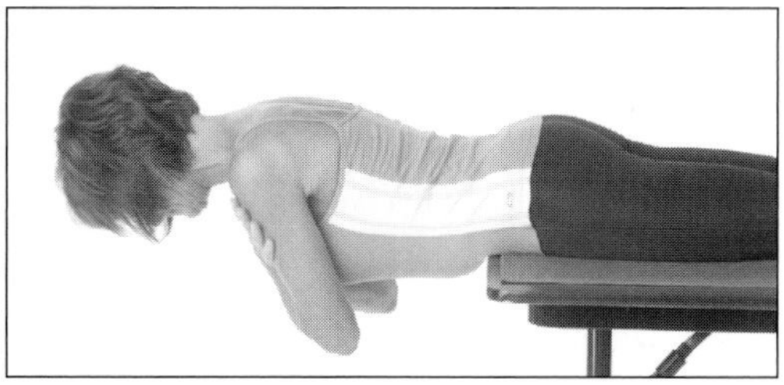

Figure 14-20
Back extensor endurance test

Lateral Musculature Endurance Test

- The client assumes a full side bridge position on the floor with both legs extended, placing the top leg in front of lower leg for support (Figure 14-21).
- The client supports the upper extremity on the lower elbow, which is positioned directly under the shoulder, and places the uninvolved hand across the chest to the opposite shoulder or at the side.
- The client elevates the torso off the floor, maintaining a rigid, straight posture.
- The ACE-AHFS records the time until fatigue—when that position can no longer be held—and then repeats to the opposite side.

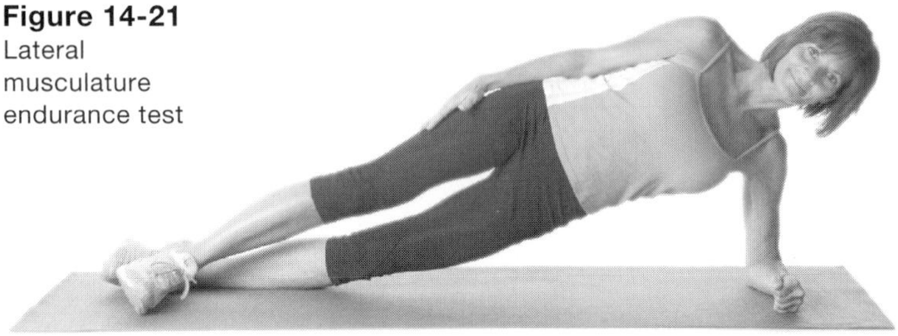

Figure 14-21
Lateral musculature endurance test

Interpreting Core Function Assessment Scores

McGill (2002) believes that interpreting the absolute scores is secondary to the relationships between the muscle-group scores. He identified optimal relationships between these scores for healthy individuals, demonstrating that the relationships become altered with back pain and potentially remain altered even after back-pain issues have been resolved. Typically, extensor endurance shows greater losses than the endurance of the flexor and lateral muscles. Table 14-2 presents his findings from different research studies, illustrating differences in absolute and relative scores between normal individuals without back problems and those with a history of back problems (McGill, 2002).

McGill (2002) suggests the following ratios indicate balanced endurance among the muscle groups:

- Flexion:extension ratio should be less than 1.0
  - ✔ For example, a flexion score of 120 seconds and an extension score of 150 seconds generates a ratio score of 0.80
- Right-side bridge (RSB):left-side bridge (LSB) scores should be no greater than 0.05 from a balanced score of 1.0
  - ✔ For example, a RSB score of 88 seconds and a LSB score of 92 seconds generates a ratio score of 0.96, which is within the 0.05 range from 1.0
- Side bridge (either side):extension ratio should be less than 0.75
  - ✔ For example, a RSB score of 88 seconds and an extension score of 150 seconds generates a ratio score of 0.59

Based on McGill's research, it appears that muscle imbalance is a contributor to low-back pain. Demonstrated deficiencies in the muscle ratios should be addressed as part of the foundational exercises for a client with a goal to create ratios consistent with McGill's recommendations.

Other Assessments

Diagnosis and Treatment of Movement Impairment Syndromes by Shirley Sahrmann, Ph.D. (2002), offers screening tools to identify movement impairments within the lumbar spine and hip. While an ACE-AHFS is not qualified to make any diagnoses or treat movement impairment syndromes, familiarization with some of the protocols offered in this reference will help an ACE-AHFS better understand the roles these muscles play across the lumbo-pelvic region in stabilizing the spine and improving balance. *Therapeutic Exercise for Musculoskeletal Injuries* (2nd ed.) by Peggy Houglum, Ph.D. (2005), and *Muscles: Testing and Function with Posture and Pain* (5th ed.) by Kendall et al. (2005) are additional references that offer valuable insight.

Gait Analysis

The detailed analysis of gait is a complicated process ideally performed by a qualified professional, although the ACE-AHFS can perform some basic evaluations of walking patterns, as illustrated in Figure 14-22. An ACE-AHFS should be able to recognize postural deviations and muscle imbalances, and identify the impact they might potentially have on movement efficiency. An ACE-AHFS can also identify compensations at the joints and within the kinetic chain, distinguish

Table 14-2
Mean Absolute Endurance Times and Relative Ratios Between Normal Individuals and Those With Low-back Pain (Expressed Relative to the Extensor Score)

Test	Men		Women		Combined Sexes	
	Mean Time	Ratio	Mean Time	Ratio	Mean Time	Ratio
Extension*	161 seconds		185 seconds		173 seconds	
Extension†					103 seconds	
Extension‡					90 seconds	
Flexion*	136 seconds		134 seconds		134 seconds	
Flexion†					66 seconds	
Flexion‡					84 seconds	
Right side bridge (RSB)*	95 seconds		75 seconds		83 seconds	
Right side bridge (RSB)†					54 seconds	
Right side bridge (RSB)‡					58 seconds	
Left side bridge (LSB)*	99 seconds		78 seconds		86 seconds	
Left side bridge (LSB)†					54 seconds	
Left side bridge (LSB)‡					65 seconds	
Flexion:extension ratio*		0.84		0.72		0.77
Flexion:extension ratio†						0.71
Flexion:extension ratio‡						1.15
RSB:LSB ratio*		0.96		0.96		0.96
RSB:LSB ratio†						1.05
RSB:LSB ratio‡						0.93
RSB:extension ratio*		0.59		0.40		0.48
RSB:extension ratio†						0.57
RSB:extension ratio‡						0.97
LSB:extension ratio*		0.61		0.42		0.50
LSB:extension ratio†						0.58
LSB:extension ratio‡						1.03

*Mean age of subjects = 21 years (n = 229; 92 men, 137 women)
†Mean age of subjects = 34 years (n = 24)
‡Mean age of subjects = 34 years (n = 26, suffered lost work due to low-back pain)

Source: McGill, S.M. (2001). Low back stability: From formal description to issues for performance and rehabilitation. *Exercise and Sports Science Review,* 29, 1, 26–31.

Instructions:
The client walks toward the ACE-AHFS along a 10-to 15-yard (9.1- to 13.6-m) hallway, following a straight line marked on the floor or carpeting, or walks toward a full-length mirror (repeat as needed).

1.	Does the gait follow a straight line?	❑
2.	Do the two hemispheres of the body appear symmetrical?	❑
3.	Does the body appear to maintain extension?	❑
4.	Are the hips and shoulder level?	❑
5.	Do the knees point forward?	❑
6.	Do the arms swing rhythmically and appear to swing symmetrically (observe for rotation)?	❑
7.	Do the step lengths appear equal?	❑
8.	Does the foot appear to make initial contact in supination, then pronate during load response?	❑
9.	After heel strike, do the toes have a controlled eccentric movement toward the floor?	❑

The client walks 10 to 15 yards (9.1 to 13.6 m) from left to right along a line or parallel to a full-length mirror (repeat as needed).

1.	Do the heels make initial contact with the floor after the swing phase?	❑
2.	Does the foot follow from heel-off to toe-off?	❑
3.	Is the knee almost fully extended immediately prior to heel strike?	❑
4.	Does the torso maintain good extension with alignment of the head and torso?	❑
5.	Are the steps of equal length?	❑
6.	Are the arms swings of equal length?	❑

Figure 14-22
Basic evaluation of walking patterns

correctible from non-correctible deviations, and then apply his or her knowledge of neuromuscular physiology and biomechanics to help the client restore anatomical joint neutrality, which in turn might improve balance and gait efficiency. For example, if excessive pronation is identified at the subtalar joint, the ACE-AHFS can direct the client to find the neutral subtalar position while standing. If the client is able to correct the position without further compensations along the kinetic chain and hold this position free of pain or discomfort, it is likely that a program of stretching **hypertonic** (tight) muscles and strengthening **latent** (weakened) muscles, coupled with neural reeducation and conscious awareness of posture, can help restore neutrality at the joint. However, the ACE-AHFS must understand the limitations of this approach and respect the scope of practice. Structural deviations or limitations within the skeletal systems may limit the client's ability to restore or correct joint position (e.g., anteversion/retroversion due to an abnormal rotational angle of the femoral neck in relation to the femur's long axis alters knee alignment and the forces acting throughout the lower kinetic chain). If a client presents with a structural deviation and/or persistent pain, a referral to the appropriate medical professional is warranted.

Programming

Traditional programming has generally focused on the health-related components of physical fitness, yet children, athletes, and rehabilitation specialists continue to place emphasis on skill-related components of fitness as well (Figure 14-23).

All programs should first address the prerequisites to these parameters to develop a solid foundation for effective programming. These prerequisite goals include:

- Restoring good posture (restorative exercises addressing correctable compensations through stretching and strengthening)
- Reeducating faulty neural pathways of the core musculature
- Developing static and basic dynamic balance*
- Enhancing sensory acuity and postural control strategies*
- Improving gait patterns and more advanced dynamic balance*

**These elements might require some prerequisite lower-extremity strengthening and improvements in flexibility.*

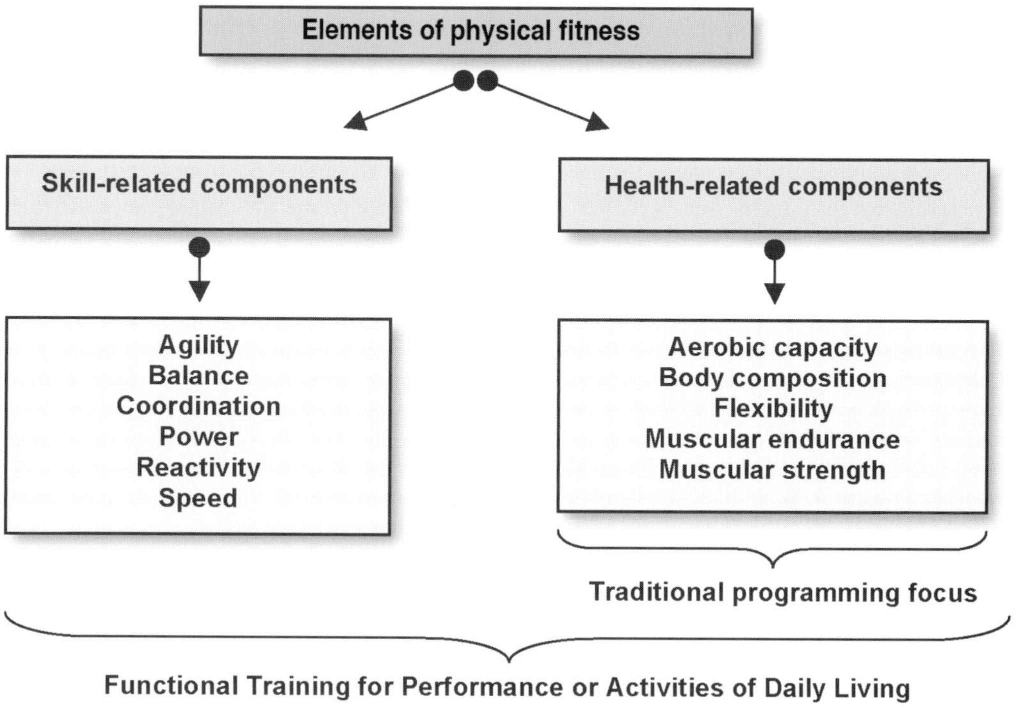

Figure 14-23
Components of physical fitness

programming and should therefore be emphasized early in all conditioning programs (Yaggie & Campbell, 2006). While good posture and muscle balance across joints helps restore movement efficiency, balance does require strength, power, and sensorimotor integration. Clients may need to develop adequate levels of strength, power, and flexibility to improve their balance and postural control strategies.

Balance, in turn, facilitates the development of muscular endurance, additional strength and power, flexibility, agility, coordination, reactivity, and perhaps even aerobic capacity. Balance not only enhances physical performance, but also contributes to the cognitive and affective (emotional) domains by building self-efficacy and confidence.

The learning of motor skills like balance occurs in stages, and several motor-learning models explain the cognitive and behavioral changes that occur. Fundamentally, the learning process should first help the client understand the goals of the basic exercises, providing opportunities to practice and explore fixed movement-pattern responses before training the body to adapt to changing environments with diversified movement patterns. Fixed movement patterns are performed in closed, or unchanging, environments (fixed control of regulatory conditions). The ACE-AHFS should allow multiple repetitions of the same movement to fine-tune the response. Diversified movement patterns are performed in open, or frequently changing, environments requiring spatial and temporal modifications to the movement response. Regulatory conditions are those characteristics of the performance environment that influence how the skill is performed and include surfaces, COG, BOS, and the height and weight of an object relative to the body when reaching.

As mentioned previously, the core functions reflexively in response to movement or loading of the spine. Any movement altering the COG, line of gravity, or BOS challenges balance and channels motor patterns to promote a stable spine (McGill, 2002). Diversified movement activates that reflexive core response and constitutes core training. A core program, therefore, involves the application of appropriate balance challenges in a progressive manner and improves both core responses and postural-control strategies.

Unstable surfaces result in greater muscle activity in the lower abdominal region than stable surfaces. Unilateral pushing and pulling movements demonstrate greater transverse abdominis activity than movements performed bilaterally. However, force production in the upper and lower extremities is significantly reduced on destabilized surfaces, given the need for synergistic force-producing muscles to act as stabilizers (Behm et al., 2005; Anderson & Behm, 2004). In reality, however, few sports and activities require the degree of instability presented with unstable training devices. While these tools provide a good medium for increasing the challenge to the body's balance centers, programs should ultimately become more specific and incorporate closed-kinetic, multiplanar movements performed on stable surfaces at real-time speeds.

As balance training involves action of the core musculature, it is important that the reflexive action of this group functions effectively. Many fitness professionals make the mistake of incorporating unstable surfaces too soon in client training. The unstable challenge, coupled with faulty neural pathways, can potentially trigger compensated muscle action, as the prime movers increase their role as spinal stabilizers and compromise their force-generating capacity (e.g., over-reliance on the abdominal muscles to function as the primary stabilizer of the spine while simultaneously generating forces in the abdominal region to move the trunk). When working with deconditioned individuals and those cleared for activity following low-back pain, programming should first emphasize re-education of the neural pathways, and then follow a progressive program that gradually increases the loading and the balance challenges.

Table 14-3 and Figure 14-24 present a suggested template that the ACE-AHFS can follow for developing a progressive core-conditioning program. The first stage involves re-education of the neural pathways through a simple series of exercises aimed at reactivating core muscles in

Table 14-3
Suggested Template for Progressing Core-conditioning Stages

Conditioning Stage	Objective	Duration	Exercises
Muscle activation and isolation	Reactivate neuromuscular pathways; centering or drawing-in action	Daily, 1–2x/day for 1–2 weeks	Static positions, supported, unloaded or minimally loaded; activation and co-contraction of the core muscles
Core stabilization	Spinal stabilization under minimal loading; improve proprioceptive awareness and reflexive responses	2–3x/week for 10–15 minutes for 2–3 weeks	Static positions (5–20 seconds), minimal loading (seated or quadruped position)
Whole-body stabilization	Introduce bracing action; spinal stabilization under increased loading; static and dynamic standing exercises	2–3x/week for 10–15 minutes for 2–3 weeks	Static (15–20 seconds) and dynamic (1 set x 10 reps) standing exercises
Core conditioning	Develop muscular endurance and strength of both layers	2–3x/week, 4–6 exercises for 4–12 weeks, or as core maintenance	Traditional set-rep program for endurance and strength; multiple exercise modalities and planes of movement
Core power	Develop power under full postural and recovery control	2x/week, 3–4 exercises for 2–4 weeks	Set-rep program for power, emphasizing postural and recovery control

Figure 14-24
Core-conditioning stages

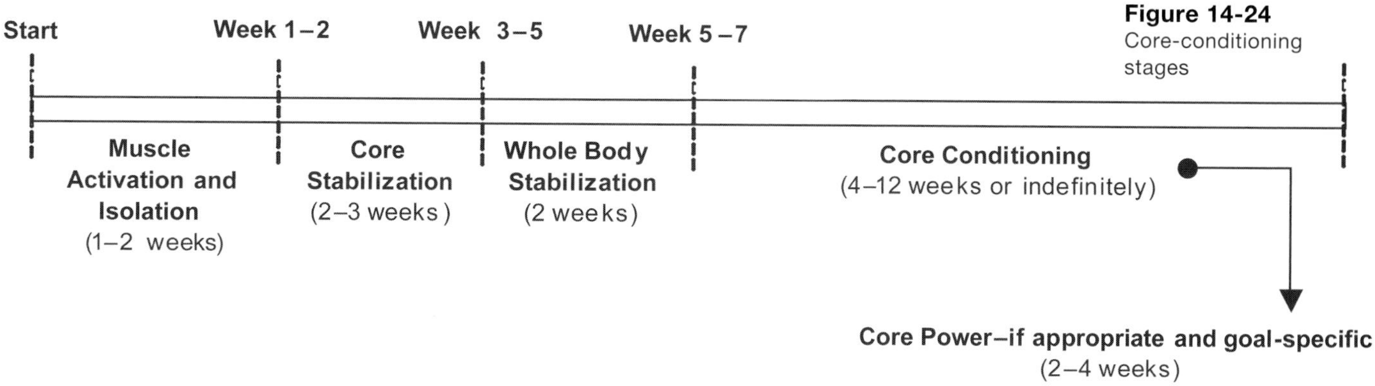

isolation, using supported surfaces to minimize spinal loading. The emphasis is on low-intensity, high-volume repetitions to re-educate the neural pathways. The ACE-AHFS should encourage clients to perform these exercises frequently throughout the day to facilitate the development of a correct reflexive response. The second stage involves a series of static exercises, each progressively challenging the body's balance in seated or quadruped positions to develop static balance. Full-standing static and dynamic movements are introduced in the third stage, increasing the stabilizing and postural-control challenges to the body. The fourth stage involves the traditional set- and rep-based exercises typically practiced by fitness professionals who frequently omit the previous three levels with clients. The fifth and final stage involves more explosive movements that generate power under postural and recovery control. This stage is suggested only for individuals with those specific needs (e.g., athletes, some fitness enthusiasts, and people with certain occupations).

Stage 1: Muscle Activation and Isolation

During this stage, the objective is to re-educate the neural pathways and activate the core muscles with no, or minimal, engagement of the rectus abdominis or hip flexors (i.e., no movement of the hips and torso). The goal is to learn the concept of centering, or "drawing in." The exercises are performed in a supine, bent-knee position, progressing to a quadruped position on stable surfaces to minimize loading on the spine. The emphasis is placed on volume and lower-intensity exercises with short recovery intervals between sets. Examples of exercise progressions include the following.

Exercise Step 1: Supine Drawing-in

The client will lie supine in a bent-knee position and place the index finger of each hand immediately medial to the iliac crest (over the transverse abdominis) (Figure 14-25). Have the client breathe normally and instruct him or her to start by performing a light-to-moderate "Kegel" squeeze (contraction to resist urination) at end-tidal volume to engage the muscles of the pelvic floor. Progress the repetitions as indicated below. Next, instruct the client to engage the transverse abdominis muscle at end-tidal volume by drawing the belly button in toward the spine. This may initially prove difficult to perform for some individuals, given the dominance of the rectus abdominis. The use of a string wrapped around the waist and cueing the client to reduce the diameter of the waistline to loosen the string may facilitate kinesthetic awareness of this muscle action. Progress to first integrating both contractions simultaneously, then incorporate a sustained contraction with breathing rather than breath holding.

Figure 14-25
Supine drawing-in

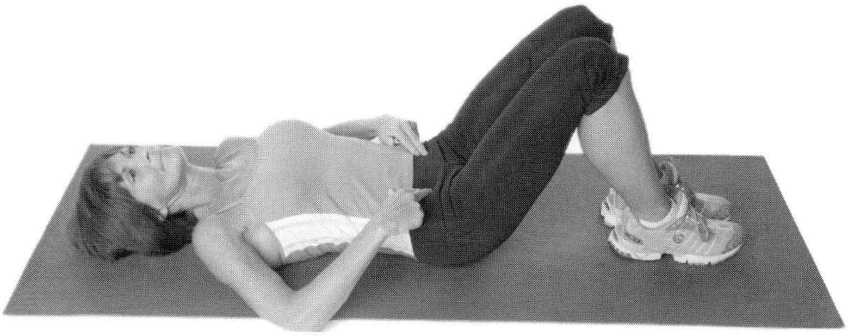

Training tips to emphasize:

- Encourage light-to-moderate intensity contractions.
- Avoid rectus abdominis engagement that will result in movement of the pelvis or ribcage.

Progression of exercises:

- 1–2 sets x 10 repetitions of pelvic floor contractions with a 2-second tempo; 15-second rest intervals between sets
- 1–2 sets of 10 repetitions of transverse abdominis contractions with a 2-second tempo; 15-second rest intervals between sets
- 1–2 sets of 10 repetitions of co-contraction of pelvic floor and transverse abdominis with a 2-second tempo; 15-second rest intervals between sets
- 1–2 sets of 5 or 6 repetitions of co-contraction of pelvic floor and transverse abdominis with slow, 10-second counts and independent breathing;15-second rest intervals between sets
- Expand this last progression to 3–4 sets x 10–12 repetitions, each with a 10-second count; 15-second rest intervals between sets

Exercise Step 2: Supine Drawing-in With Lower-extremity Movement

Repeat the step 1 progression, but add a sequence of small, slow, controlled leg movements [3-inch (7.6 cm) bent-knee leg draws or heel slides, 3-inch (7.6 cm) foot lifts, and 3-inch (7.6 cm) foot lifts with slight abduction), executed under core muscle activation with a stable pelvis and torso (Figure 14-26).

Training tips to emphasize:

- Encourage light-to-moderate intensity contractions.
- Avoid rectus abdominis engagement that will result in movement of the pelvis or ribcage.
- The tendency is to exaggerate the amount of movement. Cue the client to perform small movements to control the loading across the lumbo-pelvic region.

Progression of exercises:

- Progress each exercise from 1 set x 8–10 reps to 2–3 sets x 10–12 repetitions per leg; 15-second rest intervals between sets

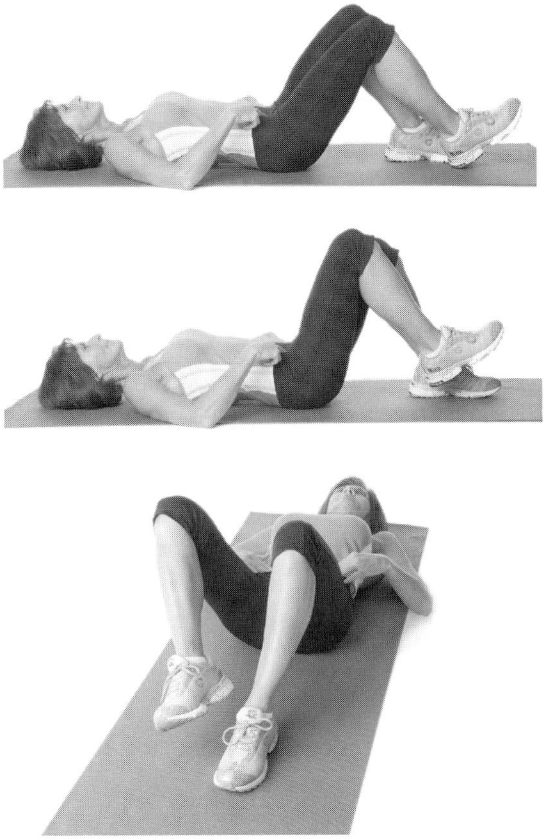

Figure 14-26
Co-contraction with lower-extremity movements

Exercise Step 3: Quadruped Drawing-in

The client assumes a quadruped position with the hands placed directly under the shoulders, and the knees placed directly under the hips. He or she should try to position the spine in neutral or as close to neutral as possible as determined by discrepancies in limb length. The quadruped position allows greater muscle activation against the force of gravity while still maintaining minimal loading along the spine. The client will repeat the co-contraction of the pelvic floor and transverse abdominis with independent breathing, ensuring that the position of the spine does not change during muscle activation (Figure 14-27).

Training tips to emphasize:

- Encourage light-to-moderate intensity contractions.
- Avoid rectus abdominis engagement that will result in movement of the pelvis or ribcage.

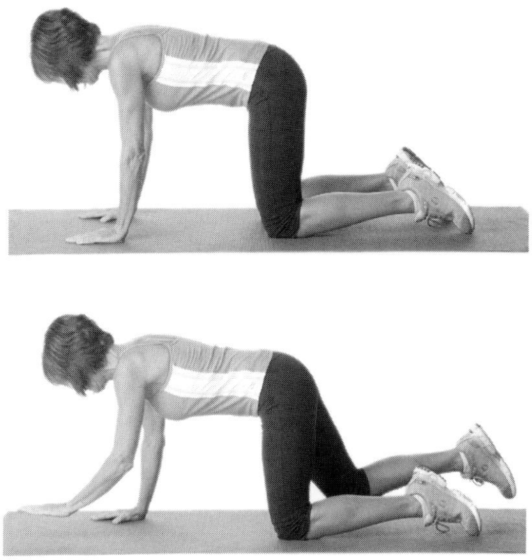

Figure 14-27
Quadruped position with co-contraction under lower- and upper-extremity movements

- The tendency is to exaggerate the amount of movement. Cue the client to perform small movements to control the loading across the lumbo-pelvic and scapulothoracic regions.

Progression of exercises:

- From the stable quadruped position, start with 1–2 sets of 5–6 repetitions of co-contraction of the pelvic floor and transverse abdominis with slow, 10-second counts and independent breathing; 15-second rest intervals between sets
- Progress the exercises by adding a sequence of controlled independent leg and arm movements, completing 1 set x 8–10 reps per movement; 15-second rest intervals between sets
- Continue to progress each exercise to 3–4 sets x 10–12 repetitions; 15-second rest intervals between sets
- Next, add contralateral limb movements following the same set and repetition progressions indicated above.

Stage 2: Spinal Stabilization

In stage 2, the exercises should introduce small balance challenges that reflexively engage the muscles under smaller spinal loads while the body is held in a static position. These exercises are best performed in seated positions using unstable devices. These static positions are generally held under core engagement for between five and 20 seconds for a few repetitions, while the client is maintaining full postural and recovery control. As new variables are introduced, others may be temporarily removed until postural control is restored. Examples of the variables include:

- Increasing the duration of the repetition (1–2 reps x 5–10 seconds to 2–4 reps x 15–20 seconds)
- Narrowing the BOS (Figure 14-28)
- Raising COM
- Creating asymmetrical loads to shift the line of gravity
- Utilizing sensory alteration or removal (visual, vestibular) (e.g., eyes open to closed; head tilts; visual tracking to head tracking; shifting points of focus, as when moving the focus from static reference points to distracting or moving objects or having clients focus on busy patterns)
  - ✔ Exercises performed with the eyes open rely predominately on visual feedback.
  - ✔ Exercises performed with the eyes closed, or where visual feedback is distracting, force reliance on somatosensory feedback.
  - ✔ Exercises performed on unstable surfaces with reduced, absent, or distracted vision force a reliance on vestibular feedback. Although somatosensory feedback is still involved, the unstable nature of the surface distorts its effectiveness.
  - ✔ Tracking progression: Hand movements to eye tracking to head tracking to eye-hand tracking

Figure 14-28
Narrowing the base of support

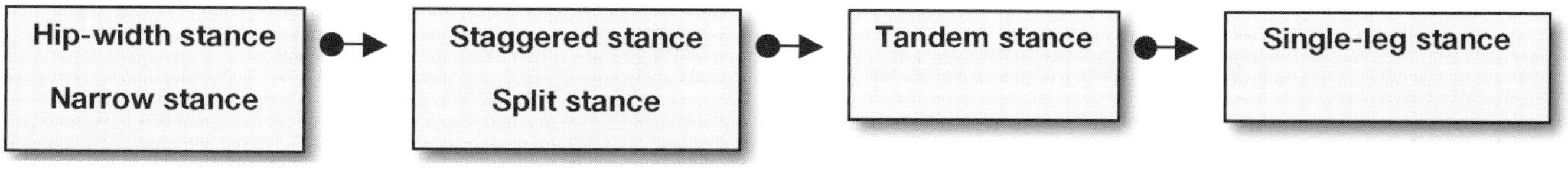

- Introduce a deviation of body position: sagittal, then frontal, then transverse (e.g., forward and backward leans, lateral flexion of five to 10 degrees to one side, lateral torso rotations)
- Adding slight external perturbations or resistance (partner or external resistance) (e.g., holding a weighted cable handle or having a partner apply a constant low-grade push to a stability ball)
- Reducing the points of contact (e.g., heel lifts, toe raises, raising one foot off the floor)
- Including additional unstable surfaces (under points of contact)

Stage 3: Whole-body Stabilization

At this stage, the exercises introduce the concept of bracing for greater spinal stability in both static and dynamic environments. The exercises transition from static to dynamic movement through various stance positions and with various surfaces (e.g., Airex pads, BOSU®). The balance challenge is gradually increased by appropriately advancing the exercise complexity through manipulation of the programming variables, again temporarily removing some variables as others are introduced until postural control is restored (Figure 14-29). Note that many of the dynamic exercises are the same exercises used in training dynamic balance for gait.

Static Exercises

Static balance challenges can be increased by changing the BOS as illustrated in Figure 14-28, or by altering many of the same variables described previously as well as these additional variables:

- Tolerating external forces (e.g., ball catches)
- Holding and moving external perturbations or resistance [e.g., arm circles, figure-8s with 1- to 4-pound (0.5 to 1.8 kg) medicine balls]
- Upper-extremity movements in all three planes (e.g., torso rotations, single-leg squat-touches, dynamic arm/leg reaches or movements). The client should begin with sagittal plane movements before progressing to frontal plane movements and then transverse plane movements.
- Altering surface stability (e.g., ground, Airex pad, disc, or BOSU)

Exercise volume for static positions are the same as for the previous stage (1–4 repetitions x 15–20 seconds) and dynamic upper-extremity movements can progress from 1–2 sets x 4–6 repetitions to 2–3 sets x 8–10 repetitions.

Exercise Example 1: Single-leg Stand With Reaches and Touches (Partner-assisted)

Working first to ensure a correct single-leg stand, have the client stand facing a mirror, feet together, hands on hips (iliac crest), and the fingers extended and lightly brushing the hips (hands-in-pocket position). He or she engages the hip abductors and adductors in the right leg and slowly lifts the left heel, then lifts the left foot 3 inches (7.6 cm) off the ground while avoiding any excessive hip adduction [i.e., the space between the left hip and left fingers

Figure 14-29
Surface and movement progressions

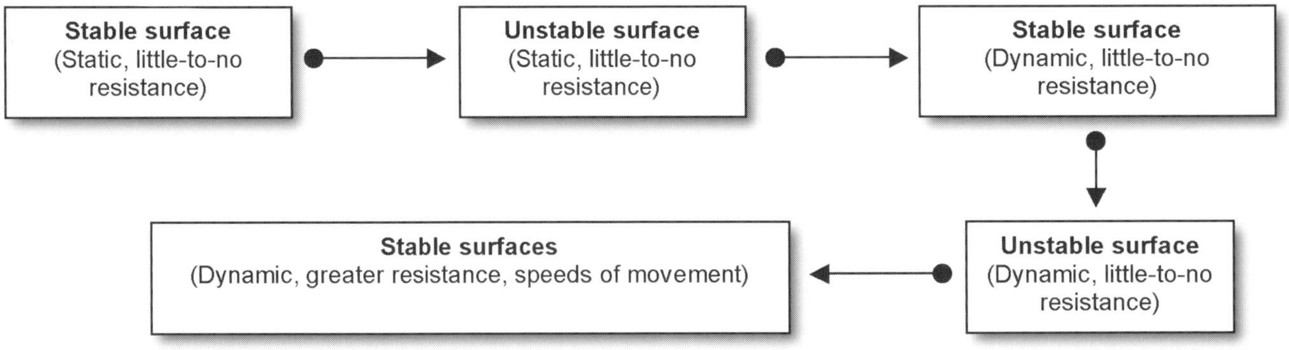

should remain within 1 to 2 inches (2.5 to 5 cm)]. The client should also avoid:

- Excessive frontal plane deviation in the hips (>5 degrees of adduction) and lateral torso leans
- Excessive transverse plane deviations (excessive internal or external rotation at the knee that is best observed by placing the right hand on the front of the right thigh and noting rotation)
- Excessive sagittal plane deviations or a forward or backward torso lean, or pelvic tilting

Have the client hold a light ball and slowly perform single-leg squats reaching across the body to touch the floor on the outside of the body while maintaining postural control and body alignment and minimizing rotation (Figure 14-30). The exercise can be progressed to include more dynamic movements. From the single leg-stand position a trainer or partner can lightly touch his or her hand to various regions of the client's body in quick succession, cueing the client to react by touching both hands to the targeted region (creating movement in all three planes). An alternative exercise is to add arm reaches to partner-positioned targets (e.g., the ACE-AHFS can give the client a ball to hold in both hands, which he or she will use to reach toward targets in quick succession).

Tip to emphasize:

- Control movement speeds and avoid loss of single-leg balance.

Exercise Example 2: Triplanar Balance Sequence

Sagittal Plane Movement (Figure 14-31)

The client assumes a static single-leg stance with the right leg as instructed in the previous exercise and maintains erect posture and control with his or her arms at the sides. The client slowly drives the left leg forward to touch the floor (hip flexion) and backward to touch the floor (hip extension) without any torso lean. The client then repeats the movement, but the leg driver must not touch the floor during this repetition. Next, the ACE-AHFS can introduce one or two arm drivers moving out of sync with the leg driver (i.e., the arms drive forward as the leg drives backward), reaching low in front and high behind while maintaining postural control. The client then repeats the movement, but with the arm drivers moving in synchronization with the leg driver (i.e., the arms drive

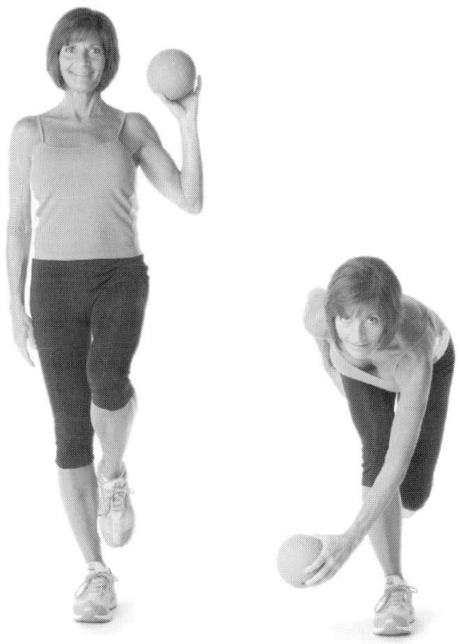

Figure 14-30
Single-leg reaches and touches

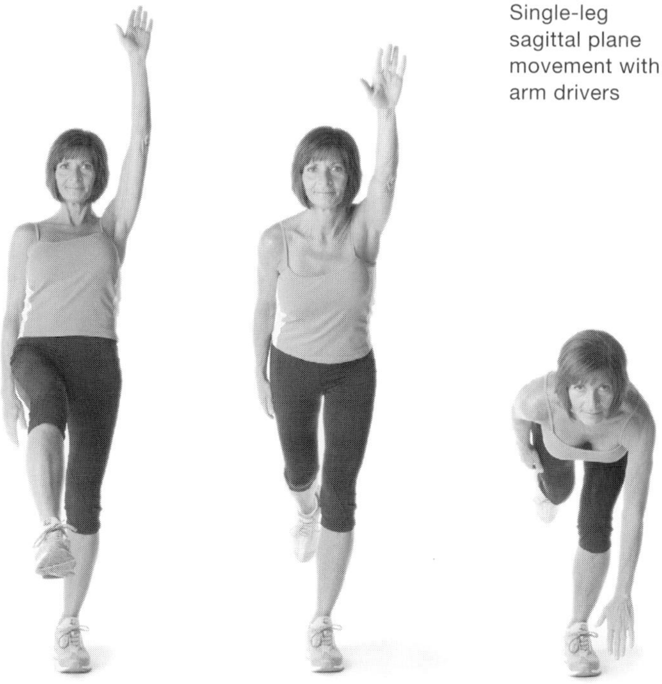

Figure 14-31
Single-leg sagittal plane movement with arm drivers

overhead and backward as the leg drives backward). Progress the exercise challenge by adding quarter or half squats to the movement. Repeat this same sequence with the opposite leg, performing 1 set x 5–10 repetitions per leg per movement.

Frontal Plane Movement (Figure 14-32)

The client assumes a static right single-leg stance as instructed previously and maintains erect posture and control with his or her arms at the sides. The client slowly drives the left leg across the body to touch the floor without any torso lean, then abducts the hip to position the leg away from the body to the side. The client then repeats the movement, but the leg driver must not touch the floor with this repetition. The ACE-AHFS can then introduce one or two arm drivers moving out of synchronization with the leg driver (i.e., the arms drive left as the leg drives right), reaching high (or low) while maintaining postural control.

Figure 14-32
Single-leg frontal plane movement

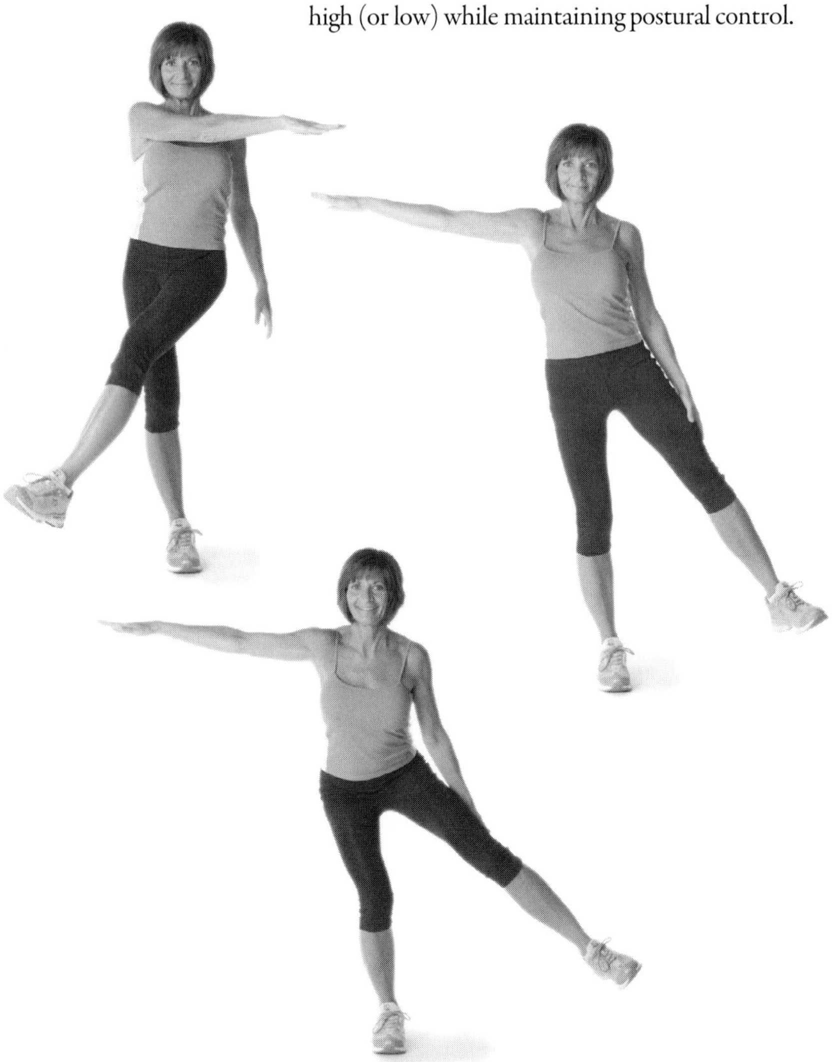

The client repeats the movement with the arm drivers moving in sync with the leg driver (i.e., the arms drive right as the leg drives right). The intensity can be progressed by adding a quarter or half squat to the movement. The client should always repeat the movement with the opposite leg.

Transverse Plane Movement (Figure 14-33)

The client assumes a static single-leg stance with the right leg as instructed previously and maintains erect posture and control with his or her arms at the sides. The client slowly rotates the left leg across and around the body to the right to touch the floor without any torso lean, then

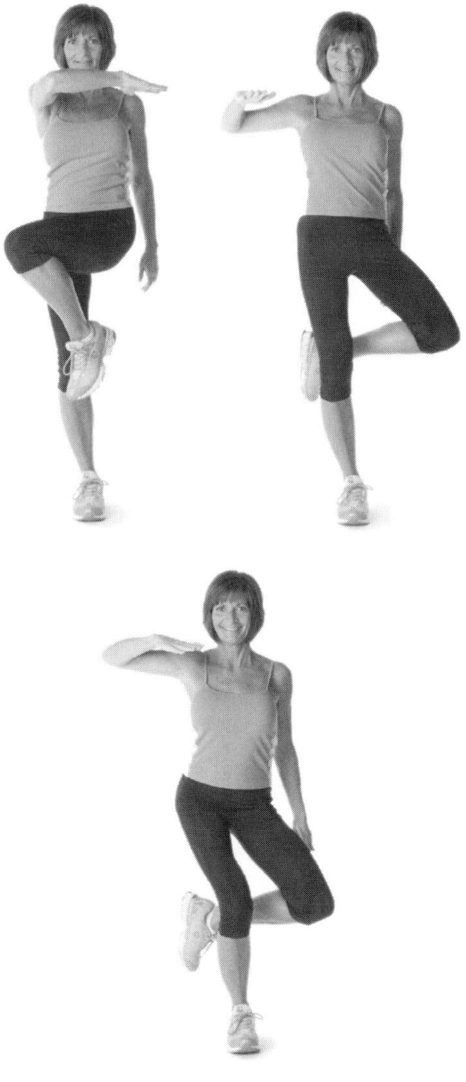

Figure 14-33
Single-leg transverse plane movement with arm drivers

rotates the right leg back to the left and behind the body to touch the floor. He or she repeats the movement, but the leg driver must not touch the floor with this repetition. The ACE-AHFS can introduce one or two arm drivers moving out of synchronization with the leg driver (i.e., the arms drive left as the leg drives right), reaching high (or low) while maintaining postural control. The client then repeats the movement with the arm drivers moving in sync with the leg driver (i.e., the arms drive right as the the leg drives right). The intensity can be progressed by adding a quarter or half squat to the movement. The client should always repeat the movement with the opposite leg.

Dynamic Exercises

The ACE-AHFS next introduces dynamic exercises, again progressing from stable to unstable surface as available and deemed appropriate. The progression of dynamic exercises that are the same as those used for training the gait in older adults should follow the sequence outlined in Figure 14-34.

The ACE-AHFS should appropriately manipulate the same programming variables discussed previously to increase the balance challenge. As new variables are introduced, others may be temporarily removed until postural control is restored. Additional variables for dynamic balance may include:

- Increasing exercise volume (sets x repetitions x duration or tempo)
- Deceleration and force dissipation through triple-flexion (e.g., body movement, tolerating external perturbations such as forces applied to a stability ball in multiple directions)
- Multiplanar stepping over obstacles (e.g., hurdles)
- Range and speed of motion
- Movement sequence:
    - ✔ Forward linear movements
    - ✔ Lateral movements
    - ✔ Backward movements or backpedaling
    - ✔ Rotational movements (crossovers)
    - ✔ Curving and cutting movements (more skill-specific and normally performed at faster rates)

Dynamic balance is a foundational skill for sports conditioning and often includes jumping and hopping. Given the impacting forces associated with these movements, jumping technique that includes alignment between the hips, knees, and foot is critical to avoid injury. This is especially true for females, who have a greater propensity for knee injuries given their larger Q-angles, joint laxity, smaller ligaments, and potentially weaker muscles. The alignment of the knee over the second toe, with minimal deviation from the ASIS is important during sit-to-stand or squat movements, any directional single-leg lunge movements, lateral shuffles, and the landing phase of a jump movement.

Jumping and Hopping Tips

- Individuals should *not* jump unless they know how to land. The ACE-AHFS should initially teach landing techniques using small, low-intensity jumps.
- Clients should land on the mid-foot, and then roll forward to push off the balls of the feet. They must avoid heel and ball landing, as these errors increase impact and ground-reaction forces. It is essential that clients know how to land softly. Landing on the mid-foot also shortens the amortization phase for power development if another jump follows.
- Ensure alignment of hip, knees and toes, especially in women due to the potential for injury.
- The ACE-AHFS should encourage clients to drop the hips to absorb the forces and develop gluteal dominance. Clients must avoid absorbing landing impacts by locking out the knees and developing

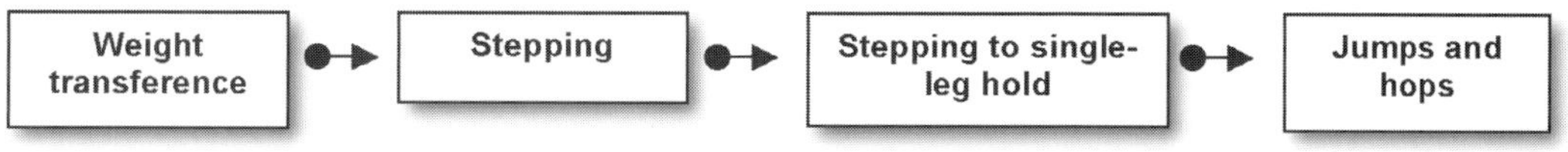

Figure 14-34
Progression of dynamic exercises

quad dominance. Poor landing technique may lead to knee injuries.
- Clients should land with the trunk inclined slightly forward, the head up, the core engaged, the torso rigid, and the knees slightly flexed.

The ACE-AHFS can progress exercise volume by increasing sets and repetitions from 1 set x 8–10 repetitions to 2–3 sets x 10–15 repetitions. The ACE-AHFS needs to keep in mind that as movements become more dynamic, consideration must be given to the energy system used and to fatigue. This implies an understanding of when each anaerobic system contributes (determined by intensity and duration), appropriate work-to-rest ratios, and mode of recovery for each.

Exercise Example 1: Lateral Shuffles With External Resistance

The client holds a stability ball close to his or her chest and begins shuffling left and right, bringing both feet together at each end. The ACE-AHFS introduces external resistance by gently pushing on the stability ball in the direction of the movement, forcing the client to eccentrically decelerate by engaging the core and lower-extremity muscles (Figure 14-35).

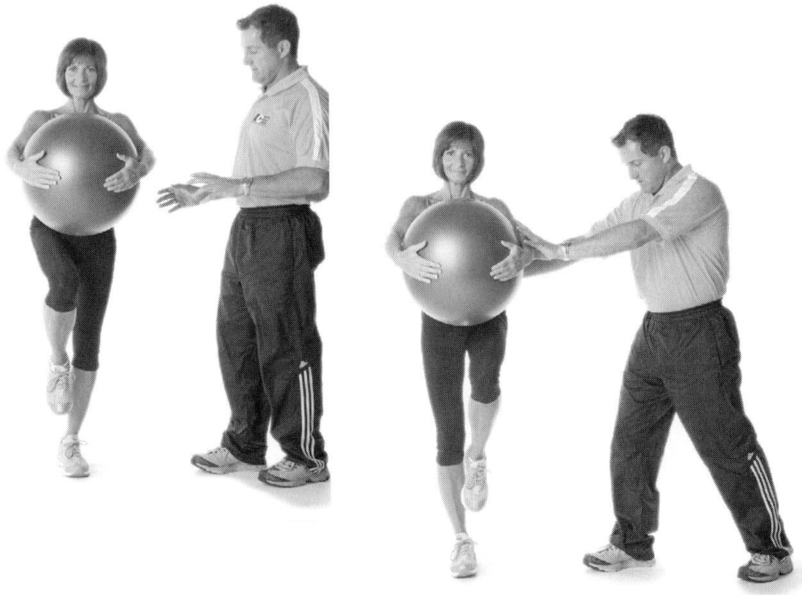

Figure 14-35
Lateral shuffles with external resistance

The exercise can be progressed by manipulating or adding several variables, including the following:
- Closing the eyes
- Decelerating at either end to stand on one leg
- Increasing the speed and range of movement
- Stepping over obstacles

Exercise Example 2: Multidirectional Lunges With Bilateral Arm Drivers

The client stands with the feet together and then proceeds to slowly lift the right foot off the ground until the thigh is parallel to the floor in a stork-stand position (i.e., 70 to 90 degrees of hip flexion without compensation in standing posture, including excessive hip adduction on the lift). The client then proceeds to perform a series of directional lunges as illustrated in Figure 14-36, ensuring alignment of the right knee over the second toe in each direction (tweaking foot and body position is encouraged as a progression or in more conditioned and stable individuals). The client should perform lunges in the following directions, repeating the pattern with the opposite leg:
- Forward
- Lateral
- Right rear-rotational
- Backward
- Crossover
- Left rear-rotational

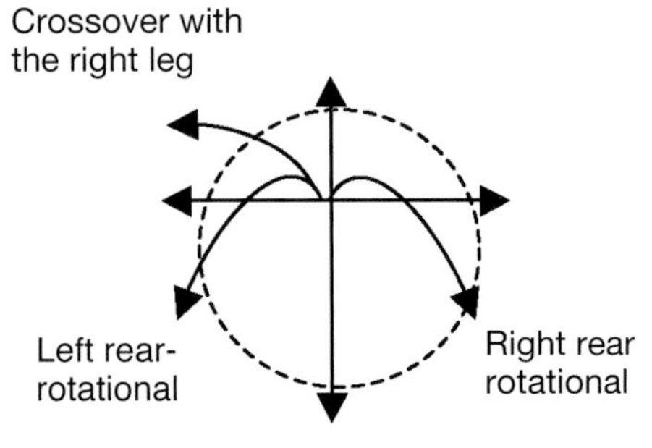

Figure 14-36
Five-point lunges from the stork-stand position

Stage 4: Core Conditioning

The goal in this stage is to develop endurance of the core musculature and strength within the outer muscle layers to effectively tolerate dynamic forces in multiple planes of movement. As most core-conditioning exercises involve dynamic movement on unstable surfaces, the ACE-AHFS must always educate clients on the safest and most effective means of maintaining postural control, exercise technique, and recovery control without risk of injury. The ACE-AHFS must only select exercises that are skill- and conditioning-level appropriate, yet consistent with client goals. It is important to incorporate a balanced mix of exercises targeting core endurance and abdominal strength, and to train the abdominal and lumbopelvic regions in all three planes via both isolated and integrated movements. Training for muscular endurance of the core muscles involves high volumes (e.g., performing two or three sets of 12 to 25 repetitions with shorter recovery intervals for endurance and three to five sets of five to 12 repetitions with longer recovery periods for strength). Remember, effective programming exists where common sense meets creative programming, especially during this stage, where exercises can take on many forms. This rule applies to all supine, prone, incline, decline, standing, seated, and kneeling exercises.

The ACE-AHFS can gradually and appropriately advance the exercise challenge by manipulating programming variables, temporarily removing variables as others are introduced until postural control is restored. Some of the programming variables include:

- Modality: stability balls, BOSU, pods, the ground, or any combination
- Planes of motion
- Isolation to whole-body integration
- Sets, repetitions, and time-under-tension
- Recovery intervals
- Force reduction, emphasizing the eccentric or deceleration phase of the movement to reduce the potential for injury

McGill (2002) recommends three basic exercises (with variations) to develop muscular endurance and protect the body from low-back injury: a curl-up movement (Figure 14-37), a side-bridge movement (Figure 14-38), and a quadruped contralateral lift ('birddog") (Figure 14-39).

Additionally, torso rotations, wood chops (high-to-low), and hay-bailers (lift, low-to-high) have become popular rotational exercises given their functional basis and engagement of many of the major core and abdominal muscles. As rotation is a primary movement, it should therefore be trained, but the ACE-AHFS must keep in mind that rotation may involve flexion and rotation if moving diagonally, potentially compromising spinal integrity. The ACE-AHFS should gradually add these exercises, and only after time has been spent conditioning the core and strengthening the abdominal muscles. These two triplanar movements require diagonal and spiral movement

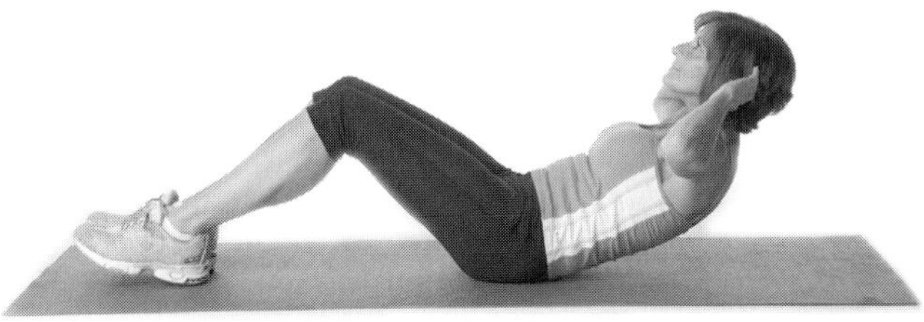

Figure 14-37
Curl-up

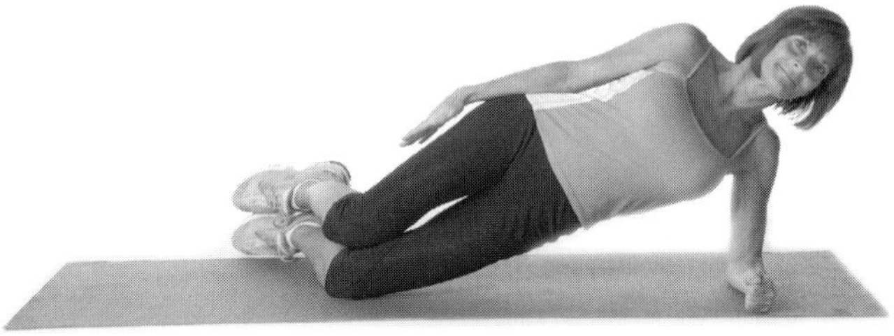

Figure 14-38
Side bridge

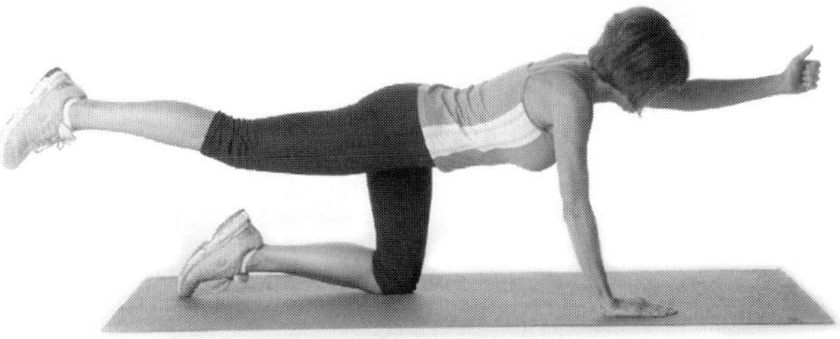

Figure 14-39
Birddog

of the arms, shoulders, trunks, hips, and legs. The wood chop involves a pull action followed by a push action in the upper extremity, stabilization of the trunk in all three planes (flexion, rotation, and side bending), and weight transference for leverage and dynamic balance. The hay bailer (lift) involves a pull action followed by a push action in the upper extremity, stabilization of the trunk in all three planes (extension, rotation, and side bending), and weight transference for leverage and dynamic balance.

These exercises should be introduced and first instructed in a sitting or half-kneeling position before progressing to a split-stance and full-standing rotational movement. The full-standing position (most advanced) allows for a functional, closed-chain movement where the body attempts to maintain a neutral lumbar spine, therefore relying upon muscular support in the trunk to maintain this neutral position at the mid-range of movement, but also minimize stresses along the joints of the spine at the end-range of movement. When training true sports movements, however, a neutral lumbar spine is rarely ever maintained. Therefore, movements toward the end-range of motion will need to be taught.

Exercise Example: Wood Chops and Hay Bailers

The client starts in a sitting or half-kneeling position to initially reduce overall lower-extremity involvement. The clients should maintain arm extension to optimally engage the torso in the spiral (diagonal) movement (Figures14-40 and 14-41). Arms positioned close to the body will involve a greater degree of elbow and shoulder movement. A chop motion is performed across to the rear leg while a lift motion is performed across to the front leg. Unstable surfaces such as sitting on a stability ball or kneeling on a disc, Airex pad, or BOSU increase the stabilization challenge. The ACE-AHFS can progress the exercise to a split-stance position prior to full rotational movements with weight transference from the inside to the outside leg. The placement of a small ball between the legs is for instructional purposes, to control motion of the lower extremity.

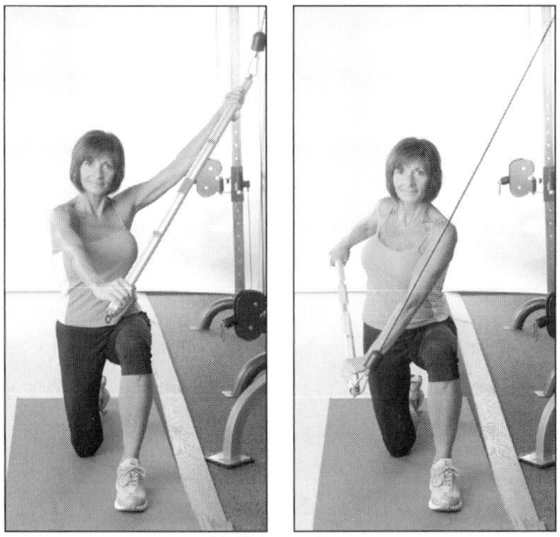

Half kneeling

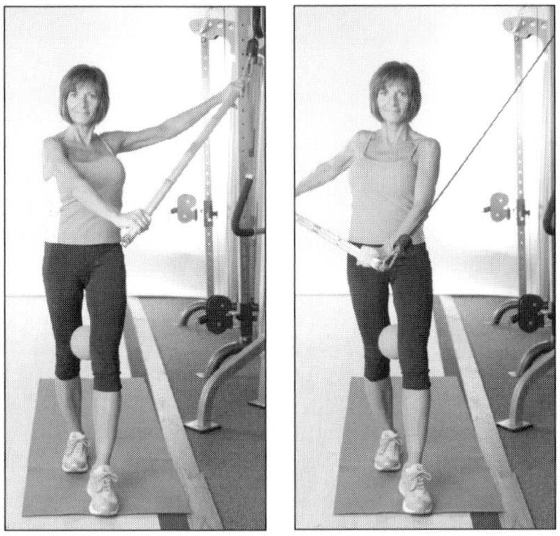

Split stance

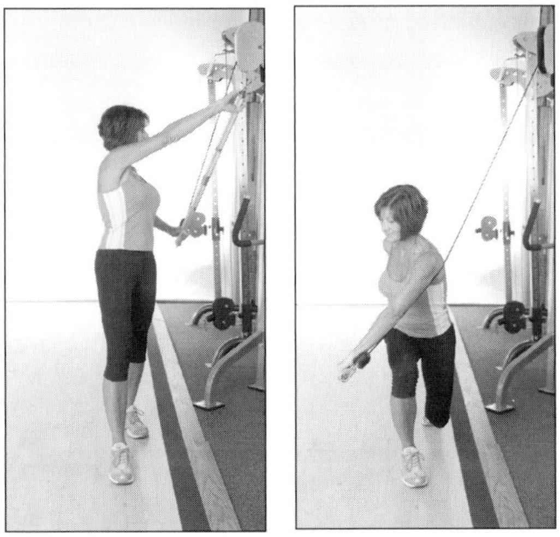

Full rotation

Figure 14-40
Wood chops

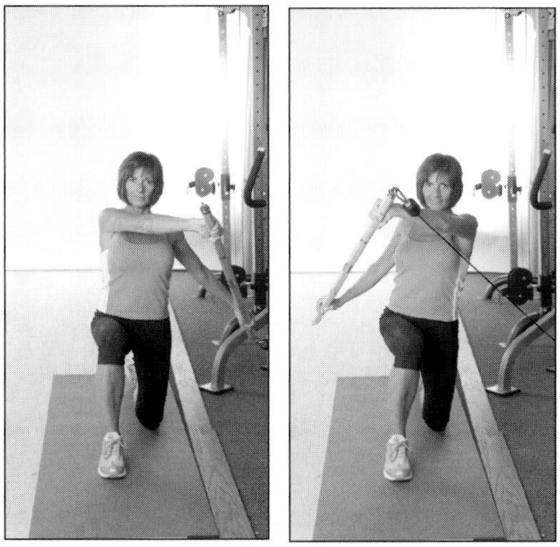

Half kneeling

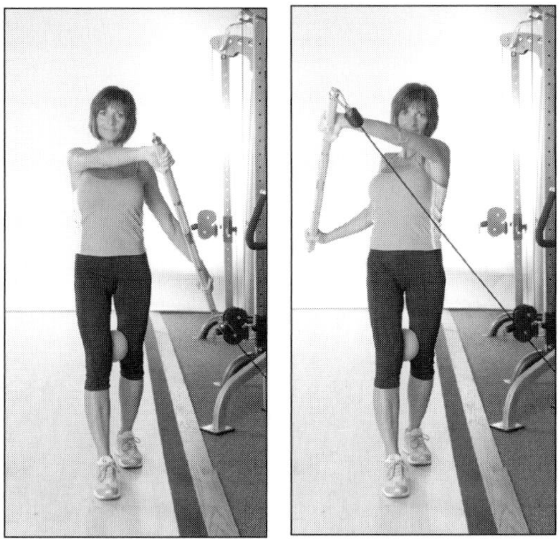

Split stance

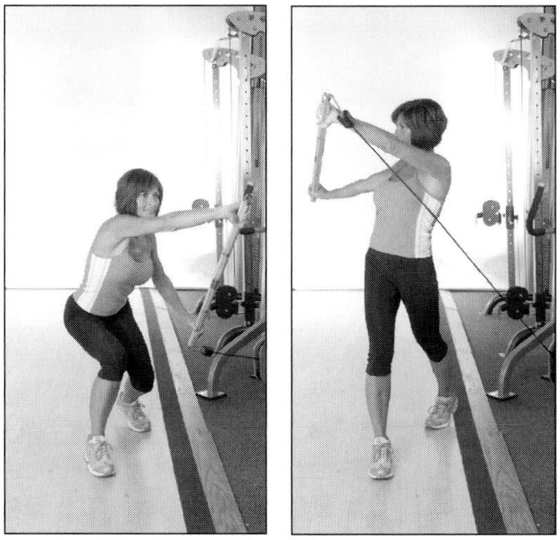

Full rotation

Figure 14-41
Hay bailers

Stage 5: Core Power

The overall goal of this stage is to improve neuromuscular control of the core during explosive movements, which are introduced during this stage and are generally *only* recommended for well-conditioned individuals. A key component in this phase is the eccentric deceleration of movement to reduce the potential for injury. Exercises may use both stable surfaces to mimic daily activities and unstable surfaces to elicit exaggerated reactive forces. While unstable surfaces exaggerate the need for deceleration and control, they decrease force output. All movements should ultimately progress to stable ground surfaces to mimic daily activities.

Upper-extremity core power can be trained using a variety of equipment including stability balls, medicine balls, kettle bells, partners, walls, the floor, or rebounders. Lower-extremity core-power training involves movements from three basic positions:

- Squat or standing stance
- Lunge stance
- Single-leg or hurdle stance

Given the specific nature of this stage, exercise examples are not provided, but the ACE-AHFS is encouraged to read further on power training if this training stage is appropriate and consistent with a client's goals.

Gait Exercises

Gait is perhaps the most functional movement in humans, yet people face significant challenges in maintaining gait function and mobility as they age and develop disorders, functional limitations, or impairments. As gait function is vital to functional independence, people must continue to train the necessary parameters that contribute to gait, including balance, agility, strength, power, flexibility, coordination, reactivity, and sensorimotor integration. Once good posture is restored, faulty core neural pathways are re-educated, confidence and efficiency with static balance is achieved, and sensory acuity and postural-control strategies are enhanced. Assuming there is no need for prerequisite lower-extremity strengthening and flexibility, the programming focus should turn to improving gait. Basic gait exercises begin with static balance and progress to dynamic balance (discussed previously in stages 2 and 3) and include:

- Static weight shifting (weight transference) in anterior-posterior and lateral directions
- Stepping in anterior-posterior and lateral directions
- In-place marching (progress in-place marching to include 90-degree turns)
- The ACE-AHFS can introduce directional walking, directional changes, and directional changes with abrupt stops and starts as the next progression (Figure 14-42).

Curving movements generally involve stepping into the curve with the inside leg, dropping the inside shoulder and arm toward the marker, and pushing off the outside leg through the curve. Cutting movements generally involve eccentric deceleration and loading on the outside leg while maintaining foot, knee, hip, and shoulder alignment, followed by a push-off of the outside leg while stepping in the new direction with the inside leg.

To lead a client through directional walking drills, the ACE-AHFS should:

- Create a 10- to 15-foot (3.0- to 4.6-m) walking pathway using cones as markers
- Instruct the client to walk through the drill as quickly as possible while maintaining postural control
- Gradually increase repetitions from two to five per exercise
- Observe efficiency in executing directional changes, offering feedback and correction as needed (Figure 14-43)

The development of agility and coordination are essential skill elements for efficient movement. Traditional exercises and drills for these skill parameters are usually performed at high speeds with athletes, but can be simplified and slowed down with individuals seeking gait improvement. Predetermined agility drills with predesignated foot placements are taught before introducing reactionary drills, a more advanced exercise format in which the client reacts to stimuli and instructions. The ACE-AHFS can teach drills in a segmented or part-to-whole format to facilitate learning and mastery.

When training for agility, the ACE-AHFS can use the same exercise equipment used for sports-conditioning drills (e.g., cones, risers, agility ladders, and hurdles). While agility ladders are an effective learning tool for developing agility, these drills need to progress to hurdles and risers that emphasize leg lift and clearance, mimicking true gait patterns, as opposed to the foot shuffles with minimal ground clearance used when working with the ladders. Agility ladder drills for foot patterns can be simple, unidirectional, slow-walking exercises that gradually increase to more advanced, faster, multidirectional, runs, jumps, and hops incorporating obstacles and simultaneous coordination drills often used with more athletic individuals. Examples of agility ladder drills include:

- Forward walks or runs (single-foot step into each square, double-foot step into each square)
- Forward jumps or hops (double hops, single hops, jumping jacks, hopscotch patterns)
- Lateral shuffles (basic, crossovers, carioca, grapevines)
- Lateral hops (double hops, single hops, split jumps)
- Backpedaling (single-foot step into each square, double-foot step into each square)
- Multidirectional (lateral-forward patterns, zigzags, slaloms or "Ickey shuffles," double slalom, Ws, Ms, machine gunners, multidirectional hops) (Figure 14-44)

Gait exercises can be advanced further with the addition of walking with altered bases of support, and by changing the speed, distance, and complexity of the exercise by introducing the following tasks:

- Narrow, wide, or alternating narrow-wide step widths

Figure 14-42
Directional progression of gait drills

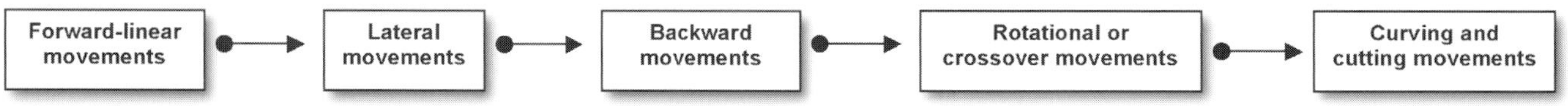

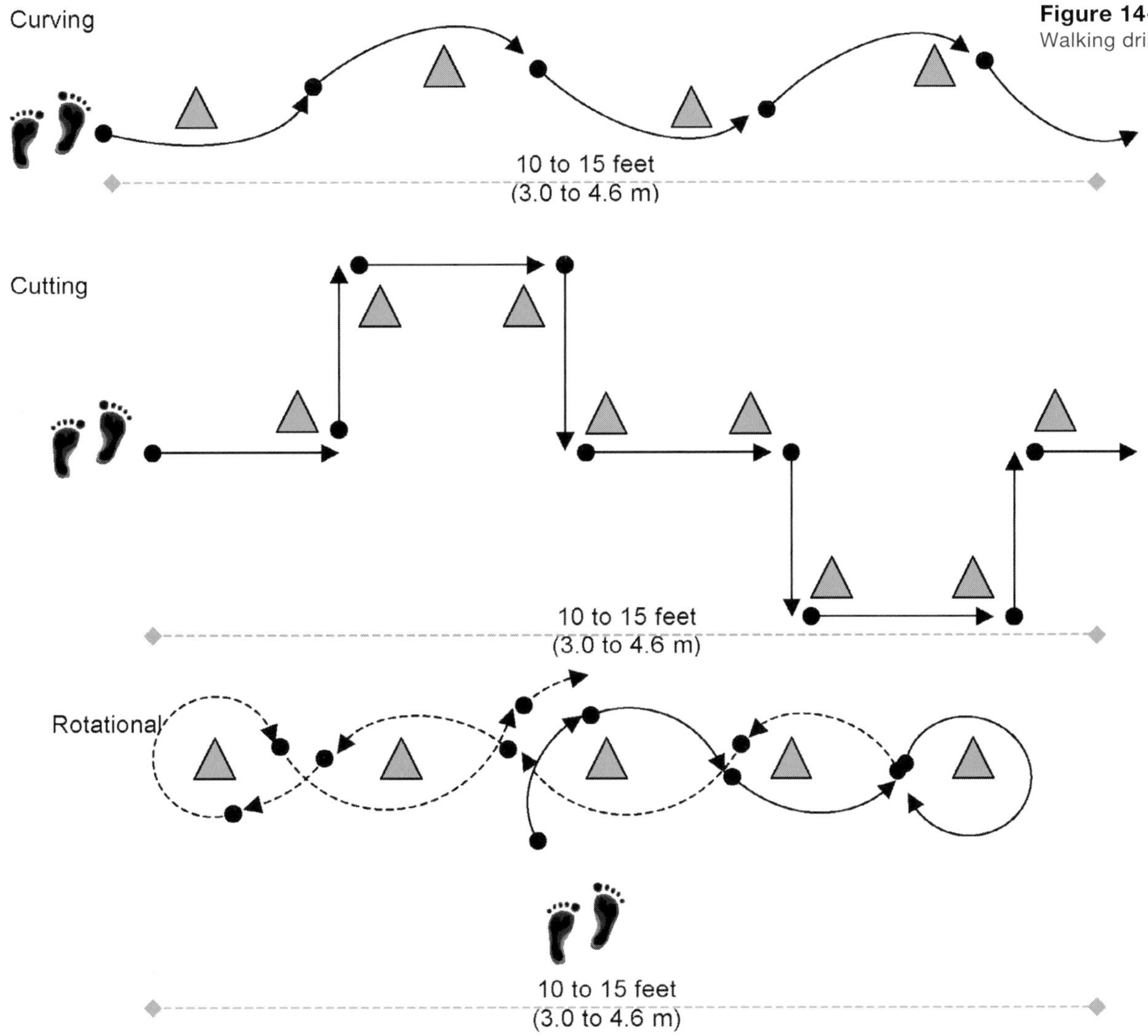

Figure 14-43
Walking drills

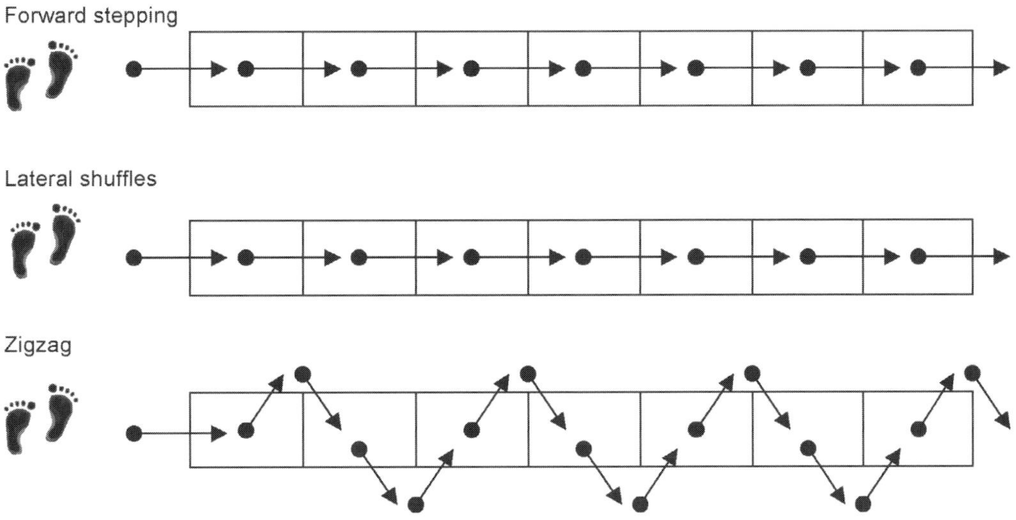

Figure 14-44
Agility drills

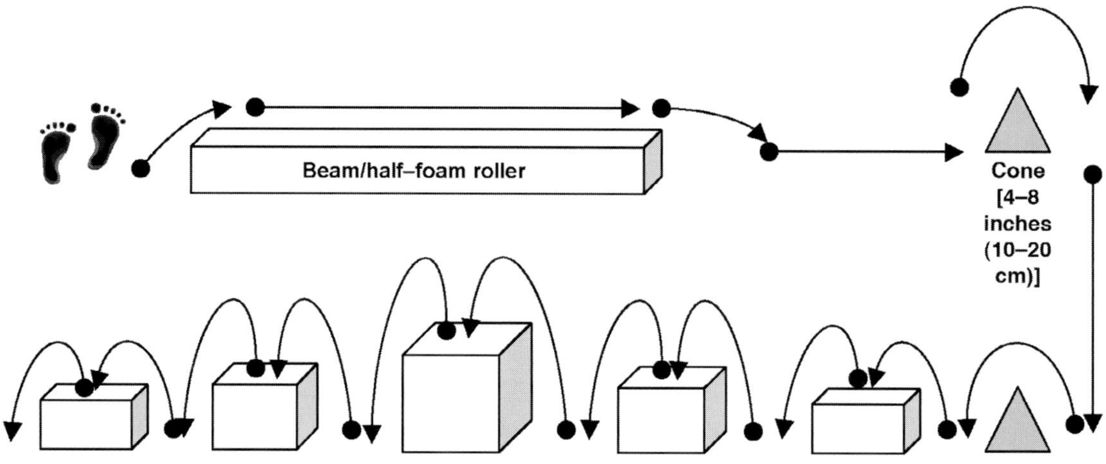

Figure 14-45
Obstacle walking using different equipment as props

- Tandem or heel-to-toe walks
- High-knee, stiff-legged march walks
- Heel-off or toe-off walks
- Crossover walks

They can also be advanced by adding obstacle walks using risers, steps, and even unstable surfaces for more advanced individuals (Figure 14-45). Obstacle walking involves walking along narrow beams or inverted half–foam rollers or performing step-up, step-over, or step-down exercises over the same height or pyramiding heights on similar or different surfaces. The ACE-AHFS should begin with a forward-linear direction, introducing directional changes as mastery is achieved. The treadmill is also an effective training modality for gait, although clients may experience a little instability at first if unfamiliar with the device. Allow adequate opportunities for each client to develop confidence and balance on a treadmill before using it as a training tool.

Coordination is the ability to train the body to enable each muscle involved in a movement to provide an accurate response in both timing and intensity. There are specific requirements for coordinated movement:

- Perception of the activity or awareness of volitional muscle activity, joint position, and movement. This element originally stems from visual feedback (a slower process), but with repetition and mastery it may originate from proprioceptive feedback (a more rapid process).
- Feedback during and following activity, as the cognitive and nervous systems evaluate performance and make any necessary adjustments
- Perfect repetitions with increasing accuracy as mastery increases, potentially decreasing the required effort and overflow from other muscles (overstimulation of muscles compensating for weaker muscles that decrease response accuracy in both timing and intensity)
- The ability to inhibit undesired muscle activity and response is facilitated by precise, slow and controlled movement until **engrams** are developed, after which speed and intensity can be increased.

Training the skill of coordination involves advancing the complexity of the more basic gait and agility drills and/or simultaneously integrating motor and cognitive tasks (e.g., having a client process questions or tasks cognitively while performing motor tasks, such as having them perform simple mathematical calculations while moving through the agility ladders or around cones).

Exercises for the Myofascial Slings

While gait may be the most functional movement in humans, functional training aims at improving overall movement efficiency, which is contingent on the efficiency of all the applicable health- and skill-related parameters of fitness, including posture. As the five primary movements can essentially define human movement, it stands to reason that a comprehensive functional training program should effectively condition the myofascial slings. This conditioning may necessitate isolated training of the weak links, or sources of "energy leaks" within the slings, prior to integrated movement training.

- The single-leg movements rely predominantly on the lateral system. Single-leg movement exercises include any single-leg stabilization and mobilization exercises (e.g., static stork stands, single-leg clock squats, or single-leg squat touches).
- Squatting movements rely predominantly on the deep longitudinal system. Squatting exercises involve extension through the posterior compartment (e.g., cobra, upward-facing dog, supine bridging, squats, and dead lifts).
- Pushing and pulling movements rely predominantly on the longitudinal and lateral systems, although the anterior oblique system contributes to pushing, while the posterior oblique system contributes to pulling movements. Pushing-movement exercises can be performed as isolated upper-extremity exercises or integrated multijoint exercises (e.g., push- and lunge-presses from a squat, split-stance, or single-leg position). Pulling-movement exercises can also be performed as isolated upper-extremity exercises or as integrated multijoint exercises (e.g., reverse squat- or lunge-pulls from a squat, split-stance, or single-leg position).
- Rotational movements rely predominantly upon the anterior and posterior oblique systems. Rotational movement exercises integrate rotation or stabilization against rotational forces [e.g., wood chops, hay bailers (see Figures 14-40 and 14-41), and sprinter pulls (Figure 14-46).

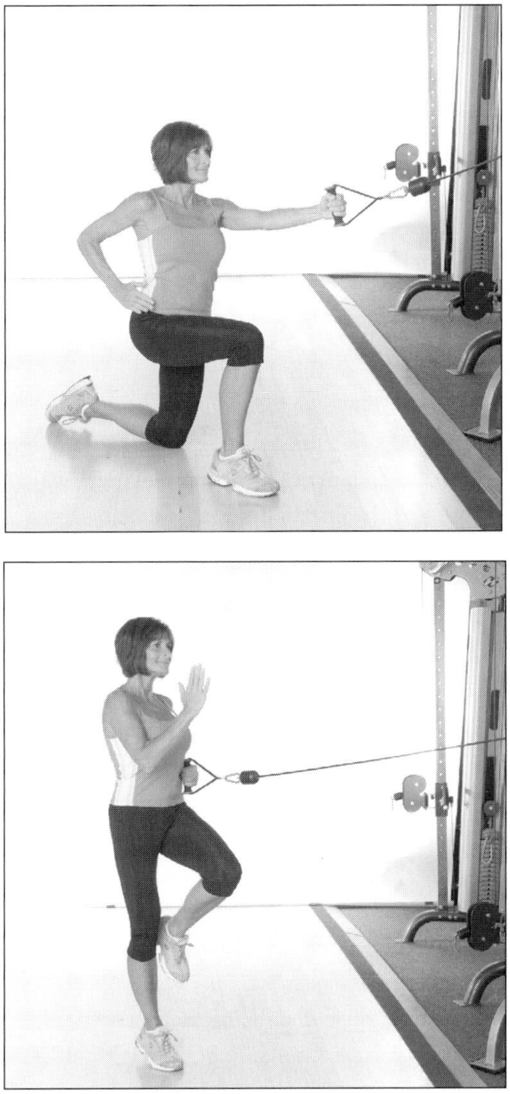

Figure 14-46
Sprinter pulls

Case Study

Joe is a 42-year-old business executive who hires an ACE-AHFS after he decides that he would like to start participating in a recreational basketball league with some of his coworkers. He was physically active throughout college and has maintained sporadic bouts of activity since he turned 35. He appears to be 20 pounds (9 kg) overweight. His current activity involves infrequent walks with his wife and golfing two or three times a month with clients. His health history reveals no significant risks factors and he has obtained clearance from his physician to exercise. His current complaints include some mild low-back discomfort, a general lack of conditioning, and a lack of power with his golf drives, which he would like to improve. The ACE-AHFS completes the initial assessments (static postural assessment, movement screens, core activation, body composition, aerobic capacity, and balance) that reveal a need to improve Joe's core conditioning, balance, and posture as foundational components. After the ACE-AHFS briefs Joe on these findings and shares recommendations, Joe agrees to focus on these parameters as his initial goal. He makes a commitment to train with the ACE-AHFS three times per week in addition to following the programming recommendations when at home and while traveling. The following outlines the core-conditioning portion of Joe's overall program.

Week 1: Muscle isolation and activation exercises
- Introduction of drawing-in
- Instruction of supine drawing-in exercises during the first 20 minutes of each session with instructions to perform exercises once or twice each day outside of the training sessions
- Progress volume from 1 set x 10 repetitions to 3 sets x 10 repetitions over the week

Week 2: Muscle isolation and activation exercises
- Instruction of new quadruped exercises during the first 15 minutes of each session with instructions to perform exercises once or twice each day outside of the training sessions
- Progress volume from 2 sets x 10 repetitions to 4 sets x 10 repetitions over the week

Week 3: Spinal stabilization
- Instruction and participation in seated stability ball exercises during the first 15–20 minutes of each session with demonstrations on how to progress the balance challenge
- Progress the duration of each exercises from 2 repetitions x 5–10 seconds to 3 repetitions x 10–15 seconds

Weeks 4–5: Spinal stabilization
- Progress seated stability ball exercises during the first 15 minutes of each session while continuing to increase the balance challenge
- Progress the duration of each exercises from 3 repetitions x 10–15 seconds to 4 repetitions x 10–15 seconds

Week 6: Whole-body stabilization
- Introduction of bracing
- Instruction and participation in static standing balance exercises on stable surfaces, progressing to unstable, static standing balance exercises toward the end of the week
- Begin with an exercise volume with 2–4 repetitions x 5–10 seconds each for static positions and 1–3 sets x 6–10 repetitions for upper-extremity dynamic moving (in static standing positions)
- Focus on sagittal plane movements and introduce frontal plane and transverse plane exercises

Week 7: Whole-body stabilization
- Progress to instruction and participation in dynamic standing balance exercises on stable surfaces
- Begin with an exercise volume of 1–2 sets x 8–10 repetitions, progressing to 2–3 sets x 10–15 repetitions
- Focus on frontal plane and transverse plane exercises

Week 8: Core conditioning
- Introduce core endurance and abdominal strengthening exercises following traditional set x repetition formats for each

Week 9: Core conditioning
- Progress the volume of core endurance exercise and the intensity of abdominal strengthening exercises
- Introduce core power exercises specific to the client's needs

Summary

Movement is essential to complete all ADL, and static and dynamic balance are critical to efficient movement. Older adults generally suffer losses to multiple senses that impact balance and, consequently, their movement efficiency. Balance, therefore, is the foundational skill element to all programming, whether functional or sports-related. It enhances physical performance, but also contributes to improving the cognitive and affective (emotional) domains and building self-efficacy and self-confidence. Improvements to balance result from increased postural stability, a key function of the core musculature. Core conditioning is a critical component of balance training and must therefore be considered a prerequisite to effective training. While the science of the core is generally well understood, a sequential approach to programming for the core is not. The five-stage model presented in this chapter will help the ACE-AHFS progress clients from neural re-education to power. Balance training improves movement and the most functional of all movement is gait. While gait is briefly reviewed, the myofascial slings involved in gait are discussed to help the ACE-AHFS understand the involvement of the entire kinetic chain. All movement can essentially be described by the five primary movements, and training programs should aim to initially target these movements prior to mimicking the specific movement patterns.

References

Anderson, K.G. & Behm, D.G. (2004). Maintenance of EMG activity and loss of force output with instability. *Journal of Strength and Conditioning Research,* 18, 637–640.

Arokoski, J.P. et al. (2001). Back and abdominal muscle function during stabilization exercises. *Archives Physical Medicine and Rehabilitation,* 82, 1089–1098.

Behm, D.G. et al. (2005). Trunk muscle electromyographic activity with unstable and unilateral exercises. *Journal of Strength and Conditioning Research,* 19, 193–201.

Bergmark, A. (1989) Stability of the lumber spine: A study in mechanical engineering. *Acta Orthopedia Scandinavia*, 230 (Suppl.), 20–24.

Bruijn, S.M. et al. (2007) Coordination of leg swing, thorax rotations and pelvis rotations during gait: The organization of total body angular momentum. *Journal of Gait and Posture,* 10, 1016.

Cook, G. (2003). *Athletic Body in Balance*. Champaign, Ill.: Human Kinetics.

Cresswell, A.G. & Thorstensson, A. (1994). Changes in intra-abdominal pressure, trunk muscle activation and force during isokinetic lifting and lowering. *European Journal of Applied Physiology,* 68, 315–321.

Gambetta, V. (2007). *Athletic Development: The Art and Science of Functional Sports Conditioning.* Champaign, Ill.: Human Kinetics.

Gracovetsky, S., Farfan H.F., & Helleur C. (1985). The abdominal mechanism. *Spine,* 10, 317–324.

Gracovetsky, S., Farfan, H.F., & Lamy, C. (1992). The mechanisms of the lumbar spine. *Spine,* 6, 1, 249–262

Gray, G.W. (2007). *Chain Reaction Transformation.* Adrian, Mich.: Winn Marketing , Inc..

Hausdorff J.M., Rios D.A., & Edelber H.K. (2001). Gait variability and fall risk in community-living older adults: A 1-year prospective study. *Archives of Physical Medicine and Rehabilitation,* 82, 8, 1050–1056.

Hodges, P.W. & Richardson, C.A. (1996). Inefficient muscular stabilization of the lumbar spine associated with LBP: A motor control evaluation of the TVA. *Spine,* 21, 2640–2650.

Hodges, P. et al. (1996). Evaluation of the relationship between laboratory and clinical tests of transversus abdominis function. *Physiotherapy Research International,* 1, 1, 30–40.

Hornbrook, M.C. et al. (1994). Preventing falls among community-dwelling older persons: Results from a randomized trial. *The Gerontologist,* 34, 1, 16–23.

Houglum, P.A. (2005) *Therapeutic Exercise for Musculoskeletal Injuries* (2nd ed.). Champaign, Ill.: Human Kinetics.

Kendall, F.P. et al. (2005). *Muscles: Testing and Function with Posture and Pain* (5th ed.). Baltimore, Md.: Lippincott Williams & Wilkins.

Lehmann J.F. & DeLater, B.J. (1990). *Gait analysis: Diagnosis and management*. In: Kottke, F. (Ed.) *Krusen's Handbook of Physical Medicine and Rehabilitation* (4th ed.). Philadelphia: Saunders.

McGill, S.M. et al. (2003). Coordination of muscle activity to assure stability of the lumbar spine. *Journal or Electromyography and Kinesiology,* 13, 353–359.

McGill, S.M. (2007). *Low Back Disorders: Evidence-based Prevention and Rehabilitation* (2nd ed.). Champaign, Ill.: Human Kinetics.

McGill, S.M. (2001). Low back stability: From formal description to issues for performance and rehabilitation. *Exercise and Sports Science Review,* 29, 1, 26–31.

McGill, S.M. et al. (1999). Endurance times for stabilization exercises: Clinical targets for testing and training from a normal database. *Archives of Physical Medicine and Rehabilitation,* 80, 941–944.

Myers, T. (2001). *Anatomy Trains: Myofascial Meridians for Manual and Movement Therapists*: New York: Churchill-Livingston.

Nagi, S.S. (1991). Disability concepts revisited: Implication for prevention. In: Pope, A.M. & Tarlov, A.R. (Eds.) *Disability in America: Toward a National Agenda for Prevention*. Washington, D.C.: National Academy Press.

Panjabi. M.M. (1992a). The stabilizing system of the spine. Part I. Function, dysfunction, adaptation and enhancement. *Journal of Spinal Disorders,* 5, 380–389.

Panjabi. M.M. (1992b). The stabilizing system of the spine. Part II. Neutral zone and instability hypothesis. *Journal of Spinal Disorders,* 5, 390–397.

Premier Training International (2005). Personal Training Solutions. London.

Richardson C. et al. (1999). *Journal of Therapeutic Exercise for Spinal Segmental Stabilization in Low Back Pain: Scientific Basis and Clinical Approach*. London: Churchill Livingstone.

Rikli, R.E. & Jones, J.C. (2001). *Senior Fitness Tests*. Champaign, Ill.: Human Kinetics.

Rose, D.J. (2003). *Fall Proof*. Champaign, Ill.: Human Kinetics.

Sahrmann, S. (2002). *Diagnosis and Treatment of Movement Impairment Syndromes.* St. Louis, Mo.: Mosby.

Sherlock, J. (1996). Getting into balance. *Physical Therapy,* Dec/Jan, 33–36.

Shumway-Cook, A. & Woollacott, M.H. (2001). *Motor Control: Theory and Practical Applications* (2nd ed.). Philadelphia: Lippincott Williams & Wilkins.

Spirduso, W.W., Francis, K.L., & MacRae, P.G. (2005). *Physical Dimensions of Aging* (2nd ed.). Campaign, Ill.: Human Kinetics.

Vleeming, A. et al. (2007). *Movement, Stability & Lumbopelvic Pain: Integration of Research and Therapy* (2nd ed.). London: Churchill Livingstone.

Vleeming A. et al. (1990a). Relation between form and function in the sacroiliac joint. Part 1: Clinical anatomical concepts. *Spine,* 15, 2, 130–132.

Vleeming A. et al. (1990b). Relation between form and function in the sacroiliac joint. Part 2: Biomechanical concepts. *Spine,* 15, 2, 133–136.

Voss, D.E., Ionta, M.K., & Myers, B.J. (1985). *Proprioceptive Neuromuscular Facilitation: Patterns and Techniques.* (3rd ed.). Philadelphia: Harper and Row.

Whiting W.C. & Rugg, S. (2006). *Dynatomy: Dynamic Human Anatomy*. Champaign, Ill.: Human Kinetics.

Willardson, J.M. (2007) Core stability training: Applications to sports conditioning programs. *Journal of Strength and Conditioning Research,* 21, 3, 979–985.

Yaggie, J.L. & Campbell, B.M. (2006). Effects of Balance Training on Selected Skills. *Journal of Strength and Conditioning Research,* 20, 2, 4227.

Suggested Reading

McGill, S.M. (2007). *Low Back Disorders: Evidence-based Prevention and Rehabilitation* (2nd ed.). Champaign, Ill.: Human Kinetics.

Rikli, R.E. & Jones, J.C. (2001). *Senior Fitness Tests.* Champaign, Ill.: Human Kinetics.

Rose, D.J. (2003). *Fall Proof*. Champaign, Ill.: Human Kinetics

Whiting W.C. & Rugg, S. (2006). *Dynatomy: Dynamic Human Anatomy.* Champaign, Ill.: Human Kinetics.

Whittle, M.W. (2007). *Gait Analysis - An Introduction* (4th ed.). Edinburgh, Scotland.: Butterworth Heinemann Elsevier

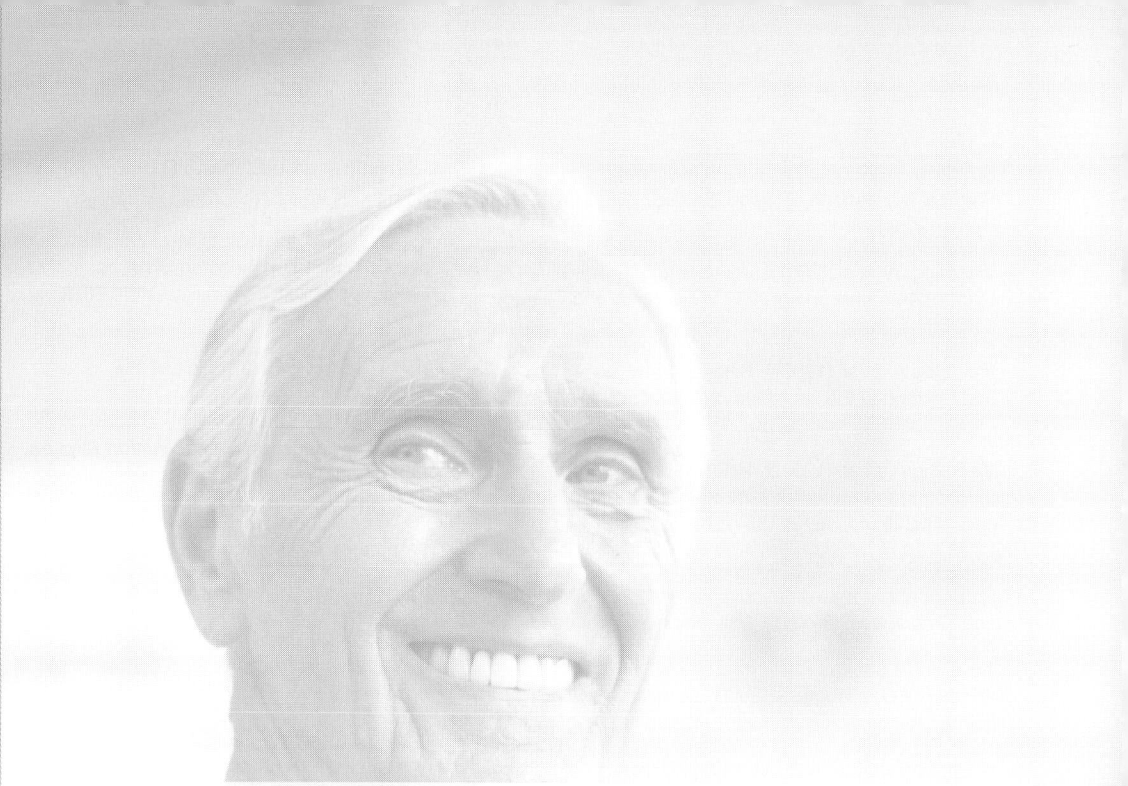

In This Chapter

About The Authors

John G. Aronen, M.D., FACSM, is an orthopedic sports medicine specialist. Retired from the Navy in 1996, Dr. Aronen is a consultant for the Center for Sports Medicine, Saint Francis Memorial Hospital in San Francisco. Dr. Aronen is a selected member of the American Orthopedic Society for Sports Medicine and the American Medical Society for Sports Medicine, and a fellow of the American College of Sports Medicine. Following two years of specialty training in sports medicine, Dr. Aronen founded and served as the head of the Sports Medicine Division of the Department of Orthopedic Surgery at the United States Naval Academy and head team physician from 1979 to 1987. Dr. Aronen then founded and directed a four-week CME/GME course for primary care providers and second-year physician assistant students in the “Evaluation and Management of Musculoskeletal Injuries Commonly Seen in Military Personnel.”

Kent A. Lorenz, M.S., CSCS, NSCA-CPT, is an exercise physiologist and program coordinator with the Center for Optimal Health and Performance at San Diego State University. He is also a lecturer and researcher within the School of Exercise and Nutritional Sciences, and uses his strength and conditioning and personal training background to develop exercise programs and classes for adults to help them maintain functional capacity and independence.

CHAPTER 15

Arthritis

John G. Aronen

Kent A. Lorenz

Arthritis is a general term that refers to joint inflammation. The two primary forms are **osteoarthritis (OA)** and **rheumatoid arthritis (RA).** OA results from a degeneration of synovial fluid and generally progresses into a loss of **articular cartilage**, which typically presents itself as localized joint pain and a reduction of **range of motion (ROM)** (Buckwalter & Martin, 2006). Buckwalter and Martin (2006) report that approximately 20 million Americans have OA, and the World Health Organization (WHO) estimates that about 10% of the world's population over the age of 60 has the disease. Of those who have OA, 80% will have limitations of movement and 25% cannot perform major **activities of daily living (ADL),** with the most common sites affected being the knees, hips, spine, hands, and feet (Buckwalter & Martin, 2006).

While OA is the most common affliction of the joints, RA is another condition the ACE-certified Advanced Health & Fitness Specialist (ACE-AHFS) may see among his or her clientele. RA is a chronic autoimmune disease that results in inflammation of the **synovium,** leading to long-term joint damage, chronic pain, and loss of function or disability (Arthritis Foundation, 2007). RA progresses in three stages, with the first being a swelling of the synovial lining, resulting in pain, warmth, stiffness, redness, and swelling of the joint. The second phase is a rapid division and growth of cells, which causes the synovium to thicken. In the third and final stage, the inflamed cells release **enzymes** that break down bone and cartilage, causing the affected joint to lose structure and alignment, leading to more pain and a further decrease in function. RA is a chronic disease that typically worsens with time, resulting in further physical limitations of the involved joints. In comparison to osteoarthritis, RA, being an autoimmune disease and having a more systemic effect, may manifest itself in the development of heart and lung disease and **diabetes.** As with OA, the quality of life for individuals with RA can be improved with exercises that are designed to maintain muscle strength, joint range of motion, and cardiovascular function. The exercise recommendations that are presented in this chapter are specific to OA, but people with RA are encouraged to perform low levels of activity that does not increase inflammation. Certain modifications, such as the use of wrist straps or ankle or wrist weights and the performance of lower-intensity and higher-duration activities, may be needed to accommodate certain clients. Helmick et al. (2008) estimate that 1.3 million Americans suffer from RA, down from 2.1 million in 1995, suggesting a reduction in the prevalence of the disease.

While this chapter introduces both forms of arthritis, the focus from this point on will be on the identification and treatment of OA. As with all chronic conditions, the ACE-AHFS should communicate with his or her clients to discuss what types of activities they are able to do—and how much. If someone presents with some of the signs and symptoms of OA or RA, and he or she has not sought medical advice, the ACE-AHFS should refer the individual to a medical professional before working with him or her. In more severe cases, where the majority of weightbearing activity is painful or limited, the ACE-AHFS may want to refer to a physical therapist or occupational therapist.

Medical conditions (e.g., illnesses, injuries) are typically placed into one of two categories based on their suspected cause, or **etiology**—primary or secondary. The determination of a condition's category is based on whether the underlying cause for the problem can be identified. If the underlying cause for a problem cannot be identified, the problem falls into the primary category (i.e., the individual has the problem, but physicians cannot determine why or what is causing or contributing to the problem). For primary problems, treatment and management must be directed at the symptoms associated with the condition. Unfortunately, while this approach may provide resolution of the symptoms, the underlying cause will continue to contribute to the natural progression of the problem.

If the underlying cause that contributed to the onset of the condition and/or continues to contribute to the condition can be identified, the condition is categorized as secondary. With a problem that is secondary, the emphasis of the treatment and management program must be directed at eliminating or minimizing the underlying cause. Failure to recognize that proper management of a secondary condition includes management of both the symptoms and, more importantly, the underlying cause(s) of the symptoms, will result in only short-term relief from the presenting symptoms, as the underlying cause is allowed to continue to contribute to the natural progression of the problem.

Injuries to a joint occur either acutely or insidiously (i.e., over a prolonged period of time). Any injury to a joint that causes detrimental changes to its structural integrity becomes the starting point for the onset and progression of osteoarthritic changes. Because there are typically detrimental changes to the structural integrity of the knee with an acute injury, such as a sprain of the anterior cruciate ligament, a tear of a meniscus, or patellar dislocation, the starting point for the onset of osteoarthritic changes is the time of the injury. In many acute injuries, due to the severity of the initial changes to the structural integrity of the joint, the starting point for osteoarthritic changes is also the starting point for the discomfort and/or swelling associated with the osteoarthritic changes, constant reminders to the individual that he or she no longer has an entirely healthy or normal joint. For others, the initial changes to the structural integrity of the joint are not severe enough to result in the onset of discomfort and/or swelling from the time of the injury. The starting point for changes to the structural integrity with an injury of insidious onset, as may be seen in the knees and hips with a steady regimen of distance running, is ill defined, as it does not come on acutely, but rather over time. Unfortunately, with the normal progression of degenerative changes that occurs in osteoarthritic joints, discomfort and/or swelling will become evident sooner or later in the majority of cases.

Structural integrity of a joint refers primarily to the following:

- Articular cartilage, which consists of hyaline cartilage, is free of pain fibers and covers the portions of bone that articulate with each other within a joint. Articular cartilage is also referred to as chondral cartilage.
- Subchondral bone, which underlies the articular cartilage, must be healthy to provide appropriate structural support to the articular cartilage overlying it.
- Discomfort and/or swelling are the earliest symptoms or physical findings that indicate that changes have occurred to the structural integrity and that the joint is no longer an entirely healthy or normal joint. Typically, the amount of discomfort and/or swelling is an indicator of the severity of changes to the structural integrity of the joint.

Epidemiology

Prior to the 1980s, OA, often referred to as **degenerative joint disease (DJD),** was believed to occur only in men who suffered an injury to a joint, most commonly the knee, while involved in a contact sport. Because the onset of OA was thought to be caused by the initial injury to the knee, the OA that occurred following a documented knee injury was classified as a secondary problem. Additionally, little concern was given to the initial treatment and long-term management of the etiology, which would have slowed down the progression of the undesirable changes to the structural integrity. Typically, the athlete would remain active in sports, only expediting the "unavoidable" progression of the acute changes, resulting in a chronically painful and functionally deficient knee. Unfortunately, due to an avid desire to return an athlete to all activities rather than be realistic and make modifications in lifestyle that may prolong the life of the injured joint, too little progress has been made in the appropriate initial treatment and long-term management.

Two other factors came into play regarding OA in the late 1970s and early 1980s, the first being the sudden surge of adolescent and teenage girls into injury-producing sports. As the number of participants in sport dramatically increased, the number of significant acute injuries, not only to the knee but to other joints as well, resulted in a large increase of symptoms and findings compatible with osteoarthritis in younger and middle-aged athletes. Additionally, it was noted that not only could the onset of OA [through findings noted on **arthroscopy, magnetic resonance imaging (MRI),** or symptoms compatible with OA] occur following an acute injury to a joint, but it could also occur following persistent microtrauma to the structural integrity of a joint, as seen in distance runners. In the early 2000s (approximately 20 to 25 years following the surge in female participation in sports), a dramatic increase in individuals with physical and radiographic findings compatible with significant osteoarthritic changes in the knees and hips began to appear. The following characteristics were common in this group:

- A female participating in sports that were only sparsely available to the female community prior to 1980, but sprang into popularity in the 1980s (e.g., basketball, volleyball, softball, soccer, distance running)
- An individual incurring a knee/hip injury or simply having a history of following a compulsive daily running regimen
- An individual treated with one of the increasing number of surgical procedures designed to address these injuries, followed by aggressive rehabilitation programs

With emphasis placed on early surgical intervention and aggressive rehabilitation, the high rate of attrition from sports entirely due to injuries at an early age suddenly came more into focus. Experts had assumed that injured joints would naturally degenerate with time and that lifestyle modifications of young athletes would have little or no effect on the outcome of the process of degeneration.

It is slowly becoming understood that the progression of the initial changes to the structural integrity of a joint can be "slowed down" through alterations in the individual's daily lifestyle and through rehabilitation programs designed to regain and maintain normal strength and flexibility of the muscles surrounding the joint. These programs are designed to slow the progression of the degenerative changes already existing in the joint. Each exercise incorporated into a rehabilitation program for an individual with OA must be evaluated for the amount of force it places on the vulnerable joint, because, although the individual may be able to perform the exercise without any pain, this is no guarantee that the exercise is not doing more harm than good over an extended period of time.

Another factor in the increase in prevalence of OA was the changing of dietary and exercise habits. Since the 1980s, the United States went from being one of the leanest and fittest countries in the world to the other end of the spectrum. It soon became apparent that people were living longer and presenting with significant arthritic changes in hips and/or knees that had never experienced acute trauma. Although from this group it appeared that a primary form of OA was associated with normal aging, 52% of patients who required total knee **arthroplasty** and 36% of those who required total hip arthroplasty were **overweight** or obese (Namba et al., 2005).

Although there are some individuals who will develop OA with no identifiable underlying causes, the vast majority of OA is secondary in nature—secondary to trauma and/or **obesity.** Therefore, exercise programs for individuals with OA must keep forces on the osteoarthritic joint to a minimum, as clients strive to retain the strength and flexibility necessary for a joint to function normally.

Physical Symptoms and Findings Associated With Osteoarthritis

To understand the symptoms experienced with OA, the ACE-AHFS must have knowledge of the anatomical structures of a joint. Furthermore, the ACE-AHFS must understand the role each structure plays in normal joint functioning and the contributions each makes to the physical symptoms experienced and the physical findings noted on examination).

The role of a joint, or **articulation,** is to allow motion between bones at a specific site. Because of its high frequency of injury and because it is a common site of OA, the knee will be used in this discussion.

A **capsule** fully encloses each joint, so that fluid produced in the joint is retained in the joint. Lining the capsule is a **synovial membrane** that consists of **synovial cells.** There are two types of synovial cells, type A and type B. The lubrication system, which sounds very simplistic, is actually very sophisticated. The type A cells are secretory in that they produce the **synovial fluid** that acts as a lubricant for the joint. The natural viscosity of the synovial fluid minimizes the degenerative process normally seen between two healthy structures that repetitively articulate with each other. The type B cells are phagocytic, in that they are responsible for the debridement (removal) of the "worn out" synovial fluid and any excess fluid (synovial fluid and/or blood) that may have accumulated in the joint. The articular cartilage of the knee is entirely separate from the two **menisci,** which are made up of fibrocartilage and function to provide shock absorption and stability to the knee.

The articular cartilage is unquestionably a key anatomical structure. Osteoarthritis begins and ends with changes to the structural integrity of the articular cartilage. There are a few properties unique to articular cartilage:

- It has no blood supply and thus cannot heal if injured.
- Because it lacks a blood supply, the role of providing nourishment to the articular cartilage is carried out by the synovial fluid, which is able to enter and exit the articular cartilage at will through microscopic pores in the surface.
- The articular cartilage is void of pain fibers.

The contributions of the articular cartilage to a normal, healthy joint include the following:

- When the surface of the articular cartilage is pristine and covered with synovial fluid, the **coefficient of friction** between the two articulating surfaces is almost zero.
- Because it lacks pain fibers, the articular cartilage prevents the subchondral bone, which has an abundance of pain fibers, from experiencing pain related to the normal transmission of force across joints on a daily basis. Without articular cartilage, the joint would be basically bone on bone—which would be very painful.
- It has been determined clinically that healthy articular cartilage can tolerate approximately seven times the person's body weight before undesirable and often silent detrimental changes begin to compromise the structural integrity of the articular cartilage, which is why it is so important to avoid activities that place unnecessarily high forces on the joints (Repo & Finlay, 1977).

Initial changes to the articular cartilage involve the changing of the once pristine surface into an uneven, incongruous surface. These changes can occur quickly from acute trauma, such as a torn anterior cruciate ligament, meniscal tear, or dislocated patella. Each of these injuries produce **shear forces** in the joint that damage the articular cartilage. The rating of the severity of damage is based on the amount of articular cartilage involved and the depth of the disruption, which ranges from grade 1 to grade 4. Grade 1 implies only superficial changes to the articular cartilage, while grade 4 implies damage to the point where subchondral bone is exposed. The loss of the pristine surfaces leads to an increase in the coefficient of friction, which hastens damage due to wear and tear on the remaining articular cartilage.

Along with the loss of the pristine surface, the once microscopic pores that allowed the synovial fluid to flow freely into the articular cartilage become enlarged, allowing the escape of chemicals from inside the articular cartilage into the joint. These chemicals are direct irritants to the synovial cells and cause them to become inflamed (chemical synovitis). Once inflamed, the cells produce soreness throughout the knee as well as an excessive amount of synovial fluid, which is experienced as tightness in the knee. The inflammation from the chemicals, with the resultant discomfort and excessive synovial fluid production, typically takes 10 to 14 hours. Thus, the individual can be physically active on the knee in the evening, but will note the diffuse discomfort and tightness the next day.

With the continuous wear-and-tear changes due to the increased coefficient of friction, the articular cartilage becomes thinner, allowing the subchondral bone to experience more of the forces transmitted across the joint. Forces experienced by the subchondral bone result in pain, the amount and frequency of which is dependent on many factors:

- The location of the site of exposed subchondral bone (weightbearing vs. nonweightbearing areas)
- The amount of force placed on the site with physical activity (e.g., minimal with swimming, highest with weightbearing activities)
- The weight of the individual, as higher body mass can increase joint **compressive forces** that are excacerbated by misalignment of the femoral-tibial joint (Felson et al., 2004)

The pain can start out as minimal following activity, but progresses in accordance with the amount and frequency of undesired forces placed on the site, typically to the point where the individual's lifestyle is greatly altered by the pain. Unfortunately, most individuals will not consider making changes in their level of physical activity until they are experiencing constant bone pain.

Normal Course of Symptoms in an Osteoarthritic Joint

In the earliest stages, there may be no symptoms or findings until continued forces are placed on the joint and the degenerative changes subsequently progress. Initial symptoms are next-day discomfort and/or stiffness of the joint from chemical synovitis.

As the changes to the structural integrity increase, the next-day discomfort and/or stiffness will increase in intensity and frequency. As the articular cartilage becomes thinner, forces are transmitted and experienced by the subchondral bone, resulting in bone pain during and after activity. Further progression leads to bone-on-bone contact and constant pain.

Because it is relatively silent in nature in its early stages, OA is comparable to **hypertension** in that they are both silent diseases that continue to worsen without telltale signs. These silent changes frequently have dramatic effects on an individual's health and lifestyle activities if he or she fails to recognize them in the early stages. The diagnostic criteria that are used to identify individuals with OA of the knee as outlined by the Agency for Healthcare Research and Quality are joint pain plus five of the following criteria (Samson et al., 2007):

- Client over 50 years of age
- Less than 30 minutes of morning joint stiffness
- **Crepitus**
- Bony tenderness
- Bony enlargement
- No palpable warmth of synovium
- Erythrocyte sedimentation rate (ESR) <40 mm/hr
- Rheumatoid factor <1:40
- Non-inflammatory synovial fluid

It is highly recommended that the ACE-AHFS speak in detail with his or her client to get a full history before developing an exercise program. If the ACE-AHFS or the client is unsure of the status or progression of OA, the client should be referred to a medical professional.

The task for an ACE-AHFS is to recommend specific exercises for clients with OA that will allow them to remain physically active without doing harm to their existing problem. The ACE-AHFS must understand which individuals are at risk for osteoarthritis and who will therefore need exercise programs designed to protect the joints.

Any individual who has had surgery on a joint involved in the exercise program: The initial injury requiring surgical intervention in the vast majority of cases disrupts the structural integrity of the joint (i.e., the articular cartilage and subchondral bone). This situation must be recognized in the development of an exercise program for these individuals.

Individuals who state that they experience discomfort and/or tightness the day following physical activity: Chemical synovitis is the number-one reason for these symptoms to occur and persist. Temporary relief can be achieved with over-the-counter anti-inflammatory medications, but the symptom and not the etiology itself is being treated. Also, the concern over the possible significant side effects of all anti-inflammatory medications often outweighs the palliative benefits. A safer route to control the discomfort may be the use of a glucosamine sulfate with a low-molecular chondroitin (only found in CosaminDS®). A study by the National Institutes of Health (Clegg et al., 2006) reported better relief of pain and no known side effects with the use of the ingredients found only in CosaminDS when compared to Celebrex® 200 mg a day or a placebo.

Overweight individuals: The excessive forces associated with overweight and obesity result in undesirable changes to the articular cartilage. The ACE-AHFS must not do anything to hasten these changes.

Individuals who walk with an altered gait, especially following participation in a weightbearing activity: This can result in an asymmetrical loading of the joint, which increases the risk of joint degeneration (Buckwalter & Martin, 2006).

Individuals who feel the need to wear a brace with activity: Bracing is often a result of a previous injury or current joint pain, which may have resulted in alterations of the articular structures and can increase the risk of the development of OA (Buckwalter & Martin, 2006).

Osteoarthritis and Exercise

By increasing muscular strength and endurance, enhancing the stability of the joints, improving range of motion, and reducing passive tension of the soft tissue surrounding joints, an ACE-AHFS can help his or her clients improve their quality of life, maintain normal function, and prevent deconditioning. One of the secondary outcomes of OA is a development of other diseases, such as **coronary artery disease,** diabetes, and hypertension, as physical activity becomes too painful to attempt, cardiovascular function declines, and the client becomes **sedentary.** For the high number of overweight or obese clients with OA, a further reduction in physical activity can increase the risk for the development of comorbidities. By encouraging clients to maintain cardiovascular fitness by doing exercise that does not increase joint pain, combined with exercises and treatments to help reduce joint pain, an ACE-AHFS can reduce the impact of OA on pain, day-to-day function, cardiovascular health, and quality of life.

Of the randomized, controlled trials exploring the effects of exercise on OA symptoms, some have used hydrotherapy, tai chi, or other low-impact exercises to reduce the stress on the joints (Ettinger et al., 1997; Fransen et al., 2007; Hinman, Haywood, & Day, 2007; Lund et al., 2008; Wang et al., 2007). This outcome is certainly recommended for individuals who experience pain throughout the day, but for those who are relatively pain free, weightbearing exercise and resistance training can be beneficial in not only reducing pain and disability, but also in maintaining normal everyday function. A study examining the effects of different exercise modes on pain, disability, and performance measures found that 60 minutes of light- to moderate-intensity walking three days per week [50 to 70% **heart-rate reserve (HRR)**], or light- to moderate-intensity resistance training three days per week (two sets of 12 repetitions of nine exercises) had significantly better results than the control group over an 18-month intervention (Ettinger et al., 1997). Similar results were obtained in a study that showed that individuals performing three days per week of light- to moderate-intensity resistance training (three sets of eight to 10 repetitions) had lower pain scores and higher functional abilities compared to those who performed only passive range-of-motion exercises (Mikesky et al., 2006). There was also a dose-response relationship between those who did more exercise (75 to 100% of programmed sessions) and those who did less activity (<40% of programmed sessions), with those in the former group experiencing lower pain and disability scores and having greater performance and fitness scores (Ettinger et al., 1997). However, as with all exercise programs for individuals with limitations, the ACE-AHFS must always be cognizant of the client. If the client is hurting, he or she will not do the exercise, so the ACE-AHFS must base decisions on individual feedback, not general guidelines.

Unfortunately, exercise is not a cure for OA, but maintaining a regular exercise program of resistance and aerobic training can reduce the pain and rate of decline in functional capacity (Ettinger et al., 1997; Mikesky et al., 2006). No evidence exists that properly programmed and managed exercise will increase the rate of joint degeneration, as measured by joint-space narrowing (Mikesky et al., 2006) or pain scores (Ettinger et al., 1997; van Baar et al., 1999). Exercise can help reduce some of the risk factors associated with the progression of OA, including weak quadriceps (Bennell & Hinman, 2005; Mikesky et al., 2006), **valgus** or **varus** knee alignment (knock-kneed or bow-legged), weak hip abductors, and obesity (Issa & Sharma, 2006). By selecting exercises or developing programs that address these conditions, an ACE-AHFS can help reduce pain and functional limitations, as well as slow the progression of OA to keep clients active. Further reductions in quadriceps strength, as well as in the hip abductors and extensors, will accelerate the deterioration of the joint by reducing the ability of the individual to control anterior-posterior motion of the knee, as well as exacerbating structural alignment problems that may lead to asymmetrical wear on the articular cartilage.

Programming Guidelines and Considerations

Contraindications and precautions

- Stop immediately if any feelings of joint pain occur during exercise.
- Reduce volume and intensity if next-day tightness or pain is present.
- More frequent, lower-intensity exercise is preferred to a single longer or higher-intensity session.

Guidelines

- Clients should always perform an adequate warm-up (10 minutes) to ensure joint lubrication and increased elasticity of tissues (Hedrick, 1992).
  - ✔They should start with light aerobic exercise to increase systemic blood flow and body temperature.
  - ✔They should perform activation exercises to target specific areas (knees, hips), such as unloaded knee flexion and extension focusing on full ROM.
  - ✔Dynamic flexibility exercises should be performed to maintain elasticity and further increase lubrication (static stretching will cool the body down; the goal is to keep it warm and moving).

Progressions and recommendations

- *Aerobic exercise:* Three to five days per week of light- to moderate-intensity training (50–70% HRR) of lower-impact exercises (e.g., walking, swimming, cycling, inline skating, rowing) for 30 to 60 continuous minutes
  - ✔Multiple, shorter sessions per day may help reduce joint pain.
  - ✔Aqua-therapy or swimming can reduce joint stress while maintaining cardiovascular function and muscular endurance.
  - ✔Clients should gradually progress to longer sessions (increases of 5–10% in duration) when able to comfortably exercise without any fatigue or increasing joint pain, keeping intensity low to avoid higher joint forces.
  - ✔If exercising on consecutive days, clients should switch modes to avoid overuse injuries.
  - ✔The ACE-AHFS should remind clients that proper footwear and softer terrain are important to reduce joint forces during weightbearing exercise.
- *Resistance training:* Two to three days per week of light- to moderate-intensity training

- ✔ Clients should perform one to three sets of eight to 12 repetitions.
- ✔ They should follow a full-body program using machines or free weights.
- ✔ The program should include functional exercises to develop **synergists** as well as overall coordination of the musculature to control and stabilize the joint.
- ✔ Clients should begin with isometrics and unloaded movements to increase ROM and develop proper movement patterns.
- ✔ Exercise in the water allows for light resistances to help condition muscles through a full, pain-free ROM, while also reducing joint stresses.
- ✔ Clients can progress to light resistance (cuff weights, tubing/bands, dumbbells) or bilateral exercises (bodyweight squats).
- ✔ Clients should work toward moderate-resistance exercises with as much ROM as can be tolerated, or to unilateral exercises (lunges, step-ups).

- *Flexibility and stress reduction:* ROM exercises daily to keep joints mobile and compliant
  - ✔ Clients should perform dynamic flexibility exercises to increase ROM and keep joints lubricated, and static stretching to decrease passive tension (emphasis on the hamstrings, quadriceps, gluteals, gastrocnemius, soleus, and adductors for the lower extremity, and the pectorals, trapezius, latissimus dorsi, deltoids, rhomboids, rotator cuff muscles, biceps, and triceps for the upper extremity).
  - ✔ Pilates, yoga, tai chi, and meditation can improve overall flexibility, reduce stress, improve mood or psychological outlook, and reduce pain.
  - ✔ **Myofascial release** (foam rollers, massage) can decrease passive tension and break down soft-tissue adhesions that impair normal muscular function.

Osteoarthritis of the knee

- Clients can begin with isometric exercises or light resistance (ankle weights) to strengthen the quadriceps, hamstrings, and gluteals without putting undue pressure on the joint. These exercises can be performed in a pool to further reduce joint pressures.
- Clients can move to bodyweight bilateral exercises (e.g., squats) to develop overall muscular and joint control while encouraging full ROM.
  - ✔ Clients can add external resistance to increase muscular strength and endurance if they are pain free.
- Clients can progress to unilateral exercises (lunges, step-ups) to develop muscular control of the joint complex.
  - ✔ They should focus on proper control and technique to make sure the patella and femur track correctly.

Osteoarthritis of the hip

- Clients can begin with passive ROM exercises to increase circulation and synovial lubrication, which helps reduce joint compression. Also, aqua-therapy can be used to reduce pressure on the joint.
- Clients can perform exercises lying on the ground to avoid putting to much load on the hips. They should begin with limited-ROM lying hip abduction and extension exercises, plus ROM exercises to strengthen the hip and increase flexibility.
- Clients can progress to bilateral weightbearing exercises with limited ROM (e.g., wall slides, bodyweight squats) to develop the hip complex. They can perform ROM exercises at the end of the session to keep the joint flexible and reduce joint compression and passive tension.
- When the client is able to perform bilateral exercises with limited pain through a larger ROM, he or she can progress to unilateral exercises (e.g., single-leg squat) to further develop the gluteals and hamstrings.

Sample Exercises

All programs should be tailored to meet the individual needs and experiences of each client, but free-weight or body-weight exercises are generally preferred for clients with OA, as they allow for the development of neuromuscular control and conditioning of **antagonists** and synergists to help control and stabilize the joint.

Note that this list of exercises is not meant to be a complete exercise program, but is instead intended to provide sample exercises that can be beneficial in reducing symptoms of OA and ameliorating the progression of the disease.

At the beginning stages of exercise, individuals need to increase quadriceps strength without increasing the risk of joint degeneration. The open-chain terminal 30 degrees knee extension exercise (Figure 15-1) is an effective means of doing just that. This exercise allows for the strengthening of the knee extensors, but by performing only the final 30 degrees the client avoids the high compression forces of the full-ROM knee extension. *Note:* One exercise that should be removed from all exercise programs of those with OA (and for those who want to avoid developing OA) is the full-ROM knee extension. This exercise places tremendous compression forces on the underside of the patella, accelerating the degeneration of the joint.

Once the client has progressed to where he or she can create adequate force and endurance to sustain the contraction shown in Figure 15-1 for 15 to 30 seconds, the client can progress to the closed-chain terminal knee extension (Figure 15-2). This exercise allows for the development of the quadriceps, but also develops the hip extensors and abductors in a stabilizing capacity.

As the client progresses, the addition of bodyweight exercises to condition the lower body is recommended. The isometric or small-ROM wall slide or wall squat (Figure 15-3) is the first exercise that should be added to the program, as it develops the strength of the knee extensors, hip extensors, and abductors, and also helps the client develop the neuromuscular control to help move on to dynamic exercises.

After the client is able to perform the wall slide comfortably, he or she can progress to the bodyweight squat to develop the musculature surrounding the hips and knees (Figure 15-4). The

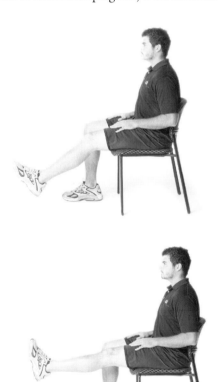

Figure 15-1
Terminal 30-degrees knee extension (open chain). Starting the knee at 30 degrees of flexion and moving to full extension reduces the compression forces on the underside of the patella, minimizing wear and preventing further degeneration of the articular cartilage. This exercise can be performed with ankle weights or as an isometric hold at the terminal range of motion.

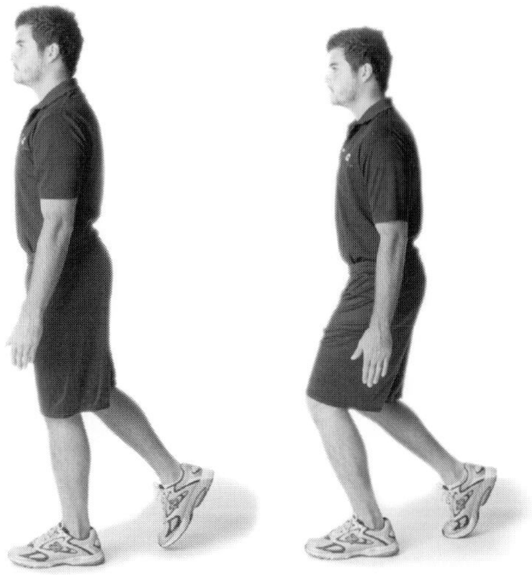

Figure 15-2
Terminal knee extensions (closed chain). The client starts by standing on one leg with the non-supporting leg resting toes-down for support. The client then moves the support leg into 30 degrees of flexion, keeping the shoulders and hips over the heel, and then presses the knee of the supporting leg backward, actively contracting the quadriceps to move into full extension. Resistance bands can be added to increase difficulty.

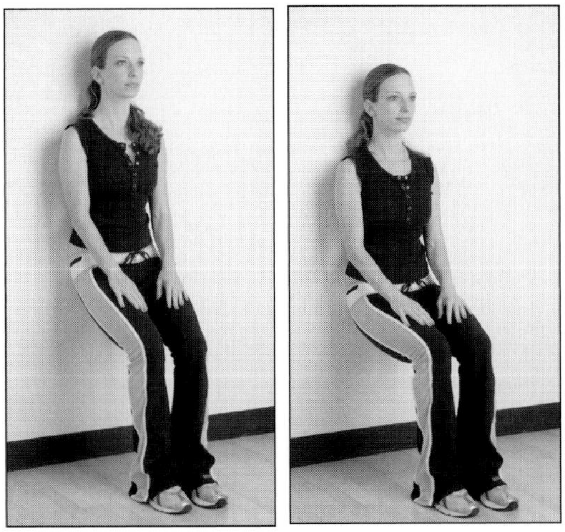

Figure 15-3
Wall slide/squat. The client begins with the feet comfortably under the hips and the back flat against the wall and slides down the wall until the knees are flexed (staying above 90 degrees or to tolerance) and holds for 2–30 seconds. The client presses through the heels and returns to the starting position.

ACE-AHFS must pay particular attention to the client's knees as he or she performs the exercise. Many clients will allow the knees to move medially (inward), which places strain on the joint and leads to uneven wear of the articular cartilage.

The next progression is the single-leg squat, which places greater demand on the client, especially on the quadriceps, to control the leg and the hip muscles to control and stabilize the pelvis and femur (Figure 15-5). Many people will have difficulty with this exercise, as they do not have the hip strength to maintain proper pelvic alignment or the strength and balance of the legs to maintain correct form. Two common errors are to allow the knees to move laterally (outward) during the eccentric phase of the exercise (descent) and medially (inward) during the concentric phase (ascent). *Note:* Individuals displaying medial motion of the knee often have poorly functioning external hip rotators and extensors (gluteal group) or tight adductors.

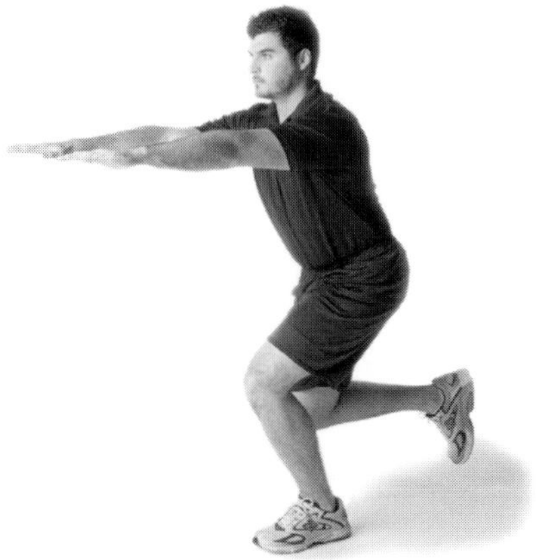

Figure 15-5
Single-leg squat. The client begins by balancing on one foot with the other leg flexed behind for counterbalance. The client initiates the movement by pulling the hips back, and then sinks the weight downward over the support-leg heel. It is essential that the patella tracks straight and the knee does not move medially.

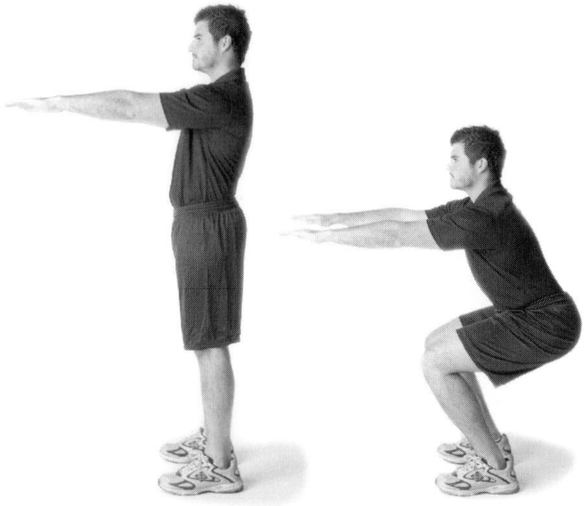

Figure 15-4
Bodyweight squat. The client starts with the feet under the hips and the arms out for balance. The client begins the movement by contracting the glutes and hamstrings to pull the hips backward. The ACE-AHFS should remind the client to allow the body to bend naturally at the hips and allow the knees to flex until comfortable. The client must keep the knees in line with the hips and ankles.

One factor that may contribute to both knee and hip pain is the inability to control the hips and pelvis, potentially leading to poor femur-tibia alignment, altered gait patterns, and weakness of the hip abductors. Therefore, development of the spinal, pelvic, and hip stabilizers is important. A simple exercise to accomplish this objective is the hip bridge (Figure 15-6). Particular emphasis should be placed on training the deep spine stabilizers to provide adequate support of the spine and pelvis when engaging in single-leg balance or locomotion activities. Dysfunction in this region often prevents the appropriate recruitment of the prime movers, as the pelvis is unstable and does not provide a good foundation for movements.

Exercises such as the side plank (Figure 15-7), prone plank (Figure 15-8), and prone hip

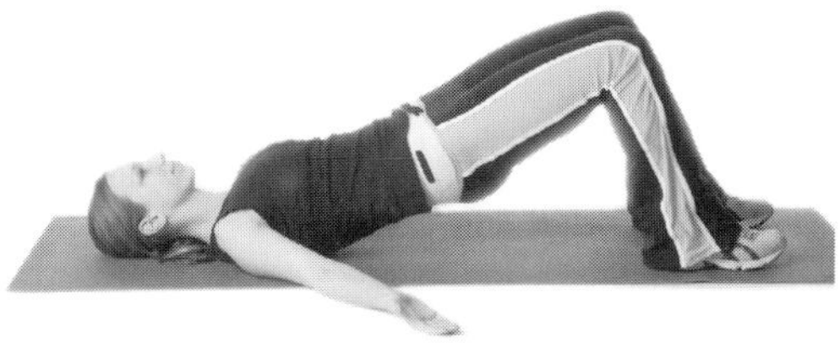

Figure 15-6
Hip bridge. The client lies supine with the feet about hip-width apart and the shoulders down with the arms out for support. The client presses through the heel and elevates the hips so that they are in a straight line with the knees and shoulders. The client engages the lower back, glutes, and hamstrings to help develop strength and endurance of the hip extensors.

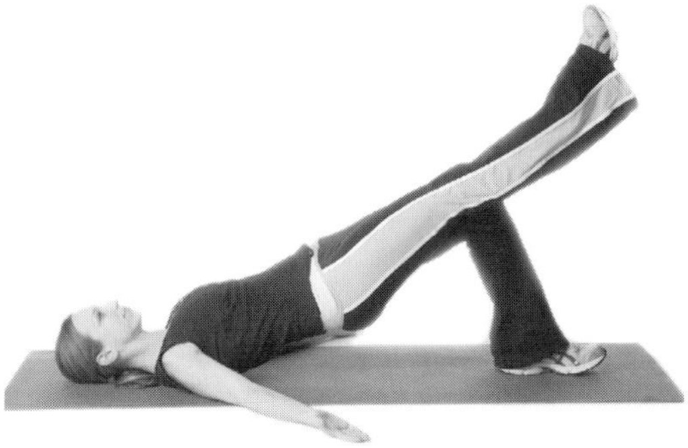

An advanced single-leg version of the hip bridge

extension (Figure 15-9) develop strength and endurance of these muscles. Not only is stability important, flexibility and adequate ROM are as well, as reducing passive tension along the kinetic chain can reduce tissue stress surrounding the joint, which may be contributing to uneven muscle-recruitment patterns. Using a foam roller or massage is effective, but doing simple hip ROM exercises (Figure 15-10) can be beneficial as well.

It is important to identify any potential muscular dysfunctions that can contribute to the development of OA. By having the client perform calf raises to full plantarflexion (Figure 15-11), perform a standing single-leg balance (Figure 15-12), and walk on the heels and toes (Figure 15-13), an ACE-AHFS can get a basic idea of any muscle-recruitment difficulties. If the client is unable to perform a full-ROM calf raise, he or she may have an underdeveloped gastrocnemius, which may limit the ability to control the knee joint during locomotion. Similarly, the performance of a

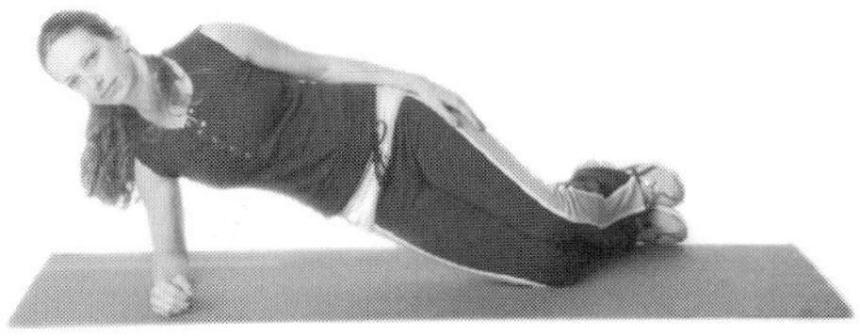

Figure 15-7
Side plank. The client positions the elbow under the shoulder and the knees in line with the hips so that the body is straight, and then lifts the hips off the ground by engaging the deep muscles of the spine (quadratus lumborum). It is important the hips are straight and not "sagging" below the level of the shoulders.

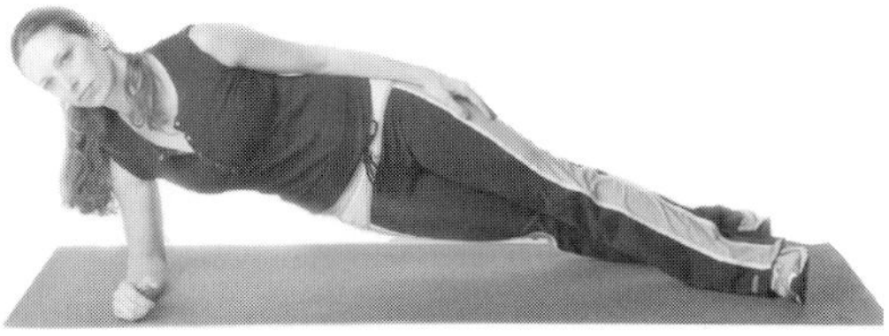

For a more advanced and challenging exercise, the client can support him- or herself on the elbow and toes, again with the hips raised so that they are level with the line of the shoulders.

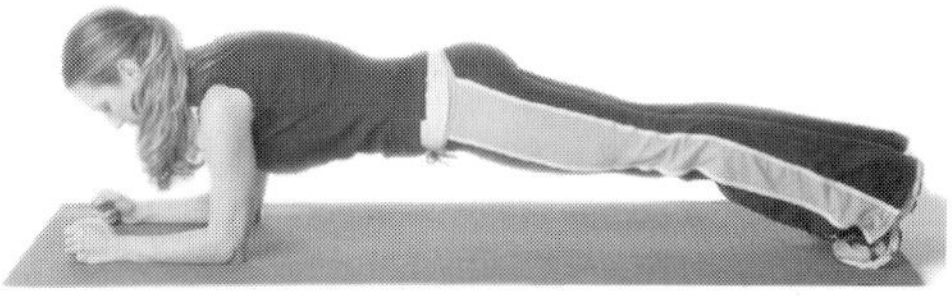

Figure 15-8
Prone plank. The client lies prone with the elbows under the shoulders and the feet flexed for support. He or she then lifts the hips off the ground by engaging the gluteals, hamstrings, and spinal extensor muscles so that the hips are level with the shoulders and knees.

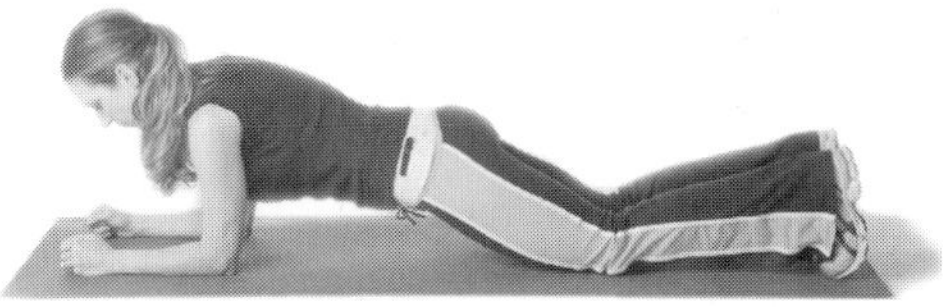

The ACE-AHFS can modify this exercise by having the client put the knees down while keeping the hips level with the shoulders.

standing single-leg balance exercise can identify any hip or pelvic stability problems, as there is increased demand on these muscles during unilateral support tasks. Often, weakness of the spine stabilizers will present itself as a leaning of the hips away from the stance leg, which results

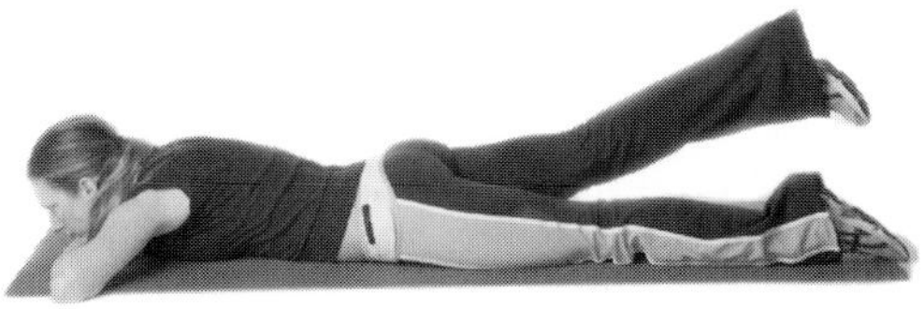

Figure 15-9
Prone hip extension. The client lies in a prone position with the hands under the chin for support and then lifts the leg with the knee straight by engaging the gluteals and hamstrings. The ACE-AHFS should watch for a "roll" of the torso away from the leg being lifted, as this is a sign of dysfunction of the hip extensors and of the pelvic/spine stabilizers.

Figure 15-10
Hip ROM complex

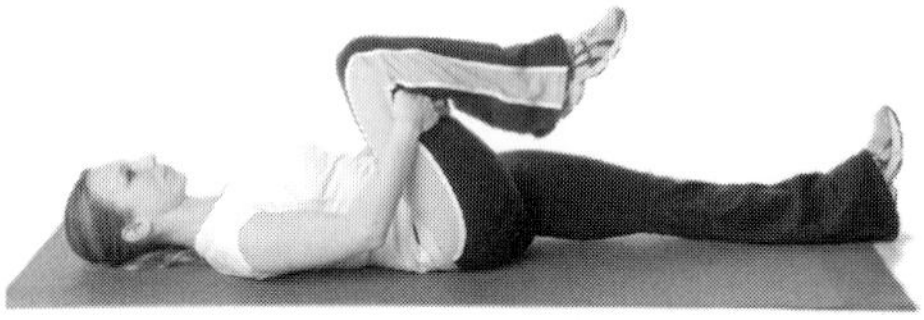

The client lies on his or her back and pulls the knee to the chest to feel the stretch in the gluteals and hamstrings.

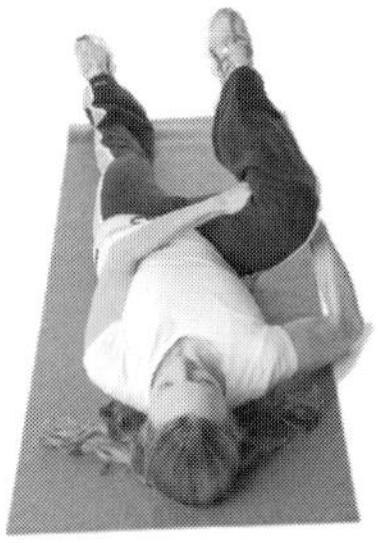

The client pulls the knee to the same-side shoulder, stretching the hips and hamstrings while also targeting the adductors.

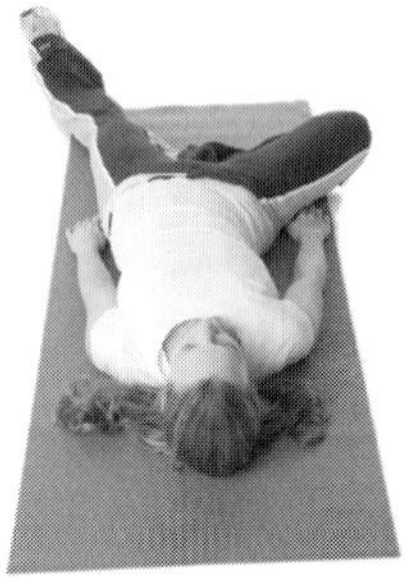

The foot is returned to the center and the knee is dropped to the outside to stretch the adductors. The ACE-AHFS should ensure that the opposite hip is kept stable and does not roll toward the side being stretched.

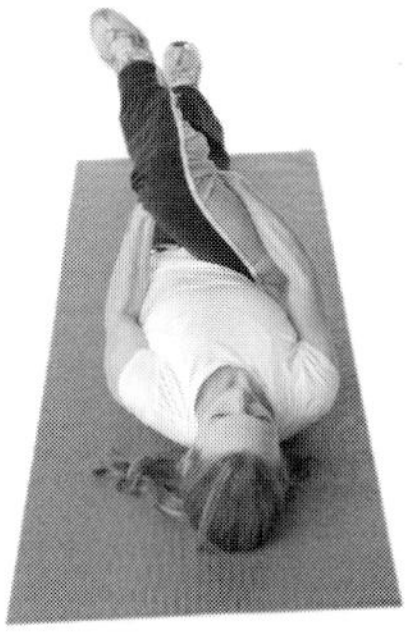

The client then pulls the knee to the opposite-side shoulder, focusing on the hip extensors and abductors.

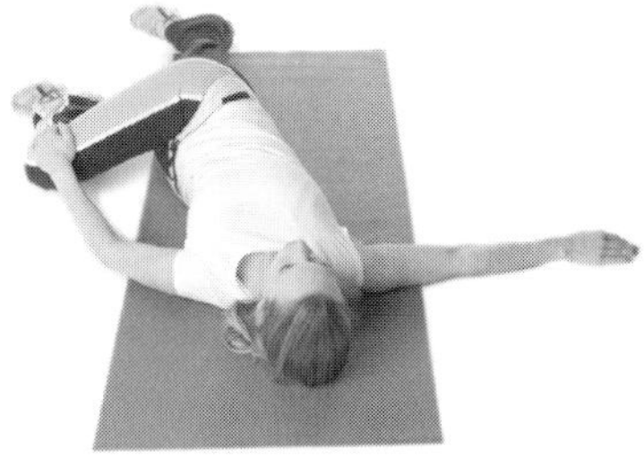

The client pulls the leg across the body, stretching the lower back and hip abductors and extensors. Note that the shoulders are kept down and the arm is extended to the side for support.

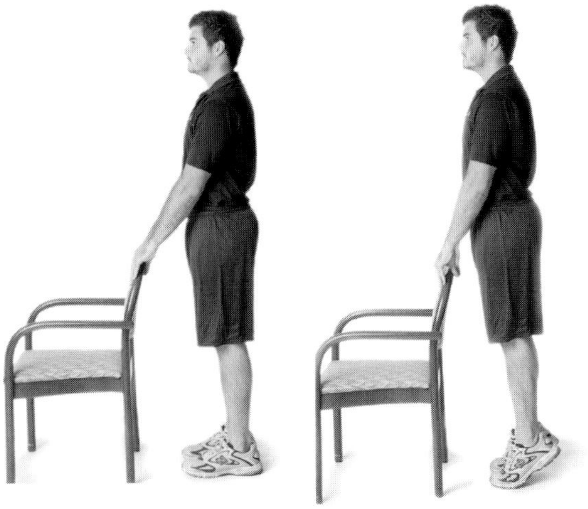

Figure 15-11
Calf raises. Using a chair or other stable object for support, the client rises onto the balls of the feet, coming to full plantarflexion and pausing to fully engage the gastrocnemius. Clients with stronger calves can perform this exercise on one leg at a time.

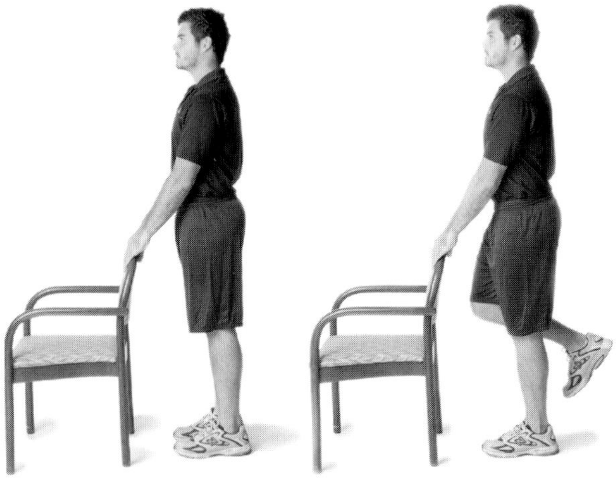

Figure 15-12
Standing single-leg balance. To test the ability of the client to engage the deep spinal stabilizers, obliques, and hip extensors and abductors, the ACE-AHFS can have the client stand facing a table or other stable surface with the feet comfortably under the hips. The client lifts one leg at a time while trying to keep the pelvis level and then holds that position for as long as possible.

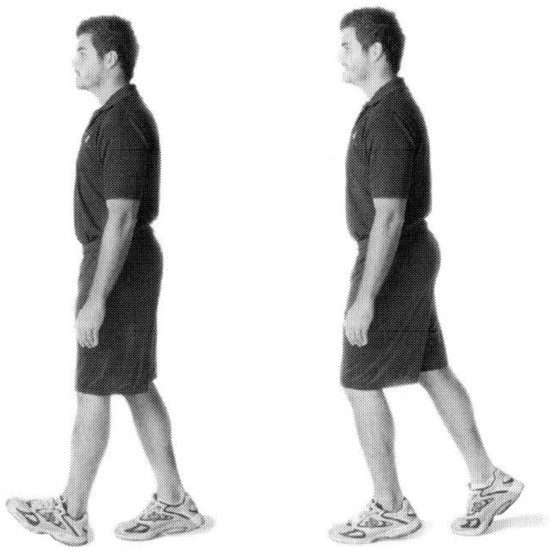

Figure 15-13
Heel and toe walking. To assess any potential neurological difficulties created by osteoarthritis of the spine or hip, the ACE-AHFS can have the client walk on the heels and then on the toes. If the client is unable to walk in these positions, this may be evidence of muscle weakness that is caused by joint pain resulting in dysfunction. It may also be evidence of neurological disorders caused by degeneration of the intervertebral discs or the hip joint that leads to pressure on the nerve, resulting in muscular atrophy. These types of diagnoses should be made formally by a physician, but they can give an ACE-AHFS an indication of whether there is some dysfunction.

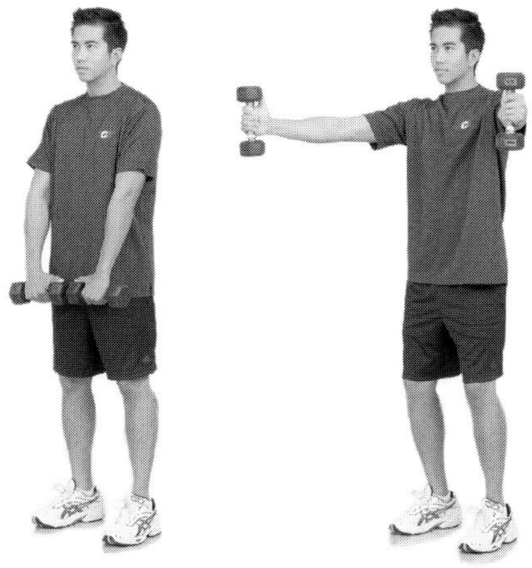

Figure 15-14
Diagonal arm raise. The client holds a dumbbell in each hand slightly below waist level. He or she then abducts the arm from the shoulder, with the arms at approximately 45 degrees in relationship to the torso until the arm reaches shoulder height. The client can then slowly return to the starting position.

in the loss of balance. Also, weakness of the hip abductors will often result in a rotation of the hips. Finally, any neurological troubles stemming from degeneration of the lumbar discs or nerve compression along the sciatic nerve can be identified if the client has difficulty walking on the heels and toes. Also, conditioning the rotator cuff muscles using the diagonal arm raise exercise (Figure 15-14), along with direct internal and external rotation of the humerus using exercise bands, can reduce the loss of shoulder function that may occur with later development of OA in the cervical spine.

Case Study

A 46-year-old male Navy Seal presents with a history of bilateral knee pain that has been increasing in intensity and frequency over the past four years. There is no history of a significant injury or surgery to either knee. At the time of initial evaluation, his daily activities of lifting weights and running in hard-soled boots on asphalt for 2 miles (3.2 km) [was running 6 miles (9.7 km) a day but steadily decreased his distance over time due to increasing knee pain], were losing appeal to him due to the bilateral knee pain, with swimming being his only well-tolerated activity.

The client was well known for more than 20 years for putting 130 pounds in a rucksack and running in the mountains until bilateral knee pain forced him to stop. Although he attempted to keep running the mountains without the weighted rucksack, the pain was a persistent problem. The client had noted **atrophy** of his quadriceps for years and attempted to build them up with knee extension exercises, squats, and lunges, only to experience more knee pain and visible atrophy of his quadriceps. Finally, he committed himself to seek medical attention. Examination revealed a disproportionate 6'3" 230-pound male (1.9 m; 103.5 kg) with an extremely well-developed upper body, while his lower extremities, most notably his quadriceps, showed significant atrophy. He has very little flexibility of the quadriceps, iliotibial band, adductors, hamstrings, and low-back muscles. The initial interview revealed no history of injuries to his knees. The client could walk a quarter-mile

(0.4 km) if necessary, but running is entirely out of the question. He admittedly avoids stairs and anything that requires him to squat.

He is on a permanent limited duty status until his scheduled retirement date from the Navy due to chronic bilateral knee pain. On examination, his vastus medialis obliques (VMO) are found to be flaccid bilaterally. Other than the gross quadriceps atrophy, the remainder of the examination is non-contributory. X-rays reveal multiple **exostosis** of both the tibiofemoral and patellofemoral joints bilaterally compatible with severe osteoarthritis.

In discussion with the client, he has no desire for total knee replacements except as a "last ditch measure." He has been on a plethora of anti-inflammatories over the years with minimal relief from pain. The treatment regimen is based on many changes in his daily lifestyle, with the end goals of decreasing the pain he experienced and regaining the size and the tone of his quadriceps via low-force, pain-free exercises, and enhancing the flexibility of the muscles of the lower extremities and lower back.

- In accordance with recommendations from his attending physician, he can manage the pain initially with Celebrex, 200 mg a day, along with CosaminDS, three tablets three times a day for the first two months. He and his physician have decided to discontinue the use of Celebrex after the initial two months over concerns of potential significant side effects, while continuing the CosaminDS at two tablets three times a day.
- The client should eliminate boots from his daily life and replace them with soft-soled shoes.
- The client should discontinue all running until he is 100% pain free, and then consider resuming a low-intensity, short-duration running program with input from his physician.
- He can use a bicycle with the seat in a high position for transportation around the base and for exercise.
- The client should avoid stairs and any activity that causes knee pain (such as full squats and lunges) due to the increased forces these movements place on the knee, especially during the descent phase.
- The client should perform exercises with an emphasis on developing strength in the quadriceps and external hip rotators. Terminal knee extensions are appropriate as long as the knee is kept within the final 30 degrees of extension. In this exercise, the client should hold the knee in full extension to see and feel the quadriceps and external hip rotators contract for 10 seconds (see Figure 15-2). Squats performed within the 30-degree range of motion with the back against the wall are encouraged. The squats should be held for 10 seconds with an emphasis on an isometric quadriceps contraction. Aquatic exercise, such as floating on the back and kicking in a pool with fins while not allowing the knees to break the surface of the water, is also indicated. Exercising through a pain-free ROM on elliptical and stair climbing machines is acceptable, since both feet are on a surface (i.e., weightbearing) at all times. He should not use a treadmill, as only one foot is on a surface at all times, thereby forcing one leg to accept the entire body weight with each step. The client should be encouraged to participate in yoga classes as frequently as possible.
- The client should undergo a trial of bilateral Bauerfeind Genutrain knee braces to be worn during waking and non-swimming hours.
- He should double the time spent in the pool, with a portion devoted to kicking on his back with fins.
- The client should have a goal of weight reduction via a modification in dietary habits so that the weight will not simply be regained once his goal of 200 pounds (90 kg) is reached.
- The ACE-AHFS should follow up in two weeks for evaluation specifically of the quadriceps and external hip rotators.

The client was very cooperative due to frustration with prolonged and increasing pain. At the two-week follow up, although his pain was significantly reduced, little gain had been made in the size and strength of his quadriceps and external hip rotators, and thus the client was scheduled for physical therapy daily for 30 sessions of quadriceps electrical stimulation for 20 minutes.

Follow-up at four weeks showed improvement in the size and tone of both quadriceps, along with a decrease in pain. Follow up at six weeks showed much improvement in the size and development of the quadriceps, along with decreased discomfort.

Summary

Osteoarthritis is the most common degenerative joint disease and, if left untreated, can reduce the quality of life for an individual. When used in combination with medical interventions, exercise can help maintain function and reduce pain in an affected joint. Exercises that focus on developing the strength and endurance of muscles that surround the joint can reduce mechanical loading and lessen symptoms. Individual selection of progressive exercises that begin with unloaded isometrics and end with full weightbearing exercises can be an effective method for maintaining joint range of motion, strength, and endurance, and reducing joint pain. The ACE-AHFS must take care to not introduce exercises or activities that have high loads or high strain rates, especially if the client is overweight.

References

Arthritis Foundation (2007). *Rheumatoid Arthritis.* http://www.arthritis.org/disease-center.php?disease_id=31.

Bennell, K. & Hinman, R. (2005). Exercise as a treatment for osteoarthritis. *Current Opinion in Rheumatology,* 17, 5, 634–640.

Buckwalter, J.A. & Martin, J.A. (2006). Osteoarthritis. *Advanced Drug Delivery Reviews*, 58, 150–167.

Clegg, D.O. et al. (2006). Glucosamine, chondrointin sulfate, and the two in combination for painful knee osteoarthritis. *New England Journal of Medicine,* 35, 8, 795–808.

Ettinger, W.H. et al. (1997). A randomized trial comparing aerobic exercise and resistance exercise with a health education program in older adults with knee osteoarthritis: The Fitness Arthritis and Seniors Trial (FAST). *Journal of the American Medical Association,* 277, 1, 25–31.

Felson, D.T. et al. (2004). The effect of body weight on progression of knee osteoarthritis is dependent on alignment. *Arthritis and Rheumatism*, 50, 12, 3904–3909.

Fransen, M. et al. (2007). Physical activity for osteoarthritis management: A randomized controlled clinical trial evaluating hydrotherapy or Tai Chi classes. *Arthritis and Rheumatism*. 57, 3, 407–414.

Hedrick, A. (1992). Exercise physiology: Physiological responses to warm-up. *National Strength & Conditioning Association Journal,* 14, 5, 25–27.

Helmick, C.G. et al. (2008). Estimates of the prevalence of arthritis and other rheumatic conditions in the United States. *Arthritis and Rheumatism.* 58, 1, 15–25.

Hinman, R.S., Haywood, S.E., & Day, A.R. (2007). Aquatic physical therapy for hip and knee osteoarthritis: Results of a single-blind randomized controlled trial. *Physical Therapy*, 87, 1, 32–43.

Issa, S.N. & Sharma, L. (2006). Epidemiology of osteoarthritis: An update. *Current Rheumatology Reports,* 8, 1, 7–15.

Lund, H. et al. (2008). A randomized controlled trial of aquatic and land-based exercise in patients with knee osteoarthritis. *Journal of Rehabilitation Medicine*, 40, 2, 137–144.

Mikesky, A.E. et al. (2006). Effects of strength training on the incidence and progression of knee osteoarthritis. *Arthritis and Rheumatism,* 55, 5, 690–699.

Namba, R.S. et al. (2005). Obesity and perioperative morbidity in total hip and total knee arthroplasty patients. *Journal of Arthroplasty,* 20, 7, Suppl. 3, 46–50.

Repo, R.U. & Finlay, J.B. (1977). Survival of articular cartilage after controlled impact. *Journal of Bone & Joint Surgery,* 59, 3, 1068–1076.

Samson, D.J. et al. (2007). *Treatment of Primary and Secondary Osteoarthritis of the Knee.* Rockville, Md.: Agency for Healthcare Research and Quality, U.S. Department of Health and Human Services. Publication No. 07-E012.

van Baar, M.E. et al. (1999). Effectiveness of exercise therapy in patients with osteoarthritis of the hip or knee: A systematic review of randomized clinical trials. *Arthritis and Rheumatism,* 42, 7, 1361–1369.

Wang, T.J. et al. (2007). Effects of aquatic exercise on flexibility, strength and aerobic fitness in adults with osteoarthritis of the hip or knee. *Journal of Advanced Nursing*, 57, 2, 141–152.

Suggested Reading

American College of Sports Medicine (2003). *ACSM's Exercise Management for Persons With Chronic Diseases and Disabilities* (2nd ed.). Champaign, Ill.: Human Kinetics.

Arthritis Foundation (1999). *PACE: People with Arthritis Can Exercise: Instructor's Manual.* Atlanta: Arthritis Foundation.

Ettinger, W.H. et al. (1997). A randomized trial comparing aerobic exercise and resistance exercise with a health education program in older adults with knee osteoarthritis: The Fitness Arthritis and Seniors Trial (FAST). *Journal of the American Medical Association,* 277, 1, 25–31.

Helmick, C.G. et al. (2008). Estimates of the prevalence of arthritis and other rheumatic conditions in the United States. *Arthritis & Rheumatism,* 58, 1, 15–25.

van Baar, M.E. et al. (1999). Effectiveness of exercise therapy in patients with osteoarthritis of the hip or knee: A systematic review of randomized clinical trials. *Arthritis and Rheumatism,* 42, 7, 1361–1369.

In This Chapter

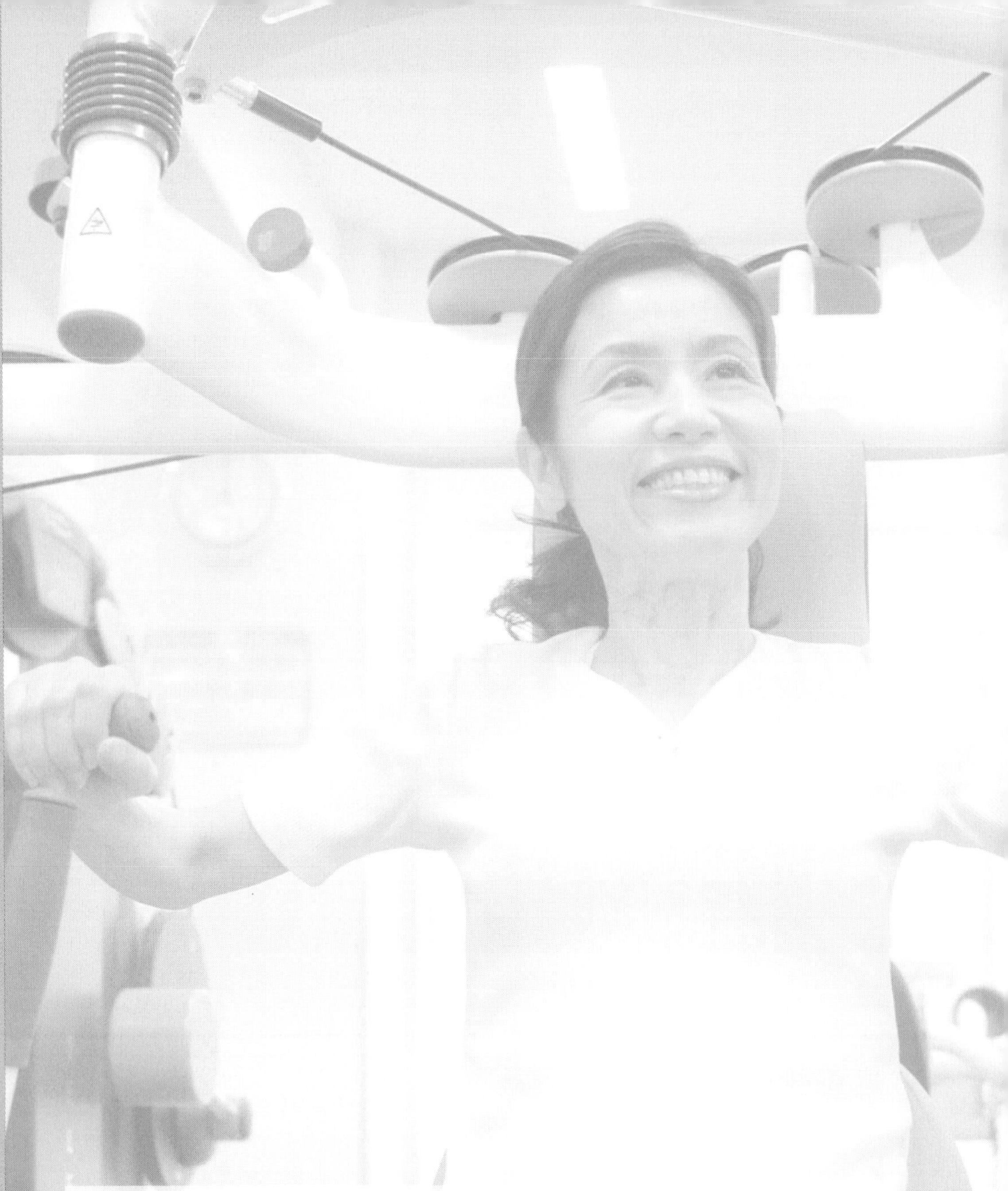

About The Author

Kara A. Witzke, Ph.D., is an associate professor and chair of the Department of Kinesiology at California State University, San Marcos in San Diego County. She has worked in industry and various wellness venues around the country and has promoted wellness and lifestyle management to children and adults of all ages through education, research, and community involvement. Dr. Witzke serves as a subject matter expert for the ACE certification and exam-development department and is an ACE media spokesperson. Her current research focuses on the effects of both diabetes and exercise on bone health.

CHAPTER 16

Osteoporosis and Osteopenia

Kara A. Witzke

Osteoporosis is defined conceptually as a condition of generalized skeletal fragility (very low bone mass) that increases the risk of fracture with minimal trauma. **Osteopenia** refers to reduced skeletal mass (low bone mass) that, while not as severe as osteoporosis, may still warrant close monitoring to ensure that the condition does not worsen.

Epidemiology of Osteoporosis and Fractures

Osteoporosis is the most prevalent disease affecting the skeleton. It is characterized by low bone mass and deterioration of the microarchitecture of the bone, resulting in structural weakness and an increased risk for fracture. It is one of the most important public health issues in America because of its prevalence. It is estimated that more than 50% of all women and 20% of all men over the age of 50 will suffer an osteoporotic fracture at some time in their lives (U.S. Department of Health and Human Services, 2004). One in six women will experience a hip fracture, the most devastating type of osteoporotic fracture, compared with only a one-in-nine risk of developing breast cancer (van Staa et al., 2001).

Osteoporotic fractures are most common in the proximal femur (hip), vertebrae (spine), and distal forearm (wrist). However, osteoporosis is really a systemic disease, and individuals with low bone mass are at an increased risk of all types of fractures. Adults who fracture are 50 to 100% more likely to fracture again in a different location (Wu et al., 2002). Hip fractures are by far the most devastating type of fracture due to their strong association with low bone mass, the cost to repair, and the level of disability that often accompanies them even post-surgery. Hip fracture incidence rates increase exponentially with age in both men and women, due to both age-related declines in bone density (a surrogate measure for bone fragility) and an increase in falls, which are responsible for more than 90% of all hip fractures.

In 1990, it was estimated that 1.7 million people worldwide suffered a hip fracture, with annual direct and indirect costs associated with these fractures exceeding $131.5 billion. In the United States alone, these hip fractures imposed costs of more than $20 billion, and these numbers are expected to rise. It is estimated that the number of worldwide hip fractures alone may exceed 6.3 million by the year 2050 (Cummings & Melton, 2002). In addition, an estimated 33.6 million Americans (80% of them women), have osteopenia, a condition of low, but not very low, bone mass. The usefulness of labeling such individuals, whose **bone mineral density (BMD)** may actually be within a "normal" range, has been questioned, but osteopenia can be viewed not unlike **prehypertension,** impaired fasting glucose, and borderline high cholesterol in defining an intermediate-risk group with somewhat uncertain boundaries. Although fracture risk is still greater in individuals with osteoporosis rather than osteopenia, the much larger number of persons with osteopenia means that this group represents a substantial portion of the population at risk for fracture (Khosla & Melton, 2007).

Because women live longer and experience more age-related bone loss and falls than men, their incidence of hip fracture is also about two to three times that seen in men (Cummings & Melton, 2002). Age-adjusted rates of hip fracture are highest in Scandinavian and North American populations, and seven times lower in southern European countries and in Asian or African populations (Melton & Cooper, 2001). It should be noted that although Asian populations are at an increased risk for osteoporosis, they suffer relatively few fractures, probably due to decreased rates of falling.

The epidemiology of vertebral fractures is different than that of hip fractures. While only about one-third of all vertebral fractures identified by x-ray come to a specialist's attention, less than 10% result in hospital admissions. These fractures do cause pain, disability, and increased **kyphosis** of the upper spine. Most vertebral fractures do not result from falls, but rather from routine activities such as bending or lifting light objects (Cooper et al., 1992).

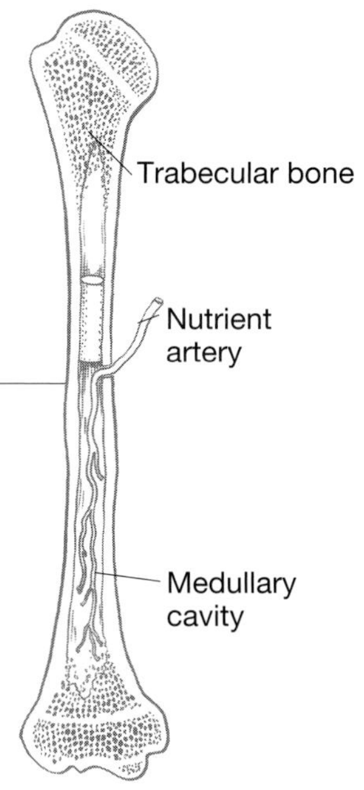

Figure 16-1
Trabecular and cortical bone

Organization of Bone

Bone is a unique tissue with enormous responsibilities. The simple task of supporting loads imposed on it requires that bone have incredible strength and resilience, while also being lightweight and adaptable so that locomotion is not a metabolic burden. Bone consists of an organic component (20 to 25% by weight), an inorganic component (70 to 75% by weight), and a water component (5% by weight). The organic component is primarily composed of type I collagen and some bone cells, while the inorganic component is almost all mineral (crystalline calcium hydroxyapatite).

The human skeleton is composed of two types of bone: cortical (compact) and trabecular (spongy). An important difference between **cortical** and **trabecular bone** is in the way the bone matrix and cellular components are arranged. Calcium comprises 80 to 90% of cortical bone volume, but only 15 to 25% of trabecular bone volume. Cortical bone forms a dense shell around all bones and constitutes the thick shafts of long bones, while trabecular bone is found in the vertebrae and in the ends of long bones (Figure 16-1). Trabecular bone forms a lattice-like network, which greatly increases its surface area for metabolic activity. As a result, trabecular bone undergoes far more remodeling cycles during an individual's lifetime than does cortical bone (Marcus, 1987). A remodeling cycle consists of a bone **resorption** (removal) stage that is followed by a period of new bone formation. Through this coupled process, bone is constantly renewed.

During growth and young adulthood, the rate of bone formation is faster than the rate of bone resorption, leading to an overall gain in bone mineral. This is called **bone modeling.** Modeling improves bone strength not only by adding mass, but also by expanding the inner and outer diameters of bone. This allows bone to adapt its shape according to the loads imposed, which maximizes its strength and resistance to fracture. **Bone remodeling,** on the other hand, is a locally coordinated activity of **osteoclasts** (bone resorption cells) and **osteoblasts** (bone formation cells), whereby bone can both prevent and repair damage caused by everyday loading. A key feature of remodeling is that it replaces damaged tissue with an equal amount of new bone tissue.

In the aging and osteoporotic skeleton, however, the balance between the amount of bone being resorbed and the amount begin formed is unequal, favoring bone resorption. This causes a net loss of bone that eventually causes bone strength and integrity to be compromised (Figure 16-2).

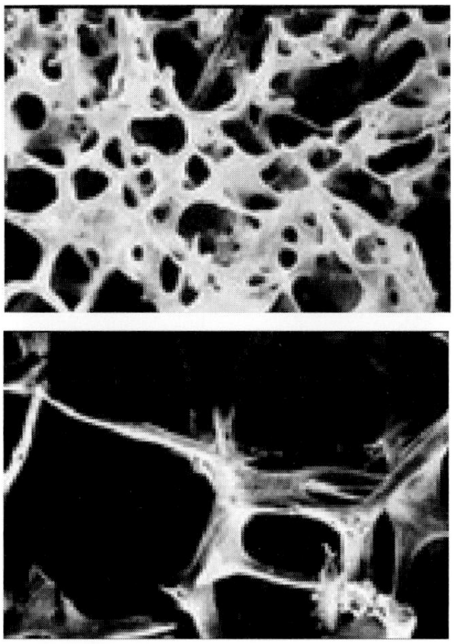

Figure 16-2
Normal versus osteoporotic trabecular bone

Source: Images courtesy of GE Healthcare.

Questions	Yes	No
Do you have a small, thin frame and/or are you Caucasian or Asian?		
Have you or a member of your immediate family broken a bone as an adult?		
Are you a postmenopausal woman?		
Have you had an early or surgically induced menopause?		
Have you taken high doses of thyroid medication or used glucocorticoids ≥5 mg a day (e.g., prednisone) for three or more months?		
Have you taken, or are you taking, immunosuppressive medications or chemotherapy to treat cancer?		
Is your diet low in dairy products and other sources of calcium?		
Are you physically inactive?		
Do you smoke cigarettes or drink alcohol in excess?		

Note: The more times an individual answers "yes," the greater the risk for developing osteoporosis.

Figure 16-3
Osteoporosis risk assessment questionnaire

Source: Reprinted with permission from *Osteoporosis: Can It Happen to You?* (2008). National Osteoporosis Foundation, Washington, DC, 20037. All rights reserved.

Factors That Affect Bone

While the effects of physical activity on bone are undeniable, these positive effects only account for approximately 10% of bone mineral in the population as a whole. The remaining 90% of bone mineral is accounted for by a combination of other factors such as genetics, gender, age, race, hormones, lifestyle factors (e.g., smoking, alcohol, caffeine), nutrition, medication, and soft-tissue composition (i.e., lean and fat mass). These factors interact with each other and their degree of influence varies based on the stage of life and the skeletal site. Figure 16-3 provides a osteoporosis risk assessment questionnaire.

Age, Sex, Genetics, and Race

Bone mineral is accrued at various rates throughout early childhood and adolescence, and then diminishes with aging. This normal, age-related process causes a net loss of approximately 5 to 10% of bone mineral per decade and begins some time after the cessation of longitudinal growth and the achievement of peak bone mass (in the third decade) (Snow-Harter & Marcus, 1991). Bone resorption in women is especially rapid during the first five years following menopause (if pharmacotherapy is not implemented), and may cause a loss of 3 to 5% of overall bone mass per year. These age-related bone mineral decrements are not as pronounced in men, primarily because men reach a higher peak BMD, have larger bones that afford a biomechanical resistance to fracture, and do not experience the same rapid postmenopausal bone loss as women. For individuals diagnosed with osteoporosis, it is often impossible to expect to build back significant amounts of bone mineral.

BMD appears to be controlled by a combination of several genes, which may also display important interactive effects with environmental factors (such as physical activity and calcium intake). Nevertheless, familial studies have shown that BMD is strongly influenced by parental bone mass (McKay et al., 1994; Tylavsky et al., 1989), and these assumptions are supported by research that shows very little variation between identical twins (Krall & Dawson-Hughes, 1993). Although various genes [such as those encoding the vitamin-D receptor, collagen Ia1, LDL receptor-related protein 5 (LRP5), and estrogen receptor] have some relation to BMD, attempts to relate them to fracture risk have generally been unsuccessful (Sambrook & Cooper, 2006).

Race implies similar genetic characteristics in a population, perhaps even among individuals in a similar environment, that interact with genes to cause the expression of a particular trait. Studies have confirmed that compared with whites, black adults have higher BMD at both the hip and spine and an increased cortical thickness. Lower fracture rates at both the hip and spine have also been reported in many studies (Aloia et al., 1996; Griffin et al., 1992). Although rates of bone loss appear similar for black and white individuals, it is estimated that African-American women have a 50% lower risk of fracture than Caucasian women (Bohannon, 1999). Similar lower fracture rates have also been shown for Hispanic and Asian populations (Maggi et al., 1991).

Hormones

The endocrine system is highly involved in the regulation of the biologic processes that control bone. The hormones involved in these processes belong to one of two classes, either "controlling" or "influencing" serum calcium levels and the levels of other agents related to bone. Controlling hormones include **parathyroid hormone (PTH),** vitamin D, and **calcitonin.** These hormones induce responses based on plasma concentrations of calcium. Influencing hormones, such as **estrogen, progesterone, testosterone, growth hormone, insulin-like growth factor I (IGF-I), corticosteroids,** and **thyroid hormone,** also modify calcium metabolism, but in response to other factors besides plasma calcium concentrations.

Estrogen has both direct and indirect effects on bone. Directly, estrogen decreases bone remodeling (turnover) through a complex interaction with the estrogen receptor on osteoblasts and by inhibiting other hormones that would normally stimulate osteoclast production. In this way, estrogen maintains bone mass by limiting resorption. Estrogen may also exhibit indirect effects on bone through the parathyroid gland, gut, and kidneys. Specifically, estrogen may lower the sensitivity of PTH to serum calcium levels that would promote mineralization by reducing bone turnover. It may also increase reabsorption of calcium via the kidneys by stimulating vitamin D and calcitonin production, which would also limit bone turnover.

Evidence has been presented about the influence of oral contraceptives on bone mass. In a systematic review of 86 studies published between 1966 and August 2005 that reported on fracture or BMD outcomes by use of combined hormonal contraceptives, researchers report that studies of adolescent and young adult women generally found lower BMD among users of combined oral contraceptives than among non-users. Evidence for premenopausal adult women suggested no differences in BMD between oral contraceptive users and non-users, and use in perimenopausal and postmenopausal women generally preserved bone mass, while non-users lost BMD (Martins, Curtis, & Glasier, 2006). Oral contraceptive pills are often prescribed to female athletes for treatment of menstrual irregularities, but it is still fairly unclear whether BMD improves in these women. It seems as though estrogen-containing pills are more beneficial (or less harmful) to bone in premenopausal women than progesterone-only derivations such as depot medroxyprogesterone acetate (Depo Provera®) (Curtis & Martins, 2006).

During the third trimester of pregnancy, estrogen levels are high, but during lactation, mothers become hypoestrogenic as prolactin becomes a dominant hormone. Maternal bone lost as a result of breastfeeding seems to be recoverable upon weaning (Eisman, 1998). However, in women with low bone mass prior to pregnancy, additional calcium supplementation during pregnancy and lactation is warranted (Funk, Shoback, & Genant, 1995).

Lifestyle Factors

Lifestyle factors such as smoking and alcohol consumption may adversely affect bone. Smoking seems to have a detrimental effect on both pre- and postmenopausal bone density via an increase bone resorption and decreased calcium absorption (Tudor-Locke & McColl, 2000).

Excessive alcohol consumption also appears to exert a direct toxic effect on bone. While studies consistently show bone irregularities in alcoholics, moderate alcohol consumption may be associated with a slight increase in bone via increases in **estradiol** concentrations. It does not appear that moderate alcohol consumption is deleterious to bone density, but women should always be cautioned against the potential effects of an alcoholic lifestyle on bone (Tudor-Locke & McColl, 2000).

Caffeine increases urinary excretion of calcium for at least three hours after ingestion and has been associated with changes in bone remodeling (Massey & Whiting, 1993). It does appear that calcium balance decreases with every cup of coffee ingested, but that these effects are offset by calcium intake. Carbonated cola beverages, on the other hand, do not appear to adversely affect short-term calcium balance, although more studies are needed in this area, since it is possible that the phosphorus contained in these beverages may adversely affect bone (Calvo & Park, 1996; Smith et al., 1989).

The effects on bone of positive lifestyle factors such as exercise are discussed later in the chapter.

Nutrition

Dietary calcium provides the essential building blocks for bone formation. Calcium also plays an important role in muscle contraction and intra- and extracellular ion **homeostasis.** Without an adequate daily intake, calcium is withdrawn from the bones to maintain normal blood levels (9 to 11 mg/dL). Adequate calcium intake is especially important during growth, when the skeleton is still forming and prior to the fourth decade of life when peak bone mass may still be influenced (Recker et al., 1992).

Availability of calcium for absorption is a result of many factors. Calcium from dairy products is highly absorbable, whereas some plant forms are less so. Large intakes of dietary **fiber** can interfere with calcium absorption and dietary protein and sodium intake can increase excretion of calcium. If vitamin D levels are insufficient, parathyroid hormone secretion is increased, which increases activity of the bone resorbing osteoclasts. The **Dietary Reference Intake (DRI)** for both calcium and vitamin D are reported in Table 16-1. Dietitians recommend food as the primary source of calcium and vitamin D. Dairy products and fortified foods such as bread, cereals, and orange juice are good sources of both nutrients. Table 16-2 lists some of the most common dietary sources of calcium.

Table 16-1
Dietary Reference Intakes (DRI) for Calcium and Vitamin D Across the Lifespan

Age (males and females)	Calcium (mg/day)	Vitamin D (IU/day)
1–3	500	200
4–8	800	200
9–18	1300	200
19–50	1000	200
51–70	1200	400
71 and over	1200	600

Source: American Dietetic Association (2006). *Nutrition Fact Sheet: Calcium and Vitamin D: Essential Nutrients for Bone Health.* Chicago: American Dietetic Association.

Table 16-2
Common Sources of Dietary Calcium and Vitamin D

Foods and Beverages	Calcium (mg)	Vitamin D (IU)
Milk, low-fat or non-fat, 1 cup	301	98
Calcium- and vitamin D–fortified orange juice, 1 cup	350	100
Fruit yogurt, low-fat, 1 cup	372	100
Cheddar cheese, low-fat, 2 oz.	236	*
Salmon, pink, canned with soft bones, 3 oz.	208	530

*Not a significant source of the nutrient indicated.

Note: Sunlight causes the skin to make Vitamin D and, for most people, 15 minutes of sunlight several days a week (with the hands and face exposed) is enough.

Source: American Dietetic Association (2006). *Nutrition Fact Sheet: Calcium and Vitamin D: Essential Nutrients for Bone Health.* Chicago: American Dietetic Association.

While dietary sources of calcium are the most bioavailable forms in the body, supplements may provide a primary source of these nutrients in individuals who are unable to achieve adequate dietary intakes. Supplements should be evaluated on the basis of their elemental calcium content (usually between 200 and 600 mg per tablet or chew), and not on the overall milligrams of calcium compounds, such as calcium carbonate or calcium citrate. Calcium carbonate supplements (e.g., Tums®, Viactiv®) may be less expensive and are best taken with food, which promotes an acidic environment in the gastrointestinal tract that aids calcium absorption. Calcium citrate or calcium citrate malate supplements (e.g., Citracal®), while sometimes more expensive, do not cause constipation, a side effect experienced by some individuals using calcium carbonate supplements. Many of these forms also contain vitamin D, which aids in the intestinal absorption of calcium.

Although it is widely accepted that dietary intake of calcium is related, at least in part, to optimal bone health, an association between calcium intake and BMD and fracture is not necessarily so straightforward. Part of the complexity lies in the fact that not all calcium ingested passes directly into the bone reservoir. Calcium retention efficiency in children peaks at about 30% for girls and 36% for boys. Retention rates are inversely related to intake, however, so that when intakes are low, retention rates are relatively higher to compensate for the reduced amount of mineral coming into the body. In randomized controlled trials that show increased bone mineral accrual in children supplementing with calcium, benefits achieved are soon lost when supplementation is withdrawn (Lee et al., 1996). Thus, bone changes following supplementation in children may be transient.

During the pre- and postmenopausal years in women, and throughout men's lives, dietary calcium may have a smaller influence on BMD than genetic and other environmental factors. Part of the problem in interpreting the research in this area is in the difficulty of measurement of lifetime dietary intake and the confounding effects of other nutrients. It is reasonably clear, however, that dietary calcium supplementation has a greater positive effect on BMD than no treatment (postmenopausally), but it probably has less of an effect on bone than either hormone replacement therapy or pharmacological interventions (Khan et al., 2001).

Special Considerations

The Female Athlete Triad

The term "female athlete triad" describes a condition consisting of a combination of disordered eating, menstrual irregularities, and decreased bone mass in athletic women. This combination of factors may increase a woman's risk of osteoporosis and premature fracture. The pattern of the triad is more typical in athletes who believe that they will receive a performance advantage by having lower body weight (e.g., gymnasts, dancers). Dieting behavior usually becomes very restrictive and the pathogenic weight-control behaviors predispose a woman to menstrual dysfunction and eventually compromised bone mass. In this way, the triad disorders are interrelated and the existence of one component is linked, directly or indirectly, to the others (Beals & Meyer, 2007).

The mechanism of bone loss in athletic women with menstrual disturbances has been debated and the original position stand published in 1997 by the American College of Sports Medicine (ACSM) has been revised. ACSM's October 2007 position stand reflects newer evidence that estrogen deficiency is probably not the primary mechanism of bone loss in these athletes, but rather a combination of low estrogen and, more importantly, chronic undernutrition that reduces the rate of bone formation (Nattiv et al., 2007). A well-designed study by Zanker and Swaine (1998) evaluated biochemical markers of bone turnover in active women. Their work showed that women distance runners with long-term amenorrhea have reduced bone formation, compared to eumenorrheic runners and sedentary age-matched eumenorrheic women. Low BMD appears to be much less responsive to estrogen therapy in premenopausal amenorrheic women. This work helps explain why treatment with estrogen in amenorrheic women has not led to the same gains in bone mass as it has with postmenopausal women.

Screening for the triad requires an understanding of the relationships among the three components. Athletes who present with one of the components of the triad should always be evaluated for the others. If an ACE-certified Advanced Health & Fitness Specialist (ACE-AHFS) suspects that a client may have an eating disorder (or restrictive/purging behaviors) and/or menstrual dysfunction, the client should be referred to the appropriate healthcare provider for follow-up.

Menopause

Menopause marks a time of dramatic change in reproductive hormone secretion in women, characterized by estrogen and progesterone deficiency that causes menstrual cycles to cease. The average onset of natural menopause is about 45 to 50 years of age. Clinically, menopause is retrospectively diagnosed when a woman has not had a menstrual period for one year. Changes and symptoms, which usually start several years earlier, as marked by the "perimenopausal" period, include:

- A change in periods—shorter or longer, lighter or heavier, with more or less time in between
- Hot flashes and/or night sweats
- Trouble sleeping
- Vaginal dryness
- Mood swings
- Trouble focusing
- Less hair on the head and more on the face

The early phase of postmenopausal estrogen and progesterone withdrawal that occurs during the first three to five years after menopause is characterized by rapid bone loss (up to 3 to 5% of total bone mass per year), increased circulating plasma levels of calcium, and increased renal calcium excretion (Borer, 2005). Estrogen replacement therapy is most effective at reducing bone loss during this early menopausal period, while calcium supplementation is less effective. After the first five years following menopause, the rate of bone loss decreases back to premenopausal rates of loss (about 1% of total bone mass per year).

Clinical Criteria and Diagnostic Testing

The operational definitions of osteoporosis and osteopenia relate to BMD scores, which are usually measured by **dual-energy x-ray absorptiometry (DEXA)** (Table 16-3).

The National Osteoporosis Foundation guidelines indicate that BMD testing should be performed on:

- All women aged 65 and older regardless of risk factors
- Younger postmenopausal women with one or more risk factors (other than being white, postmenopausal, and female)
- Postmenopausal women who present with fractures (to confirm the diagnosis and determine disease severity).

Note: Medicare covers BMD testing for the following individuals aged 65 and older:

- Estrogen-deficient women at clinical risk for osteoporosis
- Individuals with vertebral abnormalities
- Individuals receiving, or planning to receive, long-term **glucocorticoid** (steroid) therapy
- Individuals with primary **hyperparathyroidism**
- Individuals being monitored to assess the response or efficacy of an approved osteoporosis drug therapy

Medicare permits individuals to repeat BMD testing every two years.

Table 16-3
Diagnostic Categories of Bone Mineral Density

Diagnostic Category	Criterion
Normal	A value for BMD or BMC that is within 1.0 SD of the reference mean for young adults
Low bone mass (osteopenia)	A value for BMD or BMC that is more than 1.0 but less than 2.5 SD below the mean for young adults
Osteoporosis	A value for BMD or BMC that is 2.5 SD or more below the mean for young adults.
Severe osteoporosis (established osteoporosis)	A value for BMD or BMC that is 2.5 SD or more below the mean for young adults in combination with one or more fragility (low-trauma) fractures.

Note: BMD = Bone mineral density; BMC = Bone mineral content; SD = Standard deviation

Source: World Health Organization

Scientists and researchers are interested in the measurement of bone's shape and size (anatomy), strength (biomechanics), and metabolic activity (biochemistry), and the development and adaptation capabilities of bone. Clinicians see bone a little differently, because they view bone as tissue that provides structure and permits the body to move. They generally are interested in preserving or reestablishing those functions and in predicting fracture risk. In this case, bone imaging *in vivo* provides the most important information about bone. The most commonly used methods for imaging bone for clinical purposes include DEXA, **quantitative ultrasound (QUS)**, and **quantitative computed tomography (QCT).**

DEXA is probably the most widely used method of clinical evaluation of BMD and risk for fracture. DEXA uses a low-dose x-ray that emits photons at two different energy levels. BMD is calculated based on the amount of photon energy attenuated (absorbed) by the different body tissues (bone, muscle, and fat). Bone attenuates the most energy, followed by muscle and then fat, based on their relative tissue densities. In this way, DEXA can not only measure bone density, but also **body composition,** and is arguably the new "gold standard" against which other techniques are compared. Regional sites such as the lumbar spine, proximal femur (hip), and distal wrist are the most commonly measured sites for assessment of fracture risk. BMD is reported in units equal to bone mineral content divided by the area of the region of interest (g/cm^2). In this way, BMD is not a true "volumetric" density, but rather an "areal" density. The advantages of DEXA, when compared to other methods, includes its ease of measurement (five to 10 minutes), low radiation exposure (about equal to the amount received flying across the country), high accuracy and precision, and the ability to measure small changes in BMD over time. Disadvantages of DEXA include the fact that it provides no measure of bone architecture, because it does not distinguish between trabecular and cortical bone. It is therefore difficult to determine material properties of bone, including bone strength, using DEXA.

QUS is another popular method of determining bone status, especially as a "field test" due to its portability and the fact that no ionizing radiation is used. Two ultrasound transducers are positioned on each side of the tissue to be measured (commonly the heel). QUS does not measure bone density, but rather speed of sound (SOS) and broadband ultrasound attenuation (BUA). SOS is expressed as the quotient of the time taken to pass through the bone and the dimension that it passed through (expressed in m/s). Exactly what QUS measures is still a bit of a puzzle, but it is thought that the parameters measured relate to bone density and bone microarchitecture, including trabecular number, connectivity, and orientation. Prospective studies have shown that calcaneal QUS measurement can predict fracture risk in postmenopausal women (Huang et al., 1998; Thompson et al., 1998), and it could be argued that QUS measures characteristics of bone strength that are potentially independent of bone density.

QCT provides two advantages over DEXA in that it can provide a three-dimensional measure (true volumetric density; mg/cm^3) of trabecular and cortical bone. For this reason, it can also be used to study the anatomical structure of trabeculae, which makes it quite attractive for researchers in particular, though it is also useful for clinicians to monitor age-related bone loss and to follow patients with osteoporosis or other metabolic bone diseases. However, this technology has several disadvantages, including poor precision and accuracy and radiation doses 125 times higher than a standard regional DEXA scan. It is also limited to peripheral regions and the lumbar spine, so it not useful for determining qualities of bone at the hip. Newer peripheral quantitative computed tomography (pQCT) units that are typically used in research to measure bone in the tibia/fibula region have improved precision and accuracy, but still expose the patient to higher radiation doses than DEXA and cannot be used at clinically relevant fracture sites such as the hip and spine.

Treatment of Osteoporosis and Osteopenia

Since most fractures occur as a result of falls, reduction in the risk for falls is an important goal of clinicians, as well as the ACE-AHFS. Strategies to reduce fracture risk should emphasize lifestyle modifications such as optimal nutrition, smoking cessation, moderate alcohol and caffeine intake, and exercise that provides adequate bone loading. Emphasis should also be placed on reducing the risk of falls, including improving home safety by reducing tripping hazards; maintaining eyesight through regular vision check-ups and updates for prescription lenses; and improving muscle strength, power, and balance. Hip protector pads are sometimes used to help dissipate the forces sustained in a fall, although compliance in wearing the hip pads is an issue. On a mechanistic level, drugs can be used to help reduce bone resorption or increase bone formation, and, although they do nothing to mediate fall risk, they could help prevent a fracture in the case of a fall.

Non-pharmacological Treatments

An optimal diet to improve the prevention and management of osteoporosis includes adequate caloric intake (to avoid malnutrition), and adequate calcium and vitamin D intake. Adults should follow the American Dietetic Association's (ADA) DRI guidelines for dietary calcium that generally recommend calcium intakes between 1000 and 1200 mg/day and vitamin D intakes of 200 to 600 IU (see Table 16-1). Many women diagnosed with osteoporosis take some form of calcium and vitamin D supplement. A meta-analysis of studies using vitamin D to reduce fracture risk concluded that vitamin D reduced the risk of hip fracture by 26% and non-vertebral fracture by 23% in those individuals with vitamin D deficiency (Bischo-Ferrari et al., 2005). There is some controversy regarding whether the appropriate level of serum vitamin D needed for bone health is 50 or 80 nmol/L, but in those with serum levels lower than 50 nmol/L, doses higher than 1000 IU vitamin D per day could be needed to reach serum levels of 80 nmol/L (Sambrook & Cooper, 2006). Regardless, the ACE-AHFS should always refer clients to a registered dietitian or physician for recommendations regarding vitamin supplementation.

Pharmacological Treatments

Most of the drugs with current Federal Drug Administration (FDA) approval for the management of postmenopausal osteoporosis are called "antiresorptives." These include estrogens, calcitonin, bisphosphonates, selective estrogen receptor modulators (SERMs), and others, including isoflavones and parathyroid hormone (Table 16-4).

After the publication of the Women's Health Initiative study in 2002 (Rossouw et al., 2002), the role of long-term postmenopausal hormone therapy (both estrogen alone and estrogen and progesterone in combination) for the prevention and management of osteoporosis became controversial. The study population consisted of women 50 to 79 years old, many of whom had cardiovascular risk factors. Women were not specifically selected for low bone mass, as is the case in most osteoporosis trials. While both trials did find substantial reductions in subsequent osteoporotic fractures, controversy arose when the results showed an elevated risk for stroke and cardiovascular events with combined hormone therapy, especially if women over the age of 70 began treatment. Although the data suggest a different risk profile for combination therapy versus estrogen alone, the results support the recommendation that hormone therapy should be avoided in favor of alternative antiresorptive agents, and that hormone therapy should remain an option only for short-term early use around menopause in symptomatic women at risk for fracture (Sambrook & Cooper, 2006).

It is worth noting that isoflavones, plant-derived compounds with a chemical structure similar to estrogen (e.g., soy), also have physiological effects similar to estrogen. Women interested in using isoflavones in lieu of estrogen for hormone replacement therapy should be referred to their healthcare providers. Like estrogen, isoflavones exert an acute vasodilatory action and may alter physiological responses to exercise, although studies confirming this effect used larger doses of isoflavones than is commonly used in estrogen replacement therapy (Rosano et al., 1993).

Table 16-4
Antiresorptive Medications Used to Prevent Bone Loss

Drug class	Name of Drug	Brand Name
Estrogens	Estrone sulfate	Ogen®
	Conjugated estrogen	Premarin
	Transdermal estrogen	Estraderm®
	Estropipate	Ortho-Est®
	Esterified estrogen	Estratab®
	Conjugated estrogen + medroxyprogertone acetate	Premphase® Prempro®
Calcitonin	Synthetic salmon calcitonin	MiaCalcin® Calcimar®
Bisphosphonates	Alendronate	Fosamax®
	Risedronate	Actonel®
	Etidronate	Didronel®
	Ibandronate	Boniva®
	Zolendronate	Zometa® Reclast®
	Tiludronate	Skelid®
	Pamidronate	Aredia®
SERMs	Raloxifene	Evista®
	Tamoxifene	Nolvadex®
	Droloxifene (in phase III trial)	
	Levormeloxifene (in phase III trial)	
	Arzoxifene (in phase III trial)	
	Lasofoxifene (in phase III trial)	
Others	Stronitium ranelate (in phase III trial)	Protelos® (in Europe)
	Isoflavones (plant-derived)	
	Tibolone or Ipriflavone (synthetic)	Livial®
	Calcitriol	Rocaltrol®
	Sodium fluoride	
	Parathyroid hormone	Forteo®

Calcitonin is a hormone that inhibits osteoclastic activity, thus reducing bone resorption. Calcitonin derived from human, pig, salmon, and eel have all been used in studies of osteoporosis and have shown effectiveness in both increasing low bone mass and decreasing fracture risk in postmenopausal women (Iwamoto et al., 2002). Side effects may include headaches and flushing. Calcitonin is commonly administered via nasal spray in 200 IU dosages.

Bisphosphonates, another class of antiresorptives, arguably represent one of the most significant advances in the treatment of osteoporosis since the mid-1990s. Oral bisphosphonates are generally well tolerated, although they may cause gastrointestinal intolerance in some individuals. It is very important that clients remain upright for at least 30 minutes following oral dosing to avoid esophageal discomfort. This class of drugs has been shown to reduce the risk of vertebral fractures by 40 to 50% and non-vertebral fractures (including hip fractures) by 20 to 40% (Guyatt et al., 2002). They function by inhibiting the action of osteoclasts (formation remains the same), thereby slowing bone resorption. Despite their impressive potential to reduce fractures, new studies are questioning their safety. These drugs remain in the skeleton for decades, and bone turnover can be affected for up to five years after the drugs are discontinued. Since the natural purpose of bone remodeling is to repair microdamage sustained as a result of everyday wear and tear, it is suspected that bone not permitted to resorb and renew may become brittle. While the fracture data is positive, these studies have only followed patients three to five years into treatment and the optimum duration of therapy remains unclear (Keen, 2007). Furthermore, there have been reports of the rare but serious disorder of **osteonecrosis** of the jaw associated with bisphosphonate use, mainly in patients receiving high doses in combination with cancer treatment. This area needs more investigation to understand the mechanism of this disease.

SERMs represent a class of agents that, while similar in structure to estrogen, exert their effects only on target tissues. The most studied is raloxifene (Evista®) and its effects on markers of bone turnover have been more modest than with bisphosphonates, and its effect on non-vertebral fractures such as the hip have not been marked. For this reason, it is recommended for use in women with milder osteoporosis or in those with osteoporosis primarily in the spine. Side effects include hot flashes and an increased risk of venous thrombosis similar to that associated with hormone therapy.

Parathyroid hormone is an anabolic hormone that, unlike antiresorptive drugs that reduce bone resorption, acts mainly to stimulate bone formation. Although clinical trials showed a 65% risk reduction for new vertebral fractures and a 53% reduction for non-vertebral fractures, benefits to BMD receded after discontinuation. Therefore, this drug is recommended for short durations of less than two years (Sambrook & Cooper, 2006).

Strontium ranelate is an antiosteoporotic agent that is used in the European Union but is not yet approved for use in the U.S., though it is undergoing **phase III clinical trials**. Although its exact mechanism is unclear, it is the first drug that apparently increases bone formation while also reducing bone resorption. Vertebral fracture rates are reduced by about 50% and non-vertebral rates by about 16%, with even higher rates of fracture reduction seen in individuals with the weakest bones (Reginster et al., 2005).

Surgical Intervention

While surgical procedures for treatment of osteoporosis are not available, once fracture has occurred, surgery is often needed to repair damage to the bones. Despite advances in orthopedic surgery, anesthesia, and perioperative care, hip fracture surgery is still associated with complications in up to one-third of patients. The risk of nonunion (failure of the fracture to heal) and osteonecrosis are of particular concern. Data from well-designed outcome studies indicate that the most predictable, durable, and cost-effective procedure for an active older patient with a femoral neck fracture is total joint **arthroplasty.** However, not all patients are candidates for this procedure. In addition, the potential complications of such an invasive surgery, including mortality, may be more difficult to manage and more severe than those associated with less radical procedures (Schmidt et al., 2005).

A newer treatment option for vertebral fractures involves the injection of a special bone cement into the compressed body of the vertebrae. Studies have shown increased bone strength (Steens et al., 2007) and pain relief (Afzal et al., 2007; Steens et al., 2007) in patients treated with this technique.

Exercise

Weightbearing exercise provides one of the most viable, potent tools for both prevention and management of osteopenia and/or osteoporosis. In addition to the ability to improve indices of falling that may lead to fracture, properly planned weightbearing exercises also provide a direct stimulus to bone that improves its strength and structure. Clearly, a well-planned exercise program should provide the foundation from which the disease can be effectively addressed. This topic is discussed in greater detail in the remaining sections of this chapter.

Physiological/Physical Responses to Exercise Training

In general, cross-sectional research demonstrates that physically active individuals of all ages enjoy better skeletal mass than their inactive peers. The magnitude of this difference depends on the mode and intensity of the activity, when the activity was initiated during the lifetime, and for how many years it was performed. The data clearly show that loading exercises performed prior to puberty have the greatest influence on bone. Likewise, increases in bone mass of pre- and postmenopausal women have usually been modest, and the best adaptations occur in those with the lowest starting bone mass values.

Physical Activity and Bone Response in Children and Adolescents

Childhood (prior to puberty) appears to be the time when the skeleton is most responsive to bone-loading activities. Sports that require participants to begin physical training at an early age provide useful information about the role of physical activity in bone growth and mineral accretion. The volume and intensity of training performed by highly motivated young athletes often exceeds five to 24 hours per week. Studies on young gymnasts, whose bodies regularly experience ground reaction forces of 15 times bodyweight, confirm that these types of forces can induce a change in BMD that is between 30 and 85% higher than controls for the whole body, spine, and legs (Bass et al., 1998). Randomized controlled trials in prepubescent children have similarly shown that jumping exercises performed for as little as seven months can confer large differences in bone mineral content of 3 to 4% at the spine and hip between exercise and control groups (Fuchs, Bauer, & Snow, 2001). Furthermore, there is evidence that impact exercise performed during the years before puberty may produce changes in bone that are sustained into adulthood (Fuchs & Snow, 2002). Even weightlifting activities that produce high skeletal loads via muscular pull in the absence of impact have the potential to positively influence bone. In a cross-sectional study of 15- to 20-year-old Olympic weightlifters, forearm bone mineral content was 40 to 50% higher in these athletes versus controls (Virvidakis et al., 1990).

Longitudinal studies also support the observation that children who are generally more physically active than their sedentary counterparts, even in the absence of targeted bone-loading exercise, display higher BMD. A six-year study following the bone mineral accrual in children passing from childhood into adulthood found a 9% and 17% greater total body bone mineral content for active boys and girls, respectively, over their inactive peers (Bailey et al., 1999).

Physical Activity and Bone Response in Premenopausal Women

Not unlike active children, active adults tend to have higher BMD than sedentary adults. These differences have been observed for all regions of the skeleton, regardless of the measurement device used. Some activities may not incorporate loads that apply a sufficient stimulus to bone to produce an adaptive response. Those who participate in activities with high force and load magnitudes, such as gymnastics, jumping, and power lifting, display higher BMD than those who participate in low-intensity or non-weightbearing activities like swimming and cycling. Even though swimming provides muscular pull on bones, it does not appear that this level of loading is adequate to offset the many hours of skeletal *unloading* individuals experience while buoyant in the water (Bellew & Gehrig, 2006).

The most successful exercise interventions in this age group have incorporated jumping exercises that create ground reaction forces of up to six times body weight. These data also suggest that exercises must be performed for a minimum of six months to elicit a significant bone response, but it may take up to nine months or longer (Khan et al., 2001). Another important feature of bone-loading exercises done during the adult years is that unlike results observed in children, these activities must be continued if the individual is to maintain the increases in bone mass. The principle of **reversibility** definitely applies to adult bone mass. There are no studies in premenopausal women that have demonstrated permanent bone gain as a result of short-term training.

Physical Activity and Bone Response in Postmenopausal Women

Bone mineral density of the hip predicts an individual's risk for fracture, and most intervention studies in postmenopausal women have found small, positive effects on hip BMD. Many of the "benefits" to bone described in these studies are due to an observed maintenance of bone in the exercise group with a concomitant decrease in bone in the control group. In this age group, however, even maintenance of bone is a very positive thing, as it may translate into a reduced fracture risk. Intervention studies using only strength training in postmenopausal women have shown mixed results. Nelson and colleagues (1994) had 50- to 70-year-old, previously untrained, estrogen-depleted women train at 80% of **one-repetition maximum (1 RM)** for one year. They showed a 0.9% and 1% gain in BMD in the strength-training group for the hip and spine, respectively, compared to –2.5% and –1.8% BMD losses in controls. Furthermore, they showed that indices of falling, such as muscle mass, muscle strength, and dynamic balance, also improved, which may have implications for fracture risk as well, especially if the exercises are maintained. These results have since been replicated by others and suggest that exercise intervention in this age group can maintain BMD, but rarely serves to add substantial amounts of bone. Similar results have been found for hip BMD using high-impact exercises. Kohrt, Ehsani, and Birge (1997) conducted a study comparing the effects of strength training versus high-impact training on bone. They found that while both programs improved lumbar spine BMD, only the impact group augmented hip BMD. They concluded that it may be better to recommend exercises that generate impact forces on bone over those that generate muscle forces. However, because strength training reduces risk factors for falling, both types of activities should be considered when designing programs for individuals at risk for fracture.

During the late postmenopausal years, when the rate of bone loss has slowed compared to early postmenopause (if estrogen is not replaced), calcium supplementation becomes more important as a way to compensate for reduced estrogenic actions on intestinal calcium absorption and renal calcium excretion (Borer, 2005). There is also evidence that exercise has a synergistic effect on calcium retention in the skeleton and may help to ameliorate bone loss (Specker, 1996). Clients should be encouraged to obtain at least 1200 mg of calcium per day, through either dietary or supplement sources.

Physical Activity and Bone Response in Men

There is a surprising lack of intervention studies on the effects of exercise on bone in men. This is unfortunate, since the number of men with osteoporosis and related fractures is increasing. The few intervention studies that do exist indicate that the response of the male skeleton to exercise is similar to that of women, but is not complicated by the abrupt withdrawal of reproductive hormones in late adulthood. Similar to the results of studies in women, more rigorous training conveys more benefit to the skeleton, while low-intensity exercises, such as walking and moderate-intensity running, afford little benefit (Beck & Snow, 2003).

Summary of Bone's Response to Loading, Hormonal Intervention, and Dietary Intervention

The literature in this area supports eight basic principles related to how bone responds to exercise loading, hormonal intervention, and dietary intervention, which are summarized as follows (Borer, 2005):

- The best time to load bone is prior to puberty. Improvements in bone mass during this time are more dramatic and evidence suggests that they may cause an increase in peak bone mass that persists into adulthood.
- Bone requires dynamic, rather than static, loads to improve its size, shape, and/or density.
- Bone requires loads over and above normal daily loading to improve its size, shape, and/

or density. Bone must sense an overload stimulus if it is to adapt. Higher stresses produce higher bone strains, and these can be accomplished by higher force magnitudes and/or faster application of force. This may partially explain the ineffectiveness of walking programs and low-to-moderate intensity weight-training programs in producing positive gains in bone mass.

- Bone's response is proportional to strain frequency. Bone is maintained both with less frequent mechanical loads of higher intensity and with higher frequency loads at lower intensity.
- Bone's response is improved with brief, intermittent exercise, and may require six to eight hours of recovery between intense loading sessions. The number of loads need not be high (anywhere from five to 50 impacts can be beneficial) to produce the desired response.
- Bone requires an unusual loading pattern to improve. Exercise that loads the skeleton in unusual, uncustomary ways, produces more dramatic responses than those using normal loading patterns.
- Bone requires abundant available nutrient energy if it is to respond. Caloric restriction negatively impacts bone via suppression of key **anabolic** hormones.
- Bone requires abundant calcium and vitamin D availability. This is more important before puberty and after menopause, when the anti-resorptive effects of estrogen are suppressed and vitamin D intake may be inadequate. Evidence also suggests synergistic effects of exercise and calcium and vitamin D on bone during these times.

Programming and Progression Guidelines

Recommendations for Children and Young Adults

- Choose weightbearing activities such as basketball, soccer, volleyball, and gymnastics over non-weightbearing activities such as swimming and cycling. Although these weightbearing activities specifically target bone, it should be understood that a well-rounded program should also contain activities to promote cardiovascular health.
- Emphasize activities and movements that develop muscular strength and power, such as running, hopping, skipping, and jumping. These activities are easily incorporated into games and regular physical-activity classes and should maximize movement and minimize inactive time.
- Remember the principles of **specificity** and **overload.** The skeletal response to exercise is greatest at the site of maximum stress, and the training load must be greater than that encountered on an everyday basis.
- Adequate energy intake is essential for proper growth and bone development. Girls especially should be educated about the importance of a healthy diet and the dangers of menstrual dysfunction.
- Youth should avoid substituting soft drinks for milk. Calcium intake during growth is essential for healthy bones.

The FITT principle for children and young adults is as follows:

Frequency: Several bouts of bone-loading exercise are more effective than one long bout.

Intensity: High-intensity activities with high strain rates promote stronger bones than endurance-type activities.

Time: The number of strain cycles can be small (e.g., 50 to 100), so the duration can be short (five to 10 minutes depending on the types of activities chosen).

Type: A variety of loading patterns applied in unusual ways is more beneficial than activities that mimic everyday activities. Static loads (e.g., isometrics) do not promote increased bone accrual.

Recommendations for Premenopausal Women and Middle-aged Adult Men

- Choose weightbearing activities such as running, group fitness classes (including aerobic and/or muscle-conditioning classes), basketball, soccer, volleyball, and martial arts over non-weightbearing activities such as swimming, cycling, and rowing. Although these weightbearing activities specifically target bone, it should be understood that a well-rounded program should also include activities to promote cardiovascular health.

- Emphasize activities and movements that develop muscular strength and power, such as running, hopping, skipping, and jumping. These are easily incorporated into games and regular physical-activity classes and should maximize movement and minimize inactive time.
- Remember the principles of specificity and overload. The skeletal response to exercise is greatest at the site of maximum stress, and the training load must be greater than that encountered on an everyday basis.
- Simple jumping seems to provide an adequate stimulus for bone, and is a safe and appropriate loading modality for younger women and older nonosteoporotic women (Bassey & Ramsdale, 1994; Bassey et al., 1998; Heikkinen et al., 2007; Winters & Snow, 2000). Studies in premenopausal women using 50 daily jumps (two-footed, using arms for propulsion, bare/stocking feet, bent-knee landing) have shown positive gains in bone mass at the hip. This is a very simple, yet effective method for incorporating high-impact activity into an existing exercise program (Bassey & Ramsdale, 1994).
- High intensity strength-training exercises (8 RM) should also be included in a well-rounded exercise program, as they have been shown to benefit bone and multiple indices of falling and fracture risk.
- These clients should perform strength-training exercises in a standing (weightbearing) position, using free weights and/or a weighted vest when possible. Doing so will challenge the **vestibular system,** involve stabilizing muscles, and translate to **activities of daily living (ADL)** much more effectively than seated activities. Weighted vest loads of 7 to 15% of the client's body weight are an effective means of loading the skeleton during exercises performed while standing (e.g., lunges, squats, stair steps, calf raises).

Recommendations for Non-osteoporotic Postmenopausal Women and Older Men

Based on the available research, it is not only advisable to recommend exercises that will directly benefit bone, but also those that will reduce the risk for falling. Because falls cause more than 90% of hip and 50% of spine fractures, fall prevention should be central to an exercise program for older adults in general. Muscle weakness, postural instability, and poor functional mobility are important risk factors for falls.

- Any program should be individualized based on the physician's recommendations and the client's current health/fitness status, joint concerns, medication use, and ability level. Having the results from a bone density test is valuable to help determine risk for osteoporosis and fracture.
- Low-intensity activities, such as walking, impart very low bone loads and are not recommended as an effective strategy for the prevention of osteoporosis in postmenopausal women. If walking is performed as a primary exercise modality, it should definitely be accompanied by high-intensity strength training (using 8 RM as a guide).
- Older adults can perform high-intensity strength-training exercises (8 RM), as they have been shown to benefit bone and multiple indices of fracture risk.
- These clients can perform strength training exercises in a standing (weightbearing) position, using free weights and/or a weighted vest when appropriate and possible. Doing so will challenge the vestibular system, involve stabilizing muscles, and translate to improvements in ADL much better than seated activities. Heavy loads (>10% of body weight) in a weighted vest should be avoided if spine BMD status is unknown.
- Clients should focus on lower-body muscles groups, but must not neglect the upper body, as these muscles are important for daily living and maintaining independence.
- High-impact jumping (>2.5 times body weight) and other plyometric exercises should probably be avoided in these individuals, especially if bone status is unknown.

Plyometrics

Plyometric exercises provide a means for incorporating a variety of different movements, including medial/lateral movements that overload the skeleton. **Plyometrics** are specialized jumping exercises associated with high-impact loads and forceful muscular takeoffs, and include various exercises specifically designed to increase muscular strength and power. They are based on the premise that increasing eccentric preload on a muscle will induce the **myotatic stretch reflex,** thereby causing a more forceful concentric contraction. Plyometrics range in difficulty and intensity level from simple stationary jumping to traveling drills, such as hopping and bounding, to high-intensity box jumps (Chu, 1998; Radcliffe & Farentinos, 1999). An inherent benefit of utilizing these types of activities is that they require little equipment, small blocks of time, and are generally safe for adolescents and healthy adults to perform. Care should be taken to make sure clients have adequate leg strength to land properly before incorporating these types of high-intensity plyometric activities.

A proper progression of plyometric exercises is important to ensure adequate muscular strength to maintain proper body mechanics during execution and landing. A plyometric program should begin with one to two sets of 10 repetitions of five to seven different exercises and progress slowly to the more strenuous activities, adding sets and repetitions as tolerated. All exercises should be performed on a medium-hard surface such as grass (preferred), group fitness room floor, or carpet.

It is important to note that plyometrics should not be performed by osteoporotic individuals or by older adults with joint concerns. Clients can perform the sample exercises presented in Figures 16-4 through 16-10 in succession, minimizing time spent on the floor. This method maximizes muscle preload and ensures optimal gains in power.

There are also several more advanced plyometric exercises that can be used with more fit clientele. When performing alternating leg bounds, the knee on the lead leg drives up and forward, lands, and then the opposite knee drives up and forward. The client should emphasize maximum height and distance, and

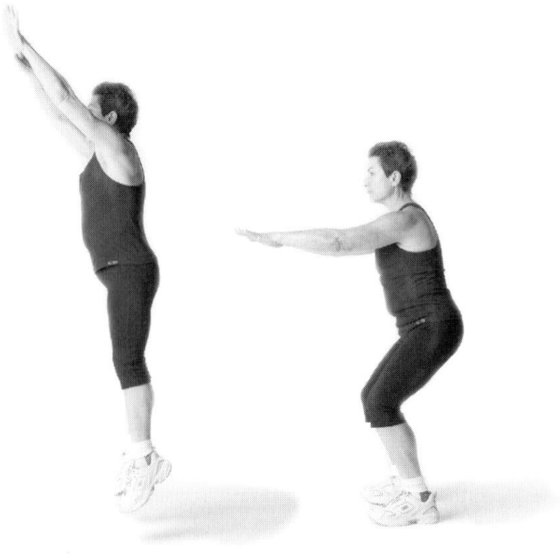

Figure 16-4
Squat jump—The client jumps as high as possible, using the arms for propulsion, and then lands in a squat position.

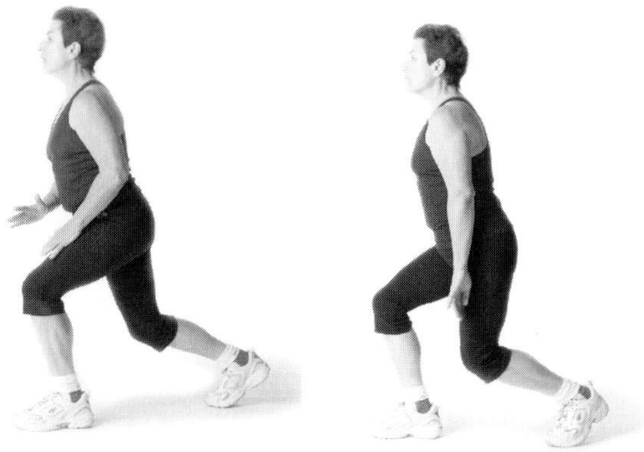

Figure 16-5
Stride jump—Starting from a front lunge position, the client drives the hips upward and lands with the opposite leg forward, again in a lunge position.

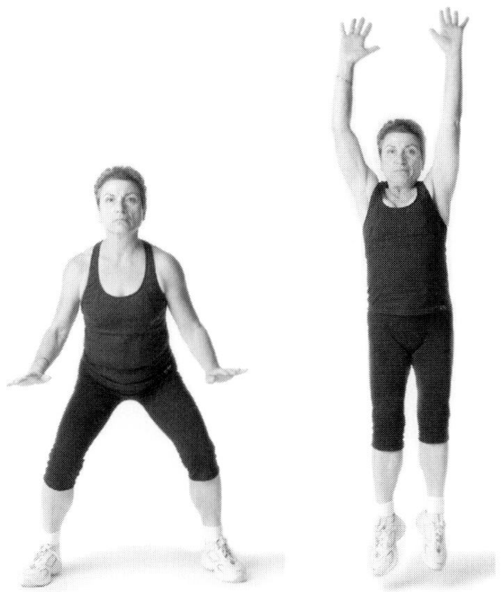

Figure 16-6
Split jump—Starting from a standing straddle position, the client jumps up, quickly brings the legs together, and lands in the same standing straddle position.

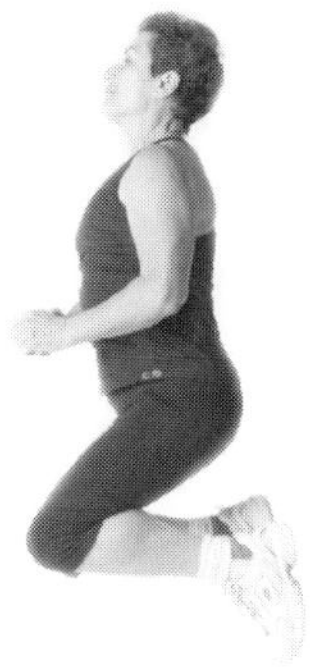

Figure 16-7
Double-leg butt kicks—From a standing position, the client jumps with both legs, kicks the buttocks, and lands on both feet, emphasizing maximum distance.

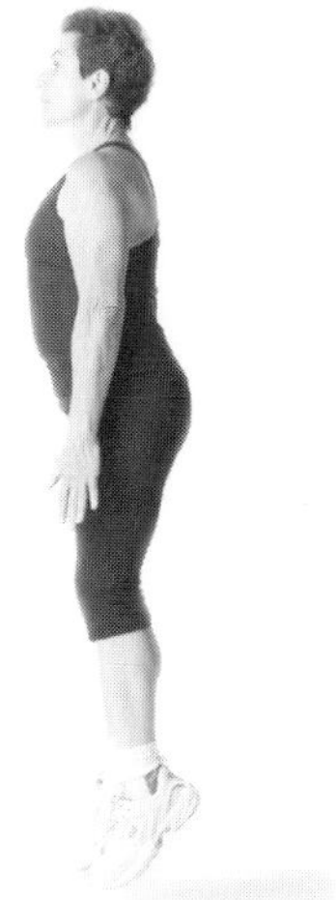

Figure 16-8
Ankle hops or hop progressions—The client performs basic, small, double-leg hops as quickly as possible.

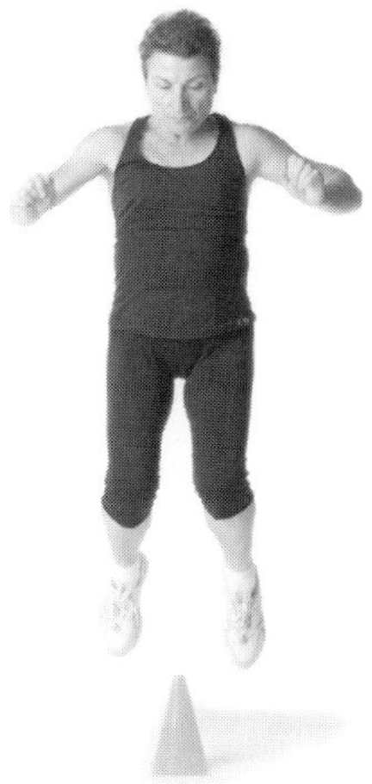

Figure 16-9
Cone or hurdle hops—The client performs large, high, two-footed hops over barriers such as cones or low hurdles. The goal is to minimize the time spent on the ground.

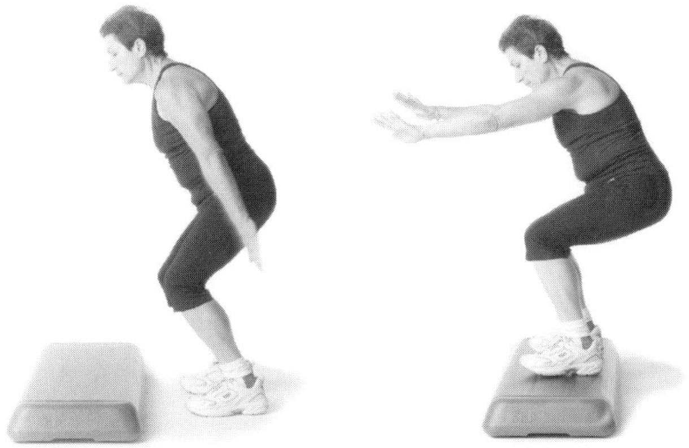

Figure 16-10
Box jump progression—Using several 4- to 8-inch steps (group fitness benches work well) spaced two to three feet apart, the client jumps onto and off of the succession of steps, spending as little time on the floor as possible. Pauses, if any, should be made on top of the bench rather than on the floor.

move the bent arms in a backward circular motion for added propulsion. This exercise also can be performed as a same-leg bound, where the lead leg cycles around and is the only leg to touch the ground.

A variety of advanced plyometric exercises can be performed on a flight of stairs, ranging from standard running, "bounding" (skipping several stairs at a time) a sideways approach. To perform a sideways stair exercise, the client stands sideways on two successive steps, with the trailing leg straight, and pushes the lead leg up to the next step. He or she then moves the trailing leg up to the next step, pushes off, and so on. This exercise represents a sort of "seesaw" motion and strengthens the hip abductors and adductors.

Recommendations for the Osteoporotic Client

To date, there have been very few intervention studies in people with osteopenia or osteoporosis, so specific recommendations are difficult for this group. Clients diagnosed with osteoporosis, with or without a history of vertebral fractures, should not engage in jumping activities or deep forward trunk flexion exercises such as rowing, toe touches, and full sit-ups (Beck & Snow, 2003). In this group of individuals, a regular walking program, combined with resistance training that targets balance and upper- and lower-body muscle strength, may help to improve muscle strength and coordination, thereby reducing fall risk.

The body-weight resistance exercises shown in Figures 16-11 through 16-24 may be useful for osteoporotic clients. The exercise session should begin with an eight- to 15-minute warm-up of gentle stretching and range-of-motion exercises, followed by five to 10 minutes of aerobic activity at 60 to 75% of maximum predicted heart rate.

If osteoporotic clients are limited by severe pain, exercise options may be limited. It may be advantageous to begin exercise with a warm pool-based program, which, while non-weight-bearing, can improve flexibility and muscle strength in deconditioned clients. These clients may also want to discuss with their physicians the use of calcitonin (a hormone beneficial to bone, administered via nasal spray that has been shown to help reduce pain).

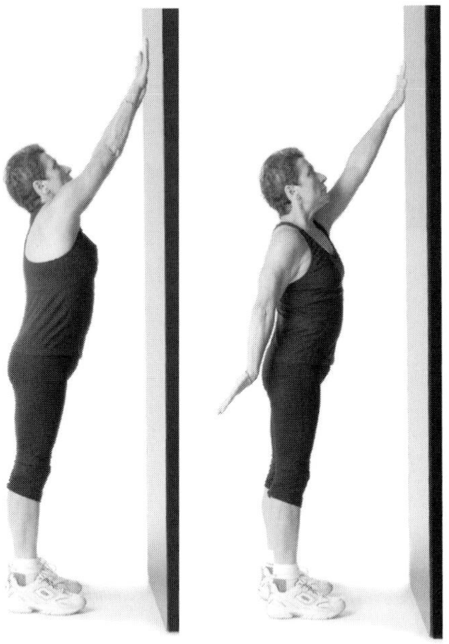

Figure 16-11
Wall arch

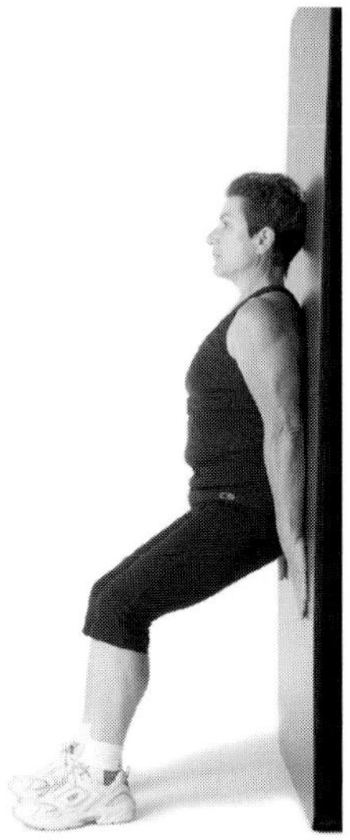

Figure 16-13
Wall slide/wall sit

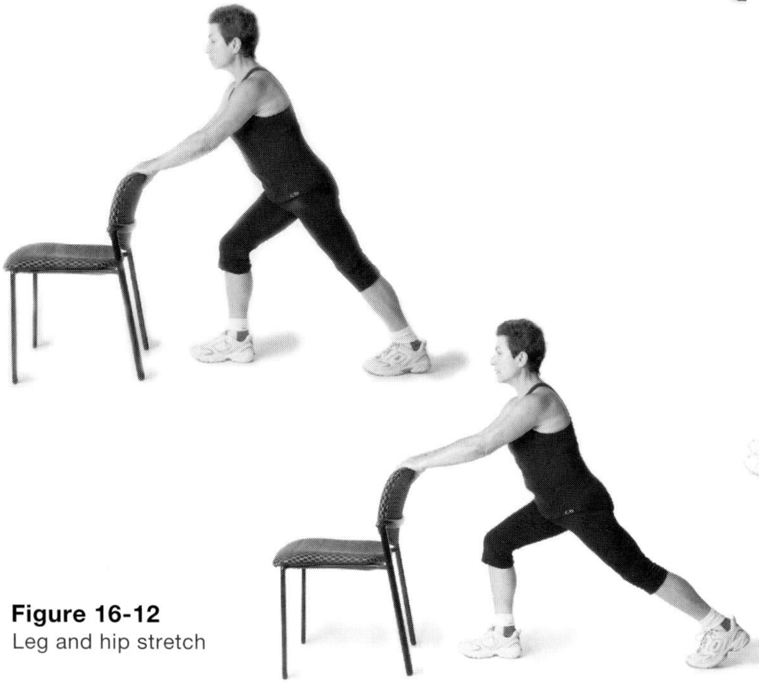

Figure 16-12
Leg and hip stretch

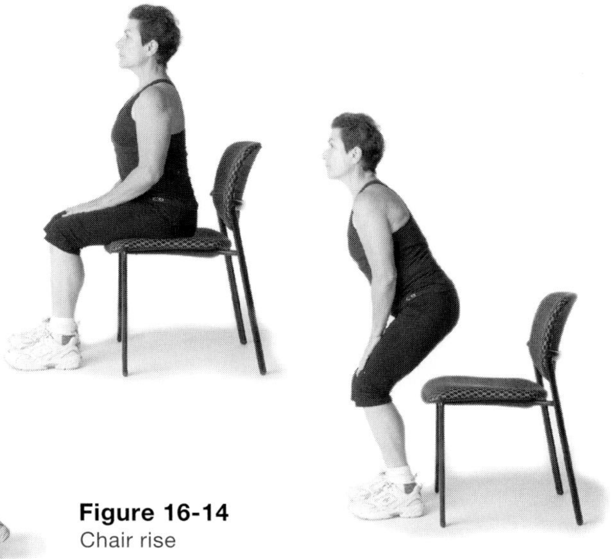

Figure 16-14
Chair rise

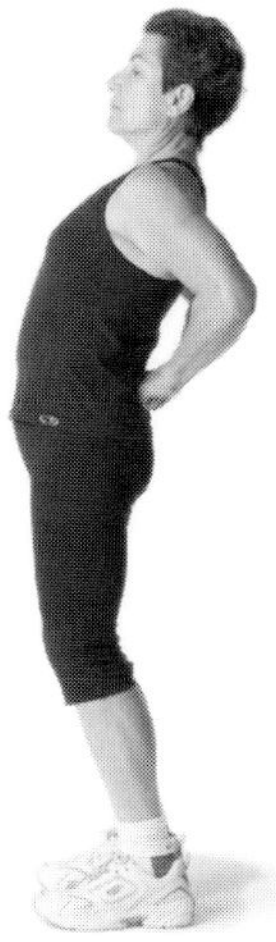

Figure 16-15
Standing back bend

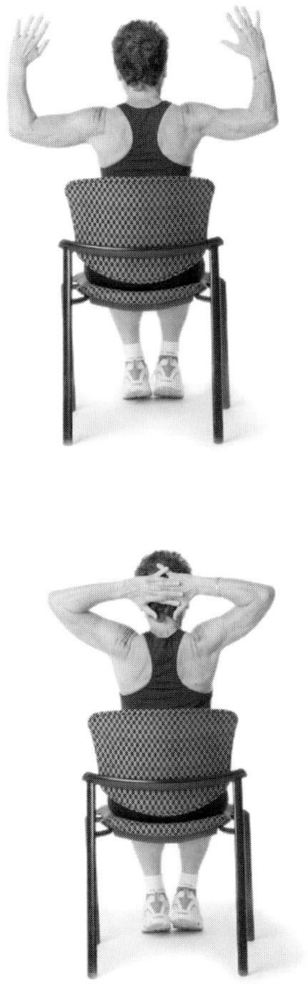

Figure 16-16
Seated posture correction

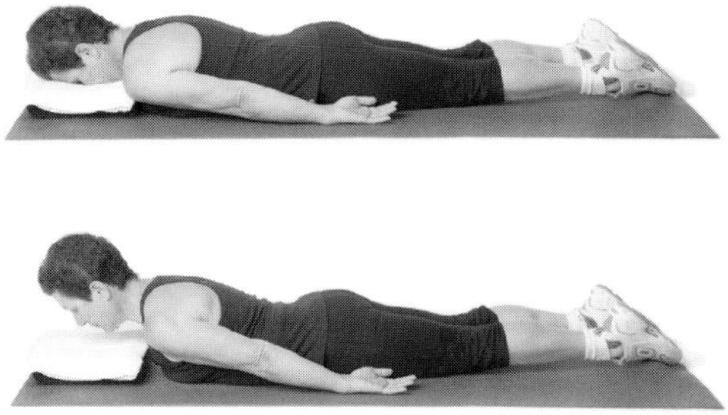

Figure 16-17
Prone trunk lift

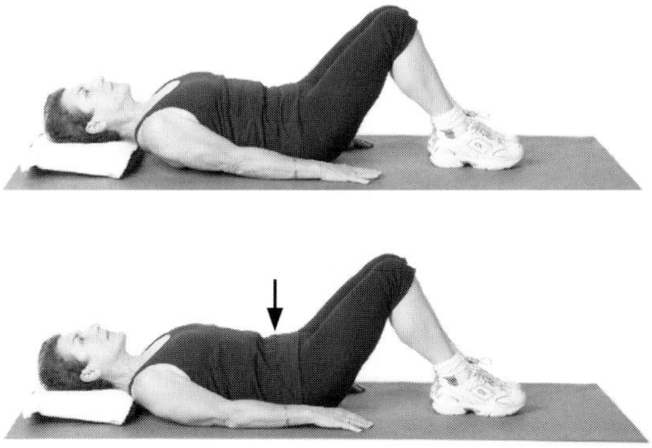

Figure 16-18
Abdominal strengthening

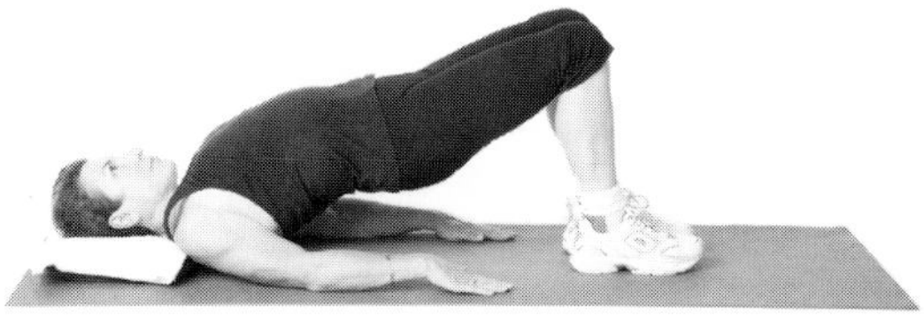

Figure 16-19
The glute bridge

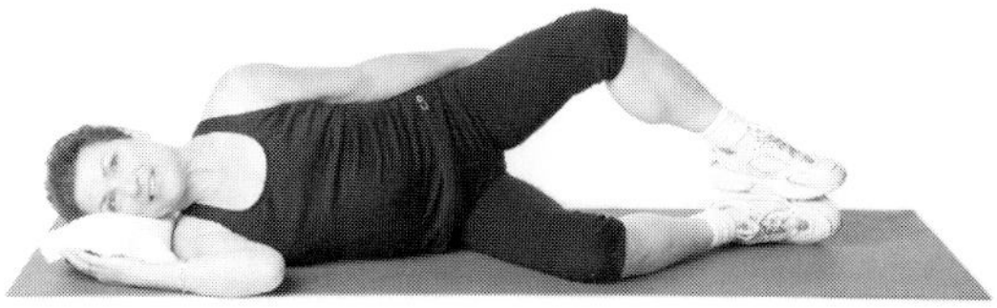

Figure 16-20
Side-lying knee lift

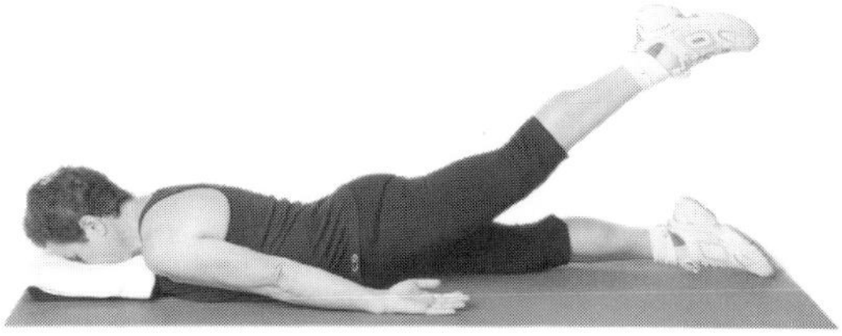

Figure 16-21
Prone leg lift

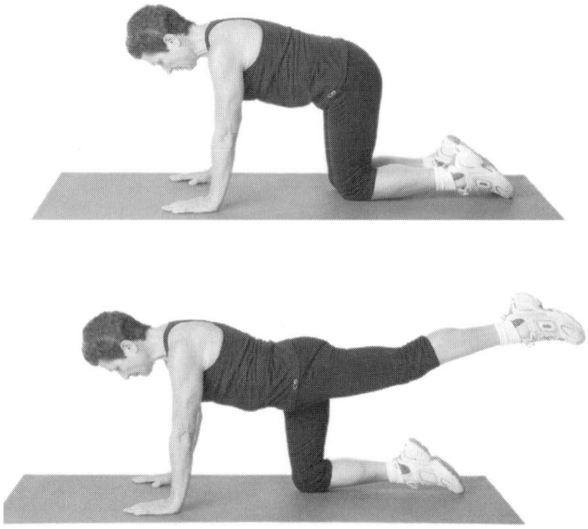

Figure 16-22
All-fours leg lift

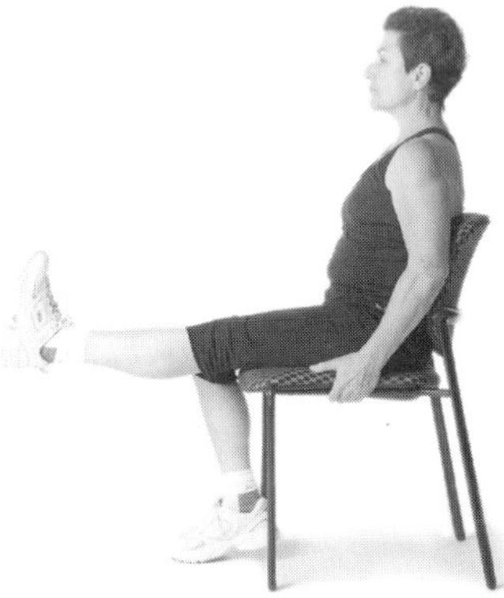

Figure 16-21
Sitting stretch

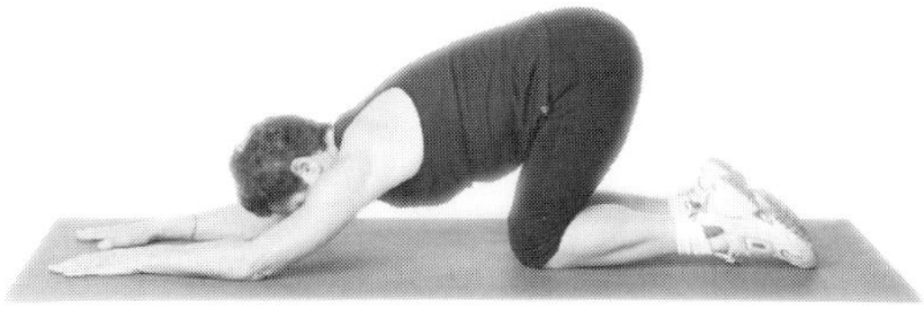

Figure 16-22
Cat stretch

Case Studies

Case Study 1

Rhonda is a thin, fair-skinned, 35-year-old marathon runner who has come to an ACE-AHFS for a strength-training program after finding out that her 50-year-old mother has osteoporosis. She currently runs about 75 miles per week (121 km/week), but would like to add a weightlifting regimen if it will help reduce her risk for osteoporosis. In the pre-screening assessment, the ACE-AHFS asks Rhonda to complete an osteoporosis risk questionnaire (see Figure 16-3) , which shows that she is at high risk. The ACE-AHFS also discovers that Rhonda has not had a menstrual period for two years (since she increased her training volume to compete in marathons) and only had a period every other month for three years prior to that. She has had two stress fractures in the past 12 months, but managed to continue her physical activity with non-weightbearing exercise while they healed. She is very concerned about her dietary fat intake, and claims that she consumes about 1200 calories per day. She is very eager to begin her strength-training program.

Rhonda is probably displaying characteristics of the female athlete triad. The ACE-AHFS should immediately be concerned that she has not menstruated in two years, and had irregular periods for some time before that. Her high training volume and low caloric intake probably have contributed to her **amenorrhea.** A visit to her physician is definitely in order before the ACE-AHFS can begin working with her. The ACE-AHFS should talk to Rhonda about concern over her training volume and associated stress fractures, and discuss amenorrhea, but must not diagnose the problem. The ACE-AHFS should also educate Rhonda on the usefulness of a bone-density assessment so that she may talk with her physician about getting one. The ACE-AHFS should also ask Rhonda about her dietary intake and recommend that she consult with a qualified nutritionist.

Once Rhonda returns with her physician release and the results from her bone-density assessment, the ACE-AHFS is ready to design a training program for Rhonda. If her bone mass is below normal (osteopenic), the ACE-AHFS should implement a conservative program of strength training and stationary jumping. Additional plyometric exercises should not be added for at least three months to ensure that Rhonda tolerates the jumping without injury. She can begin with upper- and lower-body resistance exercises for the major muscle groups using a weighted vest or dumbbells for resistance. Since she is in good physical condition, she can begin with two sets of 10 repetitions, using 8% of her body weight in the vest, or 75% of her 1 RM. Every two to three weeks, Rhonda can gradually increase her resistance. The ACE-AHFS should recommend that Rhonda weight train two days per week, substituting one of her running days for a weight-training day.

Case Study 2

Fiona is a 70-year-old, postmenopausal woman with a small build who has just been told by her physician that she has osteoporosis. She has lost 1.5 inches (3.8 cm) in height and has upper-back pain, but has been cleared by her physician to begin an exercise program. She performed some upper-body rubber tubing exercises with a physical therapist, but is more concerned about a hip fracture. She is otherwise sedentary and has chosen not to use estrogen replacement therapy, although she has heard positive things about "these new bone drugs" from her friends. She wants the ACE-AHFS to tell her which bone drug she should begin taking, and to start her on a strength-training program to help slow her bone loss. She is on an antidepressant drug that sometimes makes her dizzy, especially when she forgets to wear her glasses. She took a bad fall in her home last month when she tripped over her small dog, and is concerned that she is having trouble climbing the stairs in her home.

Since Fiona has a physician's release to begin working with the ACE-AHFS, she is ready for screening and program development. Although the ACE-AHFS can educate Fiona about the new anti-resorptive drugs, all questions about whether or not they are right for her should be directed to Fiona's physician. She should continue performing the regimen her physical therapist prescribed for her to help maintain upper-back flexibility and strength. Since she has a recent history of falling and experiences episodes of dizziness, the ACE-AHFS should assess her functional mobility using an older adult fitness battery (see Chapters 14 and 21 and Appendix F) (Rikli & Jones, 2001). The ACE-AHFS also should help Fiona assess safety in her home and suggest that she wear stable shoes and her glasses while inside to prevent another tripping incident. A bell on her dog might also be a good idea. She also should secure all area rugs in her house and might consider installing handrails in the bathroom. Fiona definitely needs lower-body strength training, especially if she is to continue to climb the stairs in her home. The ACE-AHFS should implement the exercises presented in this chapter for osteoporotic adults, but should not include any jumping activities, since Fiona's osteoporosis is already established. It is important to make sure that Fiona has her eyeglasses on while training to maximize her safety and minimize her fear and risk of falling.

Summary

Bone is a dynamic, metabolically active tissue that responds to both use and disuse by adapting the amount of mineral to accommodate daily loading patterns. Of the two types of bone in the human body, trabecular bone is more susceptible to the deleterious effects of osteoporosis. Because of its high trabecular content, the neck of the femur is a common osteoporotic fracture site; hip fractures often cause a loss of independence and death in many cases. Osteoporosis prevention and treatment strategies include estrogen replacement therapy or other pharmacological agents, increased calcium intake, and exercise.

Bone is most responsive to mechanical loading during growth, and is progressively less responsive as an individual ages. Bone-loading exercises are beneficial to the skeleton at all stages of life and should be incorporated into a well-rounded program for all clients, especially those at risk for osteoporosis. The types of exercise that are most beneficial to bone are those that sufficiently overload bone using high-force magnitude rather than a high number of low-force repetitions. High-force magnitude can be produced through direct impact loading of the bone, as with jumping, or through strong muscular contractions that bend bone, as with strength training. Nonweightbearing, non-impact exercises such as swimming and rowing do not sufficiently overload bone to increase bone formation or slow bone loss. Similarly, weightbearing exercises that are not significantly different from daily loading patterns (in normally ambulating individuals), such as walking, also do not provide a stimulus for new formation.

The frequency and intensity of the exercises should take into account the client's bone status (preferably from a bone density scan), physical and functional status, medication use, and hormonal status, as well as the overall goals for the program. If the client is at risk for osteopenia or osteoporosis, it is wise for the ACE-AHFS to obtain a physician's clearance for strength-training exercises and/or any type of impact exercise prior to beginning a program.

References

Afzal, S. et al. (2007). Percutaneous vertebroplasty for osteoporotic fractures. *Pain Physician,* 10, 4, 559–563.

Aloia, J.F. et al. (1996). Risk for osteoporosis in black women. *Calcified Tissue International,* 59, 6, 415–423.

Bailey, D.A. et al. (1999). A six-year longitudinal study of the relationship of physical activity to bone mineral accrual in growing children: The University of Saskatchewan bone mineral accrual study. *Journal of Bone Mineral Research,* 14, 10, 1672–1679.

Bass, S. et al. (1998). Exercise before puberty may confer residual benefits in bone density in adulthood: Studies in active prepubertal and retired female gymnasts. *Journal of Bone Mineral Research,* 13, 3, 500–507.

Bassey, E.J. & Ramsdale, S.J. (1994). Increase in femoral bone density in young women following high-impact exercise. *Osteoporos International,* 4, 2, 72–75.

Bassey, E.J. et al. (1998). Pre- and postmenopausal women have different bone mineral density responses to the same high-impact exercise. *Journal of Bone Mineral Research* 13, 12, 1805–1813.

Beals, K.A. & Meyer, N.L. (2007). Female athlete triad update. *Clinical Sports Medicine,* 26, 1, 69–89.

Beck, B.R. & Snow, C.M. (2003). Bone health across the lifespan: Exercising our options. *Exercise and Sport Science Review,* 31, 3, 117–122.

Bellew, J.W. & Gehrig, L. (2006). A comparison of bone mineral density in adolescent female swimmers, soccer players, and weight lifters. *Pediatric Physical Therapy,* 18, 1, 19–22.

Bischo-Ferrari H.A. et al. (2005). Fracture prevention with vitamin D supplementation: A meta-analysis of randomized controlled trials. *Journal of the American Medical Association,* 293, 2257–2264.

Bohannon, A.D. (1999). Osteoporosis and African-American women. *Journal of Women's Health and Gender-based Medicine,* 8, 5, 609–615.

Borer, K.T. (2005). Physical activity in the prevention and amelioration of osteoporosis in women: Interaction of mechanical, hormonal and dietary factors. *Sports Medicine,* 35, 9, 779–830.

Calvo, M.S. & Park, Y.K. (1996). Changing phosphorus content of the U.S. diet: Potential for adverse effects on bone. *Journal of Nutrition,* 126, 4 Suppl., 1168S–1180S.

Chu, D.A. (1998). *Jumping into Plyometrics.* Champaign, Ill.: Human Kinetics.

Cooper, C. et al. (1992). Incidence of clinically diagnosed vertebral fractures: A population-based study in Rochester, Minnesota, 1985–1989. *Journal of Bone Mineral Research,* 7, 2, 221–227.

Cummings, S.R. & Melton, L.J. (2002). Epidemiology and outcomes of osteoporotic fractures. *Lancet,* 359, 9319, 1761–1767.

Curtis, K.M. & Martins, S.L. (2006). Progestogen-only contraception and bone mineral density: A systematic review. *Contraception,* 73, 5, 470–487.

Eisman, J. (1998). Relevance of pregnancy and lactation to osteoporosis? *Lancet,* 352, 9127, 504–505.

Fuchs, R.K., Bauer, J.J., & Snow, C.M. (2001). Jumping improves hip and lumbar spine bone mass in prepubescent children: A randomized controlled trial. *Journal of Bone Mineral Research,* 16, 1, 148–156.

Fuchs, R.K. & Snow, C.M. (2002). Gains in hip bone mass from high-impact training are maintained: A randomized controlled trial in children. *Journal of Pediatrics,* 141, 3, 357–362.

Funk, J.L., Shoback, D.M.. & Genant, H.K. (1995). Transient osteoporosis of the hip in pregnancy: Natural history of changes in bone mineral density. *Clinical Endocrinology (Oxford),* 43, 3, 373–382.

Griffin, M.R. et al. (1992). Black-white differences in fracture rates. *American Journal of Epidemiology,* 136, 11, 1378–1385.

Guyatt, G.H. et al. (2002). Summary of meta-analyses of therapies for postmenopausal osteoporosis and the relationship between bone density and fractures. *Endocrinology Metabolism Clinics of North America,* 31, 3, 659–679, xii.

Heikkinen, R. et al. (2007). Acceleration slope of exercise-induced impacts is a determinant of changes in bone density. *Journal of Biomechics,* 40, 13, 2967–2974.

Huang, C. et al. (1998). Prediction of fracture risk by radiographic absorptiometry and quantitative ultrasound: A prospective study. *Calcified Tissue International,* 53, 5, 380–384.

Iwamoto, J. et al. (2002). Effects of five-year treatment with elcatonin and alfacalcidol on lumbar bone mineral density and the incidence of vertebral fractures in postmenopausal women with osteoporosis: A retrospective study. *Journal of Orthopedic Science,* 7, 6, 637–643.

Keen, R. (2007). Osteoporosis: Strategies for prevention and management. *Best Practice & Research Clinical Rheumatology,* 21, 1, 109–122.

Khan, K. et al. (2001). *Physical Activity and Bone Health.* Champaign, Ill.: Human Kinetics.

Khosla, S. & Melton III, L.J. (2007). Clinical practice: Osteopenia. *New England Journal of Medicine,* 356, 22, 2293–2300.

Kohrt, W.M., Ehsani, A.A., & Birge, Jr., S.J. (1997). Effects of exercise involving predominantly either joint-reaction or ground-reaction forces on bone mineral density in older women. *Journal of Bone Mineral Research,* 12, 8, 1253–1261.

Krall, E.A. & Dawson-Hughes, B. (1993). Heritable and life-style determinants of bone mineral density. *Journal of Bone Mineral Research,* 8, 1, 1–9.

Lee, W.T. et al. (1996). A follow-up study on the effects of calcium-supplement withdrawal and puberty on bone acquisition of children. *American Journal of Clinical Nutrition,* 64, 1, 71–77.

Maggi, S. et al. (1991). Incidence of hip fractures in the elderly: A cross-national analysis. *Osteoporosis International,* 1, 4, 232–241.

Marcus, R. (1987). Normal and abnormal bone remodeling in man. *Annual Review of Medicine,* 38, 129–141.

Martins, S.L., Curtis, K.M., & Glasier, A.F. (2006). Combined hormonal contraception and bone health: A systematic review. *Contraception,* 73, 5, 445–469.

Massey, L.K. & Whiting, S.J. (1993). Caffeine, urinary calcium, calcium metabolism and bone. *Journal of Nutrition,* 123, 9, 1611–1614.

McKay, H.A. et al. (1994). Familial comparison of bone mineral density at the proximal femur and lumbar spine. *Bone and Mineral,* 24, 2, 95–107.

Melton, L.J. & Cooper C. (2001). Magnitude and impact of osteoporosis and fractures. In: Marcus, R., Feldman, D., & Kelsey, J. (Eds.) *Osteoporosis.* San Diego, Calif.: Academic Press.

Nattiv, A. et al. (2007). American College of Sports Medicine position stand: The female athlete triad. *Medicine & Science in Sports & Exercise,* 39, 10, 1867–1882.

Nelson, M.E. et al. (1994). Effects of high-intensity strength training on multiple risk factors for osteoporotic fractures: A randomized controlled trial. *Journal of the American Medical Association,* 272, 24, 1909–1914.

Radcliffe, J.C. & Farentinos, R.C. (1999). *High-powered Plyometrics*. Champaign, Ill.: Human Kinetics.

Recker, R.R. et al. (1992). Bone gain in young adult women. *Journal of the American Medical Association,* 268, 17, 2403–2408.

Reginster, J.Y. et al. (2005). Strontium ranelate reduces the risk of nonvertebral fractures in postmenopausal women with osteoporosis: Treatment of Peripheral Osteoporosis (TROPOS) study. *Journal of Clinical Endocrinology Metabolism,* 90, 5, 2816–2822.

Rikli, R.E. & Jones, C.J. (2001). *Senior Fitness Test Manual*. Champaign, Ill.: Human Kinetics.

Rosano, G.M. et al. (1993). Beneficial effect of oestrogen on exercise-induced myocardial ischaemia in women with coronary artery disease. *Lancet,* 342, 8864, 133–136.

Rossouw, J.E. et al. (2002). Risks and benefits of estrogen plus progestin in healthy postmenopausal women: Principal results From the Women's Health Initiative randomized controlled trial. *Journal of the American Medical Association,* 17, 3, 321–333.

Sambrook, P. & Cooper, C. (2006). Osteoporosis. *Lancet,* 367, 9527, 2010–2018.

Schmidt, A.H. et al. (2005). Femoral neck fractures. *Instructional Course Lectures,* 54, 417-45.

Smith, S. et al. (1989). A preliminary report of the short-term effect of carbonated beverage consumption on calcium metabolism in normal women. *Archives of Internal Medicine,* 149, 11, 2517–2519.

Snow-Harter, C. & Marcus, R. (1991). Exercise, bone mineral density, and osteoporosis. *Exercise and Sport Science Review,* 19, 351–388.

Specker, B.L. (1996). Evidence for an interaction between calcium intake and physical activity on changes in bone mineral density. *Journal of Bone Mineral Research,* 11, 10, 1539–1544.

Steens, J. et al. (2007). The influence of endplate-to-endplate cement augmentation on vertebral strength and stiffness in vertebroplasty. *Spine,* 32, 15, E419–E422.

Thompson, P.W. et al. (1998). Quantitative ultrasound (QUS) of the heel predicts wrist and osteoporosis-related fractures in women age 45–75 years. *Journal of Clinical Densitometry,* 1, 3, 219–225.

Tudor-Locke, C. & McColl, R.S. (2000). Factors related to variation in premenopausal bone mineral status: A health promotion approach. *Osteoporosis International,* 11, 1, 1–24.

Tylavsky, F.A. et al. (1989). Familial resemblance of radial bone mass between premenopausal mothers and their college-age daughters. *Calcified Tissue International,* 45, 5, 265–272.

U.S. Department of Health and Human Services (2004). *Bone Health and Osteoporosis: A Report of the Surgeon General.* Rockville, Md.: U.S. Department of Health and Human Services, Office of the Surgeon General.

van Staa, T.P. et al. (2001). Epidemiology of fractures in England and Wales. *Bone,* 29, 6, 517–522.

Virvidakis, K. et al. (1990). Bone mineral content of junior competitive weightlifters. *International Journal of Sports Medicine,* 11, 3, 244–246.

Winters, K.M. & Snow, C.M. (2000). Body composition predicts bone mineral density and balance in premenopausal women. *Journal of Women's Health and Gender-Based Medicine,* 9, 8, 865–872.

Wu, F. et al. (2002). Fractures between the ages of 20 and 50 years increase women's risk of subsequent fractures. *Archives of Internal Medicine,* 162, 1, 33–36.

Zanker, C.L. & Swaine, I.L. (1998). Relation between bone turnover, oestradiol, and energy balance in women distance runners. *British Journal of Sports Medicine,* 32, 2, 167–171.

Suggested Reading

Bailey, D.A. et al. (1999). A six-year longitudinal study of the relationship of physical activity to bone mineral accrual in growing children: the university of

Saskatchewan bone mineral accrual study. *Journal of Bone Mineral Research,* 14, 10, 1672–1679.

Beals, K.A. & Meyer, N.L. (2007). Female athlete triad update. *Clinical Sports Medicine,* 26, 1, 69–89.

Beck, B.R. & Snow, C.M. (2003). Bone health across the lifespan: Exercising our options. *Exercise Sport Science Reviews,* 31, 3, 117–122.

Chu, D.A. (1998). *Jumping Into Plyometrics*. Champaign, Ill.: Human Kinetics.

Fuchs, R.K., Bauer, J.J., & Snow, C.M. (2001). Jumping improves hip and lumbar spine bone mass in prepubescent children: A randomized controlled trial. *Journal of Bone Mineral Research,* 16, 1, 148–156.

Khan, K. et al. (2001). *Physical Activity and Bone Health*. Champaign, Ill.: Human Kinetics.

Kohrt, W.M., Ehsani, A.A., & Birge, S.J., Jr. (1997). Effects of exercise involving predominantly either joint-reaction or ground-reaction forces on bone mineral density in older women. *Journal of Bone Mineral Research,* 12, 8, 1253–1261.

Marcus, R. (1987). Normal and abnormal bone remodeling in man. *Annual Review of Medicine,* 38, 129–141.

Nattiv, A. et al. (2007). American College of Sports Medicine position stand: The female athlete triad. *Medicine & Science in Sports & Exercise,* 39, 10, 1867–1882.

Nelson, M.E. et al. (1994). Effects of high-intensity strength training on multiple risk factors for osteoporotic fractures: A randomized controlled trial. *Journal of the American Medical Association,* 272, 24, 1909–1914.

United States Public Health Service, Office of the Surgeon General. (2004). *Bone Health and Osteoporosis : A Report of the Surgeon General*. Rockville, Md., U.S. Department of Health and Human Services, Public Health Service, Office of the Surgeon General.

In This Chapter

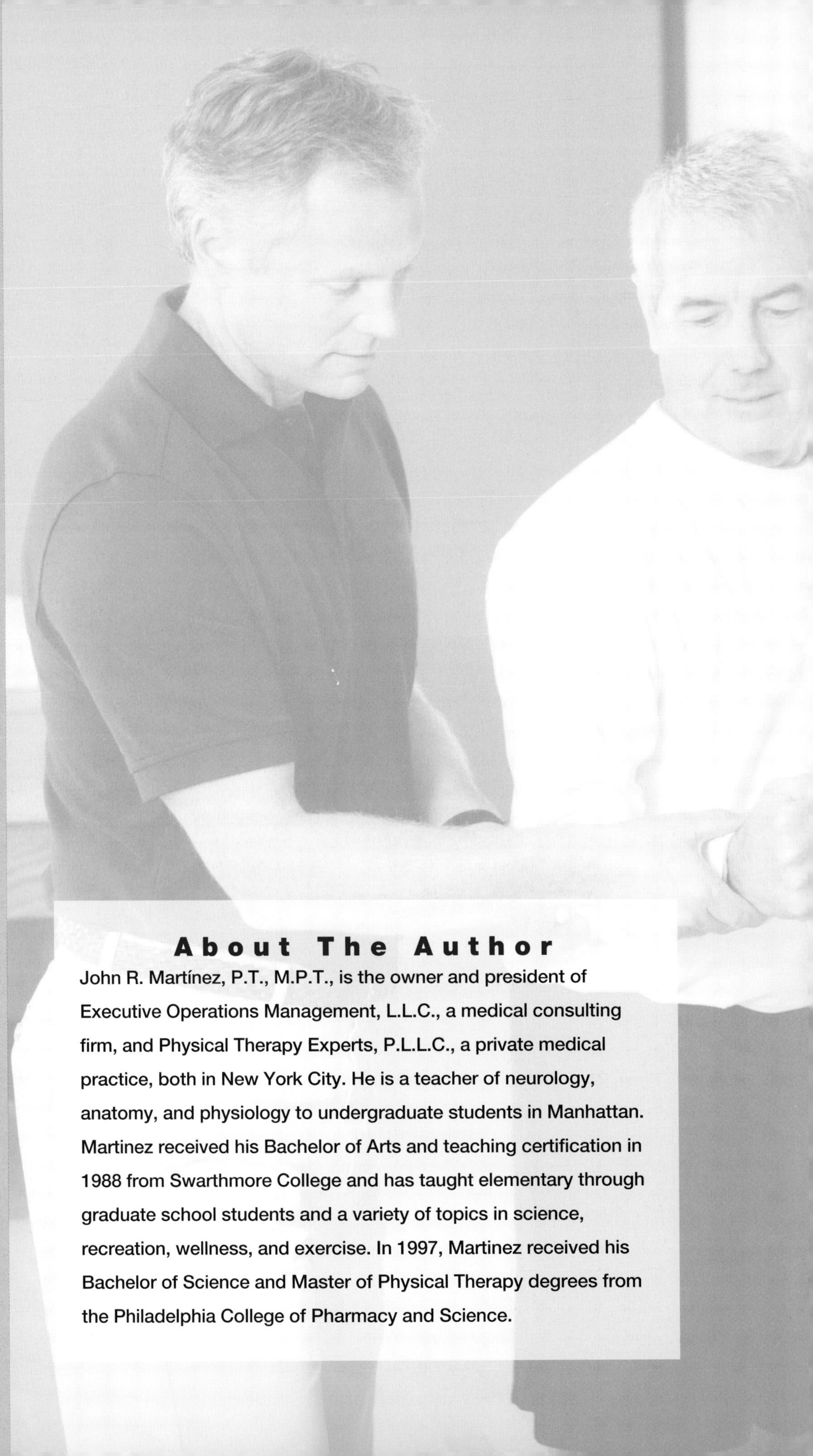

About The Author

John R. Martínez, P.T., M.P.T., is the owner and president of Executive Operations Management, L.L.C., a medical consulting firm, and Physical Therapy Experts, P.L.L.C., a private medical practice, both in New York City. He is a teacher of neurology, anatomy, and physiology to undergraduate students in Manhattan. Martinez received his Bachelor of Arts and teaching certification in 1988 from Swarthmore College and has taught elementary through graduate school students and a variety of topics in science, recreation, wellness, and exercise. In 1997, Martinez received his Bachelor of Science and Master of Physical Therapy degrees from the Philadelphia College of Pharmacy and Science.

CHAPTER 17

Principles of Post-orthopedic Rehabilitation

John Martínez

The fine line between exercise for healthy individuals and therapeutic exercise for individuals needing rehabilitation after injury, disease, illness, or other pathology can be difficult to determine. An ACE-certified Advanced Health & Fitness Specialist (ACE-AHFS) must know when it is appropriate to proceed with exercise program development for a client, rather than referring him or her to a licensed medical professional, such as a physical therapist, occupational therapist, or physician.

Considering the rather sophisticated health insurance requirements and restrictions, as well as their increasing costs, clients who need further attention from these medical professionals may have to rely on the ACE-AHFS for their continued rehabilitation. Thus, the principles of post-orthopedic rehabilitation have changed over the past few decades, requiring fitness professionals to add a strong clinical component to their educational foundation. The ability to maintain current knowledge of these medical principles and apply that knowledge successfully with the appropriate clients will be the key to an ACE-AHFS becoming an invaluable member of the modern medical team.

Communication With the Medical Team

It is impossible to overstate the importance of consistent communication with the medical team, which includes the physician or physicians involved in the medical care of the client, the physical and/or occupational therapist, any other medical or integrative medicine professional treating the client (e.g., chiropractor, acupuncturist, nutritionist), and the client him- or herself, who will have acquired a tremendous amount of information from all of these sources. Including the client as a member of the medical team is often overlooked. However, the client's understanding of his or her own body and its functions, as well as the fact that the client is in attendance at all the treatments with each of the medical professionals, makes him or her a crucial source of information regarding health history and healthcare needs. Obtaining as much information, both subjective and objective, as possible regarding the client's health will help establish a strong foundation for making exercise program development successful for the client. In particular, obtaining information from the new medical team members regarding the precautions and contraindications related to exercise is crucial, especially in orthopedic rehabilitation. Doing so will help protect the client from re-injury or any regression of the medical condition, which could damage the ACE-AHFS's relationship with not only the medical team, but also the client and future referred clients. The concept of "protection" is an important one for the ACE-AHFS to understand. Often, immediately following an acute orthopedic injury or surgical intervention, the client is placed on a status of "maximal protection" (e.g., non-weightbearing after a hip replacement). This type of information is crucial to protect the client during a time when he or she is at high risk for re-injury or worsening the medical condition. As the individual progresses, his or her status progresses to "moderate protection" (e.g., toe-touch weightbearing); to "minimal protection" (e.g., weightbearing as tolerated); and, lastly, to "unrestricted protection" (e.g., full weightbearing as risk decreases with physical recovery, both anatomically and physiologically). A clear understanding of the concept of protection and how it relates to the performance of activities that are contraindicated (higher risk) and to activities that are precautions (lower risk) is mandatory for the ACE-AHFS. The request for this specific information, along with the collection of the client's general medical history, will help to build the trust and confidence necessary from the entire medical team that will support the ACE-AHFS's work.

Initial Interview

Acquiring accurate information from any new client during the first meeting is critical to establishing a reliable history of the client's health. Clients can be a valuable source of personal health information, but since their reports often come from their untrained medical perspective, this information can have a variety of inaccuracies. Discerning which pieces of information are more or less useful requires focused listening along with targeted questioning from the ACE-AHFS. Bringing a skillful investigatory technique and style to an initial interview is crucial to the success of exercise program development for the post-orthopedic rehabilitation client. This process will provide the ACE-AHFS with the health information necessary to make informed decisions on the frequency, intensity, type, and duration of exercise that is best for the client. This is particularly true if the client must discontinue his or her medical treatment but wants to continue the recovery from injury, disease, or illness with an ACE-AHFS. To further aid in bridging the gap between the clinical and fitness settings, the ACE-AHFS should also consult with the client's rehabilitation specialist as described in the previous section.

Questioning a client regarding his or her level of pain or discomfort during this initial interview is also extremely important when developing safe exercise programming. A client's description of his or her pain will help the ACE-AHFS decipher if it is due to normal physical stress (such as muscle soreness), injury, disease, or other type of pathology. It will also lead to a discussion regarding what type of activities or circumstances exacerbate the pain or discomfort versus ones that provide relief. This type of exchange will provide valuable information on what exercises can be tolerated by the client. During post-orthopedic rehabilitation, respecting pain is important and protecting clients from further injury or exacerbation of their signs and symptoms must be a primary goal. Of course, upon exacerbation of pain or other signs and symptoms, immediate adjustments are necessary, and communication with the medical team is mandatory to formulate a plan for continued safe participation in an exercise program.

Objective Evaluation

Post-orthopedic rehabilitation clients will often come to the ACE-AHFS just short of returning to their pre-injury health status. Given a limited amount of sessions with the rehabilitation team due to health insurance and cost restrictions, clients will often be discharged from these medical services with the functional ability to return to their **activities of daily living (ADL),** but not to their normal level of activity. It is therefore important to measure a client's physical abilities before initiating a training program to establish a baseline of objective physical capabilities that can be referred to as the client progresses. It is also necessary to continue to document the client's progress overall in the transition from one medical team member to another. Documenting the role of the ACE-AHFS in the overall picture of a client's health recovery is an important component of the fitness professional's responsibilities as a member of the medical team.

The ACE-AHFS's assessment of the client's physical condition must be objective and somewhat comparable to the discharge assessment of the rehabilitation medical professionals. Acquiring an understanding of the rehabilitation specialist's measuring and assessment approaches will provide the ACE-AHFS with a solid foundation from which to build his or her own unique evaluation. Performing careful measurements from objective fitness testing techniques and activities will greatly benefit the client and the rest of the medical team by providing a consistent method for reviewing the client's progress over time and from one professional to another. Allowing the client's subjective and objective goals to guide the assessment will make the evaluation more efficient. Assessments of generalized and local joint **range of motion (ROM), muscle endurance** and **strength,** and the ability to perform important functional activities (e.g., ambulation, balance) will form a baseline of a client's initial health status. This information is crucial as the ACE-AHFS builds an effective exercise program that will continue to show rehabilitative progress compared to baseline measurements. Adding recreational activities and movements to these programs will increase a client's motivation and enthusiasm to remain compliant and show objective advances on a regular basis through comparison to a well-established evaluation, which will also make the client more committed to the program.

Professional Impression

Once the initial evaluation, interview, and testing have taken place, the ACE-AHFS's review and opinion of all this information is what makes him or her a true professional. Determining the important health issues to focus on and recognizing when a client's health status is outside one's scope of expertise are important components of any fitness professional's standard of care. Most often, the medical team's summaries are the only component of a medical report that other team members will review, given their time restraints. Trust in, and respect for, the knowledge, skills, and expertise of the ACE-AHFS will make him or her a valuable and accepted member of the team. The ACE-AHFS can develop that trust through thorough assessments of each new client's health status and professional communication to the medical team.

These assessment summaries should briefly state the client's age, gender, medical diagnosis, and history, and how the client presented to the ACE-AHFS with regard to the most important physical findings.

Sample Assessment Summary

The client is a 5'7"(1.7 m) 63-year-old female weighing 110 lb (50 kg) with a diagnosis of osteoporosis. She has had back pain for the past 3 years. She comes to the ACE-AHFS after completion of three months of physical therapy, which resulted in minimal back pain. She has a short-term goal to return to running 3–4 days per week as she did prior to her back pain and a long-term goal to run a marathon one more time.

The client's aerobic condition is diminished, with tolerance of only 10 minutes of walking on the treadmill at 3.0 mph resulting in RR 25, HR 155, BP 140/90, and RPE 18. Upper- and lower-extremity anaerobic condition is also decreased, with an ability to perform only 6–8 repetitions on all tests before fatigue and occasional loss of balance with self-correcting. Minimal back pain was reported by the client during and after testing.

The client will benefit from exercise programming to increase her aerobic condition with cardiovascular activities, elevate her extremity strength levels with resistance training, stabilize her balance during recreational activities to reduce the risk of falls through coordination and agility activities, and improve her bone strength with closed-chain exercises. Referral to a nutritional expert has been made.

Note: RR = Respiration rate; HR = Heart rate; BP = Blood pressure; RPE = Ratings of perceived exertion

These summaries provide the medical team with all the necessary information regarding an ACE-AHFS's findings and how the client will benefit from his or her services. If the medical team members disagree or feel that the ACE-AHFS needs to know additional information that will change the assessment, they will contact the ACE-AHFS with that information. This report gives them the opportunity to do so and makes them aware that their patient is actively trying to improve his or her health with the help of a qualified fitness professional. If the medical team members would like to see more details, they will be able to review the rest of the report, which should contain all of the objective activities that occurred. Therefore, the entire report should be sent to the medical team members, including a plan of what the ACE-AHFS intends to do to help the client achieve his or her goals. Additionally, the ACE-AHFS should be sure to include his or her contact information and a statement expressing a willingness to communicate further with the clinician about the client.

Plan

When preparing to work with a new post-orthopedic rehabilitation client, the ACE-AHFS should keep the process of reaching the established goals in mind. The initial evaluative report should include a written summary of the steps the ACE-AHFS plans to take to help the client reach his or her goals. Taking a broad perspective is important in visualizing how the entire program will begin, progress, and end. This will make the day-to-day planning more efficient and effective. Forecasting the exercise programming is a skill that the ACE-AHFS will develop over time with each plan he or she creates. Short-term goals that are measurable, specific, and concrete, along with long-term goals that are functional, will be helpful and can be included either in the plan or the assessment portion of the initial evaluation. Remember, health status changes and new information continues to arise. Therefore, after each month of working with a client, a new plan should be created, updating the short-term goals and fine-tuning the long-term goals in an effort to move as close as possible to a successful outcome. Signing and dating this report gives it authenticity and helps establish a level of professionalism. The ACE-AHFS should not be overly concerned about specifically achieving the original plan, as it is generally understood that components and factors may change and lead to different outcomes. It is the documentation that is important to the medical team and what makes the ACE-AHFS valuable in the post-orthopedic rehabilitation process of recovery.

Client Population

As medical technology, procedures, and skills advance, people are living longer and more functionally than ever before. This increasing **lifespan** results in a general population that is living with chronic illnesses, diseases, injuries, and other pathologies. The considerably large "Baby Boomer" population is now seeking medical attention for myriad health conditions in an effort to move forward with their active lives both with and beyond traditional medical therapies. Thus, these clients may continue seeking relief from the signs and symptoms of their conditions after considering all that the medical therapies can offer. The recommendation to significantly decrease work and recreational activities is no longer a realistic or acceptable option, creating the need for the special skills of an ACE-AHFS who can help these clients recover their functional capabilities and remain active for years into the future.

Understanding the basic medical concepts of chronic conditions in general, as well as some specific pathologies that are more common than others, will provide the ACE-AHFS with the foundation he or she will need to address clients' ongoing wellness goals. The other chapters in this manual address these needs and are the structure upon which an ACE-AHFS can build this foundation. In general, these clients will be highly ambulatory (i.e., walking in their homes and communities), and be able to accomplish functional ADL (e.g., eating, dressing, grocery shopping). They may present to the ACE-AHFS with some loss of general conditioning, complaints of consistent pain, discomfort, or **paraesthesia** from a cause either known or unknown, weakness of some muscular groups, and/or loss of ROM or flexibility. Frequently, these signs and symptoms will be affecting their daily function to some degree and be preventing them from performing at the levels they have in the past. These clients will have a strong desire, motivation, and enthusiasm to return to their past levels of function and often will have already begun this rehabilitation through participation in programs and therapies with other medical team members. An ACE-AHFS's clients usually arrive having achieved general improvement in their physical condition to a certain level, either through rehabilitation with medical experts or through their own efforts, but wish to continue advancing toward higher physical goals.

Rehabilitation Protocols

Many orthopedic medical professionals have developed rehabilitation treatment protocols that have support from scientific research regarding their effectiveness with patients. These protocols serve as treatment guidelines for the gradual process of recovery through which they and other medical team members should proceed to meet patients' rehabilitation goals. Surgeons, sports medicine physicians, physical therapists, and occupational therapists have all established such protocols for rehabilitation from a variety of diagnoses that will require their patients to exercise if they are to return to their normal ADL. Additionally, generalized protocols can be found in both the research and academic literature, particularly in the field of physical therapy rehabilitation.

Protocol for Rehabilitation After an Arthroscopic Partial Meniscectomy

Overview

Typically, damage to the meniscus results in a tear. As the torn piece begins to move in an abnormal fashion inside the joint, it can cause a great deal of pain and limitation in the knee, thereby limiting activity tolerance. Depending on the type and size of the tear, arthroscopic surgery may be recommended. The options are to perform a repair of the meniscus or a **meniscectomy,** where the damaged meniscus is removed to prevent further irritation. Since the meniscus has such a poor blood supply, a meniscectomy is often performed. Generally, following knee arthroscopy, a fairly aggressive approach can be taken and ROM and strength are progressed as tolerated.

Phase I (Weeks 1–4)

The emphasis is on regaining full knee extension so the patient can ambulate with a normal gait pattern. This requires facilitating neuromuscular control of the quadriceps, controlling swelling, emphasizing normal gait pattern, and achieving knee ROM of 0 to 90 degrees.

Strengthening: Quad sets (isometric quadriceps contractions); straight-leg raise (SLR) in all planes of motion; standing heel raises on the Total Gym®; stretching (pain-free range) of the hamstrings, gastrocnemius, iliotibial band (ITB), and piriformis

ROM: Manual patellar mobilizations; heel slides using a towel or wall if needed; prone hangs as needed to gain full extension

Balance: Weight shifting; single-limb stance

Gait: Move to single crutch when the patient is able and then discontinue (D/C) the use of crutches when the patient is able to ambulate with a normal gait pattern

Modalities: **Electrical muscle stimulation (EMS)** may be needed to facilitate the quadriceps if voluntary muscle contraction is difficult. Ice should be used following exercise and initially every hour for 20 minutes. A clinically directed home exercise program (HEP) should be performed three times a day.

Phase II (Weeks 5–11)

The criteria to progress to this phase is minimal pain and swelling to allow sufficient healing, full weightbearing with normalized gait mechanics, and good control of lower-extremity musculature. By the end of this phase, the patient should independently ambulate with a normal gait, have good quadriceps control and controlled swelling, and be able to ascend and descend stairs.

Strengthening: Quad sets should be continued until swelling is gone and quadriceps tone is restored. SLR in all planes should be continued with progression to ankle weights when ready. Leg presses, both bilateral and unilateral, should be performed with the body weight on the heels to avoid too much load on the patellar tendon. Step-ups, step-overs, wall slides, mini squats, calf raises, and hamstring curls are also appropriate strengthening exercise choices.

ROM: Biking should not be performed until 110 degrees of knee flexion is achieved. Patients must not use the bike to gain ROM. Biking should be performed daily with a focus on increasing resistance as the patient is able to work the quadriceps.

Stretching: Continue with hamstring, calf, iliotibial band, and piriformis stretching. The goal for ROM is 0 to 125 degrees. Additionally, aggressive scar massage at incision sites, prone hangs, and seated or supine heel slides are appropriate for stretching enhancement.

Balance

Single-leg stance on even and uneven surfaces focusing on knee flexion; medicine ball toss; lateral cone walking with single-leg balance between each cone; foam roller or biomechanical ankle platform system (BAPS) board balance work

Gait: Cone walking forward and lateral; D/C crutches when normal gait pattern is achieved

Modalities: Continue to use ice after exercise

Phase III (Weeks 12–18)

The criteria to progress to this phase includes a good tolerance for the previous phase, full ROM, normal muscle strength, good closed-chain control in linear and multidirectional activities, and **isokinetic** strength of 70% of the uninvolved extremity. Goals for this phase are full quadriceps control and good quadriceps tone, ability to perform ADL without difficulty, a return to pre-injury sport and recreational activities, and the establishment of an ongoing training program.

Note: Exercises will be progressed based on the patient's quadriceps tone. A client who continues to have poor quadriceps tone must not be advanced to activities that require high quadriceps strength, such as squats and lunges.

Strengthening: Continue with the previous exercises, increasing the intensity as much as the client can tolerate. Appropriate exercises during this phase include slow and controlled forward and lateral step-ups using dumbbells as needed to increase intensity; free squats or squats using the Smith machine; forward and reverse lunges using dumbbells as needed to increase intensity; hip flexion with elastic resistance; single-leg squats and single-leg wall squats; and Russian dead lifts (unilateral and bilateral).

An ACE-AHFS can often obtain these protocols through literature reviews, a simple request with a written letter, or even a telephone conversation with medical team members. Maintaining a current file of these protocols by diagnosis will be an invaluable resource to the ACE-AHFS, who can learn from them and refer to them while working with clients. Rehabilitation protocols provide structure for a client's exercise program, as well as guidance for progressing the program at any point in a client's recovery. Additionally, these protocols can effectively serve as conversation "icebreakers" with medical professionals if a client is not able to see the medical professionals due to a lack of insurance or because of other prohibitive reasons. Requesting advice and accepting it from fellow medical team members by obtaining these protocols promotes trust and support and demonstrates a commitment to the best interests of the client. The ACE-AHFS will earn respect from all involved and will receive an increase in client referrals because of the high level of professionalism displayed by adopting such an approach.

Concepts of Healing

During any phase of these protocols, or at any time during the ACE-AHFS's relationship with a post-orthopedic rehabilitation client, there may be an active process of healing taking place within the client's body. Whether the client comes to exercise training with a chronic disease, acute injury, new illness diagnosis, or existing condition, the body is always in a process of trying to achieve a state of balance, or **homeostasis** (Marieb & Hoehn, 2006). Simply in the course of improving a client's health through the development of flexibility, endurance, and strength, the body will be involved in a type of healing and rebuilding process as it adjusts to new activities (Table 17-1). One of the most common signs of healing from a tissue injury is inflammation, which usually brings symptoms of pain, redness, swelling, and warmth. This inflammation occurs in either a specific or general area of the body due to increased blood flow that brings in oxygen and nutrients and removes harmful wastes. This is one way the body signifies that healing is taking place and, although it often evokes concern, it is generally a positive process and a normal component of healing. The ACE-AHFS should immediately recognize these signs and symptoms and decide if they are significant enough to warrant a minor or major change in the course of the program. Resting the affected area is usually a beneficial option, as is controlling the inflammatory response so that it does not overly restrict the mobility of a joint or body part. Although joint movement and light muscular activity can sometimes enhance the healing process, the general rule of rest, ice, compression, and elevation (RICE) of an injured body part is the most appropriate action until further evaluation can be made by the client's primary care physician. However, this often does not restrict the continuation of a client's exercise program for the uninvolved parts of the body since maintenance of physical activity may produce positive physiological systemic effects.

Tissue injury and the advancement of a disease process, infection, illness, or other type of pathology can result in a variety of responses from the body's immune system. Given this fact, when the ACE-AHFS observes a noticeable objective change in a client physically, biologically, psychologically, emotionally, or even subjectively by report from him or her directly, the ACE-AHFS should consider making some change to the programming for that session. This change can simply be a discontinuation of one particular exercise, a decrease in the intensity and/or duration of the session, an adjustment of focus from one type of conditioning to another, or a complete cancellation of all exercises for that session. The range of options available to the ACE-AHFS is wide, but documentation of the change in the client and the response by the fitness professional is mandatory to facilitate comparison to past and future sessions and for communication to the medical team.

Table 17-1
Phases of Tissue Healing

Phase	Description	Objective	Duration
Inflammation	Immediately post-injury, the area shows signs of warmth, redness, swelling, and pain	Care for injury and control inflammation	1 day–1 week
Proliferation	Development of scar tissue that lays down with random orientation; increased girth due to edema	Clear necrotic tissue; begin tissue and cell regeneration to improve circulation	1–4 weeks
Remodeling	Scar tissue edema decreases, but density increases; signs and symptoms reduce; tissue fully fuses	Reestablish function of tissue, skeletal muscle, and joint in the area	1–12 months

Source: Denegar, C.R., Saliba, E., & Saliba, S. (2005). *Therapeutic Modalities for Musculoskeletal Injuries* (2nd ed.). Champaign, Ill.: Human Kinetics.

Although exercise is healthy for the body and its functions in general, under certain conditions it can place the immune system at a disadvantage. For example, exercising an upper extremity that is hosting a blood infection may result in an increase in blood flow to the area of infection, resulting in a more rapid spread throughout the body. Thus, the ability to recognize changing conditions in clients and then respond appropriately is a critical skill.

Systematic Progression of Programming

Following injury, disease, illness, or other pathology, clients regularly experience a decline in a series of physiological functions that affect their lives. Typically, a loss of normal joint ROM is the most debilitating to clients, as it affects their daily functional movements. The inability to perform these natural movements, which are often taken for granted, is of significant concern. The next most noticeable loss is a decline in an individual's general condition, resulting in feelings of malaise and fatigue. This occurs due to the decrease in activity secondary to injury or disease and will affect the individual's recreational activities in addition to his or her normal ADL. Often, this issue is combined with a psychological component of longing for a return to these activities. Finally, muscular weakness becomes evident to the client as everyday activities that require some strength become difficult or impossible to perform. During medical rehabilitation treatments, clients will regain some function in these areas, but most likely not return to the full functional state that was enjoyed prior to diagnosis. Following a basic process toward improved biomechanical function to address these physiological issues will help the ACE-AHFS achieve successes with clients in a systematic way.

Increasing Range of Motion and Flexibility

Developing programs to initially address losses in a client's active range of motion should be an early focus of the ACE-AHFS. Regaining age-related normal joint range of motion through stretching and exercise will result in quick gains in functional activities that are challenging for the client due simply to loss of movement. Increasing a client's flexibility usually involves stretching of the tissues surrounding the affected joints. These tissues often have become shortened due to a decrease in activities that would normally stretch the tissues on a regular basis. Healthy tissue with less structural stiffness responds differently to stretching activities than unhealthy contracture, or scar, tissue. In general, tissue (e.g., muscle, connective tissue, and skin) increases in length when it undergoes a static stretch of low magnitude for a prolonged period of time (15 to 30 seconds), when it reaches the **plastic** range and remodels to a new length. Shorter-duration stretches result in a return of this tissue to its original, pre-stretch length, as it only reaches its **elastic** range. Tissue that has been lacerated, either surgically or non-surgically, and has scar tissue forming around it will benefit from a significantly longer period of low-load, static stretching lasting minutes, due to increased bonding of collagen fibers. This effect on the tissue—called "creep"—elongates the tissue over time, influencing the scar tissue to deform permanently, resulting in greater flexibility. A tissue generally responds best to stretching when its temperature is elevated (Kisner & Colby, 2007)—a concept often overlooked by less skilled fitness professionals. Thus, an ACE-AHFS's understanding of the mechanical, physical, and neurological properties of tissue will prepare him or her to skillfully apply a variety of stretching techniques to clients' programs and quickly have a positive impact on their lives.

The phase of recovery an exercise client is currently experiencing will determine the types of stretching activities an ACE-AHFS may choose. The safest type of activity to increase a client's flexibility is a static stretch, which is a prolonged (15 to 30 seconds), low-resistance hold of a position that will bring the tissues surrounding a joint into the plastic range and change their length. Other techniques commonly used by fitness professionals include passive, active-assisted, and active range of motion activities. These techniques are effective at maintaining the current degree of movement and length of tissues at a joint, as well as maintaining joint health by promoting the progress of fluids in and out of the joint. Ballistic stretching involves a quick, dynamic, bouncing movement at the end range of joint motion and is often used by athletes to prepare them to achieve this extended flexibility during a sporting event for a short time period. Ballistic stretching has a much higher risk for injury to the tissues surrounding the joint and is usually not used during a post-orthopedic rehabilitation phase. Another popular stretching technique that is appropriate for clients during their recovery is active inhibition/**proprioceptive neuromuscular facilitation (PNF).** The body's neuromuscular system works to balance the activities of **agonist** and **antagonist** muscle groups. For example, overloading an agonist muscle using an **isometric** contraction to the point of fatigue causes its antagonist muscle to readily contract while the agonist relaxes after the isometric hold (Kisner & Colby, 2007) (Figure 17-1). An astute ACE-AHFS can take advantage of this principle to stretch a client's agonist muscle, joint, and tissues by facilitating this response and holding the agonist in a stretched position (contract-relax), and even asking the client to help by contracting the antagonist during the hold (contract-relax-contract). This broader knowledge of techniques to improve a client's flexibility through increased range of motion will help the ACE-AHFS in his or her preparations to work with a wide range of clients, including those undergoing post-orthopedic rehabilitation.

Improving Aerobic Condition

Increased flexibility sets a strong foundation for further fitness improvements by reestablishing a normalized physical structure upon which to build. Greater elasticity of both skeletal and smooth muscle tissue lends itself to a greater capacity to generate increasing forces (Marieb & Hoehn, 2006). Specifically, if the smooth muscle of the heart is able to contract with greater force, more blood will be pumping through the body with fewer heart beats per minute, bringing more oxygen and nutrients throughout the body more efficiently. Thus, improving a client's basic cardiovascular condition through a variety of aerobic endurance exercises will improve the health of various physiologic systems (e.g., cardiovascular, digestive, immune, respiratory). In addition, the client's heart rate, blood pressure, and respiratory rate will decrease, while muscle tone, energy storage, and aerobic system capacity will increase. This aerobic enhancement will also improve a client's perception of well-being by increasing his or her functional abilities, as well as psychological and emotional stability.

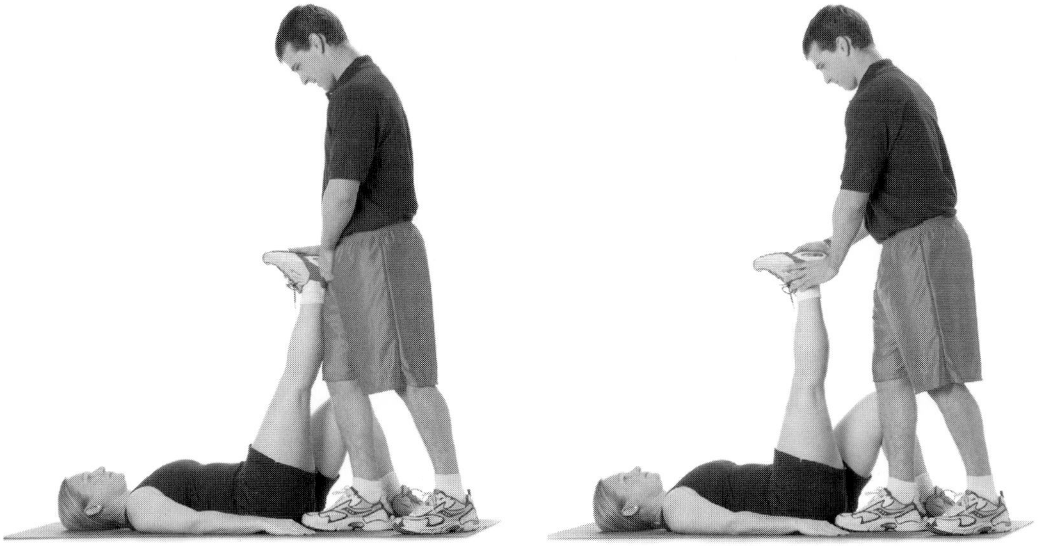

Figure 17-1
Proprioceptive neuromuscular facilitation (PNF): contraction followed by relaxation and a slow, passive stretch

Returning to Physical Activities

After seeing improvements in a client's flexibility and aerobic condition, an ACE-AHFS should continue advancing physical activities through exercise programming that distinctively mimics these movements and focuses on building the strength of the specific muscles used in performing them. Clients will benefit significantly from being able to return to their favorite recreations more often and with greater ease, whether it is bicycling , walking with a pet, or playing in the park with their children. The proprioceptive component of the body's nervous system supports the movements of a client's favorite activities through receptors in the joints (i.e., **proprioceptors**). Additionally, this system, through these peripherally (joints of the extremities) and centrally (vertebrae) located receptors, assists in the coordination of movement. Using activities requiring balance and agility, and coordinated movement patterns such as quick and repetitive upper- or lower-extremity movements, will enhance proprioception and make it easier for clients to participate in their recreational activities. Gradually building these abilities, for example, by having a client stand on one foot for 15 seconds and then progressing to a goal of standing for 60 seconds while tossing a ball, will build a client's self-confidence and clearly demonstrate a progression toward overall goals. A successful return to recreational activities is one of the most important components of exercise programming for a client with any injury, illness, disease, or other pathology, as it symbolizes a regaining of "normalcy." Improving clients' flexibility, aerobic condition, and recreational function will often effectively return them to their health status prior to diagnosis. At this point, continuing to enhance their health through strength-training activities will promote injury prevention and a life of improved wellness.

Building Strength and Power

Lastly, building the strength and power necessary in competitive sports and in some personal and career activities will offer clients the option of taking on new challenges in their lives or advancing their skills and talents in current activities. Some resistance-training activities may have been started earlier to slowly rebalance the strength of very specific muscles surrounding a client's diagnosis. These exercises may have been part of a treatment program directed by one of his or her rehabilitation medical professionals. Reviewing the home exercise program provided to the client by one of the medical team members will reveal a basic structure for building a strength program. In general, isometric exercises are safe to improve strength early after a post-orthopedic rehabilitation program and can be used at various degrees in the full range of motion of a joint. Since the tissues are not moving with resistance, there is less chance for irritation. The next step would be active-assisted resistance exercise in which the ACE-AHFS would assist the client with the resistance exercise, followed by active resistance exercise during which the client moves on his or her own. However, if the client has received any medical therapy treatments at all, he or she would likely come to the ACE-AHFS with the ability to safely and effectively perform light resistive exercise.

Understanding the various philosophies of strength exercise is important so that an appropriate program can be developed to avoid any exacerbations of signs and symptoms of a client's condition. For example, a post-surgical client may need to avoid a specific program of eccentric contractions to avoid tearing the surgical repair due to the higher stress on muscle fibers that are contracting while they are elongating. Additionally, longer periods of soreness may prevent clients from using one approach versus another, therefore requiring the ACE-AHFS to review and adjust the program more frequently. Even activities that are oriented toward a closed kinetic chain (i.e., upper and lower extremities in contact with a stable surface) need to be considered carefully and applied with purpose. Using alternative exercise equipment and environments may be necessary to create the most appropriate surroundings for the continued rehabilitation of the post-orthopedic client. Yoga or tai chi classes can improve flexibility and static strength, Pilates can help a client develop core stability, and aquatic exercise classes can be used to introduce resistance exercises in a slower, more controlled medium. A detailed understanding of the principles and applications of strength training is crucial to the successful development of the final phases of rehabilitation for post-orthopedic clients and their transition back into exercise as healthy individuals.

Overall, progressing post-orthopedic rehabilitation clients through a system of activities and exercises that do the following provides a consistent structure that will be highly successful for both the client and the ACE-AHFS:

- Improve the body's active range of motion and flexibility
- Enhance general conditioning and endurance
- Reintegrate clients into physical activity, recreation programs, and wellness
- Improve strength for competitive sports and manual labor challenges

Case Studies

Case Study 1

Having recently been discharged from physical therapy, Dorothy makes an appointment to see a "P.T." (physical therapist) to continue her recovery after surgery to simultaneously replace both of her hips. She ambulates into the facility at a pace within normal limits for a woman 62 years of age, using a cane but not heavily relying on it. She is energetic, friendly, and excited to get started on an exercise program that will help her return to her daily walks, recreational activities, and even occasional jogging.

Upon reviewing Dorothy's medical history (from standard forms that she was asked to complete), the ACE-AHFS discovers that her surgery was only six weeks ago and that she is living with her daughter in the immediate urban neighborhood where the exercise facility is located. She has been extremely active all of her life and a consistent exerciser through a variety of activities, including running. After physical testing, it becomes evident that she is more limited in her strength, cardiovascular endurance, and active range of motion than initially perceived. She also complains of pain, tightness, and fatigue that seem inconsistent with her presentation.

The first "red flag" in the initial assessment of this client are the inconsistencies with what she can achieve and how she initially presents. The ACE-AHFS should ask more questions and seek more information regarding this client.

Upon inquiry into her physical therapy treatment history and her precautions after surgery, it is discovered that Dorothy had been discharged from inpatient physical therapy and referred to outpatient physical therapy, with full hip active range of motion contraindications (i.e., no hip flexion past 90 degrees, no hip adduction beyond midline, and no hip internal rotation beyond neutral). She entered the health and wellness center seeking the "P.T." with whom she was given an appointment. Even though her remarkable presentation at this time is extremely impressive, Dorothy's hips have not fully healed and she is at risk for ruining her surgery if she neglects her contraindications and is progressed too intensely. This client should be referred to outpatient physical therapy immediately.

On the other hand, consider a situation in which this individual comes to the ACE-AHFS, who subsequently discovers that she does not have health insurance. Dorothy is able to pay for personal-training services and not physical therapy, in which case the ACE-AHFS may need to take on the client. Communication with Dorothy's physical therapist and medical doctor is crucial. Physical therapists are extremely helpful in these situations and contacting the physician's nurse with Dorothy's written permission may be the fastest way to get her surgical information from the physician. Additionally, contacting physical therapists in situations such as this is a great way to develop a relationship with them for future clients. Obey all contraindications [i.e., avoid sitting in low chairs to keep hip flexion (or trunk flexion) less than 90 degrees, avoid crossing legs with exercise to not adduct the hip past midline]; be mindful of the client getting in and out of machines or exercise positions so that hip internal rotation does not go beyond the neutral point; follow advice from the physical therapist; progress slowly while being mindful of pain, soreness, and tightness; and keep everyone informed with monthly progress reports and secure email or telephone communication. The ACE-AHFS should begin by focusing on increasing passive and active range of motion as allowed and gradually increasing Dorothy's strength to perform functional activities such as walking, carrying groceries, climbing stairs, and standing for prolonged periods of time. As Dorothy achieves these goals, she can progress to more intense community and recreational activities.

Case Study 2

Steven, a 63-year-old retired banker, enters the club and requests information about the services of an ACE-AHFS. Since he retired 10 years ago, he has been an avid golfer, going to the course about three times a week. However, a recent painful low-back episode has prevented him from participating in many of the physical activities he enjoys. His primary care physician diagnosed him with a severe muscle strain of the lumbar region and prescribed six weeks of physical therapy to reduce pain and improve the faulty posture habits that presumably caused the incident. Steven completed his physical therapy last week and has been cleared for regular physical activity. He claims to be pain free, but is hesitant to start golfing again due to his fear of becoming re-injured.

A program of general fitness should be initiated with Steven considering his goals of resuming golf and becoming more physically active again. Careful attention should be paid to Steven's subjective assessment of his pain and function during his exercise sessions with the ACE-AHFS. Low-back pain sufferers often have a strong fear of experiencing another painful episode, so this psychological component should be factored into the program by making it clear that Steven can address any concerns about any of the exercises with the ACE-AHFS.

Initially, the program should focus on functional range-of-motion activities that will enhance his ability to perform ADL and eventually play golf. Of high importance is conditioning Steven's core posture muscles and reeducating him about proper spinal alignment during all activities. After reviewing the home exercise program prescribed by his physical therapist, the ACE-AHFS can build the exercises through increases in complexity and intensity. As the client begins to feel strong and stable, reintroduction of golf-specific movements should be a priority, along with exercises to address the opposite muscles to maintain a healthy musculoskeletal balance (e.g., practicing golf swings with the opposite upper extremity).

Summary

Clients who utilize the services of an ACE-AHFS in continuing their rehabilitation after traditional medical treatments require an approach that is more attentive to the subtle, yet significant, changes that their recovering bodies present. Progressing any of the components of an exercise program too quickly can lead to re-injury, relapse, or exacerbation of signs and symptoms in the post-orthopedic rehabilitation client. The human body requires energy and physiologic support in the process of recovery and appropriate levels of stretching and exercise can help meet this requirement. Increases in the function of the cardiovascular system will enhance the transportation of oxygen and nutrients to the recovering areas of the body, and mild loading of the musculature involved will also assist in developing strength and health. However, excessive increases in stress to these systems due to overloading can rob the body of the energy it needs, resulting in a slowing of the healing process. The ACE-AHFS must understand that working with post-orthopedic rehabilitation clients involves a skillfully patient approach to exercise programming that requires recognition of subtle external changes that may represent significant internal reactions. A gradual progression and sound application of knowledge and skills, with focused attention on a client's physiologic response followed by sensitive and reasoned adjustments in programming, will result in the ACE-AHFS being singled out as an expert for post-orthopedic rehabilitation clientele.

Developing the ability to communicate this expertise through verbal and written interaction with the traditional medical team will result in the ACE-AHFS becoming a respected and trusted member. Having this support structure will lead to the opportunity to help more clients with medical conditions achieve a higher health status. Bringing enhanced wellness to post-orthopedic rehabilitation clients using these higher-level skills will enrich the lives of the clients, as well as the ACE-AHFS's life and career.

References

Denegar, C.R., Saliba, E., & Saliba, S. (2005). *Therapeutic Modalities for Musculoskeletal Injuries* (2nd ed.). Champaign, Ill.: Human Kinetics.

Kisner, C. & Colby, L.A. (2007). *Therapeutic Exercise Foundations and Techniques* (5th ed.). Philadelphia: F.A. Davis Company.

Marieb, E. & Hoehn, K. (2006). *Human Anatomy & Physiology* (7th ed.). San Francisco: Pearson Benjamin Cummings.

Suggested Reading

American Council on Exercise (2007). *Clinical Exercise Specialist Manual*. San Diego: American Council on Exercise.

American Council on Exercise (2003). *ACE Personal Trainer Manual* (3rd ed.). San Diego: American Council on Exercise.

Brimer, M. & Moran, M. (2003). *Clinical Cases in Physical Therapy* (2nd ed.). Boston: Butterworth-Heinemann.

Brotzman, S.B. & Wilk, K.E. (2003). *Clinical Orthopaedic Rehabilitation* (2nd ed.). St. Louis: Mosby.

Callahan, L. (2004). *The Fitness Factor.* New York: Lyons

Fox, S.I. (2007). *Human Physiology* (10th ed.). New York: McGraw-Hill.

Frownfelter, D. & Dean, E. (1996). *Principles and Practice of Cardiopulmonary Physical Therapy* (3rd ed.). St. Louis: Mosby.

Kendall, F., McCreary, E. & Provance, P. (2005). *Muscles: Testing and Function with Posture and Pain* (5th ed.). Philadelphia: Lippincott Williams & Wilkins.

Kisner, C. & Colby, L.A. (2007). *Therapeutic Exercise Foundations and Techniques* (5th ed.). Philadelphia: F.A. Davis Company.

Levangie, P.L. & Norkin, C.C. (2005). *Joint Structure & Function* (4th ed.). Philadelphia: F.A. Davis Company.

Magee, D. (2008). *Orthopedic Physical Assessment* (5th ed.). Philadelphia: W.B. Saunders.

McArdle, W.D., Katch, F.I., & Katch, V.L. (2006). *Exercise Physiology: Energy, Nutrition and Human Performance* (6th ed.). Philadelphia: Lippincott Williams & Wilkins.

O'Sullivan, S.B. & Schmitz, T.J. (2006). *Physical Rehabilitation Assessment and Treatment* (5th ed.). Philadelphia: F.A. Davis Company.

Reid, D.C. (2008). *Sports Injury Assessment and Rehabilitation* (2nd ed.). New York: Churchill Livingstone.

Torg, J.S. & Shephard, R.J. (1995). *Current Therapy in Sports Medicine* (3rd ed.). St. Louis: Mosby.

In This Chapter

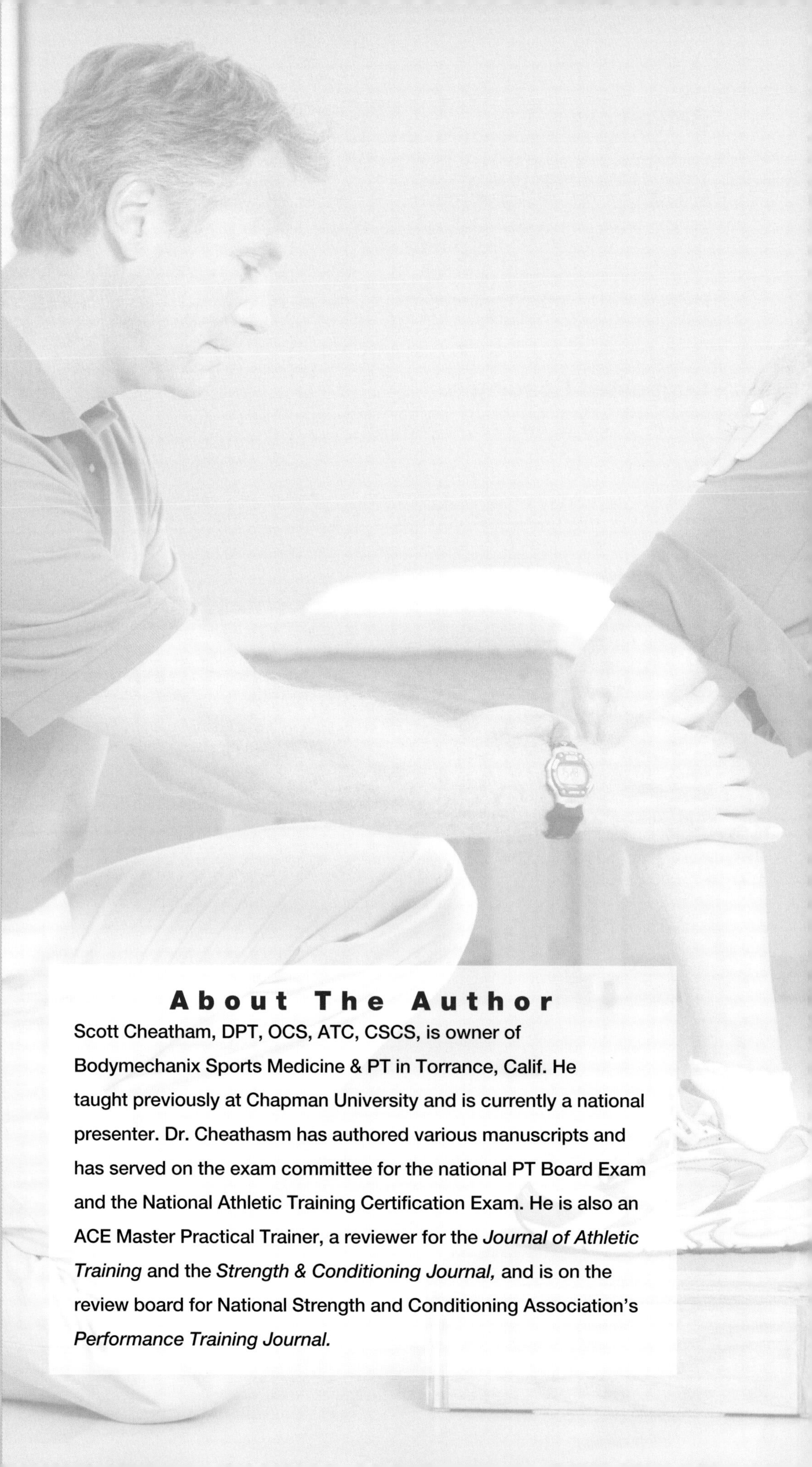

About The Author

Scott Cheatham, DPT, OCS, ATC, CSCS, is owner of Bodymechanix Sports Medicine & PT in Torrance, Calif. He taught previously at Chapman University and is currently a national presenter. Dr. Cheathasm has authored various manuscripts and has served on the exam committee for the national PT Board Exam and the National Athletic Training Certification Exam. He is also an ACE Master Practical Trainer, a reviewer for the *Journal of Athletic Training* and the *Strength & Conditioning Journal,* and is on the review board for National Strength and Conditioning Association's *Performance Training Journal.*

CHAPTER 18

Musculoskeletal Injuries of the Lower Extremity

Scott Cheatham

The fitness industry has evolved tremendously in recent years due to changes in America's healthcare system. Patients are being discharged from rehabilitation early and are being referred to fitness professionals for further guidance. The current demands require the ACE-certified Advanced Health & Fitness Specialist (ACE-AHFS) to have a broad base of knowledge about common medical and post-operative conditions to create safe, effective programs.

This chapter focuses on common musculoskeletal injuries of the lower extremity. Particular attention will be placed on recognition, management, and restorative exercise guidelines for the selected topics. A thorough understanding of common non-operative and post-operative musculoskeletal conditions is necessary to make accurate assessments and to know when to refer to other healthcare professionals.

Screening the Client

In addition to the general health information obtained from questionnaires such as the **Physical Activity Readiness Questionnaire (PAR-Q)**, more specific screening questions are needed to obtain a complete history from the client. It is important to understand what interventions have been done and at what stage in the healing process the client is currently. The following screening questions are recommended prior to designing a restorative program:

- How did the injury happen (i.e., the mechanism of injury)?
- Did the client see his or her physician? If yes, what treatment has been done (e.g., surgery, physical therapy, oral medications, cortisone injection)?
- Did the physician issue any exercise precautions or contraindications (e.g., limit walking to 15 minutes)?
- What type of symptoms is the client feeling (e.g., "sharp" pain when walking on the treadmill)?
- Does the client have any functional limitations (e.g., unable to lift objects overhead)?
- What is the client's tolerance to activity (e.g., "feeling fatigue" after 10 minutes of treadmill walking)?

These questions will help guide the ACE-AHFS in answering the single most important question: Is this client appropriate for exercise at this time?

Principles of Restorative Exercise

The design of a restorative exercise program needs to be specific to the client's goals and functional abilities. Typically, when a client is recovering from an injury or is post-surgical, restorative exercise programs can help him or her regain flexibility, strength, **proprioception,** and endurance, and provide positive progress toward more functional or sport-specific activities. There are many different approaches to designing a restorative exercise program. The most effective programs take into account the individual's functional abilities, recovery status (e.g., stage of healing), prior activity level, comorbidities (e.g., **diabetes**), and goals (Brotzman & Wilk, 2003). If a post-injury or post-surgical client undergoes rehabilitation, the physical therapist typically addresses these principles. Typically, the role of the ACE-AHFS is to progress what has been done in rehabilitation and help the client transition back to full function. The timelines given for returning to fitness activities are general recommendations and may be different among individuals due to the doctor's guidelines. In fact, the ACE-AHFS may see these clients earlier in the timeline based on their unique situation. For each topic discussed in this chapter, exercise recommendations are categorized into flexibility, strengthening, and functional integration. These categories are given for organization and ease of reference.

Flexibility

Flexibility is defined as the **range of motion (ROM)** of a joint, which can be limited by joint structure, neuromuscular coordination, muscle strength of opposing groups, and the mobility of the soft tissues (e.g., muscles, ligaments, and connective tissue) associated with the joint (Brotzman & Wilk, 2003). Most flexibility programs utilize various forms of stretching and **myofascial release** to achieve the desired level of flexibility. Common techniques include static stretching, **proprioceptive neuromuscular facilitation (PNF)**, and myofascial release using a foam roller.

Strengthening

Strengthening of the post-injury or post-surgical client is very important to the success of the program. When an individual is recovering, there may be a decline in neuromuscular control, muscular strength, and local muscular endurance. Utilizing **progressive resistive exercises (PREs)** will ensure adequate progression of strength and endurance. This technique uses the **overload** principle to challenge the client as he or she gets stronger. Increasing the weight by 5% with each set is an example of PREs. The goal is to safely overload the tissue in a progressive fashion.

Strengthening exercises can be classified into two main categories: open kinetic chain (OKC) and closed kinetic chain (CKC). OKC exercises are non-weightbearing, with the distal end (e.g., the foot) free, and involve isolating a specific muscle group. The leg extension machine and sidelying hip abduction are examples of open chain activities. CKC exercises have the distal end fixed and are typically more functional. Examples include squats and lunges. CKC exercises are often thought to be superior due to joint compression, muscle co-contraction, and increased functionality (Manske, 2006).

Functional Integration

Functional training describes specific activities that help to train the body for activities performed in life (Brotzman & Wilk, 2003). This term is used here to describe the integration of restorative exercise principles, which include flexibility, strength training, and proprioception.

Proprioception can be defined as a person's awareness of his or her body in space. Proprioception is part of the sensory system that detects joint movement (**kinesthesia**) and joint position (proprioception). Balance is dependent on sensory receptors, which are located in muscles, skin, tendons, ligaments, and joints. The **central nervous system (CNS)** receives input from these receptors along with visual and vestibular input, which are used to control body position and balance (Anderson, Hall, & Parr, 2008). When injury occurs, these pathways can be diminished due to trauma or disuse, which leads to poor balance and increased risk for injury. Retraining these pathways is necessary to maintain adequate neuromuscular control during functional and athletic activities. Proprioceptive exercises must be specific to the activity and should follow a graduated progression that includes the following principles: slow to fast, low force to high force, and controlled to uncontrolled movement (Anderson, Hall, & Parr, 2008).

Therefore, functional integration represents exercises that are specific to the activity or sport and reflect the client's physical abilities and performance goals. Specific functional integration strategies are discussed along with cardiovascular recommendations for the specific topics covered in this chapter.

Hip Pathologies

The Iliotibial Band Complex

The iliotibial band (ITB) complex is a band of fibrous connective tissue (**fascia**) on the outside of the femur that goes from the hip to the knee. Proximally, the gluteals and tensor fasciae latae (TFL) both blend into the upper fibers of the ITB. This is the region where **trochanteric bursitis** occurs. The lower fibers of the ITB attach distally to the proximal anterolateral tibia (Gerdy's tubercle) and also attach to the patella and biceps femoris via fascial connections (Brotzman & Wilk, 2003). This is also the region where **iliotibial band friction syndrome (ITBFS)** occurs. The function of the ITB complex is to serve as a shock absorber and lateral stabilizer. Problems in this complex are common among both active and sedentary individuals (Brotzman & Wilk, 2003). Acute or repetitive overuse can tighten the ITB complex, resulting in microtears of the fascia that can lead to scar tissue and functional shortening of the ITB over time (Brotzman & Wilk, 2003; Foye & Stitik, 2006).

Trochanteric Bursitis

Trochanteric bursitis is characterized by painful inflammation of the trochanteric bursa between the greater trochanter of the femur and the gluteus medius/iliotibial complex (Bierma-Zeinstra et al., 1999). This condition is becoming more common; approximately 10 to 20% of patients seeing their doctors for hip problems have pain over the trochanteric region (Bierma-Zeinstra et al., 1999). This condition is more common in female runners, cross country skiers, and ballet dancers (Lievense, Bierma-Zeinstra, & Schouten, 2005; Anderson, Hall, & Parr, 2008). Inflammation of the bursa may be due to an acute incident or repetitive (cumulative) trauma. Acute incidents may include trauma from falls, contact sports (e.g., football), and other sources of impact. Repetitive trauma may be due to excessive friction by the ITB. Factors such as prolonged running, an increase or change in activity, leg-length discrepancy, and lateral hip surgery have been described as causes of repetitive trauma (Foye & Stitik, 2006). Research shows a higher prevalence rate of trochanteric bursitis with low-back pain and **osteoarthritis** of the hip (Lievense, Bierma-Zeinstra, & Schouten, 2005; Foye & Stitik, 2006).

Iliotibial Band Friction Syndrome

Iliotibial band friction syndrome (ITBFS) is a repetitive overuse condition that occurs when the distal portion of the iliotibial band rubs against the lateral femoral epicondyle (Brotzman & Wilk, 2003; Anderson, Hall, & Parr, 2008). As the knee moves from full extension to approximately 30 degrees of flexion, the ITB moves from an anterior position to the lateral femoral epicondyle to a posterior position. The repeated flexion and extension of the knee causes the ITB to pass back and forth over the lateral femoral epicondyle, leading to irritation and inflammation (Brotzman & Wilk, 2003). ITBFS is common among active individuals 15 to 50 years of age and is primarily caused by training errors during running, cycling, playing volleyball, and weightlifting (Martinez & Honsik, 2006; Anderson, Hall, & Parr, 2008). Risk factors may include overtraining, changes in running surface, structural abnormalities (**pes planus,** bow-legs, and leg-length discrepancy), muscle imbalance, and muscle tightness (Martinez & Honsik, 2006; Brotzman & Wilk, 2003). Signs and symptoms, precautions, and restorative exercise strategies for both pathologies are discussed in the following sections.

Signs and Symptoms of Trochanteric Bursitis and ITBFS

Trochanteric bursitis pain and/or parasthesias (i.e., tingling, prickling, and numbness) often radiate from the greater trochanter to the posterior lateral hip, down the iliotibial tract, to the lateral knee (Little, 1979). Symptoms are most often related to an increase in activity or repetitive overuse. Aggravating activities may include lying on the affected side, prolonged walking/running, and certain hip movements (internal and external rotation). Deficits in hip strength, ROM, and gait may be present secondary to the pain. The client may walk with a limp (i.e., **Trendelenburg gait**) due to pain or weakness. He or she may develop a compensation pattern through the painful limb that directly affects the lower kinetic chain. This may result in decreased muscle length (e.g., in the quadriceps or hamstrings), myofascial tightness (e.g., in the ITB complex), and weak, inhibited muscles.

Clients with ITBFS often report a gradual onset of tightness, burning, or pain at the lateral aspect of the knee during activity. The pain may be localized, but generally radiates to the outside of the knee and/or up the outside of the thigh. Snapping, popping, or pain may be felt at the lateral knee when it is flexed and extended (Brotzman & Wilk, 2003; Anderson, Hall, & Parr, 2008; Martinez & Honsik, 2006). Aggravating factors may include any repetitive activity such as running (especially downhill) or cycling. Symptoms often resolve with rest but can increase in intensity and frequency if not properly treated. The client may present with weakness in the hip abductors, ITB shortening, and tenderness throughout the ITB complex (Martinez & Honsik, 2006; Brotzman & Wilk, 2003).

Precautions

There are no direct precautions for either trochanteric bursitis or ITBFS. Clients are advised to avoid any aggravating activities and return to activity in a slow, systematic manner. When a client is ready to return to fitness activities, a written clearance from his or her physician may be necessary. More specifically, clarification from the physician or physical therapist regarding what the client can and cannot do would help guide the ACE-AHFS when designing the restorative exercise program.

Early Intervention

Conservative treatment of trochanteric bursitis and ITBFS often includes avoiding aggravating activities, physical therapy, modalities (e.g., ice, heat), assistive devices (e.g., a cane), oral anti-inflammatory medication, cortisone injections, or surgery (Foye & Stitik, 2006). Once the client is cleared for more advanced activity, the restorative exercise program should progress from what has already been done in treatment and rehabilitation.

Restorative Exercise Program for Trochanteric Bursitis and ITBFS

When designing the program, the ACE-AHFS should include client education. Important components include proper training techniques, appropriate footwear, and early injury recognition. The client should be pain free with activity and should be reminded to use ice after the workouts to prevent any latent discomfort or inflammation. The following restorative exercise principles are recommended.

Flexibility

For trochanteric bursitis and ITBFS, muscle tightness and myofascial restrictions should be addressed to restore proper length and symmetry to the hip and thigh region. Particular emphasis should be placed on the ITB complex and the surrounding muscles. Due to their fascial connections, tightness or decreased length in the biceps femoris, vastus lateralis, and gluteus medius can directly impair mobility. Tightness often leads to friction over the proximal greater trochanteric bursa or the distal femoral epicondyle. These muscle and fascial connections are often called the mechanical interface to the ITB complex. Stretching should target these areas and may include static stretching, assisted PNF stretching, and myofascial release of the ITB complex using a foam roller (Figure 18-1).

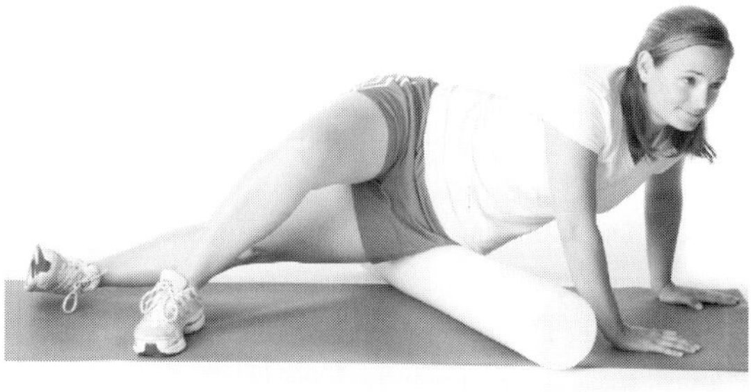

Figure 18-1
Self–myofascial release of the ITB complex with foam roller

Strengthening

For both conditions, the focus of strengthening should be to restore proper neuromuscular control throughout the hip region and abdominal core. The gluteals, hip abductors, adductors, and external rotators should be the focus of strengthening. At this point, isolated open-chain strengthening may still be necessary due to local weakness, endurance deficits, and poor muscle recruitment. Examples of isolated hip exercises include side-lying abduction and adduction, and side-lying hip abduction/external rotation "clams" (Figure 18-2).

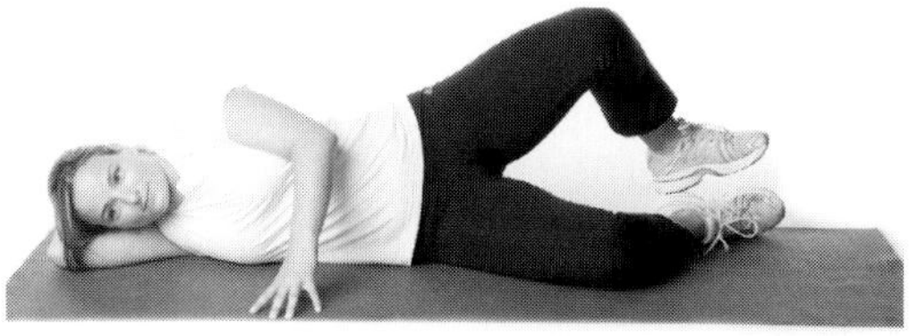

Figure 18-2
Side-lying "clams" for hip external rotator muscles

Functional Integration

For both pathologies, the functional program should focus on challenging the abdominal core and hip complex. CKC exercise can be introduced to integrate more functional activity, which can be progressed in all planes of motion (Table 18-1). Challenging the client through functional exercise will help to prepare him or her for more advanced activity or sport-specific training.

Deficits in general balance may be evident due to disuse of the kinetic chain. Basic progression of balance activities can be combined with CKC activities to challenge the client. For example, a single-leg squat on an air-filled disc combines CKC and proprioceptive exercise. Simply combining an unstable surface with different modes of exercise can be an efficient way of challenging a client (Table 18-2).

Cardiovascular conditioning is essential for recovery and overall health. The client should return to cardiovascular activity in a slow, progressive manner. Running, prolonged walking, and cycling have been associated with both trochanteric bursitis and ITBFS. Cardiovascular activities such as riding a stationary bike or using an elliptical trainer can be alternatives until the client is cleared to continue with higher-loading activities.

Table 18-1
Suggested Close Kinetic Chain Progression for the Lower Extremity

Plane of Motion	Exercise Progression (Easy → Hard)
Sagittal plane	Leg press machine → wall squats with ball → forward lunges → stair walking → bilateral squats on a foam pad → bilateral squats on air-filled discs or a BOSU® → single-leg squats on the ground → single-leg squats on a foam pad → single-leg squats on an air filled disc or BOSU
Frontal plane	Side stepping on a level surface → side stepping up onto a step → side stepping with bands → side stepping (fast) with ball passing → slide board
Combined planes	Multidirectional lunges → single-leg balance with multidirectional toe touch → single-leg reach → multidirectional hops (bilateral) → multidirectional hops (single leg)

Table 18-2
Suggested Balance Progressions

Difficulty Level	Exercise Progression (Easy→Hard)
Level I (bilateral balance)	Ground → mini-trampoline → foam pad → air-filled discs → BOSU® → wobble board
Level II (single limb—basic)	Ground → mini-trampoline → foam pad → air-filled discs → BOSU → wobble board
Level III (single limb—advanced)	Level II progression with ball tossing → head turning (up/down or side/side) → head diagonals → eyes closed Manipulate time and speed of movement

Hip Osteoarthritis

Osteoarthritis Facts

Osteoarthritis (OA), or **degenerative joint disease,** is the most common form of arthritis. Buckwalter and Martin (2006) report that approximately 20 million Americans have OA, and the World Health Organization (WHO) estimates that about 10% of the world's population over the age of 60 has the disease. The disease affects men and women equally; however, women tend to have earlier, more severe symptoms (Lawrence et al., 1998).

OA develops from the degeneration of joint cartilage and supporting structures, and changes in the underlying bone structure. This leads to stiffness, pain, mobility problems, and limited physical activity [Arthritis Foundation/Centers for Disease Control & Prevention (CDC), 1999]. This degeneration is caused by a physiologic imbalance between the stress applied to the joint and the ability of the joint to endure the stress. Simply put, osteoarthritis develops when breakdown (i.e., **catabolism**) exceeds regrowth (i.e., cartilage synthesis).

OA commonly affects joints of the hand, knee, hip, foot, and spine. The true or cause of osteoarthritis is unknown. However, certain risk factors are present (Hinton et al., 2002):

- Obesity
- Prior injury
- Age (older than 50)
- Immobilization
- Hypermobile or unstable joints
- Peripheral neuropathy (e.g., from diabetes)
- Muscle weakness
- Prolonged mechanical joint stress (e.g., sports or occupational)

Signs and Symptoms of Hip Arthritis

A client with hip arthritis may complain of a "deep aching" pain in the anterior hip with weightbearing activity and "stiffness" after inactivity (less than 30 minutes). The client may have activity limitations due to restricted, painful motion or a feeling of instability. The hip joint may be tender to touch, swollen, and have **crepitation** (i.e., grinding or crackling sensation) (Brotzman & Wilk, 2003).

Precautions

These clients must limit prolonged weightbearing activities, shock loading (e.g., running), and repetitive squatting. Specific activities to avoid include deep squats or lunges, knee extensions, and plyometric activity. Light-to-moderate activity is recommended due to the diminished shock-absorbing capacity of the joint.

Early Intervention

Early intervention includes patient education, physical therapy (e.g., ROM exercises, strengthening), weight loss, supportive devices (e.g., cane or bracing), oral anti-inflammatory medication, cortisone injections, and modalities (e.g., heat, ice) (Brotzman & Wilk, 2003).

Restorative Exercise Program

Management of hip OA includes progressing what was done in the early intervention. The focus of the program should be on light- to moderate-loading exercises that are specific to the client's needs.

Flexibility

Due to the stiffness of the hip joint and surrounding tissues, clients may have global restrictions, as opposed to restrictions related to one specific movement such as hip internal or external rotation. Flexibility exercises should be done at a level that does not elicit pain and is within a comfortable ROM. Stretching should focus on the surrounding hip muscles, including the gluteals, hamstrings, hip adductors, hip abductors, and hip external rotators.

Strengthening

The focus of strengthening should be to restore proper strength throughout the hip region and abdominal core. Specific OKC exercises, such as side-lying hip abduction, side-lying hip adduction, clams, prone hip extension, and seated internal or external rotation with a band can help to isolate the muscles that control the hip (Figures 18-3 and 18-4). CKC exercises should be progressed with caution. As mentioned earlier, light- to moderate-loading exercises are best for these clients. Exercises such as deep squatting or lunging can excessively load the joint and elicit pain. Midrange activity such as partial squats or lunges may be tolerable and can be progressed to single-leg movements.

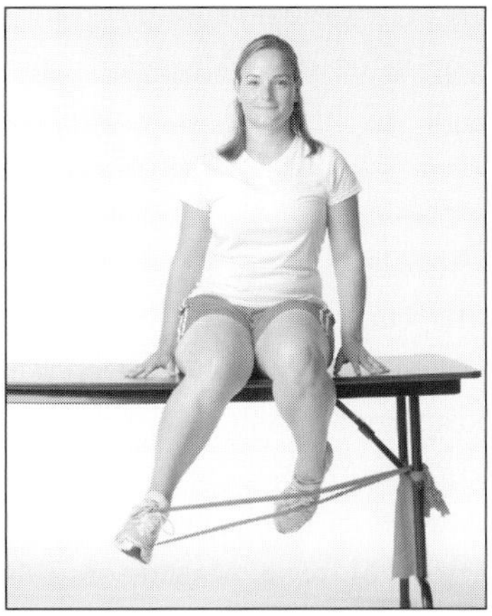

Figure 18-3
Seated hip external rotation

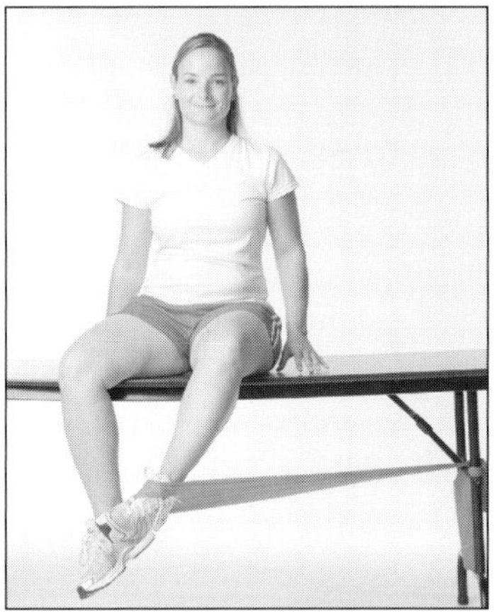

Figure 18-4
Seated hip internal rotation

Functional Integration

The combination of adequate flexibility, strength, and aerobic conditioning is vital for the success of the client. Functional activity should integrate all of these principles, but needs to follow the precautions mentioned earlier. Aquatic exercise is a great way to integrate basic functional activity while de-weighting the joint. The warmth and buoyancy of the water creates a great medium for exercise for these clients. A greater understanding of the science behind aquatic exercise is essential for the ACE-AHFS when working with individuals who have arthritis (Bonelli, 2001).

Deficits in general balance may be evident due to disuse of the kinetic chain. Basic progression of balance activities would be appropriate if no pain is elicited. Table 18-2 highlights a progressive program for balance.

Cardiovascular activity should be included to build cardiovascular and local muscular endurance. The bike or elliptical trainer is preferred over treadmill walking due to their mild-to-moderate joint loading. Other low-loading activities include swimming and water walking.

Total Hip Replacement

Total hip replacement or total hip arthroplasty is a surgical procedure where the head of the femur and the surface of the acetabulum are replaced with a prosthetic "ball and socket." The "ball" replaces the head of the femur and the "socket" is the cup-shaped form of the acetabulum. Total hip replacement is one of the most common surgical procedures performed in the United States. In 2004, 234,000 procedures were done, with patients at an average of 66 years of age (U.S. Department of Health and Human Services, 2004).

This procedure is commonly done to correct intractable damage from osteoarthritis, **rheumatoid arthritis,** hip fractures, **avascular necrosis,** and **cerebral palsy** (Maxey & Magnusson, 2007). Contraindications, or factors that would prevent the surgical procedure, may include **osteoporosis,** ligament **laxity,** infection, medical risk factors (e.g., diabetes), and poor patient motivation (Maxey & Magnusson, 2007). It is important for the ACE-AHFS to understand that a total hip replacement is an end-stage procedure for the client. Typically, the client has suffered with a painful, stiff joint for some time and may have tried conservative treatment such as oral medications, injections, and physical therapy. When these conservative approaches have failed, replacing the joint is often the best option. The primary goals of the procedure are to replace the diseased joint and to decrease or eliminate pain.

There are three commonly used procedures conducted by surgeons. First, primary total hip replacementis when the whole joint is replaced with three components: a synthetic cup that replaces the acetabulum (plastic, ceramic, or metal); a ball that replaces the femoral head (highly polished metal or ceramic material); and a metal stem that is secured in the medullary canal of the proximal femur (Maxey & Magnusson, 2007). Second, a **hemiarthroplasty,** or partial hip replacement, involves only half of the joint and includes replacing the ball portion of the joint, but not the socket portion. This procedure is commonly used to treat hip fractures or avascular necrosis of the hip (Maxey & Magnusson, 2007). Third, for younger active individuals (less than 55 years of age), hip resurfacing can be done. This procedure includes resurfacing and reshaping only the femoral head with a shell or cap. Hip resurfacing is a common alternative to primary total hip replacement because it leaves more of the bone in place and does not remove the femoral neck shaft. Therefore, the procedure may give the patient more time before having to replace the whole joint (Cioppa-Mosca et al., 2006).

Primary total hip replacement is the most common among the three procedures. The success of the surgery depends on factors such as surgical technique, patient selection, type of implant, and method of fixation (Cioppa-Mosca et al., 2006). There are three main surgical procedures for primary total hip replacement currently used by surgeons. It is important for the ACE-AHFS to have a working knowledge of these procedures.

Posterior Lateral Approach

This technique includes cutting the hip external rotators (i.e., piriformis, gemelli, obturators, quadratus femoris, and gluteus maximus) and posterior hip capsule with an incision between the gluteus maximus and medius (Maxey & Magnusson, 2007). This technique spares the hip abductors but makes the hip susceptible to posterior dislocation, because the posterior supporting structures are cut to perform the surgery. Due to this trauma, surgeons require individuals to follow specific movement precautions. In general, the individual should avoid the following (Maxey & Magnusson, 2007):

- Hip flexion greater than 90 degrees
- Hip adduction past the midline of the body
- Hip internal rotation past neutral

Typically, these precautions are followed for the first eight weeks, but can last up to one year depending on the individual and the surgeon's preference (Cioppa-Mosca et al., 2006). The reported benefits of this approach include preservation of the hip abductors and surgeon familiarity. The primary risk of this procedure is posterior dislocation (Maxey & Magnusson, 2007).

Anterior Lateral Approach

This surgical procedure utilizes a lateral curved incision that cuts through the gluteus minimus, gluteus maximus, tensor fasciae latae, vastus lateralis, and anterior capsule. The technique spares the posterior elements of the hip (i.e., hip external rotators, posterior capsule), but does violate the hip abductors (Maxey & Magnusson, 2007). Movement restrictions also apply with this procedure. In general, the patient should avoid the following (Maxey & Magnusson, 2007):

- Combined hip external rotation and flexion
- Hip adduction past the midline of the body
- Hip internal rotation beyond neutral

As with the posterior lateral approach, these restrictions are followed for the first eight weeks, but can last up to one year depending on the individual and the surgeon's preference (Maxey & Magnusson, 2007). The reported benefits of this procedure are preservation of the posterior elements and a decreased dislocation rate (Maxey & Magnusson, 2007). However, the risks include the onset of a post-operative limp due to disruption of the abductor tendon or injury to the superior gluteal nerve (Maxey & Magnusson, 2007).

Anterior Approach

This surgical procedure is more current and has fewer post-operative restrictions. The procedure utilizes an anterior incision between the tensor fasciae latae and sartorius, which affects only the anterior capsule (Kennon et al., 2004; Matta, Shahrdar, & Ferguson, 2005). The anterior incision does not violate the contractile (e.g., hip external rotators and abductors) and connective tissues (e.g., hip capsule) around the hip, except for the surgical site. The procedure is done on a special table that positions the patient supine, allowing clear access to the hip joint. This procedure has two general movement precautions. The patient should avoid the following (Kennon et al., 2004; Matta, Shahrdar, & Ferguson, 2005):

- Hyperextension of the hip
- Extreme hip external rotation

These precautions may only be relative depending on the surgeon. In fact, some surgeons have given no post-operative precautions with this procedure. The reported benefits include preservation of the hip muscles, decreased dislocation rate, normal hip mechanics, and true pelvic and leg alignment. Negligible post-operative complications have been reported with this procedure (Kennon et al., 2004; Matta, Shahrdar, & Ferguson, 2005).

Precautions

High-impact activities such as running, football, basketball, soccer, karate, waterskiing, and racquetball should be avoided following total hip replacement (Maxey & Magnusson, 2007). These activities may cause abnormal stress to the prosthetic joint. As mentioned earlier, there may be certain movement restrictions depending on the procedure.

Early Intervention

Typically, the client has been discharged from the hospital and is transitioning from home therapy to outpatient rehabilitation. Outpatient physical therapy will help the client move back to more functional activities. It is not uncommon for clients to be severely deconditioned and have post-operative pain during this phase. The focus is on improving basic strength, functional ability, range of motion, and endurance within the precautions prescribed by the physician. Management of the scar and soft-tissue restrictions will often be addressed through massage, stretching, and myofascial release.

Restorative Exercise Program

The ACE-AHFS may begin to see the client between six and 12 weeks after surgery. Typically, the client may do a combination of physical therapy and fitness activities. Prior to working with these clients, it is important for the ACE-AHFS to talk with the physician and/or physical therapist to find out the client's status. Specific questions to ask include the following:

- Does the client have any movement restrictions or medical precautions?
- Did the client attend physical therapy? If yes, what types of exercises were performed for aerobic and anaerobic activity?
- Does the client have any functional limitations?

A restorative program needs to progress systematically to avoid unnecessary pain or possible re-injury. When the client is still under movement restrictions, it is important to program exercises that do not violate the prescribed hip precautions (Table 18-3). If precautions are lifted, the client may be progressed as tolerated. The client should be monitored

Table 18-3
Movement Restrictions Following Total Hip Replacement

Hip Precautions	Posterior Lateral Approach	Anterior Lateral Approach	Anterior Approach
Flexion >90 degrees	Deep squats, lunges, yoga poses	Deep squats, lunges, yoga poses	—
Adduction (past midline)	Side-lying adduction, stretching the leg across midline	Side-lying adduction, stretching the leg across midline	—
Internal rotation	Yoga poses	Yoga poses	—
External rotation	—	Yoga poses, seated groin stretch, sitting with legs crossed	Yoga poses, seated groin stretch, sitting with legs crossed
Hyperextension	—	—	Lunges, prone hip extension

for surgical-site pain during and after training sessions. This pain is often described as "sharp or stabbing" rather than the typical low-grade "muscle ache" [i.e., **delayed onset muscle soreness (DOMS)**] that is often felt following a vigorous workout session.

The ACE-AHFS must remember that factors such as age, pre-existing medical conditions, nutritional status, prior fitness level, and client motivation will influence the client's program. There are many published post-operative protocols for primary total hip replacement. However, most surgeons have developed their own protocols based on the type of surgery, their own preferences, and available research. Reviewing specific protocols is beyond the scope of this text. The specific recommendations presented here for each category are based on the idea that the client has no motion restrictions and is cleared for fitness activities.

Flexibility

General stretching should be included to address any muscle tightness or myofascial restrictions. Static stretching, assisted PNF stretching, and self–myofascial release may be done at a mild-to-moderate level that does not stress the surgical site or hip prosthesis. A good rule is for the client to stretch into "slight or mild discomfort" but not into "pain." Particular emphasis should be placed on the gluteals, ITB complex, hamstrings, and quadriceps. Self–myofascial release should not cause "pain" that is more intense that the typical "discomfort" that is felt with this technique. Muscle groups that should be targeted include the gluteals/external rotators (Figure 18-5), ITB complex (see Figure 18-1), hamstrings (Figure 18-6), and quadriceps (Figure 18-7).

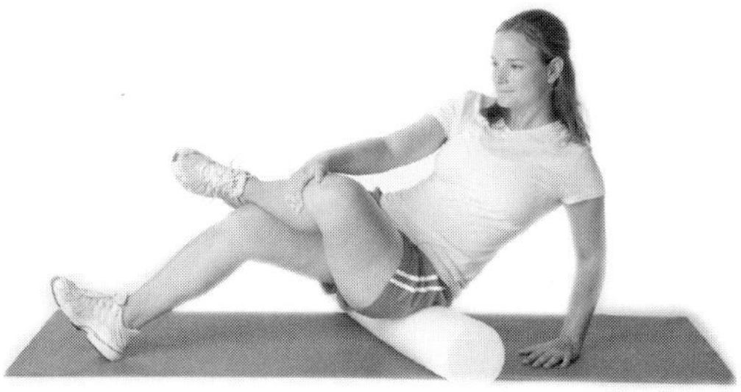

Figure 18-5
Myofascial release for gluteals/external rotators

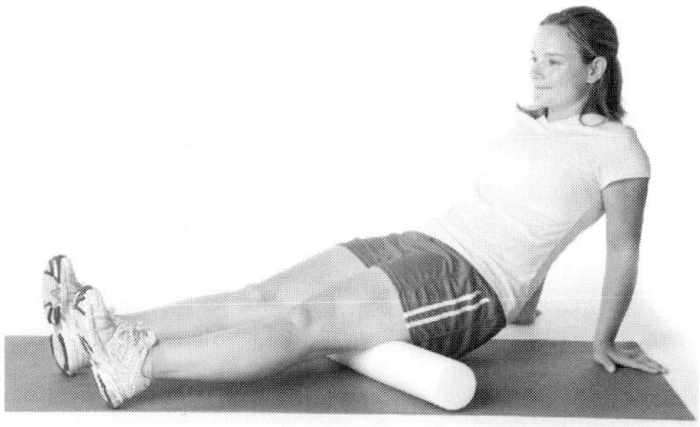

Figure 18-6
Myofascial release for the hamstrings

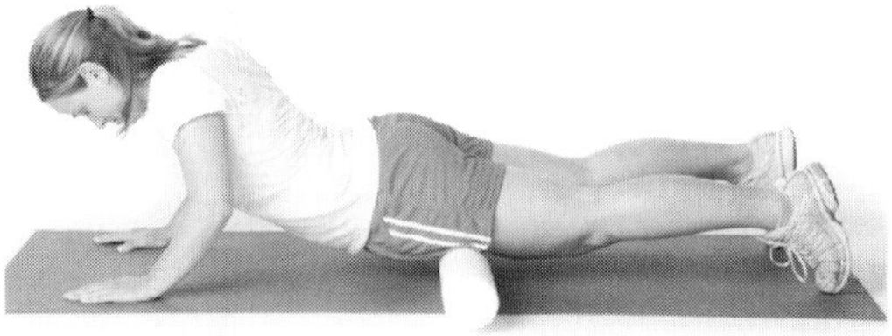

Figure 18-7
Myofascial release for the quadriceps

Strengthening

These clients are generally deconditioned and may need an initial program that focuses on building local strength and endurance throughout the hip region and abdominal core. Early fitness activity may include isolated hip open-chain strengthening using lighter resistance with higher repetitions to improve local strength, endurance, and muscle recruitment. The goal should be to restore proper strength and neuromuscular control prior to advancing to functional activity.

Functional Integration

The functional program should challenge the abdominal core and lumbo-pelvic-hip complex in all planes of motion, but must be progressed from basic functional activities. The post-operative client may be at a lower functional level than a relatively healthy client. Basic functional tasks such as sit-to-stand, rolling in bed, stair climbing, and picking up objects may still be difficult. The client may need to master these basic skills prior to progressing with the CKC exercises.

Deficits in general balance may be evident due to disuse of the kinetic chain. Remember, basic functional ability should be obtained prior to implementing balance activity. Early balance activity can be combined with basic functional tasks. For example, the client can do the sit-to-stand exercise with a foam pad under his or her feet or pick up objects while standing on two air-filled discs. When appropriate, the client can be progressed with balance activity.

Cardiovascular conditioning is essential for recovery in the post-operative client. Cardiovascular activity should be within physician guidelines and general precautions. Low-loading activities such as water aerobics, stationary cycling, and elliptical training are all good alternatives to higher-loading activities such as running.

Knee Pathologies

Patellofemoral Pain Syndrome

Patellofemoral pain syndrome (PFPS) is often called "anterior knee pain" or "runner's knee." This syndrome has been found to be the most common knee diagnosis in the outpatient setting and to have the highest prevalence among runners. In fact, PFPS makes up 16 to 25% of all running injuries (Dixit et al., 2007). The etiology of PFPS is often considered multifactorial and can be classified into three primary categories: overuse, biomechanical, and muscle dysfunction.

Mechanism of Injury

Overuse

PFPS is often classified as an overuse syndrome when repetitive loading activities (e.g., climbing and/or descending stairs or hills) or sports (e.g., running) are the cause of symptoms. These repetitive activities cause abnormal stress to the knee joint, which leads to pain and dysfunction. The excessive loading exceeds the body's physiological balance, which leads to tissue trauma, injury, and pain (Dixit et al., 2007). Recent changes in intensity, frequency, duration, and training environment (e.g., surface) may contribute to this condition.

Biomechanical

Biomechanical abnormalities can alter tracking of the patella and/or increase patellofemoral joint stress (Dixit et al., 2007). Pes planus, or flat foot, has been associated with PFPS because it alters the alignment of the knee. Loss of the medial arch flattens the foot, causing a compensatory internal rotation of the tibia or femur that alters the dynamics of the patellofemoral joint (Dixit et al., 2007). Conversely, **pes cavus,** or high arches, causes less cushioning compared to a normal foot. This leads to excessive stress to the patellofemoral joint, particularly with loading activities such as running (Dixit et al., 2007). Also, an abnormally large **Q-angle** has been associated with PFPS. The Q-angle is the angle formed by lines drawn from the anterior superior iliac spine (ASIS) to the central patella and from the central patella to the tibial tubercle. The Q-angle is an estimate of the effective angle at which the quadriceps group pulls on the patella (Brotzman & Wilk, 2003). A normal Q-angle is considered to be below 12 degrees, and angles greater than 15 degrees are considered pathological (Dixit et al., 2007; Brotzman & Wilk, 2001). *Note:* On average, the Q-angle is several degrees greater in women than in men. It is believed that this increased Q-angle places more stress on the knee joint and leads to increased foot pronation in women (Naslund et al., 2006).

Muscle Dysfunction

Muscle tightness and length deficits have been associated with PFPS. Tightness in the ITB complex (e.g., gluteals) causes an excessive lateral force to the patella via its fascial connection. Tightness in the hamstrings can cause a posterior force on the knee, leading to increased contact between the patella and femur. Also, tightness in the gastrocnemius/soleus complex can lead to compensatory pronation and excessive posterior force that result in increased patellofemoral contact pressure (Juhn, 1999; Brotzman & Wilk, 2001).

Muscle weakness in the quadriceps and hip external rotators have been associated with PFPS. In particular, quadriceps weakness has been associated with patellofemoral maltracking. For years, weakness of the vastus medialis oblique (VMO) muscle has been thought to cause patellar maltracking and increased patellofemoral contact pressure. This theory of VMO weakness has been questioned based on more recent evidence. The current thought points to training the quadriceps as a group, versus isolated training of the VMO. In fact, studies that have tried to isolate the VMO resulted in the entire quadriceps group being strengthened instead of just the VMO (Manske, 2006). Also, weakness of the hip external rotators can cause femoral internal rotation, abnormal knee **valgus,** and compensatory foot pronation (Juhn, 1999; Robinson & Nee, 2007; Brotzman & Wilk, 2003). Weakness in the external rotators and all of the resultant malalignments can affect patellofemoral tracking, which may lead to pain and dysfunction. Other contributing factors to consider include improper footwear, a history of injuries, patellar instability, direct trauma, and prior surgery (Juhn, 1999; Brotzman & Wilk, 2003).

Signs/Symptoms

Commonly reported symptoms include pain with running, stair climbing, squatting, or prolonged sitting (e.g., theater sign). The client will typically describe a gradual "achy" pain that occurs behind or underneath the knee cap and may be immediate if trauma has occurred (Dixit et al., 2007). Clients may also report knee stiffness, giving way, clicking, or a popping sensation during movement (Juhn 1999; Brotzman & Wilk, 2003).

Precautions

The client is encouraged to avoid high-stress activities such as running, repetitive squatting, prolonged sitting, and stair climbing (Brotzman & Wilk, 2003; Manske 2006). Also, certain OKC exercises (e.g., leg extensions) have been known to cause abnormal stress on the patellofemoral joint.

Early Intervention

Early intervention for PFPS includes the following (Brotzman & Wilk, 2003; Dixit et al., 2007):

- Avoiding aggravating activities (e.g., prolonged sitting, deep squats, and running)
- Modifying training techniques (e.g., frequency, intensity)
- Proper footwear
- Physical therapy
- Patellar taping
- Knee bracing
- Arch supports
- Foot orthotics
- Patient education
- Oral anti-inflammatory medication
- Modalities (e.g., ice, heat)

If non-surgical intervention fails, surgery would be the next option and is often considered the last resort (Juhn, 1999).

Restorative Exercise Program

With regard to the knee, the choice between closed and open kinetic chain activity has been debated for years. The primary concern is the stresses that are imposed on the knee joint and patella during exercise. With CKC exercises, the patellofemoral contact pressure increases as the knee bends closer to 90 degrees of flexion. In fact, the joint force begins to rise between 30 and 60 degrees and peaks at 90 degrees of flexion (Manske, 2006). These findings support the current standard of avoiding exercises that force the knee to bend beyond 90 degrees of flexion (e.g., squats). Extreme ranges of knee flexion can put the client at risk for injury due to the increased joint stress. Thus, CKC exercises between 0 and 45 degrees have been suggested as a safe range for clients with knee pathology (Kisner & Colby, 2007).

Consequently, when the foot is not fixed (as in open kinetic chain activity) the opposite occurs—the lowest force across the patella is at 90 degrees of flexion. As the knee moves toward extension, the joint forces increase and the patellar contact area decreases, producing a large increase in joint stress. The joint stress peaks between 25 and 0 degrees (Manske, 2006). These findings also support the standard that OKC exercises, such as the leg extension, need to be done with caution for certain knee pathologies [e.g., PFPS, post-operative anterior cruciate ligament (ACL) injury]. Some experts have suggested that an exercise range between 90 and 60 degrees may be safe due to low joint stress (Manske, 2006). OKC exercises that are done with the knee straight are the best option. Examples include the straight-leg raise and prone hip extension. These exercises isolate the muscle groups that cross the knee but do not impose any abnormal stress.

There has been some debate in the literature regarding the application of OKC and CKC exercises. A study by Cohen et al. (2001) measured the knee joint forces in subjects while they were doing OKC exercises (i.e., knee extension 90 to 0 degrees) and CKC exercises (partial squat 20 to 60 degrees). The authors found that during OKC exercises joint stresses were not significantly higher than with CKC exercises. Another study series by Witvrouw et al. (2000) looked at subjects with patellofemoral pain after a five-week intervention program, and again at a five-year follow-up. The goal was to assess the efficacy of OKC versus CKC exercises. At five weeks, both the open and closed kinetic chain groups showed improved function and decreased pain. At the five-year follow-up, both groups still reported functional improvements and decreased pain. The authors concluded that both OKC and CKC exercises have long-term benefits in individuals with patellofemoral pain. These studies lack clear-cut evidence regarding which type of exercise is the best. The choice to use CKC or OKC exercises should be based on a thorough assessment, the client's physical abilities, exercise tolerance, and physician clearance. Further studies are needed to confirm which exercises are safer and more effective for specific populations.

The focus of the restorative program is to progress what was done in the early stages. The ACE-AHFS must remember that restoring proper strength and flexibility is the key with PFPS.

Flexibility

Deficits in muscle length and myofascial mobility have been associated with PFPS. More specifically, addressing tightness in the ITB complex through stretching and myofascial release (e.g., on a foam roller) can have a major impact on the dynamics of the patellofemoral joint. Stretching of the hamstrings and calves will also help to restore muscle-length balance across the knee joint. Clients with PFPS may have tightness in these muscle groups from compensatory patterns that developed in response to pain. For example, the client may limp or avoid certain movements due to pain. This results in a tight, shortened muscle group that is unable to contract or relax through a full range of joint motion.

Strengthening

The focus should be to restore proper strength and neuromuscular control throughout the hip, knee, and ankle. Strengthening the quadriceps group should be the priority. The ACE-AHFS should use a combination of OKC and CKC exercises to train the quadriceps group. OKC exercises can be used to isolate the quadriceps muscle group and are often utilized in the early stages. Examples of OKC exercises include straight-leg raises and leg extensions from 90 to 60 degrees. Once local strength is obtained, CKC exercises can be introduced to progress toward more functional movements. Examples of CKC exercises include bilateral quarter squats, single-leg squats, step-ups, and side-stepping. The ACE-AHFS is again reminded to have the client do these exercises in a pain-free ROM to avoid re-injury. Exercises for the hip and ankle complex should be included due to their effects on the knee joint. Improving femoral control through strengthening of the hip muscles will help to control the forces imposed on the knee joint. The muscles that control the ankle complex may need to be strengthened if they are to have distal control. See "Ankle and Foot Pathologies" later in this chapter for further discussion.

Functional Integration

For a client with PFPS, the return to function should be a systematic process that follows the precautions mentioned earlier in this chapter. The client should have adequate flexibility, strength, and neuromuscular control prior to progressing toward more advanced movements. Slowly returning to full activity while monitoring for changes in symptoms (e.g., pain) is recommended. Refer to Table 18-1 for further examples of functional CKC exercises.

Deficits in general balance may be evident due to disuse of the kinetic chain. Basic progression of balance activities would be appropriate if no pain is elicited. Table 18-2 highlights a progressive program for balance. Low-loading cardiovascular activity such as water aerobics, riding a stationary bike, and using an elliptical trainer is preferred over higher-loading activities such as running or treadmill walking.

Meniscal Injuries

Meniscal tears are one of the most commonly reported knee injuries. Meniscal tears can be either acute or degenerative. Studies have reported that acute meniscal tears occur in 61 of out every 100,000 people. In individuals older than 65 years, the prevalence of degenerative meniscal tears is 60%. The primary age range for meniscal tears for males is 31 to 40 years and for females is 11 to 20 years (Bhagia et al., 2006; Baker & Lubowitz, 2006).

The menisci have an important role within the knee through their multiple functions. First, both the medial and lateral menisci act as shock absorbers and assist with load bearing of the joint. Second, the menisci work together to assist with joint congruency of the femur and tibia during motion. Third, they act as secondary restraints to give the joint more stability. Fourth, the menisci assist with joint lubrication by helping to maintain a synovial layer inside the joint. Fifth, nerve endings within the menisci are thought to give proprioceptive feedback during motion and compression (Manske, 2006; Bhagia et al., 2006; Baker & Lubowitz, 2006). It is important to note that the menisci only receive blood in 10 to 25% of the outer periphery, which is called the vascular zone. Due to its blood supply, this region may heal better that the non-vascular inner region of the meniscus (Manske, 2006; Bhagia et al., 2006). This can be a factor in determining when surgery is necessary.

Mechanism of Injury

Meniscal injuries often occur from trauma or degeneration. Traumatic injuries can occur from a combination of loading and twisting of the joint. For example, a tear can occur when an individual suddenly decelerates and twists on a flexed knee during running. The combination of axial loading with pivoting of the femur on the tibia causes a **shear force** across the meniscus that exceeds the strength of the tissue, resulting in injury (Manske, 2006). Older individuals with degenerative menisci are more predisposed to meniscal tears (Goldstein & Zuckerman, 2000). Meniscal tears can also occur with other traumatic injuries such as acute ACL tears (e.g., lateral meniscus) or medial collateral ligament injury (e.g., medial meniscus) (Manske, 2006).

Signs and Symptoms

When a client has a meniscal tear, he or she may complain of symptoms during activity. Commonly reported symptoms include stiffness, clicking or popping with joint loading, giving way, catching, and locking (in more severe tears). Other signs include joint pain, swelling, and muscle weakness (e.g., quadriceps) (Manske, 2006; Baker & Lubowitz, 2006).

Precautions

Frequently with non-operative management, clients will be cleared to resume activity once symptoms have diminished, but they are encouraged to avoid deep squats, cutting, pivoting, or twisting for as long as symptoms are present (Manske, 2006). Post-surgical procedures have specific precautions that are discussed later in this chapter.

Non-operative Management

Indications for non-operative management include absent or diminished symptoms, and small or degenerative tears (Manske, 2006). Typically, the client will be sent to physical therapy to improve strength and ROM. Modalities (e.g., ice, heat), compression, bracing, and oral anti-inflammatory medication often accompany physical therapy. If conservative management fails, surgical intervention may be the next step.

Surgical Considerations

In the past, total meniscectomy (removal of the greater part of the meniscus) was commonly done to relieve symptoms. Over time, this procedure has become less popular due to the progressive joint degeneration that it causes. Arthroscopic (e.g., with a camera) partial meniscectomy and meniscal repairs are now the two most common procedures. When choosing which procedure is appropriate, the surgeon must consider several factors, including age, location, severity, associated ligament injury, and type of tear (Maxey & Magnusson, 2007).

With a partial meniscectomy, the surgeon only removes the unstable, torn fragments and leaves the viable, healthy tissue intact. This is typically done when there is a large tear that enters the avascular inner zone (Maxey & Magnusson, 2007). The goal is to preserve as much of the meniscus as possible and allow the remaining meniscus to still serve its function without causing early degeneration.

A meniscal repair involves suturing the torn fragment back in place. The ideal location for repair is a tear that occurs in the outer vascular zone. This procedure preserves the meniscal tissue, but requires a slower rehabilitation due to healing of the repair versus extracting the torn tissue. Common candidates include active individuals under the age of 50 who have a small tear in the outer vascular zone (Baker & Lubowitz, 2006).

Early Intervention

Early intervention after partial meniscectomy or meniscal repair may involve specific precautions for the first two to eight weeks, depending on the surgeon's preference. With partial meniscectomy, there is no anatomical structure that needs to be protected, so rehabilitation can be progressed more aggressively with immediate partial or full weightbearing. The client may still have to use crutches and a brace. The meniscal repair often involves a slower progression with partial or non-weightbearing activities with crutches and a brace. The client may also have ROM restrictions for knee flexion (e.g., 60 degrees) for the first four to six weeks to protect the healing tissue (Manske, 2006; Brotzman & Wilk, 2003).

For both procedures, the patient is typically sent to outpatient physical therapy for six to 12 weeks, depending on the physician's plan of care and the patient's insurance constraints. During this time, the goal is to increase ROM, improve lower-extremity strength, control pain and swelling, and progress to more functional activity.

Restorative Exercise Program

The ACE-AHFS may begin to see the client for fitness activities as soon as four weeks after a meniscectomy and eight to 12 weeks after a meniscal repair (Manske, 2006; Brotzman & Wilk, 2003). The client may do a combination of physical therapy and fitness activities. As noted earlier, it is important to consult with the doctor or physical therapist regarding exercise precautions or contraindications. The strategies presented in the following sections take into account clearance by the physician and the client's ability to load the knee with no symptoms.

Flexibility

At this point, the client will have done stretching for a period of time. However, fitness activities can be more demanding than general rehabilitation on a weakened lower extremity. With both the partial meniscectomy and meniscal repair, progressive stretching of the muscle groups that cross the knee should be done. Specifically, stretching of the quadriceps and hamstrings should be emphasized to help maintain adequate flexibility.

Strengthening

When recommending exercises after both the meniscectomy and meniscal repair, exercises that require deep squatting, cutting, or pivoting should be avoided until cleared by the client's physician. Examples of exercises to avoid include bar squats, leg presses or lunges with greater than 90 degrees of flexion, full ROM on the leg-extension machine, and plyometric or agility drills that include cutting or pivoting. These exercises may impart high shear forces to the healing tissues, which can result in re-injury. In fact, deep squatting and hyperflexion of the knee are discouraged for the first six months following a meniscal repair (Manske, 2006).

Most exercises are safe if progressed appropriately by the ACE-AHFS. CKC activities such as squats, leg presses, and lunges can be performed initially from 0 to 45 degrees and progressed to 90 degrees once the client is cleared by his or her physician. OKC activities such as the straight-leg raise, side-lying abduction, and side-lying adduction are encouraged to isolate the hip musculature. Initially, knee extensions are advised from 90 to 60 degrees and progressed once cleared. More advanced, double- and single-leg multiplanar activity should be safe once adequate healing has taken place and proper clearance is obtained.

Functional Integration

Functional integration back into athletic activity should be relatively easy for these clients. In general, a client with a partial meniscectomy can return to basic activity after two to four weeks and return to athletic and sports activity between six and 12 weeks after surgery. For a client with a meniscal repair, running may begin at three to four months after surgery, and full return to athletic and sports activity may begin five to six months after surgery (Manske, 2006).

Deficits in general balance may be evident due to disuse of the kinetic chain. Basic progression of balance activities would be appropriate at this stage (see Table 18-2).

Anterior Cruciate Ligament Injuries

ACL injuries are the most common sports-related injury of the knee (Boden & Garrett, 1996). Seventy to 80% of ACL injuries are non-contact, with only 20 to 30% resulting from direct contact (Griffin, 2000). Injuries often occur in relatively young athletic individuals 15 to 45 years of age (Mankse, 2006). Females are two to eight times more likely to injure their ACL than males (Arendt & Dick, 1995). Also, female basketball players are 7.8 times more likely to injure their ACL than male basketball players (Pearl, 1993).

The ACL has a primary role in preventing anterior translation of the tibia on the femur. The ACL and posterior cruciate ligament (PCL) work together to control excessive rotary motion (Manske, 2006). An intact ACL can resist forces between 1725 and 2195 Newtons (N) prior to failing. Typical running and cutting maneuvers only create approximately 1700 N of force (Brotzman & Wilk, 2003; Manske, 2006). However, injury will occur if the forces imposed on the knee exceed its strength.

Mechanism of Injury

The mechanism of injury often involves a maneuver of deceleration combined with twisting, pivoting, or side-stepping. The combined multiplanar movements cause a traumatic shearing force that exceeds the tensile strength of the ACL, resulting in injury (Griffin, 2000; Kirkendall & Garret, 2000; Yu et al., 2002; Colby et al., 2002).

Signs/Symptoms

An ACL injury is often traumatic. The client will often report hearing a "pop" during the activity, followed by immediate swelling, instability, decreased ROM, and pain. This typically requires immediate medical care to immobilize and protect the joint, followed by a visit to the orthopedic doctor for further diagnosis and intervention (e.g., non-operative versus operative approaches) (Maxey & Magnusson, 2006).

Non-operative Management

Non-operative treatment may be beneficial for older, sedentary individuals, but it may be problematic for younger, active individuals. The ACL-deficient knee may still cause instability with activity and may lead to further injury to knee structures such as the menisci or articular cartilage (Brotzman & Wilk, 2003). The focus of treatment is to maintain adequate ROM, gait, proprioception, and strength of the muscles around the knee. Specifically, strengthening the hamstrings has been shown to help prevent anterior translation of the tibia. Modalities including ice and compression wrapping may be used to control swelling (Brotzman & Wilk, 2003).

Non-operative Precautions

With non-operative management, the client may be cleared to slowly resume activity once symptoms have diminished, but may be restricted from performing jumping, cutting, pivoting, or twisting motions (Manske, 2006). Wearing a protective knee brace is recommended to protect the deficient knee during activity. After rehabilitation, some individuals attempt to return to their activity or sport despite the presence of instability. If this proves unsuccessful, surgery may be the next option. Post-surgical procedures have specific precautions that will be discussed in subsequent sections. Prior to surgery, the physician may prescribe pre-operative rehabilitation to restore ROM, muscle strength, and proper gait.

Surgical Considerations

There are several procedures currently used by surgeons to repair the ACL. Surgery involving the medial third of the patellar tendon and the medial hamstring (i.e., semitendinosus) are the two most common procedures. Both of the procedures have good short- and long-term functional outcomes (Aglietti et al., 1994; Marder et al., 1991; Eriksson et al., 2001; Spindler et al., 2004).

The Patellar Tendon Graft

This procedure involves taking the middle third of the patellar tendon (autograft) to replace the damaged ACL. This procedure, which has been done since the 1920s, has been referred to as the "gold standard" (Maxey & Magnusson, 2003). The procedure has consistently demonstrated excellent surgical outcomes with a 90 to 95% success rate in individuals returning to pre-injury levels of activity (Maxey & Magnusson, 2003; Spindler et al., 2004). The procedure is recommended for athletes in high-demand sports and individuals with occupations that do not require large amounts of kneeling or squatting (Spindler et al., 2004). This procedure may not be indicated for people with a history of patellofemoral pain, arthritis, or patellar tendinitis, or for smaller individuals with a narrow patellar tendon (Allen, 2007). Reported problems with the procedure include post-operative pain behind the kneecap, pain with squatting, and a low risk of patellar fractures (Freedman et al., 2003; Sachs et al., 1989). The patellar graft has an initial failure rate of 2300 N, which is stronger than a healthy, intact ACL (Manske, 2006, Brotzman & Wilk, 2003).

The Hamstring Tendon Graft

With this procedure, the surgeon typically harvests strands of tendons from the medial semitendinosus to reconstruct the ACL. Surgeons also use additional tendons from the gracilis muscle, which creates a combined four-strand tendon graft that has an estimated failure rate of 4108 N (Manske, 2006; Brotzman & Wilk, 2003). This procedure may be especially beneficial for younger patients who still have open growth plates. With the hamstring tendon graft, there are no graft bone ends that could violate the growth plate and stimulate early closure, as may occur with a patellar graft (Brown, 2007). This procedure has fewer problems with pain behind the kneecap, better cosmesis (no anterior incision), decreased post-operative stiffness, and faster recovery (Manske, 2006). Reported problems with the procedure include increased laxity of the new ligament due to graft elongation (stretching), slower healing of the tendon graft, and loosening of the graft at the anchoring site in the bone (Manske, 2006).

The Allograft

Surgeons also use cadaveric or **allograft** grafts from the Achilles tendon, tibialis anterior, and patellar tendon to replace the torn ACL (Manske, 2006; Noyes & Barber-Westin,1996). The allograft procedure may be beneficial for patients who have failed prior ACL reconstruction or who have multiple ligaments that need repair. Advantages include decreased morbidity at the donor site, decreased surgical time, and less post-operative pain. Problems with the allograft procedure include risk of infection and graft elongation (Maxey &Magnusson, 2003; Noyes & Barber-Westin, 1996; Nikolaou et al., 1986). *Note:* The client's physician is always in the best position to make the most appropriate recommendation regarding the choice of a given surgical technique.

Post-operative Precautions

It is common for clients who return to higher-level activity to develop anterior knee pain. The prevalence ranges from 15 to 25%, with reported incidences as high as 55% (Manske, 2006). The healing patellar graft has been linked to anterior knee pain. The knee should be gradually introduced to activity to allow adaptation and adequate healing. To protect the graft, the physician may have the client wear a protective brace for the first year after surgery or permanently during activity. Activity should be stopped if any of the following occurs: increased pain at the surgical site, increased swelling, loss of ROM, and increased exercise pain (Manske, 2006).

Early Intervention

Typically, the client will be in physical therapy for the first three to four months, depending on the physician's preferences and the client's insurance constraints. The client is generally able to perform full weightbearing with crutches and a brace for the first two to six weeks. The client may also get a custom brace later on to wear during workouts and athletic activity (Manske, 2006).

During the first six to 12 weeks after surgery, the fixation of the graft into the bone is the weakest point (Brotzman & Wilk, 2003; Manske, 2006). Exercise programming during this time must take this weakness into account. Also, the graft goes through a sequence of **avascular necrosis** (i.e., breakdown), revascularization, and remodeling. This sequential process helps to change the properties, or "ligamentize," the graft so that it will eventually resemble the original ACL that was replaced. The implanted graft begins to resemble the original ACL after around six months to one year. Full maturation has been reported to occur after one year (Brotzman & Wilk, 2003; Manske, 2006).

There are a vast amount of published protocols on ACL rehabilitation. Early protocols developed in the 1970s and 1980s stressed more protection of the knee, limited weightbearing, and immobilization with a cast or brace for the first six to 12 weeks. The client was then slowly progressed with strength and ROM, and then began running between nine and 12 months post-surgery (Manske, 2006). As researchers began to understand more about the ACL, the protocols began to mature between the late 1980s and the 1990s with the development of the "accelerated protocol" in which early mobility is stressed while still protecting the graft through bracing. Researchers found that early, safe activities that loaded the graft site helped to stimulate healing (Manske, 2006). Most current protocols are based on milestones that the individual must meet before continuing to the next phase. For example, the individual needs to have adequate quadriceps strength, proprioception, and ROM before being able to unlock the brace and walk without crutches. Common among protocols is a return to functional activity between 12 and 16 weeks after surgery and a return to sporting activities around six months (Manske, 2006; Maxey & Magnusson, 2003; Brotzman & Wilk, 2001; Cioppa-Mosco et al., 2006). Most orthopedic surgeons have developed their own protocols based on the type of surgery, personal preferences and experience, and available research. Reviewing specific protocols is beyond the scope of this text, though the following sections cover specific recommendations within each category that are based on the idea that the client is cleared to do fitness activities.

Restorative Exercise Program

The ACE-AHFS may begin to see the client as soon as 12 to 16 weeks after surgery. The client may do a combination of physical therapy and fitness activities. It is important for the ACE-AHFS to consult the physician or physical therapist regarding what procedure was done and the post-operative protocol, as well as to obtain clearance for fitness activities.

Flexibility

Stretching the muscles around the knee is a priority for the client. One important principle is that weak muscles can become tight and tight muscles can become weak. Weakened muscles may not be able to generate adequate force due to poor strength and endurance. This may create tightness due to the inability to generate the needed force for movement. A tight muscle has a poor length-tension relationship and cannot generate adequate force for movement. Specifically, the quadriceps, hamstrings, and calves should be targeted to maintain adequate flexibility around the knee.

Strengthening

The choice between closed and open kinetic chain activity is of utmost importance for the client who is post-surgical. The goal is to progressively strengthen the leg without risking injury to the graft site. It is recommended that OKC knee extension be limited to 90 to 30 degrees, while flexion can be full ROM. With CKC exercise, 0 to 60 degrees is recommended as a safe range (Manske, 2006). It is important to understand that limiting the ROM helps protect the healing graft by preventing excessive force to the joint. OKC exercises with the knee straight and CKC exercises within the appropriate ranges are recommended to protect the surgical site. The ROM precautions can be lifted once adequate healing has taken place.

Strengthening of the quadriceps, hamstrings, and hip musculature is important. Both the hamstrings and quadriceps play a key role in prevention of further injury. Training should focus on developing symmetrical strength between muscle groups, which has been shown to be effective in preventing ACL tears (Manske, 2006). Hip strengthening should be implemented due to its effect on the knee joint during CKC exercises.

Functional Integration

Functional integration may begin with basic activity as early as 12 weeks post-surgery and can be progressed toward athletic activity between four and six months. The goal during this time (i.e., 12 weeks to six months) is to safely load the knee in all planes of motion without compromising the graft site. Refer to Table 18-1 for a description of CKC progression.

Clients who have undergone ACL reconstruction will have deficits in balance. Balance activity should have been implemented in the early stages of rehabilitation. At the time of fitness activity, the client should have good balance with basic single-leg activities. Progressively challenging the knee in multiple planes will help prepare the joint for higher-level activity (see Table 18-2).

Low-loading cardiovascular activity, such as water aerobics, stationary cycling, and elliptical training, is preferred over higher-loading activity until the client is cleared by his or her physician.

Total Knee Replacement

Total knee replacements (TKR), or total knee arthroplasty, were first performed in 1968. Since then, improvements in surgical materials and procedures have greatly increased its success. Approximately 300,000 knee replacements are performed annually in the United States (Brotzman & Wilk, 2003). TKR is indicated when conservative treatment fails to restore mobility or reduce arthritic pain, chronic knee inflammation, or swelling. Similar to a client coping with an arthritic hip, the TKR client has suffered with a painful joint for some time and may have tried conservative treatment such as oral medication, injections, and physical therapy (Maxey & Magnusson, 2007; Brotzman & Wilk, 2003). When these conservative approaches have failed, replacing the joint is often the best option. With joint replacement, the primary goals are to replace the diseased joint and eliminate knee pain (Maxey & Magnusson, 2007). Contraindication to the procedure may include osteoporosis, ligament laxity, infection, medical risk factors, **morbid obesity**, and poor patient compliance (Maxey & Magnusson, 2007). There are two common procedures conducted for total knee replacement: primary TKR and partial knee replacement.

Primary Total Knee Replacement

Primary TKR commonly consists of three components: the femoral component (e.g., highly polished metal), the tibial component (e.g., durable plastic often held in a metal tray), and the patellar component (e.g., durable plastic). The aggregate of these components make up the prosthetic knee joint. Primary TKR is recommended for candidates who have arthritis throughout the knee joint, as well as for young, active people. The primary TKR has the ability to withstand high levels of activity (Maxey & Magnusson, 2007; Brotzman & Wilk, 2003).

Partial Knee Replacement

Another alternative to primary TKR is the partial, or unicompartmental, knee replacement. The knee joint consists of three compartments: the medial compartment, the lateral compartment, and the patellofemoral compartment. This procedure is used for a knee joint that is relatively healthy with only one damaged (e.g., arthritic) compartment. If two or more compartments are damaged, partial knee replacement is not recommended [American Academy of Orthopedic Surgeons (AAOS), 2007; Manske, 2006). This technique is used to replace the medial or lateral compartment, but not the patellar component. This procedure is generally not recommended for younger, active individuals because the partial components tend to have less durability than the primary components and can break down faster. Candidates tend to be older individuals with a fairly sedentary lifestyle. Only six to eight out of 100 patients with arthritic knees are appropriate candidates for this procedure (AAOS, 2007).

Precautions

There are no specific movement precautions for these procedures. The client is encouraged to avoid high-stress activities such as jogging, skiing, tennis, racquetball, jumping, repetitive squatting, and contact sports (e.g., football, basketball). Until cleared, lifting is typically limited to no more than 40 pounds (18 kg) and heavy weightlifting is discouraged (AAOS, 2007; Brotzman & Wilk, 2003; Maxey & Magnusson, 2007).

Early Intervention

The client is typically sent to outpatient physical therapy for six to 12 weeks, depending on the physician's plan of care and the client's insurance constraints. During this time, the goal is to increase ROM, improve lower-extremity strength, enhance balance, control pain and swelling, and progress to more functional activity (AAOS, 2007; Brotzman & Wilk, 2003; Maxey & Magnusson, 2007). It is not uncommon for these clients to still have post-surgical knee pain and be deconditioned. The recommendations in the following sections are based on the idea that the client has been cleared for fitness activities.

Restorative Exercise Program

The client may be cleared to return to progressive fitness activities as soon as six to eight weeks after surgery. The client may still be attending physical therapy during this time. It is important to consult the physician or physical therapist regarding any post-operative guidelines and obtain clearance for exercise.

Flexibility

Post-operative muscle tightness is common with patients who underwent TKR. Stretching the muscles around the knee will be important to restore adequate flexibility. In particular, the quadriceps group can become tight at the incision site and throughout the muscle group. Specific stretching and myofascial release with a foam roller has shown to be beneficial for restoring flexibility (Brotzman & Wilk, 2003). General stretching and myofascial release of the hip muscles, hamstrings, and calves will also help to maintain flexibility throughout the kinetic chain. Flexibility exercises should be done at a level that does not elicit pain and is within a comfortable ROM.

Strengthening

Most exercises are safe, if they are gradually progressed. OKC exercises can still be implemented for isolated strengthening. Particular attention should be placed on the quadriceps and hamstrings to regain knee stability. Basic guidelines for OKC exercises can be applied. The ACE-AHFS must remember that even though the client has a prosthetic knee, he or she still has a patella. Therefore, OKC exercises with the knee straight or from 90 to 60 degrees will prevent excessive loading of the patella. CKC exercises (see Table 18-1) can be progressed appropriately within the acceptable range of 0 to 45 degrees with a progression to 90 degrees. General conditioning of the hip and ankle muscles should be included to address any deficits.

Functional Integration

The client should have adequate strength, ROM, and basic proprioception before progressing to more functional activities. Functional activity should progress what has been done in rehabilitation and must follow any precautions. The client should master basic functional skills before progressing to higher-level activity. For these clients, aquatic exercise is a great way to progress functional activity while de-weighting the joint. Aquatic exercise often is used to transition clients to higher-intensity land-based activity. The buoyancy of the water unloads the joint, allowing for more activity with lower amounts of pain.

Deficits in general balance may be evident due to disuse of the kinetic chain. Basic progression of balance activities would be appropriate if no pain is elicited (see Table 18-2). Low-level cardiovascular activity is indicated for these clients. Exercising on a bike or elliptical trainer is preferred over jogging or walking long distances.

Ankle and Foot Pathologies

Ankle Sprains

Ankle sprains are very common in the athletic population. They account for 10 to 30% of sports-related injuries in young athletes. Each year, an estimated 1 million people visit the physician with an acute ankle injury and 20 to 40% develop chronic problems (Brotzman & Wilk, 2003; Perlman et al., 1987). Ankle sprains are most common in sports such as basketball, volleyball, soccer, and ice skating (Ivins, 2006). There is little data regarding risk factors for ankle sprains, though a history of ankle sprains has been found to be a risk factor. Foot type, general laxity, and gender have also been linked to the incidence of ankle sprains (Ivins, 2006).

Mechanism of Injury

Lateral, or inversion, ankle sprains are the most common type of ankle sprain. In fact, 85% of ankle sprains are to the lateral structures of the ankle (Garrick, 1982; Balduini & Tetzlaff, 1982). The mechanism is typically inversion with a plantarflexed foot. The lateral ankle ligaments are the most common structures involved, including the anterior talofibular ligament (ATFL), calcaneofibular ligament (CFL), and posterior talofibular ligament (PTFL).

Medial, or eversion, ankle sprains account for approximately 10 to 15% of all ankle injuries and result from forced dorsiflexion and eversion of the ankle. The medial deltoid ligament is the most common structure involved and injury often requires further examination to rule out a fracture (Anderson, Hall, & Parr, 2008).

Signs/Symptoms

With lateral ankle sprains, the individual can often recall the mechanism and hearing a "pop" or "tearing" sound. Specific signs and symptoms for lateral ankle sprains are described in the next section. Medial ankle sprains rarely happen in isolation. The individual is often unable to recall the specific mechanism, but can reproduce discomfort by dorsiflexing and everting the ankle. There may be medial swelling with tenderness over the deltoid ligament (Anderson, Hall, & Parr, 2008).

Classification

Lateral ankle sprains are often described using a specific grading system (Table 18-4). A Grade I (first degree) ankle sprain involves

Table 18-4
Grading System for Lateral Ankle Sprains

	Grade I	Grade II	Grade III
Ligament involved	ATFL	ATFL and CFL	One or more
Stretched or ruptured	Stretched	Stretched	Ruptured
Pain/swelling	Mild	Moderate	Severe
Weightbearing	Full	Partial	Unable

Note: ATFL = Anterior talofibular ligament; CFL = Calcaneofibular ligament the ATFL ligament, with pain and mild swelling over the lateral aspect of the ankle. Typically, weightbearing is tolerable after injury. A Grade II (second degree) ankle sprain involves both the ATFL and CFL ligaments, with more severe pain and swelling over the lateral ankle. Weightbearing may be limited due to pain. A Grade III (third degree) ankle sprain is considered a complete tear of one or more of the lateral ligaments. Rapid, severe pain, swelling, and discoloration occur and individuals are unable to bear weight (Anderson, Hall, & Parr, 2008).

Medial ankle sprains are often associated with fibular fractures, severe lateral ankle sprains, and fractures to the medial malleolus. To date, there is no specific grading system for medial ankle sprains (Anderson, Hall, & Parr, 2008).

Precautions

The client may be cleared to slowly resume activity once symptoms have diminished. He or she is encouraged to wear the appropriate ankle bracing and to avoid lateral and multiplane movements until cleared by a physician. These movements may put the client at risk for further injury and should be introduced when appropriate (Brotzman & Wilk, 2003).

Early Intervention

Early intervention often includes medical management. The acronym PRICE—protection, restricted activity, ice, compression, and elevation—describes a safe early intervention strategy for an acute ankle sprain (Anderson, Hall, & Parr, 2008).

- Protection includes protecting the injured ankle with the use of crutches and appropriate ankle bracing.
- Restricted activity includes limiting weightbearing activity until the client is cleared by the physician.
- Ice should be applied every two hours for 10 to 15 minutes.
- Compression can be done by applying an elastic wrap to the area. This helps to minimize local swelling.
- Elevating the ankle 6 to 10 inches (15 to 25 cm) above the level of the heart will also help to control swelling. This is done to reduce hemorrhage, inflammation, swelling, and pain.

Most often, individuals with lateral and medial ankle sprains are referred to a medical doctor for further diagnosis and treatment. Grade I and II lateral sprains are often immobilized with an ankle brace for several days. Grade III lateral sprains are often immobilized with a removable walking boot for up to three weeks (Brotzman & Wilk, 2003).

Early intervention can begin one to three weeks after injury unless a severe ankle sprain has occurred that may require further immobilization (Brotzman & Wilk, 2003). The client may be sent to physical therapy to improve strength, flexibility, proprioception, and endurance, and to control swelling.

Restorative Exercise Program

The ACE-AHFS may begin to see the client for fitness training as soon as one to two weeks post-injury for Grade I ankle sprains, two to three weeks post-injury for Grade II ankle sprains, and three to six weeks for Grade III ankle sprains (Brotzman & Wilk, 2003). During this time, the client may still be in physical therapy and be ready to transition to fitness activities. The client should be progressed according to his or her tolerance to exercise. In other words, pain should be the guide. It is common for the injured ankle to have mild to moderate discomfort and swelling after increased activity.

Flexibility

Stretching of the gastrocnemius and soleus may be beneficial if the client has tightness and decreased length after immobilization. Stretching the ankle in motions that stress the injured ligaments is not recommended. For example, stretching the ankle into inversion or eversion can stretch the healing ligaments, resulting in local pain and irritation. General stretches for the lower extremity should be included to maintain adequate flexibility throughout the whole kinetic chain.

Strengthening

Strengthening the muscles of the kinetic chain will be beneficial, with particular emphasis on the muscles that control the foot and ankle (Table 18-5). OKC exercises using resistive bands are a good way to isolate the muscles that control the ankle (Figure 18-8).

Targeting the peroneal group for inversion ankle sprains is essential for prevention. The peroneal reflex with muscle contraction has been considered the first mechanism for dynamic joint stability. Therefore, with sudden inversion ankle movements, the peroneals will be the first muscles to contract and attempt to stabilize the ankle. Delayed action of this mechanism has been associated with inversion ankle sprains (Brotzman & Wilk, 2003). Experts recommend training these muscle groups eccentrically to improve the stabilizing effect. Eccentric loading creates higher tension levels versus **isometric** or **concentric** activities at specific joint ranges. (Kaminski & Hartsell, 2002). Strength gains have been reported as soon as six weeks after initiation of a program of progressive resistive exercise (Kaminski & Hartsell, 2002). Clients with eversion ankle sprains may have more global deficits due to the fact that eversion ankle sprains are rarely seen in isolation; often they follow other trauma such as a fracture. CKC exercise progression should emphasize dynamic single-leg strengthening activities that challenge the lower kinetic chain. Strengthening programs for these injuries are often individualized and are determined by the injury. As mentioned in previous sections, exercises for the hip and knee should be included to address any strength deficits and to help maintain control of the kinetic chain during activity.

Functional Integration

Functional activity can begin once the client has adequate strength, ROM, and most importantly, proprioception. Clients who have suffered ankle sprains may have deficits in balance. The ligaments are a major source of proprioceptive feedback for balance and joint position sense throughout the kinetic chain. If ligament trauma occurs, the feedback can be lost, which results in a higher risk of reinjury (Brotzman & Wilk,

Table 18-5
Suggested Exercises for Muscles That Control the Foot and Ankle

Muscle Group	Exercises
Gastrocnemius	Calf raise with knee straight
Soleus	Calf raise with knee bent
Tibialis anterior	Resistive ankle dorsiflexion
Tibialis posterior	Resistive ankle inversion
Peroneal group	Resistive ankle eversion
Foot intrinsic group	Towel crunches with toes

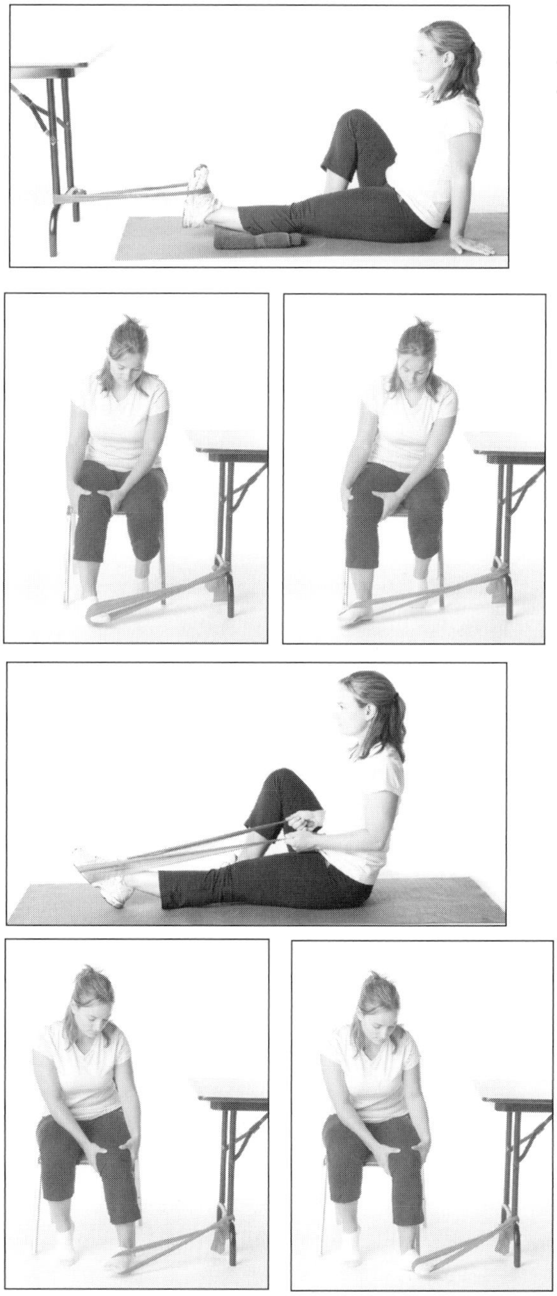

Figure 18-8
Resistive band exercises for the ankle

2003). In fact, chronic lateral ankle sprains have been associated with muscle weakness (e.g., in the hip abductors, peroneal group), delayed activation patterns in the hip and knee, and diminished postural control (Friel et al., 2006; Van Deun et al., 2007; Evans, Hertel, & Sebastianelli, 2004). Based on this evidence, one can appreciate the interaction between the muscular and proprioceptive system. If injury occurs in the lower extremity, the information to the central nervous system from the lower extremity changes, which results in delayed muscle activation patterns, weakness, and overall compensation.

The functional progression for these clients should include a combination of CKC and balance activities to achieve the optimal benefits. The client should be safely progressed though the program while wearing his or her protective bracing. OKC exercises can still be used to isolate specific muscle groups as needed. CKC exercises that integrate balance are a key element in challenging the kinetic chain and reestablishing the reactive feedback loop that is required for multiplanar activity (see Tables 18-1 and 18-2). A commonly used progression is challenging the kinetic chain with double- or single-leg activity in the **sagittal plane** first, the **frontal plane** second, and combined planes last. The frontal and combined plane activities may need to be slowly introduced to prevent re-injury.

Cardiovascular activity such as biking and elliptical training can be added to the program to build or maintain basic cardiovascular fitness. Higher-level activity such as running, sprints, or agility drills should follow the progression just described.

Plantar Fasciitis

Plantar fasciitis is an inflammatory condition of the plantar aponeurosis, or fascia, of the foot. This condition has been reported to be the most common cause of heel pain and accounts for 10% of running injuries. The prevalence is highest among individuals 40 to 60 years old. Up to one-third of injured individuals have pain in both feet. Plantar fasciitis is more common in obese individuals and people who are on their feet for long periods of time (Buchbinder, 2004; Cole, Seto, & Gazewood, 2005).

Mechanism of Injury

There have been several intrinsic and extrinsic risk factors associated with this condition. Intrinsic factors include pes planus (excessive pronation or low arch height), pes cavus (high arch height), and decreased strength and poor flexibility of the calf muscles. Extrinsic factors include overtraining, improper footwear, obesity, and unforgiving and hard surfaces (Buchbinder, 2004). Any of these factors can cause excessive loading of the plantar fascia, leading to pain and dysfunction.

Signs and Symptoms

Typically, individuals report pain on the plantar, medial heel at its calcaneal attachment that worsens after rest, but improves after 10 to 15 minutes of activity (Buchbinder, 2004). In particular, clients will commonly report excessive pain during the first few steps in the morning. Clients may also have stiffness and muscle spasms in the lower leg with tightness in the Achilles tendon (Buchbinder, 2004).

Precautions

Individuals with plantar fasciitis may be limited in their activity due to pain. Activities that excessively load the fascia, such as running or jumping, should be avoided due to exacerbation of the condition. The condition can be challenging due to the pain relief that occurs with basic activity and the recurrence of symptoms after rest. The ACE-AHFS needs to monitor changes in symptoms and refer the client to the appropriate medical professional, if necessary.

Early Intervention

Management of this condition may include modalities (e.g., ice), oral anti-inflammatory medication, heel pad or plantar arch, stretching, and strengthening exercises. The medical doctor may prescribe physical therapy, a night splint, or orthotics, or inject the area with cortisone (Buchbinder, 2004; Cole, Seto, & Gazewood, 2005). Conservative treatment of this condition has shown good long-term outcomes. A study by Wolgin and colleagues (2004) found that 80% of patients treated with conservative therapies had complete resolution of symptoms after a four-year follow-up. Some individuals may require surgery if conservative treatment fails after six to 12 months of intervention (Buchbinder, 2004; Cole, Seto, & Gazewood, 2005).

Restorative Exercise Program

The client may be cleared to exercise immediately to tolerance or he or she may have some restrictions. The role of the ACE-AHFS is to design a program that helps to meet the client's overall goals but does not excessively load the foot. Integrating specific foot exercises into the general fitness program often provides the best results, as this allows the client to work toward his or her fitness goals as well as address the foot problems.

Flexibility

Stretching of the gastrocnemius, soleus, and plantar fascia is beneficial and has been shown to help relieve symptoms (Buchbinder, 2004; Cole, Seto, & Gazewood, 2005). In fact, a study by DiGiovanni et al. (2006) found that specific plantar fascia stretching (Figure 18-9) had excellent results (94% satisfaction) in a group of 66 subjects after an eight-week program and at a two-year follow-up. Proper stretching of the calf complex will restore adequate muscle length and prevent compensatory pronation at the ankle. During gait, tight calf muscles prevent the tibia from gliding forward on the ankle, forcing the foot to excessively pronate to achieve the needed ROM for movement. Self–myofascial release techniques include rolling the foot over a baseball, golf ball, or dumbbell. This may help to break up myofascial adhesions in the plantar fascia.

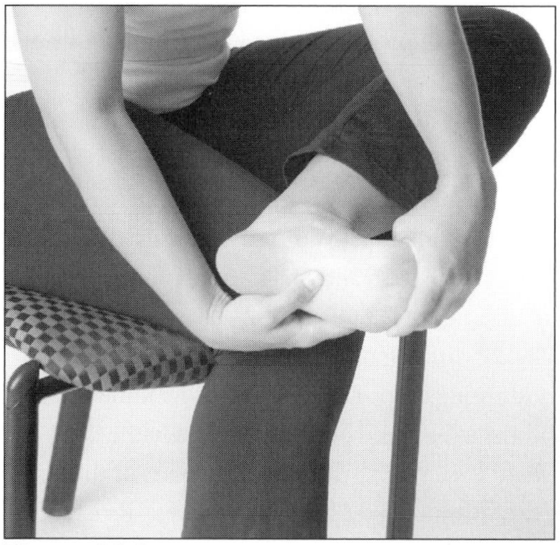

Figure 18-9
Plantar fascia stretching

Strengthening

Strengthening the foot intrinsic muscles may help to improve arch stability of the feet and help to unload the stresses imposed across the plantar fascia. Some examples of effective exercises include towel crunches (Figure 18-10) and marble pick-up (Figure 18-11). Strengthening of the gastrocnemius, soleus, peroneals, tibialis anterior, and tibialis posterior may be needed to help improve strength at the ankle. The client may have done similar exercises in physical therapy and may need to be progressed accordingly. Exercises for the hip and knee should be included as needed.

Functional Integration

Returning to functional activity may be a challenge for these clients. The nature of the condition can bring false hope due to the changes in symptoms with activity. A slow, pain-free return to activity is indicated for this condition. As mentioned earlier, high-loading activities should

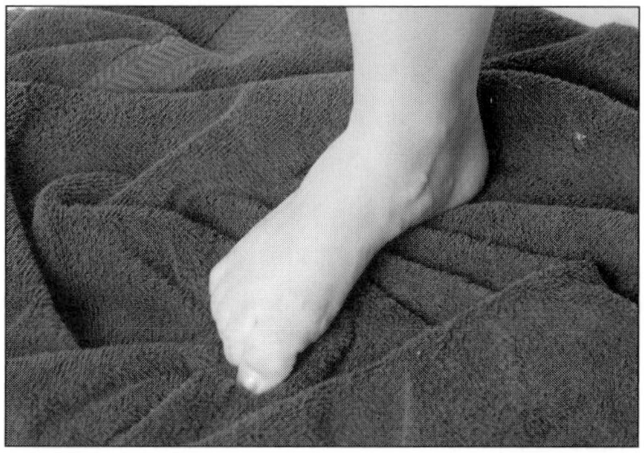

Figure 18-10
Towel crunches for foot intrinsic muscles

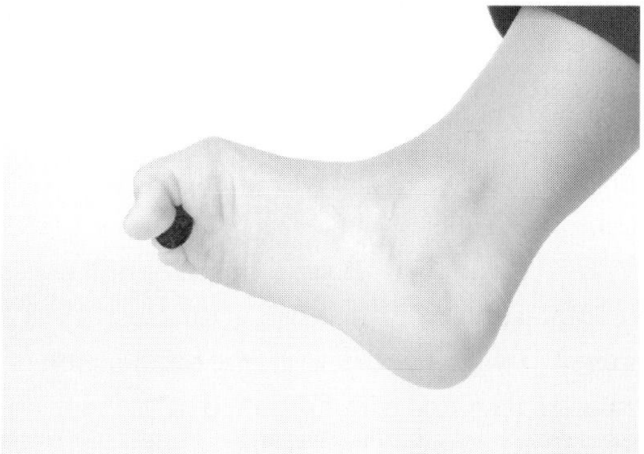

Figure 18-11
Marble pick-up for foot intrinsic muscles

be limited to avoid further exacerbation of the injury. With these clients, balance may be an issue and should be addressed, if needed. Low-loading cardiovascular activities such as biking, elliptical training, or water aerobics are preferred over higher-loading activities such as running.

Achilles Tendinopathy

Injury to the Achilles tendon is common in athletes and the active population. The prevalence of the condition is highest among runners, gymnasts, and dancers. Other sports where this injury is common include track and field, volleyball, basketball, and soccer. Typically, older athletes are more affected by the condition than teens or children (Mazzone, 2002). This condition can eventually lead to rupture if not addressed appropriately. Achilles ruptures primarily occur in males 30 to 50 years of age. The prevalence rate has increased in recent years due to the fact that more people are exercising (Mazzone, 2002).

The classification of Achilles injuries has been quite confusing due to the many names given to the condition. Terms commonly used in the past, including **Achilles tendinitis, tenosynovitis,** and **tendonosis,** have become questionable due to subsequent findings (Paavola et al., 2002; Maffulli, Khan, & Puddu, 1998; Mazzone, 2002). These studies have not found any clear sign of an inflammatory reaction in the tendon, which is often described as tendinitis and tenosynovitis. Researchers do acknowledge that there may be a prior inflammatory reaction, but no evidence has been found to date. Tendonosis or tendon degeneration is often used, but may be incorrect if not confirmed by the proper medical testing, such as biopsy, radiographic imaging, or surgical exploration (Paavola et al., 2002; Maffulli, Khan, & Puddu, 1998). Tendonosis causes a diffuse thickening of the tendon with no evidence of inflammation. This can develop from repeated microtrauma, aging, and vascular problems (Mazzone, 2002).

This confusion has led to the term **Achilles tendinopathy.** Maffulli, Khan, and Puddu (1998) suggested this term to describe the combination of pain, swelling, and poor function that accompanies this condition. Thus, Achilles tendinopathy may include both an inflammatory and degenerative process of the tendon.

Mechanism of Injury

Various intrinsic and extrinsic factors are associated with this condition. Intrinsic factors include age, bodyweight, pes cavus, pes planus, leg-length discrepancies, and lateral ankle instability. Extrinsic factors include errors in training, prior injuries, poor footwear, muscle weakness, and poor flexibility. (Paavola et al., 2002; Kader et al., 2002; Mazzone, 2002). The extrinsic factors are typically responsible for acute tendon trauma. Overuse and chronic injuries are often multifactorial and include a combination of intrinsic and extrinsic factors (Paavola et al., 2002).

Signs and Symptoms

Individuals often complain of pain that is 0.75 to 2.25 inches (2 to 6 cm) above the tendon insertion into the calcaneus. The typical pattern is initial morning pain that is "sharp" or "burning," as well as pain with more vigorous activity. Rest will often alleviate the pain, but as the condition becomes worse the pain becomes more constant and begins to interfere with **activities of daily living** (Mazzone, 2002; Brotzman & Wilk, 2003).

Precautions

Clients with this condition are encouraged to stop all aggravating activity and seek proper treatment for the condition. High-loading activities such as jumping, running, and stair climbing should be avoided until the condition has improved.

Early Intervention

Early intervention includes controlling pain and inflammation by using modalities (e.g. ice, ultrasound), rest, and oral anti-inflammatory medication (Mazzone, 2002). Management of the condition may include modified rest and the addressing of specific risk factors. Modified rest allows the injured body part to rest while the client is exercising the uninjured parts of the body (e.g., using an upper-body ergometer). Proper training techniques, losing weight, proper footwear, orthotics, strengthening, and stretching can help alleviate pain and prevent progression of the condition (Paavola et al., 2002; Mazzone, 2002). Also, the client may be sent to physical therapy to address the factors mentioned earlier. If conservative treatment fails after four to six months, then surgical intervention is indicated (Brotzman & Wilk, 2003; Mazzone, 2002).

Restorative Exercise Program

The client may be cleared to exercise immediately to tolerance, or he or she may have some activity restrictions. The role of the ACE-AHFS is to design a program that helps to meet the client's overall goals but does not exacerbate the condition. Consulting the medical doctor and physical therapist can give key information about how the client is responding to treatment and what he or she is currently doing for exercise. The following sections summarize strategies for management of this condition.

Flexibility

Restoring proper length and elasticity to the calf muscles can reduce strain to the muscle-tendon unit and decrease symptoms (Kader et al., 2002). Studies regarding stretching have suggested that stretching does stimulate the healing response (Mazzone, 2002). The goal of stretching should be to restore general lower-body flexibility, with an emphasis on calf mobility. The client should be cautioned to stretch to tolerance and avoid overexertion. Overstretching of the Achilles tendon can cause irritation to the muscle-tendon unit and should be avoided.

Strengthening

Eccentric strengthening of the calf complex has been shown to be beneficial for relieving symptoms. In fact, Wasielewski and Kotsko (2007) conducted a systematic review of research from 1980 to 2006 on eccentric strengthening of the calf muscles. Their analysis revealed that eccentric exercise may reduce pain and improve strength in Achilles tendinopathy. However, eccentric training has not been shown to be superior over other forms of therapeutic interventions for this condition (Wasielewski & Kotsko, 2007). Therefore, progressively loading the Achilles tendon with eccentric activity can benefit the client, but may be even more beneficial when combined with other interventions. Examples of eccentric activity include slowly lowering the calf while standing on a step or performing a single-leg squat with an emphasis on slowly lowering the leg.

Functional Integration

Returning to basic functional and sports activities may be challenging for these clients. The nature of the condition can bring changes in symptoms with activity. A gradual, pain-free return to activity is indicated for this condition. Modifications in training techniques and the training environment should be addressed, with an emphasis on client education. CKC exercise combined with eccentric loading can progressively challenge the Achilles tendon, but should not create pain. Any deficits in balance should be addressed as needed. Simply adding an unstable surface such as a foam pad to CKC exercises can challenge the client's balance (see Tables 18-1 and 18-2). Cardiovascular activity should be progressed with caution. Low-loading activity should precede higher-loading activity to avoid pain or reinjury.

Shin Splints

"Shin splints" is a general term used to describe exertional leg pain (Brotzman & Wilk, 2003). Shin splints are typically classified as two specific conditions: medial tibial stress syndrome (MTSS) and anterior shin splints (Figure 18-12).

MTSS, also called posterior shin splints, is an overuse injury that occurs in the active population. MTSS is an exercise-induced condition that is often triggered by a sudden change in activity (Brotzman & Wilk, 2003; Anderson, Hall, & Parr, 2008). MTSS is actually **periostitis,** or inflammation of the periosteum (connective tissue covering) of the bone. Originally, this condition was thought to be caused by posterior tibial tendinitis. It has since been related to a traction periostitis at the distal insertion of the soleus muscle or from the flexor digitorum longus muscle (Brotzman & Wilk, 2003; Anderson,

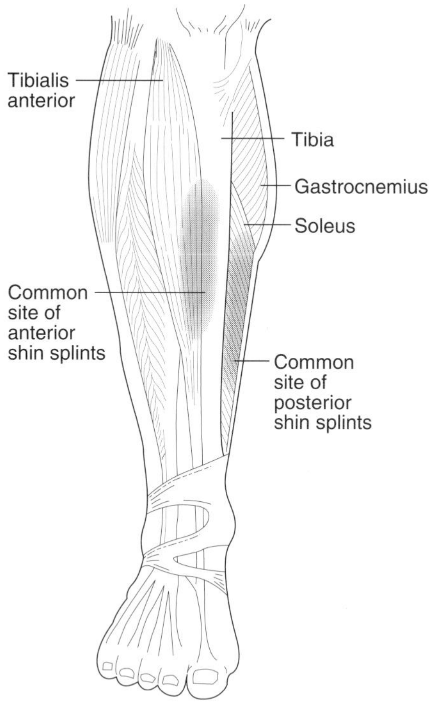

Figure 18-12
Site of pain for anterior and posterior shin splints

Hall, & Parr, 2008). MTSS is the most frequently diagnosed injury in runners and is common in dancers and in military personnel. It has a higher prevalence in female runners than male runners (Anderson, Hall, & Parr, 2008).

Anterior shin splints are also common in the active population and pain often occurs in the anterior compartment. The anterior compartment muscles (i.e., tibialis anterior, extensor digitorum longus, and extensor hallucis longus), fascia, and periosteal attachments are most commonly affected. Anterior shin splints are also common in runners and among military personnel (Brotzman & Wilk, 2003).

Mechanism of Injury

MTSS has been most frequently associated with pes planus, or flat foot. Excessive overpronation of the foot during activity produces an eccentric stress to the muscles that results in a painful periostitis. The etiology of anterior shin splints is not completely known, but the condition is often associated with exertional activity (Brotzman & Wilk, 2003). Both MTSS and anterior shin splints have been associated with overtraining, poor footwear, changes in running surface, muscle weakness, and poor flexibility (Anderson, Hall, & Parr, 2008).

Signs and Symptoms

Clients commonly complain of a "dull ache" along the distal two thirds of the posterior medial tibia for MTSS and the distal anterior shin for anterior shin splints (Brotzman & Wilk, 2003). The pain is elicited by initial activity, but diminishes as activity continues. The pain typically returns hours after activity. If the condition progresses, the pain becomes constant and tends to restrict performance (Anderson, Hall, & Parr, 2008).

Precautions

Clients are encouraged to stop all aggravating activity and rest. Repetitive loading activities such as running and jumping are discouraged until symptoms have resolved. The client should be referred to his or her physician if this condition has not resolved within one or two months after initiation of modified activity and proper intervention. It is important for the ACE-AHFS to monitor symptoms during activity and refer the client to the doctor if there is no improvement, as a stress fracture must be ruled out. Stress fractures of the tibia can have similar signs and symptoms as shin splints. For example, stress fractures can elicit pain along the posterior medial tibia (Metzl, 2005).

Early Intervention

Management of both conditions includes modifying training with lower-impact conditioning and **cross-training** (e.g., aquatic exercise). However, the best intervention may just be to rest. Five to seven days of rest has been suggested to help relieve acute symptoms (Anderson, Hall, & Parr, 2008). Modalities (e.g., ice, ultrasound), oral anti-inflammatory medication, cortisone injections, heel pads, and bracing may also be beneficial to relieve symptoms (Anderson, Hall, & Parr, 2008). The client may need to be referred to physical therapy to address these issues.

Restorative Exercise Program

The client may be restricted with activity or may be limited due to pain. The role of the ACE-

AHFS should be to slowly progress the client back to full unrestricted activity without exacerbating the symptoms. Cross-training to maintain adequate levels of fitness is indicated in the early stages. Consulting the client's physician and physical therapist can give key information about how the client is responding to treatment and what he or she is currently doing for exercise. The following sections summarize strategies for management of this condition.

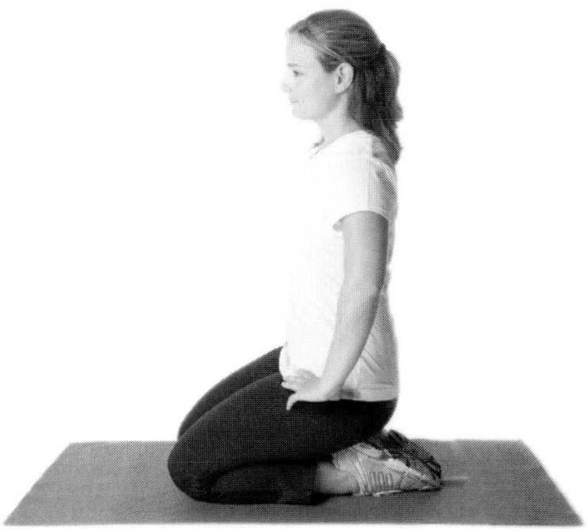

Figure 18-13
Sitting stretch for the anterior compartment

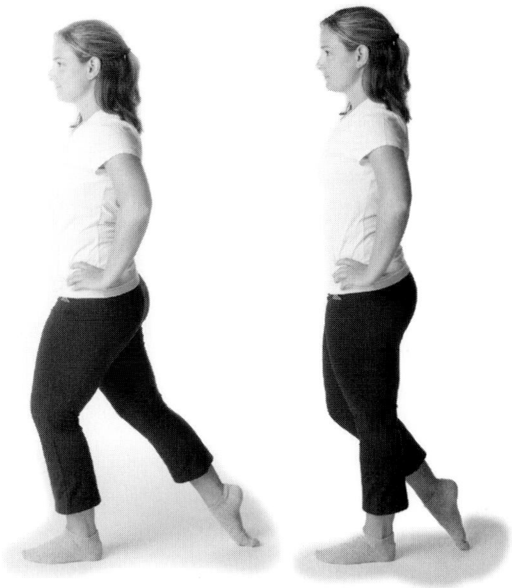

Figure 18-14
Standing "toe drag" stretch for the anterior compartment

Flexibility

Pain-free stretching of the calf muscles, especially the soleus, has been shown to be effective in relieving symptoms related to MTSS. Stretching the anterior compartment has been shown to help relieve the symptoms of anterior shin splints (Figures 18-13 and 18-14) (Anderson, Hall, & Parr, 2008; Brotzman & Wilk, 2003). The goal of stretching should be to restore proper length and elasticity to the muscle and reduce strain in the muscle-tendon unit (Kader et al., 2002). A general lower-body stretching program should accompany more specific stretching to address any secondary muscle-length deficits that may affect the foot and ankle.

Strengthening

Rest and modified activity are the primary interventions for symptom relief. However, there may be some residual strength deficits in the muscles that control the ankle. Targeting the muscles that control the ankle is the goal, especially the calf and anterior tibialis muscles. Exercises for the hip and knee should be added as needed.

Functional Integration

A gradual return to athletic and sports activity is best for these clients. Strengthening exercises should be related to the client's functional goals, but needs to be low-impact to avoid any excessive stress. Both OKC and CKC exercises can be integrated throughout the program as tolerated by the client. Progression should begin with low-loading activities and systematically progressed to higher-loading activities such as jumping or running, as long as the client is pain free. Balance exercises can also be integrated into the program as needed.

Cross-training can be utilized throughout the program to maintain adequate cardiovascular fitness. Examples of low-impact activities include water jogging, stationary biking, and elliptical training. Clients should avoid running, jumping, and shock-loading activities that stress the affected region.

Muscle Strains

Muscle strains are injuries in which a muscle works beyond its capacity, resulting in a tear of the muscle fibers. In mild strains, the client may report tightness or tension (Anderson, Hall, & Parr, 2008). In more severe cases, the client may report feeling a sudden "tear" or "pop" that leads to immediate pain and weakness in the muscle. Swelling, discoloration (**ecchymosis**), and loss of function often occur after the injury (Anderson, Hall, & Parr, 2008). Strains of the lower extremity primarily occur in the hamstrings, groin muscles, and calves.

Muscle strains of the hamstring group are often caused by a severe stretch to the muscle or a rapid, forceful contraction (e.g., during sprinting). The hamstrings have the highest frequency of strains in the body; hamstring strains are common in running and jumping sports (Anderson, Hall, & Parr, 2008). The client will often report a "sharp" posterior thigh pain that occurs after insult. Pain may also be felt with contraction or stretching of the muscle. Risk factors include poor flexibility; poor posture; muscle imbalance among the gluteals, quadriceps, and hamstrings; improper warm-up; errors in training; and prior injury (Anderson, Hall, & Parr, 2008).

Groin or adductor strains are common in sports such as ice hockey and figure skating that require explosive acceleration, deceleration, and change of direction. With injury, the client may report an initial "pull" of the groin muscles, followed by intense pain and loss of function. Pain may be felt with contraction of the muscles with the hip in adduction, passive stretching with the hip in abduction, or when crossing the leg over the midline of the body. In more severe cases, increased pain and weakness occurs, which may limit specific motions. Jogging straight may be tolerable, but any side-to-side motion tends to elicit pain. Muscle imbalance between the adductors and abductors is the most prevalent risk factor for this type of injury (Anderson, Hall, & Parr, 2008).

Calf strains are common in most running and jumping sports. With injury, the client will often report a sudden and painful "tearing" sensation in the medial muscle belly or at the junction between the muscle belly and the Achilles tendon. Pain, swelling, ecchymosis, and loss of function often occur after the injury. Risk factors include muscle fatigue, fluid and electrolyte depletion, forced knee extension while the foot is dorsiflexed, or forced dorsiflexion while the knee is extended.

Management

If a muscle strain does occur, all aggravating activity should be stopped and the RICE principle (rest, ice, compression, elevation) should be applied immediately. The ACE-AHFS should administer basic first-aid procedures and then refer the client to the appropriate healthcare professional. It is beyond the scope of the ACE-AHFS to attempt to diagnose a client's problem and make decisions regarding his or her care.

Structural Abnormalities

It is important for the ACE-AHFS to understand that certain structural changes in the lower-extremity kinetic chain have been associated with various musculoskeletal conditions. First, pes planus, or overpronation, is considered to be a flat mobile foot, which offers little structural support. It has been associated with plantar fasciitis, Achilles tendinopathy, posterior tibial tendinitis, shin splints, ITBFS, and patellofemoral pain. Second, pes cavus, or high arches, is considered to be a rigid foot that offers little shock absorption. It has been associated with ITBFS, plantar fasciitis, stress fractures of the tarsal and metatarsal bones of the foot, and peroneal tendinitis. Third, leg-length discrepancies have been associated with hip problems such as trochanteric bursitis and ITB syndrome (Brotzman & Wilk, 2003; Manske, 2006; Anderson, Hall, & Parr, 2008).

It is important for the ACE-AHFS to note any structural deviations, as they may be contributing factors to the pathologies discussed in this chapter. Attempting to correct these biomechanical deviations is beyond the scope of the ACE-AHFS. If an ACE-AHFS suspects that a deviation may be contributing to an undiagnosed problem, then referral to the appropriate medical professional is indicated.

Case Studies

Case Study 1

Client History

An ACE-AHFS was referred a 32-year-old male recreational soccer player who had a right knee ACL repair 12 weeks ago with a patellar tendon graft. The mechanism of injury was a planting and twisting maneuver. The client has been in physical therapy for the past 12 weeks and treatment has included a combination of strengthening, cardiovascular, and balance exercises. The physical therapist has also been doing massage, stretching, and myofascial release. The physical therapist reports that the client has responded well to physical therapy and is highly motivated. He or she is on schedule with the physician's protocol, but because of insurance constraints has been transitioned to fitness activity. Review of medications reveals the following: Vicodin® (pain) and Advil® as needed.

Client Interview

Upon meeting with the client for initial assessment, the ACE-AHFS notices that he is highly motivated and immediately talks about returning to soccer. The client does have written clearance by the medical doctor, with the precautions of wearing a brace during activity and no running until 16 weeks. His health history reveals no major medical problems or comorbities. The client does have a history of recurrent right ankle sprains and occasional low-back pain. The client is an engineer and works at a desk most of the day. His fitness goals are to return to soccer, running, and weightlifting.

When asked about his knee, the client reveals that he has been getting anterior knee pain with increased swelling for the past two weeks while working out at the gym. The client is doing 45 minutes of cardiovascular exercise on the elliptical trainer and general upper-body strengthening. Further questioning reveals that he has been doing lunges, leg presses, and leg extensions three to five times per week, including during his physical therapy program.

Fitness Assessment

At the time of fitness assessment, the client demonstrated problems with basic movements. In particular, the client demonstrated immediate pain with getting out of the chair and walking down stairs. At this time, the session was stopped and no further action was taken.

Management

Inspection of the knee revealed it to be swollen and painful to bend. The client was immediately referred back to the medical doctor for further evaluation. The ACE-AHFS recommended that the client use the RICE principle until he or she sees the doctor and receives proper clearance to resume activity. The goal was to make sure the client did not re-injure the ACL or damage any other structures. Upon hearing back from his patient, the doctor diagnosed him as having patellar tendinitis and general joint irritation. The client is restricted from fitness activity for two weeks. Upon clearance to resume activity, the following actions should be taken with this client:

- Client education: CKC vs. OKC exercises, overtraining, injury recognition
- Training modification: Reestablish program goals and training schedule
- Fitness evaluation: Baseline data for flexibility, muscular strength and endurance, body composition, and cardiovascular fitness
- Exercise program: Slow progression of sets, repetitions, and time
  - ✓Flexibility: Focus on stretching/myofascial release for the ITB complex, quadriceps, hamstrings, and calves
  - ✓Strengthening: Focus on the quadriceps and hamstrings, and general hip strengthening
  - ✓Balance: Progress to multiplane activity with a knee brace
  - ✓Functional: Focus on CKC exercises within pain-free limits with a progression toward sport-specific movements. After 16 weeks, begin basic agility and sport-specific movements.
- Safety
  - ✓Brace worn during workouts
  - ✓Recommend icing after workouts

✓ Monitor for increased symptoms: redness, pain, and swelling
✓ Monitor for signs and symptoms of overtraining

Case Study 2

Client History

An ACE-AHFS is working with a 72-year-old female who is three months post-operative after a left total hip replacement via the posterior lateral approach. The woman had a history of hip arthritis and finally elected to have the procedure. She has been attending physical therapy for strengthening, endurance, and balance activities. The physical therapist reports that the client is doing well with ROM but still has hip weakness that makes functional and balance activities difficult. Due to insurance constraints, the client has been transitioned to fitness activity.

Client Questions

Upon meeting with the client, she brings in written clearance from the medical doctor with precautions noted to avoid high-impact activity such as running. Her health history reveals **hypertension,** osteoporosis, and osteoarthritis. The client did have a left TKR three years ago with no reported problems. Review of medications are as follows: diuretic (hypertension), Fosamax® (osteoporosis), and Celebrex® (osteoarthritis). The client is retired but volunteers at the local school, where she is on her feet most of the day. Her fitness goals are to return to walking and swimming.

When asked about her right hip, the client reveals having mild to moderate pain after physical therapy that goes away after icing. The client reports being cleared by the medical doctor to resume full ROM of the hip with no restrictions. Further questioning reveals that she is still having trouble with functional movements, such as sit-to-stand actions and picking up objects.

Fitness Assessment

At this time, the fitness assessment was limited due to the global hip weakness that the client was having. The following information was obtained from the modified assessment:

- Movement screen: Limited due to weakness and fall risk
- Flexibility: Tightness in the ITB complex, hamstrings, and calves
- Functional testing: Weakness noted in the hip with sit-to-stand, side-stepping, quarter lunges, and partial-ROM step-ups
- Cardiovascular testing: Unable to do submaximal testing on the bike or step due to weakness and deconditioning
- Muscular strength: Able to establish baseline weights on exercise machines and resistive bands

Management

Due to the client's low functional level, a modified restorative program should be created that focuses on hip and abdominal core strengthening, balance, and cardiovascular endurance. The following actions should be taken with this client.

- Client education
  - ✓ Basic training principles, CKC vs. OKC exercises, injury recognition
  - ✓ Precautions and program modifications for osteoporosis and hypertension
- Training modification: Reestablish program goals and training schedule
- Fitness evaluation: Baseline data for flexibility, muscular strength and endurance, body composition, and cardiovascular fitness when tolerated by the client
- Exercise program: Slow progression of sets, repetitions, and time
  - ✓ Flexibility: Focus on stretching/myofascial release for the hip muscles, ITB complex, quadriceps, hamstrings, and calves
  - ✓ Strengthening: Focus on the gluteals, hip external rotators, quadriceps, and hamstrings
  - ✓ Balance: Slowly progress multiplane activity under close supervision
  - ✓ Functional: Focus on CKC exercises within pain-free limits with a progression toward multiplanar functional activities
    - o Basic movements: Sit-to-stand
    - o Gait: Walking over even and uneven terrain (e.g., cement vs. grass)

- Safety
    - ✓Precautions for osteoporosis and hypertension
    - ✓Choosing exercises that are safe
    - ✓Recommend icing after workouts and monitor for change in symptoms

Summary

Due to the changes in the healthcare system, the role of fitness professionals has expanded. The ACE-AHFS is required to have a deeper knowledge about non-operative and post-operative musculoskeletal conditions. This chapter has focused on the recognition, management, and restorative exercise guidelines for common musculoskeletal injuries and post-operative conditions of the lower extremity. The reader is encouraged to continue the study of these conditions to effectively design safe restorative programs for different conditions and populations.

References

Aglietti, P. et al. (1994). Patellar tendon versus doubled semitendinosus and gracilis tendons for anterior cruciate ligament reconstruction. *American Journal of Sports Medicine,* 22, 211–218.

Allen, C. (2007). ACL injury: Does it require surgery? *American Academy of Orthopedic Surgeons.* www.orthoinfo.aaos.org.

American Academy of Orthopedic Surgeons (2007). *Your orthopedic connection: Total knee replacement.* www.orthoinfo.aaos.org.

Anderson, M.K., Hall, S.J., & Parr, G.P. (2008). *Foundations of Athletic Training: Prevention, Assessment, and Management* (4th ed.). Baltimore, Md.: Lippincott Williams & Wilkins.

Arendt, E. & Dick, R. (1995). Knee injury patterns among men and women in collegiate basketball and soccer: NCAA data and review of literature. *American Journal of Sports Medicine,* 23, 6, 694–701.

Arthritis Foundation & Centers for Disease Control and Prevention (1999). *National Arthritis Action Plan: A Public Health Strategy.* www.cdc.gov/nccdphp/pdf/naap.pdf.

Baker, B. & Lubowitz, J. (2006). Meniscal injuries. *E-Medicine Online Journal* (Web MD), 1–14. www.emedicine.com.

Balduini, F.C. & Tetzlaff, J. (1982). Historical perspectives on injuries of the ligaments of the ankle. *Clinical Sports Medicine,* 1, 1, 3–12.

Bhagia, S.M. et al. (2006). Meniscal tears. *E-Medicine Online Journal* (Web MD), 1–14. www.emedicine.com.

Bierma-Zeinstra, S. et al. (1999). Validity of American College of Rheumatology criteria for diagnosing hip osteoarthritis in primary care research. *Journal of Rheumatology,* 26, 1129–1133.

Boden, B.P. & Garrett, W.E. (1996). Mechanism of injuries to the anterior cruciate ligament. *Medicine & Science in Sports & Exercise,* 28, 5, 156–168.

Bonelli, S. (2001). *Aquatic Exercise,* San Diego, Calif.: American Council on Exercise.

Brotzman, B. & Wilk, K. (2003). *Clinical Orthopedic Rehabilitation* (2nd ed.). St. Louis, Mo.: Mosby.

Brown, D.W. (2007). Anterior cruciate ligament reconstruction techniques. *Orthopedic Associates.* www.orthoassociates.com.

Buchbinder, R. (2004). Plantar fasciitis. *New England Journal of Medicine,* 350, 21, 2159–2167.

Buckwalter, J.A. & Martin, J.A. (2006). Osteoarthritis. *Advanced Drug Delivery Reviews,* 58, 150–167.

Cioppa-Mosca, J.M. et al. (2006). *Postsurgical Rehabilitation Guidelines for the Orthopedic Clinician.* St. Louis, Mo.: Mosby.

Cohen, Z. et al. (2001). Patellofemoral stresses during open and closed kinetic chain exercises: An analysis using computer simulation. *American Journal of Sports Medicine,* 29, 480–487.

Colby, S. et al. (2002). Electromyographic and kinematic analysis of cutting maneuvers: Implications for anterior cruciate ligament injury. *American Journal of Sports Medicine*, 28, 2, 234–240.

Cole, C., Seto, C., & Gazewood, J. (2005). Plantar fasciitis: Evidence-based review of diagnosis and therapy. *American Family Physician,* 72, 11, 2237–2243.

DiGiovanni, B.F. et al. (2006). Chronic plantar fasciitis: A prospective clinical trial with two-year follow-up. *Journal of Bone & Joint Surgery,* 88-A, 8, 1–15.

Dixit, S. et al. (2007). Management of patellofemoral pain syndrome. *American Family Physician,* 75,194–204.

Eriksson, K. et al. (2001). A comparison of quadruple semitendinosus and patellar tendon grafts in reconstruction of the anterior cruciate ligament. *Journal of Bone Joint Surgery*, 83, 348–354.

Evans, T., Hertel, J., & Sebastianelli, W. (2004). Bilateral deficits in postural control following lateral ankle sprain. *Foot & Ankle International*, 25, 11, 833–839.

Foye, P.M. & Stitik, T.P. (2006). Trochantaric bursitis. *E-Medicine Online Journal* (Web MD), Dec 21, 1–14. www.emedicine.com.

Freedman, K.B. et al. (2003). Arthroscopic anterior cruciate ligament reconstruction: A meta-analysis comparing patellar tendon and hamstring tendon autografts. *American Journal of Sports Medicine,* 31, 1, 2–11.

Friel, K. et al. (2006). Ipsilateral hip abductor weakness after inversion ankle sprain. *Journal of Athletic Training,* 41, 1, 74–78.

Garrick, J.G. (1982). Epidemiologic perspective. *Clinical Sports Medicine,* 1, 13–18.

Goldstein, J. & Zuckerman, J.D. (2000). Selected orthopedic problems in the elderly. *Rheumatic Disease Clinics of North America*, 26, 3, 593–616.

Griffin, L.Y. (2000). Noncontact anterior cruciate ligament injuries: Risk factors and prevention strategies. *Journal of American Academy of Orthopedic Surgeons,* 8, 141–150.

Hinton, R. et al. (2002). Osteoarthritis: Diagnosis and therapeutic considerations. *American Family Physician,* 65, 841–848.

Ivins, D. (2006). Acute ankle sprains: An update. *American Family Physician,* 74, 1714–1720.

Juhn, M. (1999). Patellofemoral pain syndrome: A review and guidelines for treatment. *American Family Physician,* 60, 2012–2022.

Kader, D. et al. (2002). Achilles tendinopathy: Some aspects of basic science and clinical management. *British Journal of Sports Medicine*, 36, 239–249.

Kaminski, T.W. & Hartsell, H.D. (2002). Factors contributing to chronic ankle instability: A strength perspective. *Journal of Athletic Training*, 37, 4, 394–405.

Kennon, R. et al. (2004). Anterior approach for total hip arthroplasty: Beyond the minimally invasive technique. *Journal of Bone and Joint Surgery,* 86, 91–97.

Kirkendall, D.T. & Garrett, W.E. (2000). The anterior cruciate ligament enigma: Injury mechanisms and prevention. *Clinical Orthopedics,* 372, 64–68.

Kisner, C. & Colby, L. (2007). *Therapeutic Exercise: Foundations and Techniques* (5th ed.). Philadelphia: F.A. Davis Company.

Lawrence R.C. et al. (1998). Estimates of the prevalence of arthritis and selected musculoskeletal disorders in the United States. *Arthritis and Rheumatology,* 41, 778–799.

Lievense, A., Bierma-Zeinstra, S., & Schouten, B. (2005). Prognosis of trochantaric pain in primary care. *British Journal of General Practice,* 55, 512, 199–204.

Little, H. (1979). Trochanteric bursitis: A common cause of pelvic girdle pain. *Canadian Medical Association Journal,* 120, 456–458.

Maffulli, N., Khan, K.M., & Puddu, G. (1998). Overuse tendon conditions: Time to change a confusing terminology. *Arthroscopy,* 14, 840–843.

Manske, R.C. (2006). *Postsurgical Orthopedic Sports Rehabilitation: Knee and Shoulder.* St. Louis, Mo.: Mosby.

Marder, R.A. et al. (1994). Prospective evaluation of arthroscopically assisted anterior cruciate ligament reconstruction: Patellar tendon versus semitendinosus and gracilis tendons. *American Journal of Sports Medicine,*19, 2478–2484.

Martinez, J.M. & Honsik, K. (2006). Iliotibial band syndrome. *E-Medicine Online Journal* (Web MD). Dec 6, 1–14. www.emedicine.com.

Matta, J.M., Shahrdar, C., & Ferguson, T. (2005). Single-incision anterior approach for total hip arthroplasty on an orthopedic table. *Clinical Orthopedics and Related Research,* 441,115–124.

Maxey, L. & Magnusson, J. (2007). *Rehabilitation for the Post Surgical Orthopedic Patient* (2nd ed.). St. Louis, Mo.: Mosby.

Mazzone, M. (2002). Common conditions of the achilles tendon. *American Family Physician,* 65, 1805–1810.

Metzl, J. (2005). A case-based look at shin splints. *Patient Care,* Nov, 39–46.

Naslund, J. et al. (2006). Comparison of symptoms and clinical findings in subgroups of individuals with patellofemoral pain. *Physiotherapy Theory & Practice,* 22, 5, 105–118.

Nikolaou, P. et al. (1996). Anterior cruciate ligament allograft transplantation: Long-term function, histology, revascularization, and operative technique. *American Journal of Sports Medicine*, 14, 5, 348–360.

Noyes, F.R. & Barber-Westin, S.D. (1996). Reconstruction of the anterior cruciate ligament with human allograft: Comparison of early and later results. *Journal of Bone and Joint Surgery,*78A, 524–537.

Paavola, M. et al. (2002). Current concepts review: Achilles tendinopathy. *Journal of Bone & Joint Surgery,* 84-A, 11, 2062–2076.

Pearl, A.J. (1993). *American Orthopedic Society for Sports Medicine: The Athletic Female.* Champaign, Ill.: Human Kinetics.

Perlman, M. et al. (1987). Inversion lateral ankle trauma: Differential diagnosis, review of the literature, and prospective study. *Journal of Foot Surgery,* 26, 95–135.

Robinson, R.L. & Nee, R.J. (2007). Analysis of hip strength in females seeking physical therapy treatment for unilateral patellofemoral pain syndrome. *Journal of Orthopedic and Sports Physical Therapy,* 37, 5, 232–238.

Sachs, R. et al. (1989). Patellofemoral problems after anterior cruciate ligament reconstruction. *American Journal of Sports Medicine,* 17, 6, 760–765.

Spindler, K.P. et al. (2004). Anterior cruciate ligament reconstruction autograft choice: Bone-tendon-bone versus hamstring: Does it really matter? A systematic review. *American Journal of Sports Medicine*, 32, 8, 1986–1995.

U.S. Department of Health and Human Services; Centers for Disease Control and Prevention; National Center for Health Statistics (2004). Number of Patients, Number of Procedures, Average Patient Age, Average Length of Stay. *National Hospital Discharge Survey 1998–2004.* www.cdc.gov/nchs/

Van Deun, S. et al. (2007). Relationship of chronic ankle instability to muscle activation patterns during the transition from double-leg to single-leg stance. *American Journal of Sports Medicine*, 35, 274–281.

Wasielewski, N.J. & Kotsko, K.M. (2007). Does eccentric exercise reduce pain and improve strength in physically active adults with symptomatic lower extremity tendinosis? A systematic review. *Journal of Athletic Training,* 42, 3, 409–422.

Witvrouw, E. et al. (2000). Open versus closed kinetic chain exercises for patellofemoral pain: A prospective, randomized study. *The American Journal of Sports Medicine,* 28, 687–694.

Wolgin, M. et al. (2004). Conservative treatment of plantar heel pain: Long-term follow-up. *Foot & Ankle International,* 5, 97–102.

Yu, B. et al. (2002). Lower extremity motor control-related and other risk factors for noncontact anterior cruciate ligament injuries. *Instructional Course Lecture,* 51, 315–325

Suggested Reading

Anderson, M.K., Hall, S.J., & Parr, G.P. (2008). *Foundations of Athletic Training: Prevention, Assessment, and Management* (4th ed.). Baltimore: Lippincott Williams & Wilkins.

Brotzman, B. & Wilk, K. (2003). *Clinical Orthopedic Rehabilitation* (2nd ed.). St. Louis, Mo.: Mosby.

Kisner, C. & Colby, L. (2007). *Therapeutic Exercise: Foundations and Techniques* (5th ed.). Philadelphia: F.A. Davis Company.

Manske, R.C. (2006). *Postsurgical Orthopedic Sports Rehabilitation: Knee and Shoulder.* St. Louis, Mo.: Mosby

In This Chapter

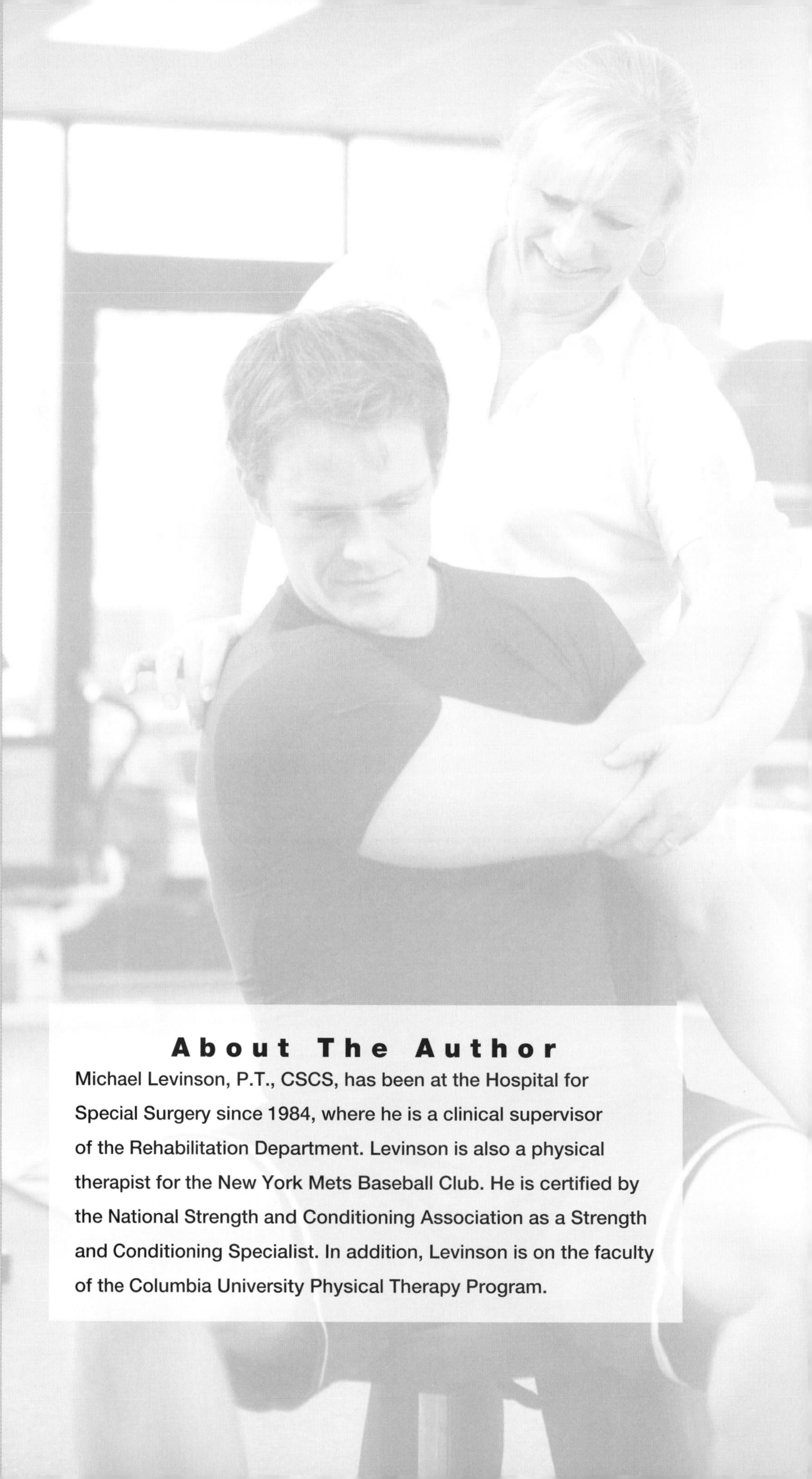

About The Author

Michael Levinson, P.T., CSCS, has been at the Hospital for Special Surgery since 1984, where he is a clinical supervisor of the Rehabilitation Department. Levinson is also a physical therapist for the New York Mets Baseball Club. He is certified by the National Strength and Conditioning Association as a Strength and Conditioning Specialist. In addition, Levinson is on the faculty of the Columbia University Physical Therapy Program.

CHAPTER 19

Musculoskeletal Injuries of the Upper Extremity

Michael Levinson

When training an individual following an upper-extremity musculoskeletal injury, it is important that the ACE-certified Advanced Health & Fitness Specialist (ACE-AHFS) is aware of several factors, including the mechanism of injury, the structures involved, the healing constraints of the structures involved, exacerbating activities, and **range-of-motion (ROM)** issues. Pain is the most important guideline when designing a training program. Communication with the client's physical therapist and physician can be extremely valuable in preventing re-injury. Symptoms such as recurrent pain, instability, or loss of ROM should be communicated.

Acromioclavicular Joint Injuries

The acromioclavicular joint consists of the articulation of the distal end of the clavicle and the acromion, which is a portion of the scapula. The joint is covered with cartilage and is stabilized by the coracoclavicular and acromioclavicular ligaments. The clavicle rotates upward 40 to 50 degrees as the arm is fully elevated. Without rotation of the clavicle, it has been demonstrated that the arm can only be elevated to approximately 110 degrees. Injuries to the acromioclavicular joint can present as either traumatic or chronic. The most common mechanism of injury is a direct force on the point of the shoulder or a fall on an outstretched arm. If the clavicle does not fracture, the acromion is driven inferiorly and medially in relation to the clavicle. The ligaments are then stretched or torn, depending on the severity of the injury. This injury is often referred to as a "separated shoulder" and occurs commonly in contact sports such as football, hockey, lacrosse, and rugby. The injury is classified by six different degrees of severity (Rockwood & Matsen, 2004). Patients with acromioclavicular joint pathology often present with pain during passive horizontal adduction or have pain during an O'Brien active compression test, which consists of resistance of the shoulder in flexion, internal rotation, and horizontal adduction (O'Brien et al., 1998) (Figure 19-1). More severe cases will present with a "step-off" deformity where the separation of the clavicle and the acromion can be seen.

Treatment varies greatly and is partially dependent on the severity of the injury. The current trend is toward conservative treatment without surgery. However, in certain severe cases, a surgical procedure is the treatment of choice. Surgical procedures vary greatly and are utilized for individuals that present with persistent pain, joint instability, or an undesirable and visible deformity at the joint sight. Especially among the female population, cosmesis, or a concern for appearance, is often a rationale for surgery. In addition, athletes who perform overhead movements and individuals who perform a great deal of highly physical work may find conservative treatment unsatisfactory. There are numerous surgical techniques available. However, there is no true "gold standard." Surgical treatment includes resection of the distal clavicle, ligament transfer, ligament reconstruction, and internal fixation. Patients undergoing clavicle resection often must modify certain activities such as push-ups and the bench press. Reconstructions that are successful can theoretically return

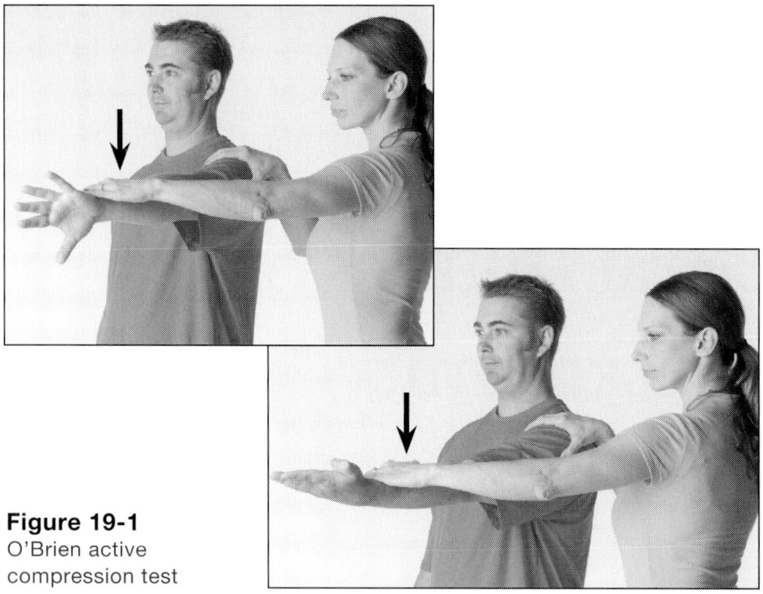

Figure 19-1
O'Brien active compression test

the individual to a normal exercise level. However, screws or pins utilized for internal fixation run the risk of breaking.

Injury to the acromioclavicular joint can lead to chronic degenerative changes at the joint. Abnormal mechanics or instability at the joint can result in a wearing away of the cartilage and **arthrosis.** In addition, people with poor mechanics who have done a great deal of bench pressing or push-ups can cause degenerative changes at the joint.

Pathomechanics following injury to this joint vary. First, there may be a loss of clavicle rotation, which can result in a loss of shoulder **elevation.** Secondly, the structural suspension of the entire shoulder girdle may be compromised. Most critical are the pathomechanics of the scapula. The scapula provides a stable platform for shoulder motion and any deviation may result in other shoulder problems. Inferior and medial **rotation** of the scapula is often a consequence of this injury.

Conservative treatment of this injury varies, but the trend is moving away from extended periods of immobilization. Initially, an immobilizer may be utilized for pain control, reduction of muscle spasm, and reduction of soft-tissue damage. Reduction of the injury with strict immobilization for extended periods has not been demonstrated to be an effective treatment plan. Patient compliance has often been a limiting factor. **Cryotherapy** for reduction of pain, swelling, and spasm is a key component of the early stages of recovery.

The goal of the initial stages of recovery is to restore pain-free ROM. Matheson and Price (2006) advise avoiding active-ROM and passive-ROM exercises in the supine position. The rationale is that the client's body weight prevents scapula ROM and thus results in greater clavicle rotation, which may result in exacerbation of the injury. Seated or standing is the preferred position.

Strengthening should be initiated with submaximal isometrics for abduction, flexion, extension, internal rotation, and external rotation. When progressing a strengthening program, several precautions should be followed:

- Traction through the shoulder joint should be avoided or minimized. For example, when a client is performing shrugs or curls, the ACE-AHFS should provide a weight that can be controlled. Also, weights should not be carried around the gym. Beginning exercise with elastic resistance or tubing is often the safest choice.
- Resistive exercises in horizontal abduction or adduction should be avoided or minimized secondary to stress on the joint.
- When performing scapula strengthening exercises, extremes of scapula **retraction** and **protraction** should be avoided.
- Internal and external rotation exercises for the rotator cuff are tolerated best with the arm in adduction.
- Overhead resistive activity, such as the military press and incline bench press, should be minimized or avoided. These activities should be initiated only when the client is asymptomatic and has a good proximal strength base.

Shoulder Instability

Shoulder instability is a very common pathology. The glenohumeral joint consists of the head of the humerus and the glenoid fossa, which is a portion of the scapula. Together they form a "ball and socket." Unlike the true ball-and-socket joint of the hip formed primarily by bony structures, the motion at the glenohumeral joint is controlled by the capsule and ligaments that surround the joint and the four rotator cuff muscles. This joint requires a great deal of ROM to perform many athletic activities. For this reason, the glenohumeral joint is an inherently unstable joint. Shoulder instability can be a result of an acute, traumatic event such as a dislocation. It can also be a chronic condition that results from overuse activities, especially overhead activities such as when throwing or playing tennis or volleyball, where the shoulder experiences various forces related to acceleration and deceleration. These powerful repetitive activities can cause excessive **laxity** in the capsule and ligaments that surround the shoulder joint. In addition, certain individuals are born with congenital joint laxity, which may predispose them to shoulder instability.

When the head of the humerus actually comes out of the socket, it is considered a dislocation. At times, it will go back in by itself. However, it often has to be **reduced** by a physician in the emergency room or on the field. Resultant trauma can cause soft-tissue damage and muscle spasm. The shoulder capsule and a structure called the **labrum** are often injured. The labrum is fibrocartilage that helps to increase the stability of the shoulder joint (Levine, 2000). Bony damage or loss can also result from recurrent instability. In addition, with instability, the humerus may **translate** excessively, but not completely come out of the socket. This is referred to as a **subluxation,** which is often a chronic condition. The most common instability is anterior. It usually occurs during some combination of shoulder external rotation, abduction, and extension. Common mechanisms of injury are falling on an outstretched arm, planting a ski pole and falling forward, or trying to arm-tackle someone. In each case, the humeral head is levered out the front of the shoulder. The recurrence rate for shoulder dislocations is extremely high, especially in the younger population (Hovelius, 1987). Clients with anterior shoulder instability may present with a positive apprehensive sign. That is, the client may become apprehensive about, or not allow the joint to be brought into, abduction and external rotation (Figure 19-2). When performing this test, the ACE-AHFS must be cautious to avoid dislocating the joint.

Following an initial dislocation, there is a period of immobilization in a sling. This allows for soft-tissue healing and reduction of pain and spasm. The trend is moving toward shorter periods of immobilization to prevent loss of ROM and excessive muscle **atrophy.**

During the initial phase of recovery, the goals are to decrease pain, inflammation, and spasm and gradually restore shoulder ROM in a safe manner. Positions of abduction, external rotation, and extension are avoided. Elevation of the arm is initiated in the plane of the scapula. This plane is 30 to 45 degrees anterior to the **frontal plane** (Figure 19-3). This plane provides the greatest amount of joint

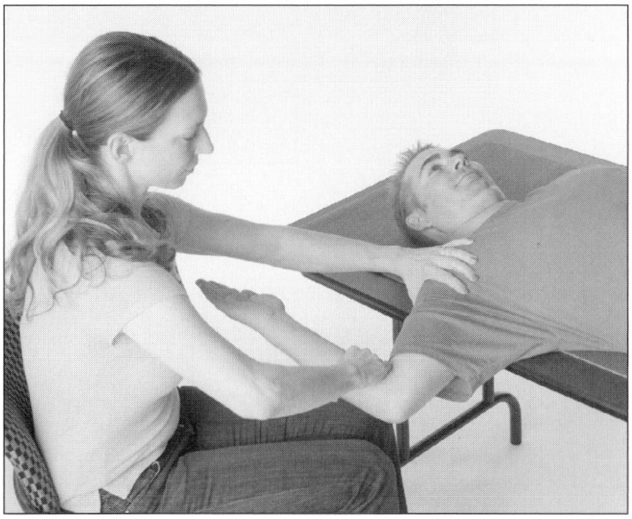

Figure 19-2
Anterior apprehension test

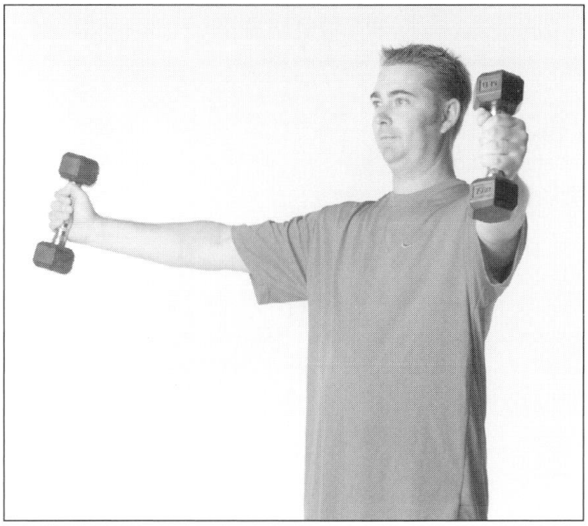

Figure 19-3
Diagonal arm raise in the plane of the scapula

congruity and the least amount of stress to the shoulder capsule (Saha, 1983).

When initiating a strengthening program, submaximal, pain-free isometrics are performed for the rotator cuff and the deltoid to help reestablish stability of the shoulder joint. Precautions should be taken for the rotator cuff when performing internal and external rotation (IR/ER) exercises. The rotator cuff is often inflamed with a shoulder dislocation or instability. Isolated IR/ER exercises can increase the inflammation and thus reflexively inhibit the rotator cuff (Timm, 1998). As external rotation ROM improves and inflammation is reduced, isotonic IR/ER exercises may be incorporated using elastic resistance.

A key component of restoring shoulder stability is to restore the strength of the muscles associated with the scapula. A normal scapula provides a stable base for shoulder rotation and maintains the proper length-tension relationship of the rotator cuff and deltoid muscles. When initiating scapula musculature strengthening, the ACE-AHFS should continue to protect the shoulder capsule and labrum. External rotation and extension should be limited to neutral. For individuals with anterior instability, closed-chain exercises are often utilized. These exercises are performed with the distal end of the limb fixed and provide a compressive load to the shoulder joint and promote stability (Tippett, 1992). Examples include ball stabilization, wall push-ups, quadruped stabilization, and dips or seated press-ups (Figures 19-4 through 19-8). As the client becomes less symptomatic and more stable, open-chain exercises are incorporated for scapula musculature strengthening. These exercises are performed with the distal end of the limb free and can be considered more functional, as most **activities of daily living (ADL)** take place in this mode. Scapula-muscle exercises may include rowing (retraction), shrugs (elevation), and serratus punches (protraction) (Figures 19-9 through 19-11). In addition, these exercises have

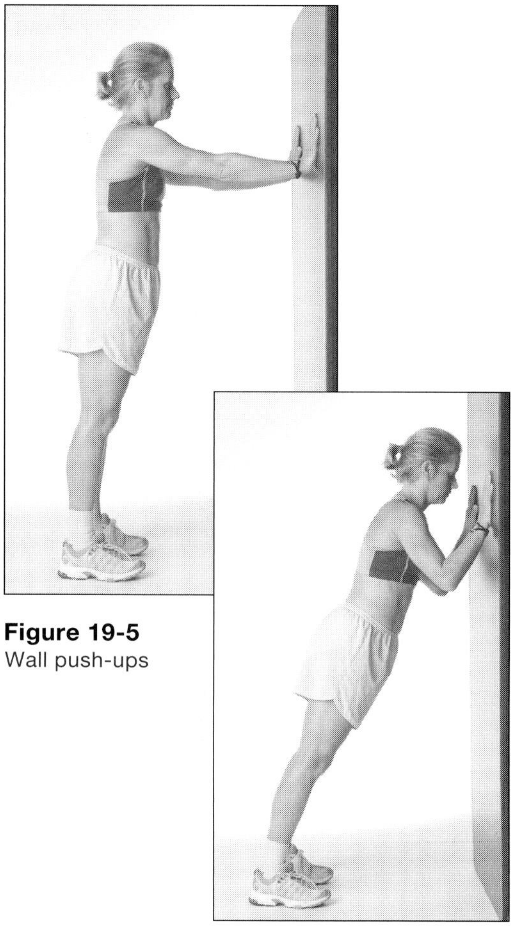

Figure 19-5
Wall push-ups

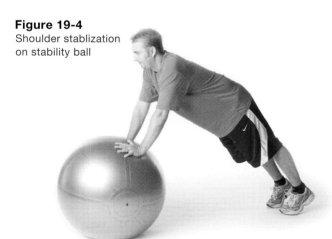

Figure 19-4
Shoulder stablization on stability ball

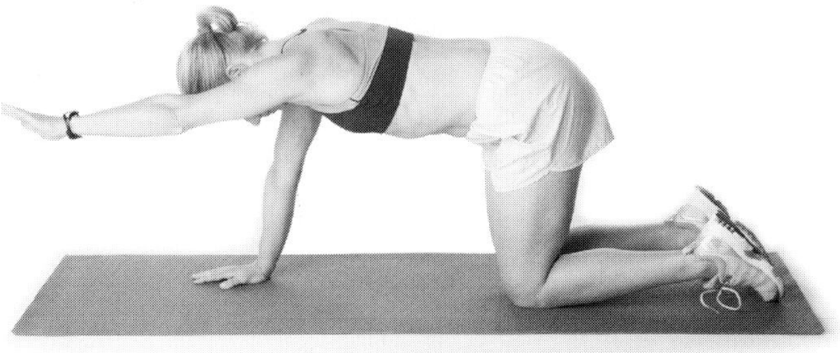

Figure 19-6
Quadruped shoulder stablization

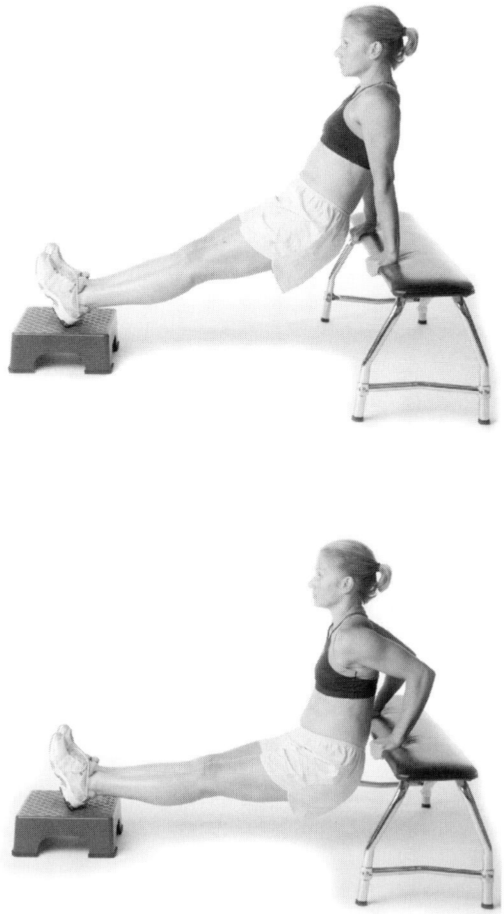

Figure 19-7
Bench dips

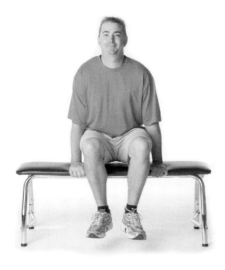

Figure 19-8
Seated press-ups

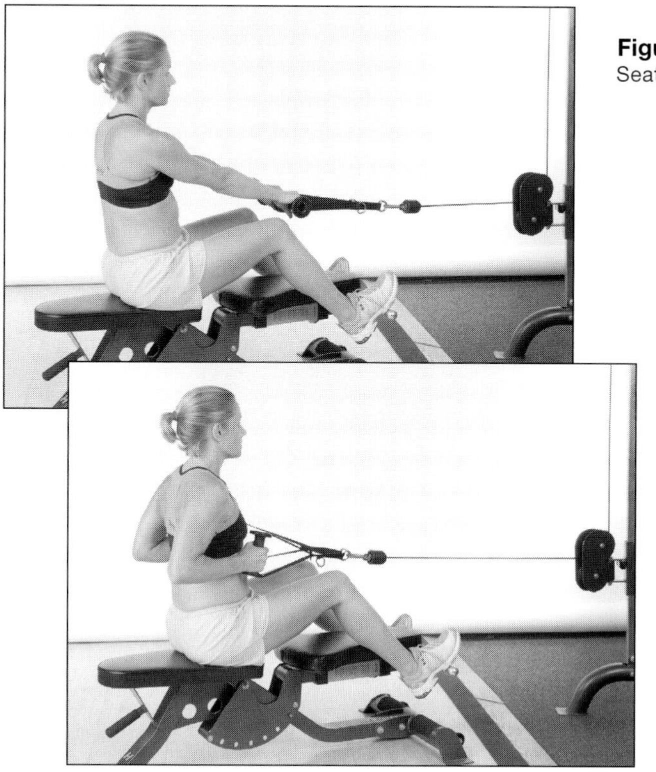

Figure 19-9
Seated rowing

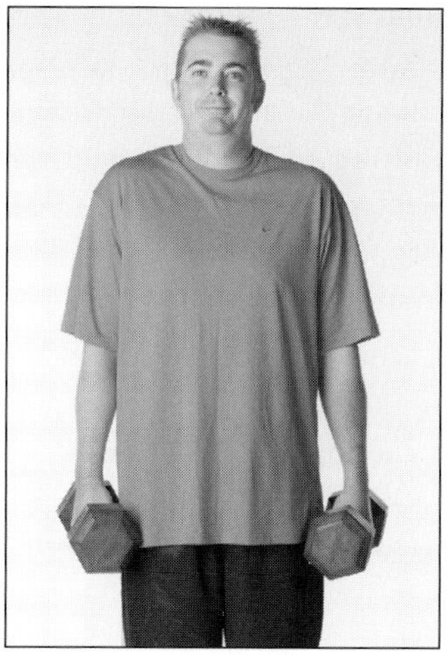

Figure 19-10
Shoulder shrugs

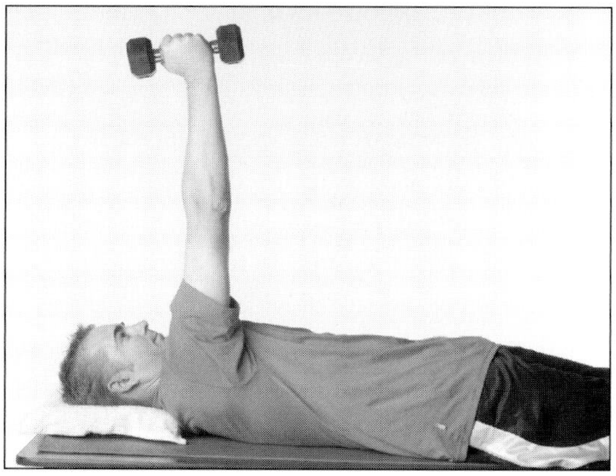

Figure 19-11
Serratus punches

been shown to indirectly strengthen the rotator cuff. The scapula initially sets during the first 60 degrees of elevation of the arm. Following this phase, there should be a 2:1 ratio of glenohumeral motion to scapulothoracic motion. Any deviation from this ratio may manifest itself as shoulder pathology.

The latissimus dorsi also contributes significantly to the stability of the shoulder by providing a compressive force to the glenohumeral joint (Bassett et al., 1988). When initiating strengthening, the ACE-AHFS should limit the ROM from below 90 degrees of forward flexion to neutral extension. This may be accomplished with elastic resistance or a cable column (Figure 19-12). When progressing, the lat pull-down should never be performed in the behind-the-neck position. This position places the shoulder in abduction and external rotation, thus increasing the stress on the shoulder capsule and ligaments (Gross et al., 1993). The pull-down should be performed in front and in a reclined position with the trunk in slight extension (Figure 19-13). The bar is pulled down to the chest. Aside from reducing the chance of injury, this position provides a greater mechanical advantage for the latissimus dorsi and the scapular retractors (Fees et al., 1998).

A client with shoulder instability may return to performing biceps curls, a very popular exercise in most health clubs and gyms. However, the ACE-AHFS must be aware that the long head of the biceps has an attachment at the labrum. One particular labral tear is referred to as a SLAP lesion (superior labrum from anterior to posterior) (Snyder et al., 1990). This injury occurs in the region where the biceps originate. If there has been any damage to the labrum, excessive biceps activity may cause **traction** and exacerbate the injury. In addition, the ACE-AHFS should monitor the client for any increased anterior/superior shoulder pain. Pain in this region with resistive forearm supination or resistive shoulder forward flexion with the forearm in supination may be an indication of **bicipital tendinitis** (Figure 19-14). In this case, the activity should be stopped and the physician or physical therapist should be informed.

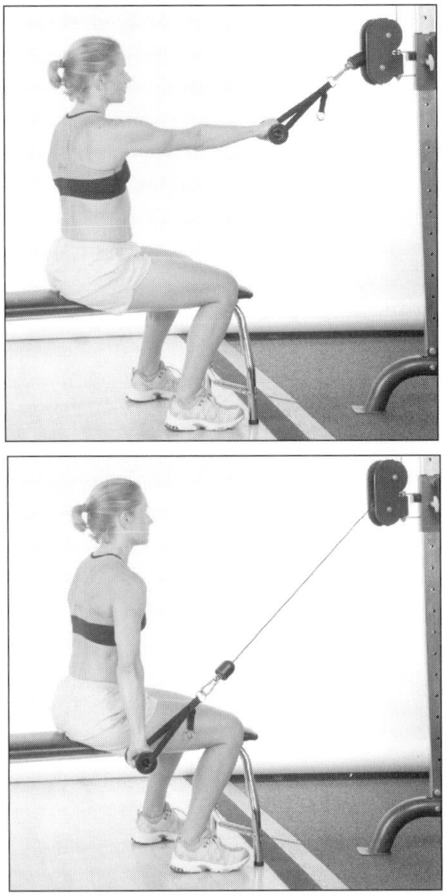

Figure 19-12
Shoulder extension

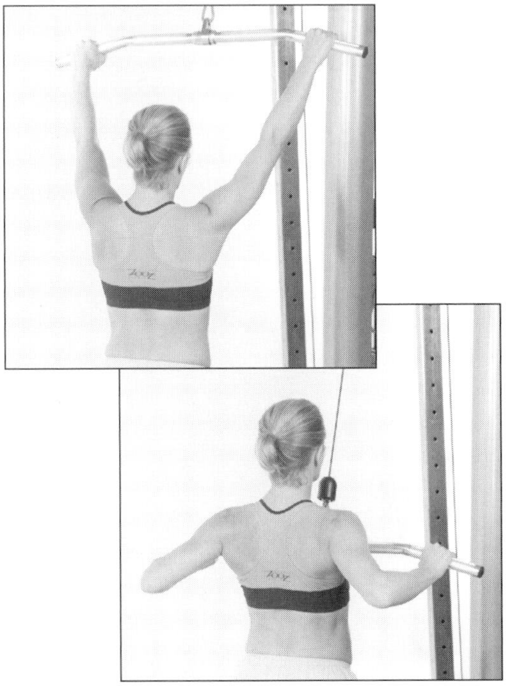

Figure 19-13
Lat pull-down

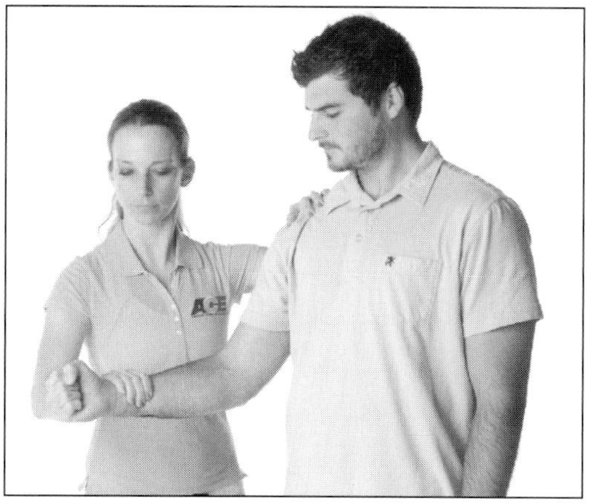

Figure 19-14
Resistive forearm supination

Biceps curls performed in a seated, supported position may reduce the chances of exacerbation. Also, avoiding end ranges of elbow extension may reduce the traction on the labrum. In addition, performing curls with a neutral forearm position will reduce the load on the biceps.

Modifications should be made for a client who wants to return to the bench press. First, there should be a mandatory "handoff" and spot. Second, shoulder position should be limited to below 90 degrees of forward flexion, 45 degrees of abduction, and neutral external rotation (Fees et al., 1998). These restrictions eliminate performance of the incline bench press, which would increase the stress on the capsule and ligaments. Repetitions should also be limited to avoid excessive fatigue, which can result in a loss of dynamic shoulder stability. Finally, weight machines such as a chest press, in which range of motion can be controlled, may be a safer option.

The shoulder press or military press is another popular exercise. It is best to discourage clients with shoulder instability from performing this exercise. An effective initial strategy for the ACE-AHFS is to advise the client to substitute other exercises in its place. Those who want to continue the shoulder press must avoid the behind-the-neck position. This position places significant stress on the shoulder capsule and ligaments and places the shoulder in a tenuous position for instability. Bringing the shoulder into a more anterior position or closer to the scapular plane significantly reduces the stress to the shoulder capsule and ligaments and provides better joint conformity between the humeral head and the glenoid fossa. Again, weight machines may provide a safer alternative to free weights.

Posterior instability is less common, but it does occur. Posterior dislocations are rare. The mechanism of injury is usually a fall on an outstretched hand in a position of shoulder flexion, adduction, and internal rotation. Other mechanisms include seizures, car accidents, and electric shock. More common are subluxations, or excessive translation, often related to overhead activities such as throwing or tennis. Clients will often complain of pain while following through during these activities. Also, repetitive activities such as bench pressing or push-ups can stretch the posterior shoulder capsule.

During the early stages of rehabilitation, the goals and treatment are similar to those used when working with a client with anterior instability. Again, the rotator cuff may be inflamed and care should be taken in restoring IR/ER strength. Conversely, positions of shoulder flexion, internal rotation, and horizontal adduction must be avoided or minimized. When restoring strength, the program is often biased to the posterior musculature to provide secondary restraints to the posterior stabilizers of the shoulder. Rowing with scapular retraction, external rotation, shoulder extension, and horizontal abduction are important exercises with posterior instability.

Contrary to anterior instability, closed-chain or weightbearing activities must be minimized or modified to avoid excessive stretch to the posterior capsule. Activities such as push-ups, which drive the humeral head posteriorly, are often contraindicated. Any exercises that may force the humeral head posteriorly should be performed with posterior support or in the plane of the scapula to avoid excessive stretching of the capsule (Figure 19-15).

Bench pressing is often contraindicated. However, clients who want to continue performing this exercise should use a wider grip and avoid full elbow extension. This will limit the amount of horizontal adduction and decrease stress on the posterior capsule.

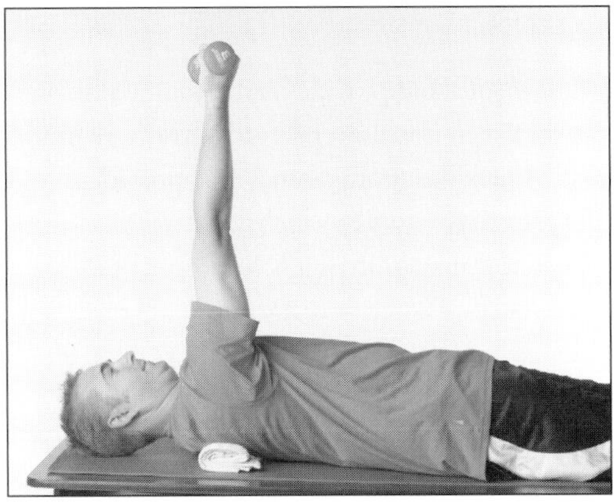

Figure 19-15
Supine serratus punch or chest press with a towel roll under the shoulder to avoid excessive posterior translation

Rotator Cuff Pathology

The rotator cuff is a group of four muscles that surround the glenohumeral joint. The muscles function to rotate the shoulder and contribute to stability by forming a dynamic "sling" for the joint. They consist of the subscapularis (anteriorly), the supraspinatus (superiorly), and the infraspinatus and teres minor (posteriorly). Injuries of the rotator cuff are common and may be chronic conditions or the result of trauma. Traumatic injuries are more common in the older population and are often related to a fall with an indirect force on an abducted arm. **Tendinitis** of the rotator cuff is very common and can be a result of repetitive overhead activities or incorrect body mechanics during weight training. Activities such as tennis, swimming, and throwing can eccentrically overload the rotator cuff and cause tendinitis. Carrying and lifting heavy bags in daily life is another common mechanism of injury. In addition, excessive shoulder laxity or instability can predispose a person to this pathology by making the rotator cuff work much harder.

A common diagnosis of the rotator cuff is referred to as **impingement syndrome.** This refers to the impingement of the soft tissues between the humeral head and the archway that is formed by the acromion and the coracoacromial ligament. Conditions that narrow this archway, such as soft-tissue swelling, bone spurs, or arthritic changes, can predispose an individual to impingement. For some individuals, the acromion is congenitally hooked or curved in shape—as opposed to flat—which may predispose the client to an impingement syndrome as the acromion rubs on the rotator cuff.

The most common structures affected are the supraspinatus, the infraspinatus, the long head of the biceps, and the subacromial **bursa.** A bursa is a sac of fluid that is present in areas of the body that are potential sites of friction. With overuse, a bursa can become swollen and inflamed, resulting in **bursitis.** As the tendons become inflamed, they may rub on the bone and become frayed and eventually lead to chronic rotator cuff tears, which can vary greatly in terms of size, thickness, and location. These tears may continue to get larger until surgical intervention may be required. Surgical intervention is determined by several factors such as pain, loss of function, activity level, and the amount of repairable tissue available.

The presentation of clients with rotator cuff injuries will vary greatly depending on the location and severity of the injury. The duration of the injury is also often a factor. A person with a torn or inflamed rotator cuff may present with pain or weakness with resistive external rotation. Supraspinatus pathology is often consistent with pain and/or weakness with resistive flexion with internal rotation in the plane of the scapula (i.e., the "empty can" position) (Jobe & Jobe, 1983). In addition, passive full forward flexion (Neer test) and passive forward flexion and internal rotation (Hawkins-Kennedy test) may elicit pain (Hawkins & Kennedy, 1980). Weakness is sometimes a function of the severity of the injury, but there is a great deal of variability. Individuals with massive tears of the rotator cuff may have difficulty initiating elevation of the arm or maintaining it in an abducted position, but this is not always the case. These clients may not be appropriate for training and need to be referred back to their therapist or physician. Finally, individuals with rotator cuff pathology may describe a "painful arc" of range of motion. As they approach 90 degrees of elevation of the shoulder, they reach the impingement zone and complain of pain that then resolves as they move beyond that zone.

The initial stages of training individuals with rotator cuff injuries focus on reducing inflammation and promoting healing. This is a stage of "active rest" in which the exacerbating activities are eliminated or modified. Common causes of injury are overhead sports, military press, incline bench press, and lateral raises in the frontal plane. Restoring flexibility is also an important goal of this phase. Individuals with rotator cuff pathology often lose flexibility of the posterior structures of the shoulder. Loss of horizontal adduction is often an indication of a contracture of the posterior capsule, while loss of internal rotation is often an indication of a contracture of the posterior rotator cuff. Both of these situations can contribute to an increased chance of rotator cuff impingement. Flexibility exercises are initiated to restore range of motion (Figures 19-16 and 19-17). As always, the ACE-AHFS should have the client avoid ranges that are painful.

As in the case of shoulder instability, strengthening should be initiated with the scapula, especially in the case of a significantly inflamed rotator cuff. Any deviation in scapular function can have a negative effect on the shoulder. For example, if the scapula is elevated too high, the mechanical advantage of the rotator cuff is altered. By restoring normal scapula function, the proper length-tension relationship of the rotator cuff is restored. In addition, many of the scapula strengthening exercises (e.g., rowing, shrugs, serratus punches, push-ups with a plus) indirectly strengthen the rotator cuff (Hintermeister et al., 1998).

As inflammation decreases, IR/ER exercises may be cautiously introduced. As mentioned previously, the ACE-AHFS should carefully monitor symptoms to avoid an inhibition of the rotator cuff. It should be noted that not everyone can tolerate these exercises. Strengthening can be introduced as submaximal isometrics. Clients can then progress to using elastic resistance. When performing external rotation exercises, the client can position a towel roll at his or her side, which places the shoulder in a slightly abducted position (Figure 19-18). This will improve the blood supply to the shoulder and enhance the mechanical advantage of the external rotators.

For those who want to continue deltoid strengthening, scapular plane elevation is preferred to performing lateral raises in the frontal plane (Figure 19-19). The exercise in the scapular plane affords the least amount of stress on the shoulder. It is also a more functional plane in which to work. Finally, this exercise also recruits much of the scapula musculature, and to some extent the supraspinatus (Moseley, Jobe, & Pink, 1994). The "empty can" position described

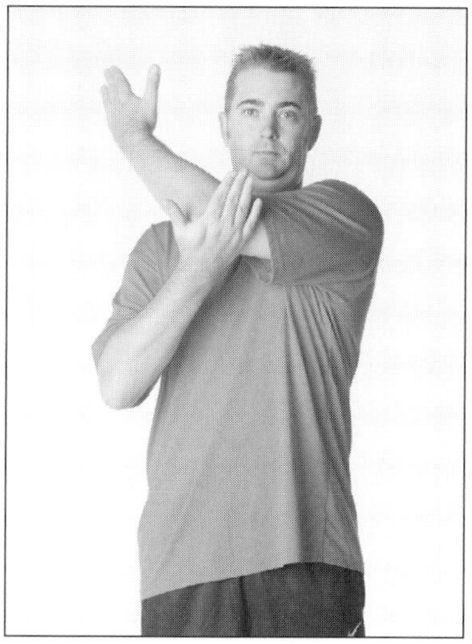

Figure 19-16
Posterior capsule stretch

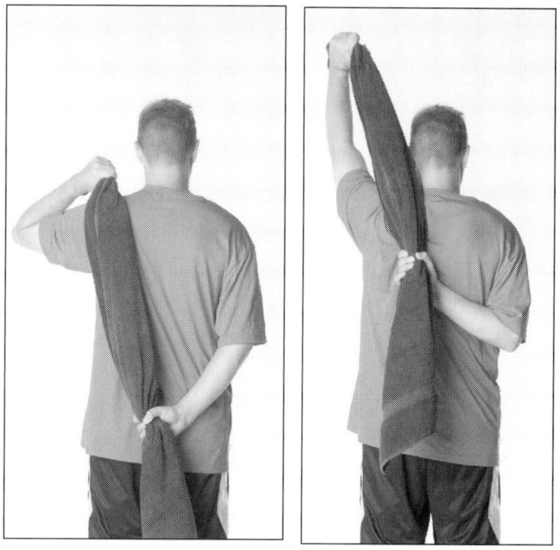

Figure 19-17
Medial rotation stretch using a towel

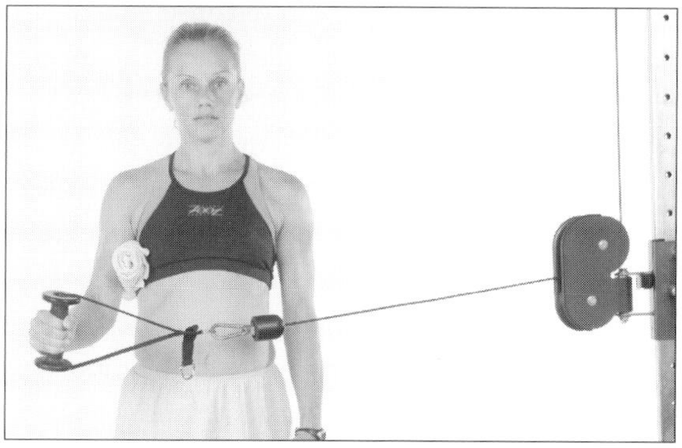

Figure 19-18
External rotation

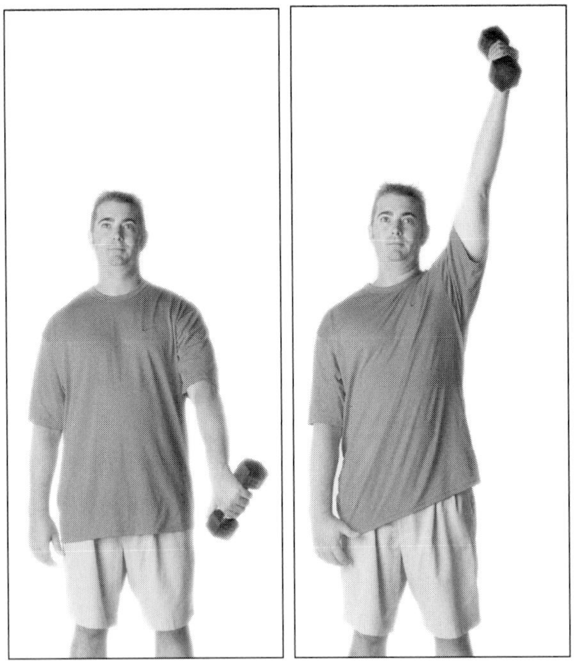

Figure 19-19
Shoulder abduction in scapular plane

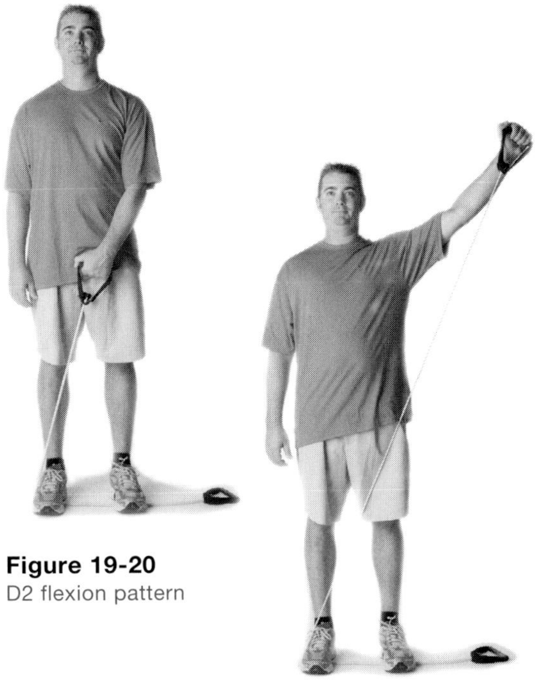

Figure 19-20
D2 flexion pattern

by Jobe and Jobe (1983) for strengthening the supraspinatus is not advised, as the internally rotated position significantly increases the chance of shoulder impingement and is a common source of shoulder pain.

When designing a strength-training program, the ACE-AHFS should consider that many athletic or functional demands require a significant amount of eccentric muscle activity. Therefore, the eccentric or negative phase of each exercise should also be emphasized. However, the ACE-AHFS should closely monitor these exercises, as they are often a cause of **delayed onset muscle soreness (DOMS).** Many clients with rotator cuff injuries will want to return to overhead activities such as tennis, swimming, or throwing. In such cases, multijoint activities such as **proprioceptive neuromuscular facilitation (PNF)** patterns are useful to reproduce these demands. In particular, the D2 flexion pattern, which consists of shoulder flexion, abduction, and external rotation, reproduces the neuromuscular demands of many overhead activities (Figure 19-20).

When a client is returning to performing a bench press, a narrower hand spacing should be utilized to minimize the peak shoulder torque in the pressing motion and reduce the rotator cuff and biceps tendon requirements for stabilization of the humeral head (Fees et al., 1998).

Lateral Epicondylitis

Lateral epicondylitis is often referred to as "tennis elbow." It results from the repetitive tension overloading of the wrist and finger extensors that originate at the lateral epicondyle. Traditionally, the mechanism of injury takes place during the backhand of a novice tennis player who has poor mechanics. For example, not getting the racquet back fast enough and hitting the ball in front of the body or having a poor weight shift can result in greater stresses on the lateral aspect of the elbow. A change in the frequency of activity or a poorly fitted racquet can also contribute to injury. Tennis players who have a deficit in their proximal strength, such as in the scapula muscles or the rotator cuff, may be more susceptible to developing lateral epicondylitis. A lack of proximal stability may manifest itself further down the chain at the elbow. In addition, poor mechanics reduces the use of the lower body and core in the tennis stroke. This can result in increased stress on the elbow.

"Tennis elbow" is often a misnomer, as this injury it is not always a result of tennis. Carrying heavy bags or performing manual labor, especially with the elbow in extension, can result in lateral epicondylitis. In addition, excessive computer work can lead to increased stress to the extensor tendons. Ergonomic adjustments are often a key aspect of treatment.

Regardless of the mechanism of injury, the overload can result in inflammation of the tendons that attach at the lateral epicondyle. In later stages, a mass may form in the tendon and even result in a tear. This injury is often very resistant to treatment, as it is not often detected until latter stages of the pathology. At those stages, clients will complain about activities such as shaking hands, holding a coffee cup, or carrying something with the elbow in extension. Pain is elicited with resistive wrist extension, especially with the elbow in extension and passive wrist flexion (Figure 19-21).

The goals of the initial stage of treatment are to reduce the symptoms and promote healing. Various modalities are utilized to reduce symptoms and a period of active rest is encouraged. The causative activity must be eliminated or modified. For example, a client may be encouraged to avoid tennis or make ergonomic adjustments. In the gym, lifting weights is avoided or modified, depending on the severity of symptoms. Lifting weights with the elbow extended is certainly to be avoided. A wrist splint may be used to rest the extensor mechanism. In addition, a counterforce brace may be used around the elbow to dissipate forces away from the injured site and reduce pain.

As symptoms begin to subside, the ACE-AHFS should help the client restore normal flexibility. Loss of passive wrist flexion is a common finding, and can be restored with passive wrist flexion with the elbow in extension (Figure 19-22). As always,

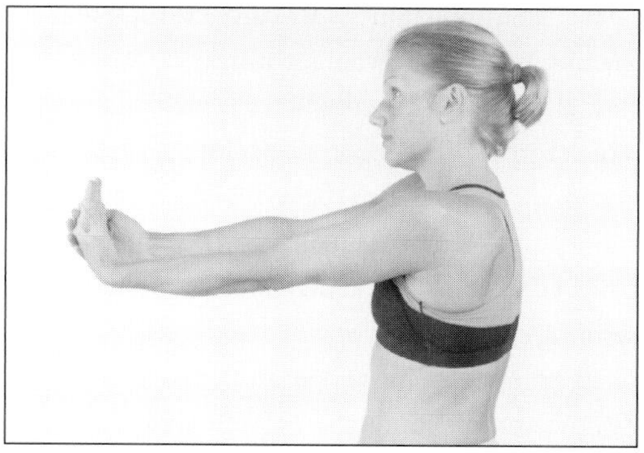

Figure 19-21
Resistive wrist extension

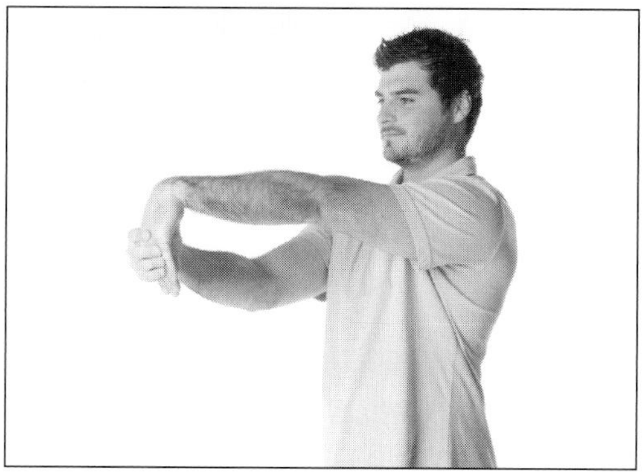

Figure 19-22
Passive wrist flexion

stretching should be performed slowly and gradually, and be maintained in a pain-free range. Slow, progressive stretching allows the muscle to relax instead of reflexively guarding the area. These types of stretches have a longer-lasting effect.

When initiating a strengthening program, the ACE-AHFS should assess the shoulder and scapula for any underlying deficits. With tennis elbow, proximal strength deficits, especially in the shoulder rotators, are often found. Initially, attempting to isolate the wrist extensors can exacerbate the symptoms. The client should be relatively asymptomatic in normal ADL prior to performing wrist extension exercises. Tolerance to a firm handshake has been described as a prerequisite to these exercises. When initiating wrist extension strengthening, the elbow should be supported and be in flexion to reduce the stress (Figure 19-23).

One approach to initiating a strengthening program is to use functional, multijoint exercises such as rowing, shrugs, lat pull-downs, and PNF patterns. These exercises allow some strengthening of the wrist and forearm without trying to isolate them. They also provide a more global approach to strengthening the entire upper extremity and establishing proximal strength. These exercises should be performed while avoiding the end ranges of elbow extension. When a client is performing any activity, increasing the grip size of resistive equipment or a tennis racquet can reduce the amount of wrist extensor activity and the amount of stress on the lateral epicondyle.

As symptoms subside, the wrist extensors and forearm supinators can gradually be exercised in greater degrees of elbow extension. Movement patterns such as a tennis stroke or a golf swing can be reproduced using elastic resistance. Novice

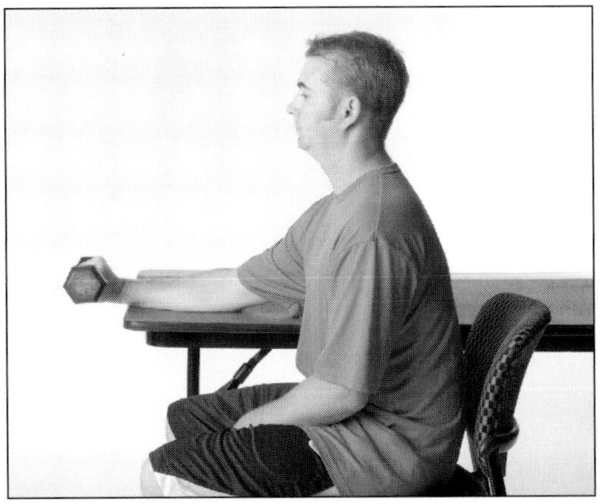

Figure 19-23
Dumbbell wrist extension

tennis players are encouraged to take lessons to improve mechanics. As weight training is progressed, the ACE-AHFS should continue to closely monitor the client for any recurrence of lateral elbow pain. Finally, when performing cardiovascular activities, the client should avoid gripping the apparatus too tightly with the affected hand.

Medial Epicondylitis

Medial epicondylitis occurs due to an overload of the wrist flexors and forearm pronators. Golf, throwing, and swimming are common mechanisms of injury. Overuse or poor mechanics may lead to tendinitis or small tears of these muscles near the origin at the medial epicondyle. "Golfer's elbow" refers to an injury to the medial side of the right elbow (for a right-handed golfer). Novice golfers who fail to use their larger body parts and do not weight shift correctly are more susceptible. Beginners tend to throw the club down at the ball or hit too far behind the ball and put greater stress on the medial aspect of the elbow. Participating in throwing sports also tends to place a great deal of stress on the medial aspect of the elbow. The ACE-AHFS must be aware that injuries to the ulnar nerve are often associated with this area. Any numbness or tingling along the ulnar aspect of the forearm or the fourth and fifth fingers should alert the ACE-AHFS to this possibility. Clients will present with tenderness over the medial epicondyle or the proximal wrist flexors and pronator teres. Resistive wrist flexion or forearm pronation may elicit symptoms. In addition, performing high-load biceps curls often exacerbates symptoms.

Remember, the goals of the early stages of rehabilitation are to reduce symptoms and promote healing. During these stages, causative activities are modified or eliminated, golfers are encouraged to take lessons, throwing mechanics are reviewed, and swimming strokes are assessed. Proximal shoulder and scapular strength are assessed for any underlying deficits.

Strengthening is again initiated with multijoint, functional exercises, as opposed to isolating the wrist flexors and forearm pronators. Exercises such as biceps curls may be better tolerated in a neutral forearm position than in a pronated position. Full elbow extension should be avoided when performing resistive exercises. Flexibility should be initiated by stretching into wrist extension and forearm supination (Figure 19-24). Once again, the range should be basically pain free. Isolated wrist flexion and forearm pronation exercises should be avoided until the client is asymptomatic. When initiating these exercises, they should be done with the elbow supported and in flexion. The ACE-AHFS should proceed cautiously with isolated pronation exercises, as they can often be a source of pain or injury. Strengthening can often be achieved with multijoint exercises. Prior to a return to activity, functional exercises such as PNF patterns may be helpful. Note that repetitive activity at the computer can result in medial epicondylitis. The etiology of this injury is rapid, repetitive finger flexion with a fixed wrist as the individual clicks and drags the mouse.

Hand and Wrist Injuries

There are numerous types of pathologies of the wrist and hand. Two of the most common injuries are **carpal tunnel syndrome** and **De Quervain's syndrome.** Carpal tunnel syndrome occurs when the median nerve, which extends from the forearm into the hand, becomes compressed at the wrist. The carpal tunnel is formed by ligaments and bones at the base of the hand. Thickened tendons or other swelling can cause the nerve to become impinged or compressed. Some people are congenitally predisposed to this condition. However, common causes are wrist trauma, arthritis, work stress, and fluid retention. Symptoms include burning,

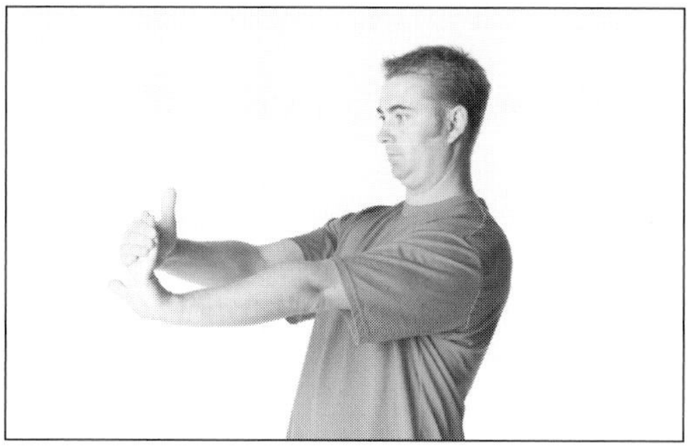

Figure 19-24
Passive wrist extension

tingling, and numbness in the palm, thumb, index, and middle fingers. As the condition worsens, grip strength may be affected. When a client presents with any of these symptoms, the ACE-AHFS should refer him or her to a hand specialist.

De Quervain's syndrome affects the two tendons that move the thumb away from the hand. Some experts believe the tendons become inflamed from overuse; however, the cause is not always clear or well-understood. Symptoms may include pain and or swelling over the thumb side of the wrist. Gripping may also become difficult. When testing for this syndrome, the thumb is tightened as in a closed fist and the hand is tilted toward the ulna side (Finkelstein's test) (Figure 19-25). If the syndrome is present, this position will produce pain at the wrist below the thumb. Any of these symptoms that last for one to two weeks should be addressed by the client's healthcare provider.

Finally, there are numerous ligamentous sprains and fractures that can occur in the small bones of the hand and wrist. While the possibilities are far too extensive to discuss specifically,

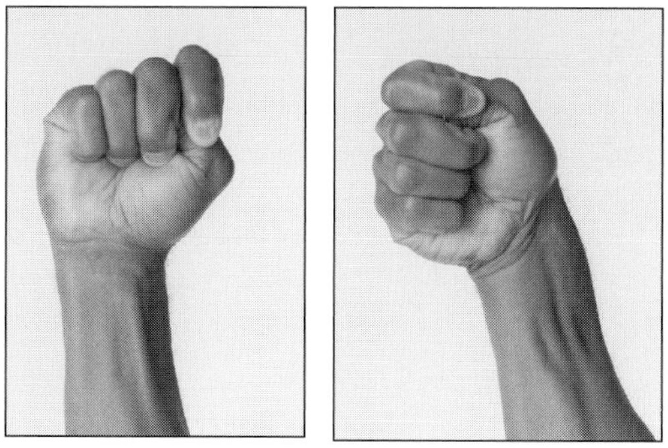

Figure 19-25
Finkelstein's test

some general precautions and adjustments for the injured hand and wrist are as follows:

- Any point tenderness at one of the small bones of the wrist or hand may indicate a fracture. If these symptoms persist, a referral to a hand specialist is advised.
- A change in positioning is often helpful for individuals with hand or wrist pain. When exercising, the wrist is often most comfortable in a neutral position. A good guideline is to avoid wrist flexion and extension greater than 30 degrees. In addition, avoid radial or ulnar deviation. Pain on the ulnar side of the wrist is often exacerbated by forearm pronation or supination.
- The grip size of exercise equipment can be adjusted. The ACE-AHFS may add padding to a piece of exercise equipment to create a larger grip. Often, a larger grip will reduce stress on the wrist, hand, or fingers.

Case Studies

Case Study 1

John is 49-year-old recreational tennis player who has been unable to play for approximately six months after developing lateral elbow pain. Upon seeing an orthopedist, he was diagnosed with lateral epicondylitis. He was treated with **nonsteroidal anti-inflammatory drugs (NSAID)** and physical therapy for three months. Following discharge, he was relatively asymptomatic. His occupation requires him to perform a great deal of computer work and travel often. He comes to an ACE-AHFS to get himself back into "tennis shape," as this is his primary exercise activity.

The ACE-AHFS should contact John's physical therapist to discuss his home exercise program and any ergonomic precautions he was given. The ACE-AHFS should incorporate the exercises into a comprehensive general program that addresses the entire kinetic chain. Shoulder and scapula strength and flexibility should be emphasized, using functional, multijoint exercises. John's lateral elbow symptoms should be monitored regularly to identify any exacerbating exercises. This is especially important if

John is performing wrist extension exercises. When designing John's exercise program, the ACE-AHFS should avoid resistive training in the end ranges of elbow extension. John should also avoid carrying weights around the gym whenever possible. When performing conditioning exercises such as cycling or treadmill walking, John should avoid excessive gripping on the handles or handrails.

Prior to returning to tennis, John should be encouraged to begin hitting with a tennis professional or taking some lessons. This will reinforce the need for him to use his entire body when hitting and develop a good weight shift to reduce the forces at the elbow. He should also be advised to have his tennis pro check his racquet for the proper tension and grip size. In addition, John should be advised to avoid carrying heavy bags when traveling.

Case Study 2

Steve is a 32-year-old recreational skier who suffered a Grade II separation of his acromioclavicular joint while skiing six weeks ago. He was immobilized for two weeks and then underwent a four-week course of physical therapy that restored his shoulder range of motion. He presents with mild, intermittent AC joint discomfort and a slight palpable defect at the joint. Prior to the injury, Steve lifted weights three times a week and is eager to resume his exercise program. He comes to the ACE-AHFS to begin a safe exercise program and avoid exacerbation of the injury. The ACE-AHFS should contact Steve's physical therapist to discuss his current home exercise program and any contraindications or safety precautions. When initiating a strength-training program, the ACE-AHFS should carefully monitor Steve's symptoms at his AC joint. Steve should be encouraged to ice after his workout, even if he is asymptomatic at the time. This may help to prevent any residual symptoms. When using free weights, Steve should be encouraged to begin with weights that he can control well to avoid any traction at the AC joint. He should also be advised to not carry the weights around the gym. Scapula strengthening exercises should be performed in the middle of the range of motion to avoid excessive retraction and protraction. This will prevent excessive stress to the AC joint. Steve should be extremely cautious with exercises that create a great deal of stress at the AC joint, such as bench pressing or push-ups. He should never perform any bench presses without a spotter.

Summary

The key to working with the post-injury client is to understand the pathology and structures involved, as well as the underlying mechanism of injury. In addition, the ACE-AHFS should understand the positions and activities that may exacerbate the condition. Listening to the subjective complaints and symptoms and being proactive in communicating with the client's clinician is critical to preventing re-injury.

References

Bassett, R. et al. (1988). Glenohumeral muscle force and movement mechanics in a position of shoulder instability. *Journal of Biomechanics,* 23, 401–415.

Fees, M. et al. (1998). Upper extremity weight-training modifications for the injured athlete. *American Journal of Sports Medicine,* 26, 5, 732–742.

Gross, M.L. et al. (1993). Anterior shoulder instability in weight lifters. *American Journal of Sports Medicine,* 21, 599–603.

Hawkins R.J. & Kennedy J.C. (1980). Impingement syndrome in athletes. *American Journal of Sports Medicine,* 8, 151–158.

Hintermeister, R.A. et al. (1998). EMG activity and applied load during shoulder rehabilitation exercises using elastic resistance. *American Journal of Sports Medicine,* 26, 210–220.

Hovelius, L. (1987). Anterior dislocation of the shoulder in teenagers and young adults. *Journal of Bone and Joint Surgery,* 69, 393.

Jobe, F.W. & Jobe, C.M. (1983). Painful athletic injuries of the shoulder. *Clinical Orthopedics,* 173, 117–125.

Levine, W.M. (2000). The pathophysiology of shoulder instability. *American Journal of Sports Medicine,* 28, 910–917.

Matheson, J.W. & Price, C.R. (2006). *Postsurgical Orthopedic Sports Rehabilitation: Knee and Shoulder.* St. Louis, Mo.: Mosby Elsevier.

Moseley, J.B., Jobe, F.W., & Pink, M. (1994). EMG analysis of scapular muscles during a shoulder rehabilitation program. *American Journal of Sports Medicine,* 20, 128–134.

O'Brien, S.J. et al. (1998). The active compression test: A new and effective test for diagnosing labral tears and acromioclavicular joint abnormality. *American Journal of Sports Medicine,* 26, 610–613.

Rockwood, C.A. & Matsen, F.A., III. (2004). *The Shoulder* (3rd ed.). Philadelphia: Saunders.

Saha, K. (1983). Mechanism of shoulder movements and plea for recognition of the zero position of the glenohumeral joint. *Clinical Orthopedics,* 173, 3–10.

Snyder, S.J. et al. (1990). SLAP lesions of the shoulder. *Arthroscopy,* 6, 274–279.

Timm, K. (1998). The isokinetic torque curve of shoulder instability in high school baseball pitchers. *Journal of Orthopedic and Sports Physical Therapy,* 26, 150–154.

Tippett, S. (1992). Closed chain exercise. *Orthopedic Physical Therapy Clinics of North America,* 1, 253–268.

Suggested Reading

Altchek, D.W. & Andrews, J.R. (2001). *The Athlete's Elbow.* Philadelphia: Lippincott Williams & Wilkins.

Andrews, J.R. & Wilk, K.E. (2008). *The Athlete's Shoulder* (2nd ed.). New York: Churchill Livingstone.

Baechle, R.T. & Earle, R.W. (2008). *Essentials of Strength Training and Conditioning* (3rd ed.). Champaign, Ill.: Human Kinetics.

Cioppa-Mosca, J. et al. (2006). *Postsurgical Rehabilitation Guidelines for the Orthopedic Clinician.* St. Louis, Mo.: Mosby Elsevier.

Fees, M. et al. (1998). Upper extremity weight-training modifications for the injured athlete. *American Journal of Sports Medicine,* 26, 5, 732–742.

Knott, M. & Voss, D. (1985). *Proprioceptive Neuromuscular Facilitation* (3rd ed.). New York: Harper & Row.

Leach, R.E. & Miller, J.K. (1987). Lateral and medial epicondylitis of the elbow. *Clinics in Sports Medicine* 6, 259–272.

Magee, D.J. (2007). *Orthopedic Physical Assessment* (5th ed.). Philadelphia: Saunders .

Manske, R.C. (2006). *Postsurgical Orthopedic Sports Rehabilitation: Knee & Shoulder.* St. Louis, Mo.: Mosby Elsevier.

Voight, M. & Draovitch, P. (1991). *Eccentric Muscle Training in Sports and Orthopedics.* New York: Churchill Livingstone.

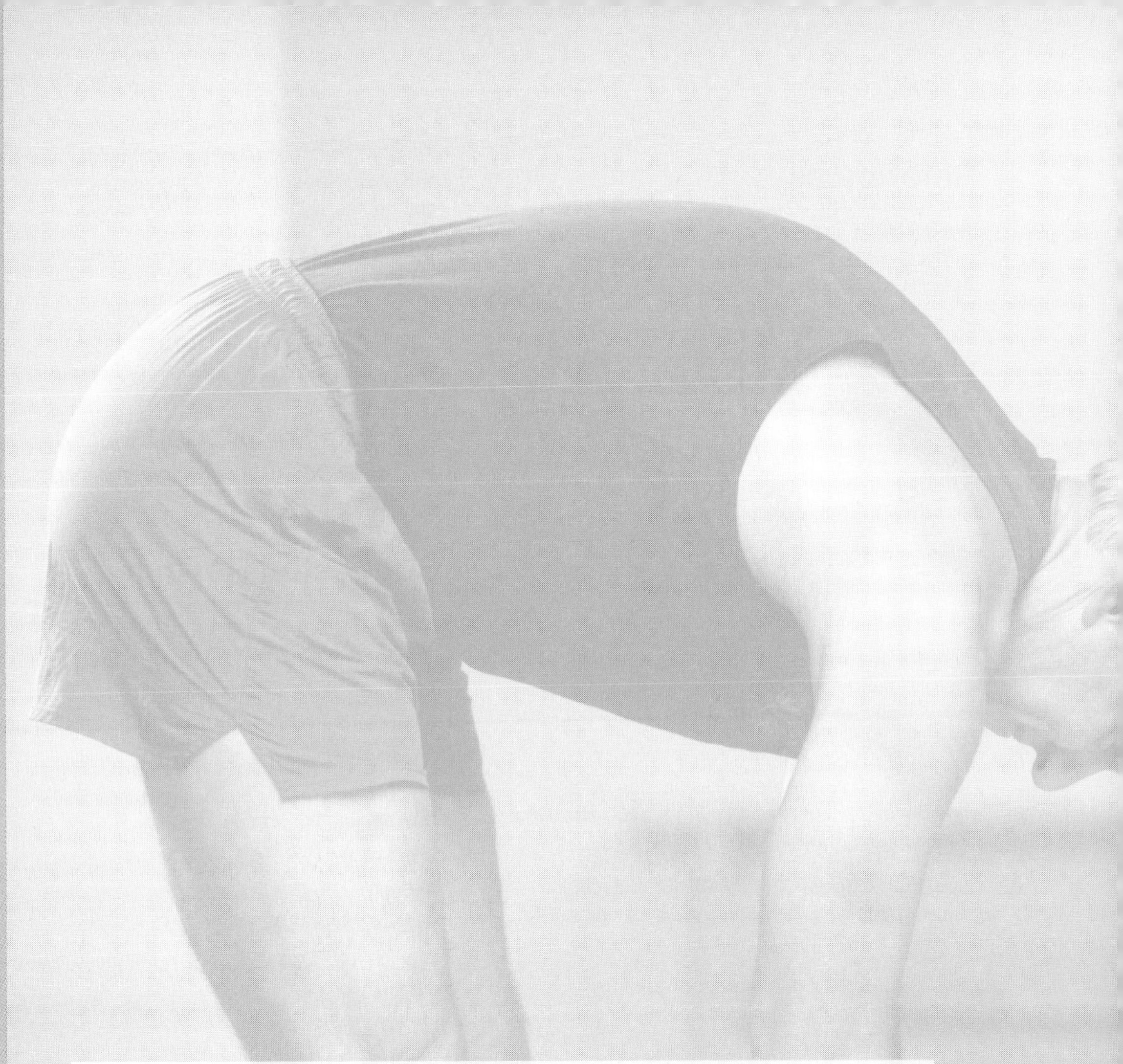

In This Chapter

ACE would like to acknowledge the contributions to this chapter made by Sabrena Merrill, M.S., fitness-industry consultant, author, and educator.

About The Author

Jennifer Solomon, M.D., is board certified in Physical Medicine and Rehabilitation and fellowship trained in Spine and Sports Medicine. She specializes in non-operative treatments for sports and spine injuries, including electrodiagnostics. Dr. Solomon is assistant attending physiatrist at the Hospital for Special Surgery's Women's Sports Medicine Center and clinical instructor at the Weill Medical College of Cornell University. She serves as team physician for St. Peter's College and has covered several sporting events, including the NYC Marathon, tennis tournaments, and various races. Dr. Solomon is also a team physician for the United States Federation Cup Tennis Team and a medical consultant for La Palestra Center for Preventative Medicine. Dr. Solomon is a member of the American Academy of Physical Medicine and Rehabilitation, the North American Spine Society, and the American Association of Electrodiagnostic Medicine. She has published more than 15 articles and chapters on a variety of spine and sports medicine topics.

CHAPTER 20

Low-back Pain

Jennifer Solomon

Epidemiology

Low-back pain (LBP) plagues modern society and is a significant source of cost and disability. Estimates from the National Health Interview Survey (NHIS), which surveyed more than 31,000 adults, revealed that about 25% experienced LBP in the past three months (Deyo et al., 2006). Studies have shown that more than 80% of Americans suffer from at least one episode of back pain during their lifetime (Anderson, 1997). While these episodes vary in length and intensity, historical records estimate that at any one time there are 1.2 million adults disabled as a result of their LBP (Wong & Transfeltd, 2007). A significant proportion of these individuals seek assistance from a healthcare professional. In fact, back pain is the second most common complaint heard in doctors' offices.

While the majority of acute back pain improves over time, some people develop recurrences, while others experience continuous pain. Acute pain can be thought of as pain resulting from a specific trauma or disease that responds to traditional modes of treatment, such as pain relievers. In contrast, chronic pain represents the lasting effects once an inciting event has faded, and is generally resistant to usual treatments (Wong & Transfeltd, 2007). Acute pain and chronic pain not only have individual physiologic mechanisms, but may also have varying psychological, societal, and economic implications. People with LBP report symptoms of **depression, anxiety,** and insomnia more frequently than those without it (Morris, 2006). LBP is the second leading cause of work absenteeism, following upper respiratory infections (Wong & Transfeltd, 2007). In an analysis of total healthcare expenditures in 1998, $90.7 billion was spent on individuals with back pain, which was 60% more than was spent on their back pain–free counterparts (Luo et al., 2004).

Factors Contributing to LBP

Researchers have attempted to discern specific factors that contribute to the onset and persistence of LBP, and while there is much discrepancy, some consistencies exist. These risk factors can be divided into individual, activity, and psychological categories.

Individual Factors

Age and Sex

LBP occurs most commonly in the 30- to 55-year-old age group (Wong & Transfeltd, 2007). Herniated disks are most common in those between the ages of 30 and 40, a time when the water content of intervertebral disks has decreased. However, many individuals will have had at least one episode of back pain earlier in life (Rubin, 2007). In fact, LBP in adolescence appears to be a risk factor for similar symptoms in adulthood. The prevalence of back pain increases with age until age 60, with older individuals experiencing greater rates of chronic or intermittent pain (Rubin, 2007).

Overall, men and women appear to be equally affected. However, older women have a higher prevalence of back pain than older men, which may be secondary to the greater rates of

osteoporosis of the spine seen in women (Bressler et al., 1999). In contrast, men are more involved in heavy work, and therefore have higher rates of occupational back pain.

Body Type

While body weight may play some role in the development of back pain, the data to prove a strong association is currently lacking (Leboeuf-Yde, 2000). Likewise, height and body build have not been shown to have a strong correlation with LBP.

Conditions affecting posture such as **scoliosis, kyphosis,** and leg-length discrepancies are not predisposing factors for LBP (Wong & Transfeltd, 2007). It is unclear, however, how congenital vertebral abnormalities such as **spina bifida occulta** or **transitional vertebra** contribute to LBP.

Smoking

Smoking is thought to be a significant risk factor, though the exact mechanism remains unclear. It is thought that smoking may decrease blood flow to the intervertebral discs, leading to a deficit of nutrients and/or a lack of sufficient oxygen, which may lead to accelerated cell death. Other effects of smoking may include an increase in the rate of development of osteoporosis, fractures, and degenerative changes in the spine (Manek & MacGregor, 2005). In addition, chronic coughing may be an indirect link between smoking and back pain.

Activity-related Factors

Occupation

Certain types of occupational activities appear to predispose individuals to LBP, including heavy lifting, carrying, pulling, pushing, prolonged walking or standing, driving, and working night shifts (Hurwitz & Morgenstern, 1997). High exposure to whole-body vibration is also a risk factor for back pain. Specific professions that are at higher risk include sales, clerical work, repair service, and transportation (Bahr et al., 2004). Work-related stress and dissatisfaction are also associated with the development of LBP.

Exercise

Studies that have surveyed athletes to determine which sports have higher rates of back pain have yielded conflicting results. However, athletes involved in certain activities, such as cross-country skiing and rowing, may have higher rates of LBP than non-athletes (Borenstein, Wiesel, & Boeden, 2004).

The protective role of specific exercise regimens in preventing LBP is less clear, as are associations with **overweight** and **obesity** (Leboeuf-Yde, 2000). In general, those who engage in regular recreational physical activity appear to be less likely to have back pain at any given time and are less likely to develop future pain (Rubin, 2007). Not surprisingly, some high-intensity or repetitive exercises (i.e., golf and tennis) may, in fact, predispose or worsen an existing condition. While physical fitness does not completely prevent LBP, it may improve functional outcomes by decreasing recovery time. Unfortunately, many people with LBP choose not to exercise and actually believe that doing so would be detrimental to their condition.

Psychological Factors

In general, depression, anxiety, and insomnia are strongly correlated with back pain. They can be both predisposing (e.g., psychogenic muscle tension, work distress) and resulting factors of existing back pain. Chronic back pain sufferers are six times more likely to be depressed than individuals without pain (Currie & Wang, 2004). Depression may affect an individual's ability to cope with pain. Fear-avoidance personality variables (exaggerated pain or fear that activity will cause permanent damage) and passive coping techniques (avoidance, withdrawal, wishful thinking) are positive predictors of chronic back pain symptoms. The inability to determine an exact cause of pain or to effectively relieve symptoms may result in further depression.

Overview of Conditions

The possible etiologies of LBP are numerous. Mechanical causes account for approximately 97% of cases, whereas 2% of cases are "visceral disease," or disease of the internal organs and structures, such as

pancreatitis, prostatitis, and **aortic aneurysm.** The remaining 1% of back pain results from non-mechanical spinal conditions such as tumors, infections, and rheumatologic disorders (Deyo & Weinstein, 2001). This section describes some of the most common mechanical back pain diagnoses, along with their causes and typical symptoms.

Lumbar **strain** or **sprain** is a non-specific term often used to describe mechanical LBP. Typically, a strain refers to a muscle injury in which the fibers are abnormally stretched, while a sprain refers to a torn ligament. A more descriptive and accurate term for most of these cases is **discogenic back pain**, which refers to dysfunction or degeneration of lumbar intervertebral discs. This phenomenon is a universal process of aging that leads to chemical and physical changes in the disc. Discs are comprised of an outer ring, the **annulus fibrosus,** and an inner gel, the **nucleus pulposus.** Over time, discs lose their water content and acquire gradual fibrotic changes that limit mobility.

While these changes occur in everyone, the presence of symptomatic back pain is multifactorial. Microtrauma may lead to small tears or cracks in the annulus and result in inflammation and pain around annular nerves. Also, gradual narrowing of the disc height may cause an unstable surface where the facet joints articulate, leading to an overloading of those structures and, ultimately, pain. Generally, discogenic pain is caused by activities that increase pressure within the disc, such as coughing, sneezing, sitting, and bending forward. Discogenic pain can be acute or chronic.

Herniated discs account for approximately 4% of all mechanical LBP (Deyo & Weinstein, 2001). As previously noted, aging affects discs by decreasing the nearly 80% water content of the nucleus and making the annulus more prone to tears. A herniation occurs when there is a tear in the annulus and a subsequent extrusion of the nucleus through this annular defect. Individuals with herniated discs complain of sharp or throbbing LBP, which is worse with movement but improved with lying down. Herniated material may extend out far enough to compress the nerve roots that exit the spinal cord at that level, causing pain, numbness, tingling, or weakness. These are signs and symptoms of lumbar **radiculopathy,** or nerve root impairment. **Sciatica** refers to radicular symptoms that follow the path of the sciatic nerve, down the posterior aspect of the thigh, lower leg, and foot. Generally, there is no acute event associated with the onset of sciatica, which may be exacerbated by standing, sitting, sneezing, heavy lifting, or having a bowel movement. In some cases, the sciatic symptoms may be equivalent to, or worse than, the LBP itself.

Another 3% of mechanical pain is secondary to **spinal stenosis,** which results from narrowing of the central spinal canal, either by bone or soft tissue (Deyo & Weinstein, 2001). Degenerative changes of the facet joints and intervertebral discs are largely responsible for this process. Thus, spinal stenosis typically arises in persons over age 50. Symptoms arise when the narrowing causes compression of the spinal cord or spinal nerves. Most commonly, spinal stenosis sufferers complain of cramping, pain, numbness, or weakness in their back or legs. However, some will report leg pain only. The typical pattern is termed **pseudoclaudication,** which refers to pain in the buttock, thigh, or leg that occurs with standing or walking and is relieved by rest in a lying or sitting position, or by flexing forward at the waist.

Approximately 4% of mechanical LBP occurs from osteoporotic **compression fractures** (Deyo & Weinstein, 2001). Spinal fractures generally result from major trauma, such as a fall from a great height or a motor vehicle accident. However, individuals with **osteopenia** or osteoporosis, in which bone density is reduced, can acquire compression fractures from less significant trauma, even from something as simple as a sneeze or cough. Up to 20% of the time, compression fractures due to osteopenia or osteoporosis may be asymptomatic and found incidentally on imaging performed for other reasons (Wong & Transfeltd, 2007). The remaining 80% of osteoporotic compression fracture cases experience a sudden onset of pain that is usually diffuse in nature.

Spondylolysis, another type of fracture, is a common asymptomatic finding in 5% of the general population (Yu & Garfin, 1994). Spondylolysis is essentially a stress fracture in the posterior aspect of the spine, the **pars intrarticularis**, where the vertebral body and posterior elements join together. The fifth lumbar vertebra is the most common location for spondylolysis. The condition typically occurs in children or young adults involved in sports and is a result of compressive forces or hyperextension. Symptoms can be unilateral or bilateral, acute or chronic, and range in severity from mild to immobilizing.

Spondylolysis can lead to **spondylolisthesis,** which is an anterior displacement of a vertebra relative to the one below it. The most common symptom is LBP, which may or may not be associated with an acute injury and is worse with flexion but relieved by extension. Leg pain can also occur with spondylolisthesis if spinal nerve roots are irritated as they leave the canal.

Diagnostic Testing

Generally, all clients with back pain should receive a thorough physical exam from a physician. In all of the previously described conditions, there are common warning signs that necessitate immediate attention, including fever, loss of bowel or bladder control, unexplained weight loss, history of cancer or recent infection, and intravenous drug use.

After careful evaluation, the physician may choose to pursue further evaluation with an imaging study. Plain radiographs or x-rays are often used as an initial test, as they are the best option for evaluating bony changes such as fracture, tumor, spondylolisthesis, and disc-space narrowing. **Computed tomography** (CT) and **magnetic resonance imaging** (MRI) are used to visualize spinal stenosis and herniated discs and may be used to rule out conditions such as infection or cancer. However, CT and MRI may also detect asymptomatic abnormalities. Therefore, careful correlation with the individual's subjective history and physical exam is essential when using any imaging technique.

Treatment

Since the natural history of LBP is variable, treatment goals depend on the specific condition. Even though studies have shown that one-third of patients presenting to primary care offices with non-specific back pain significantly improve within one week, and two-thirds improve within seven weeks, up to 40% will experience a recurrence within six months (Carey & Garrett, 1999). Thus, a significant proportion of back-pain patients experience a relapsing and remitting course of pathology. Still others may develop a chronic disabling or persistent condition. Multiple factors may determine the overall prognosis, but each diagnosis also inherently includes general expectations for the extent and timing of recovery. For example, pain from acute herniated discs has a favorable prognosis, with only 10% of patients having significant pain after six weeks. However, painful symptoms in approximately 70% of patients with spinal stenosis remain stable, while only 15% improve and the remaining 15% gradually worsen (Deyo & Weinstein, 2001).

Treatment options for patients with LBP have evolved and, in some cases, become a source of much debate. Because of the ubiquitous nature of LBP in modern society, many patients approach their diagnosis with several preconceived ideas about treatment, formed from a combination of lay press articles and recounted experiences from friends and relatives. However, for almost all conditions, current thinking among health professionals is one of active recovery. Bed rest is contraindicated, as it has been shown to not only delay recovery, but also worsen symptoms. Understanding a client's condition is essential for him or her to actively participate in improving current symptoms and preventing future recurrences.

The following sections present an overview of current treatment options, with a focus on non-surgical choices.

Non-pharmacologic Therapy

In the acute setting, clients often fear that the pain they feel with activity is a sign of further injury, or even permanent disability. However, clients can be reassured that returning to daily activities has actually been shown to be an integral part of treatment and recovery. Basic recommendations include avoiding specific movements or activities that provoke pain and limiting bed rest to times of severe pain only. Because there is little evidence that specific back exercises are useful in the acute setting, clients are generally encouraged to engage in low-stress aerobic activities such as walking. Heavy lifting and prolonged sitting and standing should be avoided. In cases of **subacute** and chronic LBP a physical therapist can design specific exercises that focus on conditioning the core musculature in an attempt to improve current symptoms and avoid future recurrences. Physical therapy serves to reeducate patients on proper posture and alignment as well as correct current muscle imbalances. Using popular exercise modalities, such as yoga and Pilates, as maintenance therapy may be appropriate for certain individuals. Exercise is covered in more depth later in the chapter.

Application of ice in patients with acute back pain is thought to decrease inflammation and swelling, while the rationale for heat application is to reduce muscle spasms. Other modalities such as ultrasound and **transcutaneous electrical nerve stimulation (TENS)** have conflicting evidence for effectiveness (Brosseau et al., 2002).

Many LBP sufferers turn to alternative therapies such as massage and acupuncture. While these therapies may aid in pain control for some individuals, they are not substitutes for exercise for ultimate symptom relief and prevention. However, as they generally have few side effects, those who are interested in these techniques may be encouraged to integrate massage or acupuncture into their treatment plans.

Spinal manipulation refers to adjustment of the spine using twisting, pushing, or pulling movements and is performed predominantly by chiropractors. Individuals interested in chiropractic services should have a thorough evaluation of their symptoms by their primary care physician and have an understanding of their diagnosis before choosing to try this modality.

Pharmacologic Therapy

Pain relievers such as acetaminophen (Tylenol®) and **nonsteroidal anti-inflammatory drugs (NSAIDs)** are often used in the short-term for acute cases of LBP. Narcotics and muscle relaxants are also options for pain, especially night-time symptoms, but their side effects and dependence profiles make them more appropriate for cases of severe pain. Occasionally, chronic pain may also be treated with antidepressants.

Neuropathy or neuropathic pain, which clients may experience as burning, "pins and needles," or "electric shock" sensations, can be treated with two newer drugs, gabapentin (Neurontin®) and pregabalin (Lyrica®). These medications work directly on the **central nervous system** and serve as nerve stabilizers. The mechanisms of action of gabapentin and pregabalin are unknown, but it is believed that they involve binding to voltage-dependent calcium ion channels.

Injections

Spinal injections, another option for chronic pain relief, can also be used as a diagnostic tool to localize symptoms. Typically, local anesthetics and/or **corticosteroids** are used to relieve pain and decrease inflammation. Injections can target several different structures:

- Trigger point injections target areas of muscle that are painful and fail to relax.
- Facet injections target facet joints on the posterior aspect of the spine that form where one vertebra overlaps another. Pain from facet joints can cause localized spinal pain or refer pain to adjacent structures.
- Epidural injections target the epidural space inside the spinal canal that contains, among other structures, spinal nerve roots.

These injections are thought to be particularly helpful for patients with radicular signs and symptoms such as sciatica. Sacroiliac joints are also occasionally injected in patients with accompanying buttock and thigh pain or sacroiliac dysfunction. Both facet and epidural injections can be done under **fluoroscopy,** or x-ray guidance, to ensure that the medications reach the correct location.

Surgery

Rarely, if conservative treatments have failed or patients develop progressive and limiting neurologic symptoms, spinal surgery is considered. The two most common types of lumbar surgery are decompression and spinal fusion. Decompression surgery, either a **laminectomy** or a **microdiscectomy,** aims to relieve impingement of the nerve root by removing a small piece of bone and/or disc material. These procedures, which are most commonly used for spinal stenosis or herniated discs, create a wider spinal canal and, therefore, more space for the spinal nerves. Spinal fusion surgery uses a bone graft to fuse two vertebral segments together. This, in turn, stops abnormal or excessive motion at the joint that is thought to be generating pain. Fusion is most often used for degenerative disc disease, spondylolysis, and spondylolisthesis.

Role of Exercise in Managing LBP

For most individuals with LBP, exercise will be the cornerstone of their treatment program. However, clients with LBP, especially chronic sufferers, may have developed fear-avoidance behaviors and negative beliefs about their abilities to exercise or perform certain activities. Therefore, clear communication between the ACE-certified Advanced Health & Fitness Specialist (ACE-AHFS) and the client is essential for facilitating a positive outcome from the exercise program. The overall goals of symptom relief and return to function must be discussed, and expectations must be set prior to beginning exercise. In some cases, complete resolution of all symptoms is not a realistic goal. In such cases, clients must view exercise as a way of overcoming their LBP rather than eradicating it. Discussing specific physical-activity objectives [e.g., work duties, **activities of daily living (ADL),** sport skills] allows the client and ACE-AHFS to create long-term goals.

Rehabilitation

Specific back exercises in the setting of acute LBP are generally not considered to be effective, and may even be detrimental to the healing process (Malmivaara et al., 1995). Instead, the exercise program for those with acute pain focuses on walking and resuming normal daily activities as soon as possible. While modifications to avoid strenuous activities such as running and heavy-lifting are reasonable, periods of immobility, including bed rest and prolonged sitting or standing, are not recommended.

Once the acute phase is over, exercise becomes a central focus of physical therapy. Chronic back pain sufferers can learn basic, life-long adjustments that both improve current symptoms and decrease the chance of recurrence. Examples include being mindful of maintaining posture, creating ergonomically correct work spaces, and committing to frequent movement and position changes when behind a desk or on a long car ride.

In the rehabilitation setting, the goal of physical therapy is to focus on specific exercises that are designed to increase strength, endurance, flexibility, and **aerobic capacity.** Physical therapy provides an opportunity to not only perform exercises, but also to learn correct technique, as exercise will be a life-long requirement for the back pain sufferer to maintain the benefits of therapy. In a meta-analysis of specific exercise strategies on outcomes in chronic LBP, programs that had the greatest impact on pain and function were individually designed, at least partially supervised, and included greater than 20 total hours (Hayden, van Tulder, & Tomlinson, 2005). The authors also found that stretching had the greatest impact on pain, while strengthening resulted in the greatest functional improvements.

Therapeutic exercises for LBP generally are classified as spinal flexion, extension, or stabilization. The theoretical goals of flexion exercises are to open the intervertebral **foramina** and facet joints, strengthen the abdominal muscles, and stretch the back extensors (Wendell, 2001). Extension exercises aim to improve motor coordination, strengthen the back extensors, improve mobility, and, perhaps, shift disrupted nuclear material to a more normal position (Borenstein, Wiesel, & Boeden, 2004). Isometric stabilization exercises promote abdominal strength and co-contraction of trunk muscles by a series of moves that ultimately result in a posterior pelvic tilt. While individual assessment of each client presenting with LBP is the key to a successful program, some commonalities among LBP sufferers exist. For example, while individuals without LBP generally have 30% greater spinal extensor strength than spinal flexor strength, those with LBP often have extensors that are weaker than flexors (Borenstein, Wiesel, & Boeden, 2004).

Aerobic fitness is thought to impede the onset of LBP, as several studies show a link between low levels of physical activity and symptoms of back pain (Leboeuf-Yde, 2000). The exact mechanism by which aerobic fitness improves overall spine health is not known. One theory is that aerobic exercise leads to increased diffusion of nutrients into the avascular space of the intervertebral disk. In addition, increases in the capillary network of the surrounding tissues as a result of aerobic fitness may increase disc nutrition (Borenstein, Wiesel, & Boeden, 2004). Aerobic exercise may also increase pain tolerance by increasing endorphins, which leads to a decreased incidence of depression. Within the first two weeks of an acute painful attack, the individual should begin a regimen of low-stress aerobic exercise. Activities such as walking, stationary biking, and swimming are good initial options for increasing physical stamina.

Core stability training is emphasized in LBP programs. The trunk, or core, of the body refers to the musculoskeletal structures associated with the cervical, thoracic, and lumbar spine, as well as the shoulder and pelvic girdles. Exercise training aims to develop the strength, coordination, and endurance of the core muscles, which in turn leads to more stability and efficiency during dynamic movements. Individuals without these competencies have excess movements in individual vertebrae and are more likely to generate greater forces, which can lead to low-back injury.

Wendell (2001) describes three stages of exercise programs: centralization, lumbar stabilization, and dynamic stabilization. Centralization is said to occur when active motion of the lumbar spine causes symptoms to either resolve or move from the periphery to the lumbar spine. Symptoms most commonly localize with either flexion, usually in individuals with degenerative or stenotic conditions, or extension, usually in individuals with lumbar disc herniation. For these patients, the rehabilitation program can focus on exercises using the centralizing movement (either flexion or extension) with the goals of decreasing the severity of symptoms and increasing activity level.

Much debate exists regarding the efficacy of choosing these types of patient-specific exercises over using a generalized program for all patients with LBP. A randomized control trial by Long, Donelson, and Fung (2004) placed 230 subjects in three separate groups after they were assessed for centralization to determine their "directional preference." Subjects were taught lumbar exercises that either matched their directional preference or opposed their directional preference, or were given a generalized program of commonly used exercises. The group that performed matched exercises had more symptom improvement and higher activity levels, among other variables. The authors concluded that these patient-specific exercises were most effective in providing pain control, thus giving weight to the popular clinical practice of creating tailored treatment plans, especially in the centralization, or early phase, of rehabilitation (Long, Donelson, & Fung, 2004).

In the second stage, lumbar stabilization, the goals of treatment are to further increase activity level and decrease disability. Exercises focus on the muscles that provide support and stabilization of the lumbar spine: transverse abdominis, erector spinae, multifidus, quadratus lumborum, and oblique abdominals. While each muscle has a specific function, they all work in concert to stabilize the lumbar spine during everyday activities.

This concept of lumbar instability causing LBP is based on the hypothesis that instability is a result of three interdependent components: structural changes, muscular changes, and ineffective neural control (Barr, Griggs, & Cadby, 2007). Bone and ligamentous structures provide passive restraint toward the end of the **range of motion (ROM)**, muscles provide support and stiffness at the intervertebral level to sustain common forces, and the neural control system coordinates muscle activity to respond to expected and unexpected forces. Instability can be a result of damage to tissues, insufficient muscular strength or endurance, or poor muscular control—or a combination of all three. Lumbar-stabilization programs are based on the belief that subjects with LBP have different biomechanics than those without back pain, such as dysfunctional superficial and deep stabilizing muscles. Studies have found that subjects with these biomechanical deficits include decreased proprioception, balance, and reaction times (Barr, Griggs, & Cadby, 2007).

Finally, patients progress to dynamic stabilization after developing core strength and endurance in stage 2. The goals of dynamic stabilization therapy are to return the client to full activity. Exercises in this stage are performed on an unstable surface such as a stability ball. Exercises can progress through balancing on a ball while performing upper- and lower-extremity movements holding weights to standing exercises incorporating a trampoline, wobble board, or foam roller. In this stage, clients are reminded to engage their core muscles as learned in stage 2 to maintain spinal stability while performing all dynamic exercises.

The final stages of rehabilitation are geared toward previously set activity goals. The unique actions used in the client's daily activities or desired sports are incorporated into the therapeutic exercises. The movements may be more complex, encompassing sport-specific actions such as catching, throwing, swinging, and lifting.

Post-rehabilitation

Creating an individualized exercise program for a person with a history of LBP requires consideration of his or her specific clinical diagnosis. Initially, an assessment of the client's overall fitness level is also important, as an athlete will have a different starting point than a **sedentary** person. Additionally, understanding the duration and severity of symptoms, as well as any activity limitations, will allow the ACE-AHFS to establish a baseline from which to observe progress.

Precautions

The following are contraindications and modifications to consider when designing an exercise program for clients with a history of LBP:

- Clients should be encouraged to obtain clearance from their physicians before beginning a program, as exercise may not be appropriate for certain individuals with serious conditions such as tumor, fracture, or progressive neurologic deficits.
- Although walking is generally a good choice for aerobic fitness in clients with LBP because it places low compressive loads on the lumbar structures, it may not be suitable for all clients. Because walking places the lumbar spine in a more extended position, clients with spinal stenosis who have symptoms while walking that are relieved with rest, should avoid prolonged walking.
- As previously described, the progression of exercises can be as important as the exercises themselves. In general, the ACE-AHFS should consider working on the muscles that stabilize the spine prior to the muscles that move the spine, to decrease the likelihood that unsupported exercises will cause damage to ligaments.
- Keep in mind that clients in beginning stages may not need additional weight added to exercises. Initially, the weight of their limbs may provide enough of a challenge.
- Know each client's limitations as set forth by his or her physician or physical therapist prior to designing the exercise program. Avoid extreme postures or actions that take the individual beyond his or her normal range of motion. Although creativity is an important motivational factor when designing a program, performing exercises outside of normal body mechanics is not useful and may be detrimental.
- Respect the client's normal spinal curvature when performing trunk exercises. Avoid hyperextension of the spine, which would cause clients to exceed their normal **lordosis.**
- Many of the exercises used in LBP rehabilitation require only subtle movements, such as **abdominal hollowing.** Using extreme movements or momentum is usually unwarranted for individuals with a history of LBP.
- Although a hands-on approach can be beneficial to provide adjustments and guidance, the ACE-AHFS must never physically force a client into a position. Providing extra force to bring a client "deeper" into a stretch can cause serious injury.

Exercise Program Guidelines and Considerations

The balance of this chapter is based on the work of Stuart M. McGill, Ph.D., a renowned expert in spine biomechanics and kinesiology whose books *Low Back Disorders,* Second Edition, and *Ultimate Back Fitness and Performance,* Third Edition, can be purchased through his website: www.backfitpro.com.

Clients with a history of back troubles may desire pain relief and spinal stability (a health objective), while others may seek a performance objective (which may be counterproductive to optimal back health). Some clients may need more stability, while others may need more mobility. Certain exercises will exacerbate the back troubles of some people but may help others. Because each individual has different needs, proficient exercise professionals will need an understanding of the issues, and of the myths and realities pertaining to each issue, to form a foundation for the decision-making process.

The scientific foundation for many "common sense" recommendations offered for back health yield no, or very thin, evidence. For example, it is widely believed that stretching the back and increasing the ROM is beneficial and reduces back problems—however, the scientific evidence shows that, on average, those who have more range of motion in their backs have a greater risk of future troubles (Biering-Sorensen, 1984). Clearly there is a tradeoff between mobility and stability; the optimal balance is a very personal and individual variable. Indeed, the "stability/mobility balance" may shift during a progressive exercise program as symptoms resolve, with advancing age, or as rehabilitation or training objectives change.

Another generally perceived goal of training the back is to increase strength. Strength has little association with low-back health (Biering-Sorensen, 1984). In fact, many people hurt their backs in an attempt to increase strength. It could be argued that this is an artifact, in that some exercise programs intended to enhance strength contained poorly chosen exercises such as sit-ups. Performing sit-ups both replicates a potent injury mechanism (i.e., posterior disc herniation) and results in high loads on the spine. On the other hand, muscle endurance, as opposed to strength, has been shown to be protective against future back troubles (Luoto et al., 1995). Further, for many people, it is better to train for stability rather than stretching to increase range of motion (Saal & Saal, 1989). Investigations into injury mechanisms have revealed that many back-training practices actually replicate the loads and motions that cause parts of the low back to become injured (Axler & McGill, 1997). For example, disc herniations need not have excessive loading on the back to occur; rather, repeated forward flexion motion of the spine is a more potent mechanism. Thus, if full flexion or deviation is avoided in the spine, the risk of herniation is remote.

Injury is caused by damage to supporting tissues. This damage reduces the normal stiffness in the spine, resulting in unstable joints. Thus, while injury results in joint instability, an event characterized by improper muscle activation can cause the spine to "buckle" or become unstable. There is no question that excessive loading can lead to back injury, but instability at low loads is also possible and problematic. For example, it is possible to damage the passive tissues of the back while bending down and picking up a pencil, if sufficient stability is not maintained. Some people recommend that when training, the client should exhale upon exertion. In terms of grooving stabilizing motor patterns for all tasks, this is a mistake. Breathing in and out should occur continuously, and not be trained to a specific exertion effort. This continuous breathing helps the client maintain constant abdominal muscle activation and ensure spine stability during all possible situations.

Further, specific muscle-activation patterns are essential to avoid injury, but have also been documented to become perturbed following injury (Hodges & Richardson, 1996). Pain is a powerful instigator in the deprogramming of normal/healthy motor patterns and the creating of perturbed patterns. The exercises and programs described in this section are based on the latest scientific knowledge of how the spine works and how it becomes injured. In addition, they have been quantified for spine load, resultant spine stability, and muscle oxygenation. These are only a few examples to begin a program. The goals are to enhance spine stability by grooving motion and muscle-activation patterns to prepare for all types of challenges. Of course, other exercises may be required subsequently to enhance daily functioning, but once again, these will depend upon the characteristics and objectives of the individual.

Two other concepts must be emphasized. First, training approaches intended to enhance athletic performance are often counterproductive to the approaches used when training for health. Too many patients are rehabilitated using athletic philosophies or, worse yet, "bodybuilding" approaches designed primarily to isolate and **hypertrophy** specific muscles, and progress is thwarted. Many bad backs are created due to inappropriate performance philosophies. Identifying the training objectives is paramount.

The emphasis should be on enhancing spine health; training for performance is another topic. Second, many of the training approaches that are used at joints such as the knee, hip, or shoulder are mistakenly applied to the back. The back is a very different and complex structure, involving a flexible column with complex muscle and ligamentous support. The spine contains the spinal cord and lateral nerve roots, and musculature intimately involved in several other functions, including breathing mechanics, to give just one example. Many of the traditional approaches for training other joints in the body are not appropriate for the back—either they do not produce the desired result or they create new LBP patients.

Caveats for Designing Exercise Programs for Back Health

- While there is a common belief that exercise sessions should be performed at least three times per week, it appears low-back exercises have the most beneficial effect when performed daily.
- The "no pain, no gain" axiom does not apply when exercising the low back in pained individuals, particularly when applied to weight training.
- General exercise programs that combine cardiovascular components (like walking) with specific low-back exercises have been shown to be more effective in both rehabilitation and for injury prevention. The exercises shown in this chapter comprise only a component of the total program.
- Diurnal variation in the fluid level of the intervertebral discs (i.e., discs are more hydrated early in the morning after rising from bed) changes the stresses on the discs throughout the day. Specifically, they are highest following bed rest and diminish over the subsequent few hours. It would be very unwise to perform full-range spine motion while under load shortly after rising from bed.
- Low-back exercises performed for maintenance of health need not emphasize strength; rather, more repetitions of less-demanding exercises will assist in the enhancement of endurance and strength. There is no doubt that back injury can occur during seemingly low-level demands (such as picking up a pencil) and that motor control error can increase the risk of injury. While it appears that the chance of motor control errors, which can result in inappropriate muscle forces, increases with fatigue, there is also evidence documenting the changes in passive tissue loading with fatiguing lifting. Given that endurance has more protective value than strength, strength gains should not be overemphasized at the expense of endurance.
- There is no such thing as an ideal set of exercises for all individuals. An individual's training objectives must be identified (be they rehabilitation specifically to reduce the risk of injury, optimize general health and fitness, or maximize athletic performance), and the most appropriate exercises chosen. While science cannot evaluate the optimal exercises for each situation, the combination of science and clinical experiential "wisdom" must be utilized to enhance low-back health.
- Clients should be encouraged to be patient and stick with the program. Increased function and pain reduction may not occur for three or more months.

Exercise Program Progressions

In Dr. McGill's *Ultimate Back Fitness and Performance,* Third Edition, a variety of LBP prevention solutions and training progressions are presented. This evidence-based approach for enhancing back health involves five distinct stages, beginning with corrective exercise and building a foundation and ultimately progressing to high-performance training.

The Five Stages for Building the Ultimate Back

According to McGill, building the ultimate back consists of a five-stage process that ensures a foundation for eventual strength, speed, and power training. The five stages are as follows:

- Groove motion/motor patterns, and corrective exercise
- Build whole-body and joint stability
- Increase muscle endurance
- Build muscle strength
- Develop power and agility

Stage 1: Groove Motion/Motor Patterns and Corrective Exercise

The first stage involves identifying disrupted motion patterns and developing appropriate corrective exercises. Determining where to begin the process of finding the most appropriate and suitable exercises for a client with a history of LBP starts with an assessment of the client's current fitness status and an evaluation of which, if any, movements produce pain.

A natural consideration when selecting appropriate exercises is to determine a course of action if an exercise or movement produces pain. Any exercise that causes pain is inhibiting and detracts from proper exercise technique or form. Attempting to "work through the pain" with the back is almost never beneficial. If an individual has pain, he or she is probably doing the exercise incorrectly, or more likely, doing the wrong exercise. The ACE-AHFS should prompt clients to describe tasks, postures, and movements that exacerbate their LBP. After determining which movements are problematic for a client, the ACE-AHFS should develop an exercise program to minimize the exacerbating movements.

Proper motor patterns of the muscles that support the spine enhance the back's ability to withstand the various loads and directional forces that it encounters during daily activities and physical exertion. A client's awareness of his or her lumbar spine, **abdominal bracing,** and gluteal complex activation are all elements in improving motor patterns for appropriate spine function.

An awareness of proper spine position allows a client to adopt a neutral spine wherein the tissues supporting the vertebrae have minimal elastic stress. Teaching clients how to adopt and maintain a neutral spine is one of the first important lessons for those with LBP. Neutral spine may be modified by clients who find relief with slightly more lumbar flexion or extension. This modified position becomes their neutral spine.

Abdominal bracing, or maintaining a mild contraction of the abdominal wall, can help ensure sufficient spine stability. Many fitness professionals mistakenly believe that activating the transverse abdominis and intentionally sucking in the abdominal wall toward the spine (a technique known as hollowing) increases spinal stability and is therefore helpful for back-pain sufferers. However, training the transverse abdominis in this manner actually compromises stability and creates spine dysfunction.

It is not uncommon for individuals to possess sufficient levels of torso flexion and extension strength, but fail tests indicative of torsional, or rotational, control. A simple, low-level test for torsional control starts in the modified push-up position (Figure 20-1a), with one hand placed directly over the other hand (Figure 20-1b). The client's pelvis and ribcage should remain locked throughout the movement. An elevated pelvis, as illustrated in Figure 20-1c, is indicative of poor lumbar torsional control. It would be contraindicated to recommend a rotational cable-pulling exercise, such as the wood-chop exercise, to a client with poor torsional control because of the high level of twisting torque it produces.

For many individuals, learning to "lock" the ribcage on the pelvis is essential for enhancing torsional control, resulting in a reduced potential for injury and optimal functional performance during rotational or twisting movements. Locking the ribcage on the pelvis involves abdominal bracing—or the co-contraction of the abdominal wall muscles without pulling in the navel.

Figure 20-1
Test for lumbar torsional control

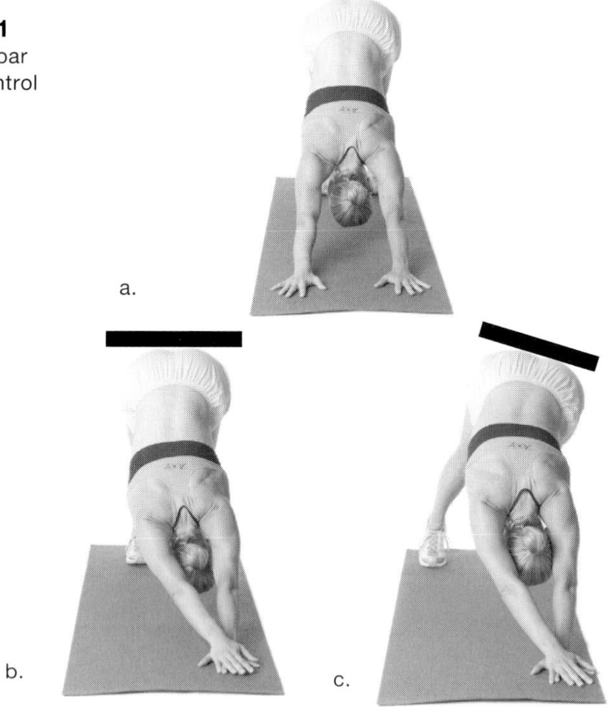

To enhance lumbar torsional control, Dr. McGill developed and used an exercise progression that begins with the wall roll exercise to improve an individual's level of torsional control. The wall roll begins with the client in the plank position with both elbows planted on the wall (Figure 20-2a). The abdominals are braced and the ribcage is locked on the pelvis. The client pivots on the balls of his or her feet while pulling one elbow off the wall (Figure 20-2b). No spine motion should occur throughout the movement.

Figure 20-2
Wall roll

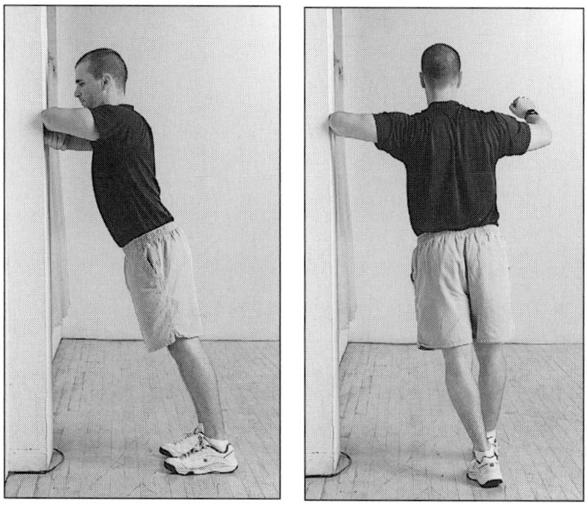

a. Starting position b. Ending position

The torsional control exercise progression continues with the floor roll and scramble-up exercise. This exercise begins with the client in contact with the floor with both hands and feet (Figure 20-3a). The ribcage is locked to the pelvis with an abdominal brace. The client pivots, rolls completely (360 degrees), and eventually moves into a sprinting or bounding motion (Figures 20-3b and 20-3c). A neutral spine should be maintained throughout the floor roll and scramble-up movements—no spine motion should occur.

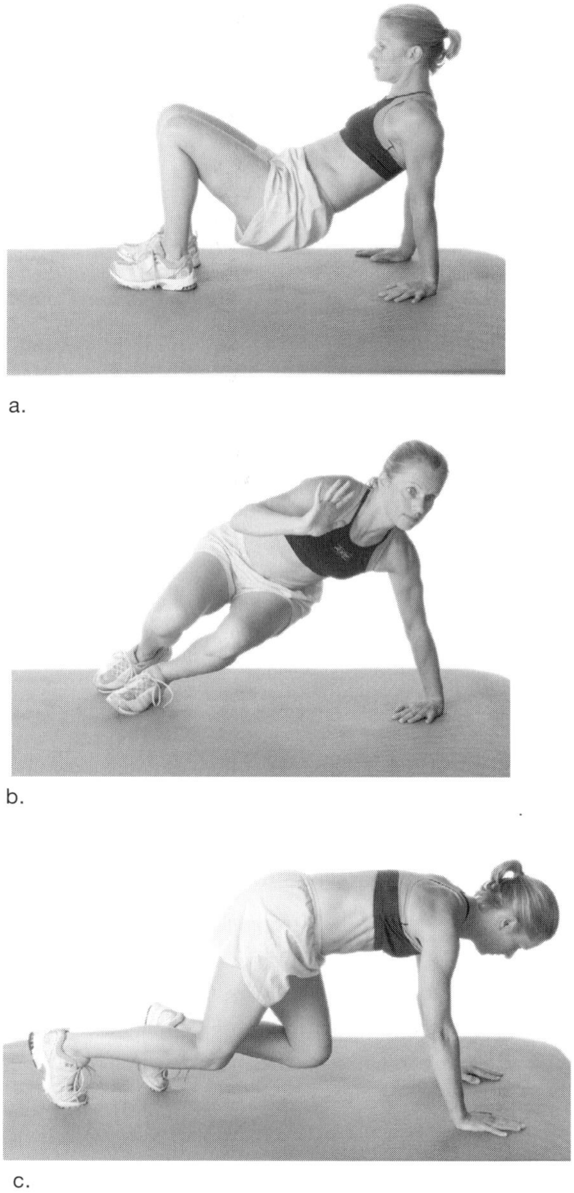

Figure 20-3
Floor roll and scramble-up exercise

A healthy back also requires healthy gluteal muscle function, since the performance and safety of many movements are dependent on balanced hip power production. The "crossed-pelvis syndrome" is a phenomenon that occurs when the gluteal complex is inhibited during squatting patterns. It is very common in individuals with a history of back problems. Interestingly, it is not known if the crossed-pelvis syndrome exists prior to back problems or is a consequence of having back problems. Regardless of whether the syndrome is a cause or an outcome, individuals with impaired gluteal motor patterns are unable to spare their backs during squatting patterns since they rely on their hamstrings and erector spinae to drive the extension motion. In turn, the erector spinae forces create loads that compress the lumbar spine. It is impossible to achieve optimal squat performance without well-integrated hip-extensor or gluteal patterns. One of the more common reasons individuals fail to properly rehabilitate their backs is due to an emphasis on strength development without first effectively addressing the impaired gluteal patterns.

Retraining of the gluteals cannot be achieved with conventional barbell squat exercises. Performing a conventional squat requires relatively little hip abduction. As a result, gluteus medius activation is minimized and activation of the gluteus maximus is delayed during the traditional barbell squat until lower squat angles are reached. McGill argues, as many other experts do, that the barbell squat is primarily a quadriceps exercise and not a gluteal exercise in the truest sense. Unlike the conventional barbell squat, the single-leg squat elicits almost immediate activation of the gluteus medius and more rapid integration of the gluteus maximus during the squat descent to assist in the **frontal plane** hip drive needed for common activities such as running and jumping.

The ACE-AHFS should begin by instructing unfit clients to learn how to activate the gluteus medius by performing the clamshell exercise. During the clamshell exercise, the client lies on his or her side while anchoring the thumb on the anterior superior iliac spine and reaching around with the fingertips, positioning them to land on the gluteus medius. Opening the knees like a clamshell will allow the individual to feel the gluteus medius activation (Figure 20-4).

The single-leg squat matrix is an example of a more advanced corrective exercise for retraining the gluteals. During the single-leg squat matrix progressions with the leg to the front (Figure 20-5a), side (Figure 20-5b), and rear (Figure 20-5c), the

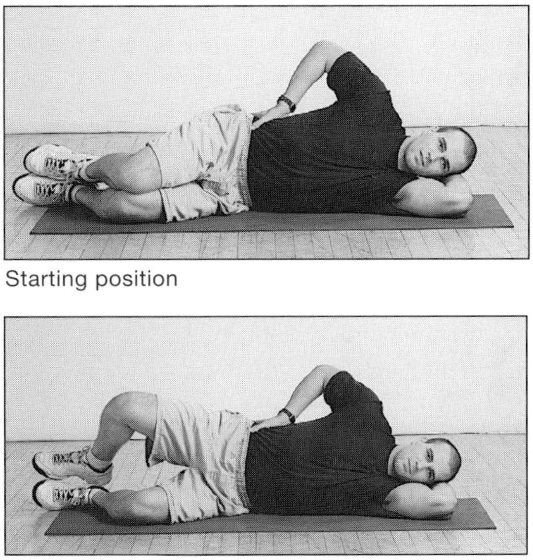

Starting position

Ending position

Figure 20-4
Beginner-level corrective exercise for retraining the gluteals—clamshell exercise

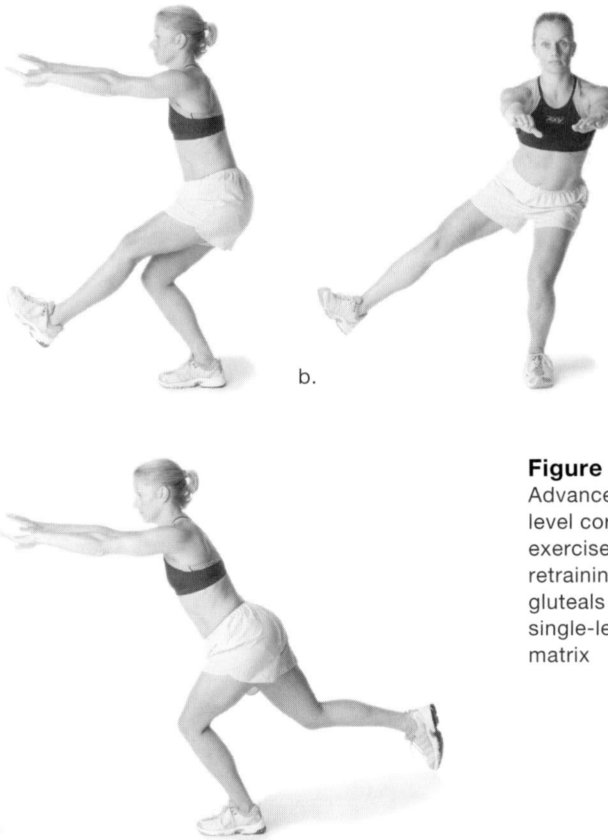

a. b. c.

Figure 20-5
Advanced-level corrective exercise for retraining the gluteals—single-leg squat matrix

abdominals are braced, the lumbar spine is neutral, and the mental focus of the individual should be on the development of hip torque.

Stage 2: Build Whole-body and Joint Stability—The "Big Three"

McGill recommends that after individuals successfully learn how to groove motion and motor patterns, they should begin focusing on developing whole-body and joint stability. An exercise program consisting of the "big three" (modified curl-ups, side bridge, and birddog) is an excellent choice for spine stabilization during the early stages of training or rehabilitation and for simply enhancing low-back health.

The modified curl-up is an exercise for the rectus abdominis. In a supine position, the client places the hands or a rolled towel under the lumbar spine and flexes one knee. He or she then raises the head and shoulders off the floor while maintaining a neutral spine, pauses, and then returns to the starting position (Figure 20-6). Clients should not flatten the back to the floor, as flattening the back flexes the lumbar spine, eliminates the neutral spine, and increases the loads on the discs and ligaments. By flexing one knee and keeping the other one straight, a neutral lumbar spine is maintained throughout the exercise movement. The bent leg should be alternated midway through each set of repetitions.

The lateral muscles of the torso (quadratus lumborum and abdominal obliques) are important for optimum spinal stability, and are targeted with the side bridge exercise. The beginner level of this exercise involves bridging the torso between the elbow and the knees (Figure 20-7). Once this is mastered and well tolerated, the challenge can be increased by bridging between the elbow and the feet (Figure 20-8). An even more advanced variation involves placing the upper leg and foot in front of the lower leg and foot to facilitate longitudinal "rolling" of the torso (Figures 20-9). This variation is far superior to exercises such as performing a sit-up with a twist because it produces greater levels of muscle activation with lower tissue loads.

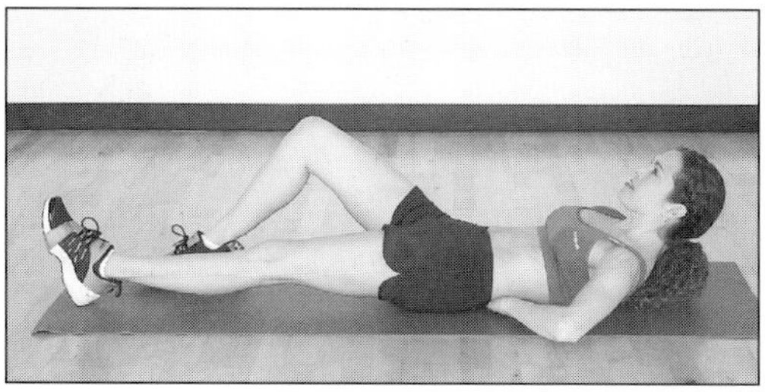

Figure 20-6
Curl-up

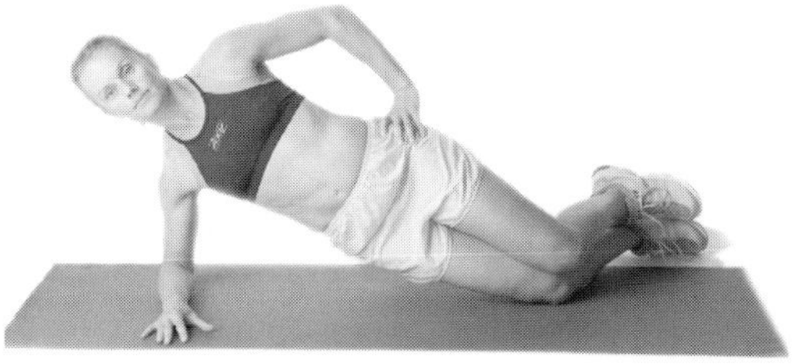

Figure 20-7
Modified side bridge

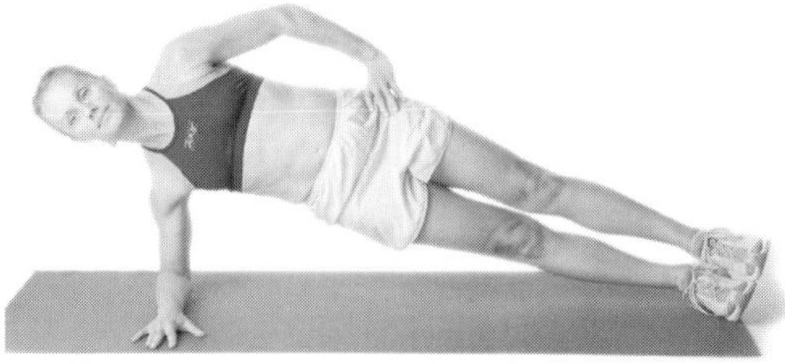

Figure 20-8
Side bridge

The birddog is a safe and effective exercise for developing the spinal extensors. It is performed by extending one leg and the opposite arm, from an all-fours position, so that they are parallel to the floor (Figure 20-10). The extended position should be held for seven to eight seconds, and then repeated with the opposite arm and leg.

More challenging exercise progressions for developing whole-body and joint stability include performing the conventional pushup with a staggered hand placement or with labile balls under the hands (Figures 20-11 and 20-12). These advanced exercises facilitate torso stabilization. As with any exercise, abdominal bracing and good torsional control should be maintained throughout the activity.

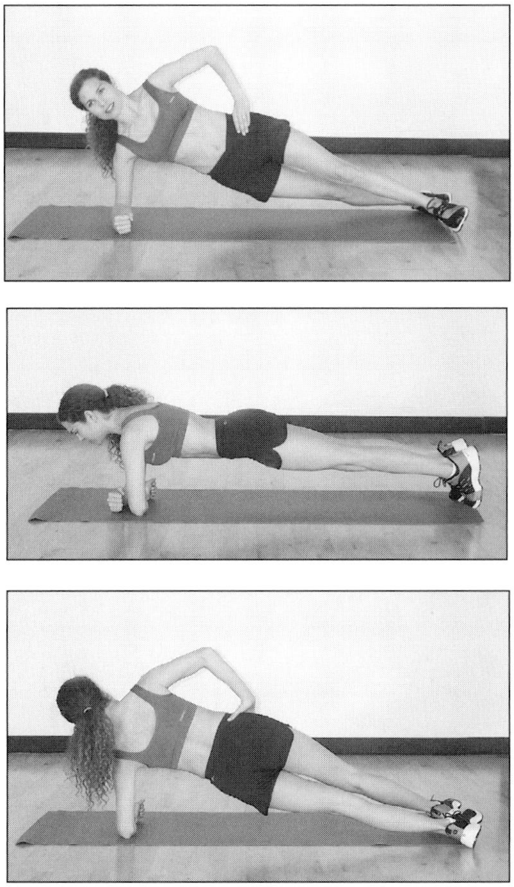

Figure 20-9
Rolling bridge

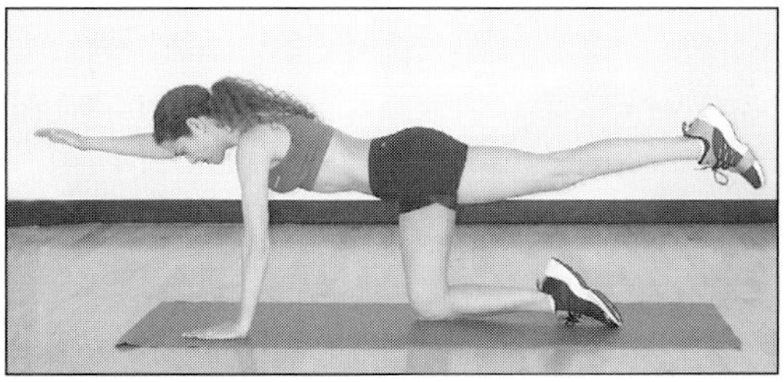

Figure 20-10
Birddog

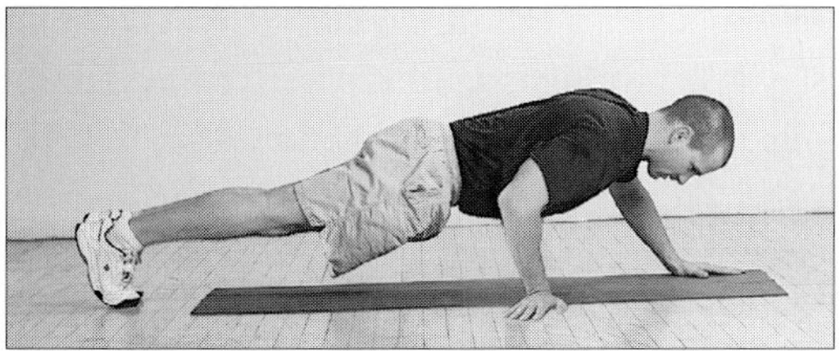

Figure 20-11
Performing the push-up with staggered hand placement (one hand forward of the shoulder and one hand beside the lower ribs) enhances shoulder and abdominal muscle activation, thereby promoting the stabilizing functions of these muscles.

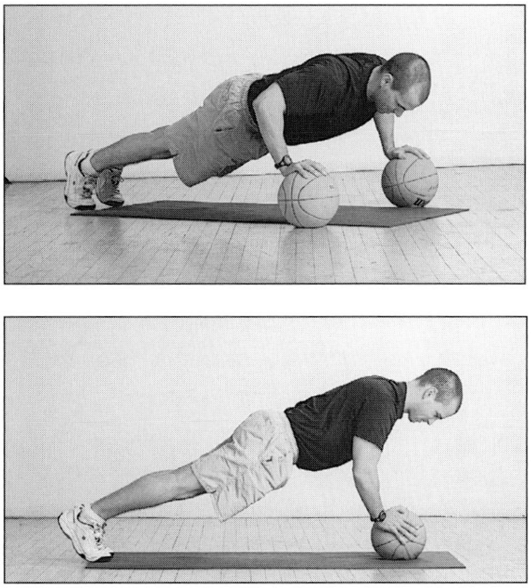

Figure 20-12
Placing both hands on a single ball or each hand on one ball while performing a push-up significantly enhances the rectus abdominis and internal and external obliques activation on both sides of the torso.

Stage 3: Increase Muscle Endurance

During stage 3, the focus is on improving muscle endurance. Endurance is typically developed first with repeated sets or repetitions of exercises. The client then progresses to longer-duration workouts for an overall increase in total work volume. Endurance progression should generally begin with isometric holds, such as curl-ups, side bridges, and birddog exercises. It is recommended that individuals continue to progress by increasing the number of repetitions completed rather than extending the "hold time."

The "reverse pyramid for endurance training" is an approach to designing endurance sets based on the Russian tradition of maintaining excellent exercise technique and form. For example, an endurance workout involving the side bridge exercise might consist of:

- Five repetitions on the right side followed by five on the left
- Rest
- Four repetitions on the right side followed by four on the left
- Rest
- Three repetitions on the right side followed by three on the left

The basic rationale behind this approach is that the exerciser does as much as possible while he or she is least fatigued. That is, it is easier to maintain proper exercise technique as the repetitions are reduced with each fatiguing set.

Stage 4: Build Strength

The fourth stage in the progression to building the ultimate back emphasizes strength development. Training for maximum back strength without injury is a difficult challenge that requires a delicate balance. A one-size-fits-all recipe for back-strength development does not exist. However, several basic considerations exist for strengthening the back:

- Develop general fitness and balancing ability to train safely and effectively
- Consider the matching of a client's fitness level and motor abilities to the skill demands of the planned training program
- Develop the foundation of proper motor and motion patterns to protect any potential weak links
- Consider the balance of strength around a joint and between adjacent joints, as well as the balance of strength to endurance
- Consider the range of motion required by the task and whether the client's motion capability is appropriately matched

Stage 5: Power

Power development represents the fifth and final stage in Dr. McGill's recommended progression to building the ultimate back. Developing spine power can potentially compromise both safety and performance. Power is the product of force and velocity.

Power = Force x Velocity

Therefore, if either force or velocity is high, then the other should generally be kept low. Power is developed in the extremities and transferred through the torso. Efficient and effective power transfer through the torso requires spine posture control, spine stiffness and stability, and strength.

For clients who have successfully progressed through the first four stages, abdominal plyometric exercises can be incorporated into the training programs to enhance their abilities to effectively and efficiently transfer power through their torsos. The medicine ball toss, performed either while standing or while supine on the floor or a stability ball, is an example of an effective abdominal plyometric exercise that provides excellent progression to power (Figure 20-13).

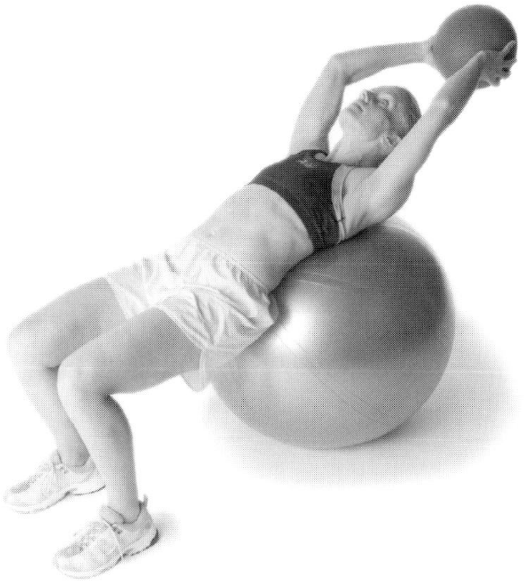

Figure 20-13
Medicine ball toss

Case Study

Amy, a 37-year-old overweight female with chronic low-back pain has decided to begin an exercise program to improve her overall conditioning and lose weight on the advice of her physician and physical therapist. She has no previous exercise history and has become increasingly inactive due to her low-back pain. Physical therapy reduced her symptoms to localized discomfort and she is afraid of making her back worse again by doing the wrong things at the gym. Amy was released from therapy with a home exercise program that includes supine pelvic tilts, modified curl-ups, several dynamic stabilization exercises (e.g., modified side bridge, modified birddog), wall squats, hamstring and piriformis stretches, and 10 minutes of cycling. She has hired an ACE-AHFS to help her achieve her weight-loss goal without exacerbating her low-back pain.

All the exercises on Amy's home exercise program are clearly described with illustrations, verbal cues, and intensity and frequency guidelines. Additional programming is developed by the ACE-AHFS to address Amy's conditioning and weight-loss goals. The ACE-AHFS initially tries aerobic exercise on a recumbent cycle; however, Amy reports some increased pain with prolonged sitting. Several other modes of activity are then tested, including stair climbers and elliptical trainers. Treadmill walking on a cushioned deck provides the most comfortable aerobic exercise for Amy and is chosen as the primary modality. The speed is kept below Amy's stride maximum to ensure that she can maintain postural alignment throughout her workout. Incline is introduced as tolerated by her conditioning as well as her low back.

A total-body strength program supplements the aerobic work for weight loss and promotes more complete conditioning. Initially, weights are low and repetitions are moderate to high due to Amy's deconditioned state and to promote her learning of exercise technique. Supine or standing exercises replace seated exercises whenever possible. In the event that a seated exercise is used, posture is closely monitored. Strengthening of the core muscles is emphasized, along with stability of the lower back. Back extension exercises are cautiously introduced because Amy's physical therapist did not recommend them and it is not clear if they are appropriate. Any complaints of pain, weakness, radicular symptoms, or increased low-back discomfort indicate that a given exercise should be discontinued.

Stretching concentrates on the iliopsoas, hamstrings, piriformis, gluteal complex, quadriceps, and quadratus lumborum.

As Amy progresses, the frequency, intensity, and duration will increase as tolerated. Her low-back comfort is continuously monitored. More functional exercises can be introduced as her fitness improves. Proper exercise technique and postural maintenance are always a critical concern during Amy's workouts.

Summary

LBP is a significant source of cost and disability, as more than 80% of Americans suffer from at least one episode of back pain during their lifetimes. A significant proportion of these individuals seek assistance from a healthcare professional. While the majority of acute back pain improves over time, some people develop recurrences, and still others experience continuous pain. The onset and persistence of LBP is related to individual, activity, and psychological factors.

Mechanical causes account for the majority of LBP cases. Discogenic pain can be attributed to conditions such as a herniated disc, sciatica, spinal stenosis, spondylolysis, and spondylolisthesis. Treatment options for individuals with LBP have evolved and, in some cases, become a source of much debate. However, for almost all conditions, current thinking among health professionals is one of active recovery. Exercise is a central focus in the treatment of LBP.

The back is a very unique and complex structure involving a flexible column with complex muscle and ligamentous support. The spine contains the spinal cord and lateral nerve roots, and musculature intimately involved in several other functions (e.g., breathing mechanics). Many of the traditional approaches used to train other joints in the body are not appropriate for the back—either they fail to produce positive results or they result in injury. The ACE-AHFS can play a vital role in the prevention of LBP and maintenance of back health through designing evidence-based exercise programs that address the important structures and functions of the spine.

References

Anderson, G.B.J. (1997). The epidemiology of spinal disorders. In: Froymoyer J.W. (Ed.) *The Adult Spine: Principles and Practice* (2nd ed.). Philadelphia: Lippincott Raven.

Axler, C. & McGill, S.M. (1997). Low back loads over a variety of abdominal exercises: Searching for the safest abdominal challenge. *Medicine & Science in Sports & Exercise,* 29, 6, 804–811.

Bahr, R. et al. (2004). Low back pain among endurance athletes with and without specific back loading: A cross-sectional survey of cross country skiers, rowers, orienteers, and nonathletic controls. *Spine,* 29, 449–454.

Barr, K.P., Griggs M., & Cadby, T. (2007). Lumbar stabilization: A review of core concepts and current literature, part 2. *American Journal of Physical Medicine and Rehabilitation,* 86, 72–80.

Biering-Sorensen, F. (1984). Physical measurements as risk indicators for low-back trouble over a one-year period. *Spine,* 9, 106–119.

Borenstein, D., Wiesel, S., & Boeden, S. (2004). *Low Back and Neck Pain: Comprehensive Diagnosis and Management* (3rd Ed.). Philadelphia: Elsevier.

Bressler, H.B. et al. (1999). The prevalence of low back pain in the elderly: A systematic review of the literature. *Spine*, 24, 1813–1819.

Brosseau L. et al. (2002). Efficacy of the transcutaneous electrical nerve stimulation for the treatment of chronic low back pain. *Spine,* 27, 596–603.

Carey, T.S. & Garrett, J.M. (1999). Recurrence and care seeking after acute back pain: Results of a long-term follow-up study. *Medical Care,* 37, 157–164.

Currie, S.R. & Wang, J.L. (2004). Chronic back pain and major depression in the general Canadian population. *Pain*, 107, 54–60.

Deyo, R.A. & Weinstein, J.N. (2001). Primary care: Low back pain. *New England Journal of Medicine,* 344, 363–370.

Deyo, R. et al. (2006). Back pain prevalence and visit rates. *Spine*, 31, 2724–2727.

Hayden, J., van Tulder, M., & Tomlinson, G. (2005). Systematic review: Strategies for using exercise therapy to improve outcomes in chronic low back pain. *Annals of Internal Medicine,* 142, 776–785.

Hodges, P.W. & Richardson, C.A. (1996). Inefficient muscular stabilization of the lumbar spine associated with low back pain. *Spine,* 21, 2640–2650.

Hurwitz, E.L. & Morgenstern, H. (1997). Correlates of back problems and back related disability in the United States. *Journal of Clinical Epidemiology,* 50, 669–681.

Leboeuf-Yde, C. (2000). Body weight and low back pain. *Spine,* 25, 2, 226–237.

Long, A., Donelson, R., & Fung T. (2004). Does it matter which exercise? A randomized control trial of exercise for low back pain. *Spine,* 29, 23, 2593–2602.

Luo, X. et al. (2004). Estimates and patterns of direct health care expenditures among individuals with back pain in the United States. *Spine,* 29, 79–86.

Luoto, S. et al. (1995). Static back endurance and the risk of low back pain. *Clinical Biomechanics*, 10, 323–324.

Malmivaara, A. et al. (1995). The treatment of acute low back pain: Bed rest, exercises, or ordinary activity? *New England Journal of Medicine,* 332, 351.

Manek N., & MacGregor, A.J. (2005). Epidemiology of back disorders: Prevalence, risk factors and prognosis. *Current Opinion in Rheumatology,* 17, 134–140.

McGill, S. (2008). *Ultimate Back Fitness and Performance* (3rd ed.). Waterloo, Ont.: Backfitpro Inc.

McGill, S. (2007). *Low Back Disorders* (2nd ed.). Champaign, Ill.: Human Kinetics.

Morris C. (2006). *Low Back Syndromes.* New York: McGraw-Hill.

Rubin, D. (2007). Epidemiology and risk factors for spine pain. *Neurologic Clinics,* 25, 353–371.

Saal, J.A. & Saal, J.S. (1989). Nonoperative treatment of herniated lumbar intervertebral disc with radiculopathy: An outcome study. *Journal of Biomechanics,* 14, 431–437.

Wendell, L. (2001). *Exercise Presciption and the Back*. New York: McGraw-Hill.

Wong, D & Transfeltd, E. (2007). *Macnab's Backache* (4th ed.). Philadelphia: Lippincott Williams & Wilkins.

Yu, C. & Garfin, S.R. (1994). Recognizing and managing lumbar spondylolisthesis. *Journal of Musculoskeletal Medicine,* 11, 55–63.

Suggested Reading

Barr, K.P., Griggs M., & Cadby, T. (2007). Lumbar stabilization: A review of core concepts and current literature, part 2. *American Journal of Physical Medicine and Rehabilitation,* 86, 72–80.

Barr, K.P., Griggs M., & Cadby T. (2005). Lumbar stabilization: A review of core concepts and current literature, part 1. *American Journal of Physical Medicine and Rehabilitation,* 84, 473–480

Borenstein, D., Wiesel, S., & Boeden, S. (2004). *Low Back and Neck Pain: Comprehensive Diagnosis and Management.* Philadelphia: Elsevier.

Deyo, R.A. & Weinstein, J.N. (2001). Primary care: Low back pain. *New England Journal of Medicine,* 344, 363–370.

Malmivaara, A. et al. (1995). The treatment of acute low back pain: Bed rest, exercises, or ordinary activity? *New England Journal of Medicine,* 332, 351.

Morris C. (2006). *Low Back Syndromes.* New York: McGraw-Hill.

Rubin, D. (2007). Epidemiology and risk factors for spine pain. *Neurologic Clinics,* 25, 353–371.

Saal, J.A. & Saal, J.S. (1989). Nonoperative treatment of herniated lumbar intervertebral disc with radiculopathy: An outcome study. *Journal of Biomechanics,* 14, 431–437.

Wendell, L. (2001). *Exercise Presciption and the Back.* New York: McGraw-Hill.

Wong, D & Transfeltd, E. (2007). *Macnab's Backache* (4th ed.). Philadelphia: Lippincott Williams & Wilkins.

Yu, C. & Garfin, S.R. (1994). Recognizing and managing lumbar spondylolisthesis. *Journal of Musculoskeletal Medicine,* 11, 55–63.

Part Five

Considerations for Specialized Population Groups

Chapter 21
Older Adults

Chapter 22
Youth

Chapter 23
Pre- and Postnatal Exercise

In This Chapter

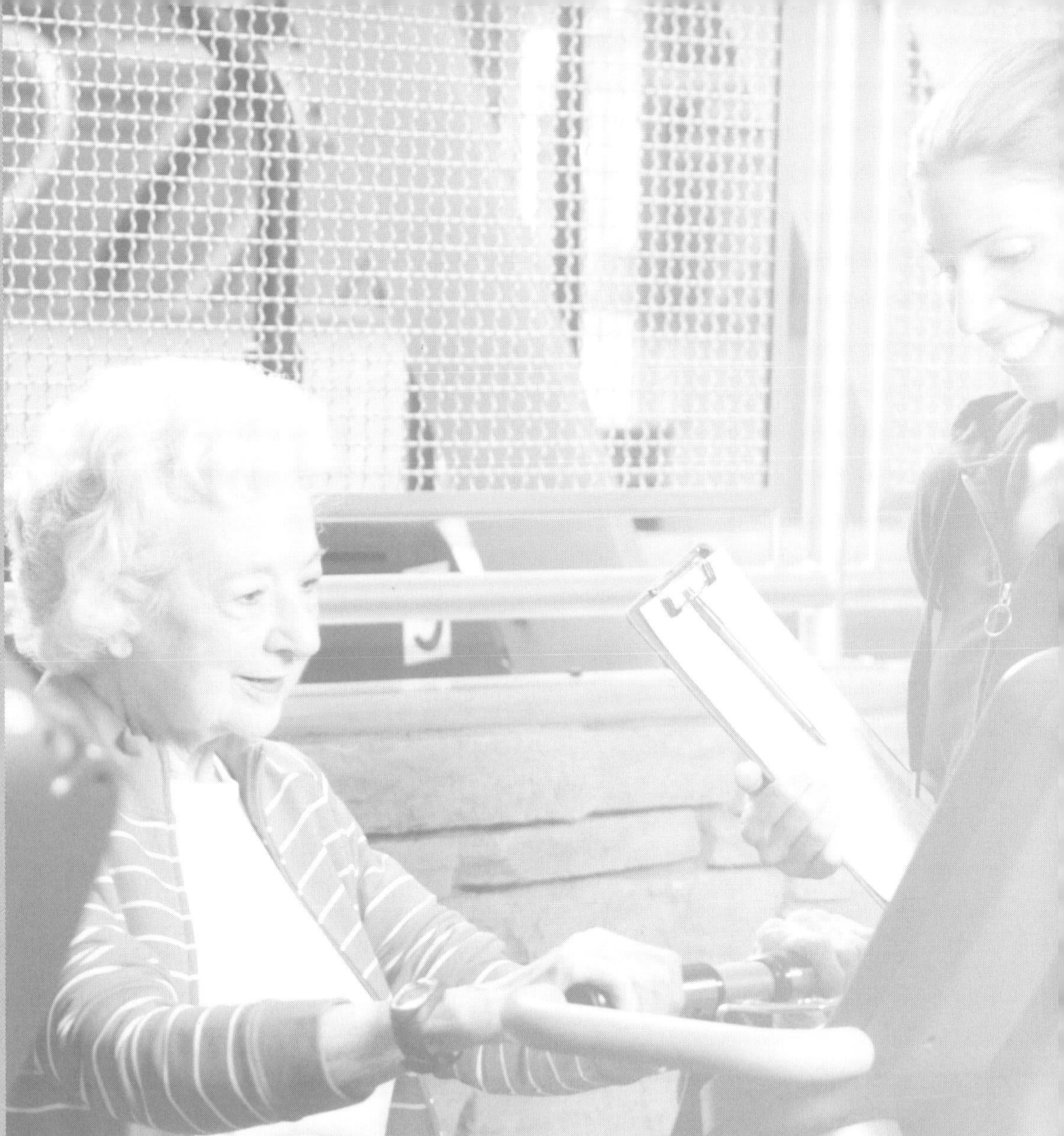

About The Author

Sabrena Merrill, M.S., has been actively involved in the fitness industry since 1987. An ACE-certified Group Fitness Instructor and Personal Trainer, Merrill teaches group exercise, owns and operates her own personal training business, has managed fitness departments in commercial facilities, and lectured to university students and established fitness professionals. She has a bachelor's degree in exercise science as well as a master's degree in physical education from the University of Kansas, and has numerous certifications in exercise instruction. Merrill acts as a spokesperson for the American Council on Exercise (ACE) and is involved in curriculum development for ACE continuing education programs. Additionally, Merrill presents lectures and workshops to fitness professionals nationwide.

CHAPTER 21

Older Adults

Sabrena Merrill

In 1974, Congress created the National Institute on Aging (NIA) as part of the National Institutes of Health (NIH) to provide leadership in aging research, training, health information dissemination, and other programs relevant to aging and older people. Much of the research in **gerontology,** which has grown considerably in the last 30 years, has been conducted or supported by the NIA. Where gerontologists once looked for a single, all-encompassing theory to explain aging, they are now finding multiple processes that combine and interact on many levels. Cells, tissues, and organ systems are all involved, and gerontologists now understand many more of the mechanisms by which these components cause or react to aging.

Among older adults, chronic diseases and their associated health limitations are a major problem that can reduce seniors' health-related quality of life. These conditions can cause years of pain, disability, and loss of function and independence. Currently, at least 80% of older Americans are living with at least one chronic condition, and 50% have at least two [Centers for Disease Control and Prevention (CDC), 2003]. The percentage of older adults who report very good or excellent health decreases with age. Based on research collected from the 2001 National Health Interview Survey, the CDC reports that 43% of men and women aged 65 years and older reported very good or excellent health, compared with 34% of those aged 75 to 84 and only 28% of those 85 or older (CDC, 2007).

Since **life expectancy** in the United States has risen dramatically in the twentieth century, from about 47 years in 1900 to about 75 years for males and 80 years for females in 2003, older adults are living for an extended period with chronic ailments that tend to appear in the fourth decade of life (Arias, 2006). Conditions such as **cardiovascular disease,** cancer, **diabetes, arthritis,** and cognitive impairment are challenges that many seniors must manage as they advance in age. Regardless of age and health limitations, older adults can expect to experience significant physiological and psychological benefits from regular physical activity. This chapter addresses the unique concerns related to exercise-program development and implementation for older adult clients.

Quantity and Quality of Life

The maximum number of years an organism from a given species can live is called its **lifespan.** For humans, the accepted maximum lifespan is 122 years, achieved by Jeane Clament of France (NIH, 2006). Lifespan is different from life expectancy, which is the average number of years a person can expect to live. The work of gerontologists focuses on closing the gap between life expectancy and lifespan, as well as improving health-related quality of life in the final years.

In general, aging refers to changes that occur throughout the lifespan. This natural, complex process potentially involves every molecule, cell, and organ in the body. Some changes due to aging are harmless and superficial, such as gray hair and wrinkles, whereas others bring about deterioration of many of the body's systems. When speaking of the progressive loss of function that increases the risk of disease, disability, or death, gerontologists use a more precise term—**senescence**—to describe aging. Experts on aging disagree, however, about when senescence begins. Some argue that it begins at birth, while others contend that it sets in after the peak reproductive years. Whether senescence begins at birth or at age 20, 30, or 40, the natural processes of aging lead to an accumulating loss of bodily functions, which ultimately increases the probability of death.

The rate and progression of the aging process vary greatly from person to person and depend on several personal and environmental factors. Because of the complex nature of aging, it is impossible to pinpoint a person's functional capabilities based solely on **chronological age.** Many gerontologists believe that to increase the understanding of senescence, chronological age must be supplemented by other measures designed to index function. **Functional age** measures take into account a person's biological, psychological, and social characteristics to create a picture of aging as whole. For example, a healthy individual who is aging successfully may have biological traits 10 years younger than his or her chronological age. On the other hand, a person experiencing multiple medical problems in old age may be older biologically than chronologically.

The concept of functional age reinforces the fact that each individual ages differently. These differences may affect the quality of life from person to person. Factors such as physical, social, cognitive, and emotional functioning can influence the overall quality of an individual's life (Rejeski, Brawley, & Shumaker, 1996). Regular physical activity has a positive impact on many of these domains (Table 21-1). The benefits

Table 21-1
Health Domains Positively Influenced by Regular Physical Activity in Older Adults

Physiological well-being	Lower overall mortality Lower risk of coronary heart disease Lower risk of colon cancer Lower risk of diabetes Lower risk of developing high blood pressure; decreased blood pressure in individuals who have hypertension Lower risk of obesity Lower risk of certain cancers
Physical well-being	Improved dyspnea Decreased fatigue Decreased pain Improved symptom perception Improved appetite Improved sleep patterns Improved quality of life Improved performance of ADL Lower risk of falls and injury
Psychological well-being	Improved self-concept Increased self-esteem Improved mood Reduced anxiety Lower risk of developing depression
Social function (in group programs)	Increased social interaction Increased social support Decreased social isolation

Note: ADL = Activities of daily living

Sources: Centers for Disease Control (2002). *Physical Activity and Older Americans: Benefits and Strategies*. Agency for Healthcare Research and Quality and the Centers for Disease Control. http://www.ahrq.gov/ppip/activity.html; Shephard, R.J. (1997). *Aging, Physical Activity and Health.* Champaign, Ill.: Human Kinetics.

of physical activity are especially important for older adults, since they are more likely to develop chronic diseases and to have conditions that can affect their physical function (CDC, 2002). For example, one study of older men demonstrated that leisure time physical activity was more important for protecting against heart disease in men over age 65 than in younger men (Talbot et al., 2002).

One of the most significant factors of quality of life for older adults is the ability to live independently. Research has shown that the mobility and functioning of frail and very old adults can be improved by regular physical activity (CDC, 2002). For midlife and older adults of all ages and abilities, adopting regular physical activity as part of a healthy lifestyle may extend years of active independent life, reduce or prevent chronic disease and disability, and improve overall quality of life (Atienza, 2001; Eakin, 2001; Linnan & Marcus, 2001, Stewart, 2001; U.S. Department of Health and Human Services, 1996). Clearly, few factors contribute as much to successful aging as maintaining a physically active lifestyle.

Physical Changes Associated With Aging

A wide variety of age-related changes occur simultaneously in different systems throughout the body (Figure 21-1). The cumulative effect of these changes results in a decrease in the body's ability to respond appropriately to the stresses of everyday life. At the cellular level, disruptions occur that cause gross morphological changes, such as decreased tissue elasticity and compliance, demyelination, and neoplastic growth. The structural decay and functional decline associated with aging organ systems exhibit reduced strength and stability and decreased coordination and endurance.

Cardiovascular System

Cardiovascular function depends on the structure and function of the heart and blood vessels, and the components and volume of blood. Aging alone does little to alter the heart's structural integrity. However, since many older adults have **hypertension**—by age 60, high blood pressure affects one in every two Americans—deterioration of the heart is most likely due to

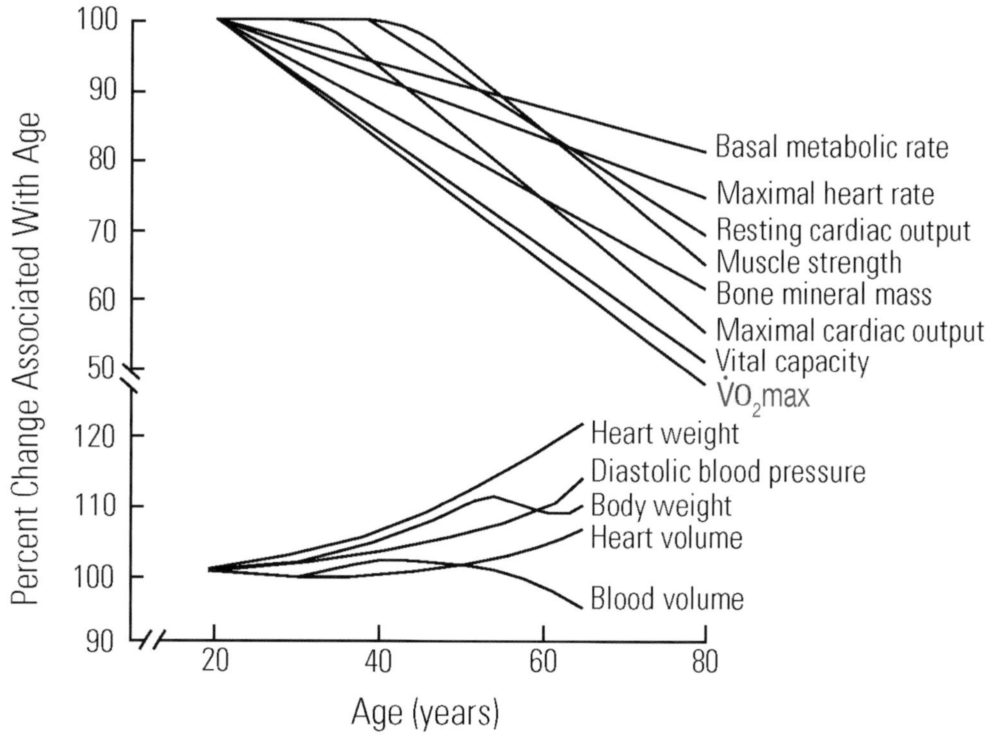

Figure 21-1
Changes in physiological function with age

Source: Bryant, C.X., Franklin, B.A., & Newton-Merrill, S. (2007). *ACE's Guide to Exercise Testing and Program Design* (2nd ed.). Monterey, Calif.: Healthy Learning. Modified from Nieman, D.C. (1995). *Fitness and Sports Medicine: An Introduction* (3rd ed.). Palo Alto, Calif.: Bull Publishing Company.

chronic disease processes and lifestyle change (NIH, 2005). The left ventricle of the heart increases in wall thickness by approximately 30% between the ages of 25 and 80, probably as a compensatory measure for age-related increases in **systolic blood pressure** (Fleg, 1986; Lakatta, 1990). As blood pressure increases, the heart has to work harder, which leads to left ventricular **hypertrophy.** Although regular exercise is also associated with a thickening of the left ventricle wall, left ventricular hypertrophy due to hypertension is a negative adaptation because the ventricular cavity dimensions do not increase as is typically seen with exercise. A smaller cavity and a thicker ventricle wall result in more strain on the heart.

While resting and submaximal heart rates show very little change due to aging, maximum heart rate declines significantly, advancing at a rate of about five to 10 beats per minute per decade (Shepard, 1997). Although not fully understood, the reasons for the age-related decline in maximum heart rate could include alterations in **catecholamine** response (Fleg et al., 1994) and increased stiffness of the heart wall. **Epinephrine** and **norepinephrine** (catecholamines), which act through the **sympathetic nervous system,** increase the contractility of the heart muscle. With aging, the heart and blood vessels become less sensitive to catecholamine stimulation. Thus, the aging heart cannot achieve the maximum heart rate levels that were possible during youth.

Similar to heart rate, both **stroke volume** and **cardiac output** are minimally affected by advancing age, whereas stroke volume and cardiac output during maximal exertion decrease significantly in older adults. The decrease in maximal effort stroke volume in older adults may be due, in part, to impaired coronary flow due to myocardial ischemia, decreased myocardial sensitivity to catecholamines, and lower blood volume typically seen in older individuals (Shepard, 1997; Spirduso, Francis, & MacRae, 2005). Maximal cardiac output in an older person is reached at a lower work rate and lower peak heart rate than in a younger person. Thus, a 65 year old exhibits a peak cardiac output that is 20 to 30% less than a younger adult (Fagard, Thijs, & Amery, 1993).

Age-related structural changes in the blood vessels are contributing factors to the higher blood pressures exhibited by older adults. The aorta and arterial tree become thicker and stiffen with age. Noncompliant vessels and increased peripheral resistance are the major contributors to the development of hypertension in older adults (Fleg, 1986; Safar, 1990). The older heart, in turn, needs to create more force to propel the blood through the less elastic arteries. The development of **coronary artery disease,** combined with hypertension, forces the cardiovascular system to work under a substantial stress, even during light physical work. Vigorous exercise overwhelms an aged, diseased heart, rendering it incapable of supplying the muscles with the oxygen and nutrients they need to perform the task.

Aging is also associated with changes in blood **lipids.** Namely, both total **cholesterol** and serum **triglycerides** are elevated in older adults compared to younger adults. In the U.S., hypertension and **hypercholesterolemia** go hand in hand. Individuals with high blood cholesterol have a higher than expected prevalence of hypertension, and those with hypertension have a higher than expected prevalence of high blood cholesterol. It is estimated that 40% of individuals with hypertension (blood pressure ≥140/90 mmHg or currently taking antihypertensive medications) have total cholesterol levels ≥240 mg/dL, and 46% of those with total cholesterol levels ≥240 mg/dL have hypertension (Lerner & Kannel, 1986). In older adults with both elevated cholesterol and high blood pressure, cardiovascular disease risk is synergistically increased. Conversely, reducing blood pressure, like cholesterol lowering, decreases the risk for cardiovascular disease (MacMahon et al., 1986).

Elevated serum triglycerides (≥150 mg/dL) are considered an independent risk factor for cardiovascular disease. Findings from the Third National Health and Nutrition Survey (NHANES III) demonstrate that elevated triglycerides affect a considerable proportion of the U.S. adult population (CDC, 1996). Among persons aged 50 years or older, the proportion with triglyceride levels of at least 150mg/dL is approximately 43%. Elevated triglycerides are also a feature of the

metabolic syndrome. In the NHANES III subset of Americans aged 50 years or older, the prevalence of triglyceride levels of at least 150mg/dL was 77.8% among individuals with the metabolic syndrome alone and 72.1% among those with both the metabolic syndrome and type 2 diabetes (CDC, 1996).

Respiratory System

The respiratory, or pulmonary, system relies, in part, on the structure and function of the chest wall, lungs, and bronchial tree. With aging, the elasticity of the chest wall decreases and the joints about which the ribs rotate stiffen, requiring an increased effort during breathing (D'Errico et al., 1989; Crapo, 1993). Thus, for a given physical activity, older people have a higher respiratory work rate. Similar to the chest wall, the lungs progressively lose elasticity with advanced age. This leads to an increase in **residual volume** (i.e., the volume of air remaining in the lungs at the end of maximal expiration), with a corresponding decrease in the **expiratory reserve volume** (i.e., the maximal volume of air that can be expelled from the lungs after normal expiration). In young adults, residual volume is about 20% of total lung capacity, whereas in persons over age 60, it increases to about 40% (Spirduso, Francis, & MacRae, 2005). Disadvantages of having an enlarged chest volume include a decrease in mechanical efficiency of the respiratory muscles, a reduction of **vital capacity** (i.e., the maximum volume of air that can be expelled from the lungs after a maximal inspiration), and a resulting tendency for **dyspnea** during exercise (Shepard, 1997).

In the bronchial tree, age-related changes include a progressive decrease in ciliary function and an increased risk of aspiration of food due to altered swallowing reflexes and impaired coughing (Tockman, 1994). Together, these changes increase the likelihood of viral and bacterial infections in the older adult, but do not seem to directly affect physical performance. Despite the natural degeneration caused by aging, respiratory function generally remains adequate for the needs of exercise in the elderly. However, dyspnea appears to become more common during physical exertion in older adults (Shepard, 1997).

Aerobic Capacity

Maximal oxygen consumption declines, on average, by about 1% each year of a sedentary adult's life. It also declines in masters athletes and individuals who have been physically active throughout their lives, but to a lesser extent. Typically, by the age of 65, aerobic power is 30 to 40% less than that of a young adult (Shepard, 1987). Possible reasons for age-related decreases in **$\dot{V}O_2$max** include a reduction in maximum heart rate with advancing age, decreases in muscle tissue and its ability to use oxygen, and a diminished ability to redirect blood flow from organs to working muscles (Spirduso, Francis, & MacRae, 2005). Although the muscle loss that occurs with aging affects both genders, women lose a higher percentage of their lean mass than do men. Also, body fat is up to two and a half times higher in women than in men. These gender-specific changes in **body composition** could explain the observation that age-related loss in **aerobic capacity** is greater in women than in men (Shepard, 1987).

The decline in aerobic capacity that occurs with aging tends to accelerate from ages 65 to 75 and again from 75 to 85. Very low aerobic capacity leads to constant fatigue in older adults, especially the frail elderly. It is estimated that a minimum functional capacity of 13 mL/kg/min (or nearly 4 METs) is needed for independent living (Shepard, 1987). The functioning of the structures responsible for oxygen delivery and utilization in many low-fit older adults falls below the minimum necessary to maintain an independent lifestyle. Thus, many 65-year-old sedentary people are dangerously close to becoming disabled (Shepard, 1987). Regular physical activity can increase functional capacity and stamina and prevent or correct many of the fatigue-related problems of the elderly.

Musculoskeletal System

Maintaining a minimum amount of muscular strength and endurance is essential for the performance of a variety of **activities of daily living (ADL).** Carrying groceries, lifting boxes, climbing stairs, and rising from a chair all require a certain level of muscular function. Both strength and endurance have been shown to decrease with age (Spirduso, Francis, & MacRae, 2005; Shepard,

1997). Bone mineral density and flexibility are other important components of the musculoskeletal system that show declines due to the aging process.

Sarcopenia

Loss in muscle function is likely due to the muscle **atrophy** that accounts for a significant decrease in lean mass with aging. In sedentary individuals, it is estimated that muscle mass declines 22% for women and 23% for men between the ages of 30 and 70 (NIH, 2006). Muscle atrophy that occurs as a natural part of the aging process is called **sarcopenia** and reflects both a decrease in the average fiber size and a decrease in the number of muscle fibers (Aoyagi & Shephard, 1992). Since the amount of force an individual can produce depends, in part, on the amount of working muscle mass, sarcopenia has a dramatic negative effect on strength (Figure 21-2).

Cross-sectional and longitudinal research data have shown that muscle strength declines by approximately 15% per decade in the sixth and seventh decades, and about 30% thereafter (Danneskoild-Samsoe et al., 1984; Harries & Bassey, 1990; Larsson, 1978; Murray et al., 1985). Age-related decreases in muscular strength, particularly in the lower body, are associated with a decreased ability to maintain dynamic balance, walk, prevent falls, and move quickly (i.e., produce power). Results from laboratory testing and clinical observations reveal that muscle strength of the lower body declines more quickly with age than does muscle strength of the upper body (Asmussen & Heebol-Neilsen, 1961; Larsson, Grimby, & Karlsson, 1979; Murray et al., 1985; Murray et al., 1980). Furthermore, isometric strength appears to be maintained better than dynamic strength, and strength during eccentric, lengthening contractions is better maintained in the elderly than strength during concentric, shortening contractions. As a result, many older adults find it easier to lower themselves into a chair, which requires a lengthening contraction of the quadriceps, than to rise from a chair, which requires a shortening contraction of these same muscles.

As noted earlier, sarcopenia plays a significant role in the decline of strength due to aging. Although controversial, many researchers contend that aging causes a selective loss of **fast-twitch muscle fibers.** One hypothesis contends that more fast-twitch than **slow-twitch muscle fibers** are lost because of a progressive and selective death of the large motor neurons that activate fast-twitch motor units (Engel, 1970; Larsson, 1978). Another theory claims that fast-twitch motor

Figure 21-2
Gradual decline of muscle strength

Source: Bryant, C.X., Franklin, B.A., & Newton-Merrill, S. (2007). *ACE's Guide to Exercise Testing and Program Design* (2nd ed.). Monterey, Calif.: Healthy Learning.

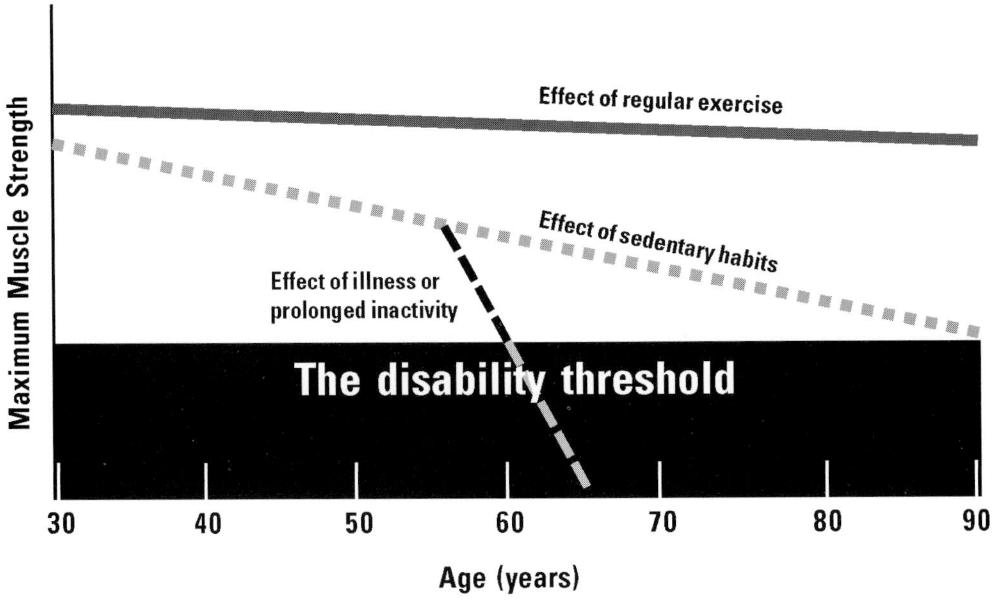

units transform, mainly through disuse, into slow-twitch units, altering the slow- to fast-twitch ratio and making it appear that fast-twitch fibers have been lost (Grimby & Saltin 1983). Despite the controversy surrounding the causative mechanisms of strength loss in the elderly, it is relatively well-accepted among gerontologists that muscle fibers, and therefore strength and function, are lost with aging.

While muscle endurance also typically diminishes as people age, it is generally better maintained than muscular strength (LaForest et al., 1990; Clarke, Hunt, & Dotson, 1992). A decrease in muscular endurance results in an earlier onset of fatigue during activity and places an older adult at an increased risk for loss of balance or a fall. Muscular power is also negatively affected by advancing age. A decrease in power may alter an older adult's ability to respond quickly and effectively to an unexpected loss of balance or move rapidly in day-to-day situations.

Bone Loss

Similar to muscle loss, older adults experience a progressive loss of bone minerals with age. The process of bone mineral depletion occurs more rapidly in women (36 grams per decade) than in men (30 grams per decade). Women also are more vulnerable to the effects of bone loss because they obtain a lower lifetime peak calcium content and experience an accelerated loss of calcium for about five years around the time of menopause (Riggs & Melton, 1992). As bones lose calcium, they become increasingly vulnerable to fractures. Individuals who suffer a fracture late in life may experience significant disability and financial hardship. Considering that it is estimated that 55% of Americans age 50 and older have **osteopenia** or **osteoporosis,** bone mineral density preservation and enhancement is a major public health concern [National Osteoporosis Foundation (NOF), 2008]. Bone loss is less marked for individuals who maximize bone mineral density by consuming an adequate amount of calcium and perform vigorous exercise as a young adult and who have continued heavy-weight or load-bearing exercise into later life (Murphy et al., 1994; Slemenda et al., 1991; Suominen & Rahkila, 1991).

Flexibility

The elasticity and compliance of connective tissue is altered with aging. As muscle fibers atrophy, they are replaced by fatty and fibrous (**collagen**) tissue. Collagen is a primary component of connective tissue that exhibits a low compliance, which contributes to the stiffening and decreased mobility of aging muscle. Additionally, a significant loss (up to 15%) of body water between the ages of 30 and 80 contributes to increased stiffness in soft tissues [American Council on Exercise (ACE), 2005]. Collectively, these changes appear to be partly responsible for flexibility loss due to aging. However, it is possible that the reduction in **range of motion (ROM)** is due, in part, to lack of physical activity, since there is some evidence that not all older adults lose flexibility at the same rate (Campanelli, 1996).

The greatest losses of flexibility are typically seen in the spine and ankle joints in middle-aged and older adults. In a study looking at spinal flexibility in women ages 20 through 84, spine extension was significantly reduced between the 30- and 50-year-old age groups (Einkauf et al., 1987). The authors discussed that these results could be an indication of the types of daily activities in which most people participate. That is, most ADL involve leaning forward (spinal flexion), whereas very few occasions arise in the course of daily life to lean backward (spinal extension). A study assessing ankle range of motion and aging showed that between the ages of 55 and 85, women lose 50% of their flexibility, while men lose about 35% of the flexibility in that joint (Vandervoort et al., 1992). Age-related weakness in the dorsiflexors and an increase in resistance due to increases in collagen cross-linkages contributes to the ankle not flexing adequately during walking. Decreased use eventually leads to a loss of range of motion at the ankle joint, which, when added to the age-related strength losses, increases an older adult's risk for falling.

Nervous System

Aging is associated with changes in overall cerebral function, vision, hearing, and reaction time. Many aspects of cerebral function, such as short-term memory, cognition, and information processing, deteriorate with advanced age. Furthermore, the pace of learning new tasks becomes slower in an older adult. These declines may be a result of conditions such as **Alzheimer's disease,** but also include a lack of recent practice of specialized sensory and motor skills, a slowing in the ability to perceive the environment, **depression,** cardiovascular disease, the administration of certain sedative medications, and lack of physical activity (Schaie, 1989; McGreer & McGreer, 1980; Poitrenaud et al., 1994). Habitual physical activity appears to enhance cognitive performance, as physically fit older adults are often able to process cognitive information more efficiently than less-fit individuals of the same chronological age (Chodzko-Zajko & Moore, 1994).

The speed at which an older adult responds to a given signal decreases progressively with age. While a slowing of nerve conduction time (a decrease of approximately 4%), increased joint stiffness, and a loss of muscle power are related to the deterioration in response times as a person ages, the main contributor is the brain (Shephard, 1997; Wright & Shephard, 1978). A progressive decrease in the brain's ability to process information and complete tasks such as coding, retrieval, comparison, and selection are associated with a decreased speed of response to environmental signals (Spirduso, Francis, & MacRae, 2005). Possible causes of decreased reaction speed include a progressive death of neurons, a loss of interconnecting **dendrites,** and decreased cerebral blood flow (Feldman, 1976; Toole & Abourezk, 1989). It has been postulated that a number of mechanisms associated with regular exercise may help to enhance both cognition and reaction speed in physically fit older adults—improvements in cerebral circulation, nerve cell regeneration, and/or changes in neurotransmitter synthesis and degradation (Chodzko-Zajko & Moore, 1994).

As noted previously, short-term memory decreases with age, which limits the ability to develop new skills and concepts. If learning a new task requires a large number of items to be remembered, information that must be manipulated, or the person's undivided attention, an older adult will experience difficulty in mastering it (Ostrow, 1989). Providing written instructions, allowing an extended time period for the anticipation of performing a new task, and prolonging the inspection period of learning a new task may enhance the learning experience for an older adult.

A discussion of changes in vision and hearing in older adults might seem like an irrelevant topic for the ACE-certified Advanced Health & Fitness Specialist (ACE-AHFS). However, reduced function in these senses has a powerful impact on the daily activities of older people. As a result of progressive declines in various aspects of vision, many older adults may limit the range and extent of physical activities. Age-related changes in vision, such as a reduced visual field, difficulty focusing on nearby objects, and a decrease in visual sharpness and clarity, lead to an impaired performance of tasks that require visual skills and a greater risk of colliding with external objects. As auditory acuity decreases with aging, some older adults withdraw from social events, including those that involve physical activity, because of a decreased ability to hear and understand speech. Older adults have a particularly difficult time detecting high-frequency sounds and distinguishing a true signal from background noise (Moller, 1981). Consequently, the affected individual has a more difficult time detecting the direction from which a sound originates and exhibits a decrease in auditory reaction time.

Neuromuscular Coordination

Neuromuscular coordination is defined as the ability to activate large and small muscles with the correct amount of force in the most efficient sequence to accomplish a task. Complex motor patterns, such as those involved in walking and running, must be practiced many times before they become a skill. More complex forms of locomotion, such as skipping and galloping, require even more learning to master the increased neuromuscular coordination involved in those tasks. A specific type of neuromuscular coordination called **hand-eye coordination** is defined as the "skillful, integrated use of the eyes, arms, hands, and fingers in fine, precision movement" (Williams, 1983). Activities such as throwing and catching a ball, hitting a golf ball, bowling, sewing, and tying a shoelace all require hand-eye coordination. Large decrements are observed in many types of coordination and skills with aging. Although the effect of aging cannot be eliminated in many coordinated motor performances, older adults can improve their performance dramatically through persistence and practice.

When introduced to new tasks, older adults perform according to the complexity of the task. While older subjects may not initially perform as well as younger subjects, they learn simple skills relatively quickly so that the gap between the ages narrows rapidly with practice. However, a complex task that requires a continuous series of varied movements is more difficult for middle-aged and older adults to learn (Welford, 1985).

With advancing age, many neurons die, and those that do survive exhibit changes in the **axons,** dendrites, and **cell bodies.** Dendritic branches, the primary path by which neurons communicate with each other, become thinner and lose contact with surrounding neurons. This loss of dendrites may be responsible for the generalized slowing in reaction speeds observed in older adults as described in the previous section. Despite the age-related deterioration in the nervous system, older adults can enhance brain activity by performing repetitions (practicing) a variety of tasks. No matter what their ages, older adults make substantial improvements in physical skill with repeated practice. Tasks that include physical activity appear to improve brain function better than tasks where physical movement is restricted or limited (Gentile, Behesti, & Held, 1987; Held, Gordon, & Gentile, 1985).

Another important factor in neuromuscular coordination is the ability to focus undivided attention on the task at hand. Older adults have an increasingly difficult time keeping attention directed on a task. Background noise is a common distraction for older people and the ability to carry out two tasks simultaneously diminishes. For example, in one study, older golfers did not perform as well as younger golfers when a meaningful noise, such as a news broadcast, was played as background noise during a putting competition. The younger golfers were able to block out irrelevant stimuli and concentrate on the putt, whereas the older golfers listened to the broadcast instead of fully concentrating on the game. The researchers suggested that the background increased the cognitive demands of the older golfers, decreasing their ability to selectively focus on the task (Backman & Molander, 1991).

Although consistent practice of specific tasks can help maintain some types of motor function into late adulthood, reduced efficiency and speed of performance eventually lead individuals to develop compensatory strategies to cope with these losses. These coping strategies include anticipation, simplification, and trading speed for accuracy (Spirduso, Francis, & MacRae, 2005). Anticipation is helpful for older adults, as they plan their movements for selected tasks well before the task is performed. When the time comes to initiate the task, such as grabbing a suitcase off of a luggage carousel at the airport, the older person has had time to anticipate the upcoming required movements so that they can be made quickly and efficiently. Simplification is used by older adults to compensate for losses in coordination by making complex movements less complicated. Breaking movements into simpler tasks to achieve the same end result compensates for the decline in coordination. For example, older people may sit on a stool to pull weeds from a garden, whereas younger people bend over and stand up many times while performing the same chore. Lastly, choosing accuracy over speed is another tactic that helps compensate for decreased coordination. By choosing to move slower, older subjects allow more time for visual and proprioceptive feedback to detect and correct errors, which could help explain the tendency for older adults to move slower and proceed more cautiously while performing physical tasks than younger adults.

Body Composition

On average, a person's body weight increases from the ages of 25 to 50, and thereafter shows a slow, progressive decline (Shephard, 1997).

Middle-age weight gain usually reflects an accumulation of body fat and a concomitant reduction in lean mass. While men and women retain their basic **android** and **gynoid** characteristics, they both experience a body-fat distribution shift from subcutaneous sites to more internal and intramuscular fat.

Increased body-fat accumulation and decreased lean mass contribute to the decrease in metabolic rate associated with aging. Potential factors tied to this negative trend in body composition include a decrease in habitual physical activity, a decrease in resting energy expenditure, and a decrease in the **thermic effect of food.** Combined, these factors result in a substantial decrease in daily energy requirements, which, without a modification in caloric intake, may lead to **overweight** or **obesity.**

Lean mass that is lost in old age is mainly from muscle, liver, kidney, and adrenal gland tissue, with a significant decrease of brain tissue occurring in the very old (Shephard, 1997). Average-health adults tend to sustain a plateau of lean tissue mass through the age of 40, and then experience an accelerated loss thereafter. Masters athletes, however, have shown little or no change in lean tissue until the seventh or eighth decade of life (Pollock et al., 1987; Shephard, 1991).

Balance and Gait Challenges in Older Adults

As adults mature and advance into old age, the constant pull of gravity on their upright postures begins to take its toll. Balance becomes more difficult, the chances of falling increase, and the quick, youthful actions of jogging, running, and jumping are replaced with walking. Maintaining an adequate sense of balance into old age is crucial for preventing trips and falls in the last decades of life. Gait and balance disorders stem from multiple factors and

Table 21-2
Medical Conditions That Cause Gait and Balance Disorders in the Elderly

Cardiovascular Conditions			
orthostatic hypotension	vertebrobasilar insufficiency intermittent claudiction	chronic lower-extremity edema	
Neurological Conditions			
Parkinson's disease stroke etat lacunaire peripheral neuropathy dementia chronic subdural hematoma	normal pressure hydrocephalus cerbellar ataxia posterior column degeneration cervical spondylosis vitamin B_{12} myelopathy deficiency	frontal lobe syndrome encephalopathy progressive supranuclear palsy peripheral neuropathy spinal cord lesions	
Musculoskeletal Conditions			
osteoarthritis osteoarthroses	status post-ortho surgery	foot problems osteomalacia	unsuspected fractures
Psychological Conditions			
depression	fear of falling		
Endocrinological Conditions			
hypothyroidism			
Other Conditions			
general weakness drug intoxication/ overdose	benzodiazepines tricyclic antidepressants	anticonvulsants salicylates antivertigo agents	senile gait idiopathic gait disorders

Sources: Tinetti, M.E., Williams, T.F., Mayewski, R. (1986). Fall risk index for elderly patients based on number of chronic disabilities. *American Journal of Medicine,* 80, 429-434; Cunha, U.V. (1988). Differential diagnosis of gait disorders in the elderly. *Geriatrics,* 43, 34.

may be caused by any number of deteriorations due to aging, disease conditions, and alterations due to medications (Table 21-2). The most effective approach to dealing with gait and balance disturbances in older clients includes communicating directly with the client's primary physician to obtain precise information specific to the individual.

Static Balance

Balance is the ability to maintain the body's position over its **base of support** within stability limits, both statically and dynamically. Stability limits are boundaries of an area of space in which the body can maintain its position without changing the base of support (i.e., without taking a step). Efficient standing balance requires that the body's **center of gravity (COG)** be kept within stability limits, as defined by the length of the feet and the distance between them. The extent to which an older adult is willing or able to lean in any direction without having to change the base of support by taking a step defines his or her stability limits.

Good posture is critical for ensuring adequate balance. Posture refers to the biomechanical alignment of the individual body parts and the orientation of the body to the environment. Standing efficiently requires the vertical alignment of each body part to expend the least amount of muscular energy. Although standing in one place requires no visible movement, a number of muscles are active in maintaining an upright posture and resisting the force of gravity. These muscles include the soleus, gastrocnemius, tibialis anterior, gluteus medius, tensor fasciae latae, iliopsoas, erector spinae, and abdominals.

Static balance refers to an individual's ability to control postural sway during quiet standing. Even when a young, fit individual who has excellent balance capabilities attempts to stand quietly on both feet, the body sways over its base of support. Given that it is impossible for someone to stand absolutely motionless, postural sway is the path of the body's movement in the anterior/posterior (i.e., sagittal) and lateral (i.e., frontal) planes while standing still. Postural sway is functionally significant because it is related to the risk of falling—specifically for older people who fall without warning and without a loss of consciousness, as opposed to those who trip and fall. This aspect of static balance is of interest because it may identify individuals at a higher risk for falling, and for whom behavioral and physiological strategies can be developed and implemented to help prevent falls.

When older people stand quietly, the amount of postural sway is greater than in younger individuals, and greater in women than in men (Brocklehurst, Roberston, & James-Groom, 1982; Overstall et al., 1977). When standing quietly with the eyes closed, postural sway is exaggerated in all individuals, but especially in the elderly. Additionally, maintaining static balance on one foot is much more difficult than maintaining stability over two feet, because the base of support is smaller and the available neuromuscular response is much more limited. Not surprisingly, postural sway in elderly subjects is much more pronounced when balancing on one foot than in younger subjects. In fact, one of the most sensitive measures of aging is the ability to stand on one leg with the eyes closed.

Explanations for the reduced stability limits seen in older adults include weakness in the muscles of the ankle joint, reduced range of motion about the ankles, neurological trauma (e.g., **stroke, Parkinson's disease**), and a fear of falling. A significant reduction in an older adult's stability limits, especially in the lateral and backward directions, increases his or her risk for falling.

Dynamic Balance

During physical activity, an individual must maintain control of the body's COG while moving over the base of support. The act of maintaining postural control while moving is called dynamic balance. It is required when upper-body movements shift the COG (e.g., reaching for objects, opening doors), or when the position of the body changes from one location to another, as in locomotion.

Results from tests used to determine age-related differences in dynamic balance have revealed that elderly subjects' area of stability over the base of support is smaller than the area found in younger subjects (Spirduso, Francis, & MacRae, 2005).

In other words, any small disruption to standing balance (e.g., a support surface on which an individual is standing moves unexpectedly) will quickly move older adult subjects beyond their limits of stability and require that they reach for something nearby or take a step to prevent a fall.

When the support surface of the subjects unexpectedly moves forward, the response of younger individuals is to sequentially contract the tibialis anterior, quadriceps, and abdominals. A sequential contraction of the gastrocnemius, biceps femoris, and erector spinae takes place in young people when an unexpected backward movement of the support surface occurs.

Compared to the muscle sequences exhibited by young people, older individuals show significant differences in the order of muscle contraction and timing when their base of support moves unexpectedly (Woollacott, Inglin, & Manchester, 1988). Older people exhibit a delay in contracting the balance support muscles, and sometimes the optimal sequence of muscle contractions is impaired in the aged. In addition, the balance of the elderly is more affected compared to younger individuals when a source of information about the balance process is lost (e.g., vision impairment).

Balance-related Sensory Systems

The **central nervous system (CNS)** holds the key to successful balance. The CNS must have an accurate picture of where the body is in space and whether it is stationary or moving. Peripheral inputs from three sensory systems—the **visual, vestibular,** and **somatosensory systems**—provide the CNS with information related to the body's position in space with respect to gravity and the environment. The visual system provides information related to where the body is in space, how fast it is moving, and what obstacles are likely to be encountered. The somatosensory system relays information from the skin, joints, and vibratory sensors, all of which help to detect body position. The vestibular system, located in the inner ear, provides information related to movements of the head. Although no separate system provides the CNS with all of the sensory information necessary to determine the body's position in space, each of the three systems contributes its own specific information about body movement and position. The sensory and motor systems are the key components of every balance-related effort, as they are inextricably linked to provide kinesthetic input and then select appropriate movements based on this input. In addition, the cognitive system is crucial for interpreting incoming sensations and planning motor responses related to balance. The cognitive system, which is composed of the processes of attention, memory, and intelligence, presents the ability to anticipate or adapt the body's actions in response to changing task demands and the environment.

Visual System

Humans rely heavily on visual inputs for balance. Visual information gives a reference for verticality, as many things in the environment, like doors and windows, are aligned vertically. The visual system also relays information regarding head motion, because as the head moves forward, surrounding objects move in the opposite direction. Furthermore, studies have suggested that peripheral vision is the most significant component of vision with regard to maintaining balance because it makes a very important contribution to the control of anterior-posterior sway (Woollacott, Inglin, & Manchester, 1988). In fact, it has been suggested that older adults rely more on peripheral vision than young adults do and that the absence of peripheral vision leads to a greater frequency of falls.

Although vision is a significant component used by the CNS to maintain balance, it is not absolutely necessary. Most people can keep their balance with their eyes closed or when standing in a dark room. In addition, visual inputs are not always accurate sources of spatial information. For example, when an individual sits at a stoplight in a car, and the car next to him or her moves slightly, a likely response is to apply even more pressure on the brake. In this situation, visual inputs signal motion, which the brain initially interprets as self-motion; in other words, the person thinks his or her car is rolling. The brain signals the motor neurons of the leg and foot to apply the brake to stop motion, even though the car is sitting still. Thus, visual input may be misinterpreted by the brain because it has a difficult time distinguishing between object-motion (i.e., exocentric motion) and self-motion (i.e., egocentric motion).

Throughout the aging process, vision becomes degraded and provides decreased or distorted information. As a result, poor visual acuity is associated with an increased number of falls in the elderly. With aging, most individuals lose the ability to detect the spatial information that is important for balance. For example, older adults need three times more contrast to see some stimuli at slow frequencies, and their depth perception and peripheral vision decline (Sekular, Hutman, & Owsley, 1980). These changes impair the quality of visual input received and will result in slower processing of the incoming sensory feedback, poor integration of sensory inputs, and an altered kinesthetic awareness. Consequently, an older adult's ability to avoid obstacles, negotiate terrain, and efficiently move about in low-light conditions will be negatively affected. Although age-related vision impairments make it difficult for the elderly to use visual inputs for balance control, information from the somatosensory and vestibular systems can be called upon to compensate for the declining visual system in most cases.

Vestibular System

The system of receptors located in the inner ear that is responsible for providing directional information as it relates to the position of the head is called the vestibular system. When the head moves, fluid rushes over hair cells within this system, causing them to bend, which signals the head's position with respect to gravity (i.e., upside down, sideways, or tilted) as well as any turning of the head. The vestibular system has a powerful influence over the motor neurons in the spinal cord that activate postural muscles (especially extensors) and thus contributes substantially to balance.

As early as age 30, hair cells within the vestibular system begin to decline in density, resulting in a reduced sensitivity to head movements. Individuals over age 70 may have lost 40% of the sensory cells within the vestibular system (Spirduso, Francis, & MacRae, 2005). Consequently, an increase in sway and risk of falling, especially when the visual and the somatosensory systems are impaired, are likely. Decreases in vestibular function also have been associated with visual problems and dizziness in older adults.

When individuals are moving around in a very dark environment and on an unstable surface, they primarily call on the vestibular system for balance. Additionally, the vestibular system helps to resolve conflicts that arise between the other sensory systems while in complex visual environments (e.g., crowded public places, traffic). Sensory conflict occurs when information provided by one or more sensory systems is not in agreement with one or both of the other sensory systems. Many older adults have reported that they dislike venturing into crowded malls or grocery stores because they feel unsteady due to people constantly moving in and out of their visual field. To compensate for this unsteadiness, they may push shopping carts for increased stabilization or simply avoid these types of sensory situations altogether. Undoubtedly, they are unable to resolve the conflict among the three sensory systems because they have lost their ability to identify and then quickly ignore the conflicting input from the visual and somatosensory systems.

Somatosensory System

The CNS receives information from the somatosensory system regarding body position in space with reference to supporting surfaces as well as the relationship of body segments to one another. Somatosensory receptors include cutaneous and pressure receptors, and joint and muscle proprioceptors. In the absence of vision, the somatosensory system becomes the primary source of sensory information for maintaining upright balance and moving about in dark environments.

When any mechanical stimulus is applied to the body's surface, cutaneous receptors in the skin relay this information to the CNS. Therefore, when the skin is contacted and changes in pressure on the skin occur, neural impulses are directed to the CNS. To exemplify the importance of this system as it relates to balance, think of the difficulty of standing up and walking after sitting in one position for a long time, which restricts the blood supply to the lower limbs. This causes a temporary loss of function of the cutaneous receptors. Consequently, the feet and lower legs feel numb and the sensation of contact of the skin with the shoes and the changes in pressure that occur as the body weight rolls through the foot during walking are no longer available and balance becomes threatened. The process of aging brings about a decline in an individual's ability to sense cutaneous inputs, which results in a reduced ability to feel the quality of contact between the feet and the supporting surface. To measure the decline in cutaneous receptor activity due to aging, researchers test how accurately individuals can detect vibration of the skin, as vibration sense in the legs is used to control postural sway (Brocklehurst, Roberston, & James-Groom, 1982). The ability to detect vibratory stimuli has been shown to decrease significantly with age as the speed with which vibration information reaches the CNS and the amplitude of this information decreases. Additionally, older adults lose some sensitivity to touch as they age (Bolton, Winkelman, & Dyck, 1966).

Muscle and joint proprioceptors provide information about the mechanical displacements of muscles and joints. Stretch receptors (i.e., muscle spindles) in the muscle signal a change in length when the muscle is stretched. Reflexively, the muscle contracts so that the desired muscle length and tension are obtained. For example, when the body leans forward, the calf muscles are stretched. This brings about a reflex contraction of the soleus and gastrocnemius to return the body to a more upright position and maintain balance within stability limits. Similarly, when a joint angle is changed, this information is relayed to the CNS via joint receptors. Muscle spindle activity and, to a lesser degree, joint receptor inputs are impaired with aging.

Confidence and Balance

Unlike the other characteristics that contribute to an individual's balance ability that are physical in nature, the fear of falling is a mindset that has been shown to increase an older adult's risk for suffering a fall. Many older adults lack confidence in their mobility and, as a result, are constantly afraid of falling. In fact, research has shown that some older adults will avoid certain activities to prevent falling and rate their fear of falling to be greater than their fear of robbery, forgetting appointments, or financial difficulties (Walker & Howland, 1991).

The fear of falling manifests itself physically in older adults when they habitually stiffen their joints, causing unnecessary contraction of muscles and a flexed-forward posture. Many elderly people have an exaggerated fear of falling backward and hitting their heads or breaking their backs and hips. Consequently, the flexed-forward posture puts them at a more advantageous position to fall forward if a disruption in balance occurs, thereby resulting in potential fractures to the wrists and arms, but protecting their backs and hips. A flexed posture does place the body in a more stable position, but because it requires more muscular force to maintain, there is an increased reliance on muscular strength and endurance.

Impaired mobility contributes to a fear of falling, which in turn can contribute to further decrements in mobility. If an individual is haunted by a fear of falling, he or she is likely to avoid walking and being physically active, which minimizes the use of the musculoskeletal system, thereby weakening the muscles that play such an important role in maintaining balance. This reluctance to be active leads to more immobility and heightens an elderly person's lack of self-confidence in ambulation. Ironically, family and friends of older adults who fall often compound the problem by discouraging walking after a fall. Ultimately, a perceived sense of insecurity related to balance may actually increase the likelihood of a traumatic fall.

Gait Changes

Walking is cyclical in nature and can be described via the **gait cycle**—the time between the first contact of the heel of one foot with the ground and the next heel-ground contact with the same foot. The decline in neuromuscular fitness associated with aging carries with it significant consequences related to gait, including a loss of walking speed. Age-related declines in strength result in failure to lift the foot high enough during the swing phase of gait and, as a result, tripping is more likely. Strength losses, particularly in the lower body, are associated with a degraded ability to maintain dynamic balance, walk, prevent falls, and move quickly. This directly affects an individual's ability to maintain balance and, therefore, prevent a fall.

Research has shown that the muscles that exert force against the ground during walking and provide stabilization around the ankle joint are considerably weakened with aging (Vandervoort & Hayes, 1989; Whipple, Wolfson, & Amerman, 1987). In addition, a decline in strength of the musculature that supports the knees has been associated with a greater risk for falling. A significant correlation between muscle strength and preferred walking speed in adults over age 65 has been reported (Bassey, Bendall, & Pearson, 1988). In frail institutionalized individuals over the age of 85, a strong relationship between quadriceps strength and habitual gait speed has been found (Fiatarone et al., 1990). In older, frail women, leg power was highly correlated with walking speed (Bassey et al., 1992). These findings suggest that with the advancing age and very low activity levels seen in the frail elderly, physical fitness is a critical component of walking ability.

Slower Gait Speeds

As noted earlier, gait speeds become slower with advanced aging. Even healthy older adults with no history of falling walk at a preferred speed that is approximately 20% slower than the walking speed of younger adults. In addition, when asked to walk at a fast speed, older adults are approximately 17% slower than younger adults who are asked to do the same (Elble et al., 1991). Interestingly, the slower gait speed that accompanies aging is not due to a decreased cadence, but is the result of a decrease in stride length. This decrease in stride length has negative consequences for other aspects of the gait cycle, including reduced arm swing and rotation of the hips, knees, and ankles; increased double-support time; and a more flat-footed contact with the ground during the stance phase prior to toe-off. Thus, older adults take more steps to cover the same distance, and the time when both feet are on the ground is longer.

One explanation for the decreased gait-related function in the elderly is the theory of motion economy. Locomotion requires the expenditure of energy. Researchers theorize that in both humans and animals, gait speeds are chosen that are most economical in terms of energy consumption (Larish, Martin, & Mungiole, 1988). Humans, presumably, prefer certain speeds of walking because those speeds are the most economical for them based on their body structure, weight, muscular strength, and flexibility. Therefore, older walkers may use the strategy of increasing stride frequency instead of stride length because it maximizes their motion economy. Furthermore, the endurance of weaker lower-body muscles is maximized with shorter strides, and the energy cost of walking is minimized.

Another possible explanation is that slower gait speeds allow older adults to spend more time monitoring the progress and result of walking and to respond to changes in the environment. Additionally, limited ranges of motion in the ankles and knees are responsible for a shortened stride length. Finally, a decreased ability to balance encourages older individuals to spend less time in the single-support phase of gait, and the increased time spent in double-support ultimately slows gait speed.

Common adaptations in the gait cycle seen in older people are the tendency to load the limb more cautiously during weight acceptance, a flatter foot-to-floor contact pattern, less forward advancement of the limb during single-limb support, and reduced flexion during the pre-swing and swing phases of gait. Furthermore, older adults approach obstacles more cautiously, reducing their gait speed and clearing the obstacle using slower, shorter steps. In addition, they cross the obstacle so that it is 10% further in front of them in their crossing step as compared to younger adults' stepping strategies (Chen et al., 1991). This reduction in step length may actually decrease the risk for tripping, but it can also cause the heel of the foot to contact the object before it returns to the ground on the other side. Thus, because older adults make more obstacle contact, their risk of tripping and falling while negotiating an obstacle is higher.

Assessing the Older Adult Client

The age-related declines in physical and cognitive function described in the previous sections often require the ACE-AHFS to develop a multidimensional approach when working with older adults. Since aging is a uniquely individual process, each older client will need to be assessed to determine his or her needs and abilities. Furthermore, approximately 80% of older Americans are living with at least one chronic condition, and 50% have at least two (CDC, 2003). This means that the ACE-AHFS will have to creatively develop fitness programs that address the client's goals while also taking into account any health conditions, medications, and associated limitations.

Resnick and colleagues (2008) developed a health screening tool specifically for the older adult population that can help the ACE-AHFS identify different types of exercise and physical-activity programs that would best serve the

Figure 21-3
Exercise and Screening for You (EASY)

Source: Resnick, B. (2007). The EASY screening tool. *International Council on Active Aging, Functional U.* May–June, 9–13.

Exercise and Screening for You (EASY)

Once a person completes the EASY, a summary page provides a report based on his or her responses. The online version (www.easyforyou.info) contains the links referred to under the "yes" column. A person who answers "yes" to question 1 should NOT start exercising before consulting with a healthcare provider. There a few additional questions for those who say "yes."

People who are advised to see a healthcare provider can print out the summary and take it with them.

Question	"Yes" answer	"No" answer
1. Do you have pains, tightness, or pressure in your chest during physical activity (walking, climbing stairs, household chores, similar activities)?	• You should not start exercising. • Make sure your healthcare provider knows about the tightness or pressure in your chest during physical activity.	
2. Do you currently experience dizziness or lightheadedness?	• Make sure your healthcare provider knows about the dizziness or lightheadedness. • View these links and tips.	
3. Have you ever been told that you have high blood pressure?	• If your blood pressure has not been checked in the past six months, it is recommended that you get it checked by a healthcare provider.	• If your blood pressure has not been checked in the past six months, it is recommended that you get it checked by a healthcare provider.
4. Do you have pain, tightness, or swelling that limits or prevents you from doing what you want or need to do?	• View these links and tips.	
5. Do you fall, feel unsteady, or use an assistive devise while walking or standing?	• View these links and tips. • If you use an assistive device, it is okay that you exercise, but please continue to use it while exercising as appropriate.	• If you use an assistive device, it is okay to exercise, but please continue to use it while exercising as appropriate.
6. Is there a reason not mentioned why you would be concerned about starting an exercise program?	• View these links and tips.	

existing health conditions, illnesses, or disabilities of older clients (Figure 21-3). Developed for older individuals, their healthcare providers, and exercise professionals, the Exercise Assessment and Screening for You (EASY) includes six screening questions that serve to:

- Enable a quick assessment of health problems
- Provide initial strategies for tailoring exercise for different health conditions and problems
- Offer safety tips to further minimize any potential health risks

A unique characteristic of EASY is the philosophy that screening should be an interactive process in which participants learn to appreciate the importance of engaging in regular exercise, paying attention to personal health, recognizing signs and symptoms that might indicate potentially harmful events, and becoming familiar with simple safety tips for physical activity. The EASY tool is available as an online resource for older adults and health/fitness professionals (www.easyforyou.info). The web-based version of EASY makes recommendations based on the older adult's answers to the six screening questions and provides a summary page listing their responses and recommendations.

Medication

It is absolutely critical that the ACE-AHFS have knowledge of common medications that are prescribed for older adults. Some physical side effects of these drugs include dizziness, reduced alertness, weakness, fatigue, and postural hypotension. It has been shown that older adults who are taking four or more prescription medications are four times more likely to experience a fall than their peers who are taking fewer medications (Campbell, Borrie, & Spears, 1989). Furthermore, specific types of medications (i.e., antianxiety, antidepressants, hypnotics/sedatives, and diuretics) are more likely to cause a fall. Tables 21-3 and 21-4 describe various medications that are commonly prescribed for older adults.

The aging process also affects the absorption, distribution, metabolism, and excretion of drugs (**pharmacokinetics**). The five age-related physiological changes that slow or diminish the pharmacokinetics of medications are as follows (ACE, 2005):

- Decreased lean mass and increased body fat
- Reduction in total body water
- Decreased efficiency of the gastrointestinal tract
- Decreased cardiac output
- Decreased efficiency of the liver and kidneys

Identifying Age and Physical Function

As noted earlier, the complex nature of aging makes it impossible to pinpoint a person's functional capabilities based solely on chronological age. However, because of the relationship between time and the aging process, chronological age is used as a preliminary identification (Table 21-5). The span of the age range from "young-old" to "oldest-old" is quite large. Therefore, determining a person's physical function level based on a label of "older adult" is impossible.

One component of assessing an older client's level of function is classification based on the performance of ADL. The American Geriatrics Society classifies ADL into three levels of function: basic (BADL), instrumental (IADL), and advanced (AADL) (American Geriatrics Society, 1989). BADL include the elemental items of self-care (e.g., feeding, bathing, toileting, and dressing). IADL, also referred to as independent or intermediate ADL, include tasks vital for maintaining independence (e.g., preparing meals, managing money, shopping for groceries or personal items, performing light or heavy housework, and using a telephone). AADL include functions well beyond those at the level observed for independent living, such as recreational, occupational, and community service functions. Another method of assessing function is to categorize older adults based on their ability to function independently (Table 21-6). Assessing an older client's ADL and physical function helps the ACE-AHFS determine the individual's immediate needs and abilities so that appropriate fitness testing and program design can be developed.

Assessing Function in Older Adults

The ACE-AHFS must determine the most appropriate exercise tests to give to older clients. Some older people should not be given any

Table 21-3
Cardiac Medications: Their Use, Side Effects, and Effects on Exercise Response

Type/Trade Name	Use	Side Effects	Effects on Exercise Response
I. Antianginal Agents			
A. Nitroglycerin compounds (Amyl nitrate; Isordil; Nitrostat)	Smooth muscle relaxation; decrease cardiac output	Headache, dizziness, hypotension	Hypotension; increase exercise capacity
B. Beta blockers (Inderal; Propranolol; Lopressor; Corgard; Biocadren)	Block beta receptors; decrease sympathetic tone; decrease HR, contractility, and BP	Bradycardia, heart block, insomnia, nausea, fatigue, weakness, increased cholesterol and blood sugar	Decrease HR; hypotension; decrease cardiac contractility
C. Calcium antagonists (Verapamil; Nifedipine; Procardia)	Block influx of calcium; dilate coronary arteries; suppress dysrhythmias	Dizziness, syncope, flushing, hypotension headache, fluid retention	Hypotension
II. Antihypertensive Agents			
A. Diuretics (Thiazides, Lasix, Aldactone)	Inhibit NA+ and Cl– in kidney; increase excretion of sodium and water, and control high BP and fluid retention	Drowsiness, dehydration, electrolyte imbalance, gout, nausea, pain, hearing loss, elevated cholesterol and lipoproteins	Hypotension
B. Vasodilators (Hydralazine, Captopril, Apresoline, Loniten, Minoxidil)	Dilate peripheral blood vessels; used in conjunction with diuretics; decrease BP	Increased HR and contractility, headache, drowsiness, nausea, vomiting, diarrhea	Hypotension
C. Drugs interfering with sympathetic nervous system (Reserprine, Propranolol, Aldomet, Catapres, Minipress)	Decrease BP, HR, and cardiac output by dilating blood vessels	Drowsiness, depression, sexual dysfunction, fatigue, dry mouth, stuffy nose, fever, upset stomach, fluid retention, weight gain	Increase exercise capacity; increase myocardial contractility
III. Digitalis Glycosides, Derivatives (Digoxin, Lonoxin, Digitoxin)	Strengthen the heart's pumping force and decrease electrical conduction disturbances	Arrhythmias, heart block, altered ECG, fatigue, weakness, headache, nausea, vomiting	
IV. Anticoagulant Agents (Coumadin, Sodium Heparin, Aspirin, Persantine)	Prevent blood clot formation	Easy bruising, stomach irritation, joint or abdominal pain, difficulty in swallowing, unexplained swelling, uncontrolled bleeding	
V. Antilipidemic Agents (Cholestyramine, Lopid, Niacin, Atromid-S, Mevacor, Questran Zocor)	Interfere with lipid metabolism and lower cholesterol and low-density lipoproteins	Nausea, vomiting, diarrhea, constipation, flatulence, abdominal discomfort, glucose intolerance	
VI. Antiarrhythmic Agents (Cardioquin, Procaine, Quinidine, Lidocaine, Dilantin, Propranolol, Bretylium tosylate, Verapamil)	Alter conduction patterns throughout the myocardium	Nausea, palpitations, vomiting, rash, insomnia, dizziness, shortness of breath, swollen ankles, coughing up blood, fever, psychosis, impotence	Hypotension; decrease HR; decrease cardiac contractility

Note: HR = Heart rate; BP = Blood pressure; ECG = Electrocardiogram

Souce: McArdle, W.D., Katch, F.I. & Katch, V.L. (2007). *Exercise Physiology* (6th ed.). Baltimore: Lippincott Williams & Wilkins.

Table 21-4
Medications and Substances Affecting Balance

Medications that reduce alertness
- Narcotics
- Hypnotics
- Sedatives
- Tranquilizers
- Alcohol

Medications that retard central conduction
- Narcotics
- Hypnotics
- Sedatives
- Tranquilizers
- Analgesics

Medications that impair cerebral perfusion
- Vasodilators
- Antihypertensives
- Some antidepressants

Medications that affect postural control
- Diuretics
- Digitalis
- Some beta blockers
- Some antihypertensives

physical fitness assessments, whereas others may enjoy the process. A proper pre-exercise screening documenting medical history, current medication use, and medical clearance (if necessary) must be performed on all clients. Additionally, interviewing clients about their recreational pursuits, occupational activities, and fitness goals is an important part of the pre-exercise screening process. This information will indicate whether or not an older adult is well-suited for various forms of fitness testing. The reader is encouraged to read the test protocols and interpretation information provided by the references for each of the following tests.

There are several reliable physical function assessments that can be used to measure balance and mobility in older adult clients. These assessments are important because they may facilitate the early identification of older adults who are beginning to experience significant changes in multiple sensory systems resulting in observable changes in postural stability and mobility. After interpreting assessment results, the ACE-AHFS can determine an appropriate exercise plan to target the impaired sensory systems. Furthermore, administering the same balance and mobility tests

Table 21-5
Chronological Age Categories

Description	Age (years)
Young-old	65–74
Old	75–84
Old-old	85–99
Oldest-old	100+

Source: Spirduso, W.W., Francis, K.L., & MacRae, P.G. (2005). *Physical Dimensions of Aging* (2nd ed.). Champaign, Ill.: Human Kinetics.

Table 21-6
Hierarchy of Physical Function of the Old (75–84 years), Old-old (85–99), and Oldest-old (100+)

Physically elite
Sports competition; Senior Olympics; high-risk and power sports (e.g., hang-gliding, weightlifting)

Physically fit
Moderate physical work;
all endurance sports and games; most hobbies

Physically independent
Very light physical work; hobbies (e.g., walking, gardening);
low physical-demand activities (e.g., golf, social dance, handcrafts, traveling, automobile driving)
Can pass some AADL, all IADL

Physically frail
Light housekeeping; food preparation;
grocery shopping
Can pass some IADL, all BADL;
May be homebound

Physically dependent
Walking; bathing; dressing; eating;
transferring
Needs home or institutional care

Disability

Note: AADL = Advanced activities of daily living; IADL = Intermediate activities of daily living; BADL = Basic activities of daily living

Source: Spirduso, W.W., Francis, K.L., & MacRae, P.G. (2005). *Physical Dimensions of Aging* (2nd ed.). Champaign, Ill.: Human Kinetics.

on a regular basis allows the ACE-AHFS to use the reassessment results to guide the selection of new exercises, the progression of existing exercises, and the deletion of certain exercises from the training program. Two tests used to measure functional limitations associated with the performance of daily activities requiring balance are the Berg Balance Scale (Berg et al., 1992) and the Fullerton Advanced Balance Scale (Rose, 2003).

Berg Balance Scale

The Berg Balance Scale (BBS) represents an individual's ability to perform a series of functional tasks that require balance. Many of the tasks simulate activities likely to be encountered by older adults in their daily lives, such as transfers, object retrieval, and turning. The BBS also may be used for identifying older adults who need intervention in the way of a comprehensive functional balance-training program. The BBS is recommended for assessing lower-functioning older adults. Detailed test administration procedures, a scoring form, a list of the possible underlying sensory impairments associated with poor performance, and a set of recommended exercises to address the identified impairments can be found in Appendix F.

Fullerton Advanced Balance Scale

The Fullerton Advanced Balance Scale (FAB) is designed to measure changes in balance occurring in higher-functioning older adults. Therefore, it is appropriate for use with community-dwelling older adults who are most likely to enroll in a community-based fitness program. The FAB Scale consists of 10 items that include a combination of static and dynamic balance activities performed in different sensory environments, as well as items that may help identify those at risk for falling as a result of sensory impairments. The FAB Scale was created for use as an alternative to the BBS, as the BBS tends to produce a ceiling effect (i.e., very high scores on repeated tests) when administered to higher-functioning older adults with impaired balance. Also, the BBS has been criticized for its lack of sensitivity in identifying various sensory system impairments. An individual's performance on the FAB Scale can be interpreted and the possible underlying balance impairment identified so that exercise progressions that specifically target those impairments can be selected. Detailed test administration procedures, a scoring form, a list of the possible underlying sensory impairments associated with poor performance, and a set of recommended exercises to address the identified impairments can be found in Appendix F. Table 21-7 presents a comprehensive list of other commonly used tests to determine overall physical function for older clients.

Functional Training for Activities of Daily Living

Functional training may be described as exercise with a purpose. Purposeful exercise entails any training movement performed with the intention of enhancing one's function, whether it is in the area of sports performance, fitness development, occupational performance, or ADL. Through effective functional training, older adults may be able to avoid, postpone, reduce, or even reverse the declines in physical function associated with aging. When developing a functional training program for older clients, the ACE-AHFS should choose exercises that will enhance the individual's day-to-day real-life tasks.

Optimal performance of movement requires that the body's muscles work together to produce force while simultaneously stabilizing the joints. Typically, clients who have weak stabilizer muscles (e.g., deep abdominals, hip stabilizers, and scapula retractors) exhibit problems performing proper, efficient movement, which may lead to pain and/or injury. Because individuals with pain or injury frequently have stabilizer weakness, functional training is often incorporated into a rehabilitation and post-rehabilitation training program, but this does not mean that functional training always focuses on the body's stabilizing musculature. Instead, functional training provides a solid foundation that the client can draw from when performing movements that require the muscles and joints to move in a coordinated, efficient manner.

A biomechanical concept that is used commonly in functional training is the idea that the body's

Table 21-7
Tests of Physical Function

Category of Physical Function	Sample Tests	Sources
Physically elite	$\dot{V}O_2$max; modified Balke treadmill	ACSM, 2006
Physically fit	Bruce treadmill protocol	Bruce et al., 1973
Physically independent (some)	Resistance strength tests (dynamometry)	McArdle, Katch, & Katch, 2007
	Routine flexibility and agility tests	
	Senior fitness test	Rikli & Jones, 2001
	AAHPERD functional fitness test	Osness, 1987
	Fitness tests:	
	Jumping, hand strength, flexion	Kimura, Hirakawa, & Morimoto, 1990
	Balance, agility, power, flexibility	Kuo, 1990
	Jumping, side-step, flexion, reaction time	Tahara et al., 1990
Physically independent	AAHPERD field test	Osness, 1987
	AADL	Reuben et al., 1990
	Continuous-scale physical functional performance test	Cress et al., 1996
Physically frail	Physical performance test	Reuben & Siu, 1990
	Tinetti's mobility assessment	Tinetti, 1986
	IADL	Lawton & Brody, 1969
	Hierarchical ADL-IADL	Kempen & Suurmeijer, 1990
	Classification schema for upper-extremity function and mobility	Williams & Greene, 1990
	Geri-AIMS	Hughes et al., 1991
	Physical impairment scale	Jette, Branch, & Berlin, 1990
	Functional independence measure	Granger et al., 1986
Physically dependent	ADL	Katz et al., 1963
	Mobility test	Schnelle et al., 1995
	Physical disability index	Gerety et al., 1993
	Physical performance and mobility exam	Lemsky et al., 1991
	Physical function scale of MOS SF-36	Ware & Sherbourne, 1992

Note: ACSM = American College of Sports Medicine; AAHPERD = American Alliance for Health, Physical Education, Recreation and Dance; AADL = Advanced activities of daily living; IADL = Intermediate activities of daily living; ADL = Activities of daily living; MOS SF-36 = Medical Outcomes Short Study Form

Source: Spirduso, W.W., Francis, K.L., & MacRae, P.G. (2005). *Physical Dimensions of Aging* (2nd ed.). Champaign, Ill.: Human Kinetics.

joints make up a kinetic chain, where each joint represents a link in the chain. Drawing on this principle, exercises may be described as either open- or closed-chain movements. In a closed-chain movement, the end of the chain furthest from the body is fixed, such as in the performance of a squat where the feet are fixed on the ground and the rest of the leg chain (i.e., ankles, knees, and hips) moves. In an open-chain exercise, the end of the chain furthest from the body is free, such as in the performance of a seated leg extension. Closed-chain exercises tend to emphasize compression of joints, which helps stabilize the joint, whereas open-chain exercises tend to involve more shearing forces at the joints. Furthermore, closed-chain exercises involve more muscles and joints than open-chain exercises, which results in better neuromuscular coordination and overall stability at the joints.

An example of a program that develops functional strength and range of motion is a conditioning routine that incorporates squats, lunges, multidirectional reaches, and overhead presses to enhance an older adult's everyday activities. Squatting and lunging are essential to human movement, as these tasks are required to stand up from a chair or stoop down to pick up a pair of shoes. Multidirectional reaches (i.e., reaching one or both arms in front of, to the side of, or behind the body) are important for training balance and postural control during dynamic activities that may place a person's COG outside the typical position between the feet during standing. Unilateral or bilateral overhead shoulder presses are tied closely to function in older adults because age-associated declines in upper-body strength often make the simplest tasks, such as putting away groceries on a top shelf, a substantial effort.

One of the most important principles of incorporating functional training into clients' programs is appropriate exercise progression. The emergence of several types of functional training devices, such as stability balls, balance boards, and foam rollers, might give the impression that functional training is synonymous with training on balance-type equipment. However, this is not the case, and the ACE-AHFS should not be tempted to place all clients on devices that challenge their abilities to balance on unstable surfaces. Clients who are ready for advanced exercises such as these must first demonstrate proper functional stability and movement patterns on stable surfaces, such as the floor, chairs, and exercise benches. In other words, functional training program design is based on moving clients from a stable training environment to a less-stable training environment over time through a series of exercises that build on previous conditioning.

Programming and Progression Guidelines

Safe and effective exercise programming for older adults is based on addressing their specific health and fitness needs without exposing them to unnecessary risks. This requires knowledge of current research on physical activity and aging, along with sound exercise programming principles. Older adults should be encouraged to develop their cardiorespiratory endurance, strength, and flexibility with a special emphasis on balance training.

Warm-up and Cool-down Techniques

For older clients, transitioning from a resting state to moderate or vigorous physical activity requires more time than it does for a younger person. Similarly, the time it takes to return to the resting state after exercise is longer. With age, sudden vigorous work or abrupt cessation of strenuous activity can strain the heart. Accordingly, warm-up periods of approximately 10 to 15 minutes and post-aerobic cool-down/stretch periods of approximately 15 minutes are recommended for most older clients.

As with other populations, the warm-up should gradually prepare the body for movements that will be required during the workout. Each of the major joints and muscle groups should be gently engaged using continuous rhythmic movements. Special attention should be focused on the postural muscles, and proper body alignment and ideal posture should be emphasized. Table 21-8 lists some practical warm-up techniques that are safe and effective for older clients.

The cool-down period following aerobic exercise should allow the heart rate to gradually decrease—generally, to fewer than 100 bpm. This can be accomplished using slow, dynamic movements. In fact, the warm-up techniques described in Table 21-8 are good for including in the post-

Table 21-8
Practical Warm-up Techniques

Provide balance support, such as the wall or the back of a sturdy chair, as necessary.

- Easy-paced walking and/or marching (on a treadmill, in place, or moving about)
- Slow, non-strenuous pedaling on a stationary cycle
- Relaxed dancing at a conservative tempo (for example, the Charleston, small kicks, and toe touches to the front, back, or sides)
- Rhythmic, limbering exercises (for example, heel raises, knee lifts, arm reaches, and shoulder lifts and circles) working through a full, pain-free range of motion

aerobic cool-down as well. If after a 15-minute cool-down period the heart rate remains elevated, the cool-down should be extended using even milder movements until the heart rate approaches 100 bpm. If the workout is devoted to resistance exercise with no aerobic component, the cool-down should still include a few minutes of gentle activity (e.g., walking or slow cycling) prior to sustained stretching to allow the body to transition to the resting state. See Table 21-9 for examples of various workout formats that incorporate safe and effective warm-up and cool-down phases.

Balance Training

A comprehensive balance-training program should include activities that increase a client's awareness of his or her COG, utilize multisensory mechanisms, and enhance the gait pattern. The ultimate goal is to tailor the exercises in the balance-training program to increase the

Table 21-9
Incorporating Warm-up and Cool-down Phases into Various Workout Formats

Aerobics-only Workout
- Warm-up: at least 10 to 15 minutes
- Aerobic work: approximately 30 minutes or longer (or multiple sessions of at least 10 minutes)
- Active post-aerobic cool-down: at least five to 10 minutes (or longer if needed for heart-rate recovery)
- Stretching/relaxation: at least five to 10 minutes, longer if time permits

Muscle Strengthening–only Workout
- Warm-up: at least 10 to 15 minutes
- Strength training: approximately 30 to 40 minutes*
- Stretching/relaxation: at least five to 10 minutes, longer if time permits

Stretch-only Workout
- Warm-up: at least 10 to 15 minutes
- Stretching/relaxation: approximately 30 to 40 minutes, longer if desired

Total-body Workout With Strength Work Preceding Aerobic Work
- Warm-up: at least 10 to 15 minutes
- Strength training: approximately 15 minutes*
- Brief stretching: approximately two to five minutes
- Repeat active rhythmic warm-up activities: approximately five minutes
- Aerobic work: approximately 15 to 20 minutes
- Active post-aerobic cool-down: at least five to 10 minutes (or longer if needed for heart-rate recovery)
- Final stretching/relaxation: at least five to 10 minutes, longer if time permits

Total-body Workout With Aerobic Work Preceding Strength Work
- Warm-up: at least 10 to 15 minutes
- Aerobic work: approximately 15 to 20 minutes
- Active post-aerobic cool-down: at least five to 10 minutes (or longer if needed for heart-rate recovery)
- Brief stretching: approximately two to five minutes
- Strength training: approximately 15 minutes*
- Final stretching/relaxation: at least five to 10 minutes, longer if time permits

* Intensive strength training should be followed by a few minutes of gentle, active cool-down activity (such as walking or stationary cycling) prior to stretching.

Note: The outlines presented above represent examples of workable exercise formats, but are not intended to cover all viable training options. To keep workout length manageable, choose numbers from each range of minutes that will combine to produce a workout lasting approximately one hour (or slightly longer). Remember that balance training techniques can and should be incorporated into all workout formats.

older adult's capacity to perform activities of daily living (e.g., reaching for, picking up, and carrying objects; performing household tasks; and reacting to obstacles in the environment). Older adults can incorporate balance-training activities into the beginning of their current exercise sessions or they may choose to perform a series of balance exercises on separate days apart from other types of training. Additionally, performing balance work in a swimming pool is an excellent choice for many older adults because it can lessen the fear of falling and takes advantage of water's natural support and balance properties—buoyancy and resistance. A frequency of two to three nonconsecutive days per week is adequate for enhancing balance through training. However, fundamental balance principles can be applied on a daily basis as individuals transfer what they learn from their balance-training exercises to the functions of daily living.

When older adults develop an increased awareness of COG, they are able to maintain a better upright position during sitting and standing, lean away from and return to midline with more postural control, and move through space more quickly and confidently. Activities that enhance COG awareness are performed seated, standing, or while moving. Different levels of balance challenge can be added by manipulating the type of support surface used for the exercise and reducing or eliminating visual feedback. These tactics require the participants to use the vestibular system as the primary system for maintaining balance because both the somatosensory and visual systems are compromised.

An introductory seated balance exercise involves having the client sit in a chair with back support while keeping the feet flat on the floor. The client should practice sitting with the back against the chair and maintaining correct posture (i.e., eyes focused forward on a target, chin gently pulled back, ears directly above the shoulders, shoulders placed slightly back and down, and abdominal muscles gently pulled up and in). Have the client hold the position for 15 seconds while breathing normally and relaxing the rest of the body. Individuals who are unable to achieve correct sitting posture while seated on a stable surface are not ready to progress to a more difficult seated balance challenge. If a client successfully completes the introductory seated posture exercise, he or she is ready to try the same exercise in an unsupported sitting position before attempting to perform the exercise while seated on an unstable surface (e.g., inflatable disc or stability ball). The individual should attempt to hold correct posture for 30 seconds with the eyes focused on a forward visual target. Next, the exercise can be repeated with the eyes closed. Finally, for added balance challenges, the client can add arm and leg movements while focusing on maintaining a correct seated posture.

Beginning standing-balance activities teach clients how to maintain correct standing posture while performing various tasks. To begin, clients should check their standing postures (i.e., eyes focused forward on a target, chin gently pulled back, ears directly above the shoulders, shoulders placed slightly back and down, abdominal muscles gently pulled up and in, hips level, kneecaps, ankles, and feet facing forward, and weight evenly distributed on both feet). Have the client hold the position for 15 seconds while breathing normally and relaxing the rest of the body. Next, the client should attempt to close his or her eyes for 15 seconds and concentrate on the feeling of standing correctly. To progress the standing-balance activities, the base of support is altered so that subtle shifts of the COG are required to maintain an upright posture. A typical altered base of support challenge starts with the individual standing with the feet together, holding the position for 15 to 30 seconds. The same exercise is repeated with the eyes closed. Next, the client moves the feet to a tandem position (front foot ahead of the rear foot with a small space between the feet) and holds for 15 to 30 seconds. The same exercise is repeated with the eyes closed. Finally, the client adopts a single-leg stance and holds the position for 15 to 30 seconds. The same exercise is repeated with the eyes closed. Other ways to manipulate the balance challenge during standing exercises are to alter the position of the arms or change the support surface beneath the feet (e.g., foam pad, rocker board, inflatable disc, or half foam roller).

Adding movement to standing balance tasks is the next progression for challenging balance. These activities enhance motor coordination and adaptive postural control by requiring the client to march in place and turn the head to one side. This will help older adults improve daily activities that might require them to turn their heads during walking (e.g., to check oncoming traffic as they cross the street). To begin, the client marches in place for 30 seconds on a firm surface with emphasis on lifting the knees toward the ceiling. Correct posture should be maintained, with the upper body and head erect and the eyes directed forward. Next, the client continues marching while turning the head one-quarter turn to the right for eight counts. The client returns the head to the forward position for eight counts before turning the head one-quarter turn to the left for eight more counts. The next progression in this series is to have the client continue to march while turning the head and body together for each eight-count quarter turn. Any of these COG awareness training activities can be progressed to a more difficult level by adding any of the following: an external timing component (e.g., music, counts), a secondary task (e.g., counting backward, reaching, throwing and catching objects), reduced vision (dark sunglasses), eyes closed, or looking at a wall with a busy visual pattern (e.g., checkerboard).

The exercises used to enhance the gait pattern build on the balance activities previously described. They are intended to help older adults achieve a gait pattern that is efficient, flexible, and adaptable to changing task and environmental demands. To begin, participants should practice walking with directional changes and abrupt starts and stops. For example, the participant makes an abrupt start or stop on command (e.g., verbal, whistle, or music). Progress the difficulty by having the participant change direction on verbal command, as well as complete quarter, half, and full turns on command. The activity can be repeated using various gait patterns (e.g., backward, side step, or marching with high knees).

The next level of balance challenge involves walking with an altered base of support to develop a more flexible gait pattern. For this activity, the client begins by walking forward with a narrow step width (2 inches; 5 cm) and then changes to walking with a wide step width (8 to 12 inches; 20 to 30 cm). Participants can then combine narrow and wide steps by completing a certain number of narrow steps followed by the same number of wide steps, or by varying the number of each type of step. To progress to the next level, participants walk forward with normal-width steps, exclusively on their heels or on the balls of their feet. Heel and toe walking can then be combined by completing a certain number of heel steps followed by the same number of toe steps, or by varying the number of each type of step.

Finally, one of the best ways to challenge the gait pattern is an obstacle course. The level of challenge can be increased by manipulating the task or environmental demands. Examples of ways to increase the task demands include the following:

- Increasing the number of obstacle types that must be negotiated along the course
- Introducing an object to be carried through the course (e.g., a laundry basket or grocery bag)
- Introducing a cognitive task while negotiating the course (e.g., counting by twos)
- Introducing an external timing demand

Environmental demands that can be manipulated to alter the challenge of an obstacle course include wearing dark glasses while walking the course, walking on different support surfaces throughout the course, and having multiple participants (two to four) negotiating the same obstacle course at the same time.

Aquatic Exercise and Balance Training

As noted previously, aquatic exercise can help clients develop confidence and minimize the fears and risks associated with falling. The water's buoyancy provides support, while the water's resistance provides a medium in which to perform exercise movements slowly so that clients can rehearse balance-recovery patterns in a safe environment. In other words, balance training in a pool, where water can support a stumble or fall, allows clients to make movement errors safely and practice corrections with more confidence. Water's buoyancy and viscosity (or thickness) slow movements, thereby lowering the risk of injury.

Water's resistive properties provide a natural overload for muscular conditioning. As movement speed in the water increases, resistance increases, and is proportional to the effort applied. For the maximum balance benefit, muscular conditioning should target the core, legs, and ankles through functional ranges of motion. Combining speed and strength to work on power, especially for the lower body, can help improve quick recovery when clients lose their balance during the course of their daily activities.

Research comparing the benefits of balance training in the water with those of land-based training indicate that aquatic balance programs provide their participants with advantages on land. Older adults who participated in five- and 16-week water-based balance-training programs showed significant improvements in functional reach and static and dynamic balance measures, respectively, when tested on land (Simmons & Hansen, 1996; Sanders, Constantino, & Rippee, 1997).

The balance-training activities previously described will do much to enhance an older adult's balance and mobility capabilities as he or she ages. However, permanent losses, such as vision impairment related to eye disease (e.g., age-related macular degeneration and glaucoma), are beyond the control of exercise interventions. With regular balance training, older individuals can expect to enhance all three balance systems (visual, somatosensory, and vestibular) so that declines in any one of the systems can be compensated for by the improved functions of the other two systems. The balance activities presented in this section are by no means a comprehensive listing of available exercises for improving one's balance abilities. The reader is encouraged to review the suggested reading list to find additional information and guidelines on balance training and fall prevention.

Muscular Strength and Power

The loss of muscle mass and declines in strength and power associated with aging have a profound effect on an older adult's ability to maintain balance, walk, and perform activities of daily living. It has been reported that 28% of men and 66% of women over the age of 74 years cannot lift objects that weigh more than 10 pounds, which equates to the weight of a typical bag of groceries (Jette & Branch, 1981). Many daily functional tasks (e.g., stair climbing, rising from a seated position, and walking) demand specific levels of lower-body muscle power, and age-related declines in power are typically much greater than the declines observed for muscle strength. Therefore, activities designed to increase both strength and power should be included in a comprehensive older adult training program.

A resistance-training program for older adults should focus on exercises that load the spine and enhance posture, such as lat pull-downs, seated rows, abdominal crunches, and prone spine extensions. In addition, exercises to protect and strengthen the hips are important (e.g., squats, lunges, and hip adductor/abductor exercises). A popular mode of resistance exercise for older adults is elastic resistance. The use of elastic resistance has been shown to be appealing to older adults due to its relative safety compared with free weights and machines, effectiveness, low cost, portability, convenience, and easy storage (Dishman, Sallis, & Orenstein, 1985). Even though training with elastic resistance is considered a safe and simple form of strength exercise, there a few precautions to consider:

- Clients should keep fingernails trimmed to avoid puncturing the elastic as well as prevent discomfort while holding the band or tube.
- They should remove jewelry prior to exercise.
- The ACE-AHFS should check bands and tubing for wear, tears, and rubbing before use, and replace as needed.
- The ACE-AHFS should check connections and secure attachments prior to each use.
- Clients must protect the eyes during exercise.
- Clients should avoid stretching the band or tubing to more than 300% elongation to prevent breakage.
- Persons with latex allergies should use latex-free forms of elastic resistance.

Although current American College of Sports Medicine guidelines (ACSM, 2006) recommend that individuals over the age of 50 lift relatively light weights for 10 to 15 repetitions (Table 21-10), the ACE-AHFS should keep in mind that more resistance and fewer repetitions are required for optimal strength preservation and bone maintenance and building [i.e., 75 to 80% of **one-repetition maximum (1 RM)** for six to eight repetitions]. Therefore, starting a resistance-training program at a lower intensity is appropriate, but the ultimate goal is to get the older adult training with greater levels of resistance to promote strength gains and preserve bone mass. Keep in mind that the aging process slows the rate of healing, so more rest is usually needed between workouts as individuals get older. Thus, older adults may need two or three full days of rest between strength workouts instead of one.

For power, an older individual's exercise program should include a combination of various directional lunges to enhance reaction time and to train the lower body to respond to balance challenges in different planes of movement. Of course, multidirectional lunges require advanced skills and should be attempted only when the individual is physically and mentally prepared to take on the task.

As with any resistance-training program, the principle of gradual progression must be followed to ensure the participant's safety and the effectiveness of the workout. Older adults should choose a weight or resistance that allows them to perform between eight and 15 repetitions before fatiguing (Figure 21-4). Once they can consistently complete 15 repetitions of an exercise, they should be encouraged to increase the amount of weight or level of resistance by 2 to 5%. Many strength-training activities can be performed seated or standing. Unstable or weak clients should begin performing strength-training exercises in a seated position to minimize the stability requirements and reduce their risk of falling during the movement. Once a client is able to consistently demonstrate correct form during an exercise and exercise performance improves, he or she is ready to add a balance component. This can be achieved by first having the individual perform the strength activity while seated on a compliant, or relatively unstable, surface. The next balance progression of standing on a compliant or moving surface can be added once the client consistently demonstrates correct form and improved performance in the seated position.

Cardiorespiratory Endurance

Aerobic exercise guidelines for older adults are consistent with the current ACSM guidelines (ACSM, 2006) for the average healthy adult (see Table 21-10). It has been observed that older adults elicit the same 10 to 30%

Table 21-10
ACSM Exercise Programming Principles

	Frequency (days/week)	Intensity	Time	Type
Cardiorespiratory	3–5	(55/65)–90% HRmax, (40/50)–85% HRR, (40/50)–85% $\dot{V}O_2R$, or 12–16 RPE throughout the day	20–60 continuous minutes or three 10-minute bouts accumulated	Large muscle groups; dynamic activity
Resistance	2–3	Volitional fatigue (e.g., 19–20 RPE) or stop 2–3 reps before volitional fatigue (e.g., 16 RPE)	1 set of 3–20 reps (e.g., 3–5, 8–10, 12–15); 1 set of 10–15 reps if >50 years	8–10 exercises that include all major muscle groups
Flexibility	Minimal: 2–3 Ideal: 5–7	Stretch to tightness up to the ROM but not to pain; mild discomfort	15–30 secomds; 2–4 reps per stretch	Static stretch for all major muscle groups

Note: HRmax = Maximal heart rate; HRR = Heart-rate reserve; $\dot{V}O_2R$ = $\dot{V}O_2$ reserve; RPE = Ratings of perceived exertion; ROM = Range of motion

Source: American College of Sports Medicine (2006). *ACSM's Guidelines for Exercise Testing and Prescription* (7th ed.). Philadelphia: Lippincott Williams & Wilkins.

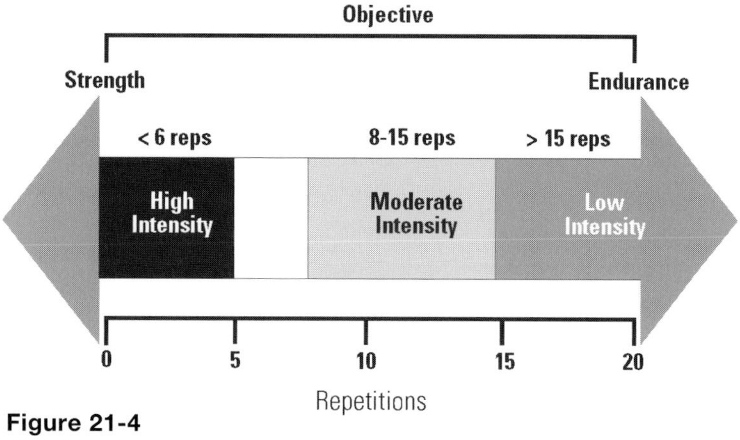

Figure 21-4
Effective repetition range for weight training in older adults

Source: Bryant, C.X., Franklin, B.A., & Newton-Merrill, S. (2007). *ACE's Guide to Exercise Testing and Program Design* (2nd ed.). Monterey, Calif.: Healthy Learning. Modified from American College of Sports Medicine (2006). *ACSM's Guidelines for Exercise Testing and Prescription* (7th ed.). Philadelphia: Lippincott Williams & Wilkins.

increases in $\dot{V}O_2max$ with prolonged endurance exercise training as young adults. Similar to young adults, the magnitude of the increase in aerobic capacity in older adults is also a function of training intensity, with light-intensity training eliciting minimal or no changes (ACSM, 1998). Aerobic exercise for older individuals should focus on a variety of low-impact weightbearing modalities to combat bone and muscle loss. For inactive individuals, 30 minutes of moderate aerobic activity, such as walking, most days of the week is sufficient for enhancing health and well-being. Gradually increasing aerobic exercise intensity and duration is an appropriate goal for those who want increased body-fat reduction and improved cardiovascular fitness.

Flexibility

With advancing age, maintaining flexibility becomes increasingly important. Loss of range of motion impairs most functions needed for good mobility. Maintaining lower-body flexibility is vital for preventing low-back pain, musculoskeletal injury, and gait abnormalities, and in reducing the risk of falling. Limited range of motion in the shoulder girdle has been associated with pain and postural instability. Both upper- and lower-body flexibility decrease with age, but can be improved through stretching. A flexibility program for an older adult should include a consistent routine of stretches for the important postural muscles of the chest, trunk, hips, and thighs. Current ASCM guidelines (ACSM, 2006) recommend stretching a minimum of two to three days per week up to seven days per week (see Table 21-10). A daily flexibility program performed after an appropriate warm-up or at the conclusion of a training session consisting of static stretches for the whole body can go a long way toward enhancing an older person's flexibility.

Physically Elite Older Adults

The very small percentage of individuals who manage to maintain remarkable physical abilities well into their 80s and 90s represent the physically elite of older adults. This group is made up of athletes who continue to train and push themselves into their 60s, 70s, and 80s, as well as individuals who keep working in occupations that require strength and endurance (e.g., firefighters, police officers, military personnel, and forest rangers) who maintain their abilities through physical training.

Most notably, record performances from events such as the World Masters Track-and-Field Championships, the World Veteran Games, the United States Amateur Union Masters Swimming Championships, and the United States Weightlifting Federation's competition provide examples of maximum human potential throughout the lifespan. Records from running events show that even at the age of 80, some men can run a 10K race in a little over 40 minutes and some 80-year-old women can run it in a little over an hour. World records from strength events, such as weightlifting and power lifting, show that a 70-year-old man can dead lift 501.5 pounds (225 kg) and a woman in her late seventies can dead lift 220.5 pounds (99 kg) (Spirduso, Francis, & MacRae, 2005).

Clearly, physically elite older adults have been able to successfully master physical aging. Apart from a unique genetic makeup that enables them to take advantage of their talent and physical stamina, physically elite older adults have inherited resistance to injury and disabling disease such as Parkinson's disease, **multiple sclerosis,** or **muscular dystrophy.** Additionally, they have been lucky and have not been involved in fatal or debilitating accidents. Furthermore, aside from good genetics and lucky circumstances, physically elite older adults have capitalized on their performance potential by maintaining healthy behaviors such as physical training and eating a good diet, and by abstaining from poor health habits such as smoking and drug and alcohol abuse.

Biomechanical Considerations for the Older Adult

The prevalence of musculoskeletal pain and joint alterations in the aging is remarkably high. About half of persons age 65 and older are affected by **osteoarthritis** (American Geriatrics Society, 2001), approximately half of adults age 80 and older experience sarcopenia (Baumgartner et al., 1998), and 55% of Americans age 50 and older have osteopenia or osteoporosis (NOF, 2008). Decreased range of motion and loss of spinal flexibility in many older adults results in a "stooped" posture that is associated with a vertical displacement of the COG backward toward the heels. This change in postural alignment can lead to lowered self-confidence, faulty balance, and an increased risk for falls (Horak, Shupert, & Mirka, 1989). These and other musculoskeletal conditions impart varying levels of discomfort and disability to older adults. The ACE-AHFS should be knowledgeable in making appropriate exercise and equipment modifications to make physical activity more comfortable for the older client.

Chair-seated Exercise

Whenever possible, training older clients in weightbearing, functional positions is preferred to chair-seated work. However, if a client has issues related to endurance, mobility, and **self-efficacy,** a chair-seated exercise routine may be appropriate. For example, when working with the frailest older-adult populations, seated exercise may be the only practical method.

Ideally, a chair used for seated exercise should not have arm rests. This will increase the potential range of movement and allow a broader variety of possible exercises. However, many individuals who are well-suited for chair exercise use wheelchairs, so it is important for the ACE-AHFS to develop the ability to work effectively using armchairs. During chair exercise, the client's back should be supported by the back of the chair or by a pillow, pad, or rolled towel if necessary. Additionally, the client's feet should be in full contact with the floor, which can be accomplished by using a book, stool, or other type of platform. Another option for clients who have good functional strength during standing, but who have low self-confidence and a fear of falling, is to include standing work using the back of the chair for balance support.

Aquatic Exercise

Exercise in the water provides a great alternative for both aerobic and resistance activities for many older adults. Because water's buoyancy negates the impact of exercise, many older adults who cannot safely jog, jump, or kick on land can successfully perform those activities in the pool. Accessories made for in-pool use, such as water bells, paddles, webbed gloves, and ankle cuffs, can be incorporated to increase intensity and challenge strength or to provide more buoyancy to help an individual float during certain activities. A water temperature of 83 to 88° F (30 to 31° C) works well for most older adults, especially those who suffer from arthritis.

The performance of ADL has been shown to improve in older adults who participate in a regular aquatic-based functional training program. Sufferers of chronic back pain who undergo therapeutic water exercise programs experience reduced pain and improved ADL performance (Landgridge & Phillips, 1988; Smit & Harrison, 1991). Furthermore, joint motion and ADL performance for individuals with arthritis and rheumatic diseases have improved after water therapy sessions (Suomi & Lindaur, 1997; Templeton, Booth, & Kelley, 1996). In addition to improved functional abilities, water exercise for older adults has also resulted in increased muscle strength and flexibility, decreased body fat, and improved self-esteem (Sanders, Constantino, & Rippee, 1997).

For older clients diagnosed with osteoporosis, land-based training is preferable to aquatic exercise for stimulating increases in bone mineral density. However, joint pain and disability may prohibit many osteoporotic clients from performing functional activities on land. In these individuals, water-based exercise will help maintain or enhance joint range of motion. Furthermore, with the use of the pool-based equipment, older adults can improve muscle strength, thereby improving functional abilities and reducing the risk of falls on land.

Strategies for Teaching Exercise to Older Adults

Strong communication and leadership skills are important traits for the ACE-AHFS to develop for working with the older adult population. The communication process in general is complex and can be further complicated by age. One of the biggest challenges the ACE-AHFS may face when dealing with older clients is that they are actually more heterogeneous than younger people. Because older clients typically have a wide range of life experiences and cultural backgrounds, communication between younger fitness professionals and older clients can be complicated (Halter, 1999). Communication can also be hindered by the normal aging process, which may involve sensory loss, decline in memory, slower processing of information, lessening of power and influence over their own lives, retirement from work, and separation from family and friends (Ostuni & Mohl, 1994).

Older people are often stereotyped or patronized by others, which makes attentive listening and understanding even more important. It has been reported that language beliefs and attitudes toward older people tend to be negatively biased (Hummert, Nussbaum, & Wiemann, 1992), which can be problematic for communication between generations. In an attempt to make themselves better understood, some younger people use tactics such as speaking more slowly and loudly, using very simple grammar, and articulating very carefully when speaking to older adults. Unfortunately, this can lead an older person to feel that he or she is being "talked down to." As when communicating with clients of any age, the ACE-AHFS should use the major keys to effective communication—attending, listening, and empathetic responding—when speaking with older clients. Table 21-11 lists important communication tips when working with older adults, and presents their application.

Exemplifying leadership in relationships with older clients is a powerful tool for enhancing communication. As a leader, the ACE-AHFS has the primary responsibility for defining how clients can best approach their health and fitness goals. Strong leadership skills, such as using feedback for educational and motivational purposes while making clients feel emotionally safe, appreciating gender and cultural differences, and using creativity in making exercise fun, will encourage clients to adhere to their exercise routines.

Psychological comfort is another important aspect of training older adults. Many older adults may have exaggerated beliefs about the risks associated with physical activity that prevent them from exercising or limit their exercise options. Most older clients will refuse to participate in physical activities they deem dangerous. To help alleviate their fears, the ACE-AHFS can help older adults safely exercise at or near their physical abilities by minimizing the physical and psychological risks of exercise. The exercise programming variables discussed previously in this chapter appropriately address minimizing the physical risks associated with exercise for older clients. Table 21-12 presents some common psychological risks of exercise for older adults, along with strategies to help overcome these risks.

Nutritional Considerations

The aging process brings about changes in the nervous and digestive systems that alter an older adult's ability to take in and absorb nutrients from food. Sensory changes include a decline in vision, hearing, smell, and taste. These losses affect nutritional intake and health status. Slowing of the normal action of the smooth muscle lining the digestive tract, as well as diminished digestive secretions, results in decreased nutrition in older people. Dietary needs start to change due to the aging process at about age 70. Older clients may

Table 21-11
Communication Tips for Working With Older Adults

Listen without interruption to your clients' questions and statements before responding.

Instructors often think they must have all of the answers—and FAST—to look competent. But fitness instructors sometimes miss part of what a client is saying because they are busy thinking about how they will answer. To avoid this problem, hear all of what your client has to say before commenting. If needed, remind yourself to take your time and think about what is being said. If you are at a loss for a response, tell your client that you need to think about the question for a moment, then formulate your answer. If you are "stumped," assure the client that you will consider the question and get back to him or her. If you do this, be sure to follow up with an answer as soon as you have researched one.

Tune out distractions.

Distractions can occur in the environment (things we see or hear around us), within ourselves (our state of mind or physical condition), or from the speaker (mannerisms or a communication style that make it difficult to pay attention). Because your clients should be the focus of your attention, eliminate or minimize distractions that make it hard for you to listen. Move to a quiet location if surrounding noise or activity is disruptive. If your mind keeps wandering to a personal issue, silently repeat to yourself everything the speaker says. If the speaker's style makes it hard to listen, respectfully work with the speaker to solve the problem (e.g., ask a soft speaker to speak more loudly).

Avoid overuse of filler words.

Sometimes, instructors feel uncomfortable with brief silences and attempt to fill pauses with words. While it often is helpful to acknowledge that you are listening with an occasional "uh-hum," overuse of filler words can become annoying and should be avoided. If you find yourself using too many filler words, take a deep breath and remind yourself that some pauses and brief silences are natural and productive. Smiling and nodding in a supportive manner can show your interest without being disruptive.

Avoid patronizing language.

Too often, older adults are spoken to as if they are children, with little regard for their dignity. For example, if a small-framed elderly female fits the "little old lady" stereotype, some adults may unthinkingly address this woman as "dear" or "honey." While the speaker may consider these terms of affection, others may find this approach condescending and offensive. Address older adults as you would any other adults—with respect—in the manner they request. It is not uncommon for older persons to prefer being addressed in a more formal manner (e.g., Mr. Smith, rather than Bill.) If in doubt about addressing an older client by first or last name, ask their preference.

Avoid using slang.

Remember that slang often is age-, gender-, and/or culturally specific. For instance, it might be appropriate for a 25-year-old woman to use the phrase "you guys" to address her close friends, both male and female. Older women, however, might find such a phrase to be disrespectful. It is best to use mainstream English (or whatever primary language your instruction is in). If you are working with an individual or with group members who are from a similar age group and background as yourself, the use of some slang may be acceptable. Be careful, however, not to patronize clients by attempting to use slang terms you would not otherwise use.

Make eye contact.

This demonstrates your interest in each client. A steady gaze can be threatening, but among most American cultures frequently making brief eye contact with clients shows concern and interest. If you are leading a group or class, be sure to make eye contact with each participant.

Speak at an appropriate volume and pace.

Nervous and/or enthusiastic leaders tend to speak quite rapidly, often not allowing time for listeners to ask about what was said. If you are a rapid speaker, be conscious of slowing your pace. Additionally, the volume of speech must be loud enough for clients to hear, especially if there is background noise. (Remember that hearing aids amplify all noise—not just your voice—so any background music must be low.) Ask your clients about volume and pace until you become familiar with their needs. Inquire whether the volume of your voice is okay. Likewise, you can ask clients, "Am I talking too fast?" and adjust accordingly. For hearing-impaired clients, it often is beneficial to slow down the rate of your speech, use some gestures or demonstrations to emphasize points, and look at clients so they can pick up visual cues about what you are saying.

Continued on next page

Table 21-11
Communication Tips for Working With Older Adults (continued)

Teach new material at an appropriate pace.

It has been noted that although the ability to learn new information remains relatively stable over time, the speed of learning may slow with aging (Spotts & Schewe,1989). There may be tremendous variation from one client to another, but a good rule of thumb is to allow older adults (and, ideally, all of your clients) to learn at their own pace. Allow clients to tell you when they are comfortable with what you have taught them and when they are ready to move on. Periodically ask individuals to demonstrate new moves or explain what you have just said. Inquire whether additional practice is desired. If the majority of a class is ready to move on, reassure those who want more practice that you will review the information again, making sure to let them know when. In groups, give clients the option of using a familiar move until they become comfortable with the new one. Provide frequent opportunities for older clients to meet with you or peers to work on new steps or exercises.

Visual communication aids should be easy to read.

Older adults' vision will vary widely. To meet the needs of those with vision difficulties, it is best to make writing on chalk boards, signs, flyers, and instruction sheets easy to read. Keep visual material uncluttered and brief. Color combinations that give maximum contrast should be used, while varying shades of the same colors (like grays) should be avoided. Pictures or diagrams can enhance some messages, but they should be simple and clear.

Remember that the best way to determine if you are meeting clients' needs is simply to ask. Most clients will appreciate your concern and will attempt to tell you how to help them. An old adage about teaching applies well to fitness instructors working with older adults: It is less important to know all the answers than to ask the right questions.

Table 21-12
Common Psychological Risks of Exercise for Older Adults

Risk of Embarrassment or Ridicule. This risk may be especially serious for older adults who never have been physically active or who are attempting to engage in exercise after an extended break. All clients may be susceptible to the risk of embarrassment, but remember that older adults are attempting to engage in an exercise plan despite societal messages that exercise is most appropriate for younger adults, and that older adults may be too frail for exercise or too old to develop new skills. (Hence the term, "You can't teach an old dog new tricks.") It is no wonder that some older adults fear criticism.

To Help Your Older Clients: Acknowledge your client's wisdom and courage in committing to their health or physical fitness by exercising. Reassure them that the vast majority of individuals in exercise programs are preoccupied with their own performance, leaving little time to worry about what others are doing. Predictions of failure from family members or others, if they occur, can be used as a motivator to succeed and to prove skeptics wrong.

Risk of Facing Diminished Physical Abilities. This problem can be especially difficult for former athletes or former regular exercisers who have not been active in a long time. Some older adults may compare their current performance to what they could do when they were younger or prior to a medical problem. Finding out that they can do less than expected can be a demotivating blow to self-esteem. Older clients who note declines in their abilities may be reluctant to continue exercise activities that painfully remind them of these changes.

To Help Your Older Clients: Encourage them to measure progress from their present starting point. You would never expect a person of any age who has not exercised for a while to be able to automatically perform as they did when they were exercising regularly. Additionally, remind clients that individuals of any age have plenty of room for substantial gains in physical abilities. With time and consistent participation in their exercise routine, they may be pleasantly surprised at how much they can improve.

Risk of Confronting Ageist Stereotypes of Physical Beauty. Given society's obsession with youth, older women may feel acutely self-conscious while exercising, particularly if the setting is a facility where slim, well-toned young women work out. Males, too, can suffer from damaged self-esteem when comparing their own physiques to those of well-conditioned young men who exercise at the same facility.

To Help Your Older Clients: Remind your clients that the only people they need to please are themselves. Suggest they concentrate on the benefits from participating in an exercise program regardless of how they fit into the visual profile of others attending a facility. Point out, too, that by actively taking steps to improve their health, appearance, and self-esteem by exercising, they are improving their own physical attractiveness.

These are just a few of a wide variety of psychological risks your clients may associate with physical activity programs. By supportively encouraging them to come to terms with these and other risks, you will free your clients of restrictive barriers to exercise and fears that may impact many aspects of their lives.

need to address these unique nutritional concerns with their primary healthcare provider.

Sensory Losses

Loss of visual acuteness may lead to a fear of cooking, especially using a stove. Inability to read food prices, nutrition labels, or recipes may affect grocery shopping, food preparation, and eating. Loss of hearing may lead to less eating out or not asking questions of the waiter or store clerk. Changes in smell and taste may make food less appetizing. If older clients have been instructed by their physicians to cut back on salt, sugar, or fat, they may tend not to eat. Combined, these factors could have an adverse effect on nutritional status.

Structural Changes

Structural changes, such as reduced lean mass, esophageal problems, and loss of teeth, affect nutritional status in older people. The most significant result of the loss of lean mass may be the decrease in basal energy metabolism. Metabolic rate declines proportionately with the decline in total protein tissue. To avoid gaining weight, older adults must reduce calorie intake or increase physical activity to promote energy balance. Loss of lean body mass also means a direct reduction in total body water. This makes proper hydration in a physically active older person a priority. The motor activity of the esophagus may be poorly coordinated in older people, and sudden movements may cause a reflux of gastric contents (Minaker & Rowe, 1982; Young & Urban, 1986). Lost teeth or improperly fitting dentures may unconsciously change eating patterns because of difficulty chewing. As a result, an older person may choose a soft, low-fiber diet without fresh fruits and vegetables. Suggestions for dealing with tooth discomfort are to have poorly fitting dentures adjusted, and to chop, steam, stew, grind, or grate hard or tough foods to make them easier to chew without sacrificing their nutritional value. Adequate dietary fiber, as opposed to increased use of laxatives, will maintain regular bowel function and not interfere with the digestion and absorption of nutrients, as occurs with laxative use or abuse.

Vitamins and Minerals

Research on nutrition and aging suggests that older adults are more vulnerable to deficiencies of calcium, the B vitamins, and vitamins C and D (Tiidus, Shephard, & Montelpare, 1989). With age, the amount of ascorbic acid produced in the stomach, which helps absorb vitamin B12, decreases. To avoid deficiency, older adults are advised to regularly eat foods rich in vitamin B12, including meat, poultry, fish, eggs, and dairy foods. Vitamin C deficiencies are linked to an inability to buy expensively priced fresh fruits and vegetables among the older population (Shephard, 1997). Deficiencies in vitamin D are attributed to the limited exposure of older people to sunlight. A lack of vitamin D, in turn, diminishes the absorption of calcium and increases the risk of developing osteoporosis. Calcium intake of many older people falls below the level recommended for protection from osteoporosis (Tiidus, Shephard, & Montelpare, 1989). Furthermore, the prolonged administration of antacids may increase calcium loss in the stool (Albanese, 1980).

Iron and zinc deficiencies may be a problem for some older people. A reduced gastric secretion of hydrochloric acid and **enzymes** may restrict the absorption of iron, which could result in **anemia.** Antacid use also interferes with iron absorption. Furthermore, medications that cause blood loss, such as anticoagulants, aspirin, and arthritis drugs, can enhance a tendency toward anemia. Iron absorption may be improved by eating iron-rich foods with vitamin C–rich fruits and vegetables. For example, clients can have juice or sliced fruit with cereal, a baked potato with roast beef, vegetables with fish, or fruit with chicken. Zinc deficiencies are common in older people. As many as 95% of older adults may not get the zinc they need (Swanson, 1988), and zinc absorption also may be less efficient in this population. Zinc deficiency, in turn, may lead to a depressed appetite and a diminished sense of taste, which may lead to lower food intakes and worsened zinc status. Regular consumption of meats, eggs, and seafood should provide adequate zinc intake.

Vitamin and mineral intakes may be affected by the use of medications. For example, drugs used to control hypertension or heart disease can alter the need for **electrolytes,** sodium, and potassium. However, even though absorption and utilization of some vitamins and minerals becomes less effective with age, higher intakes are not always necessary. As for any age group, it is important for older adults to enjoy a wide variety of foods. Furthermore, eating nutrient-dense foods becomes increasingly important when calorie needs decline but vitamin and mineral needs remain high.

Water

Dehydration is a major risk factor for older adults who may not notice or pay attention to their thirst. The thirst mechanism declines with age, causing older people to go for longer periods without drinking fluids (Rolls & Phillips, 1990). Adequate water intake reduces stress on kidney function, which also tends to decline with age. Adequate fluid intake also eases constipation. Older clients should be advised to drink plenty of water, juice, milk, and coffee or tea to stay hydrated. To get the recommended six to eight glasses of fluids every day, it may be helpful to use a cup or water bottle that has calibrated measurements on it to keep track of how much is consumed throughout the day.

Macronutrients

In general, guidelines for **carbohydrate, protein,** and **fat** consumption are the same for healthy older adults as they are for younger people. The ACE-AHFS may refer to the USDA's 2005 Dietary Guidelines for Americans when considering a healthful nutrition plan for older clients. However, since certain nutritional requirements begin to change around the seventh decade of life, questions regarding specific nutrients and nutrition-related health concerns should be referred to the client's primary healthcare physician or a registered dietitian.

In late 2007, the Friedman School of Nutrition Science and Policy at Tufts University presented an updated version of the Modified MyPyramid for Older Adults (Lichtenstein et al., 2008) (Figure 21-5). This modified version of the original MyPyramid Food Guidance System emphasizes the unique characteristics of a nutrition plan for individuals age 70 and older. Features that distinguish the Modified MyPyramid from the original include the following:

- A narrower base to reflect the lower energy needs of older adults
- Replacement of selected food icons with nutrient-dense examples to help reconcile decreased food intake with unchanged or increased recommended dietary allowances
- Addition of a fiber icon in appropriate food categories to facilitate achieving adequate intakes to promote optimal bowel function
- Inclusion of a row of glasses at the base of the pyramid to remind older adults to maintain adequate fluid intakes
- Placement of a flag at the top to alert some older adults that their healthcare provider should consider recommending vitamins B12 or D or calcium supplements

However, congruent with the USDA's 2005 Dietary Guidelines for Americans, there is continued emphasis that most, if not all, nutrients that an older adult consumes should come from food rather than supplements.

Case Study

Tim K. is an active, 76-year-old retired business executive who enjoys swimming and walking. He has been diagnosed with osteoarthritis in his knees and hips as well as hypertension. Mr. K. currently takes glucosamine and ibuprofen for arthritis and a diuretic for hypertension. His goals are to increase functional strength and improve balance. He has been cleared by his physician to incorporate resistance training into his already established program of 30 minutes of swimming and/or walking four days per week.

Frequency: Mr. K. may continue to exercise at least four days per week as dictated by his tolerance to arthritis-related discomfort. He may be encouraged to increase his physical activity to a daily routine, especially with aquatic exercise, as it may be helpful in controlling blood pressure, improving balance, and alleviating joint discomfort. However, if an increased volume of physical activity exacerbates his arthritic knees and hips, he should be instructed to reduce the volume of activity. Mr. K. should incorporate two days of resistance training into his current program. If an increased frequency of exercise is intolerable, he may need to substitute a day or two of cardiorespiratory exercise for strength-training exercise. A consideration for Mr. K.

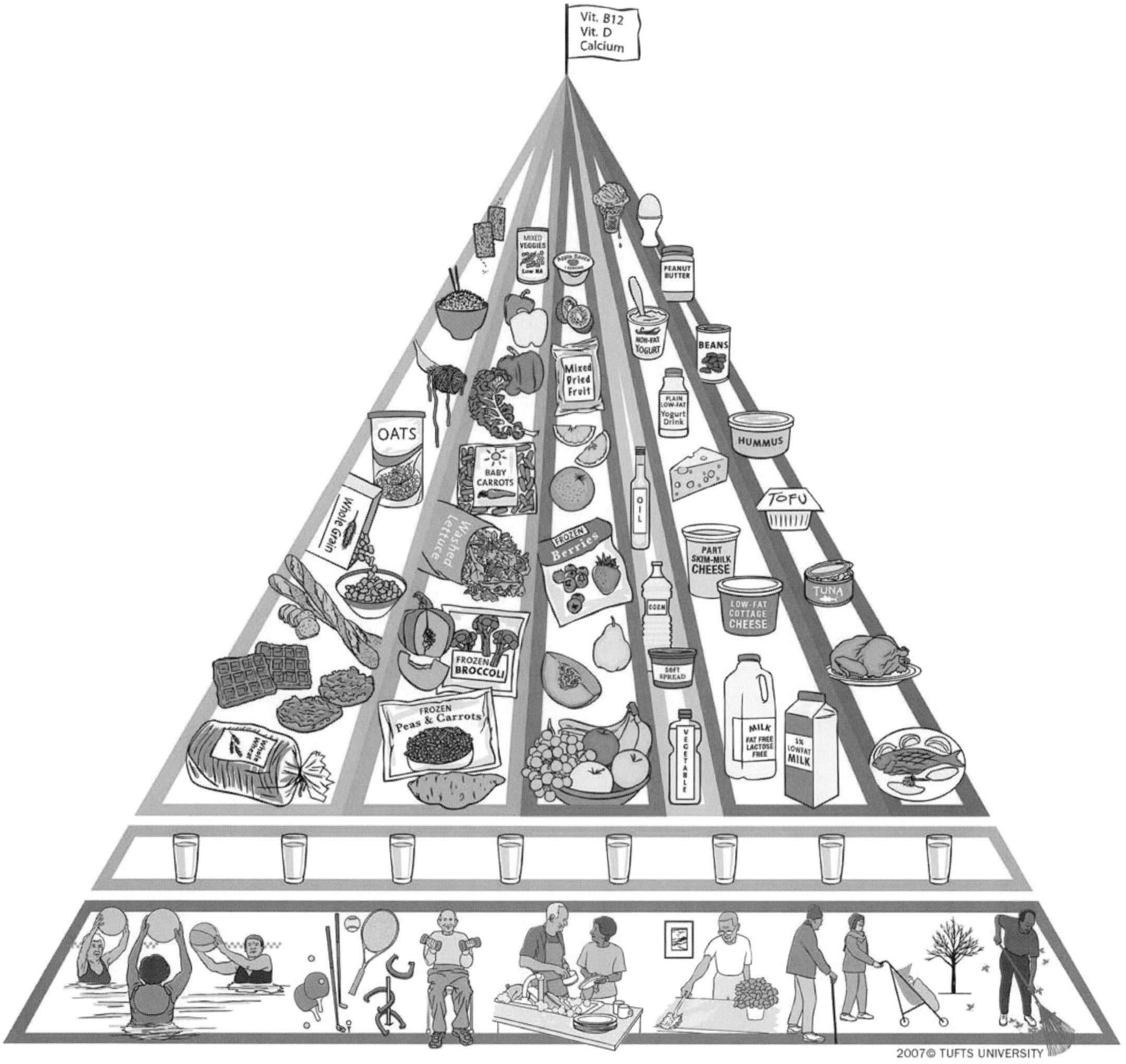

Figure 21-5
Modified MyPyramid for older adults

Source: Lichtenstein, A.H. et al. (2008). Modified MyPyramid for Older Adults. *Journal of Nutrition,* 138, 78–82.

may be to utilize his time in the pool by combining cardiorespiratory exercise and resistance training using specialized water equipment.

Intensity: Mr. K. should use RPE as a method to monitor cardiorespiratory exercise intensity and should be encouraged to maintain an average rating of 13, or "somewhat hard," on Borg's 6 to 20 scale. A warm-up period of approximately 10 to 15 minutes and a post-aerobic cool-down/stretch period of approximately 15 minutes should precede and follow the cardiorespiratory conditioning portion of his workout, respectively. For resistance training, Mr. K. should choose a weight that allows him to perform between eight and 15 repetitions before fatiguing.

Time: Mr. K. should be encouraged to continue his current program of 30-minute activity sessions, with the addition of an extra 15 minutes devoted to range-of-motion exercises for postural muscles and his arthritic joints.

Type: Mr. K. should incorporate aquatic exercise sessions that target balance, strength, and cardiorespiratory fitness. He should also be encouraged to walk as much as he can tolerate to keep a land-based, weightbearing activity in his program. His resistance-training program, whether in the water or on land, should include effective functional movements such as squats, lunges, and presses, as well as core stabilization work. Since Mr. K. is taking a diuretic for hypertension, standing, land-based exercise should be performed near a stable object (e.g., chair, wall, or railing) in the event he becomes dizzy, drowsy, or disoriented as a side effect of the medication.

Summary

The life expectancy of Americans has increased dramatically over the past century. Advancing age is characterized by a progressive decline in the functional capacity of most physiological systems. Accordingly, people are living longer with chronic conditions such as cardiovascular disease, cancer, diabetes, arthritis, and cognitive impairment. Regardless of age and health limitations, older adults can expect to experience significant physiological and psychological benefits from regular physical activity. As a health and fitness professional, the ACE-AHFS has a distinct opportunity to support older adults in their journey to a healthier lifestyle through physical activity. Understanding the unique characteristics of the older adult population will help the ACE-AHFS apply the necessary communication and leadership techniques to provide the best possible lifestyle-modification experience for older clients.

References

Albanese, A.A. (1980). *Nutrition for the Elderly*. New York: Liss.

American College of Sports Medicine (2006). *ACSM's Guidelines for Exercise Testing and Prescription* (7th ed.). Philadelphia: Lippincott Williams & Wilkins.

American College of Sports Medicine (1998). Position stand: Exercise and physical activity for older adults. *Medicine & Science in Sports & Exercise,* 30, 6, 992–1008.

American Council on Exercise (2005). *ACE's Exercise for Older Adults* (2nd ed.). San Diego, Calif.: American Council on Exercise.

American Geriatrics Society (2001). Exercise prescription for older adults with osteoarthritis pain: Consensus practice recommendations. *Journal of the American Geriatrics Society*, 49, 808–823.

American Geriatrics Society (1989). Assessments in geriatrics: Of caveats and names. *Journal of the American Geriatrics Society*, 37, 6, 570–572.

Aoyagi, Y. & Shephard, R.J. (1992). Aging and muscle function. *Sports Medicine*, 14, 376–396.

Arias, E. (2006). United States life tables, 2003. *National Vital Statistics Reports*, 54, 14.

Asmussen, E. & Heebol-Neilsen, K. (1961). Isometric muscle strength of adult men and women. *Danish National Association of Infantile Paralysis*, 11, 1–43.

Atienza, A.A. (2001). Home-based physical activity programs for middle-aged and older adults: Summary of empirical research. *Journal of Aging and Physical Activity*, 9 (Suppl.), 38–58.

Backman, L. & Molander, B. (1991). On the generalizability of the age-related decline in coping with high-arousal conditions in a precision sport: Replication and extension. *Journal of Gerontology: Psychological Sciences*, 46, 79–81.

Bassey, E.J., Bendall, M.J., & Pearson, M. (1988). Muscle strength in the triceps surae and objectively measured customary walking activity in men and women over 65 years of age. *Clinical Science*, 74, 85–89.

Bassey, E.J. et al. (1992). Leg extensor power and functional performance in very old men and women. *Clinical Science*, 82, 321–327.

Baumgartner, R.N. et al. (1998). Epidemiology of sarcopenia among the older persons in New Mexico. *American Journal of Epidemiology*, 147, 755–763.

Berg, K.O. et al. (1992). Measuring balance in the elderly: Validation of an instrument. *Canadian Journal of Public Health*, 2, S7–S11.

Bolton, C.F., Winkelman, M.D., & Dyck, P.J. (1966). A quantitative study of Meissner's corpuscles in man. *Neurology*, 16, 1–9.

Brocklehurst, J.C., Roberston, D., & James-Groom, P. (1982). Clinical correlates of sway in old age: Sensory modalities. *Age and Aging*, 11, 1–10.

Bruce, R.A. et al. (1973). Variations in responses to maximal exercise in health and cardiovascular disease. *Angiology,* 24, 691–702.

Bryant, C.X., Franklin, B.A., & Newton-Merrill, S. (2007). *ACE's Guide to Exercise Testing and Program Design* (2nd ed.). Monterey, Calif.: Healthy Learning.

Campanelli, L.C. (1996). Mobility changes in older adults: Implications for practitioners. *Journal of Aging and Physical Activity*, 4, 2, 105–118.

Campbell, A., Borrie, M.J., & Spears, G.F. (1989). Risk factors for falls in a community-based prospective study of people 70 years and older. *Journal of Gerontology: Medical Sciences*, 52, 218–224.

Centers for Disease Control and Prevention (2007). *The State of Aging and Health in America 2007*. Centers for Disease Control and Prevention and the Merck Company Foundation. www.cdc.gov/aging.

Centers for Disease Control and Prevention (2003). Public health and aging: Trends in aging—United States and worldwide. *Morbidity and Mortality Weekly Report*, 52, 6, 101–106.

Centers for Disease Control and Prevention (2002). *Physical Activity and Older Americans: Benefits and Strategies*. Agency for Healthcare Research and Quality and the Centers for Disease Control. www.ahrq.gov/ppip/activity.htm.

Centers for Disease Control and Prevention (1996). *The Third National Health and Nutrition Examination Survey (NHANES III 1988-94) Reference Manuals and Reports*. Bethesda, Md.: National Center for Health Statistics.

Chen, H. Et al. (1991). Stepping over obstacles: Gait patterns of healthy young and old adults. *Journal of Gerontology: Medical Sciences*, 46, 196–203.

Chodzko-Zajko, W.J. & Moore, K.A. (1994). Physical fitness and cognitive functioning in aging. *Exercise and Sport Science Reviews*, 22, 195–220.

Clarke, D.H., Hunt, M.Q., & Dotson, C.O. (1992). Muscular strength and endurance as a function of age and activity level. *Research Quarterly*, 63, 302–310.

Crapo, R.O. (1993). The aging lung. In: Mahler, D.A. (Ed.) *Pulmonary Disease in the Elderly* (pp. 1–25). New York: Marcel Dekker.

Cress, M.E. et al. (1996). Continuous-scale physical functional performance in a broad range of older adults: A validation study. *Archives of Physical Medicine & Rehabilitation,* 77, 12, 1243–1250.

Cunha, U.V. (1988). Differential diagnosis of gait disorders in the elderly. *Geriatrics,* 43, 34.

Danneskoild-Samsoe, B. et al. (1984). Muscle strength and functional capacity in 77–81 year old men and women. *European Journal of Applied Physiology*, 52, 123–135.

D'Errico, A. et al. (1989). Changes in the alveolar connective tissue of the aging lung. *Virchow's Archives. A. Pathological Anatomy and Histopathology*, 415, 137–144.

Dishman, R.K., Sallis, J.F., & Orenstein, D.R. (1985). The determinants of physical activity and exercise. *Public Health Reports*, 100, 2, 158–171.

Eakin, E. (2001). Promoting physical activity among middle-aged and older adults in health care settings. *Journal of Aging and Physical Activity*, 9 (Suppl.), 29–37.

Einkauf, D.K. et al. (1987). Changes in spinal mobility with increasing age in women. *Physical Therapy*, 67, 370–375.

Elble, R.J. et al. (1991). Stride dependent changes in gait of older people. *Journal of Neurology*, 238, 1–5.

Engel, W.K. (1970). Selective and nonselective susceptibility of muscle fiber types: A new approach to human neuromuscular diseases. *Archives of Neurology*, 22, 97–117.

Fagard, R., Thijs, L., & Amery, A. (1993). Age and the hemodynamic response to posture and to exercise. *American Journal of Geriatric Cardiology*, 2, 2, 23–30.

Feldman, M.L. (1976). Aging changes in the morphology of cortical dendrites. In: Terry, R.D. & Gershon, S. (Eds.) *Neurobiology of Aging*, 211–227. New York: Raven Press.

Fiatarone, M.A. et al. (1990). High-intensity strength training in nonagenarians: Effects on skeletal muscle. *Journal of the American Medical Association*, 263, 3029–3034.

Fleg, J.L. (1986). Alterations in cardiovascular structure and function with advancing age. *American Journal of Cardiology*, 57, 33–44.

Fleg, J.L. et al. (1994). Effects of acute beta-adrenergic receptor blockade on age-associated changes in cardiovascular performance during dynamic exercise. *Circulation*, 90, 2333–2341.

Gentile, A.M., Behesti, Z., & Held, J.M. (1987). Environment vs. exercise effects on motor impairments following cortisol lesions in rats. *Behavior and Neural Biology*, 47, 321–332.

Gerety, M.B. et al. (1993). Development and validation of a physical performance instrument for the functionally impaired elderly: The Physical Disability Index (PDI). *Journal of Gerontology: Medical Sciences*, 48, M33–M38.

Granger, C.V. et al. (1986). Advances in functional assessment for medical rehabilitation. *Topics in Geriatric Rehabilitation* 1, 3, 59–74.

Grimby, G. & Saltin, B. (1983). The aging muscle. *Clinical Physiology*, 3, 209–218.

Halter, J.B. (1999). The challenge of communicating health information to elderly patients: A view from geriatric medicine. In: Park, D.C., Morrell, R.W., & Shifren, K. (Eds.) *Processing of Medical Information in Aging Patients: Cognitive and Human Factors Perspectives*. Mahwah, N.J.: Lawrence Erlbaum Associates.

Harries, U.J. & Bassey, E.J. (1990). Torque-velocity relationships for the knee extensors in women in their 3rd and 7th decades. *European Journal of Applied Physiology*, 60, 187–190.

Held, J., Gordon, J., & Gentile, A.M. (1985). Environmental influences on locomotor recovery following cortical lesions in rats. *Journal of Behavioral Neuroscience*, 99, 678–690.

Horak, F., Shupert, C., & Mirka, A. (1989). Components of postural dyscontrol in the elderly: A review. *Neurobiology of Aging*, 10, 727–745.

Hughes, S.L. et al. (1991). The GERI-AIMS. Reliability and validity of the arthritis impact measurement scales adapted for elderly respondents. *Arthritis and Rheumatism,* 34, 856–865.

Hummert, M.L., Nussbaum, J.F., & Wiemann, J.M. (1992). Communication and the elderly: Cognition, language, and relationships. (Special Issue: Communication and aging: Cognition, language, and relationships). *Communication Research*, 19, 4, 413–422.

Jette, A.M. & Branch, L.G. (1981). The Framingham disability study II—Physical disability among the aging. *American Journal of Public Health*, 71, 1211–1216.

Jette, A.M., Branch, L.G., & Berlin, J. (1990). Musculoskeletal impairments and physical disablement among the aged. *Journal of Gerontology: Medical Sciences*, 45, M203–M208.

Katz, S.C. et al. (1963). Studies of illness in the aged. The index of ADL: A standardized measure of biological and psychosocial function. *Journal of the American Medical Association,* 185, 914–919.

Kempen, G.I.J.M. & Suurmeijer, T.P.B.M. (1990). The development of a hierarchical polychotomous ADL-IADL scale for noninstitutionalized elders. *The Gerontologist,* 30, 497–502.

Kimura, M., Hirakawa, K., & Morimoto, T. (1990). Physical performance survey in 900 aged individuals. In: Kaneko, M. (Ed.) *Fitness for the Aged, Disabled, and Industrial Worker* (pp. 55–60). Champaign, Ill.: Human Kinetics.

Kuo, G.H. (1990). Physical fitness of people in Taipei including the aged. In: Kaneko, M. (Ed.) *Fitness for the Aged, Disabled, and Industrial Worker* (pp. 21–24). Champaign, Ill.: Human Kinetics.

LaForest, S. et al. (1990). Effects of age and regular exercise on muscle strength and endurance. *European Journal of Applied Physiology*, 60, 104–111.

Lakatta, E.G. (1990). Changes in cardiovascular function with aging. *European Heart Journal*, 11, 22–29.

Landgridge, J. & Phillips, D. (1988). Group hydrotherapy exercises for chronic back pain sufferers. *Physiotherapy*, 74, 269–273.

Larish, D.D., Martin, P.E., & Mungiole, M. (1988). Characteristic patterns of gait in the healthy old. In: Joseph, J. (Ed.) *Central Determinants of Age-related Declines in Motor Function: Annals of the New York Academy of Sciences,* 515, 18–31.

Larsson, L. (1978). Morphological and functional characteristics of the aging skeletal muscle in man. *Acta Physiologica Scandinavica,* Suppl. 457, 1–36.

Larsson, L., Grimby, G., & Karlsson, J. (1979). Muscle strength and speed of movement in relation to age and muscle morphology. *Journal of Applied Physiology*, 46, 451–456.

Lawton, M.P. & Brody, E.M. (1969). Assessment of older people: Self-maintaining and instrumental activities of daily living. *The Gerontologist*, 9, 179–186

Lemsky, C. et al. (1991). Reliability and validity of a physical performance and mobility examination for hospitalized elderly. *Society of Gerontology (Abstracts),* 31, 221.

Lerner, D.J., & Kannel, W.B. (1986). Patterns of coronary heart disease morbidity and mortality in the sexes: A 26-year follow-up of the Framingham population. *American Heart Journal*, 111, 383–390.

Lichtenstein, A.H. et al. (2008). Modified MyPyramid for older adults. *Journal of Nutrition*, 138, 78–82.

Linnan, L.A. & Marcus, B. (2001). Worksite-based physical activity programs and older adults: Current status and priorities for the future. *Journal of Aging and Physical Activity*, 9 (Suppl.), 59–70.

MacMahon, S.W. et al. (1986). The effects of drug treatment for hypertension on morbidity and mortality from cardiovascular disease: A review of randomized controlled trials. *Progress in Cardiovascular Diseases*, 29, 99–118.

McArdle, W.D., Katch, F.I., & Katch, V.L. (2007). *Exercise Physiology* (6th ed.). Philadelphia: Lea & Febiger.

McGreer, P.L. & McGreer, E.G. (1980). Chemistry of mood and emotion. *Annual Reviews of Psychology*, 31, 273–307.

Minaker, K.L. & Rowe, J.W. (1982). The gastrointestinal system. In: Rowe, J.W. & Besdine, R.W. (Eds.) *Health and Disease of Old Age* (pp. 297–315). Boston: Little, Brown.

Moller, B.M. (1981). Hearing in 70- and 75-year-old people: Results from a cross-sectional and longitudinal population study. *American Journal of Otology*, 2, 22–29.

Murphy, S. et al. (1994). Milk consumption and bone mineral density in middle-aged and elderly women. *British Medical Journal*, 308, 939–941.

Murray, M.P. et al. (1985). Age-related differences in knee muscle strength in normal women. *Journal of Gerontology*, 40, 275–280.

Murray, M.P. et al. (1980). Strength of isometric and isokinetic contractions. *Physical Therapy*, 60, 412–419.

National Institutes of Health (2006). National Institute on Aging, *Aging Under the Microscope: A Biological Quest*. NIH Publication No. 02-2756. Bethesda, Md. www.nia.nih.gov.

National Institutes of Health (2005). National Institute on Aging, *Aging Hearts and Arteries: A Scientific Quest*. NIH Publication No. 05-3738. Bethesda, Md. www.nia.nih.gov.

National Osteoporosis Foundation (2008). www.nof.org.

Osness, W.H. (1987). Assessment of physical function among older adults. In: Leslie, D. (Ed.) *Mature Stuff.* Reston, Va.: American Association for Health, Physical Education, Recreation, and Dance.

Ostrow, A.C. (1989). *Aging and Motor Behavior*. Indianapolis: Benchmark Press.

Ostuni, E. & Mohl, G.R. (1994). Communication with elderly patients. *Dental Economics*, 84, 3, 27–32.

Overstall, P.W. et al. (1977). Falls in the elderly related to postural imbalance. *British Medical Journal*, 1, 260–264.

Poitrenaud, J. et al. (1994). Sources of individual differences in cognitive aging: A longitudinal study of an elderly French managerial population. *Facts and Research in Gerontology*, 35–50.

Pollack, M.L. et al. (1987). Effect of age and training on aerobic capacity and body composition of master athletes. *Journal of Applied Physiology*, 62, 725–731.

Rejeski, W.J., Brawley, L.R., & Shumaker, S.A. (1996). Relationships between physical activity and health-related quality of life. *Exercise and Sport Sciences Reviews*, 24, 71–108.

Resnick, B. (2007). The EASY screening tool. *International Council on Active Aging, Functional U.* May–June, 9–13. www.icaa.cc.

Resnick, B. et al. (2008). A proposal for a new screening paradigm and tool called Exercise Assessment and Screening for You (EASY). *Journal of Aging and Physical Activity*, 16, 2.

Reuben, D.B. & Siu, A.L. (1990). An objective measure of physical function of elderly outpatients: The physical performance test. *Journal of the American Geriatrics Society*, 38, 1105–1112.

Reuben, D.B. et al. (1990). A hierarchical exercise scale to measure function at the advanced activities of daily living (AADL) level. *Journal of the American Geriatrics Society*, 38, 855–861.

Riggs, B.L. & Melton, L.J. (1992). The prevention and treatment of osteoporosis. *New England Journal of Medicine,* 327, 620–627.

Rikli, R.E. & Jones, C.J. (2001). *Senior Fitness Test Manual*. Champaign, Ill.: Human Kinetics.

Rolls, B.J. & Phillips, P.A. (1990). Aging and disturbances of thirst and fluid balance. *Nutrition Reviews*, 48, 137–144.

Rose, D.J. (2003). *Fall Proof! A Comprehensive Balance and Mobility Training Program*. Champaign, Ill.: Human Kinetics.

Safar, M. (1990). Aging and its effects on the cardiovascular system. *Drugs*, 39, 1–18.

Sanders, M., Constantino, N., & Rippee, N. (1997). A comparison of results of functional water training on field and laboratory measures in older women. *Medicine & Science in Sports & Exercise*, 29, ixx.

Schaie, K.W. (1989). Perceptual speed in adulthood: Cross-sectional and longitudinal studies. *Psychology and Aging*, 4, 443–453.

Schnelle, J.F. et al. (1995). Functional incidental training, mobility performance, and incontinence care with nursing home residents. *Journal of American Geriatrics Society*, 43, 1356–1362.

Sekular, R., Hutman, L., & Owsley, C. (1980). Human aging and spatial vision. *Science*, 209, 1255–1256.

Shephard, R.J. (1997). *Aging, Physical Activity, and Health*. Champaign, Ill.: Human Kinetics.

Shephard, R.J. (1991). Fitness and aging. In: Blais, C. (Ed.) *Aging Into the Twenty-first Century* (pp. 22–35). Downsview, Ont.: Captus University.

Shephard, R.J. (1987). *Physical Activity and Aging* (2nd ed.). London: Croom Helm.

Simmons, V. & Hansen, P. (1996) Effectiveness of water exercise on postural mobility in the well elderly: An experimental study on balance enhancement. *Journal of Gerontology*, 51A, M233–M238.

Slemenda, C.W. et al. (1991). The role of physical activity in the development of skeletal mass in children. *Journal of Bone Mineral Research*, 6, 1227–1233.

Smit, T. & Harrison, R. (1991). Hydrotherapy and chronic lower back pain: A pilot study. *Australian Journal of Physiotherapy*, 37, 229–234.

Spirduso, W.W., Francis, K.L., & MacRae, P.G. (2005). *Physical Dimensions of Aging* (2nd ed.). Champaign, Ill.: Human Kinetics.

Spotts, A.E., Jr., & Schewe, C.D. (1989). Communicating with the elderly consumer: The growing health care challenge. *Journal of Health Care Marketing,* 9, 3, 36–44.

Stewart, A.L. (2001). Community-based physical activity programs for adults age 50 and older. *Journal of Aging and Physical Activity*, 9 (Suppl.), 71–91.

Suomi, R. & Lindaur, S. (1997). Effectiveness of arthritis foundation program on strength and range of motion in women with arthritis. *Journal of Aging and Physical Activity*, 5, 341–351.

Suominen, H. & Rahkila, P. (1991). Bone mineral density of the calcaneus in 70-to 81-year-old male athletes and a population sample. *Medicine & Science in Sports & Exercise*, 23, 1227–1233.

Swanson, C.A. (1988). Zinc status of elderly adults: Response to supplement. *American Journal of Clinical Nutrition,* 48, 343–349.

Tahara, J. et al. (1990). Longitudinal study on motor fitness tests for the aged. In Kaneko, M. (Ed.) *Fitness for the Aged, Disabled, and Industrial Worker* (pp. 15–17). Champaign, Ill.: Human Kinetics.

Talbot, L.A. et al. (2002) Comparison of cardiorespiratory fitness versus leisure time physical activity as predictors of coronary events in men aged ≤65 years and >65 years. *American Journal of Cardiology*, 89, 1187–1192.

Templeton, M.S., Booth, D.L., & Kelley, W.D.O. (1996). Effects of aquatic therapy on joint flexibility and functional ability in subjects with rheumatic disease. *Journal of Orthopaedic and Sports Physical Therapy*, 23, 376–381.

Tiidus, P., Shephard, R.J., & Montelpare, W. (1989). Overall intake of energy and key nutrients: Data for middle-aged and older middle-class adults. *Canadian Journal of Sport Sciences*, 14, 173–177.

Tinetti, M.E. (1986). Performance-oriented assessment of mobility problems in elderly patients. *Journal of the American Geriatrics Society,* 34, 119–126.

Tinetti, M.E., Williams, T.F., Mayewski, R. (1986). Fall risk index for elderly patients based on number of chronic disabilities. *American Journal of Medicine,* 80, 429-434.

Tockman, M.S. (1994). Aging of the respiratory system. In: Hazzard, W.R. et al. (Eds.) *Principles of Geriatric Medicine and Gerontology* (3rd ed.) (pp. 555–564). New York: McGraw-Hill.

Toole, T. & Abourezk, T. (1989). Aerobic function, information processing and aging. In: Ostrow, A.C. (Ed.) *Aging and Motor Behavior* (pp. 37–65). Indianapolis: Benchmark Press.

United States Department of Health and Human Services (1996). *Physical Activity and Health: A Report of the Surgeon General*. Atlanta, Ga.: U.S. Department of Health and Human Services, Centers for Disease Control and Prevention, National Center for Chronic Disease Prevention and Health Promotion.

Vandervoort, A.A. & Hayes, K.C. (1989). Plantarflexor muscle function in young and elderly women. *European Journal of Applied Physiology*, 58, 389–394.

Vandervoort, A.A. et al. (1992). Age and sex effects on mobility of the human ankle. *Journal of Gerontology: Medical Sciences*, 47, 17–21.

Walker, J.E. & Howland, J. (1991). Falls and fear of falling among elderly persons living in the community: Occupational therapy interventions. *American Journal of Occupational Therapy*, 45, 119–122.

Ware, J.E. & Sherbourne, C.D. (1992). The MOS 36-Item Short-Form Health Survey (SF-36®): I. Conceptual framework and item selection. *Medical Care,* 30, 6, 473–483.

Welford, A.T. (1985). Practice effects in relation to age: A review and a theory. *Developmental Neuropsychology*, 1, 173–190.

Whipple, R.H., Wolfson, L.I., & Amerman, P.M. (1987). The relationship of knee and ankle weakness to falls in nursing home residents: An isokinetic study. *Journal of the American Geriatrics Society*, 35, 13–20.

Williams, H. (1983). *Perceptual and Motor Development*. Englewoods Cliffs, N.J.: Prentice-Hall.

Williams, H.G. & Greene, L.S. (1990). *Williams-Greene Test of Physical/Motor Function.* Columbia, S.C.: Laboratory report from the Motor Development/Motor Control Laboratory, Department of Exercise Science, University of South Carolina, Columbia.

Woollacott, M.H., Inglin, B., & Manchester, D. (1988). Response preparation and posture control in the older adult. In: Joseph, J. (Ed.) *Central Determinants of Age-related Declines in Motor Function* (pp. 42–51). New York: New York Academy of Sciences.

Wright, G.R. & Shephard, R.J. (1978). Brake reaction time: Effects of age, sex and carbon monoxide. *Archives of Environmental Health*, 33, 141–150.

Young, E.A. & Urban, E. (1986). Aging, the aged and the gastrointestinal tract. In: Young, E.A. (Ed.) *Nutrition, Aging, and Health* (pp. 91–131). New York: Liss.

Suggested Reading

AARP, ACSM, American Geriatrics Society, CDC, National Institute on Aging, and the Robert Wood Johnson Foundation (2004). *National Blueprint: Increasing Physical Activity Among Adults Age 50 and Older*.

American College of Sports Medicine (1998). Position stand: Exercise and physical activity for older adults. *Medicine & Science in Sports & Exercise,* 30, 6, 992–1008.

American Council on Exercise (2005). *ACE's Exercise for Older Adults* (2nd ed.). San Diego, Calif.: American Council on Exercise.

Centers for Disease Control and Prevention (2007). *The State of Aging and Health in America 2007*. Centers for Disease Control and Prevention and the Merck Company Foundation. www.cdc.gov/aging.

National Institutes of Health (2006). National Institute on Aging, *Aging Under the Microscope: A Biological Quest*. NIH Publication No. 02-2756. Bethesda, Md. www.nia.nih.gov.

National Institutes of Health (2005). National Institute on Aging, *Aging Hearts and Arteries: A Scientific Quest*. NIH Publication No. 05-3738. Bethesda, Md. www.nia.nih.gov.

Page, P. & Ellenbecker, T. (2004). *Strength Band Training.* Champaign, Ill.: Human Kinetics.

Page, P. & Ellenbecker, T. (2003). *The Scientific and Clinical Applications of Elastic Resistance.* Champaign, Ill.: Human Kinetics.

Sanders, M.E. (Ed.) (2000). *YMCA Water Fitness for Health.* Champaign, Ill.: Human Kinetics.

Shephard, R.J. (1997). *Aging, Physical Activity, and Health*. Champaign, Ill.: Human Kinetics.

Spirduso, W.W., Francis, K.L., & MacRae, P.G. (2005). *Physical Dimensions of Aging* (2nd ed.). Champaign, Ill.: Human Kinetics.

In This Chapter

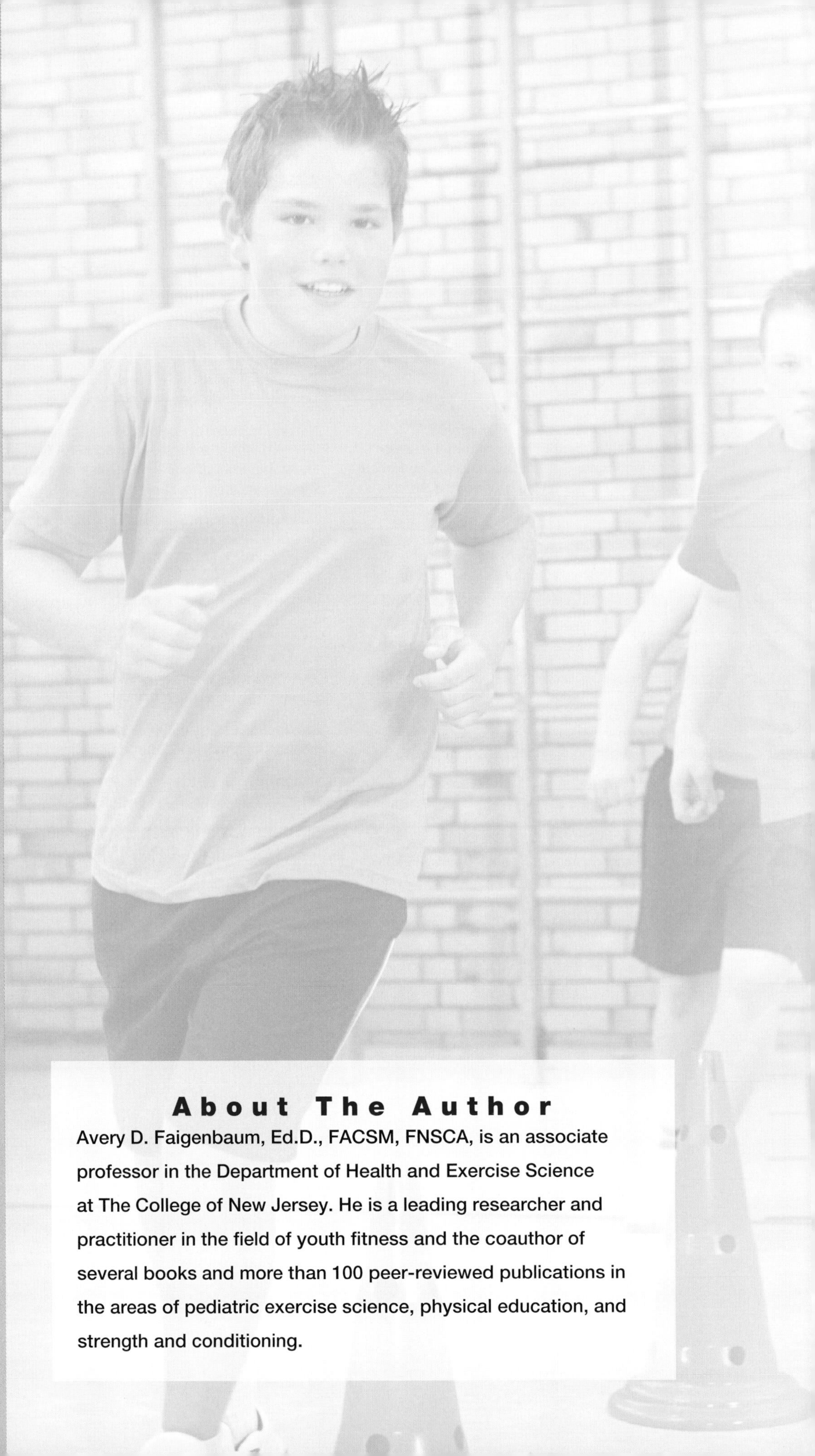

About The Author

Avery D. Faigenbaum, Ed.D., FACSM, FNSCA, is an associate professor in the Department of Health and Exercise Science at The College of New Jersey. He is a leading researcher and practitioner in the field of youth fitness and the coauthor of several books and more than 100 peer-reviewed publications in the areas of pediatric exercise science, physical education, and strength and conditioning.

CHAPTER 22

Youth

Avery D. Faigenbaum

Traditionally, children and adolescents walked or bicycled to school, participated regularly in school-based activity programs, and performed physical chores at home that kept their bodies healthy, fit, and strong. But today, fewer children walk or ride their bicycles to school and physical education and recess, sadly, are viewed as expendable in some school districts. Moreover, computers and video games have decreased youngsters' desire to move and there are fewer safe places for youngsters to play. As a result, physical inactivity among children and adolescents has become a major public health concern. Some observers suggest that unless effective interventions are developed, the youth of today may, on average, live shorter lives than their parents (Olshansky et al., 2005).

The United States spends billions of dollars each year on lifestyle-related diseases, and the likelihood of a significant increase in spending is both real and alarming (Wang & Dietz, 2002). The prevalence of childhood **obesity** in the United States has tripled in recent decades and **type 2 diabetes**—which was once called "adult onset" diabetes—is now also being diagnosed in adolescents (Narayan et al., 2003; Ogden et al., 2008). If current trends continue, the health-related consequences of physical inactivity and childhood obesity will likely pose an unprecedented burden on youth, their families, and the American healthcare system. The bottom line is that a **sedentary** lifestyle during childhood and adolescence increases a person's risk of developing major health problems such as heart disease, **diabetes,** cancer, and **osteoporosis** later in life (U.S. Department of Health and Human Services, 1996).

Due to the disturbing health trends among children and adolescents, a growing number of health clubs and YMCAs are expanding their services by providing young members with creative, enjoyable, and kid-friendly programs. Over the past five years, the number of health club members between the ages of six and 17 increased by 58%, which is the biggest growth of any age segment (International Health, Racquet and Sportsclub Association, 2006). In addition, the YMCA of the USA reported that half of their 20.2 million members are under the age of 18 years (YMCA of the USA, 2007). Since most physical activity among youth occurs outside of the school setting, there will be more opportunities for ACE-certified Advanced Health & Fitness Specialists (ACE-AHFS) to design and implement safe, effective, and enjoyable fitness programs for children and adolescents with different needs, goals, and abilities.

Since adult exercise guidelines and training philosophies are inappropriate for younger populations, this chapter explores the uniqueness of childhood and adolescence and addresses age-appropriate exercise guidelines and teaching strategies. In this chapter, "children" refers to boys and girls who have not yet developed secondary sex characteristics (roughly up to the age of 11 in girls and 13 in boys) and "adolescent" (or teenager) refers to a period of time between childhood and adulthood and includes girls aged 12 to 18 years and boys aged 14 to 18 years. For ease of discussion, "youth" is broadly defined to include both children and adolescents.

Current Health and Fitness Status

Although youth tend to be more active than adults, a significant number of children and adolescents do not participate in the recommended amount of physical activity. National survey data of children ages nine to 13 years revealed that 61% do not participate in any organized physical activity during non-school hours, and 23% do not participate in any free time physical activity [Centers for Disease Control and Prevention (CDC), 2003]. Only 33% of high school students attend physical education class daily, and a considerable number of young people do not engage in the recommend amount of physical activity on most days of the week (CDC, 2005). Of note, data from the National Health and Nutrition Examination Survey identified low fitness in 33.6% of American adolescents (Carnethon, Gulati, & Greenland, 2005). More recent findings suggest that this decline in physical activity may start during the preschool years in obese children (Gillis, Kennedy, & Bar-Or, 2006).

Instead of active, unstructured, outdoor play, children are spending more time with electronic media (e.g., video games and computers) and 38% of students watch television for three or more hours on a typical day (CDC, 2005). Less than 15% of youth ages five to 15 years walk to or from school and only 1% ride their bikes (Bureau of Transportations Statistics, 2003). Even recess has been reduced or eliminated in some elementary schools (Waite-Stupinsky & Findlay, 2001). Moreover, snack foods and beverages high in fat and sugar are now available in many elementary schools, most middle schools, and almost all secondary schools [Institute of Medicine (IOM), 2005)]. At the same time, children and adolescents are not meeting the minimum recommended serving of five fruits and vegetables daily [American Dietetic Association (ADA), 2004)].

It is becoming more apparent that the lack of regular physical activity, along with the greater accessibility to energy-dense foods, is contributing to the increasing prevalence of obesity among children and adolescents. Over the past three decades, the prevalence of childhood obesity has more than doubled for adolescents and it has more than tripled for children (Ogden et al., 2008). Data from a national survey using **body mass index (BMI)** as a main outcome measure indicate that 31.9% of American youth ages two to 19 were at or above the 85th percentile of the sex-specific BMI for age and 16.3% were at or above the 95th percentile (Ogden et al., 2008). In addition, statistics show that 24.4% of American children aged two to five years had excess body fat (Ogden et al., 2008). Some observers estimate that 20% of **overweight** four year olds, and as many as 80% of overweight adolescents, will become obese adults (Dietz, 2004).

These trends have significant ramifications for the present and future health of children and adolescents due to the increased prevalence of **cardiovascular disease** risk factors and obesity-related comorbidities, such as type 2 diabetes, heart disease, and cancer (Freedman et al., 1999; Narayan et al., 2003). The increasing incidence of type 2 diabetes in youth is particularly troubling because conditions related to diabetes (e.g., kidney failure, amputation, and blindness) will occur earlier in life. Type 2 diabetes now accounts for up to 45% of all new cases of diabetes in children and adolescents who, for the most part, remain obese throughout life (Botero & Wolfsdorf, 2005). For American children born in the year 2000, the lifetime risk of being diagnosed with diabetes is estimated to be 30% for boys and 40% for girls (Narayan et al., 2003).

The ACE-AHFS should also be aware that obesity during childhood and adolescence may be associated with psychosocial abnormalities, including **depression** and low self-esteem (Goodman & Whitaker, 2002). Obese youth tend to have fewer friends, miss more school days, and are often ostracized and teased about their weight (Gortmaker et al., 1993; Taras & Potts-Datema, 2005). In one study, researchers observed that obese children and adolescents had a lower health-related quality of life than youth who were healthy and a similar quality of life as those diagnosed with having cancer (Schwimmer, Burwinkle, & Varni, 2003).

Benefits of Youth Fitness

Since both positive and negative behaviors established at a young age have a high probability of persisting into adulthood (Epstein, Paluch, & Gordy, 1999; Janz, Dawson, & Mahoney, 2000), preventive health efforts that increase physical activity during childhood and adolescence will likely have favorable health benefits in later years. In the long run, health-promotion strategies that ensure healthy levels of physical activity among children and teenagers could help maintain the progress that has been made in reducing deaths from cardiovascular disease over the past few decades. A summary of potential health benefits of youth fitness training is presented in Table 22-1.

Table 22-1
Potential Health and Fitness Benefits of Youth Strength Training

- Enhanced muscular fitness
- Increased bone mineral density
- Improved body composition
- Improved motor fitness performance
- Enhanced sports performance
- Increased resistance to injury
- Enhanced psychological well-being
- Improved attitude toward lifelong physical activity
- Enhanced academic performance

Never before have fitness professionals been equipped with so much information to justify physical-activity programs for children and teenagers because of the numerous physical and psychosocial benefits that have been documented through research (Hills, King, & Armstrong, 2007; Strong et al., 2005; United States Department of Health and Human Services, 1996). Regular participation in moderate-to-vigorous physical activity helps reduce body fat, improve blood **lipids,** build skeletal tissue, strengthen muscles, and improve aerobic fitness (Strong et al., 2005). Moreover, regular participation in physical-activity programs can enhance motor performance skills and reduce the risk of injuries in youth sports (Faigenbaum, 2007). Although the total elimination of sports-related injuries is an unrealistic goal, Micheli (2006) suggested that both acute and overuse injuries in young athletes could be reduced by 15 to 50% if young athletes were better prepared for the demands of sports practice and competition.

Regular participation in physical activity also promotes feelings of well-being, enhances self-esteem, and simply makes boys and girls feel better about themselves (National Association of Sport and Physical Education, 2005). Well-organized youth activity programs characterized by caring and competent instruction give children and adolescents the opportunity to make new friends and experience the mere enjoyment of physical activity. Numerous studies have also shown positive relationships between academic achievement and physical activity (Sibley & Ethnier, 2003). Others have reported that in-school physical activity can improve on-task behavior during academic instruction (Mahar et al., 2006). Although the mechanisms by which students may do better in school as a result of physical activity are worthy of further study, it appears that increased activity levels may improve concentration, increase alertness, and reduce boredom (Coe et al., 2006).

Perhaps of greater importance is the observation that health-related behaviors that are acquired during childhood and adolescence are likely to be carried into adulthood (Janz, Dawson, & Mahoney, 2000; Telama, Yang, & Viikari, 2005). In fact, it appears that physical-activity habits that are established during childhood and sustained across the lifespan may provide the greatest impact on mortality and longevity (Paffenbarger et al., 1986). A youngster who enjoys physical activity and learns how to live a physically active life is more likely to become an active, healthy adult. Thus, the goal of youth fitness programs is not only to engage boys and girls in a variety of enjoyable physical activities, but also for youth to become aware of the intrinsic values and benefits of regular physical activity so they become adults who engage in desirable patterns of habitual physical activity.

Growth and Development

The ACE-AHFS should realize that youth have different needs than adults and are active in different ways. Watching boys and girls on a playground supports the premise that the natural physical-activity pattern of boys and girls is characterized by sporadic bursts of energy with brief periods of rest as needed. No matter how big, strong, or coordinated a child is, the ACE-AHFS must appreciate the fact that boys and girls are still growing and are often experiencing many activities for the very first time. Clearly, adult exercise guidelines and training philosophies should not be imposed on children and adolescents who are physically and psychologically less mature.

Because children and adolescents are still developing and maturing, their physiology is dynamic and the measures of health and fitness are in a constant state of evolution. Thus, training-induced adaptations in youth need to be considered within the context of change. There are also considerable inter-individual differences in physical development between youth of the same age. For example, a 12-year-old girl can be taller and more physically skilled than a 12-year-old boy and two adolescents of the same age can have considerable differences in height and weight (Servedio, 1997). These differences are related to the timing of puberty, which typically occurs between the ages of eight and 13 in girls and nine and 15 in boys.

Stages of maturation, or pubertal development, can be measured in terms of skeletal age, somatic (physique) maturity, or sexual maturation. In girls, the onset of menstruation (menarche) is a marker of sexual maturation, whereas in boys the best indicators of sexual maturity are facial hair, pubic hair, and deepening of the voice. The term biological age refers to a child's stage of maturation, whereas the term chronological age refers to one's age in years. Hence, two girls in an after-school fitness program can have the same chronological age, but differ by several years in their biological age. Sensitivity to inter-individual differences in abilities and physical appearance is especially important when working with children and adolescents.

The ACE-AHFS also needs to be aware of physiological differences between youth and adults. Children and adolescents have a higher breathing frequency and a lower **tidal volume** than adults at all exercise intensities (Rowland, 2005). Thus, it is normal for a healthy child to breathe rapidly during a fitness workout. In regards to the cardiovascular responses to aerobic exercise, children and adolescents exhibit lower **stroke volumes** and higher heart rates at all exercise intensities (Rowland, 2005). Maximal heart rates do not change appreciably during childhood and early adolescence, and it is not uncommon for a child's heart rate to exceed 200 bpm during a bout of vigorous physical activity. Consequently, the estimation of maximal heart rate by age-based equations (e.g., 220 – age) is inappropriate for youth between seven and 15 years of age. Researchers have also reported that heart rate recovery is generally faster in children and adolescents than in adults (Rowland, 2005).

Perhaps the most visible difference between children and adults is that children tend to be "metabolic nonspecialists" in regards to fitness performance (Bar-Or, 1983). Unlike adults who tend to specialize in such sports as weightlifting and long-distance running, the strongest child in a class is likely to be a leader in an endurance run as well. These observations are supported by laboratory data that suggest that children with a high **maximal oxygen uptake** tend to perform well during anaerobic tests (Rowland, 2005). The ACE-AHFS should appreciate the lack of metabolic specialization in children, and therefore expose youth to a variety of sports and activities during this developmental period.

Children and adolescents also have different fitness goals than adults. Enhancing one's level of aerobic fitness and improving one's blood lipid profile may be important motivating factors for adults, but most children just want to have fun, build friendships, and improve physical skills. In fact, since young children are "concrete thinkers," they need to enjoy the experience of being physically active and see little value in long-duration and/or high-intensity exercise. Thirty minutes of continuous exercise on a stepping machine may be an enjoyable experience for adults, but most children (especially if they are sedentary and overweight) do not enjoy this type of activity and often drop out due to lack of interest and boredom. The ACE-AHFS should not forget about the importance of play, which is one of the ways children learn.

Fitness Assessment

When properly administered, fitness assessments can be used to evaluate strengths and weaknesses, develop personalized programs, track progress, and motivate students. Standardized testing procedures for assessing physical fitness have been developed and normative data are available (Safrit, 1995). However, when evaluating youth, it is important to avoid the "pass-fail" mentality, as this approach may actually discourage unfit or overweight boys and girls from participating in fitness classes or other physical-activity programs. To create an environment in which boys and girls enjoy the fitness assessment and feel good about participating, the ACE-AHFS should not refer to the assessment as a test, but instead call it a "challenge." As such, fitness assessments should provide youth with an opportunity to demonstrate what they can do now that they could not do before.

While different fitness assessments are available, one good example of a comprehensive assessment for children and adolescents is the Fitnessgram (Meredith & Welk, 2004). Since the most worthwhile youth programs inspire children and teenagers to develop lifelong healthy habits, the Fitnessgram aims to help all school-age youth achieve and maintain an attainable level of fitness and good health. The Fitnessgram includes a variety of health-related measures designed to assess cardiovascular fitness, **muscle strength** and **endurance, flexibility**, and **body composition** (Table 22-2).

Table 22-2
Fitnessgram* Fitness and Health Assessments

Fitness Component	Assessment Tool
Aerobic capacity	PACER 20-meter shuttle run One-mile run Walk test
Upper-body strength and endurance	90-degree push-up†
Core strength and endurance	Curl-up Trunk lift
Flexibility	Back-saver sit-and-reach Shoulder stretch
Body composition measurements	Triceps and calf skinfold Body mass index

*For more information on each of these assessments, and for established standards for other health-related fitness components, refer to the *Fitnessgram/Activitygram Test Administration Manual* (Meredith & Welk, 2004).
†Alternatives to the 90-degree push-up include the pull-up, modified pull-up, and flexed arm hang.

Performance on each Fitnessgram measure is classified into one of two categories—the "Healthy Fitness Zone" or "Needs Improvement." For example, to attain the lower end of the "Healthy Fitness Zone" category for the push-up assessment, 12-year-old boys and girls need to perform 10 push-ups and seven push-ups, respectively. Established standards for other health-related fitness components are available in the *Fitnessgram/Activitygram Test Administration Manual* (Meredith & Welk, 2004).

The ACE-AHFS can use a variety of fitness measures to assess physical fitness in youth. In the Fitnessgram, aerobic capacity is assessed with the PACER (Progressive Aerobic Cardiovascular Endurance Run), the one-mile run, or the walk test. The PACER is a 20-meter shuttle run that is easy at the beginning and gets harder toward the end. Upper-body strength and endurance are typically assessed with the 90-degree push-up, although a pull-up, modified pull-up, or flexed arm hang are alternatives. The curl-up and trunk lift are used to assess the trunk muscles, which are important for good posture and maintenance of low-back health. The objective of the curl-up test is to perform as many curl-ups as possible at a specified pace, up to a maximum of 75. The objective of the trunk lift test is to lift the upper body off the floor from a prone position using the muscles of the upper back. Flexibility is assessed with the back-saver sit-and-reach and shoulder stretch. Body composition can be assessed with triceps and calf skinfold measurements or via BMI. Details for administering the aforementioned assessments, as well as other fitness measures, are available in youth fitness testing manuals (Meredith & Welk, 2004; Safrit, 1995).

Youth Fitness Guidelines

Children and adolescents should be encouraged to be physically active daily, or nearly every day, as part of play, recreation, sports, and school. While the intensity and duration of the activity are important considerations, the ACE-AHFS should not overlook the fact that calories are burned and a habit of physical activity is being established at an early age. This does not mean that exercising within a recommended target heart rate range is not beneficial. Rather, the ACE-AHFS should not expect youth to do what adults do. The bottom line is that physical-activity experiences need to be positive and consistent with the needs, abilities, and activity patterns of children and adolescents. To make physical activity a lifelong habit, youth should experience success, gain confidence in their physical abilities, establish a base of general fitness (not necessarily a high level of fitness), and become aware of the health benefits of physical activity (Barrett, 2001; Reynolds et al., 1990).

Over the past decade, several organizations have developed physical-activity guidelines for children and adolescents (Cavill, Biddle, & Sallis, 2001; Fulton et al., 2004; United States Department of Health and Human Services, 2005). Strong and colleagues (2005) conducted a systematic review of the literature on physical activity in school-age youth, concluding that children and adolescents should participate in 60 minutes or more of daily moderate-to-vigorous physical activity that is developmentally appropriate, enjoyable, and involves a variety of activities.

Most supervised intervention studies use programs of continuous moderate-to-vigorous physical activity of 30 to 45 minutes duration three to five days per week. However, the amount of physical activity necessary to achieve similar or greater beneficial effects with ordinary daily activities or intermittent exercise is substantially more than indicated in controlled research studies. The recommended amount of physical activity can be accumulated throughout the day by participating in physical education, recess, intramural sports, and before- and after-school programs (Strong et al., 2005).

These recommendations provide a reasonable standard that even sedentary children can achieve with a modest commitment to physical activity and support from their parents and schools. In addition to daily physical education, walks to and from school, recreational activities, sport practice and competitions, chores around the house, and physical movements on a playground are all examples of physical activities that allow youth to achieve their daily physical-activity goal. They could also increase the amount of time for physical activity by simply reducing such sedentary leisure pursuits as television or DVD viewing, computer use, telephone conversations or text messaging, and video games. If youth have been inactive for a while, they should gradually increase their amount of physical activity by about 10% per week until they reach the 60-minute goal (Strong et al., 2005).

The ACE-AHFS needs to remember the importance of focusing on the accumulation of physical activity throughout the day rather than on continuous bouts of physical activity performed at a predetermined intensity. While continuous moderate-to-vigorous physical activity is not physiologically harmful, it is not the most appropriate method of exercise for youth, who tend to enjoy non-sustained activities or games (Ratel et al., 2004). In fact, continuous moderate-to-vigorous physical activity lasting more than five to 10 minutes without rest or recovery is rare among children, because they have short attention spans and do not enjoy this type of training. Therefore, the ACE-AHFS should assess the needs and abilities of all participants, and carefully design physical-activity programs that alternate moderate-to-vigorous amounts of physical activity with brief periods of rest and recovery as needed. The following sections present specific youth physical-activity guidelines for enhancing aerobic fitness, muscle strength and endurance, and flexibility.

Aerobic Exercise

Adults typically perform continuous aerobic (or endurance) exercise to increase their maximal oxygen uptake and improve their cardiovascular disease risk profile. Although this type of training can be beneficial, most youth view prolonged periods of aerobic exercise as monotonous, boring, and discomforting. The ACE-AHFS who works with children and adolescents should modify aerobic exercise procedures to better match the physical and psychosocial characteristics of youth.

Higher-effort exercises such as circuit training are typically performed for shorter durations (e.g., 30 minutes per session), and lower-effort exercises such as rollerblading can be continued for longer durations (e.g., 60 minutes per session). Because most children will not complete a 30-minute session of continuous aerobic training, some modifications must be made to ensure exercise compliance. While most youth can remain physically active for 30 to 60 minutes, the training session must be punctuated with brief rest periods to recover and recharge. The ACE-AHFS may consider stop-and-go games or circuit-training activities that alternate higher-effort and lower-effort segments, as doing so increases a child's likelihood of completing the exercise session.

The standard means of assessing aerobic exercise intensity in adults is heart-rate monitoring (e.g., 70 to 85% percent of maximum heart rate). Heart-rate monitoring is problematic for children, who often have great difficulty finding and counting their pulse rates during exercise. Moreover, there is little need for healthy children to monitor their heart-rate response, because adult target heart rate formulas are inappropriate for youth under 16 years of age. Simple observations are usually sufficient for determining children's physical exertion during their training sessions (e.g., breathing rate or ability to pass the "talk test"). As long as youth participate in the fitness program and maintain a reasonable flow with the group activities at the desired intensity, they tend to meet the criteria for aerobic conditioning.

The aerobic segment of youth programs can include a lot of locomotion skills (e.g., running, skipping, jumping, hopping, stepping, and throwing), as well as activities that involve apparatus, including hoops, cones, playground balls, and beach balls. In addition, physically active but less-competitive games can keep children moving and motivated without fear of failure. If appropriate, the ACE-AHFS can lead group activities and perform essentially all of the aerobic exercises along with the children. This role-model approach is highly effective for eliciting enthusiastic and energetic responses from boys and girls.

The following basic aerobic-training guidelines are recommended for healthy children and adolescents and are applicable to all types of aerobic activities, including running, cycling, stepping, rowing, and swimming.

- Begin with 20 to 30 minutes of intermittent aerobic exercise.
- Gradually progress to 60 minutes or more on all or most days of the week.
- Alternate moderate and vigorous bouts of aerobic exercise with brief rest periods.
- Estimate exercise intensity by simple observation.
- Participate in a variety of developmentally appropriate aerobic activities that include locomotion skills and apparatus activities.
- Perform aerobic activities that are challenging, interesting, and fun.

Muscle Strength and Endurance Exercise

For decades, youth were discouraged from participating in structured strength-training programs. The primary reason for this precaution was a belief that strength training would damage children's bone growth plates and retard their musculoskeletal development. However, research clearly demonstrates that strength-training can be a safe, effective, and worthwhile activity for children and adolescents provided that age-appropriate training guidelines are followed (Faigenbaum, 2007; Falk & Tenenbaum, 1996; Malina, 2006). The qualified acceptance of youth strength training by medical and fitness organizations is becoming universal, as evidenced by support from the American Council on Exercise (Faigenbaum & Westcott, 2005), the American Academy of Pediatrics (2008), the Canadian Society for Exercise Physiology (Behm et al., 2008), the National Association for Sport and Physical Education (NASPE) (2005), and the National Strength and Conditioning Association (NSCA) (Faigenbaum et al., 1996).

In addition to increasing muscular strength, muscular power, and muscular endurance, regular participation in a youth strength-training program has the potential to positively influence cardiorespiratory fitness, body composition, blood lipids, bone mineral density, motor performance skills, and selected psychological measures (Faigenbaum, 2007). Moreover, some evidence suggests that carefully planned preseason strength and conditioning programs may reduce the risk of sports-related injuries in young athletes (Micheli, 2006).

Another benefit of youth strength training is its ability to improve the body composition of overweight and obese youth (Faigenbaum & Westcott, 2007). Although these children and adolescents have traditionally been encouraged to participate in aerobic activities, excess body fat hinders the abilities of weightbearing physical activities such as jogging and increases the risk of musculoskeletal overuse injuries. Conversely, youth with excess body fat seem to enjoy strength training because it is not aerobically taxing and it gives all participants a chance to experience success and feel good about their abilities. A growing body of evidence suggests that fitness programs that include strength training can improve the health and body composition of overweight and obese youth (Shabi et al., 2006; Sothern et al., 2000; Watts et al., 2004). While further study is warranted, it seems that strength training with moderate loads and a high number of repetitions may be part of the solution for long-term fat loss and weight management in overweight and obese youth.

Although there is no scientific evidence to suggest that the risks and concerns associated with youth strength training are greater than those of other sports and recreational activities in which children and adolescents participate regularly, youth strength-training programs must be competently supervised, properly instructed, and appropriately designed. The ACE-AHFS must be aware of the inherent but very manageable risk associated with strength training, and should attempt to decrease this risk by following established training guidelines.

Youth should not strength train on their own without guidance from a qualified fitness professional who should match the strength-training program to the needs, interests, and abilities of each participant. In addition, since the training-induced gains in strength during childhood are primarily due to neuromuscular factors (e.g., enhanced motor unit recruitment and firing) as opposed to muscle **hypertrophy** (Ramsay et al., 1990), the ACE-AHFS should not suggest to children that strength training will make their muscles bigger (beyond growth and maturation).

Although there is no minimum age for participating in a youth strength-training program, children and adolescents should have the emotional maturity to accept and follow directions. They should also appreciate the benefits and concerns associated with this type of training. In general, if a child is ready for participation in some type of athletic activity (generally age seven or eight), then he or she may be ready to strength train. Different types of equipment, including free weights (i.e., barbells and dumbbells), child-size weight machines, elastic bands, medicine balls, and body-weight exercises, have proven to be safe and effective for children and adolescents (Annesi et al., 2005; Faigenbaum & Mediate, 2006; Faigenbaum et al., 2005a; Falk & Mor, 1996; Faigenbaum et al., 2007).

The greatest concern for children and adolescents who strength train is the risk of an overuse soft-tissue injury, particularly to the lower back (Reynolds, 1997; Risser, 1991). Since weak musculature, improper lifting techniques, or improperly designed strength-training programs may explain these observations, the ACE-AHFS needs to be aware of the inherent risks associated with strength training and should attempt to decrease this risk with proper instruction and program design. As such, strengthening exercises for the hips, abdomen, and lower back should be included in youth strength-training programs as part of a preventative health measure. Additional youth strength-training guidelines are as follows:

- Start with one or two sets of 10 to 15 repetitions using light to moderate loads.
- Increase the resistance gradually (5 to 10%) as strength improves.
- Focus on the correct exercise technique instead of the amount of weight lifted.
- Progress to multiple sets of six to 15 repetitions on selected exercises.
- Progress from simple to more advanced movements that require balance and coordination.
- Strength train two to three times per week on nonconsecutive days.

- Use individualized workout logs to monitor progress.
- Cool down with less intense activities and static stretching.

Flexibility Exercise

While flexibility is a well-recognized component of health-related youth fitness programs (NASPE, 2005), long-held beliefs regarding the traditional practice of warm-up static stretching have been questioned (Shrier, 2004; Thacker et al., 2004). Several studies involving youth have indicated that an acute bout of static stretching can have a negative influence on strength and power performance (Faigenbaum et al., 2005b; Faigenbaum, et al., 2006; McNeal & Sands, 2003). Moreover, research findings suggest that static stretching immediately before exercise has no significant effect on injury prevention (Shrier, 2005; Thacker et al., 2004). This is not to suggest that children and teenagers should avoid regular static stretching, but rather that the ACE-AHFS should consider the immediate impact of an acute bout of static stretching on health and performance.

The ACE-AHFS should also consider the potential impact of warm-up procedures on behavior. After sitting in school for several hours, boys and girls need to move when they come to the health club or recreation center. If a warm-up is slow and monotonous, the performance during the subsequent physical activities may be lagging. However, if the warm-up is up-tempo, exciting, and offers variety, behavior during the exercise sessions will likely meet or exceed expectations. As such, it is reasonable to suggest that children and adolescents perform dynamic activities during the warm-up period and static stretching exercises during the cool-down period.

The cool-down may actually be the ideal time to perform static stretching exercises because the muscles are already warmed up and participants need to recover from the exercise session with less intense activities. The potential benefits of regular static stretching include improved **range of motion,** decreased muscle tension, better postural alignment, and greater ease of movement (NASPE, 2005). Since gains in flexibility are specific to the flexibility exercises performed at each joint, youth should perform a variety of static stretches for the upper body, lower body, and midsection. In addition, the ACE-AHFS should be aware that extreme static stretching may actually increase the risk of injury (Knudson, 2000). Thus, the goal should be to achieve and maintain normal flexibility in all joints. General guidelines for static stretching are presented in Table 22-3.

Table 22-3
General Guidelines for Static Stretching

- Perform static stretching exercises after a warm-up or exercise session.
- Stretch at least three times per week, preferably daily.
- Perform a variety of stretches for all the major muscle groups.
- Stretch a muscle to the point of mild discomfort and back off slightly.
- Hold each stretch for 15 to 30 seconds.

Fundamental Movement Skills

In addition to helping youth enhance aerobic fitness, muscle strength and endurance, and flexibility, the ACE-AHFS should also include games, activities, and exercises that enhance fundamental movement skills such as skipping, hopping, twisting, kicking, and throwing. Although children and adolescents should be encouraged to participate in a variety of physical activities, the ACE-AHFS must ensure that youngsters develop the necessary prerequisite movement skills so they can sustain the more demanding fitness programs and sports training sessions.

Youth who do not establish a sound fitness base and enhance their skill-related fitness abilities (i.e., agility, coordination, balance, reaction time, speed, and power) are likely to drop out due to frustration, embarrassment, or failure, and may suffer injuries. With competent instruction and quality practice time, children and adolescents can learn the fundamental fitness skills needed for successful and enjoyable participation in recreational activities and organized sports. Although health- and skill-related fitness components are not mutually exclusive, most youth programs focus primarily on enhancing the health-related components of fitness, and thus underemphasize the importance of developing fundamental fitness skills that are characteristic of how children move and play.

The key issue, however, is not only understanding the importance of health- and skill-related fitness for youth, but also to understand how to provide youth with the skills, knowledge, attitudes, and behaviors that lead to a lifetime of physical activity. Unlike most adult fitness programs, which isolate fitness components, youth programs should provide children and teenagers with the opportunity to improve their health and fitness with different exercises, activities, and games that enhance aerobic fitness, muscular strength and endurance, and flexibility, as well as fundamental fitness skills such as balance, agility, and speed.

For example, instead of performing 30 minutes of aerobic exercise, 20 minutes of strength training, and then 10 minutes of flexibility exercises, youth programs should integrate health- and skill-related fitness components into one comprehensive class in which all participants can learn, improve, and feel good about their performances. This type of exercise session will optimize training adaptations because participants will be more focused on what they are doing and become more engaged in class activities. Additional guidelines for developing physical-activity programs for youth are discussed in the following sections.

Program Design Considerations

Youth fitness programs are a good way for children and adolescents to learn new skills, be with friends, and feel good about themselves. Although the focus of many youth programs has traditionally been on sports performance, the ACE-AHFS should encourage youth to participate in a variety of movement experiences. Instead of focusing entirely on highly competitive activities, youth physical-activity programs should also include less-competitive, age-appropriate games and activities that keep everyone moving most of the time.

While there are many exercises, activities, and games that children and adolescents can perform, the following format works best for an ACE-AHFS who wants to work with youth on nonconsecutive days. Each 60-minute session can include a 10- to 15-minute dynamic warm-up, about 20 to 30 minutes of fitness conditioning activities, 10 to 15 minutes of games, and five minutes of cool-down static stretching. Since youth should not strength train two days in a row, alternative games and activities that focus on aerobic fitness, balance, coordination, and agility can be performed in place of strength-building exercises if sessions are scheduled on two consecutive days.

Dynamic Warm-up

Instead of static stretching, the focus of the warm-up should be the performance of dynamic movements that are designed to elevate core body temperature, enhance motor unit excitability, improve kinesthetic awareness, maximize active ranges of motion, and develop fundamental movement skills by reinforcing critical movement patterns (Faigenbaum & McFarland, 2007). A dynamic warm-up typically includes low-, moderate-, and high-intensity hops, skips, and jumps, as well as various movement-based exercises for the upper and lower body. In addition to the physiological value, these movements satisfy the need for children to move at the start of each session, which also helps focus their attention on listening and learning.

The ACE-AHFS should begin each session with a 10- to 15-minute dynamic warm-up period of 10 to 12 drills (e.g., high-knee marches, lateral shuffles) that progress from low to higher intensity. Participants should perform each dynamic movement for about 10 yards (9 m), rest for five to 10 seconds, and then repeat the same exercise for 10 yards (9 m) as they return to the starting point. The dynamic warm-up may feel like a workout, but remember that the goal is to prepare youth for the main activity segment of class without undue fatigue. When appropriate, the ACE-AHFS can ask the participants for their ideas so that they can help design the warm-up activities.

Fitness Conditioning

This phase of the program includes training exercises and activities that are specifically designed to enhance physical fitness. Following a review of proper training procedures, the ACE-AHFS should demonstrate the correct technique for any new exercise. In addition to body-weight strength exercises, different types of training equipment can be used, including child-size weight machines, dumbbells, medicine balls, elastic tubing, balance boards, aerobic steps, and agility ladders. While some boys and girls may be tempted to see how much weight they can lift on certain exercises, the ACE-AHFS should remind all participants that the focus of the program is to learn new skills and have fun, as opposed to maximal lifting. No matter how strong or fast a child is, the ACE-AHFS should keep in mind that children and adolescents are still growing and may be experiencing new types of exercise for the very first time.

Depending on individual needs, goals, and abilities, sessions can include a variety of exercises and activities to enhance both health- and skill-related fitness measures. For example, the ACE-AHFS can create a fitness circuit using body-weight exercises, medicine balls, and agility ladders that integrates all health- and skill-related fitness components into one well-designed workout (Faigenbaum & Westcott, 2000; NASPE, 2005; Ward, Saunders, & Pate, 2007).

Games

Children and adolescents enjoy games that require moderate amounts of skill and keep everyone moving. Games using balls, beanbags, hoops, and parachutes are inclusive and lots of fun. In addition, some games can be physically challenging and promote training-induced adaptations in physical fitness. The ACE-AHFS should not leave it up to youngsters to play whatever game they want, but rather explain what type of games and activities would be appropriate, and then let participants choose an activity from within that range. Games that eliminate participants or embarrass children do little to promote a lifelong interest in physical activity. Figure 22-1 presents a checklist that the ACE-AHFS can use when creating games for youth.

- ❑ Is the environment safe and free of hazards?
- ❑ Does the activity provide for differences in the skill levels of all participants?
- ❑ Are teams formed randomly or cooperatively, rather than by selecting captains?
- ❑ Can all kids experience success, and at the same time be challenged?
- ❑ Does the activity provide for maximum participation?
- ❑ Are kids encouraged to ask questions and communicate their concerns?

Figure 22-1
Summary checklist for creating games and activities

Cool-down Activities

As the games come to an end, the ACE-AHFS should begin to quiet things down by decreasing the intensity of activities and leading the participants through some static stretching. At the end of every training session, the ACE-AHFS should thank the participants for coming and provide positive feedback about their performance.

Health and Safety

Due to age, size, and maturational differences, the ACE-AHFS should address the needs and concerns of all participants in a physical-activity program. Although it is not mandatory for apparently healthy children and teenagers to have a medical examination, parents should complete a health and activity questionnaire for each participant prior to the first training session. The questionnaire should include questions about pre-existing medical ailments (e.g., asthma and diabetes), previous injuries, recent surgeries, allergies, and the participant's activity level. The ACE-AHFS should ask for a physician screen of any youngster with known or suspected health problems, including illness or injury, prior to participation.

Prior to every training session, the ACE-AHFS should do a quick "health check" by asking participants how they feel. The ACE-AHFS should pay particular attention to any signs of illness or unusual aches or pains. He or she should also remind participants of program rules, including listening and following directions, trying to give the best effort possible, and being a good sport. Additionally, providing safety tips, such as on the importance proper footwear, ensuring that children's shoes are tied, and prohibiting gum chewing are good practices. Youngsters, like adults, may occasionally come to an exercise session feeling tired or lazy. On such days, the ACE-AHFS should allow youngsters to "take it easy" by performing a modified workout that may include exercising at a lower intensity for a shorter period of time.

All youth programs should take place in a clean and clutter-free exercise environment. If the ACE-AHFS makes safety a priority, in many cases, activity-related injuries can be prevented. The ACE-AHFS should take time before every exercise session to ensure that equipment is stored appropriately, the room is well lit, and the floor is clean. Because children often like to explore, it may be necessary to remove or disassemble a broken piece of equipment from the youth-training area. Overcrowded and poorly designed fitness centers increase the likelihood that a youngster may get hurt or bump into a piece of equipment or another child.

A traditional anatomical concern associated with youth fitness programs involves the potential for injury to the **epiphysis,** or growth plate, of children's long bones. Although injury to the growth plate is a serious concern, this type of injury seems to be largely preventable if the volume and intensity of exercise are carefully programmed and children are taught how to perform exercises properly. Traditional concerns involving the potential for injury to immature skeletons are being replaced with scientific findings that suggest that appropriate weightbearing physical activity is actually a potent stimulus for bone mineralization in children (Vicente-Rodriguez, 2006).

Leadership and Instruction

The challenges associated with promoting youth fitness should be met with enthusiastic leadership, creative programming, and effective age-specific teaching strategies. The ACE-AHFS needs to respect children's feelings while appreciating the fact that their thinking is different from adults. When leading an exercise session, the ACE-AHFS should allow each child or adolescent to control the intensity of the activity and provide him or her the opportunity to choose an enjoyable activity. Youth dislike and often fear activities that they perceive to be forced upon them by an adult. The ACE-AHFS needs to make every class fun, interesting, and challenging. The tips presented in Table 22-4 may help the ACE-AHFS develop safe, worthwhile, and enjoyable youth programs.

Table 22-4
Tips for Youth Fitness Leaders

- Treat youngsters respectfully and listen to their concerns.
- Provide opportunities for boys and girls of all ages and abilities to regularly engage in physical activity.
- Play down competition and focus on intrinsic values such as skill improvement, personal successes, and excitement.
- Recognize individual differences and capabilities of all youth.
- Learn the names of all youngsters in the program.
- Give kids an opportunity to perform a new skill while observing and providing feedback. Most children and teenagers learn best by doing.
- Provide competent and caring supervision at all times.
- Offer a variety of creative activities and avoid regimentation.
- Be a good role model and lead a healthy lifestyle.
- Encourage parents to support youth physical-activity programs.

A major objective of youth fitness programming is for physical activity to become a habitual part of children's lives and hopefully persist into adulthood. With this objective in mind, the ACE-AHFS must strive to increase children's **self-efficacy** regarding their physical abilities. To achieve this objective, the ACE-AHFS must provide clear instructions so that participants can experience success and develop a sense of mastery of a specific skill. Thus, the focus of youth fitness programs should be on positive experiences instead of stressful competition in which most children fail. In some cases, overzealous parents, youth coaches, and fitness professionals may need to reevaluate their views regarding winning and competition.

Professionals who choose to work with children and adolescents need to relate to youth in a positive manner and understand how they think. In some cases, educational training sessions and youth fitness seminars may be needed to help fitness professionals learn how to effectively work with children and teenagers. In short, the ACE-AHFS needs to keep in mind that participation in a fitness class is a personal choice. Thus, it is unlikely that youth will continue in the program if they do not understand the games or are unable to perform the exercises.

Instead of forcing fitness on participants, the ACE-AHFS should teach them how to be physically active. The ACE-AHFS must also be enthusiastic about working with youth and take pride in being in the fitness industry. Along with the primary objective of engaging youth in fun physical activities, the ACE-AHFS is also responsible for class management, quality instruction, transition periods, and skill development. Needless to say, the development of successful youth fitness programs requires preparation, coordination, and a good understanding of the physical and psychosocial uniqueness of childhood and adolescence.

The following recommendations for teaching youth have proven to be effective:

- Keep instructions short and simple. Even the best fitness activities will not work if participants do not understand the rules.
- Avoid using vague terms and realize that the choice of words can influence a child's ability to understand what was said. The use of "show and tell" demonstrations can assist in explaining an exercise or game.
- If the element of fun seems to be missing, reevaluate the intellectual requirements of the game or activity.

Provide Attentive Supervision and Instruction

Sedentary youth often lack confidence in their physical abilities and are understandably reluctant to perform exercises on their own. Therefore, the ACE-AHFS should observe and encourage participants as they perform their exercises and ensure that they are performing the movements properly. Knowing that the instructor is watching is a motivating factor for most children and adolescents.

Alternate Exercise Intensity

Participants should understand that exercise does not have to be continuous to be beneficial. Intermittent bouts of low-, moderate-, and high-intensity physical activity are consistent with how youth move and play. After a vigorous game, the ACE-AHFS may choose a less intense activity to provide adequate rest and recovery.

Utilize Gradual Progression

The ACE-AHFS should take small steps in the learning process when dealing with children and adolescents who have little exercise experience. With few exceptions, an ACE-AHFS should not introduce a follow-up task until the first task has been mastered. It is much more efficient to progress slowly and steadily than progress too quickly, which can lead to discouragement or mistakes that must be unlearned and rectified at a later time.

Add Variety

Children and adolescents quickly get bored when they perform the same activity day after day. Furthermore, chronic, repetitive stress can result in an overuse injury. The ACE-AHFS must use a variety of age-appropriate games and activities when working with children and teenagers. Not only will the participants enjoy the program, but variety is key to long-term exercise adherence.

Provide Specific Feedback

Praising children for doing a good job is one of the best ways to keep them motivated and performing well. However, positive reinforcement is much more meaningful when it is coupled with specific feedback. The ACE-AHFS should try to provide relevant information that supports encouraging comments. Giving a reason for positive reinforcement increases its value as an educational and motivational tool.

Lead a Pre- and Post-exercise Dialogue

The ACE-AHFS should have an arriving and departing dialogue with the young participants. Spending a few minutes in conversation with each participant before and after each workout is time well spent. The ACE-AHFS should greet each child by name upon arrival and welcome him or her to the workout. The instructor should always say good-bye and thank each youngster for taking part in the exercise program.

Have Fun

The ACE-AHFS should utilize activities that get youth excited and maximize participation. Physical activities should be challenging without being threatening. When youth have fun and experience success, they are more likely to continue participating. The ACE-AHFS should never use fitness activities or exercises as punishment.

Enlist Parent Support

It is important to get parents involved when working with children and adolescents. Parents should be informed about the benefits of regular physical activity and support their child's participation in a physical-activity program. A newsletter or personal communication serves as a great means for parents to learn about safe exercise guidelines, healthy eating habits, and other programs offered at the health club or sports training center.

Nutrition and Hydration

In addition to promoting physical activity, the ACE-AHFS should recognize the importance of encouraging children and adolescents to eat nutritious foods to maintain their health and optimize their performance. In fact, a well-balanced, nutrient-dense diet is essential for healthy growth and development. But in more households than ever before, nutritious home-cooked meals are being replaced with fast foods that are high in fat, salt, and sugar. Poor nutrition is a major health concern affecting many children and teenagers.

According to the CDC (2006), 80% of children and adolescents in the United States do not consume the recommended five or more servings of daily fruits and vegetables. Researchers have found that less than 40% of today's youth meet the dietary guidelines for **saturated fat** [United States Department of Agriculture (USDA), 1998]; and only 39% of youth meet dietary recommendations for fiber (Lin, Guthrie, & Frazao, 2001). At the same time, the daily consumption of soft drinks continues to increase (USDA, 1998), whereas the consumption of milk, the largest source of calcium, has decreased over the past few years (Cavadini, Siega-Riz, & Popkin, 2000). Powell et al. (2007) reported that an overwhelming majority of food products advertised on television shows targeting children and adolescents were high in fat, sugar, or sodium.

Not only does poor nutrition contribute to obesity, type 2 diabetes, osteoporosis, and other health ailments, but research suggests that unhealthy eating habits can also affect children's intellectual performance (Pollitt & Matthews, 1998). Clearly, children and adolescents need to eat a nutrient-dense diet that is high in fruits, vegetables, whole grains, and low-fat dairy products, as well as consume essential vitamins, minerals, antioxidants, and fiber to gain needed energy. In addition, youth need to limit their intake of saturated fat, **trans fat, cholesterol,** salt, and added sugar. Total fat intake should be restricted to about 30% of total calories, with most fats coming from polyunsaturated and monounsaturated sources. Carbohydrates should make up 55% and proteins about 20% of the total caloric intake.

The recommended intake of five servings of fruits and vegetables may seem like a lot, but is actually easy to meet when one considers how small a serving really is. For example, one medium piece of fruit, ¼ cup of dried fruit, ½ cup of cooked vegetables, and ¾ cup of 100% fruit or vegetable juice are all equal to one serving. Youth can meet these guidelines by simply adding a piece of fruit to their morning cereal, topping lunch sandwiches with lettuce and tomatoes, and eating a salad and vegetables with dinner.

Sadly, many children and adolescents eat a diet composed of cheeseburgers, French fries, ice cream, and soda, all of which are high in fat, salt, and sugar. A diet composed of healthy foods, such as bananas, raisins, salads, cooked vegetables, fish, and chicken, is lower in fat and packed with nutrients. However, instead of eliminating any food that a youngster truly enjoys, the ACE-AHFS may want to suggest balancing foods high in fat with selections from the fruit, vegetable, and grain groups. For the ACE-AHFS, the greatest challenge is likely to be teaching youngsters how to eat for proper nutrition. In some cases, it may be appropriate for the ACE-AHFS to consult with a healthcare provider when working with a child or teenager who has special dietary needs.

Since most youth are not concerned about serious health conditions such as diabetes or heart disease, they may see little value in making healthier food selections. Furthermore, some children are fussy eaters and do not want to try new foods or spend time cutting up fruits or vegetables for a salad. Therefore, the ACE-AHFS needs to develop strategies to motivate youngsters to develop healthier eating habits. The following ideas may help foster healthier eating:

- Encourage youngsters to eat breakfast. A well-balanced meal at the start of the day can enhance cognitive performance and provide energy.
- Provide healthy "grab-and-go" foods such as raisins, air-popped popcorn, and low-fat yogurt at health clubs and recreation centers.
- Create games and fun activities that encourage healthy eating habits and invite parents to be part of the nutrition education program so they can plan healthy meals and keep healthy snacks at home.
- Give children and teenagers healthy snack ideas, such as baby carrots with low-fat dressing and celery sticks with peanut butter.
- Set a good example by choosing healthy snacks before and after class. If youngsters see an adult eating high-fat snacks, they will likely imitate the behavior.

The ACE-AHFS should also emphasize the importance of adequate hydration. Children and teenagers should be encouraged to drink water before, during, and after every fitness class. Although a decrease in body weight of only 1% through exercise-induced sweating negatively affects performance, **dehydration** levels of 2 to 3% or even higher are commonly reported in youth sports (Dougherty et al., 2006). Because youth respond to dehydration with an excessive increase in body core temperature and a greater risk of heat-related illnesses, the ACE-AHFS should make every effort to ensure that youth arrive fully hydrated and drink fluid before, during, and after the exercise session or sports competition. Although plain water is best for activities lasting less than one hour, some boys and girls may find sports drinks more palatable than water. If a youngster prefers the taste of flavored drinks, he or she may be more likely to drink regularly and avoid voluntary dehydration (Rivera-Brown et al., 1999).

The ACE-AHFS must remind participants to drink regularly, even when they are not thirsty, and take drink breaks about every 15 to 20 minutes during prolonged activities. Given that many children and teenagers often show up dehydrated for fitness classes and sports practices, it is particularly important to enforce water breaks during youth activity programs. Moreover, the ACE-AHFS should encourage purposeful drinking throughout the entire day.

Healthy food choices and adequate hydration will provide children and teenagers with the necessary energy, nutrients, and fluids to maintain an active lifestyle. Furthermore, teaching boys and girls to eat nutritious foods during childhood and adolescence will increase their likelihood of making healthy lifestyle choices as adults. Educate by example by providing healthy snacks, encouraging hydration, and recognizing that regular physical activity and proper nutrition are part of a happy and healthy lifestyle.

Case Study

Sam is a 14-year-old boy who is 5'5" (1.7 m) and weighs 148 lb (67 kg). He does not participate regularly in any type of physical activity and, according to his pediatrician, he is at risk for becoming obese. He mother states that Sam spends most of his free time watching television and "surfing" the Internet. Sam has never been on a sports team and seems to lack confidence in his ability to engage in any type of physical activity. With the support of his parents and pediatrician (*Note:* His pediatrician provided written medical clearance), Sam signed up for an after-school "kids workout" program. His parents contacted the ACE-AHFS for additional guidance and support for their son.

The ACE-AHFS should reassure Sam and his parents that his or her goal is for Sam to participate in a safe, effective, and enjoyable physical-activity program that provides an opportunity for him to make friends, learn something new, and have fun. Remind the parents that teenagers are not miniature adults, and therefore adult exercise guidelines and training philosophies are not appropriate for younger populations. Before the first day of the program, it may be helpful for the ACE-AHFS to give Sam and his parents a tour of the facility and introduce them to other fitness professionals who work with youth at the center. In addition, the ACE-AHFS can provide an overview of the program along with realistic objectives. After touring the facility, the ACE-AHFS should ask Sam what type of physical activity he may want to try in the future.

When designing the "kids workout" class, the ACE-AHFS should keep in mind that overweight youth tend to dislike prolonged periods of aerobic exercise. On the other hand, these youth tend to enjoy resistance training because it is not aerobically taxing and they are often the strongest students in class. An enthusiastic ACE-AHFS should begin each class with low- to moderate-intensity dynamic warm-up activities that enhance fundamental fitness abilities. After the warm-up, Sam and the other students should participate in a resistance-training circuit that strengthens all the major muscle groups. It is important to begin with a moderate load on each exercise and focus on developing proper form and technique. Also, the ACE-AHFS should allow for adequate rest between stations and encourage Sam to keep track of his progress on a workout log to give his efforts direction and purpose. Next, the youth can play cooperative games that integrate both health- and skill-related fitness components. Note that the games should be consistent with the interests and skill level of all students. Throughout the class, the ACE-AHFS should encourage students to help each other, ask questions, and, when appropriate, demonstrate selected exercises.

With the goal of enhancing physical fitness and improving body composition, the ACE-AHFS should consider teaching Sam and the other students about healthy eating through creative games and special events. For example, once a week the ACE-AHFS can teach students how to make fruit smoothies while providing healthy alternatives to "junk food" and soft drinks. With regular participation and attentive supervision, Sam should see noticeable gains in his muscle strength and overall physical-fitness level. The ACE-AHFS should progress the program by modifying the resistance-training circuit and adding new games and activities and keep the workout challenging and fun. It is also a good idea to encourage Sam's parents to be good role models by regularly engaging in physical activity at home or at the fitness center.

Summary

Children and teenagers are active, but in different ways than adults. It is up to the ACE-AHFS to address participants' individual needs and concerns, reinforce safety rules, foster fun and enjoyment, and understand the uniqueness of childhood and adolescence. Youth physical-activity programs should enhance both health- and skill-related components of fitness and provide boys and girls with an opportunity to establish a solid base of fundamental movement skills. With enthusiastic leadership and qualified instruction, children and adolescents can gain confidence in their physical abilities, experience success, and develop healthier eating habits. Perhaps most importantly, youth who enjoy physical activity and gain confidence in their abilities to be physically active are more likely to be active in their later years.

References

American Dietetic Association (2004). Position of the American Dietetic Association: Dietary guidance for healthy children ages 2 to 11 years. *Journal of the American Dietetic Association,* 104, 4, 660–677.

American Academy of Pediatrics (2008). Strength training by children and adolescents. *Pediatrics,* 121, 4, 835–840.

Annesi, J. et al. (2005). Effects of a 12-week physical activity protocol delivered by YMCA after-school counselors (Youth Fit for Life) on fitness and self-efficacy changes in 5–12 year old boys and girls. *Research Quarterly in Exercise and Sport*, 76, 468–476.

Bar-Or, O. (1983). *Sports Medicine for the Practitioner*. New York: Springer-Verlag.

Barrett, B. (2001). Play now, play later: Lifetime fitness implications. *Journal of Physical Education, Recreation and Dance,* 72, 8, 35–39.

Behm, D, et al. (2008). Canadian Society for Exercise Physiology position paper: Resistance training in children and adolescents. *Journal of Applied Physiology, Nutrition and Metabolism,* 33, 547–561.

Botero, D. & Wolfsdorf, J. (2005). Diabetes mellitus in children and adolescents. *Archives of Medical Research,* 36, 281–290.

Bureau of Transportation Statistics (2003). *National Household of Travel Survey*. http://www.bts.gov/programs/national_household_travel_survey

Carnethon, M., Gulati, M., & Greenland, P. (2005). Prevalence and cardiovascular disease correlates of low cardiorespiratory fitness in adolescents and adults. *Journal of the American Medical Association*, 294, 2981–2988.

Cavadini, C., Siega-Riz, A., & Popkin, B. (2000). U.S. adolescent food intake trends from 1965 to 1996. *Archives of Diseases in Childhood,* 83, 1, 18–24.

Cavill, N., Biddle S., & Sallis, J. (2001). Health-enhancing physical activity for young people: Statement of the United Kingdom Expert Consensus Conference. *Pediatric Exercise Science,* 13, 12–25.

Centers for Disease Control and Prevention (2006). Youth Risk Behavior Surveillance—United States, 2005. *Morbidity and Mortality Weekly Report,* 55 (SS-5), 1–108.

Centers for Disease Control and Prevention (2005). Participation in high school physical education—United States, 1991–2003, *Journal of School Health,* 75, 2, 47–49.

Centers for Disease Control and Prevention (2003). Physical activity levels among children aged 9–13 years: United States, 2002. *Morbidity and Mortality Weekly Report,* 52, 33, 785–788.

Coe, D. et al. (2006). Effect of physical education and activity levels on academic achievement in children. *Medicine & Science in Sports & Exercise,* 38, 1515–1519.

Dietz, W. (2004). Overweight in childhood and adolescence. *New England Journal of Medicine,* 350, 855–857.

Dougherty, K. et al. (2006). Two percent dehydration impairs and six percent carbohydrate drink improves boys basketball skills. *Medicine & Science in Sports & Exercise,* 38, 9, 1650–1658.

Epstein, L., Paluch, R., & Gordy, C. (1999). Reinforcing value of physical activity as a determinant of child activity level. *Health Psychology,* 18, 599–603.

Faigenbaum, A. (2007). Resistance training for youth: Are there health outcomes? *American Journal of Lifestyle Medicine,* 1, 3, 190–200.

Faigenbaum A. & McFarland, J. (2007). Guidelines for implementing a dynamic warm-up for physical education. *Journal of Physical Education Recreation and Dance,* 78, 25–28.

Faigenbaum, A. & Mediate, P. (2006). The effects of medicine ball training on physical fitness in high school physical education students. *The Physical Educator,* 63, 3, 161–168.

Faigenbaum, A. & Westcott, W. (2007). Resistance training for obese children and adolescents. *President's Council on Physical Fitness and Sports Research Digest,* 8, 3, 1–8.

Faigenbaum, A. & Westcott, W. (2005). *Youth Strength Training*. San Diego, Calif.: American Council on Exercise.

Faigenbaum, A. & Westcott, W. (2000). *Strength and Power for Young Athletes.* Champaign, Ill.: Human Kinetics.

Faigenbaum, A. et al. (2007). Preliminary evaluation of an after-school resistance training program. *Perceptual and Motor Skills,* 104, 407–415.

Faigenbaum, A. et al. (2006). Acute effects of different warm-up protocols on anaerobic performance in teenage athletes. *Pediatric Exercise Science,* 17, 64–75.

Faigenbaum, A. et al. (2005a). Early muscular fitness adaptations in children in response to two different resistance training regimens. *Pediatric Exercise Science,* 17, 237–248.

Faigenbaum, A. et al. (2005b). Acute effects of different warm-up protocols on fitness performance in children. *Journal of Strength and Conditioning Research,* 19, 2, 376–381.

Faigenbaum, A. et al. (1996).Youth resistance training: Position statement paper and literature review. *Strength and Conditioning Journal,* 18, 62–75.

Falk, B. & Mor, G. (1996). The effects of resistance training and martial arts training in 6- to 8-year-old boys. *Pediatric Exercise Science,* 8, 48–56.

Falk, B. & Tenenbaum, G. (1996). The effectiveness of resistance training in children: A meta-analysis. *Sports Medicine,* 22, 176–186.

Freedman, D. et al. (1999). The relation of overweight to cardiovascular disease risk factors among children and adolescents: The Bogalusa Heart Study. *Pediatrics,* 103, 6 Pt. 1, 1175–1182.

Fulton, J. et al. (2004). Public health and clinical recommendations for physical activity and physical fitness with a special focus on overweight youth. *Sports Medicine,* 34, 581–599.

Gillis L., Kennedy, L., & Bar-Or, O. (2006). Overweight children reduce their activity levels earlier in life than healthy weight children. *Clinical Journal of Sports Medicine,* 16, 1, 51–55.

Goodman, E. & Whitaker, R. (2002). A prospective study of the role of depression in the development and persistence of adolescent obesity. *Pediatrics,* 110, 497–504.

Gortmaker, S. et al. (1993). Social and economic consequences of overweight in adolescence and young adulthood. *New England Journal of Medicine,* 329, 1008–1012.

Hills, A., King, N., & Armstrong, T. (2007). The contribution of physical activity and sedentary behaviors to the growth and development of children and adolescents. *Sports Medicine,* 37, 6, 533–545.

Institute of Medicine (2005). *Preventing Childhood Obesity: Health in the Balance.* Washington, D.C.: The National Academies Press.

International Health, Racquet and Sportsclub Association (2006). *2006 Profiles of Success.* Boston: International Health, Racquet and Sportsclub Association.

Janz, K., Dawson, J., & Mahoney, L. (2000). Tracking physical fitness and physical activity from childhood to adolescence: The Muscatine study. *Medicine & Science in Sports & Exercise,* 32, 1250–1257.

Knudson, D. (2000). Current issues in flexibility fitness. *President's Council on Physical Fitness and Sports Research Digest,* 3, 1–6.

Lin, B., Guthrie, J., & Frazao, E. (2001). American children's diets not making the grade. *Food Review,* 24, 2, 8–17.

Mahar, M. et al. (2006). Effects of a classroom-based program on physical activity and on-task behavior. *Medicine & Science in Sports & Exercise*, 38, 12, 2086–2094.

Malina, R. (2006). Weight training in youth-growth, maturation and safety: An evidence-based review. *Clinical Journal of Sports Medicine,* 16, 478–487.

McNeal, J. & Sands, W. (2003). Acute static stretching reduces lower extremity power in trained children. *Pediatric Exercise Science,* 15, 139–145.

Meredith, M. & Welk G. (2007). *Fitnessgram/ Activitygram: Test Administration Manual* (4th ed.). Champaign, Ill.: Human Kinetics.

Micheli L. (2006). Preventing injuries in sports: What the team physician needs to know. In: Chan, K. et al. (Eds.) *F.I.M.S. Team Physician Manual* (2nd ed.). Hong Kong: CD Concept.

Narayan, K. et al. (2003). Lifetime risk for diabetes in the United States. *Journal of the American Medical Association,* 290, 1884–1890.

National Association for Sport and Physical Education (2005). *Physical Education for Lifetime Fitness* (2nd ed.). Champaign, Ill.: Human Kinetics. National Strength and Conditioning Association (NSCA)

Ogden, C. L. et al. (2008). High body mass index for age among US children and adolescents, 2003–2006. *Journal of the American Medical Association*, 299, 20, 2401–2405.

Olshansky, S. et al. (2005). A potential decline in life expectancy in the United States in the 21st century. *New England Journal of Medicine,* 352, 11, 1138–1145

Paffenbarger, R. et al. (1986). Physical activity and all-cause mortality and longevity of college alumni. *New England Journal of Medicine,* 314, 605–613.

Pollitt, E. & Matthews, R. (1998). Breakfast and cognition: An integrative summary. *American Journal of Clinical Nutrition,* 67 (Suppl.), 804S–813S.

Powell, L. et al. (2007). Nutritional content of television food advertisements seen by children and adolescents in the United States. *Pediatrics,* 120, 576–583.

Ramsay J. et al. (1990). Strength training effects in prepubescent boys. *Medicine & Science in Sports & Exercise,* 22, 605–614.

Ratel, S. et al. (2004). High-intensity intermittent activities at school: Controversies and facts. *Journal of Sports Medicine and Physical Fitness.* 44, 272–280.

Reynolds, N. (1997). Back injuries in the young athlete. *Orthopedic Physical Therapy Clinics of North America.* 6, 4, 491–503.

Reynolds, K. et al. (1990). Psychosocial predictors of physical activity in adolescents. *Preventative Medicine,* 19, 541–551.

Risser, W. (1991). Weight training injuries in children and adolescents. *American Family Physician,* 44, 2104–2110.

Rivera-Brown, A. et al. (1999). Drink composition, voluntary drinking, and fluid balance in exercising trained, heat-acclimatized boys. *Journal of Applied Physiology*, 86, 1, 78–84.

Rowland, T. (2005). *Children's Exercise Physiology* (2nd ed.). Champaign, Ill.: Human Kinetics.

Safrit, M. (1995). *Complete Guide to Youth Fitness Testing.* Champaign, Ill.: Human Kinetics.

Schwimmer, J., Burwinkle, T., & Varni, J. (2003). Health-related quality of life of severely obese children and adolescents. *Journal of the American Medical Association,* 289, 1813–1819.

Servedio, F. (1997). Normal growth and development: Physiological factors associated with exercise and training in children. *Orthopedic Physical Therapy Clinics of North America,* 6, 4, 417–436.

Shabi, G. et al. (2006). Effects of resistance training on insulin sensitivity in overweight Latino adolescent males. *Medicine & Science in Sports & Exercise,* 38, 1208–1215.

Shrier, I. (2005) Does stretching improve performance? A systematic and critical review of the literature. *Clinical Journal of Sports Medicine,* 14, 267–273.

Sibley, B. & Ethnier, J. (2003). The relationship between physical activity and cognition in children: A meta analysis. *Pediatric Exercise Science,* 15, 243–253.

Sothern, M. et al. (2000). Safety, feasibility and efficacy of a resistance training program in preadolescent obese youth. *American Journal of Medical Sciences,* 319, 6, 370–375.

Strong, W. et al. (2005). Evidence-based physical activity for school-age youth. *Journal of Pediatrics,* 146, 732–737.

Taras, H. & Potts-Datema, W. (2005). Obesity and student performance at school. *Journal of School Health.* 75, 291–295.

Telama, R., Yang, X., & Viikari, J. (2005). Physical activity from childhood to adulthood: A 21-year tracking study. *American Journal of Preventive Medicine,* 28, 3, 267–273.

Thacker, S. et al. (2004). The impact of stretching on sports injury risk: A systematic review of the literature. *Medicine & Science in Sports & Exercise,* 36, 371–378.

United States Department of Agriculture (1998). *Continuing Survey of Food Intakes by Individuals 1994–96.* Washington, D.C.: United States Department of Agriculture.

U.S. Department of Health and Human Services (1996). *Physical Activity and Health: A Report from the Surgeon General.* Atlanta, Ga.: U.S. Department of Health and Human Services, Centers for Disease Control and Prevention, National Center for Chronic Disease Prevention and Health Promotion.

U.S. Department of Health and Human Services and U.S. Department of Agriculture (2005). *Dietary Guidelines for Americans* (6th ed.). Washington, D.C.: U.S. Government Printing Office.

Vicente-Rodriquez, G. (2006). How does exercise affect bone development during growth? *Sports Medicine,* 36, 561–569.

Waite-Stupinsky, S. & Findlay, M. (2001). The fourth R: Recess and its link to learning. *The Educational Forum,* 66, 16–25.

Wang G. & Dietz, W. (2002). Economic burden of obesity in youths aged 6 to 17 years: 1979–1999. *Pediatrics,* 109, 5, E81–E86.

Ward, D., Saunders, R., & Pate, R. (2007). *Physical Activity Interventions in Children and Adolescents.* Champaign, Ill.: Human Kinetics.

Watts, K. et al. (2004). Exercise training normalizes vascular dysfunction and improves central adiposity in obese adolescents. *Journal of the American College of Cardiology,* 43, 1823–1827.

YMCA of the USA (2007). YMCAs expand programs to respond to nation's growing health crisis. www.ymca.net.

Suggested Reading

Bailey, R. et al. (1995). The level and tempo of children's physical activities: An observational study. *Medicine & Science in Sports & Exercise,* 27, 1033–1041.

Bar-Or, O. & Rowland, T. (2004). *Pediatric Exercise Medicine*. Champaign, Ill.: Human Kinetics.

Burdette, H. & Whitaker, R. (2005). Resurrecting free play in young children. *Archives of Pediatric and Adolescent Medicine,* 159, 46–50.

Chu, D., Faigenbaum, A., & Falkel, J. (2006). *Progressive Plyometrics for Kids*. Monterey, Calif.: Healthy Learning.

Drabik, J. (1996). *Children and Sports Training.* Island Pond, Vt.: Stadion Publishing.

Kraemer W., & Fleck, S. (2004). *Strength Training for Young Athletes* (2nd ed.). Champaign, Ill.: Human Kinetics.

Mediate, P. & Faigenbaum, A. (2007). *Medicine Ball for All Kids.* Monterey, Calif.: Healthy Learning.

National Association for Sports and Physical Education (2004). *Physical Best Activity Guide.* Elementary Level (2nd ed.). Champaign, Ill.: Human Kinetics.

National Association for Sports and Physical Education (2004). *Physical Best Activity Guide.* Middle and High School Levels (2nd ed.). Champaign, Ill.: Human Kinetics.

Pate, R. et al. (2006). Promoting physical activity in children and youth. *Circulation,* 114, 1214–1224.

Payne, V. & Issacs, L. (2007). *Human Motor Development* (7th ed.). Boston, Mass.: McGraw Hill.

Volpe, S., Sabelawski, S., & Mohr, C. (2007). *Fitness Nutrition for Special Dietary Needs.* Champaign, Ill.: Human Kinetics.

Watts, K. et al. (2005). Exercise training in obese children and adolescents. *Sports Medicine,* 35, 375–392.

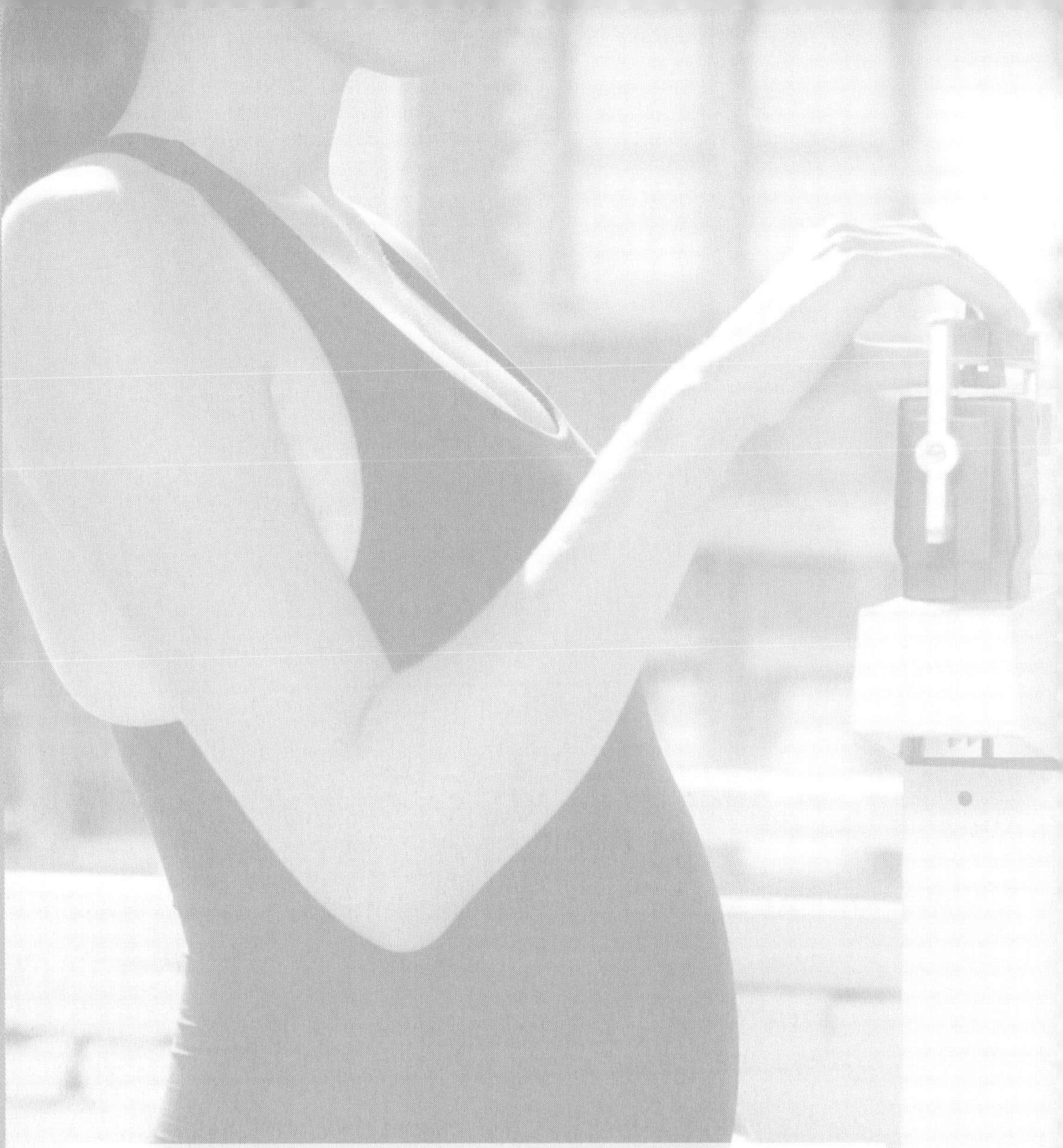

In This Chapter

About The Author

Sabrena Merrill, M.S., has been actively involved in the fitness industry since 1987. An ACE-certified Group Fitness Instructor and Personal Trainer, Merrill teaches group exercise, owns and operates her own personal training business, has managed fitness departments in commercial facilities, and lectured to university students and established fitness professionals. She has a bachelor's degree in exercise science as well as a master's degree in physical education from the University of Kansas, and has numerous certifications in exercise instruction. Merrill acts as a spokesperson for the American Council on Exercise (ACE) and is involved in curriculum development for ACE continuing education programs. Additionally, Merrill presents lectures and workshops to fitness professionals nationwide.

CHAPTER 23

Pre- and Postnatal Exercise

Sabrena Merrill

An increasing amount of research on exercise in pregnancy has led to a waning debate over the maternal and fetal risks of regular physical activity during pregnancy. There is a growing trend of women entering pregnancy with regular aerobic and strength-conditioning activities as a part of their daily routines. Many women who are not physically active view pregnancy as a time to modify their lifestyles to include more health-conscious activities, including exercise.

Traditionally, the medical community has encouraged pregnant women to reduce their habitual levels of physical exertion and refrain from starting strenuous exercise programs. These restrictive guidelines were based on concerns that exercise could negatively affect pregnancy outcomes by increasing core body temperature, raising the risk of congenital anomalies, and shifting oxygenated blood and nutrients to maternal skeletal muscles—and away from the fetus [American College of Obstetricians and Gynecologists (ACOG), 1985; Shangold, 1989]. More recent investigations, however, focusing on both aerobic training and strength conditioning in pregnancy, have shown no increase in early pregnancy loss, late pregnancy complications, abnormal fetal growth, or adverse neonatal outcomes, suggesting that previous recommendations have been overly conservative (Clapp, 1989; Klebanoff et al., 1990; Hatch et al., 1993; Kardel et al., 1998; Sternfeld et al., 1995; O'Neill, 1996).

While prenatal exercise recommendations from allied healthcare professionals are becoming more commonplace, the majority of women do not get the recommended minimum amount of daily physical activity. It is estimated that only 42% of pregnant women exercise 30 minutes or more at least three times a week, and 23% of healthy, previously active women stop exercise or reduce it significantly during pregnancy (Zhang & Savits, 1996; Ning et al., 2003). Given the current epidemic of obesity and its associated comorbidities, as well as the apparent health risks of not exercising, fitness professionals who are competent to work with this population can provide safe and effective exercise programming to promote a healthy pregnancy and healthy lifestyle after the birth.

Benefits and Risks of Exercise During Pregnancy

Evidence is increasing that regular prenatal exercise is an important component of a healthy pregnancy. Expectant mothers can maintain or even improve cardiovascular and muscular fitness. Additionally, regular exercise is associated with a lower incidence of excessive maternal weight gain, **gestational diabetes mellitus (GDM),** pregnancy-induced **hypertension,** varicose veins, **deep vein thrombosis, dyspnea,** and low-back pain (Davies et al., 2003; Weissgerber et al., 2006). Furthermore, it has been shown that women who continue regular, weightbearing exercise throughout the entire duration of pregnancy tend to have easier, shorter, and less complicated deliveries (Clapp, 2002).

Maternal Fitness

Healthy women who consistently exercise throughout pregnancy show a marked reduction in weight gain, fat accumulation, and fat retention. In one study, pregnant exercisers had average increases in weight (29 pounds; 13 kg) and skinfold thicknesses (10 mm) well within the normal range, but their body-fat mass averaged 3% lower than the control subjects who performed no exercise during pregnancy (Clapp & Little, 1995). In other words, the women who performed regular weightbearing exercise throughout their pregnancies maintained a leaner **body composition** than their **sedentary** counterparts.

Due to the many physiological adaptations that occur during pregnancy, women who continue moderate-to-high levels of endurance exercise can experience an increase in their **maximal aerobic capacity** by up to 10% postpartum, even though exercise volume is typically reduced by the added responsibility of childcare (Clapp & Capeless, 1991). Furthermore, improvements in aerobic efficiency, but not necessarily **$\dot{V}O_2$max,** are seen in women who begin a low-volume exercise program (moderate intensity for 20 minutes, three to five days per week) during pregnancy (Clapp, 2002).

Gestational Diabetes

Glucose intolerance that is first recognized or diagnosed during pregnancy is called gestational diabetes. Maternal muscular insulin resistance during mid-pregnancy is a normal response to hormonal adaptations that occur to ensure adequate glucose regulation for fetal growth and development. In women with GDM, this insulin increase is exacerbated, resulting in maternal **hyperglycemia.** Women with GDM are more likely to have complications such as a difficult labor and delivery, as well as delivery by Caesarean section (C-section).

Risk factors for GDM include a family history of diabetes, previous diagnosis of GDM, belonging to a high-risk ethnic group (Aboriginal, Hispanic, South Asian, Asian, or African descent), age ≥35 years, overweight [**body mass index (BMI)** ≥25], obesity (BMI ≥30), or a history of insulin resistance (ACOG, 2001). Once diagnosed, GDM patients are primarily treated through nutritional management by a registered dietician (R.D.). Exercise is considered an adjunct therapy for women with GDM. Preliminary studies have found that women who participated in any type of recreational activity within the first 20 weeks of gestation decreased their risk of GDM by almost half (Dempsey et al., 2004). Research has shown that even mild exercise (30% of $\dot{V}O_2$max, regardless of modality) combined with nutritional control can help prevent GDM and excessive weight gain during pregnancy (Batada et al., 2003).

Preeclampsia

A serious maternal-fetal disease called **preeclampsia** is diagnosed after 20 weeks of gestation and characterized by persistent hypertension (>140/90 mm/Hg) and **proteinuria** (24-hour urinary protein level ≥0.3 g) (ACOG, 2002a). Complications associated with preeclampsia include preterm birth, **abruptio placentae,** renal failure, pulmonary **edema,** cerebral hemorrhage, circulatory collapse, **eclampsia,** and the necessity for immediate delivery regardless of gestational age. Risk factors for preeclampsia include abnormal placental development, predisposing maternal constitutional factors, oxidative stress, immune maladaptation, and genetic susceptibility.

A review of the literature examining physical activity and preeclampsia risk reveals several epidemiological studies that indicate that regular leisure-time physical activity in early pregnancy is associated with a reduced incidence of preeclampsia (Weissgerber et al., 2004). Although not proven, several protective mechanisms associated with exercise are thought to play a role in preeclampsia prevention, including enhanced placental growth and vascularity, enhanced antioxidant defense systems, reduction of the systemic inflammatory response, and improved endothelial function (Weissgerber et al., 2006).

Traditional treatment of gestational hypertension and mild preeclampsia has focused on bed rest to prevent blood pressure increases associated with daily activity. However, up to one-third of women fail to comply with bed rest recommendations, and compliance does not affect pregnancy outcome in women who develop mild preeclampsia in the latter part of gestation (Magee, Ornstein, & von Dadelszen, 1999). More recent treatment guidelines for hypertension and mild preeclampsia have shifted toward ambulatory management with careful patient monitoring (Lenfant, 2001; Moutquin et al., 1997). Exercise intervention studies in women with gestational hypertension and preeclampsia are inconclusive, and it remains unclear whether a program of regular exercise can positively affect this population. Exercise in women with high-risk pregnancy conditions, such as preeclampsia, should be closely monitored and supervised by their physicians in a clinical setting, as these situations are outside the **scope of practice** for an ACE-certified Advanced Health & Fitness Specialist (ACE-AHFS).

Maternal Obesity

In the U.S., the percentage of women of childbearing age (20 to 39 years) who are overweight has climbed to 49% among white women and 70% among African-American women (Okosun et al., 2004). Obesity-related reproductive complications that occur before, during, and after pregnancy may be reduced through lifestyle interventions such as regular aerobic exercise.

Ovulatory infertility increases progressively with increasing BMI, as do the risks for polycystic ovarian syndrome and menstrual irregularities. The effectiveness of regular aerobic exercise (three hours per week) and educational seminars (one hour per week on weight-related topics) on restoring fertility in obese women was demonstrated by a six-month lifestyle intervention study (Clark et al., 1998). The subjects who completed the intervention lost an average of 10.2 ± 4.3 kg (22.4 ± 9.5 lb). Prior to the study, all subjects had been infertile for at least two years; however, 77% of the subjects conceived successfully during or after the lifestyle intervention. The authors hypothesized that improved fertility resulted from the beneficial effects of reduced insulin resistance and lower insulin concentrations on reproductive hormone profiles.

During pregnancy, the risk of maternal and fetal complications increases with the degree of obesity. The incidence of preeclampsia and GDM increase progressively in overweight and obese women. Additionally, overweight and obese women are more likely to deliver large-for-gestational-age infants and require C-section and instrumental delivery. Exercise performed before conception and during pregnancy may help to prevent these obesity-related complications by decreasing BMI to a healthy range, preventing GDM and preeclampsia, and reducing the likelihood of excessive gestational weight gain. Prenatal exercise also has been associated with a timely return to pre-pregnancy weight after delivery (Rooney & Schauberger, 2002).

Maternal Exercise and the Fetal Response

In uncomplicated pregnancies, fetal injuries are highly unlikely, as most of the potential fetal risks are hypothetical. However, there are several areas of theoretical concern surrounding maternal exercise and its effects on the fetus. First, the selective redistribution of blood flow away from the fetus during regular or prolonged exercise in pregnancy may interfere with the transplacental transport of oxygen, carbon dioxide, and nutrients. To address this concern, many experts recommend aquatic exercise as an excellent choice of aerobic training during pregnancy. During immersion, women experience a smaller decrease in plasma volume as compared to exercising on land. In addition, as a result of the hydrostatic pressure in aquatic exercise, maintenance of blood flow around the central organs may provide better maintenance of uterine and placental blood flow (Watson et al., 1991).

A second concern is that during exercise, transient **hypoxia** could result in fetal **tachycardia** and an increase in fetal blood pressure. These fetal responses are protective mechanisms that occur during obstetric events and allow the fetus to facilitate the transfer of oxygen and decrease the carbon dioxide tension across the **placenta.** However, there are no reports to link such adverse events with maternal exercise. A majority of studies examining fetal responses to exercise monitored fetal heart rate as an indicator of fetal stress (Collings, Curet, & Mullin, 1983; Clapp, 1985; Artal, 1990; Carpenter et al., 1988; Wolfe et al., 1988). Most of these studies show a minimum or moderate increase in fetal heart rate by 10 to 30 beats per minute over baseline during or after maternal exercise. Fetal heart rate decelerations and **bradycardia**, with a frequency of 8.9%, have also been reported to occur during maternal exercise. The causes of the alterations in fetal heart rate during maternal exercise are still unclear, and no associated lasting effects on the fetus have been reported.

A third concern is intrauterine growth restriction due to strenuous physical activity. Studies on the effect of exercise during pregnancy and resultant birth weights are inconclusive. Epidemiological studies have shown a link between strenuous physical activity, poor diet, and low birth weight. It has also been reported that mothers who perform strenuous physical work in their occupations, such as repetitive lifting, have a tendency to deliver earlier and have small-for-gestational-age infants (Naeye & Peters, 1982; Launer et al., 1990; McDonald et al., 1988). However, other studies have provided conflicting data suggesting that other variables, such as inefficient nutrition, have to be present for strenuous activities to affect fetal growth (Saurel-Cubizolles & Kaminski, 1987; Ahlborg Bodin, & Hogstedt, 1990). Overall, it appears that birth weight is not affected by exercise in women who have adequate energy intake.

Contraindications and Risk Factors

Research from the past several decades has produced valid and reliable evidence that supports participation in a regular exercise program during pregnancy because of the important maternal-fetal benefits it provides. In fact, the available studies show that adverse pregnancy or neonatal outcomes are not increased for exercising women (Clapp, 1989; Hall & Kaufmann, 1987; Hatch et al., 1993; Klebanoff et al., 1990; Kulpa, White, & Visscher, 1987). ACOG, the American College of Sports Medicine (ACSM), the Canadian Society for Exercise Physiology (CSEP), and the Society of Obstetricians and Gynaecologists of Canada (SOGC) all provided guidelines and recommendations for exercise during pregnancy and the postpartum period that indicate that, in uncomplicated pregnancies, women with or without a previously sedentary lifestyle should be encouraged to participate in aerobic and strength-conditioning exercises as part of a healthy lifestyle (ACSM, 2006; ACOG, 2002b; SOGC & CSEP, 2003). However, it is recommended that women with complicated pregnancies be discouraged from participating in exercise activities for fear of impacting the underlying disorder or maternal or fetal outcomes.

ACOG has established that there are some women for whom exercise during pregnancy is absolutely contraindicated (Table 23-1), while for other women the potential benefits of exercising may outweigh the risks (Table 23-2). Furthermore, fitness professionals and pregnant exercisers should familiarize themselves with specific signs or symptoms that may indicate a problem, including those items listed in Tables 23-3 and 23-4. It is imperative that an ACE-AHFS perform routine health screenings on all clients and require a physician's clearance before initiating an exercise program with a pregnant or postpartum woman.

In general, participation in a wide range of recreational activities appears safe during and after pregnancy. Overly vigorous activity in the third trimester, activities that have a high potential for contact, and activities with a high risk of falling should be avoided (Table 23-5). Additionally, women should refrain from activities with a risk of abdominal trauma, exertion at altitude greater than 6000 feet (1829 m), and scuba diving (ACOG, 2002b).

Table 23-1
Absolute Contraindications to Aerobic Exercise During Pregnancy

- Hemodynamically significant heart disease
- Restrictive lung disease
- Incompetent cervix/cerclage
- Multiple gestation at risk for premature labor
- Persistent second- or third-trimester bleeding
- Placenta previa after 26 weeks of gestation
- Premature labor during the current pregnancy
- Ruptured membranes
- Preeclampsia/pregnancy-induced hypertension

Source: American College of Obstetricians and Gynecologists (2002). Exercise during pregnancy and the postpartum period. ACOG Committee Opinion No. 267. *Obstetrics and Gynecology,* 99, 171–173.

Table 23-2
Relative Contraindications to Aerobic Exercise During Pregnancy

- Severe anemia
- Unevaluated maternal cardiac arrhythmia
- Chronic bronchitis
- Poorly controlled type 1 diabetes
- Extreme morbid obesity
- Extreme underweight (BMI <12)
- History of extremely sedentary lifestyle
- Intrauterine growth restriction in current pregnancy
- Poorly controlled hypertension
- Orthopedic limitations
- Poorly controlled seizure disorder
- Poorly controlled hyperthyroidism
- Heavy smoker

Source: American College of Obstetricians and Gynecologists (2002). Exercise during pregnancy and the postpartum period. ACOG Committee Opinion No. 267. *Obstetrics and Gynecology,* 99, 171–173.

Table 23-3
Reasons to Discontinue Exercise and Seek Medical Advice

- Any sign of bloody discharge from the vagina
- Any "gush" of fluid from the vagina (premature rupture of membranes)
- Sudden swelling of the ankles, hands, or face (possible preeclampsia)
- Persistent, severe headaches and/or visual disturbances (possible hypertension)
- Unexplained spell of faintness or dizziness
- Swelling, pain, and redness in the calf of one leg (possible phlebitis)
- Elevation of pulse rate or blood pressure that persists after exercise
- Excessive fatigue, palpitations, or chest pain
- Persistent contractions (more than six to eight per hour) that may suggest onset of premature labor
- Unexplained abdominal pain
- Insufficient weight gain [less than 1 kg/month (2.2 lb/month)] during last two trimesters

Source: American College of Sports Medicine (2006). *ACSM's Guidelines for Exercise Testing and Prescription* (7th ed.). Philadelphia: Lippincott Williams & Wilkins.

Table 23-4
Warning Signs to Cease Exercise While Pregnant

- Vaginal bleeding
- Dyspnea prior to exertion
- Dizziness
- Headache
- Chest pain
- Muscle weakness
- Calf pain or swelling (need to rule out thrombophlebitis)
- Preterm labor
- Decreased fetal movement
- Amniotic fluid leakage

Source: American College of Obstetricians and Gynecologists (2002). Exercise during pregnancy and the postpartum period. ACOG Committee Opinion No. 267. *Obstetrics and Gynecology,* 99, 171–173.

Table 23-5
High-risk Exercises

- Snow- and waterskiing
- Rock climbing
- Snowboarding
- Diving
- Scuba diving
- Bungee jumping
- Horseback riding
- Ice skating/hockey
- Road or mountain cycling
- Vigorous exercise at altitude (non-acclimated women)

Note: Risk of activities requiring balance is relative to maternal weight gain and morphologic changes; some activities may be acceptable early in pregnancy but risky later on.

Physiological Changes During Pregnancy

During pregnancy, a woman's endocrine system signals changes in virtually every part of her body to prepare her and the fetus for gestation, delivery, and lactation. This section covers the adaptations related to exercise performance. Understanding these factors and how they impact a woman's ability to engage in prenatal physical activity is essential for safe and effective exercise programming.

Musculoskeletal System

With the average weight gain during pregnancy in the range of 25 to 40 pounds (11 to 18 kg) (15 to 25% of pre-pregnancy weight), forces across joints are significantly increased. Such large forces may cause discomfort to normal joints and increase damage to arthritic or previously unstable joints. A woman's enlarging abdomen increases the mechanical stress on the joints of the back, pelvis, hips, and legs as her **center of gravity** moves upward and out. Because of these anatomical changes, pregnant women report a high incidence of low-back pain (up to 76%). (Brynhildsen, 1998; Kristiansson, Svardsudd, & von Schoultz, 1996).

During the first trimester, increased amounts of the hormones **relaxin** and **progesterone** are released to expand the uterine cavity. These hormones allow expansion by softening the ligaments surrounding the joints of the pelvis (hips and lumbosacral spine), thereby increasing mobility and joint laxity. Whether or not joint laxity occurs in other joints, such as the neck, shoulder, or periphery, is unclear. Theoretically, increased mechanical stress combined with joint laxity would predispose pregnant women to increased incidence of strains and sprains. However, with the exception of the reporting of low-back pain, data on the effects of increased weight of pregnancy on joint injury and pathology are lacking. While an increased incidence of falling during pregnancy has not been reported, a woman's balance may be affected by changes in posture, predisposing her to loss of balance and increased risk of falling. Despite a lack of clear evidence that musculoskeletal injuries are increased during pregnancy, these possibilities should be considered when designing prenatal exercise programs.

Cardiovascular System

During pregnancy, the entire cardiovascular system experiences dramatic changes as hormonal signals initiate relaxation and reduced responsiveness in most, if not all, the smooth muscle cells in a woman's blood vessels. In addition to causing many of the unpleasant early symptoms of pregnancy (e.g., lightheadedness, nausea, fatigue, cravings, constipation, bloating, and frequent urination), these hormonal changes result in an increase in the elasticity and volume of the entire circulatory system (i.e., a decrease in systemic vascular resistance). Initially, this creates a vascular "underfill" problem where the amount of blood returning to the heart decreases. To correct the underfill, the body triggers the release of several hormones, which cause a decrease in the excretion of salt and water by the kidneys. Ultimately, the retained extra salt and water expand plasma volume, allowing more venous return to the heart, thereby increasing cardiac output and improving arterial pressure and blood flow to the organs. Eventually, hormonal signals cause increases in heart volumes (chamber volume and **stroke volume**), blood volume, **heart rate,** and **cardiac output.**

By mid-pregnancy, cardiac outputs are 30 to 50% greater than before pregnancy (Morton, 1991). Additionally, maternal stroke volume increases by 10% by the end of the first trimester, and is followed by a 20% increase in heart rate during the second and third trimesters (Pivaranik, 1996; Morton et al., 1985). Maternal resting heart rate can be up to 15 beats per minute higher than pre-pregnancy rates near the third trimester. Mean arterial pressure decreases 5 to 10 mmHg by the middle of the second trimester before gradually increasing back to pre-pregnancy levels. These hemodynamic changes appear to establish a circulatory reserve necessary to provide nutrients and oxygen to both mother and fetus at rest and during moderate exercise. Since heart-rate response among pregnant exercisers is variable, **ratings of perceived exertion (RPE)** should be used to assess intensity instead of traditional heart rate–based methods.

As pregnancy progresses, a woman's body position can affect her cardiovascular system both at rest and during exercise. After the first trimester, the supine position results in relative obstruction of venous return, and therefore decreased cardiac output. For this reason, supine positions should be avoided as much as possible during rest and exercise. In addition, motionless standing is associated with a significant decrease in cardiac output. Therefore, this position should be avoided.

Respiratory System

The delivery of oxygen to the mother and fetus is enhanced through improvements in lung function during pregnancy. At rest, an increase in the depth of each breath increases the amount of air inhaled by up to 50% or more (Prowse & Gaensler, 1965; Artal et al., 1986). This increase is the result of elevated levels of progesterone, which stimulates "overbreathing" by increasing the brain's sensitivity to carbon dioxide. As a result, oxygen tension is increased and carbon dioxide tension is decreased in the alveoli. Ultimately, these directional changes in breathing gases widen the pressure gradients, which improve the efficiency of oxygen uptake from the lungs and the elimination of carbon dioxide from maternal and fetal blood and tissues.

Prenatal adaptations of the respiratory system cause women to experience an associated increase in oxygen uptake and a 10 to 20% increase in baseline oxygen consumption (Pivarnik et al., 1992; Sady et al., 1989). Peak ventilation and maximal aerobic capacity are maintained during pregnancy. As a result of this maintained function and the pregnancy-induced increase in alveolar ventilation, gas transfer at the tissue level may improve. This causes a "training effect" of pregnancy in women who maintain moderate-to-intense exercise programs throughout gestation, and may explain anecdotal reports of women who experience an improvement in competitive endurance performance after giving birth.

Thermoregulatory System

A woman's ability to dissipate heat improves during pregnancy. The improved ability to eliminate body heat is most likely due to a decrease of the body's set point for normal temperature in early pregnancy and a significant increase in blood flow to the skin, which increases the rate of heat loss directly into the air. Additionally, a 40 to 50% increase in tidal volume allows a pregnant woman to increase heat loss through exhalation by 40 to 50%.

During moderate-intensity aerobic exercise in thermoneutral conditions, the core temperature of non-pregnant women rises an average of 1.5° C during the first 30 minutes of exercise, and then reaches a plateau if exercise is continued for an additional 30 minutes (Soultanakis, Artal, & Wiswell, 1996). If heat production exceeds heat dissipation capacity, as is commonly the case during exercise in hot, humid conditions or during very high-intensity exercise, a woman's core temperature will continue to rise. During prolonged exercise, loss of fluid as sweat may compromise heat dissipation. Given that fetal body core temperatures are naturally about 1° C higher than maternal temperatures, maintenance of proper hydration, and therefore blood volume, is critical to heat balance. Research examining the effects of exercise on core temperature during pregnancy is limited. The results of some human studies suggest that **hyperthermia** in excess of 39° C (100° F) during the first 45 to 60 days of gestation may be **teratogenic** in humans (Milunsky et al., 1992; Edwards, 1986). However, there have been no reports that hyperthermia associated with exercise causes malformations of the embryo or fetus in humans.

Programming Guidelines and Considerations for Prenatal Exercise

Exercise programming guidelines for prenatal activity include the same elements as guidelines for non-pregnant women. Aerobic exercise consisting of any activity that uses large muscle groups in a continuous rhythmic manner (e.g., walking, hiking, jogging/running, aerobic dance, swimming, cycling, rowing, dancing, and rope skipping) may be appropriate. Some activities, such as scuba diving and prolonged exertion in the supine position, should be avoided due to the potential for fetal hypoxia. Activities that increase the risk of falls, such as skiing, or those that may result in excessive joint stress, such as jogging and tennis, should be engaged in only after evaluation and consultation with a physician.

Musculoskeletal conditioning appears to be safe and effective during pregnancy when low weights and multiple repetitions through a dynamic, controlled range of motion are performed. While research is lacking, it would be prudent to limit repetitive **isometric** or heavy-resistance weightlifting, as well as any exercises that result in a large **pressor response** (i.e., a disproportionate rise in heart rate during resistance training resulting from **autonomic nervous system** reflex activity). Additionally, maintenance of normal joint range of motion through individualized stretching exercises is acceptable. However, pregnant exercisers should be aware of increased ligamentous laxity and strive to limit excessive stretching or ballistic stretching movements during pregnancy.

Several national health and medical organizations have published recommendations and guidelines on exercise and pregnancy (ACOG, 2002b; ACSM, 2006; SOCG & CSEP, 2003). Not surprisingly, the content in the guidelines from the different organizations is similar. Specifically, the ACOG Committee Opinion on exercise during pregnancy published in 2002 recommends that, barring medical or obstetric contraindications, pregnant women engage in 30 or more minutes of moderate exercise on "most" days of the week (ACOG, 2002b). This recommendation is essentially the same as that made for the general population by the CDC and ACSM (ACSM, 2006). ACOG and ACSM jointly support recommendations stating that the mode, frequency, duration, and overload principles for cardiorespiratory, resistance, and flexibility exercise are the same for pregnant women as for non-pregnant women. According to ACSM, pregnancy-specific issues to consider when designing prenatal exercise programs focus on attaining additional calories to maintain **homeostasis**, avoiding motionless standing, preventing maternal hyperthermia and **hypoglycemia**, and avoiding high-risk exercises (Table 23-6). Furthermore, the sole use of heart-rate monitoring to assess exercise intensity is not recommended for pregnant exercisers due to the natural physiological influences of the cardiovascular system during pregnancy. The "category" RPE scale (6–20) or the "category-ratio" Borg scale (0–10) may be used. Ratings of "fairly light" to "somewhat hard" are the recommended intensity ranges for prenatal exercise (Pivernak et al., 1991; Clapp, Lopez, & Harcar-Sevcik, 1999).

Another set of guidelines, jointly sponsored by SOGC and CSEP, promote similar recommendations as those set forth by ACSM and ACOG,

Table 23-6
Special Considerations for Prenatal Exercise Programming

- Pregnancy requires an additional 300 calories per day to maintain homeostasis. Therefore, women should ingest additional calories to meet the needs of exercise and pregnancy.
- Motionless standing results in venous blood pooling, so it should be avoided.
- Heat dissipation is important throughout pregnancy. Appropriate clothing, environmental considerations, and adequate hydration should be priorities during the exercise program to prevent the possibility of hyperthermia and the corresponding risk to the fetus. Pregnant women should drink ample water to prevent dehydration and avoid brisk exercise in hot, humid weather or when suffering with a fever.
- Maternal hypoglycemia may be associated with strenuous exercise during the last trimester of pregnancy. The reduction in blood glucose may result from increased glucose uptake by the fetus and mother, decreased maternal liver glycogen stores, or reduced maternal liver glycogenolysis. Pregnant women should attenuate the opportunity for hypoglycemia with increased carbohydrate intake (e.g., 30 to 50 g/day) via food and/or a sports drink prior to exercise.
- Pregnant women should avoid exercise that involves the risk of abdominal trauma, falls, and excessive joint stress. Sport activities such as softball, basketball, and racquet sports are not recommended because of the increased risk of abdominal injury. When exercising, pregnant women should be aware of the signs and symptoms for discontinuing exercise and seeking medical advice (see Table 23-3).

Source: American College of Sports Medicine (2006). *ACSM's Guidelines for Exercise Testing and Prescription* (7th ed.). Philadelphia: Lippincott, Williams & Wilkins.

with the addition of a modified version of the conventional age-corrected heart rate target zone for pregnant exercisers (Table 23-7), and a recommendation for resistance exercise and aerobic exercise (SOGC/CSEP, 2003). Furthermore, the SOGC/CSEP position statement provides a plan for inactive women to gradually increase their activity level (i.e., previously sedentary women should begin with 15 minutes of continuous exercise three times a week, increasing gradually to 30-minute sessions four times a week). Table 23-8 presents the joint recommendations of SOGC and CSEP for exercise in pregnancy and the postpartum period.

Table 23-7
Modified Heart Rate Target Zones for Aerobic Exercise in Pregnancy

Maternal Age	Heart Rate Target Zone (beats/min)	Heart Rate Target Zone (beats/10 seconds)
Less than 20	140–155	23–26
20–29	135–150	22–25
30–39	130–145	21–24
40 or greater	125–140	20–23

Note: The most appropriate use of these modified heart rate guidelines is in conjunction with RPE, as blunted, exaggerated, and normal linear responses to exercise have been observed at different stages during pregnancy.

Source: Society of Obstetricians and Gynaecologists of Canada (SOGC) & Canadian Society for Exercise Physiology (CSEP) (2003). Joint SOGC/CSEP clinical practice guideline: Exercise in pregnancy and the postpartum period. *Journal of Obstetrics and Gynaecology Canada,* 25, 6, 516–522.

Table 23-8
Recommendations for Exercise in Pregnancy and the Postpartum Period

- All women without contraindications should be encouraged to participate in aerobic and strength-conditioning exercises as part of a healthy lifestyle during their pregnancy.
- Reasonable goals of aerobic conditioning in pregnancy should be to maintain a good fitness level throughout pregnancy without trying to reach peak fitness or train for an athletic competition.
- Women should choose activities that will minimize the risk of loss of balance and fetal trauma.
- Women should be advised that adverse pregnancy or neonatal outcomes are not increased for exercising women.
- Initiation of pelvic floor exercises in the immediate postpartum period may reduce the risk of future urinary incontinence.
- Women should be advised that moderate exercise during lactation does not affect the quantity or composition of breast milk or impact infant growth.

Validation: This guideline has been approved by the Society of Obstetricians and Gynaecologists of Canada (SOGC) Clinical Practice Obstetrics Committee, the Executive and Council of SOGC, and the Board of Directors of the Canadian Society for Exercise Physiology (CSEP).

Sponsors: This guideline has been jointly sponsored by the SOGC and the CSEP.

Source: Society of Obstetricians and Gynaecologists of Canada (SOGC) & Canadian Society for Exercise Physiology (CSEP) (2003). Joint SOGC/CSEP clinical practice guideline: Exercise in pregnancy and the postpartum period. *Journal of Obstetrics and Gynaecology Canada,* 25, 6, 516–522.

Biomechanical Considerations for the Pregnant Mother

Due to the wide range of postural and physiological adaptations that occur during pregnancy, the ACE-AHFS must be proficient at designing exercise programs geared toward making physical activity more comfortable for this population. Physiological adaptations include a profound increase in body mass, retention of fluid, and laxity in supporting structures. Postural adaptations correspond with these physiological changes and usually entail an alteration in the loading and alignment of, and muscle forces along, the spine and weightbearing joints. During pregnancy, production of the hormone relaxin increases tenfold. The hormone creates joint laxity, which not only allows the pelvis to accommodate the enlarging uterus, but also weakens the ability of static supports in the lumbar spine to withstand shearing forces. In the pelvis, joint laxity is most prominent in the symphysis pubis and the sacroiliac joints.

Typically, it is thought that advancing pregnancy produces a forward shift in the center of gravity followed by an anterior pelvic tilt and subsequent increase in lumbar **lordosis** and thoracic **kyphosis.** However, research on postural changes associated with prenatal weight gain does not confirm this line of thinking (Perkins, Hammer, & Loubert, 1998; Dumas et al., 1995; Moore, Dumas, & Reid, 1990). After the first trimester, the uterus can no longer be contained within the pelvis and moves superiorly and anteriorly. As pregnancy progresses, the biomechanical alterations of increased abdominal girth and weakened abdominal muscles were thought to increase lumbar lordosis; however, studies have shown that the lordosis remains the same or increases only slightly (Hummel, 1987). Instead, it appears that the entire spine shifts to a more posterior position and the center of gravity as a whole tends to move in a posterior and caudal direction. In fact, one study showed that 75% of women demonstrated a more posterior posture, wherein the weight of the uterus was carried posterior to the normal center of gravity (Perkins, Hammer, & Loubert, 1998).

As noted previously, a large majority of women complain of low-back pain during pregnancy (Brynhildsen, 1998; Kristiansson, Svardsudd, & von Schoultz,1996; Perkins, Hammer, & Loubert, 1998). Prenatal low-back and pelvic pain appear to be more related to pre-pregnancy postural habits that are exaggerated during gestation than to postural adaptations to pregnancy. Laxity in the supporting tissues, either pre-existing or enhanced by the hormone relaxin, becomes greater in the direction of habitual posture (Dumas et al., 1995). In other words, pronated feet may become flatter, hyperextended knees may become more pronounced, and spinal curves may soften. Increased ligament laxity has been postulated as a cause for back and pelvic pain, particularly if the pain begins early in the pregnancy before an increase in body mass is evident (Damen et al., 2002; Bullock-Saxton, 1998). During the term of their pregnancies, most women adapt to these postural and physiological changes and, following the baby's delivery, return to their pre-pregnant states.

To alleviate the postural discomforts of exercise, many pregnant women choose to work out in the water. Women who participate in a water exercise class have been shown to experience reduced symptoms of back pain during late pregnancy and miss fewer days at work compared to a control group (Kihlstrand et al., 1999). Aquatic exercise in relatively cool water decreases the rise in body temperature observed during land-based exercise, which can help minimize the risk of hyperthermia (McMurray & Katz, 1990). The hydrostatic pressure exerted on a pregnant woman's body during pool exercise may lessen fluid retention and swelling, and the buoyancy of water supports the bodyweight, relieving pressure on the weightbearing joints and allowing the muscles relief from bearing extra mechanical stress during the pregnancy. Thus, water exercise is a valuable option for women to consider, especially as advancing pregnancy makes other forms of physical activity uncomfortable or stressful on the joints.

In addition to low-back pain, common musculoskeletal complaints that arise during pregnancy include sacroiliac (SI) joint dysfunction, pubic pain, nerve compression syndromes, **diastasis recti,** and **stress urinary incontinence.** The remainder of this section covers each of these conditions in more detail.

Low-back and Posterior Pelvic Pain

The two most common sites of back pain in pregnancy are the lumbar and posterior pelvic areas. Back pain occurs most commonly after the sixth month and can last until the sixth month postpartum. After 12 weeks of pregnancy, the uterus can no longer be contained within the pelvis and the mass moves superiorly and anteriorly. As the abdominal muscles are stretched and tone is diminished, they lose their ability to contribute effectively to the maintenance of neutral posture. In the lumbar spine, joint laxity is most notable in the anterior and posterior longitudinal ligaments. This weakens the ability of static supports in the lumbar spine to withstand the shearing forces. As a result, there may be an increase in discogenic symptoms and/or pain coming from the facet joints.

Lumbar pain during pregnancy is defined as back pain from the lumbar area only, with or without radiation to the legs. **Sciatica** is rare and thought to account for only 1% of low-back pain in pregnancy (Östgaard, Andersson, & Karlsson, 1991; Hainline, 1994). In general, lumbar pain during pregnancy is similar to low-back pain experienced by non-pregnant women. This type of pain typically increases with such prolonged postures as sitting, standing, and repetitive lifting.

Exercises appropriate for pregnant women with lumbar pain include mobility and stretching movements that emphasize relaxing and lengthening the back extensors, hip flexors, scapulae protractors, shoulder internal rotators, and neck flexors. Strengthening exercises should focus on the abdominals, gluteals, and scapulae retractors to reinforce their ability to support proper alignment.

Posterior pelvic pain is four times more prevalent than lumbar pain in pregnancy and is thought to be caused by SI joint dysfunction. Sacroiliac pain is felt distal and lateral to the lumbar spine, with or without lower-extremity radiation, and can occur on one or both sides of the sacrum. Women with sacroiliac pain as their primary complaint tend to have low-back pain for a longer duration than those who simply have lumbar pain. They also tend to experience symptoms for several months after delivery (Hainline, 1994). Occupational activities that involve prolonged postures at extreme ranges, such as sitting at a computer and leaning forward or standing and leaning over a desk or workstation, increase the risk of developing posterior pelvic pain during pregnancy. Unlike other forms of low-back pain during pregnancy, a previous high level of fitness does not necessarily prevent this problem.

The hypothetical origins of SI joint dysfunction during pregnancy focus on decreased stability of the pelvic girdle. It is assumed that the stability of the pelvic girdle is provided, in part, by the coarse texture of the SI cartilage surfaces, the undulated shape of the joint, and the compressive forces of the muscles, ligaments, and thoracolumbar fascia. Muscles that generate a force perpendicular to the SI joints or increase tension on the sacroiliac ligaments or thoracolumbar fascia generate forces that may act to stabilize the SI joint. These include the internal and external abdominal obliques, the latissimus dorsi, the transversospinal parts of the erector spinae muscle (especially the multifidus), and the gluteus maximus. Therefore, functional exercise programs that target this musculature may benefit women with prenatal pelvic pain, partly by increasing muscle force and endurance (Snijders, Vleeming, & Stoeckart, 1993a; Snijders, Vleeming, & Stoeckart, 1993b; Vleeming et al., 1995; Vleeming, Stoeckart, & Snijders, 1989; Vleeming et al., 1989; Vleeming et al., 1996).

Pubic Pain

The irritation of the pubic symphysis caused by increased motion at the joint is called **symphysitis.** Symptoms include mild to severe pain in the pubic region, groin, and medial aspect of the thigh (unilateral or bilateral), frequently accompanied by sacroiliac, low-back, and suprapubic pain. Weightbearing activities, particularly those that involve lifting one leg, intensify the pain. Women also may hear or feel a clicking or grinding sensation in the joint, and there is often difficulty walking, so that a "waddling" gait is adopted.

As noted previously, it has been suggested that pelvic instability is the primary cause of pelvic (sacroiliac and symphysis pubis) joint pain during pregnancy (Fast et al., 1990; Svensson et al., 1990). Pregnancy-related connective tissue changes and the change in the center of gravity result in lengthening, and thus weakening of the ligaments of the pelvic joints, the thoracolumbar fascia, and the surrounding muscles, all of which provide stability to the pelvic ring. Normally, the pre-pregnancy width of the pubic symphysis is 0.5 mm. As pregnancy progresses, the symphysis pubis continues to widen to a maximum of approximately 12 mm. With this widening, there is the risk of vertical displacement of the pubis, and the possibility of rotatory stress on the sacroiliac joints. During delivery, partial symphyseal separations and complete dislocations are possible, resulting in a greater concern for postnatal exercisers.

Treatment of pubic symphysis dysfunction includes avoidance of weightbearing activities that intensify pain, a physician evaluation, and physical therapy. Pelvic belts, which compress the pelvis and minimize motion in the symphysis pubis and SI joint, may be prescribed.

Carpal Tunnel Syndrome

The most common neurological disorder during pregnancy is **carpal tunnel syndrome.** Symptoms include pain and **paresthesias** in the median nerve distribution (thumb, index, and middle fingers), as the nerve becomes depressed as it passes through the carpal tunnel in the wrist. Carpal tunnel syndrome is very common and most often occurs in women aged 30 to 50. Emergence or worsening of carpal tunnel syndrome may occur during pregnancy. The presumed mechanism is pressure on the median nerve within the carpal compartment at the wrist as a result of tissue swelling, secondary to the fluid retention that occurs during pregnancy. Women who develop carpal tunnel syndrome in pregnancy are not likely to develop it again, unless there is another pregnancy. The condition usually discontinues after delivery.

Treatments include ergonomic improvements, analgesia, splinting, and sometimes corticosteroid injection or surgery. Since activities or jobs that require repetitive **flexion** and **extension** of the wrist may contribute to carpal tunnel syndrome, these activities should be minimized. Care should be taken to avoid loading the wrist in hyperextension, grasping objects tightly, and repetitive flexion and extension of the wrist during exercise. Keeping the wrist in its neutral position during physical activities such as weightlifting should provide a comfortable, non-aggravating option for pregnant exercisers.

Diastasis Recti

Diastasis recti is a partial or complete separation between the left and right sides of the rectus abdominis muscle. During pregnancy, the maternal inferior thoracic diameter is increased, thus altering the spatial relationship between the superior and inferior abdominal muscle attachments. In addition, anterior and lateral dimensions of the abdomen during pregnancy increase the distance between muscle attachments, producing increases in muscle length. In some women, the rectus abdominis muscles move laterally and may remain separated in the immediate post-delivery period.

Diastasis recti is commonly seen in women who have multiple pregnancies, because the muscles have been stretched many times. Extra skin and soft tissue in the front of the abdominal wall may be the only signs of this condition in early pregnancy. In late pregnancy, the top of the pregnant uterus is often seen bulging out of the abdominal wall. Three main factors contribute to the incidence and severity of diastasis recti during pregnancy: maternal hormones (relaxin, estrogen, and progesterone), mechanical stress within the abdominal cavity due to increasing girth, and weak abdominal muscles (strong abdominal muscles are more likely to resist this condition).

While some rectus abdominis separation is a normal part of every pregnancy, too much separation may lead to diminished muscular force production and even more separation during physical exertion. The most common test for diastasis recti is performed by placing two fingers horizontally on the suspected location while the client lies supine with the knees bent and performs a curl-up. If the fingers can penetrate at the location, there is probably a split. The degree of separation is measured according to the number of fingerwidths of the split. One to two fingerwidths is considered normal, whereas greater than three fingerwidths is excessive and care should be taken to avoid placing a direct line of stress on the area. Abdominal compression exercises and curl-ups in a semirecumbent position may be helpful for strengthening the rectus abdominis in this situation.

Stress Urinary Incontinence

Stress urinary incontinence (SUI) is the involuntary loss of urine that occurs with physical exertion and a rise in abdominal pressure. Coughing, sneezing, straining, laughing, and impact activities such as jumping and running are events commonly associated with SUI. The pelvic-floor muscles are considered important in maintaining pelvic organ support and bowel and bladder continence. Several studies have shown that women with urinary incontinence have decreased pelvic floor muscle thickness and electromyographic activity, and less muscle strength compared with control subjects without urinary incontinence (Bernstein, 1997; Hoyte et al., 2004; Aanestad & Flink, 1999; Morkved, Schei, & Salvesen, 2003; Morin et al., 2004).

During pregnancy and delivery, the prolonged stretching and trauma sustained by the pelvic floor musculature and the concomitant neural damage thought to accompany this stretching can reduce the strength of the pelvic floor. These changes interfere with the normal transmission of information regarding changes in abdominal pressure to the proximal urethra, thereby predisposing the woman to SUI. Five risk factors predispose a woman to postpartum SUI: Multiple pregnancies, vaginal delivery, high infant birth weight (>8.1 lb; 3.7 kg), large infant cranial circumference (>13.8 inches; 35.5 cm), high maternal weight gain during pregnancy (>28.6 lb; 13 kg), and tearing of the perineum during delivery.

Women experiencing SUI during pregnancy and/or childbirth are generally thought to have a greater risk of developing the condition later in life.

Treatment of SUI during and after pregnancy includes the performance of **Kegel exercises** to strengthen the pelvic-floor muscles. Since the introduction of Kegel exercises in 1948, the efficacy of pelvic-floor muscle strengthening in the treatment of SUI has been supported by the findings of several randomized controlled studies and systematic reviews (Burns et al., 1993; Bo, Talseth, & Holm, 1999; Henalla et al., 1989; Goode et al., 2003; Hay-Smith et al., 2002). The benefits of an effective Kegel exercise regimen include providing support for the pelvic organs; preventing prolapse (falling) of the bladder, uterus, and rectum; supporting proper pelvic alignment; reinforcing sphincter control; enhancing circulation to the pelvic floor muscles; and providing a healthy environment for the healing process after labor and delivery (Dunbar, 1992). Women who exercise during pregnancy and resume it early in the postpartum period have a shorter duration of SUI than those who do not (Morkved & Bo, 2000).

Nutritional Considerations

After the thirteenth week of pregnancy, approximately 300 additional calories per day are required to meet the metabolic needs of pregnancy. Weightbearing exercise, such as walking, increases the energy requirement even further. Furthermore, as the pregnancy progresses, the caloric needs of the mother progressively increase in correspondence with the increase in body weight. An added concern related to nutrition during pregnancy is adequate carbohydrate intake. Pregnant women use carbohydrates at a greater rate both at rest and during exercise than do non-pregnant women (Clapp et al., 1988; Soultanakis, Artal, & Wiswell, 1996). Since maternal blood glucose is the fetus' primary energy source, there is concern that low maternal blood glucose could compromise fetal energy supply. However, intrauterine growth retardation, or other short- or long-term effects on newborns of exercising mothers, have not been reported (ACOG, 2002b; Clapp, Lopez, & Harcar-Sevcik, 1999). As a precaution to help avoid hypoglycemia, pregnant women should be reminded to consume a pre-exercise snack and eat frequent small meals throughout the day, especially later in pregnancy. Pregnant exercisers should be made aware of the signs of hypoglycemia, such as weakness, dizziness, fatigue, and nausea.

The position of the American Dietetic Association (ADA) on nutrition during pregnancy maintains that the key components of a healthy lifestyle during pregnancy include appropriate weight gain (Table 23-9); consumption of a variety of foods in accordance with the MyPyramid Food Guidance System; appropriate and timely vitamin and mineral supplementation; avoidance of tobacco, alcohol, and other harmful substances; and safe food-handling practices (ADA, 2002). The ADA recommends that pregnant women eat a total of 2500 to 2700 calories per day, and that those calories should come from a variety of healthy foods. Additionally, women considering becoming pregnant need to ensure that they are consuming adequate amounts of folic acid, iron, calcium, vitamin D, and water to sustain health before, during, and after pregnancy. The ACE-AHFS should encourage pregnant clients to consult with their physicians in the area of nutrition during pregnancy. For a more detailed analysis of nutrition concerns in pregnancy,

Table 23-9
Appropriate Weight Gain During Pregnancy

Weight Classification	Weight Gain Goal*
Underweight	About 28 to 40 pounds (13 to 18 kg)
Normal weight	About 25 to 35 pounds (11 to 16 kg)
Overweight	About 15 to 25 pounds (7 to 11 kg)
Obese	At least 15 pounds (7 kg)

* Women should talk to their healthcare providers about how much weight they should gain during pregnancy. The general weight-gain recommendations listed here refer to weight before pregnancy and are for women expecting only one baby.

Source: U.S. Department of Health and Human Services, National Institutes of Health. *Fit for Two: Tips for Pregnancy*. win.niddk.nih.gov/publications/two.htm.

refer to the American Dietetic Association's position statement: "Nutrition and Lifestyle for a Healthy Pregnancy Outcome" (ADA, 2002).

Psychological Considerations

Pregnancy is associated with increased psychological distress for many women, which includes increased **anxiety, depression,** and fatigue. Investigations that measured depressive symptoms throughout pregnancy have shown that depression is more common during the third trimester and that an overwhelming majority (97%) of women report fatigue as a concern at some point during their pregnancy (Evans et al., 2001; Zib, Lim, & Walters, 1999). In most societies, it is a long-held belief that a mother's psychological state can influence her unborn baby. Some studies have shown that babies of stressed or anxious mothers have a significantly lower average birth weight for gestational age and tend to be born early (Perkin et al., 1993; Wadwa et al., 1993; Copper et al., 1996; Hedegaard et al., 1996). This is an area of concern because low birth weight seems to be associated with health problems in later life (e.g., hypertension and ischemic heart disease) (Barker, 1995). Furthermore, ultrasound studies have shown that fetal behavior is affected by maternal anxiety (Ianniruberto & Tajani, 1981; Groome et al., 1995). It has been proposed that maternal stress or anxiety might affect the fetus through increased concentrations of maternal hormones being transported directly across the placenta (Gitau et al., 1998). In addition, blood flow to the baby may be impaired through the uterine arteries with high levels of maternal anxiety, which would contribute to the low birth weights associated with psychologically distressed mothers (Teixeira, Fisk, & Glover, 1999).

Another major psychological concern for many women is postpartum or postnatal depression. Postnatal depression affects approximately 10 to 13% of women in the early weeks postpartum, with episodes typically lasting two to six months. This depressive disorder has well-documented health consequences for the mother, child, and family. Women who have postpartum depression are significantly more likely to experience future episodes of depression (Cooper & Murray, 1995), and infants and children are particularly vulnerable to difficulties with maternal bonding and developmental problems because of impaired maternal-infant interactions and negative perceptions of infant behavior. The cause of postnatal depression is unclear. However, research suggests the influence of psychosocial and psychological risk factors, such as life stress, unemployment, marital conflict, maternal self-esteem, and lack of social support (O'Hara & Swain, 1996; Cooper & Murray, 1997; Beck, 2001; Bernazzani et al., 1997; O'Hara et al., 1991; Gotlib et al., 1991).

A disorder related to postpartum depression, but considered not as severe, is called "maternity blues." Maternity blues refers to the tearfulness, irritability, **hypochondriasis,** sleeplessness, impairment of concentration, and headache that occurs in the 10 days or so postpartum. A peak in symptoms typically occurs around the fourth to fifth day after delivery, coinciding with maximal hormonal changes, which include falling concentrations of progesterone, estradiol, and cortisol and rising prolactin concentrations. During pregnancy, progesterone concentrations slowly rise to a maximum until they reach levels several hundred times higher than normal. After delivery and the withdrawal of the placenta, there is a precipitous drop in progesterone concentration. It is hypothesized that the symptoms of maternity blues are related to progesterone withdrawal (Harris et al., 1994). Cortisol concentrations also rise during pregnancy to several times their normal values. They rise further during the stress of labor and then slowly return to normal within 15 days of delivery.

As noted earlier, many previously active women stop exercise or significantly reduce it during pregnancy (Zhang & Savits, 1996; Ning et al., 2003). Given the known links between physical inactivity and reduced mental health, it is plausible that a relationship exists between pregnancy-related reductions in physical activity and psychological distress. A small number of investigations have found that low physical activity is associated with higher scores on anxiety, depression, and fatigue scales during pregnancy (DaCosta et al., 2003; Goodwin, Astbury, & McMeeken, 2000; Koniak-Griffin, 1994; Wallace et al., 1986). In a study that measured physical activity and mood during pregnancy, it was shown that healthy women who maintain an above-average level of physical activity during the second and third trimesters enjoy more mood stability (Poudevigne & O'Connor, 2005). These findings support the theory that regular endurance exercise throughout pregnancy not only improves maternal and fetal physical health, but may enhance psychological health as well.

Benefits and Risks of Exercise Following Pregnancy

Regular exercise is as beneficial in the postpartum period as it is at other times in a woman's life. The possible benefits include the following:

- Preventing obesity (or overweight) through promotion of body fat/body weight loss
- Promoting aerobic fitness and strength, leading to an improved ability to perform activities of mothering
- Optimizing bone health by increasing bone mineral density and/or preventing lactation-associated bone loss
- Improving mood or self-esteem

Furthermore, a mother's participation in regular exercise after childbirth may encourage regular physical activity in her children.

A theoretical risk of postpartum exercise is that strenuous activity in women who breastfeed may alter the quality (e.g., macronutrient and micronutrient composition, immunological properties, accumulation of exercise by-products) or quantity of their milk. However, a review of the literature pertaining to breast milk production and composition in relation to postnatal exercise revealed that there were no remarkable differences in the breast milk of women who performed submaximal exercise, maximal exercise, or who were physically inactive (Larson-Meyer, 2002). The author of the review concluded that several studies have collectively determined that neither acute nor regular exercise has adverse effects on a mother's ability to successfully breastfeed. Another potential risk of postnatal exercise involves new mothers who deliver their babies via C-section. If physical activity is resumed prematurely, there is a risk of disrupting post-surgery healing.

Epidemiological studies have shown an association between higher levels of physical activity in the postpartum period and a return to pre-pregnancy body weight, as well as an increased loss of pregnancy-associated weight gain (Ohlin & Rossner, 1996; Sampselle et al., 1999; Harris, Ellison, & Clement, 1999). A randomized control study that compared the effect of a combination of diet (500 calories less than predicted total energy expenditure) plus exercise to no intervention on weight loss and body composition in overweight lactating women found that the combined diet and exercise intervention resulted in significantly greater weight and fat loss compared with the control group (Lovelady et al., 2000).

Research is lacking on maternal aerobic fitness and strength during the postpartum period. However, two randomized controlled trials have found a significant increase in aerobic capacity resulting from an endurance-exercise intervention during the first 10 to 12 weeks postpartum (Dewey et al., 1994; Lovelady et al., 2000). To date, studies have not assessed the effect of strength training (with or without aerobic exercise) during the postpartum period on muscle strength and endurance or the preservation of lean body mass. It seems reasonable to state, however, that the possible benefit of maternal fitness on the daily physical activities of mothering, including lifting, carrying, or running after a child, is worth the effort of beginning or maintaining regular exercise during the postpartum period.

Lactation in the two-to-six-month postpartum period is associated with axial bone loss. It is speculated that these changes result from the prolonged lactation-induced estrogen deficiency, combined with the "calcium drain" of breastfeeding (an additional 200 to 400 mg per day of calcium is required during lactation). It is unclear whether exercise can attenuate or prevent lactation-associated bone loss. Research demonstrates, however, that bone loss recovers in healthy women with the cessation of lactation and the return of normal menses (Cross et al., 1995; Sowers et al., 1993; Ritchie et al., 1998).

As noted previously, dealing with the hormonal changes and fatigue associated with becoming a new mother often results in emotional distress. Some women have trouble finding the time or energy to exercise, and some feel guilty about being away from the baby to exercise. Longitudinal studies suggest that the incidence of significant postpartum depression is lower in exercising women compared with active controls (Clapp, 2002). The author hypothesized that depression occurs less in physically active women because exercise gives them a regular break from the 24-hour, seven-day-a-week commitment that comes with a new infant. In other words, physically active postpartum women appear less overwhelmed and more ready to master motherhood. It has also been reported that exercising women have a more positive self-image during and after pregnancy than do non-exercising women (Clapp, 2002). Additionally, among postnatal women, an acute bout of aerobic exercise has been shown to lead to decreases in acute transitory anxiety and depression as well as increases in vigor (Koltyn & Schultes, 1997).

Research on the quantity and quality of breast milk in physically active women has found no affect on the volume (adjusted for infant's weight) or the energy density or energy composition (protein, lipid, and lactose) of breast milk in non-overweight women training vigorously or in overweight women randomly assigned to an exercise and calorie-restriction intervention (Lovelady, Lonnerdal, & Dewey, 1990; Lovelady et al., 2000). These investigations also found no differences in body weight or growth among infants whose mothers were in either the exercise or control groups. As a result of anecdotal reports from mothers who claimed that their babies often had a difficult time breastfeeding post-workout, researchers examined the levels of lactic acid accumulation in breast milk after exercise (Wallace, Inbar, & Ernsthausen, 1992). Lactic acid may have initially been targeted among other metabolites that increase with exercise (e.g., hydrogen ion and ammonia) because it readily diffuses into the water compartments of the body (making it likely to diffuse into breast milk). Research in this area has been inconclusive due to inconsistent reports of lactic acid concentrations in breast milk and study results showing that infant acceptance of breast milk is not reduced after submaximal or maximal exercise (Carey, Quinn, & Goodwin, 1997; Quinn & Carey, 1999; Carey & Quinn, 2001; Wright, Carey, & Quinn, 1999).

With regard to exercising after childbirth, a major consideration is the method of delivery. Women who have undergone C-section have had major abdominal surgery that results in pain and tenderness in the abdomen, as well as considerable fatigue. The current thinking on recovery and rehabilitation after C-section is that walking as soon as possible after the surgery helps to minimize muscle wasting, increase circulation, and speed the healing process. Additionally, deep breathing, abdominal compression exercises, and Kegels can be resumed early in the recovery process. Many women are ready to introduce intermittent walking or other gentle forms of exercise by two weeks postpartum, with the degree of discomfort, fatigue, and motivation guiding activity levels. Vigorous exercise is contraindicated after a C-section until the recovery and rehabilitation process is complete. Re-entry into a structured fitness program should be postponed until a physician's clearance has been obtained after the six-week postpartum check-up.

Physiological Changes Following Pregnancy

As in pregnancy, the physiological changes following pregnancy are primarily determined by the endocrine system. The hormones that dominate during pregnancy return to pre-pregnancy levels after childbirth, which results in concomitant changes in the musculoskeletal, cardiovascular, and respiratory systems.

The hormone relaxin, responsible for producing laxity in the collagenous structures of the pelvis and other areas in preparation for childbirth, rises to 10 times its normal level during pregnancy. While the research is not clear on how long it takes for relaxin to subside to pre-pregnancy levels after delivery, ligamentous overstretching can remain in a new mother for up to eight months postpartum. For this reason, a new mother should learn how to correctly lift and carry her baby, put the baby in the crib, and take the baby out of the crib to reduce the risk of back pain due to the relaxed soft-tissue structures supporting the joints.

During pregnancy, the cardiovascular system adapts by increasing blood volume, heart rate, and cardiac output. Plasma volume increases by as much as 40 to 50% and red cell volume goes up by 15 to 20% to maintain the increased circulatory need of the enlarging uterus and fetoplacental unit, fill the ever-increasing venous reservoir, and protect the mother from the blood loss at the time of delivery. It takes about eight weeks after delivery for the blood volume to return to pre-pregnancy levels. Cardiac output increases by 30 to 40% during pregnancy, with the maximum increase attained at 24 weeks of gestation. The increase in heart rate lags behind the increase in cardiac output initially, and then ultimately increases by 10 to 15 bpm by 28 to 32 weeks of gestation. Cardiac output, heart rate, and stroke volume decrease to pre-labor values 24 to 72 hours after birth and return to non-pregnant levels within six to eight weeks after delivery.

The respiratory system exhibits adaptations to pregnancy starting as early as the fourth week of gestation. A woman can expect minute ventilation to increase by about 50% above non-pregnant values and tidal volume and respiratory rate to also increase during pregnancy. Within six to 12 weeks postpartum, all respiratory parameters return to non-pregnant values.

Because of the gradual return to pre-pregnancy musculoskeletal, cardiovascular, and respiratory parameters, and the detraining effect that occurs for most women during pregnancy, postpartum exercise programs should be individualized and resumed gradually. There are no known maternal complications associated with the resumption of exercise training postpartum (Hale & Milne, 1996). Furthermore, moderate weight reduction while nursing is considered safe and does not compromise neonatal weight gain (McCrory et al., 1999).

Programming Guidelines and Considerations for Postnatal Exercise

From an analysis of the available physiological data in the perinatal period, ACOG has developed guidelines for postpartum exercise. The guidelines are very general and state that many of the physiological and morphological changes of pregnancy persist four to six weeks postpartum, and recommend that pre-pregnancy exercise routines be resumed gradually based on the woman's physical capabilities (ACOG, 2002b). A more detailed set of guidelines for postnatal exercise has been developed by Clapp (2002), who suggests that the initial goal of exercise (within the first six weeks) is to obtain personal time and redevelop a sense of control. This can be accomplished by doing the following:

- Beginning slowly and increasing gradually
- Avoiding excessive fatigue and dehydration
- Supporting and compressing the abdomen and breasts
- Stopping to evaluate if it hurts
- Stopping exercise and seeking medical evaluation if the postpartum client is experiencing bright red vaginal bleeding that is heavier than a menstrual period

Clapp goes on to suggest that after six weeks postpartum, the goal of the exercise regimen in the remainder of the first year following birth is to improve physical fitness. Other recommendations suggest that, if pregnancy and delivery are uncomplicated, a mild exercise program consisting of walking, pelvic floor exercises, and stretching may begin immediately (Kochan-Vintinner, 1999). However, if delivery was complicated or was by C-section, a physician should be consulted before resuming pre-pregnancy levels of physical activity, usually after the first postpartum check-up at six to eight weeks (Kochan-Vintinner, 1999).

One area of concern for many women after childbirth is strengthening the pelvic floor. It is estimated that up to three months after delivery, 20 to 30% of women have SUI and about 4%

have fecal incontinence (Wilson, Herbison, & Herbison, 1996; MacArthur, Lewis, & Bick, 1993; MacArthur, Bick, & Keighley, 1997; Sultan et al., 1993). The pelvic-floor muscles form the pelvic basin and help maintain continence by actively supporting the pelvic organs and closing the pelvic openings when contracting. The pelvic-floor muscles are composed of the pelvic diaphragm muscles (together known as the levator ani), which can be referred to as the deep layer; the urogenital diaphragm muscles (together known as the perineal muscles), which can be referred to as the superficial layer; and the urethral and anal sphincter muscles (Figure 23-1). The pelvic-floor muscles are encased in fascia, which is connected to the endopelvic (parietal) fascia surrounding the pelvic organs and assists in pelvic organ support.

Correct action of the pelvic-floor muscles has been described as a squeeze around the pelvic openings and an inward lift (such as the action performed during a Kegel exercise). Pelvic-floor muscle training can increase the strength of the pelvic-floor muscles, thereby enhancing the structural support, timing, and strength of automatic contraction and resulting in the reduction or elimination of leakage. Initially, Kegel exercises can be performed utilizing the following three steps:

- Tightening the pelvic floor muscles and holding a static contraction for a count of 10
- Relaxing the muscles completely for a count of 10
- Performing 10 Kegel exercise sets, three times per day

Another option is to perform the Kegel exercises quickly (tighten, lift up, and let go) to work the muscles in a way that mimics shutting off the flow of urine to help prevent accidents. Many women prefer to do these exercises while lying down or sitting in a chair, but they can be performed anywhere. After four to six weeks, there is usually some improvement, but it may take up to three months to see a significant change.

Training the pelvic-floor musculature goes hand-in-hand with performing exercises to strengthen the core. Research findings have shown that maximum pelvic-floor muscle contractions are not possible without a co-contraction of the abdominal muscles, specifically the transversus abdominis and internal oblique muscles (Bo et al., 1990; Neumann & Gill, 2002). This abdominal contraction can be observed as a small inward movement of the lower abdomen. Prior to any strenuous abdominal exercise, postnatal clients should perform transversus abdominis work (i.e., a drawing-in maneuver), pelvic tilts, and spinal stabilization exercises. Since traditional abdominal crunches compress the abdominal space and increase pressure on the pelvic floor, they should be reserved for exercise regimens after the postnatal client has had time to re-educate the pelvic floor muscles through Kegel training and core stabilization work.

Figure 23-1
Pelvic floor muscles (inferior view)

Source: © Anatomedia Pty Ltd. (www.anatomedia.com)

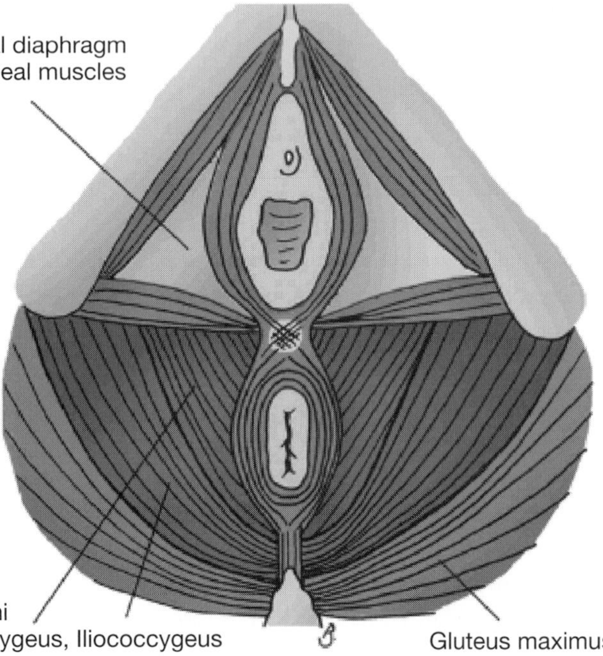

Biomechanical Considerations for the Lactating Mother

Increased weight in the breasts from lactation, coupled with the forward-rounded postures associated with holding, feeding, and cuddling the baby, may lead to upper-back pain in a new mother. Additionally, lifting car seats and pushing strollers with handles that are set too low can contribute to the back pain often reported after childbirth. Stretches for the anterior shoulder girdle, followed by scapular retraction and external shoulder rotation exercises, are appropriate for new mothers looking to improve posture post-delivery and ease the pain associated with these biomechanical concerns.

Good breast support is important for comfort during postpartum exercise. It is recommended that postnatal exercisers wear a very supportive exercise bra, or two bras together if necessary. Furthermore, breastfeeding women are advised to avoid exercise with a breast abscess or with painful, engorged breasts. Nursing or expressing milk before exercise has also been suggested to increase comfort during exercise.

Case Study

Jacki S. is 37 years old and has recently discovered she is pregnant. She is in her first trimester and would like to continue her exercise program. Currently, Mrs. S. runs 3 to 4 (5 to 6 km) miles per workout for a total of about 12 to 15 (19 to 24 km) miles per week, and lifts weights two days a week. She has been cleared by her physician to continue her current routine as long as she reduces her exercise as overall discomfort dictates. Mrs. S. has two children already, and during both pregnancies suffered from mild diastasis recti and lumbar back pain.

Frequency: Mrs. S. may continue to exercise at least three times per week following her typical exercise routine.

Intensity: Mrs. S. should use RPE to monitor the intensity of her workout and aim for a rating of "fairly light" to "somewhat hard," or 11 to 13 on Borg's 6 to 20 scale. She should also be instructed to avoid hot and humid conditions and remain properly hydrated.

Time: Mrs. S. should be encouraged to exercise in accordance with her regular exercise program. However, she should be instructed not to continue an exercise session to the point of fatigue or exhaustion.

Type: Mrs. S. may continue to perform weightbearing exercise, including running, as long as she is comfortable. As her pregnancy progresses, she may want to perform non-weightbearing exercise such as cycling or water aerobics, especially if she notices a recurrence of the low-back pain she experienced in her first two pregnancies. Mrs. S. may continue her resistance-training program, but may find lighter resistance and higher repetitions more comfortable than a higher-intensity program. She should be instructed to avoid prolonged exercise in the supine position after the first trimester.

Exercises appropriate for Mrs. S. that will help her avoid low-back pain include mobility and stretching movements that emphasize relaxing and lengthening the back extensors, hip flexors, scapulae protractors, shoulder internal rotators, and neck flexors. Strengthening exercises should focus on the abdominals, gluteals, and scapulae retractors to reinforce their ability to support proper alignment. Specifically, abdominal compression exercises and curl-ups in a semirecumbent position may be helpful for strengthening the rectus abdominis without exacerbating her diastasis recti.

Summary

An increasing amount of research on exercise in pregnancy has led to less debate regarding the maternal and fetal risks of regular physical activity during pregnancy. Women entering pregnancy with regular aerobic and strength-conditioning activities as a part of their daily routines is a growing trend, and many women who are not physically active view pregnancy as a time to modify their lifestyles to include more health-conscious activities.

Evidence that regular prenatal exercise is an important component of a healthy pregnancy is increasing. The positive affects of exercise during pregnancy on the musculoskeletal, cardiovascular, respiratory, and thermoregulatory systems have been reported. Several national health and medical organizations have published recommendations and guidelines on exercise and pregnancy (ACOG, 2002b; ACSM, 2006; SOCG & CSEP, 2003). According to ACOG (2002b), there are some women for whom exercise during pregnancy is absolutely contraindicated, and others for whom the potential benefits associated with exercise may outweigh the risks.

Due to the wide range of postural and physiological adaptations that occur during and after pregnancy, the ACE-AHFS must be proficient at designing exercise programs geared toward making physical activity more comfortable for this population. Physiological adaptations include a profound increase in body mass, retention of fluid, and laxity in supporting structures. Postural adaptations correspond with these physiological changes and usually entail an alteration in the loading and alignment of, and muscle forces along, the spine and weightbearing joints.

For more detailed information on exercise and pregnancy, refer to *Pre- and Post-Natal Fitness: A Guide for Fitness Professionals from the American Council on Exercise*, available at www.acefitness.org.

References

Aanestad, O. & Flink, R. (1999). Urinary stress incontinence: A urodynamic and quantitative electromyographic study of the perineal muscles. *Acta Obstetricia et Gynecologica Scandinavica*, 78, 245–253.

Ahlborg, G., Bodin, L.. & Hogstedt, C. (1990) Heavy lifting during pregnancy: A hazard to the fetus? A prospective study. *International Journal of Epidemiology*, 19, 90–97.

American College of Obstetricians and Gynecologists (2002a). Exercise during pregnancy and the postpartum period, ACOG Committee Opinion No. 276. *Obstetrics and Gynecology*, 99, 171–173.

American College of Obstetricians and Gynecologists (2002b). Diagnosis and management of pre-eclampsia and eclampsia. *International Journal of Gynaecology and Obstetrics*, 77, 67–75.

American College of Obstetricians and Gynecologists (2001). Clinical management guidelines for obstetrician-gynecologists: Gestational diabetes. *Obstetrics and Gynecology*, 98, 525–538.

American College of Obstetricians and Gynecologists (1985). *Exercise During Pregnancy and the Postnatal Period.* Washington, D.C.: American College of Obstetricians and Gynecologists.

American College of Sports Medicine (2006*). ACSM's Guidelines for Exercise Testing and Prescription* (7th ed.). Philadelphia: Lippincott Williams & Wilkins.

American Dietetic Association (2002). Position of the American Dietetic Association: Nutrition and lifestyle for a healthy pregnancy outcome. *Journal of the American Dietetic Association*, 102, 10, 1479–1490.

Artal, R. (1990). Exercise and diabetes mellitus: A brief review. *Sports Medicine*, 9, 261–265.

Artal, R. et al. (1986). Pulmonary responses to exercise in pregnancy. *American Journal of Obstetrics and Gynecology*, 154, 378–383.

Barker, D.J. (1995). The fetal origins of adult disease. *Proceedings of the Royal Society London Biological Sciences*, 262, 37–43.

Batada, A. et al. (2003). Effects of a nutrition, exercise and lifestyle intervention program (NELIP) on women at risk for gestational diabetes (GDM). *Canadian Journal of Applied Physiology*, 28, S29.

Beck, C.T. (2001). Predictors of postpartum depression: An update. *Nursing Research*, 50, 275–285.

Bernazzani, O. et al. (1997). Psychosocial predictors of depressive symptomatology level in postpartum women. *Journal of Affective Disorders*, 46, 39–49.

Bernstein, I. (1997). The pelvic floor muscles: Muscle thickness in healthy and urinary incontinent women measured by perineal ultrasonography with reference to the effect of pelvic floor training—estrogen receptor studies. *Neurourology and Urodynamics*, 6, 237–275.

Bo, K., Talseth, T. & Holm, I. (1999). Single blind, randomized controlled trial of pelvic floor exercises, electrical stimulation, vaginal cones, and no treatment in the management of genuine stress incontinence in women. *British Medical Journal*, 318, 487–493.

Bo, K. et al. (1990). Pelvic floor muscle exercise for the treatment of female stress urinary incontinence, II: Validity of vaginal pressure measurements of pelvic floor muscle strength and the necessity of supplementary methods for control of correct contraction. *Neurourology and Urodynamics*, 9, 479–487.

Brynhildsen, J. (1998). Follow-up of patients with low back pain during pregnancy. *Obstetrics and Gynecology*, 91, 2, 182–86.

Bullock-Saxton, J. (1998). Musculoskeletal changes in the perinatal period. In: Sapsford, R., Bullock-Saxton, J., & Markwell, S. *Women's Health: A Textbook for Physiotherapists*. pp. 134–161. London: WB Saunders.

Burns, P.A. et al. (1993). A comparison of effectiveness of biofeedback and pelvic muscle exercise treatment of stress incontinence in older community-dwelling women. *Gerontology*, 48, M167–M174.

Carey, G.B. & Quinn, T.J. (2001). Exercise and lactation: Are they compatible? *Canadian Journal of Applied Physiology*, 26, 55–74.

Carey, G.B., Quinn, T.J., & Goodwin, S.E. (1997). Breast milk composition after exercise of different intensities. *Journal of Human Lactation*, 13, 115–120.

Carpenter, M.W. et al. (1988). Fetal heart rate response to maternal exertion. *Journal of the American Medical Association*, 259, 3006–3009.

Clapp, J.F. (2002). *Exercising Through Your Pregnancy*. Champaign, Ill.: Human Kinetics.

Clapp, J.F. (1989). The effects of maternal exercise on early pregnancy outcome. *American Journal of Obstetrics and Gynecology*, 161, 1453–1457.

Clapp, J.F. (1985). Fetal heart rate responses to running in mid-pregnancy and late pregnancy. *American Journal of Obstetrics and Gynecology*, 153, 251-252.

Clapp, J.F. & Capeless, E.L. (1991). The $\dot{V}O_2$max of recreational athletes before and after pregnancy. *Medicine & Science in Sports & Exercise*, 23, 1128–1133.

Clapp, J.F. & Little, K.D. (1995). The effect of endurance exercise on pregnancy weight gain and subcutaneous fat deposition. *Medicine & Science in Sports & Exercise*, 27, 170–177.

Clapp, J.F., Lopez, B., & Harcar-Sevcik, R. (1999). Neonatal behavioral profile of the offspring of women who continued to exercise regularly throughout pregnancy. *American Journal of Obstetrics and Gynecology*, 180, 91–94.

Clapp, J.F. et al. (1988). Maternal physiologic adaptations to early human pregnancy. *American Journal of Obstetrics and Gynecology*, 159, 1456–1460.

Clark, A.M. et al. (1998). Weight loss in obese infertile women results in improvement in reproductive outcome for all forms of fertility treatment. *Human Reproduction*, 13, 1502-1505.

Collings, C.M.S., Curet, L.B., & Mullin, J.P. (1983). Maternal and fetal responses to a maternal aerobic exercise program. *American Journal of Obstetrics and Gynecology*, 145, 702–707.

Cooper, P. & Murray, L. (1997). Prediction, detection, and treatment of postnatal depression. *Archives of Disease in Childhood*, 77, 97–99.

Cooper, P.J. & Murray, L. (1995). Course and recurrence of postnatal depression: Evidence for the specificity of the diagnostic concept. *British Journal of Psychiatry*, 166, 191–195.

Copper, R.L. et al. (1996). The preterm prediction study: Maternal stress is associated with spontaneous preterm birth at less than 35 weeks gestation. *American Journal of Obstetrics and Gynecology*, 175, 1286–1292.

Cross, N.A. et al. (1995). Changes in bone mineral density and markers of bone remodeling during lactation and post-weaning in women consuming high amounts of calcium. *Journal of Bone Mineral Research*, 10, 1312–1320.

DaCosta, D. et al. (2003). Self-reported leisure time physical activity during pregnancy and relationship to psychological well-being. *Journal of Psychosomatic Obstetrics and Gynaecology*, 24, 111–119.

Damen, L. et al. (2002). The prognostic value of asymmetric laxity of the sacroiliac joints in pregnancy-related pelvic pain. *Spine*, 27, 24, 2820–2824.

Davies, G.A. et al. (2003) Joint SOGC/CSEP clinical practice guideline: Exercise in pregnancy and the postpartum period. *Canadian Journal of Applied Physiology*, 28, 330–341.

Dempsey, J.C. et al. (2004). A case-control study of maternal recreational physical activity and risk of gestational diabetes mellitus. *Diabetes Research and Clinical Practice*, 66, 203–215.

Dewey, K.G. et al. (1994). A randomized study of the effects of aerobic exercise by lactating women on breast-milk volume and composition. *New England Journal of Medicine*, 330, 449–453.

Dumas, G.A. et al. (1995). Exercise, posture, and back pain during pregnancy—part 1: Exercise and posture. *Clinical Biomechanics*, 10, 2, 98–103.

Dunbar, A. (1992). Why Jane stopped running. *The Journal of Obstetric and Gynecological Physical Therapy*, 16, 3.

Edwards, M.J. (1986). Hyperthermia as a teratogen: A review of experimental studies and their clinical significance. *Teratogenesis, Carcinogenesis, and Mutagenesis,* 6, 563–582.

Evans, J. et al. (2001). Cohort study of depressed mood during pregnancy and after childbirth. *British Medical Journal*, 323, 257–260.

Fast, A. et al. (1990). Low-back pain in pregnancy: Abdominal muscles, situp performance and back pain. *Spine*, 15, 28–30.

Gitau, R. et al. (1998). Fetal exposure to maternal cortisol. *Lancet*, 352, 707–708.

Goode, P.S. et al. (2003). Effect of behavioral training with or without pelvic floor electrical stimulation on stress incontinence in women: A randomized controlled trial. *Journal of the American Medical Association*, 290, 345–352.

Goodwin, A., Astbury, J., & McMeeken, J. (2000). Body image and psychological well-being in pregnancy: Comparison of exercisers and non-exercisers. *Australia and New Zealand Journal of Obstetrics and Gynaecology*, 40, 443–447.

Gotlib, I.H. et al. (1991). Prospective investigation of postpartum depression: Factors involved in onset and recovery. *Journal of Abnormal Psychology*, 100, 122–132.

Groome, L.J. et al. (1995). Maternal anxiety during pregnancy: Effect on fetal behaviour at 38 to 40 weeks' gestation. *Journal of Developmental and Behavioral Paediatrics*, 16, 391–396.

Hainline, B. (1994). Low-back pain in pregnancy. *Advances in Neurology*, 64, 65–76.

Hale, R.W. & Milne, L. (1996). The elite athlete and exercise in pregnancy. *Seminars in Perinatology*, 20, 277–284.

Hall, D.C. & Kaufmann, D.A. (1987). Effects of aerobic and strength conditioning on pregnancy outcomes. *American Journal of Obstetrics and Gynecology*, 157, 1199–1203.

Harris, B. et al. (1994). Maternity blues and major endocrine changes: Cardiff puerperal mood and hormone study II. *British Medical Journal*, 308, 949–953.

Harris, H.E., Ellison, G.T., & Clement, S. (1999). Do the psychosocial and behavioral changes that accompany motherhood influence the impact of pregnancy on long-term weight gain? *Journal of Psychosomatic Obstetrics and Gynaecology*, 20, 65–79.

Hatch, M.C. et al. (1993). Maternal exercise during pregnancy, physical fitness, and fetal growth. *American Journal of Epidemiology*, 137, 1105–1114.

Hay-Smith, E.J.C. et al. (2002). Pelvic floor muscle training for urinary incontinence in women. *Cochrane Database System Review*.

Hedegaard, M. et al. (1996). Do stressful life events affect the duration of gestation and risk of preterm delivery? *Epidemiology*, 7, 339–345.

Henalla, S.M. et al. (1989). Non-operative methods in the treatment of female genuine stress incontinence of urine. *Journal of Obstetrics and Gynecology*, 9, 222–225.

Hoyte, L. et al. (2004). Levator ani thickness variations in symptomatic and asymptomatic women using magnetic resonance-based 3-dimensional color mapping. *American Journal of Obstetrics and Gynecology*, 191, 856–861.

Hummel, P. (1987). *Changes in Posture During Pregnancy.* Philadelphia: WB Saunders.

Ianniruberto, A. & Tajani, E. (1981). Ultrasonographic study of fetal movements. *Seminars in Perinatology*, 1, 5, 175–181.

Kardel, K.R. et al. (1998). Training in pregnant women: Effects on fetal development and birth. *American Journal of Obstetrics and Gynecology*, 178, 280–286.

Kihlstrand, M. et al. (1999). Water-gymnastics reduced the intensity of back/low back pain in pregnant women. *Acta Obstetrica Et Gynecologica Scandinavica*, 78, 180–185.

Klebanoff, M.A. et al. (1990). The effect of physical activity during pregnancy on preterm delivery and birth weight. *American Journal of Obstetrics and Gynecology*, 163, 1450–1456.

Kochan-Vintinner, A. (1999). *Active Living During Pregnancy: Physical Activity Guidelines for Mother and Baby*. Ottawa: Canadian Society for Exercise Physiology and Health.

Koltyn, K.F. & Schultes, S.S. (1997). Psychological effects of an aerobic exercise session and a rest session following pregnancy. *Journal of Sports Medicine and Physical Fitness,* 37, 287–291.

Koniak-Griffin, D. (1994). Aerobic exercise, psychological well-being, and physical discomforts during adolescent pregnancy. *Research in Nursing and Health*, 17, 253–263.

Kristiansson, P., Svardsudd, K., & von Schoultz, B. (1996). Back pain during pregnancy: A prospective study. *Spine*, 21, 6, 702–709.

Kulpa, P.J., White, B.M., & Visscher R. (1987). Aerobic exercise in pregnancy. *American Journal of Obstetrics and Gynecology*, 156, 1395–1403.

Larson-Meyer, D.E. (2002). Effect of postpartum exercise on mothers and their offspring: A review of the literature. *Obesity Research*, 10, 841–853.

Launer, L.H. et al. (1990). The effect of maternal work on fetal growth and duration of pregnancy: A prospective study. *British Journal of Obstetrics and Gynaecology*, 97, 62–70.

Lenfant, C. (2001). Working group report on high blood pressure in pregnancy. *Journal of Clinical Hypertension*, 3, 75–88.

Lovelady, C.A., Lonnerdal, B., & Dewey, K. (1990). Lactation performance of exercising women. *American Journal of Clinical Nutrition*, 52,103–109.

Lovelady et al. (2000). The effect of weight loss in overweight, lactating women on the growth of their infants. *New England Journal of Medicine,* 342, 449–453.

MacArthur, C., Bick, D.E., & Keighley, M.R.B. (1997). Faecal incontinence after childbirth. *British Journal of Obstetrics and Gynaecology*, 104, 46–50.

MacArthur, C., Lewis, M., & Bick, D. (1993). Stress incontinence after childbirth. *British Journal of Midwifery*, 1, 207–215.

Magee, L.A., Ornstein, M.P., & von Dadelszen, P. (1999). Fortnightly review: Management of hypertension in pregnancy. *British Medical Journal*, 318, 1332–1336.

McCrory, M.A. et al. (1999). Randomized trial of short-term effects of dieting compared with dieting plus aerobic exercise on lactation performance. *American Journal of Clinical Nutrition*, 69, 959–967.

McDonald, A.D. et al. (1988). Prematurity and work in pregnancy. *British Journal of Industrial Medicine*, 45, 56–62.

McMurray, R.G. & Katz, V.L. (1990). Thermoregulation in pregnancy, implications for exercise. *Sports Medicine*, 10, 3.

Milunsky, A. et al. (1992). Maternal heat exposure and neural tube defects. *Journal of the American Medical Association*, 268, 882–885.

Moore, K., Dumas, G.A., & Reid, J.G. (1990). Postural changes associated with pregnancy and their relationship with low-back pain. *Clinical Biomechanics*, 5, 3, 169–174.

Morin, M. et al. (2004). Pelvic floor muscle function in continent and stress urinary incontinent women using dynamometric measurements. *Neurourology and Urodynamics*, 23, 668–674.

Morkved, S. & Bo, K. (2000). Effect of postpartum pelvic floor muscle training in prevention of urinary incontinence: A one-year follow up. *British Journal of Obstetrics and Gynaecology*, 107, 8, 1022–1028.

Morkved, S., Schei, B., & Salvesen, K. (2003). Pelvic floor muscle training during pregnancy to prevent urinary incontinence: A single-blind randomized controlled trial. *Obstetrics and Gynecology*, 101, 313–319.

Morton, M.J. (1991). Maternal hemodynamics in pregnancy. In: Artal, R., Wiswell, R.A., & Drinkwater, B.L. (Eds.) *Exercise in Pregnancy* (2nd ed.). Baltimore: Williams & Wilkins.

Morton, J.M. et al. (1985). Exercise dynamics in late gestation. *American Journal of Obstetrics and Gynecology*, 152, 91–97.

Moutquin, J.M. et al. (1997). Report of the Canadian Hypertension Society Consensus Conference: 2. Nonpharmalogic management and prevention of hypertensive disorders in pregnancy. *Canadian Medical Association Journal*, 157, 907–919.

Naeye, R.L. & Peters, E. (1982). Working during pregnancy, effects on the fetus. *Pediatrics*, 69, 724–727.

Neumann, P. & Gill, V. (2002). Pelvic floor and abdominal muscle interaction: EMG activity and intra-abdominal pressure. *International Urogynecological Journal of Pelvic Floor Dysfunction*, 13, 125–132.

Ning, Y. et al. (2003). Correlates of recreational physical activity in early pregnancy. *Journal of Maternal-Fetal and Neonatal Medicine*, 13, 385–393.

O'Hara, M. & Swain, A. (1996). Rates and risk of postpartum depression: A meta-analysis. *International Review of Psychiatry*, 8, 37–54.

O'Hara, M.W. et al. (1991). Controlled prospective study of postpartum mood disorders: Psychological, environmental, and hormonal variables. *Journal of Abnormal Psychology*, 100, 63–73.

Ohlin, A. & Rossner, S. (1996). Factors related to body weight changes during and after pregnancy: The Stockholm Pregnancy and Weight Development Study. *Obesity Research*, 4, 271–276.

Okosun, I.S. et al. (2004). Abdominal adiposity in U.S. adults: Prevalence and trends, 1960–2000. *Preventative Medicine*, 39, 197–206.

O'Neill, M.E. (1996). Maternal rectal temperature and fetal heart rate responses to upright cycling in late pregnancy. *British Journal of Sports Medicine*, 30, 32–35.

Östgaard, H.C., Andersson, G.B., & Karlsson, K. (1991). Prevalence of back pain in pregnancy. *Spine*, 16, 549–552.

Perkin, M.R. et al. (1993). The effect of anxiety and depression during pregnancy on obstetric complications. *British Journal of Obstetrics and Gynaecology*, 100, 629–634.

Perkins, J., Hammer, R.L., & Loubert, P.V. (1998). Identification and management of pregnancy-related low back pain. *Journal of Nurse Midwifery*, 43, 5, 331–340.

Pivarnik, J.M. (1996). Cardiovascular responses to aerobic exercise during pregnancy and postpartum. *Seminars in Perinatology*, 20, 242–249.

Pivarnik, J.M. et al. (1992). Maternal respiration and blood gases during aerobic exercise performed at moderate altitude. *Medicine & Science in Sports & Exercise*, 24, 868–872.

Pivarnik, J.M. et al. (1991). Physiological and perceptual responses to cycle and treadmill exercise during pregnancy. *Medicine & Science in Sports & Exercise*, 23, 4.

Poudevigne, M.S. & O'Connor, P.J. (2005). Physical activity and mood during pregnancy. *Medicine & Science in Sports & Exercise*, 37, 8, 1374–1380.

Prowse, C.M. & Gaensler, E.A. (1965). Respiratory and acid-base changes during pregnancy. *Anesthesiology*, 26, 381–392.

Quinn, T.J. & Carey, G.B. (1999). Does exercise intensity or diet influence lactic acid accumulation in breast milk? *Medicine & Science in Sports & Exercise,* 31, 105-110.

Ritchie, L.D. et al. (1998). A longitudinal study of calcium homeostasis during human pregnancy and lactation and after resumption of menses. *American Journal of Clinical Nutrition,* 67, 693–701.

Rooney, B.L. & Schauberger, C.W. (2002). Excess pregnancy weight gain and long-term obesity: One decade later. *Obstetrics and Gynecology*, 102, 1022–1027.

Sady, S.P. et al. (1989). Cardiovascular response to cycle during and after pregnancy. *Journal of Applied Physiology*, 66, 336–341.

Sampselle, C.M. et al. (1999). Physical activity and postpartum well-being. *Journal of Obstetrics and Gynecology in Neonatal Nursing*, 28, 41–49.

Saurel-Cubizolles, M.J. & Kaminski, M. (1987). Pregnant women's working conditions and their changes during pregnancy: A national study in France. *British Journal of Industrial Medicine,* 44, 236–243.

Shangold, M.M. (1989). Exercise during pregnancy: Current state of the art. *Canadian Family Physician*, 35, 1675–1689.

Snijders, C.J., Vleeming, A., & Stoeckart, R. (1993a). Transfer of lumbosacral load to iliac bones and legs, part I: Biomechanics of self-bracing of the sacroiliac joints and its significance for treatment and exercise. *Clinical Biomechanics*, 8, 285–294.

Snijders, C.J., Vleeming, A., & Stoeckart, R. (1993b). Transfer of lumbosacral load to iliac bones and legs, part II: Loading of the sacroiliac joints when lifting in a stooped posture. *Clinical Biomechanics*, 8, 295–301.

Society of Obstetricians and Gynaecologists of Canada (SOGC) & Canadian Society for Exercise Physiology (CSEP) (2003). Joint SOGC/CSEP clinical practice guideline: Exercise in pregnancy and the postpartum period. *Journal of Obstetrics and Gynaecology Canada*, 25, 6, 516–522.

Soultanakis, H.N., Artal, R., & Wiswell, R.A. (1996). Prolonged exercise in pregnancy: Glucose homeostasis, ventilatory and cardiovascular responses. *Seminars in Perinatology*, 20, 315–327.

Sowers, M. et al. (1993). Changes in bone density with lactation. *Journal of the American Medical Association*, 269, 3130–3135.

Sternfeld, B. et al. (1995). Exercise during pregnancy and pregnancy outcome. *Medicine & Science in Sports & Exercise*, 27, 634–640.

Sultan, A.H. et al. (1993). Anal sphincter disruption during vaginal delivery. *New England Journal of Medicine*, 329, 1905–1911.

Svensson, H.O. et al. (1990). The relationship of low back pain to pregnancy and gynecologic factors. *Spine*, 15, 371–375.

Teixeira, J.M.A., Fisk, N.M., & Glover, V. (1999). Association between maternal anxiety in pregnancy and increased uterine artery resistance index: Cohort-based study. *British Medical Journal*, 318, 153–157.

U.S. Department of Health and Human Services, National Institutes of Health-*Fit for Two: Tips for Pregnancy*. win.niddk.nih.gov/publications/two.htm.

Vleeming, A., Stoeckart, R., & Snijders, C.J. (1989). The sacrotuberous ligament: A conceptual approach to its dynamic role in stabilizing the sacroiliac joint. *Clinical Biomechanics*, 4, 201–203.

Vleeming, A. et al. (1996). The function of the long dorsal sacroiliac ligament: Its implication for understanding low back pain. *Spine,* 21, 556–562.

Vleeming, A. et al. (1995). The posterior layer of the thoracolumbar fascia: Its function in load transfer from spine to legs. *Spine,* 20, 753–758.

Vleeming, A. et al. (1989). Load application to the sacrotuberous ligament: Influences on sacroiliac joint mechanics. *Clinical Biomechanics*, 4, 204–209.

Wadwa, P.D. et al. (1993). The association between prenatal stress and infant birth weight and gestational age at birth: A prospective investigation. *American Journal of Obstetrics and Gynecology*, 169, 858–865.

Wallace, A.M. et al. (1986). Aerobic exercise, maternal self-esteem and physical discomforts during pregnancy. *Journal of Nurse Midwifery*, 31, 255–262.

Wallace, J., Inbar G., & Ernsthausen, K. (1992). Infant acceptance of post-exercise breast milk. *Pediatrics*, 89, 1245–1247.

Watson, W.J. et al. (1991). Fetal responses to maximal swimming and cycling exercise during pregnancy. *Obstetrics and Gynecology*, 77, 3.

Weissgerber et al. (2006). Exercise in the prevention and treatment of maternal-fetal disease: A review of the literature. *Applied Physiology, Nutrition, and Metabolism*, 31, 661–674.

Weissgerber, T.L. et al. (2004). The role of regular physical activity in pre-eclampsia prevention. *Medicine & Science in Sports & Exercise*, 36, 2024–2031.

Wilson, P.D., Herbison, R.M., & Herbison, G.P. (1996). Obstetric practice and the prevalence of urinary incontinence three months after delivery. *British Journal of Obstetrics and Gynaecology,* 103, 154–161.

Wolfe, L.A. et al. (1988). Fetal heart rate during maternal static exercise [abstract]. *Canadian Journal of Sport Science*, 13, 95P–96P.

Wright, K.S., Carey, G.B., & Quinn, T.J. (1999). Infant acceptance of breast milk is unaffected by maternal exercise. *Medicine & Science in Sports &* Exercise, 31, S67.

Zhang, J. & Savitz, D.A. (1996). Exercise during pregnancy among U.S. women. *Annals of Epidemiology*, 6, 1, 53–59.

Zib, M., Lim, L., & Walters, W.A. (1999). Symptoms during normal pregnancy: A prospective controlled study. *Australia and New Zealand Journal of Obstetrics and Gynaecology*, 39, 401–410.

Suggested Reading

American Council on Exercise (2007). *Group Fitness Instructor Manual* (2nd ed.). San Diego, Calif.: American Council on Exercise.

Anthony, L. (2006). *Pre- and Post-natal Fitness: A Guide for Fitness Professionals.* San Diego, Calif.: American Council on Exercise.

Clapp, J.F. (2002). *Exercising Through Your Pregnancy*. Champaign, Ill.: Human Kinetics.

Hammer, R.L., Perkins, J., & Parr, R. (2000). Exercise during the childbearing year. *Journal of Perinatal Education*, 9, 1, 1–13.

Society of Obstetricians and Gynaecologists of Canada (SOGC) & Canadian Society for Exercise Physiology (CSEP) (2003). Joint SOGC/CSEP clinical practice guideline: Exercise in pregnancy and the postpartum period. *Journal of Obstetrics and Gynaecology Canada*, 25, 6, 516–522.

Appendices

Appendix A
ACE Code of Ethics

Appendix B
Exam Content Outline

Appendix C
Cardiovascular Medications

Appendix D
10-Step Decision-making Approach

Appendix E
Framingham Risk Scoring Tables

Appendix F
Functional Ability Tests

Appendix G
ACE Position Statement on Nutritional Supplements

APPENDIX A

ACE Code of Ethics

ACE-certified Professionals are guided by the following principles of conduct as they interact with clients/participants, the public, and other health and fitness professionals.

ACE-certified Professionals will endeavor to:

- ✔ Provide safe and effective instruction
- ✔ Provide equal and fair treatment to all clients
- ✔ Stay up-to-date on the latest health and fitness research and understand its practical application
- ✔ Maintain current CPR certification and knowledge of first-aid services
- ✔ Comply with all applicable business, employment, and intellectual property laws
- ✔ Maintain the confidentiality of all client information
- ✔ Refer clients to more qualified health or medical professionals when appropriate
- ✔ Uphold and enhance public appreciation and trust for the health and fitness industry
- ✔ Establish and maintain clear professional boundaries

Provide Safe and Effective Instruction

Providing safe and effective instruction involves a variety of responsibilities for ACE-certified Professionals. Safe means that the instruction will not result in physical, mental, or financial harm to the client/participant. Effective means that the instruction has a purposeful, intended, and desired effect toward the client's/participant's goal. Great effort and care must be taken in carrying out the responsibilities that are essential in creating a positive exercise experience for all clients/participants.

Screening

ACE-certified Professionals should have all potential clients/participants complete an industry-recognized health-screening tool to ensure safe exercise participation. If significant risk factors or signs and symptoms suggestive of chronic disease are identified, refer the client/participant to a physician or primary healthcare practitioner for medical clearance and guidance regarding which types of assessments, activities, or exercises are indicated, contraindicated, or deemed high risk. If an individual does not want to obtain medical clearance, have that individual sign a legally prepared document that releases you and the facility in which you work from any liability related to any injury that may result from exercise participation or assessment. Once the client has been cleared for exercise and you have a full understanding of the client's/participant's health status and medical history, including his or her current use of medications, a formal risk-management plan for potential emergencies must be prepared and reviewed periodically.

Assessment

The main objective of a health assessment is to establish the client's/participant's baseline fitness level in order to design an appropriate exercise program. Explain the risks and benefits of each assessment and provide the client/participant with any pertinent instructions. Prior to conducting any type of assessment, the client/participant must be given an opportunity to ask questions and read and sign an informed consent. The types and order of assessments are dictated by the client's/participant's health status, fitness level, symptoms, and/or use of medications. Remember that each assessment has specific protocols and only those within your scope of practice should be administered. Once the assessments are completed, evaluate and discuss the results objectively as they relate to the client's/participant's health condition and goals. Educate the client/participant and emphasize how an exercise program will benefit the client/participant.

Program Design

You must not prescribe exercise, diet, or treatment, as doing so is outside your scope of practice and implies ordering or advising a medicine or treatment. Instead, it is appropriate for you to design exercise programs that improve components of physical fitness and wellness while adhering to the limitations of a previous injury or condition as determined by a certified, registered, or licensed allied health professional. Because nutritional laws and the practice of dietetics vary in each state, province, and country, understand what type of basic nutritional information is appropriate and legal for you to disseminate to your client/participant. The client's/participant's preferences, and short- and long-term goals as well as current industry standards and guidelines must be taken into consideration as you develop a formal yet realistic exercise and weight-management program. Provide as much detail for all exercise parameters such as mode, intensity, type of exercise, duration, progression, and termination points.

Program Implementation

Do not underestimate your ability to influence the client/participant to become active for a lifetime. Be sure that each class or session is well-planned, sequential, and documented. Instruct the client/participant how to safely and properly perform the appropriate exercises and communicate this in a manner that the client/participant will understand and retain.

Each client/participant has a different learning curve that will require different levels of attention, learning aids, and repetition. Supervise the client/participant closely, especially when spotting or cueing is needed. If supervising a group of two or more, ensure that you can supervise and provide the appropriate amount of attention to each individual at all times. Ideally, the group will have similar goals and will be performing similar exercises or activities. Position yourself so that you do not have to turn your back to any client/participant performing an exercise.

Facilities

Although the condition of a facility may not always be within your control, you are still obligated to ensure a hazard-free environment to maximize safety. If you notice potential hazards in the health club, communicate these hazards to the client and the facility management. For example, if you notice that the clamps that keep the weights on the barbells are getting rusty and loose, it would be prudent of you to remove them from the training area and alert the facility that immediate repair is required.

Equipment

Obtain equipment that meets or exceeds industry standards and utilize the equipment only for its intended use. Arrange exercise equipment and stations so that adequate space exists between equipment, participants, and foot traffic. Schedule regular maintenance and inspect equipment prior to use to ensure it is in proper working condition. Avoid the use of homemade equipment, as your liability is greater if it causes injury to a person exercising under your supervision.

Provide Equal and Fair Treatment to All Clients/ Participants

ACE-certified Professionals are obligated to provide fair and equal treatment for each client/participant without bias, preference, or discrimination against gender, ethnic background, age, national origin, basis of religion, or physical disability.

The Americans with Disabilities Act protects individuals with disabilities against any type of unlawful discrimination. A disability can be either physical or mental, such as epilepsy, paralysis, HIV infection, AIDS, a significant hearing or visual impairment, mental retardation, or a specific learning disability. ACE-certified Professionals should, at a minimum, provide reasonable accommodations to each individual with a disability. Reasonable simply means that you are able to provide accommodations that do not cause you any undue hardship that requires additional or significant expense or difficulty. Making an existing facility accessible by modifying equipment or devices, assessments, or training materials are a few examples of providing reasonable accommodations. However, providing the use of personal items or providing items at your own expense may not be considered reasonable.

This ethical consideration of providing fair and equal treatment is not limited to behavioral interactions with clients, but also extends to exercise programming and other business-related services such as communication, scheduling, billing, cancellation policies, and dispute resolution.

Stay Up-to-Date on the Latest Health and Fitness Research and Understand Its Practical Application

Obtaining ACE-certification required you to have broad-based knowledge of many disciplines; however, this credential should not be viewed as the end of your professional development and education. Instead, it should be viewed as the beginning or foundation. The dynamic nature of the health and fitness industry requires you to maintain an understanding of the latest research and professional standards and guidelines, and of their impact on the design and implementation of exercise programming. To stay informed, make time to review a variety of industry resources such as professional journals, position statements, trade and lay periodicals, and correspondence courses, as well as to attend professional meetings, conferences, and educational workshops.

An additional benefit of staying up-to-date is that it also fulfills your certification renewal requirements for continuing education credit (CEC). To maintain your ACE-certification status, you must obtain an established amount of CECs every two years. CECs are granted for structured learning that takes place within the educational portion of a course related to the profession and presented by a qualified health and fitness professional.

Maintain Current CPR Certification and Knowledge of First-aid Services

ACE-certified Professionals must be prepared to recognize and respond to heart attacks and other life-threatening emergencies. Emergency response is enhanced by training and maintaining skills in CPR, first aid, and using automated external defibrillators (AEDs), which have become more widely available. An AED is a portable electronic device used to restore normal heart rhythm in a person experiencing a cardiac arrest and can reduce the time to defibrillation before EMS personnel arrive. For each minute that defibrillation is delayed, the victim's chance of survival is reduced by 7 to 10%. Thus, survival from cardiac arrest is improved dramatically when CPR and defibrillation are started early.

Comply With All Applicable Business, Employment, and Intellectual Property Laws

As an ACE-certified Professional, you are expected to maintain a high level of integrity by complying with all applicable business, employment, and copyright laws. Be truthful and forthcoming with communication to clients/participants, co-workers, and other health and fitness professionals in advertising, marketing, and business practices. Do not create false or misleading impressions of credentials, claims, or sponsorships, or perform services outside of your scope of practice that are illegal, deceptive, or fraudulent.

All information regarding your business must be clear, accurate, and easy to understand for all potential clients/participants. Provide disclosure about the name of your business, physical address, and contact information, and maintain a working phone number and email address. So that clients/participants can make an informed choice about paying for your services, provide detailed information regarding schedules, prices, payment terms, time limits, and conditions. Cancellation, refund, and rescheduling information must also be clearly stated and easy to understand. Allow the client/participant an opportunity to ask questions and review this information before formally agreeing to your services and terms.

Because employment laws vary in each city, state, province, and country, familiarize yourself with the applicable employment regulations and standards to which your business must conform. Examples of this may include conforming to specific building codes and zoning ordinances or making sure that your place of business is accessible to individuals with a disability.

The understanding of intellectual property law and the proper use of copyrighted materials is an important legal issue for all ACE-certified Professionals. Intellectual property laws protect the creations of authors, artists, software programmers, and others with copyrighted materials. The most common infringement of intellectual property law in the fitness industry is the use of music in an exercise class. When commercial music is played in a for-profit exercise class, without a performance or blanket license, it is considered a public performance and a violation of intellectual property law. Therefore, make sure that any music, handouts, or educational materials are either exempt from intellectual property law or permissible under laws by reason of fair use, or obtain express written consent from the copyright holder for distribution, adaptation, or use. When in doubt, obtain permission first or consult with a qualified legal professional who has intellectual property law expertise.

Maintain the Confidentiality of All Client/Participant Information

Every client/participant has the right to expect that all personal data and discussions with an ACE-certified Professional will be safeguarded and not disclosed without the client's/participant's express written consent or acknowledgement. Therefore, protect the confidentiality of all client/participant information such as contact data, medical records, health history, progress notes, and meeting details. Even when confidentiality is not required by law, continue to preserve the confidentiality of such information.

Any breach of confidentiality, intentional or unintentional, potentially harms the productivity and trust of your client/participant and undermines your effectiveness as a fitness professional. This also puts you at risk for potential litigation and puts your client/class participant at risk for public embarrassment and fraudulent activity such as identity theft.

Most breaches of confidentiality are unintentional and occur because of carelessness and lack of awareness. The most common breach of confidentiality is exposing or storing a client's personal data in a location that is not secure. This occurs when a client's/participant's file or information is left on a desk, or filed in a cabinet that has no lock or is accessible to others. Breaches of confidentiality may also occur when you have conversations regarding a client's/participant's performance or medical/health history with staff or others and the client's/participant's first name or other identifying details are used.

Post and adhere to a privacy policy that communicates how client/participant information will be used and secured and how a client's/participant's preference regarding unsolicited mail and email will be respected. When a client/participant provides you with any personal data, new or updated, make it a habit to immediately secure this information and ensure that only you and/or the appropriate individuals have access to it. Also, the client's/participant's files must only be accessed and used for purposes related to health and fitness services. If client/participant information is stored on a personal computer, restrict access by using a protected password. Should you receive any inquiries from family members or other individuals regarding the progress of a client/participant or other personal information, state that you cannot provide any information without the client's/participant's permission. If and when a client/participant permits you to release confidential information to an authorized individual or party, utilize secure methods of communication such as certified mail, sending and receiving information on a dedicated private fax line, or email with encryption.

Refer Clients/Participants to More Qualified Health or Medical Professionals When Appropriate

A fitness certification is not a professional license. Therefore, it is vitally important that ACE-certified Professionals who do not also have a professional license (i.e., physician, physical therapist, dietitian, psychologist, and attorney) refer their clients/participants to a more qualified professional when warranted. Doing so not only benefits your clients/participants by making sure that they receive the appropriate attention and care, but also enhances your credibility and reduces liability by defining your scope of practice and clarifying what services you can and cannot reasonably provide.

Knowing when to refer a client/participant is, however, as important as choosing to which professional to refer. For instance, just because a client/participant complains of symptoms of muscle soreness or discomfort or exhibits signs of fatigue or lack of energy is not an absolute indication to refer your client/participant to a physician. Because continual referrals such as this are not practical, familiarize and educate yourself on expected signs and symptoms, taking into consideration the client's/participant's fitness level, health status, chronic disease, disability, and/or background as they are screened and as they begin and progress with an exercise program. This helps you better discern between emergent and non-emergent situations and know when to refuse to offer your services, continue to monitor, and/or make an immediate referral.

It is important that you know the scope of practice for various health professionals and which types of referrals are appropriate. For example, some states require that a referring physician first approve visits to a physical therapist, while other states allow individuals to see a physical therapist directly. Only registered or licensed dietitians or physicians may provide specific dietary recommendations or diet plans; however, a client/participant who is suspected of an eating disorder should be referred to an eating disorders specialist. Refer clients/participants to a clinical psychologist if they wish to discuss family or marital problems or exhibit addictive behaviors such as substance abuse.

Network and develop rapport with potential allied health professionals in your area before you refer clients/participants to them. This demonstrates good will and respect for their expertise and will most likely result in reciprocal referrals for your services and fitness expertise.

Uphold and Enhance Public Appreciation and Trust for the Health and Fitness Industry

The best way for ACE-certified Professionals to uphold and enhance public appreciation and trust for the health and fitness industry is to represent themselves in a dignified and professional manner. As the public is inundated with misinformation and false claims about fitness products and services, your expertise must be utilized to dispel myths and half-truths about current trends and fads that are potentially harmful to the public.

When appropriate, mentor and dispense knowledge and training to less-experienced fitness professionals. Novice fitness professionals can benefit from your experience and skill as you assist them in establishing a foundation based on exercise science, from both theoretical and practical standpoints. Therefore, it is a disservice if you fail to provide helpful or corrective information—especially when an individual, the public, or other fitness professionals are at risk for injury or increased liability. For example, if you observe an individual using momentum to perform a strength-training exercise, the prudent course of action would be to suggest a modification. Likewise, if you observe a fitness professional in your workplace consistently failing to obtain informed consents before clients/participants undergo fitness testing or begin an exercise program, recommend that he or she consider implementing these forms to minimize liability.

Finally, do not represent yourself in an overly commercial or misleading manner. Consider the fitness professional who places an advertisement in a local newspaper stating: Lose 10 pounds in 10 days or your money back! It is inappropriate to lend credibility to or endorse a product, service, or program founded upon unsubstantiated or misleading claims; thus a solicitation such as this must be avoided, as it undermines the public's trust of health and fitness professionals.

Establish and Maintain Clear Professional Boundaries

Working in the fitness profession requires you to come in contact with many different people. It is imperative that a professional distance be maintained in relationships with all clients/participants. Fitness professionals are responsible for setting and monitoring the boundaries between a working relationship and friendship with their clients/participants. To that end, ACE-certified Professionals should:

- Never initiate or encourage discussion of a sexual nature
- Avoid touching clients/participants unless it is essential to instruction
- Inform clients/participants about the purpose of touching and find an alternative if the client/participant objects
- Discontinue all touching if it appears to make the client/participant uncomfortable
- Take all reasonable steps to ensure that any personal and social contacts between themselves and their clients/participant do not have an adverse impact on the trainer–client or instructor–participant relationship.

If you find yourself unable to maintain appropriate professional boundaries with a client/participant (whether due to your attitudes and actions or those of the client/participant), the prudent course of action is to terminate the relationship and, perhaps, refer the client/participant to another professional. Keep in mind that charges of sexual harassment or assault, even if groundless, can have disastrous effects on your career.

APPENDIX B

Exam Content Outline

Examination Content Outline

The Examination Content Outline is essentially a blueprint for the exam. All exam questions are based on this outline.

Target Audience Statement

The ACE Advanced Health & Fitness Specialist (ACE-AHFS) works with special populations (e.g., disease, post-rehabilitation) in cooperation with other qualified healthcare professionals to enhance quality of life and manage health risk. ACE-certified Advanced Health & Fitness Specialists conduct appropriate health- and fitness-related assessments for members of special populations and develop and administer programs designed to enhance strength, muscular endurance, balance, range of motion, and cardiovascular function.

The following eligibility requirements have been established for the ACE-AHFS certification examination:

- At least 18 years of age
- Adult CPR certification, current at the time of the examination
- Hold a current ACE Personal Trainer or Lifestyle & Weight Management Consultant Certification; or an NCCA-accredited certification in health and fitness; or hold a four-year (bachelor's) degree in exercise science or a related field. Registrants holding degrees in nutrition or nursing must submit documentation supporting completion of exercise science–related coursework at the time of registration.
- 300 hours of work experience designing and implementing weight-management and exercise programs for overweight and obese individuals, as documented by a qualified professional

Domains, Tasks, and Knowledge and Skill Statements

A Role Delineation Study completed for the Advanced Health & Fitness Specialist certification first identified the major categories of responsibility for the professional. These categories are defined as Domains and it was determined that the profession could be divided into four Performance Domains, or major areas of responsibility. These Performance Domains are:

Domain I:	Assessment
Domain II:	Program Design
Domain III:	Program Implementation and Management
Domain IV:	Professional Responsibility

The Advanced Health & Fitness Specialist draws upon knowledge from four foundational sciences, or Content Domains, in his or her work. Content Domains include topics important to the competence of the Advanced Health & Fitness Specialist that apply primarily to the Assessment, Program Design, and Program Implementation and Management Domains.

The Exercise Science Domain was delineated further into three significant topics: Anatomy, Kinesiology, and Physiology. Within each Performance Domain, there is additional

Domain-specific information referring to tests, procedures, and techniques.

The Content Domains are:

- Exercise Science (Anatomy, Kinesiology, and Physiology)
- Nutrition
- Psychology
- Pathophysiology

There are two dimensions in test specifications: vertically for Assessment, Program Design, Program Implementation and Management, and Professional Responsibility. The horizontal dimension includes Exercise Science (Anatomy, Kinesiology, and Physiology), Nutrition, Psychology, and Pathophysiology.

ACE determined that the Professional Responsibility Performance Domain is managed to a large degree by its policies concerning professional discipline and certification renewal, and that 10 questions in this Domain suffice. As a result, the test specifications on the following page distribute the weighting that would otherwise be allocated beyond the eight questions among the remaining three Performance Domains.

Each Domain is composed of Task Statements that detail the job-related functions of that Domain. Each Task Statement is divided into Knowledge and Skill Statements to further detail the scope of information required and how that information is applied in a practical setting for task statement.

EXAM CONTENT OUTLINE DOMAIN I: ASSESSMENT 26%

Task 1 - Obtain health information by establishing rapport with the client, using questionnaires, and communicating with other healthcare providers, as indicated, to assess the individual's appropriateness for physical activity, facilitate program design, and identify the need for referral.

Exercise Science

Knowledge of:

Anatomy

1. General anatomy of the following systems: musculoskeletal, cardiorespiratory, neuromuscular, digestive, endocrine, reproductive, and integumentary.
2. General anatomical terminology (e.g., landmarks, planes of movement, position, muscle roles, muscle origin, and muscle insertion).

Kinesiology

3. Passive and active ranges of motion.
4. Muscle function, types of muscle contraction, and associated factors affecting movement (e.g., neurological, biomechanical, kinesthetic).
5. Appropriate exercise design to address balance (e.g., static, dynamic), muscular imbalances, and postural alignment.
6. Biomechanical concepts of human movement (e.g., Newton's laws) as applied to exercise.
7. Application of the principles related to muscular strength and endurance (e.g., resistance, overload, specificity, repetitions, sets, frequency, rest periods, progression).

Physiology

8. Types of training (cardiorespiratory, resistance, and flexibility) and the risks and benefits associated with each.
9. Health-related components of physical fitness, principles of training, and adaptations (acute and chronic) to exercise.
10. Skill-related components of physical fitness, principles of training, and adaptations (agility, balance, coordination, speed, power, and reaction time).
11. Cardiorespiratory system with respect to the carrying capacity, delivery, and extraction of oxygen.
12. Metabolism, including energy production and nutrient utilization.
13. Neuromuscular physiology (e.g., muscle fiber types, proprioceptors, motor-unit recruitment).
14. Programming guidelines to improve fitness.
15. Environmental conditions impacting exercise (e.g., heat, humidity, cold, air pollution, altitude).

Skill in:

1. Facilitating cardiorespiratory fitness, musculoskeletal strength, and flexibility.

2. Selecting appropriate exercise modalities.
3. Selecting safe exercises for all muscle groups.
4. Applying appropriate training principles (FITT).
5. Modifying programs.
6. Assessing body composition.
7. Assessing dynamic and static posture and balance.
8. Assessing gait.
9. Assessing cardiorespiratory and musculoskeletal fitness.
10. Interpreting medical history.
11. Assessing clients' lifestyles.
12. Conducting risk stratification.
13. Comparing test data to normative values.
14. Selecting appropriate assessments.
15. Referring to the appropriate healthcare professional(s).
16. Communicating with members of the healthcare team.
17. Assessing anthropometric parameters.
18. Recognizing side effects associated with common categories of medications as they relate to energy and performance.

Nutrition

Knowledge of:

1. Macronutrients, micronutrients, hydration, supplements, engineered foods, alcohol, drugs (illicit, over-the-counter, prescription), and stimulants.
2. Current, credible, and appropriate nutrition resources.
3. Nutrition guidelines, and food selection, preparation, and storage.
4. Digestion and absorption process.
5. Popular diets and associated health risks.
6. Nutrition requirements specific to each classification of disease or dysfunction.
7. Metabolic conversion of nutrients.

Skill in:

1. Assessing the quality of the client's food intake.
2. Educating the client on making appropriate food choices based on sound nutritional practices.
3. Recommending reputable resources for clients with an interest in a structured dietary management program.
4. Educating the client on appropriate food selections based on known risk reduction.
5. Recognizing deficiencies in nutrition as they relate to exercise performance.
6. Maintaining a current knowledge base of popular diets and extreme dietary measures.
7. Applying hydration guidelines as they relate to exercise duration, environmental conditions, and client status.

Psychology

Knowledge of:

1. Psychological conditions that require referral to appropriate allied health professionals.
2. Communication techniques (e.g., active listening, appropriate eye contact, non-verbal behavior).
3. Techniques that build and enhance rapport.
4. Individual differences that influence behavior (e.g., exercise history, lifestyle, gender, age, culture, ethnicity).
5. Psychological implications of chronic diseases, disabilities, and dysfunction.
6. Sources for disease-specific guidelines.
7. Theories of behavior change (e.g., stages of change, health belief model) and their implications.
8. Psychological obstacles that may interfere with the attainment of goals (e.g., self-esteem, anxiety, self-efficacy, mood).
9. Principles of adult learning (e.g., readiness, success, practice) and appropriate educational tools.
10. Psychological side effects of medications and appropriate precautions for a client taking medications and/or other substances.
11. The negative and positive impact of assessment data on motivation.
12. Motivational techniques used to optimize exercise adherence and other healthy lifestyle behaviors.
13. How chronic diseases, disabilities, and injuries will impact exercise adherence based on a client's perception of signs and symptoms.

Skill in:

1. Interviewing and communicating effectively with the client and/or healthcare team.
2. Interpreting body language and recognizing incongruities between verbal and non-verbal behaviors.
3. Building trust and rapport.
4. Assessing client's readiness, expectations, and preferences.
5. Applying principles of behavioral change.
6. Identifying barriers associated with various chronic diseases, disabilities, and injuries that may affect programming.
7. Adapting programming in accordance with identified barriers.
8. Identifying and/or addressing unrealistic expectations as they relate to underlying chronic diseases, disabilities, and injuries.
9. Establishing goals (e.g., specific, measurable, action-oriented, realistic, timed).
10. Selecting and integrating appropriate educational tools for use in client instruction.
11. Facilitating the client's acceptance, responsibility, and accountability for program goals.
12. Designing a safe, well-balanced, and comprehensive program specific to the client's health status, special needs, program preferences, and goals.
13. Instructing and/or supervising the client in the safe and proper execution of exercise.
14. Modifying motivational strategies based upon assessment and/or reassessment.
15. Making appropriate referrals.

Pathophysiology

1. General pathophysiology of chronic diseases, disabilities, and injuries as related to each organ system, including cardiovascular, respiratory, endocrine, neurological, musculoskeletal, gastrointestinal, reproductive, and integumentary.
2. Signs and symptoms of chronic diseases, disabilities, and injuries.
3. Guidelines for designing programs specific to chronic diseases, disabilities, and injuries using FITT principles as they apply to cardiorespiratory, strength, and flexibility training.
4. Influence of chronic diseases, disabilities, and injuries on exercise selection.
5. Influence of chronic diseases, disabilities, and injuries on the selection of assessment tools.
6. Predicted responses to exercise in clients with chronic diseases, disabilities, and injuries.
7. Designing safe, comprehensive, and effective programs based on the client's current health status.
8. Appropriate exercise modifications for chronic diseases, disabilities, and injuries based on the client's response to exercise.
9. Indications for modification or termination of an exercise session or activity.
10. Circumstances requiring referral to other health professionals.
11. Contraindicated activities/exercises.
12. Appropriate documentation of signs, symptoms, and responses to exercise.
13. Effect of medication on exercise selection.
14. Potential effect of exercise on medication requirements.
15. How environmental factors affect exercise for clients with chronic diseases, disabilities, and injuries.
16. Alternative medical services (e.g., chiropractic, acupuncture, naturopathy) and how they may affect exercise/activity selection for clients with chronic diseases, disabilities, and injuries.
17. Potential medical emergencies in clients with chronic diseases, disabilities, and injuries.
18. Recognized protocols (e.g., McKenzie extension exercises, rotator cuff progression) for clients with chronic diseases, disabilities, and injuries.

Skill in:

1. Assessing and reassessing the client's readiness, expectations, and limitations.
2. Administering and analyzing assessment data.
3. Interpreting the data from the referring health professional.
4. Modifying the program to meet the needs of the client.
5. Applying standard and accepted testing methods to measure current fitness status.
6. Identifying environmental factors that influence exercise performance.

7. Recognizing the need for terminating a specific activity, an exercise session, or the entire program.
8. Recognizing personal scope of practice.
9. Teaching proper alignment and execution techniques.
10. Recognizing and managing emergency situations.
11. Addressing unrealistic expectations.
12. Applying program guidelines specific to special populations.
13. Identifying problematic signs and symptoms before, during, and after the exercise session.
14. Documenting health- and fitness-related data.
15. Referring the client to appropriate health professionals.

Task 2 - Gather lifestyle information using interviews and questionnaires to facilitate program design and optimize adherence.

Exercise Science

Knowledge of:

Anatomy

1. General anatomy of the following systems: musculoskeletal, cardiorespiratory, neuromuscular, digestive, endocrine, reproductive, and integumentary.
2. General anatomical terminology (e.g., landmarks, planes of movement, position, muscle roles, muscle origin, and muscle insertion).

Kinesiology

3. Passive and active ranges of motion.
4. Muscle function, types of muscle contraction, and associated factors affecting movement (e.g., neurological, biomechanical, kinesthetic).
5. Appropriate exercise design to address balance (e.g., static, dynamic), muscular imbalances, and postural alignment.
6. Biomechanical concepts of human movement (e.g., Newton's laws) as applied to exercise.
7. Application of the principles related to muscular strength and endurance (e.g., resistance, overload, specificity, repetitions, sets, frequency, rest periods, progression).

Physiology

8. Types of training (cardiorespiratory, resistance, and flexibility) and the risks and benefits associated with each.
9. Health-related components of physical fitness, principles of training, and adaptations (acute and chronic) to exercise.
10. Skill-related components of physical fitness, principles of training, and adaptations (agility, balance, coordination, speed, power, and reaction time).
11. Cardiorespiratory system with respect to the carrying capacity, delivery, and extraction of oxygen.
12. Metabolism, including energy production and nutrient utilization.
13. Neuromuscular physiology (e.g., muscle fiber types, proprioceptors, motor-unit recruitment).
14. Programming guidelines to improve fitness.
15. Environmental conditions impacting exercise (e.g., heat, humidity, cold, air pollution, altitude).

Skill in:

1. Facilitating cardiorespiratory fitness, musculoskeletal strength, and flexibility.
2. Selecting appropriate exercise modalities.
3. Selecting safe exercises for all muscle groups.
4. Applying appropriate training principles (FITT).
5. Modifying programs.
6. Assessing body composition.
7. Assessing dynamic and static posture and balance.
8. Assessing gait.
9. Assessing cardiorespiratory and musculoskeletal fitness.
10. Interpreting medical history.
11. Assessing clients' lifestyles.
12. Conducting risk stratification.
13. Comparing test data to normative values.
14. Selecting appropriate assessments.
15. Referring to the appropriate healthcare professional(s).
16. Communicating with members of the healthcare team.
17. Assessing anthropometric parameters.

18. Recognizing side effects associated with common categories of medications as they relate to energy and performance.

Nutrition

Knowledge of:

1. Macronutrients, micronutrients, hydration, supplements, engineered foods, alcohol, drugs (illicit, over-the-counter, prescription), and stimulants.
2. Current, credible, and appropriate nutrition resources.
3. Nutrition guidelines, food selection, preparation, and storage.
4. Digestion and absorption process.
5. Popular diets and associated health risks.
6. Nutrition requirements specific to each classification of disease or dysfunction.
7. Metabolic conversion of nutrients.

Skill in:

1. Assessing the quality of the client's food intake.
2. Educating the client on making appropriate food choices based on sound nutritional practices.
3. Recommending reputable resources for clients with an interest in a structured dietary management program.
4. Educating the client on appropriate food selections based on known risk reduction.
5. Recognizing deficiencies in nutrition as they relate to exercise performance.
6. Maintaining a current knowledge base of popular diets and extreme dietary measures.
7. Applying hydration guidelines as they relate to exercise duration, environmental conditions, and client status.

Psychology

Knowledge of:

1. Psychological conditions that require referral to appropriate allied health professionals.
2. Communication techniques (e.g., active listening, appropriate eye contact, non-verbal behavior).
3. Techniques that build and enhance rapport.
4. Individual differences that influence behavior (e.g., exercise history, lifestyle, gender, age, culture, ethnicity).
5. Psychological implications of chronic diseases, disabilities, and dysfunction.
6. Sources for disease-specific guidelines.
7. Theories of behavior change (e.g., stages of change, health belief model) and their implications.
8. Psychological obstacles that may interfere with the attainment of goals (e.g., self-esteem, anxiety, self-efficacy, mood).
9. Principles of adult learning (e.g., readiness, success, practice) and appropriate educational tools.
10. Psychological side effects of medications and appropriate precautions for a client taking medications and/or other substances.
11. The negative and positive impact of assessment data on motivation.
12. Motivational techniques used to optimize exercise adherence and other healthy lifestyle behaviors.
13. How chronic diseases, disabilities, and injuries will impact exercise adherence based on a client's perception of signs and symptoms.

Skill in:

1. Interviewing and communicating effectively with the client and/or healthcare team.
2. Interpreting body language and recognizing incongruities between verbal and non-verbal behaviors.
3. Building trust and rapport.
4. Assessing a client's readiness, expectations, and preferences.
5. Applying principles of behavioral change.
6. Identifying barriers associated with various chronic diseases, disabilities, and injuries that may affect programming.
7. Adapting programming in accordance with identified barriers.
8. Identifying and/or addressing unrealistic expectations as they relate to underlying chronic diseases, disabilities, and injuries.
9. Establishing goals (e.g., specific, measurable, action-oriented, realistic, timed).

10. Selecting and integrating appropriate educational tools for use in client instruction.
11. Facilitating the client's acceptance, responsibility, and accountability for program goals.
12. Designing a safe, well-balanced, and comprehensive program specific to the client's health status, special needs, program preferences, and goals.
13. Instructing and/or supervising the client in the safe and proper execution of exercise.
14. Modifying motivational strategies based upon assessment and/or reassessment.
15. Making appropriate referrals.

Pathophysiology

1. General pathophysiology of chronic diseases, disabilities, and injuries as related to each organ system, including cardiovascular, respiratory, endocrine, neurological, musculoskeletal, gastrointestinal, reproductive, and integumentary.
2. Signs and symptoms of chronic diseases, disabilities, and injuries.
3. Guidelines for designing programs specific to chronic diseases, disabilities, and injuries using FITT principles as they apply to cardiorespiratory, strength, and flexibility training.
4. Influence of chronic diseases, disabilities, and injuries on exercise selection.
5. Influence of chronic diseases, disabilities, and injuries on the selection of assessment tools.
6. Predicted responses to exercise in clients with chronic diseases, disabilities, and injuries.
7. Designing safe, comprehensive, and effective programs based on the client's current health status.
8. Appropriate exercise modifications for chronic diseases, disabilities, and injuries based on the client's response to exercise.
9. Indications for modification or termination of an exercise session or activity.
10. Circumstances requiring referral to other health professionals.
11. Contraindicated activities/exercises.
12. Appropriate documentation of signs, symptoms, and responses to exercise.
13. Effect of medication on exercise selection.
14. Potential effect of exercise on medication requirements.
15. How environmental factors affect exercise for clients with chronic diseases, disabilities, and injuries.
16. Alternative medical services (e.g., chiropractic, acupuncture, naturopathy) and how they may affect exercise/activity selection for clients with chronic diseases, disabilities, and injuries.
17. Potential medical emergencies in clients with chronic diseases, disabilities, and injuries.
18. Recognized protocols (e.g., McKenzie extension exercises, rotator cuff progression) for clients with chronic diseases, disabilities, and injuries.

Skill in:

1. Assessing and reassessing the client's readiness, expectations, and limitations.
2. Administering and analyzing assessment data.
3. Interpreting the data from the referring health professional.
4. Modifying the program to meet the needs of the client.
5. Applying standard and accepted testing methods to measure current fitness status.
6. Identifying environmental factors that influence exercise performance.
7. Recognizing the need for terminating a specific activity, an exercise session, or the entire program.
8. Recognizing personal scope of practice.
9. Teaching proper alignment and execution techniques.
10. Recognizing and managing emergency situations.
11. Addressing unrealistic expectations.
12. Applying program guidelines specific to special populations.
13. Identifying problematic signs and symptoms before, during, and after the exercise session.

14. Documenting health- and fitness-related data.
15. Referring the client to appropriate health professionals.

Task 3 - Identify the client's readiness, expectations, and personal preferences using interviews and questionnaires to facilitate program design.

Exercise Science

Knowledge of:

Anatomy

1. General anatomy of the following systems: musculoskeletal, cardiorespiratory, neuromuscular, digestive, endocrine, reproductive, and integumentary.
2. General anatomical terminology (e.g., landmarks, planes of movement, position, muscle roles, muscle origin, and muscle insertion).

Kinesiology

3. Passive and active ranges of motion.
4. Muscle function, types of muscle contraction, and associated factors affecting movement (e.g., neurological, biomechanical, kinesthetic).
5. Appropriate exercise design to address balance (e.g., static, dynamic), muscular imbalances, and postural alignment.
6. Biomechanical concepts of human movement (e.g., Newton's laws) as applied to exercise.
7. Application of the principles related to muscular strength and endurance (e.g., resistance, overload, specificity, repetitions, sets, frequency, rest periods, progression).

Physiology

8. Types of training (cardiorespiratory, resistance, and flexibility) and the risks and benefits associated with each.
9. Health-related components of physical fitness, principles of training, and adaptations (acute and chronic) to exercise.
10. Skill-related components of physical fitness, principles of training, and adaptations (agility, balance, coordination, speed, power, and reaction time).
11. Cardiorespiratory system with respect to the carrying capacity, delivery, and extraction of oxygen.
12. Metabolism, including energy production and nutrient utilization.
13. Neuromuscular physiology (e.g., muscle fiber types, proprioceptors, motor-unit recruitment).
14. Programming guidelines to improve fitness.
15. Environmental conditions impacting exercise (e.g., heat, humidity, cold, air pollution, altitude).

Skill in:

1. Facilitating cardiorespiratory fitness, musculoskeletal strength, and flexibility.
2. Selecting appropriate exercise modalities.
3. Selecting safe exercises for all muscle groups.
4. Applying appropriate training principles (FITT).
5. Modifying programs.
6. Assessing body composition.
7. Assessing dynamic and static posture and balance.
8. Assessing gait.
9. Assessing cardiorespiratory and musculoskeletal fitness.
10. Interpreting medical history.
11. Assessing clients' lifestyles.
12. Conducting risk stratification.
13. Comparing test data to normative values.
14. Selecting appropriate assessments.
15. Referring to the appropriate healthcare professional(s).
16. Communicating with members of the healthcare team.
17. Assessing anthropometric parameters.
18. Recognizing side effects associated with common categories of medications as they relate to energy and performance.

Nutrition

Knowledge of:

1. Macronutrients, micronutrients, hydration, supplements, engineered foods, alcohol, drugs (illicit, over-the-counter, prescription), and stimulants.

2. Current, credible, and appropriate nutrition resources.
3. Nutrition guidelines, food selection, preparation, and storage.
4. Digestion and absorption process.
5. Popular diets and associated health risks.
6. Nutrition requirements specific to each classification of disease or dysfunction.
7. Metabolic conversion of nutrients.

Skill in:

1. Assessing the quality of the client's food intake.
2. Educating the client on making appropriate food choices based on sound nutritional practices.
3. Recommending reputable resources for clients with an interest in a structured dietary management program.
4. Educating the client on appropriate food selections based on known risk reduction.
5. Recognizing deficiencies in nutrition as they relate to exercise performance.
6. Maintaining a current knowledge base of popular diets and extreme dietary measures.
7. Applying hydration guidelines as they relate to exercise duration, environmental conditions, and client status.

Psychology

Knowledge of:

1. Psychological conditions that require referral to appropriate allied health professionals.
2. Communication techniques (e.g., active listening, appropriate eye contact, non-verbal behavior).
3. Techniques that build and enhance rapport.
4. Individual differences that influence behavior (e.g., exercise history, lifestyle, gender, age, culture, ethnicity).
5. Psychological implications of chronic diseases, disabilities, and dysfunction.
6. Sources for disease-specific guidelines.
7. Theories of behavior change (e.g., stages of change, health belief model) and their implications.
8. Psychological obstacles that may interfere with the attainment of goals (e.g., self-esteem, anxiety, self-efficacy, mood).
9. Principles of adult learning (e.g., readiness, success, practice) and appropriate educational tools.
10. Psychological side effects of medications and appropriate precautions for a client taking medications and/or other substances.
11. The negative and positive impact of assessment data on motivation.
12. Motivational techniques used to optimize exercise adherence and other healthy lifestyle behaviors.
13. How chronic diseases, disabilities, and injuries will impact exercise adherence based on the client's perception of signs and symptoms.

Skill in:

1. Interviewing and communicating effectively with the client and/or healthcare team.
2. Interpreting body language and recognizing incongruities between verbal and non-verbal behaviors.
3. Building trust and rapport.
4. Assessing the client's readiness, expectations, and preferences.
5. Applying principles of behavioral change.
6. Identifying barriers associated with various chronic diseases, disabilities, and injuries that may affect programming.
7. Adapting programming in accordance with identified barriers.
8. Identifying and/or addressing unrealistic expectations as they relate to underlying chronic diseases, disabilities, and injuries.
9. Establishing goals (e.g., specific, measurable, action-oriented, realistic, timed).
10. Selecting and integrating appropriate educational tools for use in client instruction.
11. Facilitating the client's acceptance, responsibility, and accountability for program goals.
12. Designing a safe, well-balanced, and comprehensive program specific to the client's health status, special needs, program preferences, and goals.
13. Instructing and/or supervising the client in the safe and proper execution of exercise.
14. Modifying motivational strategies based upon assessment and/or reassessment.
15. Making appropriate referrals.

Pathophysiology

1. General pathophysiology of chronic diseases, disabilities, and injuries as related to each organ system, including cardiovascular, respiratory, endocrine, neurological, musculoskeletal, gastrointestinal, reproductive, and integumentary.
2. Signs and symptoms of chronic diseases, disabilities, and injuries.
3. Guidelines for designing programs specific to chronic diseases, disabilities, and injuries using FITT principles as they apply to cardiorespiratory, strength, and flexibility training.
4. Influence of chronic diseases, disabilities, and injuries on exercise selection.
5. Influence of chronic diseases, disabilities, and injuries on the selection of assessment tools.
6. Predicted responses to exercise in clients with chronic diseases, disabilities, and injuries.
7. Designing safe, comprehensive, and effective programs based on the client's current health status.
8. Appropriate exercise modifications for chronic diseases, disabilities, and injuries based on the client's response to exercise.
9. Indications for modification or termination of an exercise session or activity.
10. Circumstances requiring referral to other health professionals.
11. Contraindicated activities/exercises.
12. Appropriate documentation of signs, symptoms, and responses to exercise.
13. Effect of medication on exercise selection.
14. Potential effect of exercise on medication requirements.
15. How environmental factors affect exercise for clients with chronic diseases, disabilities, and injuries.
16. Alternative medical services (e.g., chiropractic, acupuncture, naturopathy) and how they may affect exercise/activity selection for clients with chronic diseases, disabilities, and injuries.
17. Potential medical emergencies in clients with chronic diseases, disabilities, and injuries.
18. Recognized protocols (e.g., McKenzie extension exercises, rotator cuff progression) for clients with chronic diseases, disabilities, and injuries.

Skill in:

1. Assessing and reassessing the client's readiness, expectations, and limitations.
2. Administering and analyzing assessment data.
3. Interpreting the data from the referring health professional.
4. Modifying the program to meet the needs of the client.
5. Applying standard and accepted testing methods to measure current fitness status.
6. Identifying environmental factors that influence exercise performance.
7. Recognizing the need for terminating a specific activity, an exercise session, or the entire program.
8. Recognizing personal scope of practice.
9. Teaching proper alignment and execution techniques.
10. Recognizing and managing emergency situations.
11. Addressing unrealistic expectations.
12. Applying program guidelines specific to special populations.
13. Identifying problematic signs and symptoms before, during, and after the exercise session.
14. Documenting health- and fitness-related data.
15. Referring the client to appropriate health professionals.

Task 4 - Perform baseline and periodic follow-up evaluations of physical fitness levels and physical limitations using recommended guidelines and established protocols to facilitate program design, ensure safety, and monitor effectiveness.

Exercise Science

Knowledge of:

Anatomy

1. General anatomy of the following systems: musculoskeletal, cardiorespiratory, neuromuscular, digestive, endocrine, reproductive, and integumentary.
2. General anatomical terminology (e.g., landmarks, planes of movement, position, muscle roles, muscle origin, and muscle insertion).

Kinesiology

3. Passive and active ranges of motion.
4. Muscle function, types of muscle contraction, and associated factors affecting movement (e.g., neurological, biomechanical, kinesthetic).
5. Appropriate exercise design to address balance (e.g., static, dynamic), muscular imbalances, and postural alignment.
6. Biomechanical concepts of human movement (e.g., Newton's laws) as applied to exercise.
7. Application of the principles related to muscular strength and endurance (e.g., resistance, overload, specificity, repetitions, sets, frequency, rest periods, progression).

Physiology

8. Types of training (cardiorespiratory, resistance, and flexibility) and the risks and benefits associated with each.
9. Health-related components of physical fitness, principles of training, and adaptations (acute and chronic) to exercise.
10. Skill-related components of physical fitness, principles of training, and adaptations (agility, balance, coordination, speed, power, and reaction time).
11. Cardiorespiratory system with respect to the carrying capacity, delivery, and extraction of oxygen.
12. Metabolism, including energy production and nutrient utilization.
13. Neuromuscular physiology (e.g., muscle fiber types, proprioceptors, motor-unit recruitment).
14. Programming guidelines to improve fitness.
15. Environmental conditions impacting exercise (e.g., heat, humidity, cold, air pollution, altitude).

Skill in:

1. Facilitating cardiorespiratory fitness, musculoskeletal strength, and flexibility.
2. Selecting appropriate exercise modalities.
3. Selecting safe exercises for all muscle groups.
4. Applying appropriate training principles (FITT).
5. Modifying programs.
6. Assessing body composition.
7. Assessing dynamic and static posture and balance.
8. Assessing gait.
9. Assessing cardiorespiratory and musculoskeletal fitness.
10. Interpreting medical history.
11. Assessing clients' lifestyles.
12. Conducting risk stratification.
13. Comparing test data to normative values.
14. Selecting appropriate assessments.
15. Referring to the appropriate healthcare professional(s).
16. Communicating with members of the healthcare team.
17. Assessing anthropometric parameters.
18. Recognizing side effects associated with common categories of medications as they relate to energy and performance.

Nutrition

Knowledge of:

1. Macronutrients, micronutrients, hydration, supplements, engineered foods, alcohol, drugs (illicit, over-the-counter, prescription), and stimulants.
2. Current, credible, and appropriate nutrition resources.
3. Nutrition guidelines, food selection, preparation, and storage.
4. Digestion and absorption process.
5. Popular diets and associated health risks.
6. Nutrition requirements specific to each classification of disease or dysfunction.
7. Metabolic conversion of nutrients.

Skill in:

1. Assessing the quality of the client's food intake.
2. Educating the client on making appropriate food choices based on sound nutritional practices.
3. Recommending reputable resources for clients with an interest in a structured dietary management program.
4. Educating the client on appropriate food selections based on known risk reduction.
5. Recognizing deficiencies in nutrition as they relate to exercise performance.

6. Maintaining a current knowledge base of popular diets and extreme dietary measures.
7. Applying hydration guidelines as they relate to exercise duration, environmental conditions, and client status.

Psychology

Knowledge of:

1. Psychological conditions that require referral to appropriate allied health professionals.
2. Communication techniques (e.g., active listening, appropriate eye contact, non-verbal behavior).
3. Techniques that build and enhance rapport.
4. Individual differences that influence behavior (e.g., exercise history, lifestyle, gender, age, culture, ethnicity).
5. Psychological implications of chronic diseases, disabilities, and dysfunction.
6. Sources for disease-specific guidelines.
7. Theories of behavior change (e.g., stages of change, health belief model) and their implications.
8. Psychological obstacles that may interfere with the attainment of goals (e.g., self-esteem, anxiety, self-efficacy, mood).
9. Principles of adult learning (e.g., readiness, success, practice) and appropriate educational tools.
10. Psychological side effects of medications and appropriate precautions for a client taking medications and/or other substances.
11. The negative and positive impact of assessment data on motivation.
12. Motivational techniques used to optimize exercise adherence and other healthy lifestyle behaviors.
13. How chronic diseases, disabilities, and injuries will impact exercise adherence based on the client's perception of signs and symptoms.

Skill in:

1. Interviewing and communicating effectively with the client and/or healthcare team.
2. Interpreting body language and recognizing incongruities between verbal and non-verbal behaviors.
3. Building trust and rapport.
4. Assessing client's readiness, expectations, and preferences.
5. Applying principles of behavioral change.
6. Identifying barriers associated with various chronic diseases, disabilities, and injuries that may affect programming.
7. Adapting programming in accordance with identified barriers.
8. Identifying and/or addressing unrealistic expectations as they relate to underlying chronic diseases, disabilities, and injuries.
9. Establishing goals (e.g., specific, measurable, action-oriented, realistic, timed).
10. Selecting and integrating appropriate educational tools for use in client instruction.
11. Facilitating the client's acceptance, responsibility, and accountability for program goals.
12. Designing a safe, well-balanced, and comprehensive program specific to the client's health status, special needs, program preferences, and goals.
13. Instructing and/or supervising the client in the safe and proper execution of exercise.
14. Modifying motivational strategies based upon assessment and/or reassessment.
15. Making appropriate referrals.

Pathophysiology

1. General pathophysiology of chronic diseases, disabilities, and injuries as related to each organ system, including cardiovascular, respiratory, endocrine, neurological, musculoskeletal, gastrointestinal, reproductive, and integumentary.
2. Signs and symptoms of chronic diseases, disabilities, and injuries.
3. Guidelines for designing programs specific to chronic diseases, disabilities, and injuries using FITT principles as they apply to cardiorespiratory, strength, and flexibility training.
4. Influence of chronic diseases, disabilities, and injuries on exercise selection.
5. Influence of chronic diseases, disabilities, and injuries on the selection of assessment tools.
6. Predicted responses to exercise in clients with chronic diseases, disabilities, and injuries.
7. Designing safe, comprehensive, and effective programs based on the client's current health status.

8. Appropriate exercise modifications for chronic diseases, disabilities, and injuries based on the client's response to exercise.
9. Indications for modification or termination of an exercise session or activity.
10. Circumstances requiring referral to other health professionals.
11. Contraindicated activities/exercises.
12. Appropriate documentation of signs, symptoms, and responses to exercise.
13. Effect of medication on exercise selection.
14. Potential effect of exercise on medication requirements.
15. How environmental factors affect exercise for clients with chronic diseases, disabilities, and injuries.
16. Alternative medical services (e.g., chiropractic, acupuncture, naturopathy) and how they may affect exercise/activity selection for clients with chronic diseases, disabilities, and injuries.
17. Potential medical emergencies in clients with chronic diseases, disabilities, and injuries.
18. Recognized protocols (e.g., McKenzie extension exercises, rotator cuff progression) for clients with chronic diseases, disabilities, and injuries.

Skill in:

1. Assessing and reassessing the client's readiness, expectations, and limitations.
2. Administering and analyzing assessment data.
3. Interpreting the data from the referring health professional.
4. Modifying the program to meet the needs of the client.
5. Applying standard and accepted testing methods to measure current fitness status.
6. Identifying environmental factors that influence exercise performance.
7. Recognizing the need for terminating a specific activity, an exercise session, or the entire program.
8. Recognizing personal scope of practice.
9. Teaching proper alignment and execution techniques.
10. Recognizing and managing emergency situations.
11. Addressing unrealistic expectations.
12. Applying program guidelines specific to special populations.
13. Identifying problematic signs and symptoms before, during, and after the exercise session.
14. Documenting health- and fitness-related data.
15. Referring the client to appropriate health professionals.

Task 5 - Maintain detailed records of assessment data using established documentation policies and procedures to adhere to professional guidelines and facilitate program design.

Exercise Science

Knowledge of:

Anatomy

1. General anatomy of the following systems: musculoskeletal, cardiorespiratory, neuromuscular, digestive, endocrine, reproductive, and integumentary.
2. General anatomical terminology (e.g., landmarks, planes of movement, position, muscle roles, muscle origin, and muscle insertion).

Kinesiology

3. Passive and active ranges of motion.
4. Muscle function, types of muscle contraction, and associated factors affecting movement (e.g., neurological, biomechanical, kinesthetic).
5. Appropriate exercise design to address balance (e.g., static, dynamic), muscular imbalances, and postural alignment.
6. Biomechanical concepts of human movement (e.g., Newton's laws) as applied to exercise.
7. Application of the principles related to muscular strength and endurance (e.g., resistance, overload, specificity, repetitions, sets, frequency, rest periods, progression).

Physiology

8. Types of training (cardiorespiratory, resistance, and flexibility) and the risks and benefits associated with each.
9. Health-related components of physical fitness, principles of training, and adaptations (acute and chronic) to exercise.
10. Skill-related components of physical fitness, principles of training, and adaptations (agility,

balance, coordination, speed, power, and reaction time).

11. Cardiorespiratory system with respect to the carrying capacity, delivery, and extraction of oxygen.
12. Metabolism, including energy production and nutrient utilization.
13. Neuromuscular physiology (e.g., muscle fiber types, proprioceptors, motor-unit recruitment).
14. Programming guidelines to improve fitness.
15. Environmental conditions impacting exercise (e.g., heat, humidity, cold, air pollution, altitude).

Skill in:

1. Facilitating cardiorespiratory fitness, musculoskeletal strength, and flexibility.
2. Selecting appropriate exercise modalities.
3. Selecting safe exercises for all muscle groups.
4. Applying appropriate training principles (FITT).
5. Modifying programs.
6. Assessing body composition.
7. Assessing dynamic and static posture and balance.
8. Assessing gait.
9. Assessing cardiorespiratory and musculoskeletal fitness.
10. Interpreting medical history.
11. Assessing clients' lifestyles.
12. Conducting risk stratification.
13. Comparing test data to normative values.
14. Selecting appropriate assessments.
15. Referring to the appropriate healthcare professional(s).
16. Communicating with members of the healthcare team.
17. Assessing anthropometric parameters.
18. Recognizing side effects associated with common categories of medications as they relate to energy and performance.

Nutrition

Knowledge of:

1. Macronutrients, micronutrients, hydration, supplements, engineered foods, alcohol, drugs (illicit, over-the-counter, prescription), and stimulants.
2. Current, credible, and appropriate nutrition resources.
3. Nutrition guidelines, food selection, preparation, and storage.
4. Digestion and absorption process.
5. Popular diets and associated health risks.
6. Nutrition requirements specific to each classification of disease or dysfunction.
7. Metabolic conversion of nutrients.

Skill in:

1. Assessing the quality of the client's food intake.
2. Educating the client on making appropriate food choices based on sound nutritional practices.
3. Recommending reputable resources for clients with an interest in a structured dietary management program.
4. Educating the client on appropriate food selections based on known risk reduction.
5. Recognizing deficiencies in nutrition as they relate to exercise performance.
6. Maintaining a current knowledge base of popular diets and extreme dietary measures.
7. Applying hydration guidelines as they relate to exercise duration, environmental conditions, and client status.

Psychology

Knowledge of:

1. Psychological conditions that require referral to appropriate allied health professionals.
2. Communication techniques (e.g., active listening, appropriate eye contact, non-verbal behavior).
3. Techniques that build and enhance rapport.
4. Individual differences that influence behavior (e.g., exercise history, lifestyle, gender, age, culture, ethnicity).
5. Psychological implications of chronic diseases, disabilities, and dysfunction.
6. Sources for disease-specific guidelines.

7. Theories of behavior change (e.g., stages of change, health belief model) and their implications.
8. Psychological obstacles that may interfere with the attainment of goals (e.g., self-esteem, anxiety, self-efficacy, mood).
9. Principles of adult learning (e.g., readiness, success, practice) and appropriate educational tools.
10. Psychological side effects of medications and appropriate precautions for a client taking medications and/or other substances.
11. The negative and positive impact of assessment data on motivation.
12. Motivational techniques used to optimize exercise adherence and other healthy lifestyle behaviors.
13. How chronic diseases, disabilities, and injuries will impact exercise adherence based on client's perception of signs and symptoms.

Skill in:

1. Interviewing and communicating effectively with the client and/or healthcare team.
2. Interpreting body language and recognizing incongruities between verbal and non-verbal behaviors.
3. Building trust and rapport.
4. Assessing client's readiness, expectations, and preferences.
5. Applying principles of behavioral change.
6. Identifying barriers associated with various chronic diseases, disabilities, and injuries that may affect programming.
7. Adapting programming in accordance with identified barriers.
8. Identifying and/or addressing unrealistic expectations as they relate to underlying chronic diseases, disabilities, and injuries.
9. Establishing goals (e.g., specific, measurable, action-oriented, realistic, timed).
10. Selecting and integrating appropriate educational tools for use in client instruction.
11. Facilitating the client's acceptance, responsibility, and accountability for program goals.
12. Designing a safe, well-balanced, and comprehensive program specific to the client's health status, special needs, program preferences, and goals.
13. Instructing and/or supervising the client in the safe and proper execution of exercise.
14. Modifying motivational strategies based upon assessment and/or reassessment.
15. Making appropriate referrals.

Pathophysiology

1. General pathophysiology of chronic diseases, disabilities, and injuries as related to each organ system, including cardiovascular, respiratory, endocrine, neurological, musculoskeletal, gastrointestinal, reproductive, and integumentary.
2. Signs and symptoms of chronic diseases, disabilities, and injuries.
3. Guidelines for designing programs specific to chronic diseases, disabilities, and injuries using FITT principles as they apply to cardiorespiratory, strength, and flexibility training.
4. Influence of chronic diseases, disabilities, and injuries on exercise selection.
5. Influence of chronic diseases, disabilities, and injuries on the selection of assessment tools.
6. Predicted responses to exercise in clients with chronic diseases, disabilities, and injuries.
7. Designing safe, comprehensive, and effective programs based on the client's current health status.
8. Appropriate exercise modifications for chronic diseases, disabilities, and injuries based on the client's response to exercise.
9. Indications for modification or termination of an exercise session or activity.
10. Circumstances requiring referral to other health professionals.
11. Contraindicated activities/exercises.
12. Appropriate documentation of signs, symptoms, and responses to exercise.
13. Effect of medication on exercise selection.
14. Potential effect of exercise on medication requirements.
15. How environmental factors affect exercise for clients with chronic diseases, disabilities, and injuries.
16. Alternative medical services (e.g., chiropractic, acupuncture, naturopathy) and how they may affect exercise/activity selection for clients with chronic diseases, disabilities, and injuries.

17 Potential medical emergencies in clients with chronic diseases, disabilities, and injuries.
18. Recognized protocols (e.g., McKenzie extension exercises, rotator cuff progression) for clients with chronic diseases, disabilities, and injuries.

Skill in:

1. Assessing and reassessing the client's readiness, expectations, and limitations.
2. Administering and analyzing assessment data.
3. Interpreting the data from the referring health professional.
4. Modifying the program to meet the needs of the client.
5. Applying standard and accepted testing methods to measure current fitness status.
6. Identifying environmental factors that influence exercise performance.
7. Recognizing the need for terminating a specific activity, an exercise session, or the entire program.
8. Recognizing personal scope of practice.
9. Teaching proper alignment and execution techniques.
10. Recognizing and managing emergency situations.
11. Addressing unrealistic expectations.
12. Applying program guidelines specific to special populations.
13. Identifying problematic signs and symptoms before, during, and after the exercise session.
14. Documenting health- and fitness-related data.
15. Referring the client to appropriate health professionals.

DOMAIN II: PROGRAM DESIGN 26%

Task 1 - Establish realistic and appropriate goals using the client's expectations and limitations, assessment data, and the principles of exercise science to develop a safe and effective program.

Exercise Science

Knowledge of:

Anatomy

1. General anatomy of the following systems: musculoskeletal, cardiorespiratory, neuromuscular, digestive, endocrine, reproductive, and integumentary.
2. General anatomical terminology (e.g., landmarks, planes of movement, position, muscle roles, muscle origin, and muscle insertion).

Kinesiology

3. Passive and active ranges of motion.
4. Muscle function, types of muscle contraction, and associated factors affecting movement (e.g., neurological, biomechanical, kinesthetic).
5. Appropriate exercise design to address balance (e.g., static, dynamic), muscular imbalances, and postural alignment.
6. Biomechanical concepts of human movement (e.g., Newton's laws) as applied to exercise.
7. Application of the principles related to muscular strength and endurance (e.g., resistance, overload, specificity, repetitions, sets, frequency, rest periods, progression).

Physiology

8. Types of training (cardiorespiratory, resistance, and flexibility) and the risks and benefits associated with each.
9. Health-related components of physical fitness, principles of training, and adaptations (acute and chronic) to exercise.
10. Skill-related components of physical fitness, principles of training, and adaptations (agility, balance, coordination, speed, power, and reaction time).
11. Cardiorespiratory system with respect to the carrying capacity, delivery, and extraction of oxygen.
12. Metabolism, including energy production and nutrient utilization.
13. Neuromuscular physiology (e.g., muscle fiber types, proprioceptors, motor-unit recruitment).
14. Programming guidelines to improve fitness.
15. Environmental conditions impacting exercise (e.g., heat, humidity, cold, air pollution, altitude).

Skill in:

1. Facilitating cardiorespiratory fitness, musculoskeletal strength, and flexibility.
2. Selecting appropriate exercise modalities.

3. Selecting safe exercises for all muscle groups.
4. Applying appropriate training principles (FITT).
5. Modifying programs.
6. Assessing body composition.
7. Assessing dynamic and static posture and balance.
8. Assessing gait.
9. Assessing cardiorespiratory and musculoskeletal fitness.
10. Interpreting medical history.
11. Assessing clients' lifestyles.
12. Conducting risk stratification.
13. Comparing test data to normative values.
14. Selecting appropriate assessments.
15. Referring to the appropriate healthcare professional(s).
16. Communicating with members of the healthcare team.
17. Assessing anthropometric parameters.
18. Recognizing side effects associated with common categories of medications as they relate to energy and performance.

Nutrition

Knowledge of:

1. Macronutrients, micronutrients, hydration, supplements, engineered foods, alcohol, drugs (illicit, over-the-counter, prescription), and stimulants.
2. Current, credible, and appropriate nutrition resources.
3. Nutrition guidelines, food selection, preparation, and storage.
4. Digestion and absorption process.
5. Popular diets and associated health risks.
6. Nutrition requirements specific to each classification of disease or dysfunction.
7. Metabolic conversion of nutrients.

Skill in:

1. Assessing the quality of the client's food intake.
2. Educating the client on making appropriate food choices based on sound nutritional practices.
3. Recommending reputable resources for clients with an interest in a structured dietary management program.
4. Educating the client on appropriate food selections based on known risk reduction.
5. Recognizing deficiencies in nutrition as they relate to exercise performance.
6. Maintaining a current knowledge base of popular diets and extreme dietary measures.
7. Applying hydration guidelines as they relate to exercise duration, environmental conditions, and client status.

Psychology

Knowledge of:

1. Psychological conditions that require referral to appropriate allied health professionals.
2. Communication techniques (e.g., active listening, appropriate eye contact, non-verbal behavior).
3. Techniques that build and enhance rapport.
4. Individual differences that influence behavior (e.g., exercise history, lifestyle, gender, age, culture, ethnicity).
5. Psychological implications of chronic diseases, disabilities, and dysfunction.
6. Sources for disease-specific guidelines.
7. Theories of behavior change (e.g., stages of change, health belief model) and their implications.
8. Psychological obstacles that may interfere with the attainment of goals (e.g., self-esteem, anxiety, self-efficacy, mood).
9. Principles of adult learning (e.g., readiness, success, practice) and appropriate educational tools.
10. Psychological side effects of medications and appropriate precautions for a client taking medications and/or other substances.
11. The negative and positive impact of assessment data on motivation.
12. Motivational techniques used to optimize exercise adherence and other healthy lifestyle behaviors.
13. How chronic diseases, disabilities, and injuries will impact exercise adherence based on the client's perception of signs and symptoms.

Skill in:

1. Interviewing and communicating effectively with the client and/or healthcare team.

2. Interpreting body language and recognizing incongruities between verbal and non-verbal behaviors.
3. Building trust and rapport.
4. Assessing client's readiness, expectations, and preferences.
5. Applying principles of behavioral change.
6. Identifying barriers associated with various chronic diseases, disabilities, and injuries that may affect programming.
7. Adapting programming in accordance with identified barriers.
8. Identifying and/or addressing unrealistic expectations as they relate to underlying chronic diseases, disabilities, and injuries.
9. Establishing goals (e.g., specific, measurable, action-oriented, realistic, timed).
10. Selecting and integrating appropriate educational tools for use in client instruction.
11. Facilitating the client's acceptance, responsibility, and accountability for program goals.
12. Designing a safe, well-balanced, and comprehensive program specific to the client's health status, special needs, program preferences, and goals.
13. Instructing and/or supervising the client in the safe and proper execution of exercise.
14. Modifying motivational strategies based upon assessment and/or reassessment.
15. Making appropriate referrals.

Pathophysiology

1. General pathophysiology of chronic diseases, disabilities, and injuries as related to each organ system, including cardiovascular, respiratory, endocrine, neurological, musculoskeletal, gastrointestinal, reproductive, and integumentary.
2. Signs and symptoms of chronic diseases, disabilities, and injuries.
3. Guidelines for designing programs specific to chronic diseases, disabilities, and injuries using FITT principles as they apply to cardiorespiratory, strength, and flexibility training.
4. Influence of chronic diseases, disabilities, and injuries on exercise selection.
5. Influence of chronic diseases, disabilities, and injuries on the selection of assessment tools.
6. Predicted responses to exercise in clients with chronic diseases, disabilities, and injuries.
7. Designing safe, comprehensive, and effective programs based on the client's current health status.
8. Appropriate exercise modifications for chronic diseases, disabilities, and injuries based on the client's response to exercise.
9. Indications for modification or termination of an exercise session or activity.
10. Circumstances requiring referral to other health professionals.
11. Contraindicated activities/exercises.
12. Appropriate documentation of signs, symptoms, and responses to exercise.
13. Effect of medication on exercise selection.
14. Potential effect of exercise on medication requirements.
15. How environmental factors affect exercise for clients with chronic diseases, disabilities, and injuries.
16. Alternative medical services (e.g., chiropractic, acupuncture, naturopathy) and how they may affect exercise/activity selection for clients with chronic diseases, disabilities, and injuries.
17. Potential medical emergencies in clients with chronic diseases, disabilities, and injuries.
18. Recognized protocols (e.g., McKenzie extension exercises, rotator cuff progression) for clients with chronic diseases, disabilities, and injuries.

Skill in:

1. Assessing and reassessing the client's readiness, expectations, and limitations.
2. Administering and analyzing assessment data.
3. Interpreting the data from the referring health professional.
4. Modifying the program to meet the needs of the client.
5. Applying standard and accepted testing methods to measure current fitness status.
6. Identifying environmental factors that influence exercise performance.
7. Recognizing the need for terminating a specific activity, an exercise session, or the entire program.
8. Recognizing personal scope of practice.

9. Teaching proper alignment and execution techniques.
10. Recognizing and managing emergency situations.
11. Addressing unrealistic expectations.
12. Applying program guidelines specific to special populations.
13. Identifying problematic signs and symptoms before, during, and after the exercise session.
14. Documenting health- and fitness-related data.
15. Referring the client to appropriate health professionals.

*Task 2 - **Apply the principles of exercise science by integrating the specific, measurable goals and interpreting assessment and reassessment data to develop individualized, safe, and effective programs for clients with chronic disease and/or disabilities.***

Exercise Science

Knowledge of:

Anatomy

1. General anatomy of the following systems: musculoskeletal, cardiorespiratory, neuromuscular, digestive, endocrine, reproductive, and integumentary.
2. General anatomical terminology (e.g., landmarks, planes of movement, position, muscle roles, muscle origin, and muscle insertion).

Kinesiology

3. Passive and active ranges of motion.
4. Muscle function, types of muscle contraction, and associated factors affecting movement (e.g., neurological, biomechanical, kinesthetic).
5. Appropriate exercise design to address balance (e.g., static, dynamic), muscular imbalances, and postural alignment.
6. Biomechanical concepts of human movement (e.g., Newton's laws) as applied to exercise.
7. Application of the principles related to muscular strength and endurance (e.g., resistance, overload, specificity, repetitions, sets, frequency, rest periods, progression).

Physiology

8. Types of training (cardiorespiratory, resistance, and flexibility) and the risks and benefits associated with each.
9. Health-related components of physical fitness, principles of training, and adaptations (acute and chronic) to exercise.
10. Skill-related components of physical fitness, principles of training, and adaptations (agility, balance, coordination, speed, power, and reaction time).
11. Cardiorespiratory system with respect to the carrying capacity, delivery, and extraction of oxygen.
12. Metabolism, including energy production and nutrient utilization.
13. Neuromuscular physiology (e.g., muscle fiber types, proprioceptors, motor-unit recruitment).
14. Programming guidelines to improve fitness.
15. Environmental conditions impacting exercise (e.g., heat, humidity, cold, air pollution, altitude).

Skill in:

1. Facilitating cardiorespiratory fitness, musculoskeletal strength, and flexibility.
2. Selecting appropriate exercise modalities.
3. Selecting safe exercises for all muscle groups.
4. Applying appropriate training principles (FITT).
5. Modifying programs.
6. Assessing body composition.
7. Assessing dynamic and static posture and balance.
8. Assessing gait.
9. Assessing cardiorespiratory and musculoskeletal fitness.
10. Interpreting medical history.
11. Assessing clients' lifestyles.
12. Conducting risk stratification.
13. Comparing test data to normative values.
14. Selecting appropriate assessments.
15. Referring to the appropriate healthcare professional(s).
16. Communicating with members of the healthcare team.
17. Assessing anthropometric parameters.

18. Recognizing side effects associated with common categories of medications as they relate to energy and performance.

Nutrition

Knowledge of:

1. Macronutrients, micronutrients, hydration, supplements, engineered foods, alcohol, drugs (illicit, over-the-counter, prescription), and stimulants.
2. Current, credible, and appropriate nutrition resources.
3. Nutrition guidelines, food selection, preparation, and storage.
4. Digestion and absorption process.
5. Popular diets and associated health risks.
6. Nutrition requirements specific to each classification of disease or dysfunction.
7. Metabolic conversion of nutrients.

Skill in:

1. Assessing the quality of the client's food intake.
2. Educating the client on making appropriate food choices based on sound nutritional practices.
3. Recommending reputable resources for clients with an interest in a structured dietary management program.
4. Educating the client on appropriate food selections based on known risk reduction.
5. Recognizing deficiencies in nutrition as they relate to exercise performance.
6. Maintaining a current knowledge base of popular diets and extreme dietary measures.
7. Applying hydration guidelines as they relate to exercise duration, environmental conditions, and client status.

Psychology

Knowledge of:

1. Psychological conditions that require referral to appropriate allied health professionals.
2. Communication techniques (e.g., active listening, appropriate eye contact, nonverbal behavior).
3. Techniques that build and enhance rapport.
4. Individual differences that influence behavior (e.g., exercise history, lifestyle, gender, age, culture, ethnicity).
5. Psychological implications of chronic diseases, disabilities, and dysfunction.
6. Sources for disease-specific guidelines.
7. Theories of behavior change (e.g., stages of change, health belief model) and their implications.
8. Psychological obstacles that may interfere with the attainment of goals (e.g., self-esteem, anxiety, self-efficacy, mood).
9. Principles of adult learning (e.g., readiness, success, practice) and appropriate educational tools.
10. Psychological side effects of medications and appropriate precautions for a client taking medications and/or other substances.
11. The negative and positive impact of assessment data on motivation.
12. Motivational techniques used to optimize exercise adherence and other healthy lifestyle behaviors.
13. How chronic diseases, disabilities, and injuries will impact exercise adherence based on client's perception of signs and symptoms.

Skill in:

1. Interviewing and communicating effectively with the client and/or healthcare team.
2. Interpreting body language and recognizing incongruities between verbal and non-verbal behaviors.
3. Building trust and rapport.
4. Assessing client's readiness, expectations, and preferences.
5. Applying principles of behavioral change.
6. Identifying barriers associated with various chronic diseases, disabilities, and injuries that may affect programming.
7. Adapting programming in accordance with identified barriers.
8. Identifying and/or addressing unrealistic expectations as they relate to underlying chronic diseases, disabilities, and injuries.
9. Establishing goals (e.g., specific, measurable, action-oriented, realistic, timed).

10. Selecting and integrating appropriate educational tools for use in client instruction.
11. Facilitating the client's acceptance, responsibility, and accountability for program goals.
12. Designing a safe, well-balanced, and comprehensive program specific to the client's health status, special needs, program preferences, and goals.
13. Instructing and/or supervising the client in the safe and proper execution of exercise.
14. Modifying motivational strategies based upon assessment and/or reassessment.
15. Making appropriate referrals.

Pathophysiology

1. General pathophysiology of chronic diseases, disabilities, and injuries as related to each organ system, including cardiovascular, respiratory, endocrine, neurological, musculoskeletal, gastrointestinal, reproductive, and integumentary.
2. Signs and symptoms of chronic diseases, disabilities, and injuries.
3. Guidelines for designing programs specific to chronic diseases, disabilities, and injuries using FITT principles as they apply to cardiorespiratory, strength, and flexibility training.
4. Influence of chronic diseases, disabilities, and injuries on exercise selection.
5. Influence of chronic diseases, disabilities, and injuries on the selection of assessment tools.
6. Predicted responses to exercise in clients with chronic diseases, disabilities, and injuries.
7. Designing safe, comprehensive, and effective programs based on the client's current health status.
8. Appropriate exercise modifications for chronic diseases, disabilities, and injuries based on the client's response to exercise.
9. Indications for modification or termination of an exercise session or activity.
10. Circumstances requiring referral to other health professionals.
11. Contraindicated activities/exercises.
12. Appropriate documentation of signs, symptoms, and responses to exercise.
13. Effect of medication on exercise selection.
14. Potential effect of exercise on medication requirements.
15. How environmental factors affect exercise for clients with chronic diseases, disabilities, and injuries.
16. Alternative medical services (e.g., chiropractic, acupuncture, naturopathy) and how they may affect exercise/activity selection for clients with chronic diseases, disabilities, and injuries.
17. Potential medical emergencies in clients with chronic diseases, disabilities, and injuries.
18. Recognized protocols (e.g., McKenzie extension exercises, rotator cuff progression) for clients with chronic diseases, disabilities, and injuries.

Skill in:

1. Assessing and reassessing the client's readiness, expectations, and limitations.
2. Administering and analyzing assessment data.
3. Interpreting the data from the referring health professional.
4. Modifying the program to meet the needs of the client.
5. Applying standard and accepted testing methods to measure current fitness status.
6. Identifying environmental factors that influence exercise performance.
7. Recognizing the need for terminating a specific activity, an exercise session, or the entire program.
8. Recognizing personal scope of practice.
9. Teaching proper alignment and execution techniques.
10. Recognizing and managing emergency situations.
11. Addressing unrealistic expectations.
12. Applying program guidelines specific to special populations.
13. Identifying problematic signs and symptoms before, during, and after the exercise session.
14. Documenting health- and fitness-related data.

15. Referring the client to appropriate health professionals.

Task 3 - Modify the program based on reassessment data, exercise logs, and client-reported information to maximize the probability of success.

Exercise Science

Knowledge of:

Anatomy

1. General anatomy of the following systems: musculoskeletal, cardiorespiratory, neuromuscular, digestive, endocrine, reproductive, and integumentary.
2. General anatomical terminology (e.g., landmarks, planes of movement, position, muscle roles, muscle origin, and muscle insertion).

Kinesiology

3. Passive and active ranges of motion.
4. Muscle function, types of muscle contraction, and associated factors affecting movement (e.g., neurological, biomechanical, kinesthetic).
5. Appropriate exercise design to address balance (e.g., static, dynamic), muscular imbalances, and postural alignment.
6. Biomechanical concepts of human movement (e.g., Newton's laws) as applied to exercise.
7. Application of the principles related to muscular strength and endurance (e.g., resistance, overload, specificity, repetitions, sets, frequency, rest periods, progression).

Physiology

8. Types of training (cardiorespiratory, resistance, and flexibility) and the risks and benefits associated with each.
9. Health-related components of physical fitness, principles of training, and adaptations (acute and chronic) to exercise.
10. Skill-related components of physical fitness, principles of training, and adaptations (agility, balance, coordination, speed, power, and reaction time).
11. Cardiorespiratory system with respect to the carrying capacity, delivery, and extraction of oxygen.
12. Metabolism, including energy production and nutrient utilization.
13. Neuromuscular physiology (e.g., muscle fiber types, proprioceptors, motor-unit recruitment).
14. Programming guidelines to improve fitness.
15. Environmental conditions impacting exercise (e.g., heat, humidity, cold, air pollution, altitude).

Skill in:

1. Facilitating cardiorespiratory fitness, musculoskeletal strength, and flexibility.
2. Selecting appropriate exercise modalities.
3. Selecting safe exercises for all muscle groups.
4. Applying appropriate training principles (FITT).
5. Modifying programs.
6. Assessing body composition.
7. Assessing dynamic and static posture and balance.
8. Assessing gait.
9. Assessing cardiorespiratory and musculoskeletal fitness.
10. Interpreting medical history.
11. Assessing clients' lifestyles.
12. Conducting risk stratification.
13. Comparing test data to normative values.
14. Selecting appropriate assessments.
15. Referring to the appropriate healthcare professional(s).
16. Communicating with members of the healthcare team.
17. Assessing anthropometric parameters.
18. Recognizing side effects associated with common categories of medications as they relate to energy and performance.

Nutrition

Knowledge of:

1. Macronutrients, micronutrients, hydration, supplements, engineered foods, alcohol, drugs (illicit, over-the-counter, prescription), and stimulants.
2. Current, credible, and appropriate nutrition resources.
3. Nutrition guidelines, food selection, preparation, and storage.

4. Digestion and absorption process.
5. Popular diets and associated health risks.
6. Nutrition requirements specific to each classification of disease or dysfunction.
7. Metabolic conversion of nutrients.

Skill in:

1. Assessing the quality of the client's food intake.
2. Educating the client on making appropriate food choices based on sound nutritional practices.
3. Recommending reputable resources for clients with an interest in a structured dietary management program.
4. Educating the client on appropriate food selections based on known risk reduction.
5. Recognizing deficiencies in nutrition as they relate to exercise performance.
6. Maintaining a current knowledge base of popular diets and extreme dietary measures.
7. Applying hydration guidelines as they relate to exercise duration, environmental conditions, and client status.

Psychology

Knowledge of:

1. Psychological conditions that require referral to appropriate allied health professionals.
2. Communication techniques (e.g., active listening, appropriate eye contact, non-verbal behavior).
3. Techniques that build and enhance rapport.
4. Individual differences that influence behavior (e.g., exercise history, lifestyle, gender, age, culture, ethnicity).
5. Psychological implications of chronic diseases, disabilities, and dysfunction.
6. Sources for disease-specific guidelines.
7. Theories of behavior change (e.g., stages of change, health belief model) and their implications.
8. Psychological obstacles that may interfere with the attainment of goals (e.g., self-esteem, anxiety, self-efficacy, mood).
9. Principles of adult learning (e.g., readiness, success, practice) and appropriate educational tools.
10. Psychological side effects of medications and appropriate precautions for a client taking medications and/or other substances.
11. The negative and positive impact of assessment data on motivation.
12. Motivational techniques used to optimize exercise adherence and other healthy lifestyle behaviors.
13. How chronic diseases, disabilities, and injuries will impact exercise adherence based on the client's perception of signs and symptoms.

Skill in:

1. Interviewing and communicating effectively with the client and/or healthcare team.
2. Interpreting body language and recognizing incongruities between verbal and non-verbal behaviors.
3. Building trust and rapport.
4. Assessing client's readiness, expectations, and preferences.
5. Applying principles of behavioral change.
6. Identifying barriers associated with various chronic diseases, disabilities, and injuries that may affect programming.
7. Adapting programming in accordance with identified barriers.
8. Identifying and/or addressing unrealistic expectations as they relate to underlying chronic diseases, disabilities, and injuries.
9. Establishing goals (e.g., specific, measurable, action-oriented, realistic, timed).
10. Selecting and integrating appropriate educational tools for use in client instruction.
11. Facilitating the client's acceptance, responsibility, and accountability for program goals.
12. Designing a safe, well-balanced, and comprehensive program specific to the client's health status, special needs, program preferences, and goals.
13. Instructing and/or supervising the client in the safe and proper execution of exercise.
14. Modifying motivational strategies based upon assessment and/or reassessment.
15. Making appropriate referrals.

Pathophysiology

1. General pathophysiology of chronic diseases, disabilities, and injuries as related to each organ system, including cardiovascular, respiratory, endocrine, neurological, musculoskeletal, gastrointestinal, reproductive, and integumentary.
2. Signs and symptoms of chronic diseases, disabilities, and injuries.
3. Guidelines for designing programs specific to chronic diseases, disabilities, and injuries using FITT principles as they apply to cardiorespiratory, strength, and flexibility training.
4. Influence of chronic diseases, disabilities, and injuries on exercise selection.
5. Influence of chronic diseases, disabilities, and injuries on the selection of assessment tools.
6. Predicted responses to exercise in clients with chronic diseases, disabilities, and injuries.
7. Designing safe, comprehensive, and effective programs based on the client's current health status.
8. Appropriate exercise modifications for chronic diseases, disabilities, and injuries based on the client's response to exercise.
9. Indications for modification or termination of an exercise session or activity.
10. Circumstances requiring referral to other health professionals.
11. Contraindicated activities/exercises.
12. Appropriate documentation of signs, symptoms, and responses to exercise.
13. Effect of medication on exercise selection.
14. Potential effect of exercise on medication requirements.
15. How environmental factors affect exercise for clients with chronic diseases, disabilities, and injuries.
16. Alternative medical services (e.g., chiropractic, acupuncture, naturopathy) and how they may affect exercise/activity selection for clients with chronic diseases, disabilities, and injuries.
17. Potential medical emergencies in clients with chronic diseases, disabilities, and injuries.
18. Recognized protocols (e.g., McKenzie extension exercises, rotator cuff progression) for clients with chronic diseases, disabilities, and injuries.

Skill in:

1. Assessing and reassessing the client's readiness, expectations, and limitations.
2. Administering and analyzing assessment data.
3. Interpreting the data from the referring health professional.
4. Modifying the program to meet the needs of the client.
5. Applying standard and accepted testing methods to measure current fitness status.
6. Identifying environmental factors that influence exercise performance.
7. Recognizing the need for terminating a specific activity, an exercise session, or the entire program.
8. Recognizing personal scope of practice.
9. Teaching proper alignment and execution techniques.
10. Recognizing and managing emergency situations.
11. Addressing unrealistic expectations.
12. Applying program guidelines specific to special populations.
13. Identifying problematic signs and symptoms before, during, and after the exercise session.
14. Documenting health- and fitness-related data.
15. Referring the client to appropriate health professionals.

DOMAIN III: PROGRAM IMPLEMENTATION AND MANAGEMENT 40%

Task 1 - Orient the client to an individualized program using appropriate educational techniques to set the foundation for program implementation.

Exercise Science

Knowledge of:

Anatomy

1. General anatomy of the following systems: musculoskeletal, cardiorespiratory, neuromuscular, digestive, endocrine, reproductive, and integumentary.

2. General anatomical terminology (e.g., landmarks, planes of movement, position, muscle roles, muscle origin, and muscle insertion).

Kinesiology

3. Passive and active ranges of motion.
4. Muscle function, types of muscle contraction, and associated factors affecting movement (e.g., neurological, biomechanical, kinesthetic).
5. Appropriate exercise design to address balance (e.g., static, dynamic), muscular imbalances, and postural alignment.
6. Biomechanical concepts of human movement (e.g., Newton's laws) as applied to exercise.
7. Application of the principles related to muscular strength and endurance (e.g., resistance, overload, specificity, repetitions, sets, frequency, rest periods, progression).

Physiology

8. Types of training (cardiorespiratory, resistance, and flexibility) and the risks and benefits associated with each.
9. Health-related components of physical fitness, principles of training, and adaptations (acute and chronic) to exercise.
10. Skill-related components of physical fitness, principles of training, and adaptations (agility, balance, coordination, speed, power, and reaction time).
11. Cardiorespiratory system with respect to the carrying capacity, delivery, and extraction of oxygen.
12. Metabolism, including energy production and nutrient utilization.
13. Neuromuscular physiology (e.g., muscle fiber types, proprioceptors, motor-unit recruitment).
14. Programming guidelines to improve fitness.
15. Environmental conditions impacting exercise (e.g., heat, humidity, cold, air pollution, altitude).

Skill in:

1. Facilitating cardiorespiratory fitness, musculoskeletal strength, and flexibility.
2. Selecting appropriate exercise modalities.
3. Selecting safe exercises for all muscle groups.
4. Applying appropriate training principles (FITT).
5. Modifying programs.
6. Assessing body composition.
7. Assessing dynamic and static posture and balance.
8. Assessing gait.
9. Assessing cardiorespiratory and musculoskeletal fitness.
10. Interpreting medical history.
11. Assessing clients' lifestyles.
12. Conducting risk stratification.
13. Comparing test data to normative values.
14. Selecting appropriate assessments.
15. Referring to the appropriate healthcare professional(s).
16. Communicating with members of the healthcare team.
17. Assessing anthropometric parameters.
18. Recognizing side effects associated with common categories of medications as they relate to energy and performance.

Nutrition

Knowledge of:

1. Macronutrients, micronutrients, hydration, supplements, engineered foods, alcohol, drugs (illicit, over-the-counter, prescription), and stimulants.
2. Current, credible, and appropriate nutrition resources.
3. Nutrition guidelines, food selection, preparation, and storage.
4. Digestion and absorption process.
5. Popular diets and associated health risks.
6. Nutrition requirements specific to each classification of disease or dysfunction.
7. Metabolic conversion of nutrients.

Skill in:

1. Assessing the quality of the client's food intake.
2. Educating the client on making appropriate food choices based on sound nutritional practices.
3. Recommending reputable resources for clients with an interest in a structured dietary management program.
4. Educating the client on appropriate food selections based on known risk reduction.

5. Recognizing deficiencies in nutrition as they relate to exercise performance.
6. Maintaining a current knowledge base of popular diets and extreme dietary measures.
7. Applying hydration guidelines as they relate to exercise duration, environmental conditions, and client status.

Psychology

Knowledge of:

1. Psychological conditions that require referral to appropriate allied health professionals.
2. Communication techniques (e.g., active listening, appropriate eye contact, non-verbal behavior).
3. Techniques that build and enhance rapport.
4. Individual differences that influence behavior (e.g., exercise history, lifestyle, gender, age, culture, ethnicity).
5. Psychological implications of chronic diseases, disabilities, and dysfunction.
6. Sources for disease-specific guidelines.
7. Theories of behavior change (e.g., stages of change, health belief model) and their implications.
8. Psychological obstacles that may interfere with the attainment of goals (e.g., self-esteem, anxiety, self-efficacy, mood).
9. Principles of adult learning (e.g., readiness, success, practice) and appropriate educational tools.
10. Psychological side effects of medications and appropriate precautions for a client taking medications and/or other substances.
11. The negative and positive impact of assessment data on motivation.
12. Motivational techniques used to optimize exercise adherence and other healthy lifestyle behaviors.
13. How chronic diseases, disabilities, and injuries will impact exercise adherence based on the client's perception of signs and symptoms.

Skill in:

1. Interviewing and communicating effectively with the client and/or healthcare team.
2. Interpreting body language and recognizing incongruities between verbal and non-verbal behaviors.
3. Building trust and rapport.
4. Assessing client's readiness, expectations, and preferences.
5. Applying principles of behavioral change.
6. Identifying barriers associated with various chronic diseases, disabilities, and injuries that may affect programming.
7. Adapting programming in accordance with identified barriers.
8. Identifying and/or addressing unrealistic expectations as they relate to underlying chronic diseases, disabilities, and injuries.
9. Establishing goals (e.g., specific, measurable, action-oriented, realistic, timed).
10. Selecting and integrating appropriate educational tools for use in client instruction.
11. Facilitating the client's acceptance, responsibility, and accountability for program goals.
12. Designing a safe, well-balanced, and comprehensive program specific to the client's health status, special needs, program preferences, and goals.
13. Instructing and/or supervising the client in the safe and proper execution of exercise.
14. Modifying motivational strategies based upon assessment and/or reassessment.
15. Making appropriate referrals.

Pathophysiology

1. General pathophysiology of chronic diseases, disabilities, and injuries as related to each organ system, including cardiovascular, respiratory, endocrine, neurological, musculoskeletal, gastrointestinal, reproductive, and integumentary.
2. Signs and symptoms of chronic diseases, disabilities, and injuries.
3. Guidelines for designing programs specific to chronic diseases, disabilities, and injuries using FITT principles as they apply to cardiorespiratory, strength, and flexibility training.
4. Influence of chronic diseases, disabilities, and injuries on exercise selection.
5. Influence of chronic diseases, disabilities, and injuries on the selection of assessment tools.

6. Predicted responses to exercise in clients with chronic diseases, disabilities, and injuries.
7. Designing safe, comprehensive, and effective programs based on the client's current health status.
8. Appropriate exercise modifications for chronic diseases, disabilities, and injuries based on the client's response to exercise.
9. Indications for modification or termination of an exercise session or activity.
10. Circumstances requiring referral to other health professionals.
11. Contraindicated activities/exercises.
12. Appropriate documentation of signs, symptoms, and responses to exercise.
13. Effect of medication on exercise selection.
14. Potential effect of exercise on medication requirements.
15. How environmental factors affect exercise for clients with chronic diseases, disabilities, and injuries.
16. Alternative medical services (e.g., chiropractic, acupuncture, naturopathy) and how they may affect exercise/activity selection for clients with chronic diseases, disabilities, and injuries.
17. Potential medical emergencies in clients with chronic diseases, disabilities, and injuries.
18. Recognized protocols (e.g., McKenzie extension exercises, rotator cuff progression) for clients with chronic diseases, disabilities, and injuries.

Skill in:

1. Assessing and reassessing the client's readiness, expectations, and limitations.
2. Administering and analyzing assessment data.
3. Interpreting the data from the referring health professional.
4. Modifying the program to meet the needs of the client.
5. Applying standard and accepted testing methods to measure current fitness status.
6. Identifying environmental factors that influence exercise performance.
7. Recognizing the need for terminating a specific activity, an exercise session, or the entire program.
8. Recognizing personal scope of practice.
9. Teaching proper alignment and execution techniques.
10. Recognizing and managing emergency situations.
11. Addressing unrealistic expectations.
12. Applying program guidelines specific to special populations.
13. Identifying problematic signs and symptoms before, during, and after the exercise session.
14. Documenting health- and fitness-related data.
15. Referring the client to appropriate health professionals.

Task 2 - Instruct the client on safe and effective exercise techniques using appropriate educational techniques to achieve optimal program goals.

Exercise Science

Knowledge of:

Anatomy

1. General anatomy of the following systems: musculoskeletal, cardiorespiratory, neuromuscular, digestive, endocrine, reproductive, and integumentary.
2. General anatomical terminology (e.g., landmarks, planes of movement, position, muscle roles, muscle origin, and muscle insertion).

Kinesiology

3. Passive and active ranges of motion.
4. Muscle function, types of muscle contraction, and associated factors affecting movement (e.g., neurological, biomechanical, kinesthetic).
5. Appropriate exercise design to address balance (e.g., static, dynamic), muscular imbalances, and postural alignment.
6. Biomechanical concepts of human movement (e.g., Newton's laws) as applied to exercise.
7. Application of the principles related to muscular strength and endurance (e.g., resistance, overload, specificity, repetitions, sets, frequency, rest periods, progression).

Physiology

8. Types of training (cardiorespiratory, resistance, and flexibility) and the risks and benefits associated with each.

9. Health-related components of physical fitness, principles of training, and adaptations (acute and chronic) to exercise.
10. Skill-related components of physical fitness, principles of training, and adaptations (agility, balance, coordination, speed, power, and reaction time).
11. Cardiorespiratory system with respect to the carrying capacity, delivery, and extraction of oxygen.
12. Metabolism, including energy production and nutrient utilization.
13. Neuromuscular physiology (e.g., muscle fiber types, proprioceptors, motor-unit recruitment).
14. Programming guidelines to improve fitness.
15. Environmental conditions impacting exercise (e.g., heat, humidity, cold, air pollution, altitude).

Skill in:

1. Facilitating cardiorespiratory fitness, musculoskeletal strength, and flexibility.
2. Selecting appropriate exercise modalities.
3. Selecting safe exercises for all muscle groups.
4. Applying appropriate training principles (FITT).
5. Modifying programs.
6. Assessing body composition.
7. Assessing dynamic and static posture and balance.
8. Assessing gait.
9. Assessing cardiorespiratory and musculoskeletal fitness.
10. Interpreting medical history.
11. Assessing clients' lifestyles.
12. Conducting risk stratification.
13. Comparing test data to normative values.
14. Selecting appropriate assessments.
15. Referring to the appropriate healthcare professional(s).
16. Communicating with members of the healthcare team.
17. Assessing anthropometric parameters.
18. Recognizing side effects associated with common categories of medications as they relate to energy and performance.

Nutrition

Knowledge of:

1. Macronutrients, micronutrients, hydration, supplements, engineered foods, alcohol, drugs (illicit, over-the-counter, prescription), and stimulants.
2. Current, credible, and appropriate nutrition resources.
3. Nutrition guidelines, food selection, preparation, and storage.
4. Digestion and absorption process.
5. Popular diets and associated health risks.
6. Nutrition requirements specific to each classification of disease or dysfunction.
7. Metabolic conversion of nutrients.

Skill in:

1. Assessing the quality of the client's food intake.
2. Educating the client on making appropriate food choices based on sound nutritional practices.
3. Recommending reputable resources for clients with an interest in a structured dietary management program.
4. Educating the client on appropriate food selections based on known risk reduction.
5. Recognizing deficiencies in nutrition as they relate to exercise performance.
6. Maintaining a current knowledge base of popular diets and extreme dietary measures.
7. Applying hydration guidelines as they relate to exercise duration, environmental conditions, and client status.

Psychology

Knowledge of:

1. Psychological conditions that require referral to appropriate allied health professionals.
2. Communication techniques (e.g., active listening, appropriate eye contact, non-verbal behavior).
3. Techniques that build and enhance rapport.
4. Individual differences that influence behavior (e.g., exercise history, lifestyle, gender, age, culture, ethnicity).
5. Psychological implications of chronic diseases, disabilities, and dysfunction.
6. Sources for disease-specific guidelines.

7. Theories of behavior change (e.g., stages of change, health belief model) and their implications.
8. Psychological obstacles that may interfere with the attainment of goals (e.g., self-esteem, anxiety, self-efficacy, mood).
9. Principles of adult learning (e.g., readiness, success, practice) and appropriate educational tools.
10. Psychological side effects of medications and appropriate precautions for a client taking medications and/or other substances.
11. The negative and positive impact of assessment data on motivation.
12. Motivational techniques used to optimize exercise adherence and other healthy lifestyle behaviors.
13. How chronic diseases, disabilities, and injuries will impact exercise adherence based on client's perception of signs and symptoms.

Skill in:

1. Interviewing and communicating effectively with the client and/or healthcare team.
2. Interpreting body language and recognizing incongruities between verbal and non-verbal behaviors.
3. Building trust and rapport.
4. Assessing client's readiness, expectations, and preferences.
5. Applying principles of behavioral change.
6. Identifying barriers associated with various chronic diseases, disabilities, and injuries that may affect programming.
7. Adapting programming in accordance with identified barriers.
8. Identifying and/or addressing unrealistic expectations as they relate to underlying chronic diseases, disabilities, and injuries.
9. Establishing goals (e.g., specific, measurable, action-oriented, realistic, timed).
10. Selecting and integrating appropriate educational tools for use in client instruction.
11. Facilitating the client's acceptance, responsibility, and accountability for program goals.
12. Designing a safe, well-balanced, and comprehensive program specific to the client's health status, special needs, program preferences, and goals.
13. Instructing and/or supervising the client in the safe and proper execution of exercise.
14. Modifying motivational strategies based upon assessment and/or reassessment.
15. Making appropriate referrals.

Pathophysiology

1. General pathophysiology of chronic diseases, disabilities, and injuries as related to each organ system, including cardiovascular, respiratory, endocrine, neurological, musculoskeletal, gastrointestinal, reproductive, and integumentary.
2. Signs and symptoms of chronic diseases, disabilities, and injuries.
3. Guidelines for designing programs specific to chronic diseases, disabilities, and injuries using FITT principles as they apply to cardiorespiratory, strength, and flexibility training.
4. Influence of chronic diseases, disabilities, and injuries on exercise selection.
5. Influence of chronic diseases, disabilities, and injuries on the selection of assessment tools.
6. Predicted responses to exercise in clients with chronic diseases, disabilities, and injuries.
7. Designing safe, comprehensive, and effective programs based on the client's current health status.
8. Appropriate exercise modifications for chronic diseases, disabilities, and injuries based on the client's response to exercise.
9. Indications for modification or termination of an exercise session or activity.
10. Circumstances requiring referral to other health professionals.
11. Contraindicated activities/exercises.
12. Appropriate documentation of signs, symptoms, and responses to exercise.
13. Effect of medication on exercise selection.
14. Potential effect of exercise on medication requirements.
15. How environmental factors affect exercise for clients with chronic diseases, disabilities, and injuries.
16. Alternative medical services (e.g., chiropractic, acupuncture, naturopathy) and how they may affect exercise/activity selection for clients with chronic diseases, disabilities, and injuries.

17. Potential medical emergencies in clients with chronic diseases, disabilities, and injuries.
18. Recognized protocols (e.g., McKenzie extension exercises, rotator cuff progression) for clients with chronic diseases, disabilities, and injuries.

Skill in:
1. Assessing and reassessing the client's readiness, expectations, and limitations.
2. Administering and analyzing assessment data.
3. Interpreting the data from the referring health professional.
4. Modifying the program to meet the needs of the client.
5. Applying standard and accepted testing methods to measure current fitness status.
6. Identifying environmental factors that influence exercise performance.
7. Recognizing the need for terminating a specific activity, an exercise session, or the entire program.
8. Recognizing personal scope of practice.
9. Teaching proper alignment and execution techniques.
10. Recognizing and managing emergency situations.
11 Addressing unrealistic expectations.
12. Applying program guidelines specific to special populations.
13. Identifying problematic signs and symptoms before, during, and after the exercise session.
14. Documenting health- and fitness-related data.
15. Referring the client to appropriate health professionals.

Task 3 - Facilitate program adherence through education, the principles of behavior change, rapport building, etc., to achieve goals.

Exercise Science

Knowledge of:

Anatomy
1. General anatomy of the following systems: musculoskeletal, cardiorespiratory, neuromuscular, digestive, endocrine, reproductive, and integumentary.
2. General anatomical terminology (e.g., landmarks, planes of movement, position, muscle roles, muscle origin, and muscle insertion).

Kinesiology
3. Passive and active ranges of motion.
4. Muscle function, types of muscle contraction, and associated factors affecting movement (e.g., neurological, biomechanical, kinesthetic).
5. Appropriate exercise design to address balance (e.g., static, dynamic), muscular imbalances, and postural alignment.
6. Biomechanical concepts of human movement (e.g., Newton's laws) as applied to exercise.
7. Application of the principles related to muscular strength and endurance (e.g., resistance, overload, specificity, repetitions, sets, frequency, rest periods, progression).

Physiology
8. Types of training (cardiorespiratory, resistance, and flexibility) and the risks and benefits associated with each.
9. Health-related components of physical fitness, principles of training, and adaptations (acute and chronic) to exercise.
10. Skill-related components of physical fitness, principles of training, and adaptations (agility, balance, coordination, speed, power, and reaction time).
11. Cardiorespiratory system with respect to the carrying capacity, delivery, and extraction of oxygen.
12. Metabolism, including energy production and nutrient utilization.
13. Neuromuscular physiology (e.g., muscle fiber types, proprioceptors, motor-unit recruitment).
14. Programming guidelines to improve fitness.
15. Environmental conditions impacting exercise (e.g., heat, humidity, cold, air pollution, altitude).

Skill in:
1. Facilitating cardiorespiratory fitness, musculoskeletal strength, and flexibility.
2. Selecting appropriate exercise modalities.
3. Selecting safe exercises for all muscle groups.

4. Applying appropriate training principles (FITT).
5. Modifying programs.
6. Assessing body composition.
7. Assessing dynamic and static posture and balance.
8. Assessing gait.
9. Assessing cardiorespiratory and musculoskeletal fitness.
10. Interpreting medical history.
11. Assessing clients' lifestyles.
12. Conducting risk stratification.
13. Comparing test data to normative values.
14. Selecting appropriate assessments.
15. Referring to the appropriate healthcare professional(s).
16. Communicating with members of the healthcare team.
17. Assessing anthropometric parameters.
18. Recognizing side effects associated with common categories of medications as they relate to energy and performance.

Nutrition

Knowledge of:

1. Macronutrients, micronutrients, hydration, supplements, engineered foods, alcohol, drugs (illicit, over-the-counter, prescription), and stimulants.
2. Current, credible, and appropriate nutrition resources.
3. Nutrition guidelines, food selection, preparation, and storage.
4. Digestion and absorption process.
5. Popular diets and associated health risks.
6. Nutrition requirements specific to each classification of disease or dysfunction.
7. Metabolic conversion of nutrients.

Skill in:

1. Assessing the quality of the client's food intake.
2. Educating the client on making appropriate food choices based on sound nutritional practices.
3. Recommending reputable resources for clients with an interest in a structured dietary management program.
4. Educating the client on appropriate food selections based on known risk reduction.
5. Recognizing deficiencies in nutrition as they relate to exercise performance.
6. Maintaining a current knowledge base on popular diets and extreme dietary measures.
7. Applying hydration guidelines as they relate to exercise duration, environmental conditions, and client status.

Psychology

Knowledge of:

1. Psychological conditions that require referral to appropriate allied health professionals.
2. Communication techniques (e.g., active listening, appropriate eye contact, non-verbal behavior).
3. Techniques that build and enhance rapport.
4. Individual differences that influence behavior (e.g., exercise history, lifestyle, gender, age, culture, ethnicity).
5. Psychological implications of chronic diseases, disabilities, and dysfunction.
6. Sources for disease-specific guidelines.
7. Theories of behavior change (e.g., stages of change, health belief model) and their implications.
8. Psychological obstacles that may interfere with the attainment of goals (e.g., self-esteem, anxiety, self-efficacy, mood).
9. Principles of adult learning (e.g., readiness, success, practice) and appropriate educational tools.
10. Psychological side effects of medications and appropriate precautions for a client taking medications and/or other substances.
11. The negative and positive impact of assessment data on motivation.
12. Motivational techniques used to optimize exercise adherence and other healthy lifestyle behaviors.
13. How chronic diseases, disabilities, and injuries will impact exercise adherence based on the client's perception of signs and symptoms.

Skill in:

1. Interviewing and communicating effectively with the client and/or healthcare team.

2. Interpreting body language and recognizing incongruities between verbal and non-verbal behaviors.
3. Building trust and rapport.
4. Assessing client's readiness, expectations, and preferences.
5. Applying principles of behavioral change.
6. Identifying barriers associated with various chronic diseases, disabilities, and injuries that may affect programming.
7. Adapting programming in accordance with identified barriers.
8. Identifying and/or addressing unrealistic expectations as they relate to underlying chronic diseases, disabilities, and injuries.
9. Establishing goals (e.g., specific, measurable, action-oriented, realistic, timed).
10. Selecting and integrating appropriate educational tools for use in client instruction.
11. Facilitating the client's acceptance, responsibility, and accountability for program goals.
12. Designing a safe, well-balanced, and comprehensive program specific to the client's health status, special needs, program preferences, and goals.
13. Instructing and/or supervising the client in the safe and proper execution of exercise.
14. Modifying motivational strategies based upon assessment and/or reassessment.
15. Making appropriate referrals.

Pathophysiology

1. General pathophysiology of chronic diseases, disabilities, and injuries as related to each organ system, including cardiovascular, respiratory, endocrine, neurological, musculoskeletal, gastrointestinal, reproductive, and integumentary.
2. Signs and symptoms of chronic diseases, disabilities, and injuries.
3. Guidelines for designing programs specific to chronic diseases, disabilities, and injuries using FITT principles as they apply to cardiorespiratory, strength, and flexibility training.
4. Influence of chronic diseases, disabilities, and injuries on exercise selection.
5. Influence of chronic diseases, disabilities, and injuries on the selection of assessment tools.
6. Predicted responses to exercise in clients with chronic diseases, disabilities, and injuries.
7. Designing safe, comprehensive, and effective programs based on the client's current health status.
8. Appropriate exercise modifications for chronic diseases, disabilities, and injuries based on the client's response to exercise.
9. Indications for modification or termination of an exercise session or activity.
10. Circumstances requiring referral to other health professionals.
11. Contraindicated activities/exercises.
12. Appropriate documentation of signs, symptoms, and responses to exercise.
13. Effect of medication on exercise selection.
14. Potential effect of exercise on medication requirements.
15. How environmental factors affect exercise for clients with chronic diseases, disabilities, and injuries.
16. Alternative medical services (e.g., chiropractic, acupuncture, naturopathy) and how they may affect exercise/activity selection for clients with chronic diseases, disabilities, and injuries.
17. Potential medical emergencies in clients with chronic diseases, disabilities, and injuries.
18. Recognized protocols (e.g., McKenzie extension exercises, rotator cuff progression) for clients with chronic diseases, disabilities, and injuries.

Skill in:

1. Assessing and reassessing the client's readiness, expectations, and limitations.
2. Administering and analyzing assessment data.
3. Interpreting the data from the referring health professional.
4. Modifying the program to meet the needs of the client.
5. Applying standard and accepted testing methods to measure current fitness status.
6. Identifying environmental factors that influence exercise performance.

7. Recognizing the need for terminating a specific activity, an exercise session, or the entire program.
8. Recognizing personal scope of practice.
9. Teaching proper alignment and execution techniques.
10. Recognizing and managing emergency situations.
11. Addressing unrealistic expectations.
12. Applying program guidelines specific to special populations.
13. Identifying problematic signs and symptoms before, during, and after the exercise session.
14. Documenting health- and fitness-related data.
15. Referring the client to appropriate health professionals.

Task 4 - Monitor the client's progress and changing status based on subjective and objective data that includes periodic reassessments to ensure safe and effective programming.

Exercise Science

Knowledge of:

Anatomy

1. General anatomy of the following systems: musculoskeletal, cardiorespiratory, neuromuscular, digestive, endocrine, reproductive, and integumentary.
2. General anatomical terminology (e.g., landmarks, planes of movement, position, muscle roles, muscle origin, and muscle insertion).

Kinesiology

3. Passive and active ranges of motion.
4. Muscle function, types of muscle contraction, and associated factors affecting movement (e.g., neurological, biomechanical, kinesthetic).
5. Appropriate exercise design to address balance (e.g., static, dynamic), muscular imbalances, and postural alignment.
6. Biomechanical concepts of human movement (e.g., Newton's laws) as applied to exercise.
7. Application of the principles related to muscular strength and endurance (e.g., resistance, overload, specificity, repetitions, sets, frequency, rest periods, progression).

Physiology

8. Types of training (cardiorespiratory, resistance, and flexibility) and the risks and benefits associated with each.
9. Health-related components of physical fitness, principles of training, and adaptations (acute and chronic) to exercise.
10. Skill-related components of physical fitness, principles of training, and adaptations (agility, balance, coordination, speed, power, and reaction time).
11. Cardiorespiratory system with respect to the carrying capacity, delivery, and extraction of oxygen.
12. Metabolism, including energy production and nutrient utilization.
13. Neuromuscular physiology (e.g., muscle fiber types, proprioceptors, motor-unit recruitment).
14. Programming guidelines to improve fitness.
15. Environmental conditions impacting exercise (e.g., heat, humidity, cold, air pollution, altitude).

Skill in:

1. Facilitating cardiorespiratory fitness, musculoskeletal strength, and flexibility.
2. Selecting appropriate exercise modalities.
3. Selecting safe exercises for all muscle groups.
4. Applying appropriate training principles (FITT).
5. Modifying programs.
6. Assessing body composition.
7. Assessing dynamic and static posture and balance.
8. Assessing gait.
9. Assessing cardiorespiratory and musculoskeletal fitness.
10. Interpreting medical history.
11. Assessing clients' lifestyles.
12. Conducting risk stratification.
13. Comparing test data to normative values.
14. Selecting appropriate assessments.
15. Referring to the appropriate healthcare professional(s).

16. Communicating with members of the health-care team.
17. Assessing anthropometric parameters.
18. Recognizing side effects associated with common categories of medications as they relate to energy and performance.

Nutrition

Knowledge of:

1. Macronutrients, micronutrients, hydration, supplements, engineered foods, alcohol, drugs (illicit, over-the-counter, prescription), and stimulants.
2. Current, credible, and appropriate nutrition resources.
3. Nutrition guidelines, food selection, preparation, and storage.
4. Digestion and absorption process.
5. Popular diets and associated health risks.
6. Nutrition requirements specific to each classification of disease or dysfunction.
7. Metabolic conversion of nutrients.

Skill in:

1. Assessing the quality of the client's food intake.
2. Educating the client on making appropriate food choices based on sound nutritional practices.
3. Recommending reputable resources for clients with an interest in a structured dietary management program.
4. Educating the client on appropriate food selections based on known risk reduction.
5. Recognizing deficiencies in nutrition as they relate to exercise performance.
6. Maintaining a current knowledge base of popular diets and extreme dietary measures.
7. Applying hydration guidelines as they relate to exercise duration, environmental conditions, and client status.

Psychology

Knowledge of:

1. Psychological conditions that require referral to appropriate allied health professionals.
2. Communication techniques (e.g., active listening, appropriate eye contact, non-verbal behavior).
3. Techniques that build and enhance rapport.
4. Individual differences that influence behavior (e.g., exercise history, lifestyle, gender, age, culture, ethnicity).
5. Psychological implications of chronic diseases, disabilities, and dysfunction.
6. Sources for disease-specific guidelines.
7. Theories of behavior change (e.g., stages of change, health belief model) and their implications.
8. Psychological obstacles that may interfere with the attainment of goals (e.g., self-esteem, anxiety, self-efficacy, mood).
9. Principles of adult learning (e.g., readiness, success, practice) and appropriate educational tools.
10. Psychological side effects of medications and appropriate precautions for a client taking medications and/or other substances.
11. The negative and positive impact of assessment data on motivation.
12. Motivational techniques used to optimize exercise adherence and other healthy lifestyle behaviors.
13. How chronic diseases, disabilities, and injuries will impact exercise adherence based on client's perception of signs and symptoms.

Skill in:

1. Interviewing and communicating effectively with the client and/or healthcare team.
2. Interpreting body language and recognizing incongruities between verbal and non-verbal behaviors.
3. Building trust and rapport.
4. Assessing client's readiness, expectations, and preferences.
5. Applying principles of behavioral change.
6. Identifying barriers associated with various chronic diseases, disabilities, and injuries that may affect programming.
7. Adapting programming in accordance with identified barriers.
8. Identifying and/or addressing unrealistic expectations as they relate to underlying chronic diseases, disabilities, and injuries.
9. Establishing goals (e.g., specific, measurable, action-oriented, realistic, timed).

10. Selecting and integrating appropriate educational tools for use in client instruction.
11. Facilitating the client's acceptance, responsibility, and accountability for program goals.
12. Designing a safe, well-balanced, and comprehensive program specific to the client's health status, special needs, program preferences, and goals.
13. Instructing and/or supervising the client in the safe and proper execution of exercise.
14. Modifying motivational strategies based upon assessment and/or reassessment.
15. Making appropriate referrals.

Pathophysiology

1. General pathophysiology of chronic diseases, disabilities, and injuries as related to each organ system, including cardiovascular, respiratory, endocrine, neurological, musculoskeletal, gastrointestinal, reproductive, and integumentary.
2. Signs and symptoms of chronic diseases, disabilities, and injuries.
3. Guidelines for designing programs specific to chronic diseases, disabilit ies, and injuries using FITT principles as they apply to cardiorespiratory, strength, and flexibility training.
4. Influence of chronic diseases, disabilities, and injuries on exercise selection.
5. Influence of chronic diseases, disabilities, and injuries on the selection of assessment tools.
6. Predicted responses to exercise in clients with chronic diseases, disabilities, and injuries.
7. Designing safe, comprehensive, and effective programs based on the client's current health status.
8. Appropriate exercise modifications for chronic diseases, disabilities, and injuries based on the client's response to exercise.
9. Indications for modification or termination of an exercise session or activity.
10. Circumstances requiring referral to other health professionals.
11. Contraindicated activities/exercises.
12. Appropriate documentation of signs, symptoms, and responses to exercise.
13. Effect of medication on exercise selection.
14. Potential effect of exercise on medication requirements.
15. How environmental factors affect exercise for clients with chronic diseases, disabilities, and injuries.
16. Alternative medical services (e.g., chiropractic, acupuncture, naturopathy) and how they may affect exercise/activity selection for clients with chronic diseases, disabilities, and injuries.
17. Potential medical emergencies in clients with chronic diseases, disabilities, and injuries.
18. Recognized protocols (e.g., McKenzie extension exercises, rotator cuff progression) for clients with chronic diseases, disabilities, and injuries.

Skill in:

1. Assessing and reassessing the client's readiness, expectations, and limitations.
2. Administering and analyzing assessment data.
3. Interpreting the data from the referring health professional.
4. Modifying the program to meet the needs of the client.
5. Applying standard and accepted testing methods to measure current fitness status.
6. Identifying environmental factors that influence exercise performance.
7. Recognizing the need for terminating a specific activity, an exercise session, or the entire program.
8. Recognizing personal scope of practice.
9. Teaching proper alignment and execution techniques.
10. Recognizing and managing emergency situations.
11. Addressing unrealistic expectations.
12. Applying program guidelines specific to special populations.
13. Identifying problematic signs and symptoms before, during, and after the exercise session.
14. Documenting health- and fitness-related data.
15. Referring the client to appropriate health professionals.

Task 5 - Document program activity using accepted recording techniques to track progress and communicate (as necessary) with other healthcare professionals.

Exercise Science

Knowledge of:

Anatomy

1. General anatomy of the following systems: musculoskeletal, cardiorespiratory, neuromuscular, digestive, endocrine, reproductive, and integumentary.
2. General anatomical terminology (e.g., landmarks, planes of movement, position, muscle roles, muscle origin, and muscle insertion).

Kinesiology

3. Passive and active ranges of motion.
4. Muscle function, types of muscle contraction, and associated factors affecting movement (e.g., neurological, biomechanical, kinesthetic).
5. Appropriate exercise design to address balance (e.g., static, dynamic), muscular imbalances, and postural alignment.
6. Biomechanical concepts of human movement (e.g., Newton's laws) as applied to exercise.
7. Application of the principles related to muscular strength and endurance (e.g., resistance, overload, specificity, repetitions, sets, frequency, rest periods, progression).

Physiology

8. Types of training (cardiorespiratory, resistance, and flexibility) and the risks and benefits associated with each.
9. Health-related components of physical fitness, principles of training, and adaptations (acute and chronic) to exercise.
10. Skill-related components of physical fitness, principles of training, and adaptations (agility, balance, coordination, speed, power, and reaction time).
11. Cardiorespiratory system with respect to the carrying capacity, delivery, and extraction of oxygen.
12. Metabolism, including energy production and nutrient utilization.
13. Neuromuscular physiology (e.g., muscle fiber types, proprioceptors, motor-unit recruitment).
14. Programming guidelines to improve fitness.
15. Environmental conditions impacting exercise (e.g., heat, humidity, cold, air pollution, altitude).

Skill in:

1. Facilitating cardiorespiratory fitness, musculoskeletal strength, and flexibility.
2. Selecting appropriate exercise modalities.
3. Selecting safe exercises for all muscle groups.
4. Applying appropriate training principles (FITT).
5. Modifying programs.
6. Assessing body composition.
7. Assessing dynamic and static posture and balance.
8. Assessing gait.
9. Assessing cardiorespiratory and musculoskeletal fitness.
10. Interpreting medical history.
11. Assessing clients' lifestyles.
12. Conducting risk stratification.
13. Comparing test data to normative values.
14. Selecting appropriate assessments.
15. Referring to the appropriate healthcare professional(s).
16. Communicating with members of the healthcare team.
17. Assessing anthropometric parameters.
18. Recognizing side effects associated with common categories of medications as they relate to energy and performance.

Nutrition

Knowledge of:

1. Macronutrients, micronutrients, hydration, supplements, engineered foods, alcohol, drugs (illicit, over-the-counter, prescription), and stimulants.
2. Current, credible, and appropriate nutrition resources.
3. Nutrition guidelines, food selection, preparation, and storage.
4. Digestion and absorption process.
5. Popular diets and associated health risks.
6. Nutrition requirements specific to each classification of disease or dysfunction.
7. Metabolic conversion of nutrients.

Skill in:

1. Assessing the quality of the client's food intake.
2. Educating the client on making appropriate food choices based on sound nutritional practices.
3. Recommending reputable resources for clients with an interest in a structured dietary management program.
4. Educating the client on appropriate food selections based on known risk reduction.
5. Recognizing deficiencies in nutrition as they relate to exercise performance.
6. Maintaining a current knowledge base of popular diets and extreme dietary measures.
7. Applying hydration guidelines as they relate to exercise duration, environmental conditions, and client status.

Psychology

Knowledge of:

1. Psychological conditions that require referral to appropriate allied health professionals.
2. Communication techniques (e.g., active listening, appropriate eye contact, non-verbal behavior).
3. Techniques that build and enhance rapport.
4. Individual differences that influence behavior (e.g., exercise history, lifestyle, gender, age, culture, ethnicity).
5. Psychological implications of chronic diseases, disabilities, and dysfunction.
6. Sources for disease-specific guidelines.
7. Theories of behavior change (e.g., stages of change, health belief model) and their implications.
8. Psychological obstacles that may interfere with the attainment of goals (e.g., self-esteem, anxiety, self-efficacy, mood).
9. Principles of adult learning (e.g., readiness, success, practice) and appropriate educational tools.
10. Psychological side effects of medications and appropriate precautions for a client taking medications and/or other substances.
11. The negative and positive impact of assessment data on motivation.
12. Motivational techniques used to optimize exercise adherence and other healthy lifestyle behaviors.
13. How chronic diseases, disabilities, and injuries will impact exercise adherence based on the client's perception of signs and symptoms.

Skill in:

1. Interviewing and communicating effectively with the client and/or healthcare team.
2. Interpreting body language and recognizing incongruities between verbal and non-verbal behaviors.
3. Building trust and rapport.
4. Assessing the client's readiness, expectations, and preferences.
5. Applying principles of behavioral change.
6. Identifying barriers associated with various chronic diseases, disabilities, and injuries that may affect programming.
7. Adapting programming in accordance with identified barriers.
8. Identifying and/or addressing unrealistic expectations as they relate to underlying chronic diseases, disabilities, and injuries.
9. Establishing goals (e.g., specific, measurable, action-oriented, realistic, timed).
10. Selecting and integrating appropriate educational tools for use in client instruction.
11. Facilitating the client's acceptance, responsibility, and accountability for program goals.
12. Designing a safe, well-balanced, and comprehensive program specific to the client's health status, special needs, program preferences, and goals.
13. Instructing and/or supervising the client in the safe and proper execution of exercise.
14. Modifying motivational strategies based upon assessment and/or reassessment.
15. Making appropriate referrals.

Pathophysiology

1. General pathophysiology of chronic diseases, disabilities, and injuries as related to each organ system, including cardiovascular, respiratory, endocrine, neurological, musculoskeletal, gastrointestinal, reproductive, and integumentary.

2. Signs and symptoms of chronic diseases, disabilities, and injuries.
3. Guidelines for designing programs specific to chronic diseases, disabilities, and injuries using FITT principles as they apply to cardiorespiratory, strength, and flexibility training.
4. Influence of chronic diseases, disabilities, and injuries on exercise selection.
5. Influence of chronic diseases, disabilities, and injuries on the selection of assessment tools.
6. Predicted responses to exercise in clients with chronic diseases, disabilities, and injuries.
7. Designing safe, comprehensive, and effective programs based on the client's current health status.
8. Appropriate exercise modifications for chronic diseases, disabilities, and injuries based on the client's response to exercise.
9. Indications for modification or termination of an exercise session or activity.
10. Circumstances requiring referral to other health professionals.
11. Contraindicated activities/exercises.
12. Appropriate documentation of signs, symptoms, and responses to exercise.
13. Effect of medication on exercise selection.
14. Potential effect of exercise on medication requirements.
15. How environmental factors affect exercise for clients with chronic diseases, disabilities, and injuries.
16. Alternative medical services (e.g., chiropractic, acupuncture, naturopathy) and how they may affect exercise/activity selection for clients with chronic diseases, disabilities, and injuries.
17. Potential medical emergencies in clients with chronic diseases, disabilities, and injuries.
18. Recognized protocols (e.g., McKenzie extension exercises, rotator cuff progression) for clients with chronic diseases, disabilities, and injuries.

Skill in:

1. Assessing and reassessing the client's readiness, expectations, and limitations.
2. Administering and analyzing assessment data.
3. Interpreting the data from the referring health professional.
4. Modifying the program to meet the needs of the client.
5. Applying standard and accepted testing methods to measure current fitness status.
6. Identifying environmental factors that influence exercise performance.
7. Recognizing the need for terminating a specific activity, an exercise session, or the entire program.
8. Recognizing personal scope of practice.
9. Teaching proper alignment and execution techniques.
10. Recognizing and managing emergency situations.
11. Addressing unrealistic expectations.
12. Applying program guidelines specific to special populations.
13. Identifying problematic signs and symptoms before, during, and after the exercise session.
14. Documenting health- and fitness-related data.
15. Referring the client to appropriate health professionals.

DOMAIN IV: PROFESSIONAL RESPONSIBILITY 8%

Task 1 - Adhere to applicable law, regulations, industry guidelines, and sound business practices by maintaining a working knowledge of these topics and/or obtaining qualified consultation as needed to protect the interests of clients and minimize risk.

Knowledge of:

1. Risk management, including risk assessment, waiver, and informed consent.
2. Liability, including health screening, medical release forms, exercise recommendations, supervision, instruction, facilities, and equipment.
3. Negligence, both contributory and comparative.
4. Copyright law.
5. Scope of practice.
6. Standard of care.
7. Americans with Disabilities Act.
8. Standards governing confidentiality (e.g. HIPAA).

Skill in:

1. Completing an accident/injury report.

2. Completing and interpreting health-history data.
3. Safeguarding confidential information.
4. Following industry guidelines to minimize risk of injury and litigation.
5. Maintaining professionalism with employers, peers, and clients.
6. Securing copyrighted and intellectual property.

Task 2 - Adhere to the ACE Code of Ethics by upholding its principles consistently to protect the interests of clients, enhance confidence in the industry, and maintain professional responsibilities.

Knowledge of:
1. American Council on Exercise Code of Ethics.
2. Standards governing confidentiality.
3. Scope of practice for all members of the treatment team.
4. Current CPR, AED, infection control, and first-aid procedures.
5. Fair and equal treatment for all clients.
6. American Council on Exercise Professional Practices and Disciplinary Procedure.

Skill in:
1. Providing safe and effective exercise instruction/education.
2. Safeguarding confidential information.
3. Referring clients to more qualified fitness, medical, or health professionals when appropriate.
4. Administering CPR, and AED if accessible.
5. Administering basic injury-management procedures.
6. Enhancing healthcare professionals' confidence in the fitness industry.
7. Establishing and maintaining clear professional boundaries.

Task 3 - Respond to acute medical conditions and injuries as they arise by providing first aid, initiating CPR, using an AED if available, and following an emergency action plan to provide appropriate care and risk management.

Knowledge of:
1. CPR, AED, and basic first-aid procedures.
2. Signs and symptoms of injuries.
3. Factors associated with injury prevention.
4. Contraindications to exercise.
5. Facility risk management and emergency protocols, including EMS activation.
6. Facility evacuation procedures.
7. Signs and symptoms of acute medical conditions.

Skill in:
1. Administering basic first aid, CPR, and AED if accessible.
2. Completing an incident report and notifying appropriate parties.
3. Directing the evacuation process of clients in accordance with facility evacuation procedures.
4. Securing updated medical clearance.

Task 4 - Maintain appropriate insurance consistent with the characteristics of the professional setting to protect clients and other parties.

Knowledge of:
1. Professional liability insurance.
2. General liability insurance.
3. Worker's compensation insurance.
4. Health and disability insurance.
5. Property insurance.
6. Business interruption insurance.
7. Differences between an independent contractor and employee.

Task 5 - Enhance competence through ongoing education in current research and exercise modalities to optimize professional services when dealing with special populations.

Knowledge of:
1. Appropriate sources for acquiring continuing education.
2. Credible and current health and physical activity information and research as related to special populations.

Skill in:
1. Applying current information and recommendations when working with a client and/or treatment team.

APPENDIX C

Cardiovascular Medications

GENERIC NAME	BRAND NAME	EXERCISE PRECAUTIONS
Antiarrhythmic		
Quinidine	Quinidex, Quinaglute Cardioquin	May increase HR and decrease BP
Disopyramide	Norpace	
Procainamide	Pronestyl, Procan SR	Little or no effect
Moricizine	Ethmozine	Little or no effect
Mexiletine	Mexitil	Little or no effect
Phenytoin	Dilantin	Little or no effect
Tocainide	Tonocard	Little or no effect
Flecainide	Tambocor	Little or no effect
Propafenone	Rhymol	May decrease HR
Amiodarone	Cordarone	May decrease HR
Beta-blockers Acebutolol Atenolol Betaxol Bisoprolol Carteolol Metoprolol Nadolol Penbutolol Pindolol Propranolol Timolol Sotalol	Sectral Tenormin Kerlone Zebeta Cartrol Lopressor, Toprol Corgard Levatol Visken Inderal Blocadren Betapace	Decrease resting and exercise heart rate, consider using RPE to monitor exercise intensity Decrease resting and exercise BP Decrease myocardial contractility Decrease maximum oxygen uptake May cause fatigue and limit exercise capacity in non-ischemic, hypertensive individuals May exacerbate asthma in individuals with hyperactive airways May worsen claudication in individuals with PVD
Alpha- & Beta-blocker Carvedilol Labetalol	Coreg Trandate	Same as beta-blocker
Alpha-Adrenergic blocker Doxazosin Mesylate Prazosin Terazosin	Cardura Minipres Hytrin	No effect on HR Lower resting and exercise BP via peripheral vasodilation
Digitalis Digoxin	Lanoxin	May decrease HR in patients with atrial fibrillation No effect on BP May result in non-specific ST-T wave changes at rest and ST depression with exercise

GENERIC NAME	BRAND NAME	EXERCISE PRECAUTIONS
Diuretics		
Thiazides		
Chlorothiazide	Diuril	No influence on HR
Hydorchlorathiazide (HTCZ)	Esidrex, Hyodrodiuril, Microzide	May decrease BP
Metolazone	Zaroxolyn, Mykrox	Can cause hypovolemia (dehydration), reduced CO and PVC's due to hypokalemia, and/or hypomagnesemia.
"Loop"		
Furosemide	Lasix	
Ethacrynic Acid	Edecrin	
Torsemide	Demadex	
Potassium Sparing		
Spironolactone	Aldactone	
Triamterene	Dyrenism	
Amiloride	Midamor	
Combination		
Triamterene & HTCZ	Dyazide, Maxide	
Amiloride & HTCZ	Moduretic	
Calcium Channel Blockers		
Amlodipine	Norvasc	Variable effects on HR: Diltiazem, Verapamil, and Bepridil may decrease resting and exercise HR; Nifedipine may increase HR Consider using RPE to monitor exercise intensity. Decrease resting and exercise BP.
Bepridil	Vascor	
Diltiazem	Cardizem, Dilacor, Tiazac	
Felodipine	Plendil	
Isradipine	DynaCirc	
Mibefradil	Posicor	
Nicardipine	Cardene	
Nifedipine	Procardia, Adalat	
Nisoldipine	Sular	
Reserpine	Serpasil, Sandril	
Verapamil	Calan, Isoptin, Verelan, Covera	
	Nimotop	
Nimodipine		
Hyperlipidemic		
Cholestyramine	Questran, LoCholest	Dextrothyroxine may increase HR and BP and along with Clofibrate can provoke arrhythmias.
Colestipol	Colestid	
Clofibrate	Atromids	
Dextrothyroxine	Choloxin	
Gemfibrozil	Lopid	
Lovastatin	Mevacor	Nicotinic acid may decrease resting and exercise BP; be careful of hypotension following exercise.
Nicotinic Acid	Nicobid	
Pravastatin	Pravachol	
Probucol	Lorelo	
Simvastatin	Zocor	
Nitrates		
Isorbide	Isordil, Sorbitrate, Monoket, Ismo, Dilatrate	May increase resting and exercise HR, decrease resting and exercise BP, and improve exercise capacity in individuals with angina.
Nitroglycerin	Nitrostat, Nitro-bid	
Nitroglycerin Patch	Transderm Nitro, Nitrodisc, Nitro-Dur, Minitran, Deponit	

GENERIC NAME	BRAND NAME	EXERCISE PRECAUTIONS
Vasodilators Hydralazine Minoxidil	Apresoline Loniten	May cause reflex tachycardia Decrease resting and exercise BP May accentuate post-exercise hypotension
Other Dipyridamole Warfarin Pentoxifylline	Persantine Coumadin Trental	Generally no effect on exercise, except Pentoxifylline, which may increase exercise capacity in patients with peripheral vascular disease
Angiotensin-converting Enzyme (ACE) Inhibitors Benazepril Captopril Enalapril Fosinopril Lisinopril Perindopril Quinapril Rampril Trandolopril	Lotensin Capoten Vasotec Monopril Prinivil, Zestril Aceon Accupril Altace Mavik	Little or no effect on HR or BP

APPENDIX D

10-Step Decision-making Approach

10-Step Decision-making Approach

I. Introduction

A. Purpose of this module

1. To familiarize the ACE-AHFS with a step-wise approach based on the principles of exercise science and clinical medicine, to the management of clients with chronic diseases, disabilities, and special health conditions.
2. To provide the ACE-AHFS with a model for reasoning/thinking through (versus memorizing) the critical steps of exercise programming for clients with any of a variety of health conditions.

B. Model premise

1. For a client with any particular disease or disability, the ACE-AHFS must understand the effects of each of the following on all of the body's major organ systems:
   a. exercise, both acute and long-term
   b. disease/disability pathophysiology
   c. medications
2. With knowledge of the above information, the ACE-AHFS will be able to determine:
   a. Mechanisms by which the disease/disability alters the exercise response.
   b. Benefits of exercise (usually related to long-term exercise adaptations).
   c. Risks of exercise (usually related to acute exercise response).
3. Knowledge of the exercise benefits and risks for each organ system will then direct all subsequent steps in the management of clients with chronic diseases, disabilities, or special health conditions.

C. Module outline

1. Review of normal exercise physiology
2. General guidelines for modifying exercise programs when the exercise response is altered by disease or disability
3. The 10-Step Decision-making Approach

II. Review of Normal Exercise Physiology

A. Normal acute physiological responses to aerobic exercise

1. Cardiovascular responses to exercise.
   Primary purpose—to transport nutrients, remove waste products, and help maintain homeostasis at rest and during exercise.
   a. Increased heart rate.
   b. Increased stroke volume (volume of blood ejected per heart beat).
   c. Increased cardiac output (stroke volume x heart rate)
   d. Increased systolic blood pressure (force generated during ventricular contraction).
   e. Increased diastolic blood pressure with static exercise.
   f. Decreased peripheral resistance (dilation of arteries in active muscle).
2. Respiratory responses to exercise
Primary purpose—to exchange carbon dioxide and oxygen.
   a. Increased $\dot{V}O_2$ (volume of oxygen consumed).
   b. Increased respiratory rate (frequency of breathing).
   c. Increased ventilation (volume of air passing through pulmonary system).
   d. Increased tidal volume (volume of air expired per breath).
3. Metabolic responses to exercise
Primary purpose—to provide energy source to exercising tissues.
   a. Increased glucose utilization.
   b. Increased insulin sensitivity.
   c. Increased fats utilization.
   d. Increased lactic acid production (by-product of anaerobic ATP production).
4. Neuromuscular responses to exercise

Primary purpose—to produce bodily movement.

a. Increased blood flow to working muscles.
b. Increased motor unit recruitment.
c. Increased mechanical force production.

5. Thermoregulatory responses to exercise.

Primary purpose—to maintain the body's temperature within a safe zone.

a. Increased heat production.
b. Increased core temperature.
c. Increased skin temperature.
d. Increased sweating.

B. Long-term physiological adaptations to aerobic exercise training (benefits)

1. Cardiovascular adaptations to aerobic exercise training
   a. Decreased resting heart rate.
   b. Decreased submaximal exercise heart rate.
   c. Increased stroke volume (resting & exercise).
   d. Increased cardiac output.
2. Respiratory adaptations to aerobic exercise training
   a. Increased $\dot{V}O_2$max.
   b. Increased aerobic endurance.
3. Metabolic adaptations to aerobic exercise training
   a. Increased glycogen stores.
   b. Increased ability to mobilize fat from tissues.
   c. Decreased insulin resistance.
4. Neuromuscular adaptations to aerobic exercise training
   a. Dependent upon the complexity of the aerobic modality
5. Thermoregulatory adaptations to aerobic exercise training
   a. Sweating begins at a lower body temperature.
   b. Larger volumes of more dilute sweat is produced during exercise.
   c. Acclimatization to heat after approximately 10–14 days of exposure.

C. Normal physiological responses to strength training

1. Cardiovascular responses to strength training
   a. Increased heart rate.
   b. Increased stroke volume (eccentric phase).
   c. Increased cardiac output.
   d. Increased systolic blood pressure.
   e. Increased diastolic blood pressure during isometric contraction.
2. Respiratory responses to strength training
   a. Increased oxygen consumption.
   b. Increased respiratory rate.
   c. Increased ventilation.
   d. Increased tidal volume.
3. Neuromuscular responses to strength training
   a. Increased blood flow to working muscles.
   b. Increased motor unit recruitment.
   c. Increased mechanical force production.
4. Metabolic responses to strength training
   a. Increased resting metabolic rate.
5. Thermoregulatory responses to strength training
   a. Increased heat production.
   b. Increased core temperature.
   c. Increased skin temperature.
   d. Increased sweating.

D. Physiological adaptations to strength training

1. Cardiovascular adaptations to strength training
   a. Increased heart size.
2. Respiratory adaptations to strength training
   a. Generally no significant changes in respiratory system.
3. Neuromuscular adaptations to strength training
   a. Increased muscle strength and endurance.
   b. Increased anaerobic power.
   c. Increased muscle fiber size.
   d. Increased neuromuscular activation.
4. Metabolic adaptations to strength training
   a. Increased energy stores (ATP, CP, glycogen).
   b. Decreased percentage body fat.

I. Guidelines for Modifying Exercise Programs When the Exercise Response Is Altered by Disease or Disability

A. How to use these guidelines

1. The following guidelines are provided to assist the ACE-AHFS in developing a clinically based

organ-systems approach to managing clients with any of a number of diseases and disabilities.
2. Each set of guidelines pertains to an altered exercise response in one distinct organ system. Many chronic diseases coexist. Some diseases affect multiple organ systems. For the client with multiple organ system involvement, the ACE-AHFS should refer to all applicable sets of organ-system guidelines.
3. Exercise-related risks are identified for each organ system. The lists are not intended to be all-inclusive. Only the risks of greatest medical consequence are identified.
4. The guidelines are general recommendations. Not all recommendations will apply to all clients, in all cases. The ACE-AHFS should manage each client as an individual with unique characteristics and exercise needs and limitations.
5. The guidelines should be used only in conjunction with consultation from the client's physician and other appropriate health team members.
6. Guidelines are based on currently available scientific and clinical information. Because exercise medicine is a new and rapidly advancing field, the ACE-AHFS is advised of the critical necessity of staying current with the latest research in this area and of updating their program guidelines accordingly.

B. Altered central cardiovascular response

1. Examples: coronary artery disease, cardiomyopathies
2. Effect on exercise response: reduced capacity to deliver oxygen and blood to the myocardium and exercising muscles
3. Risks: myocardial ischemia, adverse cardiac event
4. Exercise modifications
   a. Reduce intensity (all modes of exercise). Exercise at levels below "symptom threshold."
   b. Prolong warm-up and cool-down periods.
   c. Avoid exercise to fatigue.
   d. Avoid exercise in extreme temperatures (hot or cold).
   e. Avoid isometric strength exercises.
   f. Progress exercise very gradually.
   g. Avoid Valsalva maneuvers.

C. Altered peripheral cardiovascular response

1. Examples: peripheral artery disease (due to arteriosclerosis)
2. Effect on exercise response: reduced capacity to deliver oxygen and blood to the exercising muscles
3. Risks: muscle ischemia and associated pain (intermittent claudication)
4. Exercise modifications
   a. Reduce intensity.
   b. Use intermittent exercise (repetitive exercise-rest periods: exercise to onset of moderate claudication pain, stop until pain resolves, and restart exercise).
   c. Prolong warm-up and cool-down periods.
5. Special considerations: Central cardiovascular disease frequently coexists in clients with peripheral artery disease.

D. Altered respiratory response

1. Examples: asthma, chronic obstructive pulmonary disease
2. Effect on exercise response:
   a. reduced oxygen supply to myocardium, exercising muscles, brain
   b. reduced capacity to eliminate excess carbon dioxide
3. Risks
   a. hypoxemia (decreased oxygenation of arterial blood) with resultant potential hypoxic effect on myocardium and central nervous system (CNS)
   b. hypercapnia (excess carbon dioxide) with potential toxic effect on CNS
4. Exercise modifications
   a. Reduce intensity. Use client's rating of perceived dyspnea (breathlessness) to monitor exercise intensity.
   b. Prolong warm-up and cool-down periods. (Prolonged cool-downs will help prevent post-exercise bronchospasm.)
   c. Use very gradual exercise progression, with emphasis on progressing duration over intensity.
   d. Use repetitive exercise-rest periods for the more dyspneic clients, especially during initial exercise sessions.

   e. Avoid exercise during periods of acute exacerbation of symptoms (e.g., increased coughing, wheezing, dyspnea).
   f. Avoid exercise in environments with poor air quality (e.g., high air pollution, automobile exhaust).
   g. Avoid exercise in climates with extreme temperatures or humidity. Especially for asthmatics, avoid exercise in cold, dry climates.
   h. Avoid exercise in the early morning hours, when pulmonary symptoms frequently are worse.
5. For advanced disease:
   a. Include exercises that improve breathing efficiency.
   b. Use pursed lip breathing technique.
   c. Use supplemental oxygen during exercise.
6. Special considerations: COPD frequently coexists with cardiovascular disease such as coronary artery disease, hypertension, and peripheral artery disease.

E. Altered metabolic response

1. Examples: diabetes
2. Effect on exercise response: varies with the specific disease pathophysiology
3. Risks: specific to the disease pathophysiology
4. Exercise modifications
   a. Dependent on the disease pathophysiology and resultant effect on the exercise response.
   b. Refer to the individual disorder guidelines.

F. Altered Neuromuscular response—joint disorders

1. Examples: arthritis, acute or overuse injuries (e.g., sprains, strains, meniscal tears)
2. Effect on exercise response
   a. reduced capacity of affected joint(s) to sustain increased or repetitive mechanical loads
   b. possible limited range of motion
3. Risks:
   a. further joint damage
   b. delayed healing of injuries
   c. increased pain and decreased function of affected joint
   d. For unstable joints, subluxations and dislocations
4. Exercise modifications
   a. Avoid exercises that place excessive or repetitive loads on affected joint (e.g., 1-RM knee extension or running for client with chronic patellofemoral syndrome).
   b. Avoid exercising affected joints during acute exacerbations of symptoms (e.g., red, hot, swollen, painful joint in client with rheumatoid arthritis).
   c. Use intermittent exercise-rest periods if exercise endurance is limited by joint pain.
   d. Include flexibility and joint range of motion exercises as key exercise components, but avoid over-stretching and hypermobility.
   e. Use caution (controlled movements, careful spotting) when exercising affected joints at extremes of motion.
   f. Avoid poorly controlled movements of the affected joints.
   g. Condition supporting muscles prior to exposing affected joints to more vigorous activity.
   h. Alternate exercise modalities to avoid overuse of affected joints.
   i. For unilateral joint involvement, use independent versus dependent exercise modalities (e.g., use unilateral heel raises and not bilateral heel raises in client with resolving ankle sprain) to provide targeted exercise effect and to prevent compensation by the unaffected side.
   j. Avoid exercise modalities that result in altered biomechanics due to the limited capacity of the affected joint (e.g., running with a limp in a client with a resolving ankle sprain). Altered biomechanics frequently lead to secondary injuries.
   k. For unstable joints, avoid exercises that place joint in vulnerable positions (e.g., shoulder abduction plus external rotation, such as in behind-the-neck lat pull-downs, in client with anterior shoulder subluxation).

G. Altered neuromuscular response—muscle, tendon, and associated soft tissue injuries

1. Examples: strains, tears, tendinitis, fasciitis
2. Effect on exercise response
   a. reduced capacity of affected tissues to sustain increased or repetitive mechanical loads
   b. reduced capacity of affected muscles to generate increased or repetitive mechanical forces
3. Risks:
   a. further tissue damage
   b. delayed healing
   c. increased pain and decreased function of affected tissue
4. Exercise modifications
   a. Avoid exercises that place excessive or repetitive loads on affected tissues (e.g., breaststroke swimming for client with hip adductor muscle strain).
   b. Use carefully controlled stretching techniques to avoid over-stretching and re-injury of the affected tissues.
   c. Use caution (controlled movements, careful spotting) when exercising affected tissues at extremes of motion.
   d. Alternate exercise modalities to avoid overuse of affected tissues.
   e. For unilateral injuries, use independent versus dependent exercise modalities (e.g., use unilateral heel raises and not bilateral heel raises in clients with right gastrocnemius strain) to provide targeted exercise effect and to prevent compensation by the unaffected side.
   f. Avoid exercise modalities that result in altered biomechanics secondary to the limited capacity of the affected tissue (e.g., running with a limp in a client with a quadriceps strain).

H. Altered neuromuscular response—systemic disease

1. Examples: multiple sclerosis, muscular dystrophy, poliomyelitis, amyotrophic lateral sclerosis
2. Note: These diseases have complex pathophysiologies. They can present with a variety of clinical manifestations, a range of degrees of disease severity, and with multiple organ-system involvement. Exercise research in these populations is very limited. For all these reasons, it is not possible to provide general guidelines for exercise management. An ACE-AHFS who manages clients with these conditions should work very closely with other members of each client's healthcare team.

I. Altered thermoregulatory response

1. Examples: obesity; diseases that can affect the autonomic nervous system (e.g., diabetes, multiple sclerosis, Parkinson's disease)
2. Effect on exercise response: reduced capacity to regulate body temperature during exercise.
3. Risks: heat and cold stress injuries
4. Exercise modifications
   a. Avoid exercise in extreme temperatures.
   b. Ensure adequate hydration before, during, and after exercise.
   c. Dress appropriately for climate.
   d. For warmer environments, utilize air-conditioners and fans, when possible.

The 10-Step Approach

A. The 10 steps

Step 1. Perform pre-exercise health risk assessment
Step 2. Obtain physician clearance
Step 3. Identify exercise benefits and goals
Step 4. Determine acute exercise risks
Step 5. Prepare for medical emergencies
Step 6. Obtain informed consent
Step 7. Plan baseline "fitness" screening and testing
Step 8. Design exercise program
Step 9. Plan exercise program implementation
Step 10. Double-check established guidelines

Critical components of each step are presented below.

B. Step 1: Perform pre-exercise health risk assessment

1. Purpose
   a. To maximize client safety by assisting in the detection of known and unknown conditions that may increase exercise-related risks

b. To assist in individualizing client's exercise program
c. To provide the ACE-AHFS with some level of protection from potential liabilities.

2. This is probably the most important step of all because it "defines the problems." All other decisions are made based upon the results of Step 1.
3. The procedures and tools used for the pre-exercise health risk assessment are covered in more detail in the Screening, Evaluation, and Programming Module.

C. Step 2: Obtain physician clearance

1. Determining requirement for a physician clearance
   a. ACSM guidelines
   b. Other established exercise guidelines from professional medical groups (e.g., American Heart Association, American College of Obstetricians and Gynecologists).
   c. As a general rule, it is prudent, from both a medical and legal perspective, to obtain a physician clearance for all clients with an identified chronic disease, disability, or injury, even if a clearance is not explicitly recommended in any of the established guidelines. When in doubt, an ACE-AHFS should be conservative with these higher risk clients.
2. Essential elements of the physician clearance
   a. Diagnosis(es)
   b. Associated conditions and disease complications
   c. Disease status (stable vs. progressing)
   d. Medications and doses
   e. MD's goals for exercise
   f. Limitations/contraindications for exercise
   g. Results of any clinical exercise screening tests
   h. Other members of the healthcare team

D. Step 3: Identify exercise benefits and goals

1. Questions to answer
   a. What are the client's goals?
   b. What are the health team's goals?
   c. What role does exercise play in the management of the disease/disability?
   d. Is there documented evidence of the benefits of exercise?
2. Recommended strategies to answer questions
   a. Client's goals
      - Use interviews, surveys, informal discussions.
   b. Health team's goals
      - Include questions on the medical clearance form.
      - Interview health team members (phone or by personal visits, if possible).

      Note: The medical team's goals will most likely relate to the health benefits gained through exercise.
   c. Role of exercise/benefits
      - Apply organ-systems model. (Based on what you know about the normal long-term effects of exercise on each organ system, and what you know about how the disease affects each organ system, how might exercise affect disease progression and/or the general health of the client?)
      - Perform medical/scientific literature reviews.
      - Refer to exercise medicine texts and journals.
      - Review any established guidelines.

E. Step 4: Determine acute exercise risks

1. Questions to answer
   a. What are the risks of exercise?
   b. Are there any absolute and/or relative contraindications to exercise?
   c. Has the physician identified any special limitations/contraindications?
2. Recommended strategies to answer questions
   a. Apply organ-systems model. (Based on what you know about each organ system's normal acute response to exercise, and what you know about how the disease affects each organ system, what risks do you think may be associated with exercise?)
      - primary disease

- associated conditions
- medications

b. Consult with healthcare team.
c. Review established guidelines.

F. Step 5: Prepare for medical emergencies

1. Questions to answer
   a. What are the potential exercise-related medical emergencies?
   b. How will an ACE-AHFS recognize a medical emergency?
   c. How should an ACE-AHFS respond?
2. Recommended strategies to answer questions
   a. Proper completion of Step 4 will identify the most common potential emergencies.
   b. Learn the signs and symptoms of the events identified in Step 4.
      - Refer to first aid, medical, and/or sports medicine texts and manuals.
      - Take a basic first aid course.
   c. Develop an emergency plan based on your qualifications. An ACE-AHFS should know, at a minimum, standard CPR and basic first aid.(ACE requires CPR certification and highly recommends basic first aid certification.)
   d. Practice the emergency plan.

G. Step 6: Obtain informed consent

1. The purpose and procedure for obtaining informed consent are the same as for apparently healthy clients.
2. Clients should be informed of the potential risks, identified in Step 4, associated with exercise. These risks should be clearly documented on the informed consent.
3. Informed consent should be obtained prior to performing fitness screening tests.

H. Step 7: Plan baseline "fitness" screening tests

1. Questions to be answered
   a. Is fitness testing safe?
   b. Is it necessary?
   c. What should an ACE-AHFS measure?
      - Fitness variables?
      - Health variables?
      - Ability to perform activities of daily living (ADL)?
2. Strategies to answer questions
   a. Refer to Steps 3 and 4 and to the appropriate "altered-organ-system exercise guidelines" (section III above) for guidance.
   b. Safety: Remember that fitness testing is exercise! The answers derived in Step 4 will provide guidance.
   c. Include measurements that will allow tracking of goals and expected benefits.
   d. Refer to any established guidelines.

I. Step 8: Design the exercise program

1. Questions to be answered
   a. What exercise program will most effectively maximize the benefits and minimize the risks?
2. Strategies to answer questions
   a. Refer to Steps 3 and 4 and to the appropriate "altered-organ-system exercise guidelines" (section III above) for guidance.
   b. Consider all components of a balanced exercise program (aerobic, muscle conditioning, flexibility, balance and gait, warm-up and cool-down). Determine frequency, intensity, mode, and duration.
   c. For clients with advanced diseases and/or disabilities, focus on improving ability to perform activities of daily living.
   d. Remember that many individuals with chronic diseases and disabilities lead sedentary lifestyles. In many cases, exercise capacity frequently will be more limited by poor general conditioning than the disease/ disability.
   e. Refer to established guidelines.

J. Step 9: Plan exercise program implementation

1. Questions to be answered
   a. What should an ACE-AHFS include in the pre-exercise session (prior to every exercise session) screen?
   b. What should an ACE-AHFS monitor during each exercise session?
   c. What program variables should an ACE-AHFS monitor over time?
      - Fitness variables?

- Health variables?
- Ability to perform ADL?

d. How quickly should I progress the client's program?

e. What are indications for
- program modification?
- referral to a physician?

f. What type of follow-up should I provide my client's physician?

2. Strategies for answering questions

a. For all questions
- Refer to Steps 3 and 4 and to the appropriate "altered-organ-system exercise guidelines" (section III above) for guidance.
- Consult members of healthcare team, as needed.
- Review established guidelines.

b. Pre-exercise session screen:
- Primarily a safety screen

c. Monitoring during exercise session
- Signs and symptoms of medical problems (e.g., ratings of perceived dyspnea in client with COPD; pre- and post-exercise session blood pressure in client with hypertension).
- Exercise variables central to program design (e.g., RPE for client with coronary artery disease on program limited to moderate intensity).

d. Monitoring long-term program variables
- Measurements, preferably objective, that will track goals and expected benefits.
- Signs and symptoms of evolving medical problems (e.g., increased severity or frequency of disease symptoms; increased medication requirements).

e. Physician follow-up

K. Step 10: Double-check established guidelines

1. Importance

a. client safety

b. liability

2. Resources

a. *ACE Advanced Health & Fitness Specialist Manual*

b. ACSM guidelines

c. Medical specialty colleges

Examples:
- American College of Obstetricians and Gynecologists
- American College of Cardiology

d. Other medical and public education groups

Examples:
- American Heart Association
- American Cancer Society
- American Diabetes Association

3. Staying current in the field

a. Most exercise research to date addresses the prevention of chronic diseases.

b. The role of exercise in the management of most chronic diseases has not been well-studied.

c. For most chronic diseases, there is insufficient scientific data for the development of specific exercise guidelines.

d. ACE-AHFS s must continually review the exercise medicine literature to stay informed of new research findings and practice guidelines.

APPENDIX E

Framingham Risk Scoring Tables

Table 1
Estimate of 10-Year Risk for Men (Framingham Point Score)

Age	Points
20–34	–9
35–39	–4
40–44	0
45–49	3
50–54	6
55–59	9
60–64	10
65–69	11
70–74	12
75–79	13

	Points				
Total Cholesterol	**Age 20–39**	**Age 40–49**	**Age 50–59**	**Age 60–69**	**Age 70–79**
<160	0	0	0	0	0
160–199	4	3	2	1	0
200–239	7	5	3	1	0
240–279	9	6	4	2	1
≥280	11	8	5	3	1

	Points				
	Age 20–39	**Age 40–49**	**Age 50–59**	**Age 60–69**	**Age 70–79**
Nonsmoker	0	0	0	0	0
Smoker	8	5	3	1	1

HDL (mg/dl)	Points
≥60	–1
50–59	0
40–49	1
<40	2

Systolic BP (mg/dl)	If Untreated	If Treated
<120	0	0
120–129	0	1
130–139	1	2
140–159	1	2
≥160	2	3

Point Total	10-Year Risk %
<0	<1
0	1
1	1
2	1
3	1
4	1
5	2
6	2
7	3
8	4
9	5
10	6
11	8
12	10
13	12
14	16
15	20
16	25
≥17	≥30

Table 2
Estimate of 10–Year Risk for Women (Framingham Point Score)

Age	Points
20–34	–7
35–39	–3
40–44	0
45–49	3
50–54	6
55–59	8
60–64	10
65–69	12
70–74	14
75–79	16

	Points				
Total Cholesterol	Age 20–39	Age 40–49	Age 50–59	Age 60–69	Age 70–79
<160	0	0	0	0	0
160–199	4	3	2	1	1
200–239	8	6	4	2	1
240–279	11	8	5	3	2
≥280	13	10	7	4	2

	Points				
	Age 20–39	Age 40–49	Age 50–59	Age 60–69	Age 70–79
Nonsmoker	0	0	0	0	0
Smoker	9	7	4	2	1

HDL (mg/dl)	Points
≥60	–1
50–59	0
40–49	1
<40	2

Systolic BP (mg/dl)	If Untreated	If Treated
<120	0	0
120–129	1	3
130–139	2	4
140–159	3	5
≥160	4	6

Point Total	10-Year Risk %
<9	<1
9	1
10	1
11	1
12	1
13	2
14	2
15	3
16	4
17	5
18	6
19	8
20	11
21	14
22	17
23	22
24	27
≥25	≥30

APPENDIX F

Functional Ability Tests

Berg Balance Scale

Source: Berg, K.O. et al. (1992). Measuring balance in the elderly: Validation of an instrument. *Canadian Journal of Public Health,* 2, S7–S11. Reprinted with permission.

Name: ______________________________ Date of Test: __________

1. Sit to stand

Instructions: "Please stand up. Try not to use your hands for support."

Grading: Please mark the lowest category that applies.

- ❑ 0 Needs moderate or maximal assistance to stand
- ❑ 1 Needs minimal assistance to stand or to stabilize
- ❑ 2 Able to stand using hands after several tries
- ❑ 3 Able to stand independently using hands
- ❑ 4 Able to stand with no hands and stabilize independently

2. Standing unsupported

Instructions: "Please stand for 2 minutes without holding onto anything."

Grading: Please mark the lowest category that applies.

- ❑ 0 Unable to stand 30 seconds unassisted
- ❑ 1 Needs several tries to stand 30 seconds unsupported
- ❑ 2 Able to stand 30 seconds unsupported
- ❑ 3 Able to stand 2 minutes with supervision
- ❑ 4 Able to stand safely for 2 minutes

If person is able to stand 2 minutes safely, score full points for sitting unsupported (item 3). Proceed to item 4.

3. Sitting with back unsupported with feet on floor or on a stool

Instructions: "Sit with arms folded for 2 minutes."

Grading: Please mark the lowest category that applies.

- ❑ 0 Unable to sit without support for 10 seconds
- ❑ 1 Able to sit for 10 seconds
- ❑ 2 Able to sit for 30 seconds
- ❑ 3 Able to sit for 2 minutes under supervision
- ❑ 4 Able to sit safely and securely for 2 minutes

4. Stand to sit

Instructions: "Please sit down."

Grading: Please mark the lowest category that applies.

- ❑ 0 Needs assistance to sit
- ❑ 1 Sits independently, but has uncontrolled descent
- ❑ 2 Uses back of legs against chair to control descent
- ❑ 3 Controls descent by using hands
- ❑ 4 Sits safely with minimal use of hands

5. Transfers

Instructions: "Please move from chair to chair and back again." (Person moves one way toward a seat with armrests and one way toward a seat without armrests.) Arrange chairs for pivot transfer.

Grading: Please mark the lowest category that applies.

- ❑ 0 Needs two people to assist or supervise to be safe
- ❑ 1 Needs one person to assist
- ❑ 2 Able to transfer with verbal cueing and/or supervision
- ❑ 3 Able to transfer safely with definite use of hands
- ❑ 4 Able to transfer safely with minor use of hands

6. *Standing unsupported with eyes closed

Instructions: "Close your eyes and stand still for 10 seconds."

Grading: Please mark the lowest category that applies.

- ❑ 0 Needs help to keep from falling
- ❑ 1 Unable to keep eyes closed for 3 seconds but remains steady
- ❑ 2 Able to stand for 3 seconds
- ❑ 3 Able to stand for 10 seconds with supervision
- ❑ 4 Able to stand for 10 seconds safely

7. *Stand unsupported with feet together

Instructions: "Place your feet together and stand without holding on to anything."

Grading: Please mark the lowest category that applies.

- ❑ 0 Needs help to attain position and unable to hold for 15 seconds
- ❑ 1 Needs help to attain position, but able to stand for 15 seconds with feet together
- ❑ 2 Able to place feet together independently, but unable to hold for 30 seconds
- ❑ 3 Able to place feet together independently and stand for 1 minute with supervision
- ❑ 4 Able to place feet together independently and stand for 1 minute safely

The following items are to be performed while standing unsupported.

8. *Reaching forward with outstretched arm

Instructions: "Lift your arm to 90°. Stretch out your fingers and reach forward as far as you can." (Examiner places a ruler at end of fingertips when arm is at 90°. Fingers should not touch the ruler while reaching forward. The recorded measure is the distance forward that the fingers reach while the person is in the most forward lean position.)

Grading: Please mark the lowest category that applies.

❑ 0 Needs help to keep from falling
❑ 1 Reaches forward, but needs supervision
❑ 2 Can reach forward more than 2 inches safely
❑ 3 Can reach forward more than 5 inches safely
❑ 4 Can reach forward confidently more than 10 inches

9. *Pick up object from the floor from a standing position

Instructions: "Please pick up the shoe/slipper that is placed in front of your feet."

Grading: Please mark the lowest category that applies.

❑ 0 Unable to try/needs assistance to keep from losing balance or falling
❑ 1 Unable to pick up shoe and needs supervision while trying
❑ 2 Unable to pick up shoe, but comes within 1–2 inches and maintains balance independently
❑ 3 Able to pick up shoe, but needs supervision
❑ 4 Able to pick up shoe safely and easily

10. * Turn to look behind over left and right shoulders while standing

Instructions: "Turn your upper body to look directly over your left shoulder. Now try turning to look over your right shoulder."

Grading: Please mark the lowest category that applies.

❑ 0 Needs assistance to keep from falling
❑ 1 Needs supervision when turning
❑ 2 Turns sideways only, but maintains balance
❑ 3 Looks behind one side only; other side shows less weight shift
❑ 4 Looks behind from both sides and weight shifts well

11. * Turn 360°

Instructions: "Turn completely in a full circle. Pause, then turn in a full circle in the other direction."

Grading: Please mark the lowest category that applies.

❑ 0 Needs assistance while turning
❑ 1 Needs close supervision or verbal cueing
❑ 2 Able to turn 360° safely but slowly
❑ 3 Able to turn 360° safely to one side only in less than 4 seconds
❑ 4 Able to turn 360° safely in less than 4 seconds to each side

12. * Place alternate foot on bench or stool while standing unsupported

Instructions: "Place each foot alternately on the bench (or stool). Continue until each foot has touched the bench (or stool) four times." (Recommend use of 6-inch-high bench.)

Grading: Please mark the lowest category that applies.

- ☐ 0 Needs assistance to keep from falling/unable to try
- ☐ 1 Able to complete fewer than two steps; needs minimal assistance
- ☐ 2 Able to complete four steps without assistance, but with supervision
- ☐ 3 Able to stand independently and complete eight steps in more than 20 seconds
- ☐ 4 Able to stand independently and safely and complete eight steps in less than 20 seconds

13. * Stand unsupported with one foot in front

Instructions: "Place one foot directly in front of the other. If you feel that you can't place your foot directly in front, try to step far enough ahead that the heel of your forward foot is ahead of the toes of the other foot." (Demonstrate this test item.)

Grading: Please mark the lowest category that applies.

- ☐ 0 Loses balance while stepping or standing
- ☐ 1 Needs help to step, but can hold for 15 seconds
- ☐ 2 Able to take small step independently and hold for 30 seconds
- ☐ 3 Able to place one foot ahead of the other independently and hold for 30 seconds
- ☐ 4 Able to place feet in tandem position independently and hold for 30 seconds

14. * Standing on one leg

Instructions: "Please stand on one leg as long as you can without holding onto anything."

Grading: Please mark the lowest category that applies.

- ☐ 0 Unable to try or needs assistance to prevent fall
- ☐ 1 Tries to lift leg, unable to hold 3 seconds, but remains standing independently
- ☐ 2 Able to lift leg independently and hold up to 3 seconds
- ☐ 3 Able to lift leg independently and hold for 5 to 10 seconds
- ☐ 4 Able to lift leg independently and hold more than 10 seconds

Total score________/56

Note: Perform only items 6 though 14 (*) in the modified version of the scale. Maximum score for modified version is 36 points.

Score Interpretation:

0–20: Wheelchair bound
21–40: Walking with assistance
41–56: Independent

Interpretation of Individual Test Item Results on the Berg Balance Scale (BBS)

Item	Possible Impairments	Recommended Exercises
1. Sit to stand	1. Lower- and/or upper-body weakness 2. Poor dynamic COG control 3. Abnormal weight distribution	Wall sits; UB and LB exercises with resistance (quadriceps, biceps/triceps, hip abductors/adductors) Seated/standing balance activities emphasizing forward weight shifts Standing balance activities with eyes closed (controlled sway in A-P and lateral directions)
2. Stand for 2 minutes	1. Poor gaze stabilization 2. Lower-body weakness 3. Abnormal weight distribution in standing	Teach gaze fixation and stabilization techniques Wall sits; LB exercises with resistance COG standing balance activities
3. Sit for 2 minutes	1. Poor trunk stabilization and/or UB weakness 2. Abnormal perception of true vertical	UB exercises with resistance (own body); seated balance activities on compliant surfaces Standing against wall with eyes closed; somatosensory cues
4. Stand to sit	1. Poor dynamic COG control 2. Lower- and/or upper-body weakness 3. Poor trunk flexibility	Seated/standing balance activities emphasizing backward weight shifts UB and LB exercises with resistance (own body/resistance band; emphasize eccentric component) Flexibility exercises emphasizing trunk rotation/flexion; seated and standing
5. Transfer (chair to chair)	1. Poor dynamic control of COG 2. Lower- and/or upper-body weakness	Seated/standing balance activities emphasizing multidirectional weight shifts UB and LB exercises with resistance
6. Stand with eyes closed (10 sec)	1. Poor use of somatosensory inputs; visual dependency and/or fear of falling 2. Lower-body weakness	Seated/standing balance activities with eyes closed; verbally emphasize use of surface cues Wall sits; LB exercise with resistance
7. Stand with feet together (1 min)	1. Poor COG control 2. Weak hip abductors/adductors	Standing balance activities with reduced BOS Lateral leg raises/weight shifts against resistance
8. Standing forward reach	1. Poor dynamic COG control (reduced limits of stability) 2. Lower-body weakness 3. Reduced ankle ROM	Seated/standing COG activities emphasizing leaning away from and back to midline LB exercises with resistance (body/resistance band); emphasize dorsiflexors; gastrocnemius/soleus muscles Flexibility exercises (emphasize dorsiflexion)

Note: A-P = anterior-posterior direction; BOS = base of support; COG = center of gravity; LB = lower body; UB = upper body.

Item	Possible Impairments	Recommended Exercises
9. Pick up object	1. Poor dynamic COG control	Seated/standing COG activities emphasizing leaning away from and back to midline
	2. Poor upper- and lower-body flexibility	Selected exercises to improve UB and LB flexion
	3. Lower-body weakness	LB exercises with resistance (body/resistance band)
	4. Vestibular impairment (dizziness)	Head and eye movements; habituation exercises
10. Turn to look behind	1. Poor dynamic COG control	Standing weight shifts in lateral direction
	2. Poor neck and/or trunk flexibility	Selected exercises emphasizing rotation of neck, shoulders, and hips
	3. Lower-body weakness	LB exercises with resistance; ball movement exercises in standing position
11. Turn in a circle	1. Poor dynamic COG control	Standing weight transfer activities; gait pattern enhancement (turns, directional changes)
	2. Possible vestibular impairment (e.g. dizziness)	Head and eye movement coordination exercises
	3. Lower-body weakness	LB exercises with resistance; emphasize hip and knee flexion; hip abduction/adduction
12. Dynamic toe touch	1. Poor dynamic COG control	Standing weight shifts in lateral/A-P directions
	2. Lower-body weakness	LB exercises with resistance; emphasize hip and knee flexion; hip abduction/adduction
13. Tandem stance	1. Poor static and dynamic COG control	Standing A-P weight shifts and transfers; reduced BOS activities
	2. Lower-body weakness	LB exercises with resistance (body/resistance band); emphasize hip abductors/adductors
	3. Poor gaze stabilization	Practice focusing on visual targets in front of and at head height during standing and moving activities
14. Stand on one leg	1. Poor static and dynamic COG control	Standing A-P weight shifts and transfers; reduced BOS activities
	2. Lower-body weakness	LB exercises with resistance (body/resistance band); emphasize hip abductors/adductors
	3. Poor gaze stabilization	Practice focusing on visual targets during standing and moving activities

Note: A-P = anterior-posterior direction; BOS = base of support; COG = center of gravity; LB = lower body; UB = upper body.

Fullerton Advanced Balance Scale

From D.J. Rose, *Fallproof!*, pages 66–71. © 2003 by Deborah J. Rose.
Reprinted with permission from Human Kinetics (Champaign, Ill.).

The Fullerton Advanced Balance Scale is designed to measure changes in multiple dimensions of balance in higher functioning community-dwelling older adults.

Test Administration Instructions for the Fullerton Advanced Balance (FAB) Scale

1. Stand with feet together and eyes closed

Purpose: Assess ability to use ground cues to maintain upright balance while standing with reduced base of support

Equipment: Stopwatch

Testing procedures: Demonstrate the correct test position and then instruct the participants to move the feet independently until they are together. If some participants are unable to achieve the correct position due to lower-extremity joint problems, encourage them to bring their heels together even though the front of the feet are not touching. Have participants adopt a position that will ensure their safety as the arms are folded across the chest and they prepare to close the eyes. Begin timing as soon as the participant closes the eyes. (Instruct participants to open the eyes if they feel so unsteady that a loss of balance is imminent.)

Verbal instructions: "Bring your feet together, fold your arms across your chest, close your eyes when you are ready, and remain as steady as possible until I instruct you to open your eyes."

2. Reach forward to retrieve an object (pencil) held at shoulder height with outstretched arm

Purpose: Assess ability to lean forward to retrieve an object without altering the base of support; measure of stability limits in a forward direction

Equipment: Pencil and 12-inch ruler

Testing procedures: Instruct the participant to raise the preferred arm to 90° and extend it with fingers outstretched. (Follow with a demonstration of the correct action.) Use the ruler to measure a distance of 10 inches from the end of the fingers of the outstretched arm. Hold the object (pencil) horizontally and level with the height of the participant's shoulder. Instruct the participant to reach forward, grasp the pencil, and return to the initial starting position without moving feet, if possible. (It is acceptable to raise the heels as long as the feet do not move while reaching for the pencil.) If the participant is unable to reach the pencil within 2–3 seconds of initiating the forward lean, indicate to the participant that it is okay to move the feet in order to reach the pencil. Record the number of steps taken by the participant in order to retrieve the pencil.

Verbal instructions: "Try to lean forward to take the pencil from my hand and return to your starting position without moving your feet from their present position." After allowing 2–3 seconds of lean time: "You can move your feet in order to reach the pencil."

3. Turn 360° in right and left directions

Purpose: Assess ability to turn in a full circle in both directions in the fewest number of steps without loss of balance

Equipment: None

Testing procedures: Verbally explain and then demonstrate the task to be performed, making sure to complete each circle in four steps or less and pause briefly between turns. Instruct the participant to turn in a complete circle in one direction, pause, and then turn in a complete circle in the opposite direction. Count the number of steps taken to complete each circle. Allow for a small correction in foot position before a turn in the opposite direction is initiated.

Verbal instructions: "Turn around in a full circle, pause, and then turn in a second full circle in the opposite direction."

4. Step up, onto, and over a 6-inch bench

Purpose: Assess ability to control center of gravity in dynamic task situations; also a measure of lower-body strength and control

Equipment: 6-inch-high bench (18- by 18-inch stepping surface)

Testing procedures: Verbally explain and demonstrate the step up, onto, and over the bench in both directions before the participant performs the test. Instruct the participant to step onto the bench with the right foot, swing the left leg directly up and over the bench, and step off the other side, then repeat the movement in the opposite direction with the left leg leading the action. During performance of the test, watch to see that the participant's trailing leg (a) does not make contact with the bench or (b) swing around, as opposed to directly over, the bench.

Verbal instructions: "Step up onto the bench with your right leg, swing your left leg directly up and over the bench, and step off the other side. Repeat the movement in the opposite direction with your left leg as the leading leg."

5. Tandem walk

Purpose: Assess ability to dynamically control center of mass with an altered base of support

Equipment: Masking tape

Testing procedures: Verbally explain and demonstrate how to perform the test correctly before the participant attempts to perform it. Instruct the participant to walk on the line in a tandem position (heel-to-toe) until you tell them to stop. Allow the participant to repeat the test one time if unable to achieve a tandem stance position within the first two steps. The participant may elect to step forward with the opposite foot on the second trial. Score as interruptions any instances where the participant (a) takes a lateral step away from the line when performing the tandem walk or (b) is unable to achieve correct heel-to-toe position during any step taken along the course. Do not ask the participant to stop until 10 steps have been completed.

Verbal instructions: "Walk forward along the line, placing one foot directly in front of the other such that the heel and toe are in contact on each step forward. I will tell you when to stop."

6. Stand on one leg

Purpose: Assess ability to maintain upright balance with a reduced base of support

Equipment: Stopwatch

Testing procedures: Instruct the participant to fold the arms across the chest, lift the preferred leg off the floor, and maintain balance until instructed to return the foot to the floor. Begin timing as soon as the participant lifts the foot from the floor. Stop timing if the legs touch, the preferred leg contacts the floor, or the participant removes the arms from the chest before 20 seconds have elapsed. Allow the participant to perform the test a second time with the other leg if he or she is unsure as to which is the preferred limb.

Verbal instructions: "Fold your arms across your chest, lift your preferred leg off the floor (without touching other leg), and stand with your eyes open as long as you can."

7. Stand on foam with eyes closed

Purpose: Assess the ability to maintain upright balance while standing on a compliant surface with eyes closed

Equipment: Stopwatch; two Airex pads, with a length of nonslip material placed between the two pads and an additional length of nonslip material between the floor and first pad if the test is being performed on an uncarpeted surface

Testing procedures: Instruct the participant to step onto the foam pads without assistance, fold the arms across the chest, and close the eyes when ready. (Demonstrate the correct standing position on foam.) Make sure the position adopted ensures the safety of the participant. Position the foam pads close to a wall in all cases and in a corner of the room if the participant appears unsteady. Begin timing as soon as the eyes close. Stop the trial if the participant (a) opens the eyes before the timing period has elapsed, (b) lifts the arms off the chest, or (c) loses balance and requires manual assistance to prevent falling. (Instruct participants to open their eyes if they feel so unsteady that a loss of balance is imminent.)

Verbal instructions: "Step up onto the foam and stand with your feet shoulder-width apart. Fold your arms over your chest, and close your eyes when you are ready. I will tell you when to open your eyes."

8. Two-footed jump for distance

Purpose: Assess upper- and lower-body coordination and lower-body power

Equipment: 36-inch ruler

Testing procedures: Instruct the participant to jump as far but as safely as possible while maintaining a two-footed stance. Demonstrate the correct movement prior to the participant performing the jump. (Do not jump much more than twice the length of your own feet when demonstrating.) Observe whether the participant leaves the floor with both feet and lands with both feet. Use the ruler to measure the length of the foot and then multiply by two to determine the ideal distance to be jumped.

Verbal instructions: "Try to jump as far but as safely as you can with both feet."

9. Walk with head turns

Purpose: Assess ability to maintain dynamic balance while walking and turning the head

Equipment: Metronome set at 100 beats per minute

Testing procedures: After first demonstrating the test, allow the participant to practice turning the head in time with the metronome while standing in place. Encourage the participant to turn the head at least 30° in each direction (e.g., "Turn your head to look into each corner of the room."). Observe how far the participant is able to turn the head during the standing head turns. A 30° head turn is required during the walking trial. Instruct the participant to walk forward while turning the head from side to side and in time with the auditory tone. Begin counting steps as soon as the participant deviates from a straight path while walking or is unable to turn the head the required distance to the timing of the metronome.

Verbal instructions: "Walk forward while turning your head from left to right with each beat of the metronome. I will tell you when to stop."

10. Reactive postural control

Purpose: Assess ability to efficiently restore balance following an unexpected perturbation

Equipment: None

Testing procedures: Instruct the participant to stand with his or her back to you. Extend your arm with the elbow locked and place the palm of your hand against the participant's back between the scapula. Instruct the participant to lean back slowly against your hand until you tell him or her to stop. Quickly flex your elbow until your hand is no longer in contact with the participant's back at the moment you estimate that a sufficient amount of force has been applied to require a movement of the feet to restore balance. You may actually begin releasing your hand while you are still giving the instructions. This release should be unexpected, so do not prepare the participant for the moment of release.

Verbal instructions: "Slowly lean back into my hand until I ask you to stop."

Score Sheet for
Fullerton Advanced Balance (FAB) Scale

Name:____ Date of Test:________________

1. Stand with feet together and eyes closed

- ❑ 0 Unable to obtain the correct standing position independently
- ❑ 1 Able to obtain the correct standing position independently but unable to maintain the position or keep the eyes closed for more than 10 seconds
- ❑ 2 Able to maintain the correct standing position with eyes closed for more than 10 seconds but less than 30 seconds.
- ❑ 3 Able to maintain the correct standing position with eyes closed for 30 seconds but requires close supervision
- ❑ 4 Able to maintain the correct standing position safely with eyes closed for 30 seconds

2. Reach forward to retrieve an object (pencil) held at shoulder height with outstretched arm

- ❑ 0 Unable to reach the pencil without taking more than two steps
- ❑ 1 Able to reach the pencil but needs to take two steps
- ❑ 2 Able to reach the pencil but needs to take one step
- ❑ 3 Can reach the pencil without moving the feet but requires supervision
- ❑ 4 Can reach the pencil safely and independently without moving the feet

3. Turn 360° in right and left directions

- ❑ 0 Needs manual assistance while turning
- ❑ 1 Needs close supervision or verbal cueing while turning
- ❑ 2 Able to turn 360° but takes more than four steps in both directions
- ❑ 3 Able to turn 360° but unable to complete in four steps or fewer in one direction
- ❑ 4 Able to turn 360° safely taking four steps or fewer in both directions

4. Step up, onto, and over a 6-inch bench

- ❑ 0 Unable to step up onto the bench without loss of balance or manual assistance
- ❑ 1 Able to step up onto the bench with leading leg, but trailing leg contacts the bench or leg swings around the bench during the swing-through phase in both directions
- ❑ 2 Able to step up onto the bench with leading leg, but trailing leg contacts the bench or swings around the bench during the swing-through phase in one direction
- ❑ 3 Able to correctly complete the step up and over in both directions but requires close supervision in one or both directions
- ❑ 4 Able to correctly complete the step up and over in both directions safely and independently

5. Tandem walk

- ❑ 0 Unable to complete 10 steps independently
- ❑ 1 Able to complete the 10 steps with more than five interruptions
- ❑ 2 Able to complete the 10 steps with five or fewer interruptions
- ❑ 3 Able to complete the 10 steps with two or fewer interruptions
- ❑ 4 Able to complete the 10 steps independently and with no interruptions

6. Stand on one leg

- ❑ 0 Unable to try or needs assistance to prevent falling
- ❑ 1 Able to lift leg independently but unable to maintain position for more than 5 seconds
- ❑ 2 Able to lift leg independently and maintain position for more than 5 but less than 12 seconds
- ❑ 3 Able to lift leg independently and maintain position for more than 12 but less than 20 seconds
- ❑ 4 Able to lift leg independently and maintain position for the full 20 seconds

7. Stand on foam with eyes closed

- ❑ 0 Unable to step onto foam or maintain standing position independently with eyes open
- ❑ 1 Able to step onto foam independently and maintain standing position but unable or unwilling to close eyes
- ❑ 2 Able to step onto foam independently and maintain standing position with eyes closed for at least 10 seconds
- ❑ 3 Able to step onto foam independently and maintain standing position with eyes closed for more than 10 seconds but less than 20 seconds
- ❑ 4 Able to step onto foam independently and maintain standing position with eyes closed for 20 seconds

8. Two-footed jump for distance

- ❑ 0 Unable to attempt or attempts to initiate two-footed jump, but one or both feet do not leave the floor
- ❑ 1 Able to initiate two-footed jump, but one foot either leaves the floor or lands before the other
- ❑ 2 Able to perform two-footed jump, but unable to jump farther than the length of their own feet
- ❑ 3 Able to perform two-footed jump and achieve a distance greater than the length of their own feet
- ❑ 4 Able to perform two-footed jump and achieve a distance greater than twice the length of their own feet

9. Walk with head turns

- ❑ 0 Unable to walk 10 steps independently while maintaining 30° head turns at an established pace
- ❑ 1 Able to walk 10 steps independently but unable to complete required number of 30° head turns at an established pace
- ❑ 2 Able to walk 10 steps but veers from a straight line while performing 30° head turns at an established pace
- ❑ 3 Able to walk 10 steps in a straight line while performing head turns at an established pace but head turns less than 30° in one or both directions
- ❑ 4 Able to walk 10 steps in a straight line while performing required number of 30° head turns at established pace

10. Reactive postural control

- ❑ 0 Unable to maintain upright balance; no observable attempt to step; requires manual assistance to restore balance
- ❑ 1 Unable to maintain upright balance; takes fewer than two steps and requires manual assistance to restore balance
- ❑ 2 Unable to maintain upright balance; takes fewer than two steps, but is able to restore balance independently
- ❑ 3 Unable to maintain upright balance; takes one to two steps, but is able to restore balance independently
- ❑ 4 Unable to maintain upright balance but able to restore balance independently with only one step

Tinetti Balance and Gait Tests

Source: Tinetti, M.E. (1986). Performance-oriented assessment of mobility problems in elderly patients. *Journal of the American Geriatrics Society,* 34, 119–126.

The test consists of two test stages; nine test items evaluating postural control in seated and standing activities, and seven test items evaluating basic tasks in gait, scoring the performance of each specific task. The scoring uses a 3-point ordinal scale with a score of 0 representing greatest impairment and 2 representing independence in performing the task. Individual item scores are combined to determine an overall balance score, overall gait score, and an overall balance and gait score.

Test purpose: Evaluate functional balance and limitations associated with performing basic seated, standing, and walking activities.

Equipment needed: Armless chair for the balance sequence.

Test instructions: Perform the sequence of balance tests and select the score that best describes the performance of each test, totaling the scores of all the tests.

Test interpretations: A maximum score for the balance and gait portions are 16 and 12 points, respectively, collectively totaling 28 points. Individuals scoring less than 19 are at high risk for falls; individuals scoring between 19 and 24 demonstrate some risk for falls, while those scoring above 24 demonstrate good balance and postural control.

Tinetti Balance Tests

Movement	Scoring	Points	Score
Sitting balance	Leans or slides in chair Steady, safe	0 1	
Arises out of a chair (movement out of a chair)	Unstable without help Able, but uses the arms to help Able, without using the arms	0 1 2	
Attempt to arise (number of attempts to arise)	Unable to arise without help Able, but requires more than one attempt (scooting, rocking) Able to arise in one attempt	0 1 2	
Immediate standing balance (within the first 5 seconds)	Unsteady (staggers, moves feet, marked trunk sway) Steady, but uses a walker or cane or grabs other objects for support Steady without walker, cane, or other support	0 1 2	
Standing balance	Unsteady Steady but wide stance [medial heels more than 4 inches (10 cm) apart] or uses cane, walker, or other support Narrow stance without support	0 1 2	
Nudging [with the subject's feet as close together as possible, the tester pushes lightly on the sternum with the palm of the hand three times (or safely pulls from behind)]	Begins to fall Staggers and grabs, but catches self Steady	0 1 2	
Eyes closed with the subject's feet as close together as possible	Unsteady Steady	0 1	
Turning 360 degrees	Discontinuous steps (stops and starts) Continuous steps and movement Unsteady (grabs and staggers) Steady	0 1 0 1	
Sitting down	Unsafe (misjudges distance, falls into chair) Uses arms or lacks smooth motion Safe, smooth motion	0 1 2	
Total:			/16

Tinetti Gait Tests

Movement	Scoring	Points	Score
Initiation of gait (after told to go)	Any hesitancy or multiple attempts to start No hesitancy	0 1	
Step length and height	Right swing foot: Foot does not pass the left stance foot with a step Foot passes the left stance foot with a step Foot does not clear the floor completely with a step Foot completely clears the floor with a step Left swing foot: Foot does not pass the right stance foot with a step Foot passes the right stance foot with a step Foot does not clear the floor completely with a step Foot completely clears the floor with a step	 0 1 0 1 0 1 0 1	
Step symmetry	Right and left step lengths are not equal Right and left step lengths appear equal	0 1	
Step continuity	Stopping or discontinuity between steps Steps appear continuous	0 1	
Path [observe over 10 feet (3 m) of walking]	Marked deviation Mild-to-moderate deviation or uses walking aid Straight line without any walking aid	0 1 2	
Trunk	Marked sway or uses walking aid No sway, but there is flexion of the knees or back; or spreads arms out while walking No sway, no flexion, no use of arms or walking aids	0 1 2	
Walking stance (width between heels)	Heels wide apart (near shoulder width) Heels almost touching while walking (normal width)	0 1	
Total			**/12**
Balance and Gait Total			**/28**

APPENDIX G

ACE Position Statement on Nutritional Supplements

It is the position of the American Council on Exercise (ACE) that it is outside the defined scope of practice of a fitness professional to recommend, prescribe, sell, or supply nutritional supplements to clients. Recommending supplements without possessing the requisite qualifications (e.g., R.D.) can place the client's health at risk and possibly expose the fitness professional to disciplinary action and litigation. If a client wants to take supplements, a fitness professional should work in conjunction with a qualified registered dietitian or medical doctor to provide safe and effective nutritional education and recommendations.

ACE recognizes that some fitness and health clubs encourage or require their employees to sell nutritional supplements. If this is a condition of employment, fitness professionals should protect themselves by ensuring their employers possess adequate insurance coverage for them should a problem arise. Furthermore, ACE strongly encourages continuing education on diet and nutrition for all fitness professionals.

GLOSSARY

Abdominal hollowing A movement that involves the "sucking in" of the abdomen to activate the transverse abdominis.

Abdominal bracing A mild contraction of the abdominal wall.

Abduction Movement away from the midline of the body.

Abruptio placentae The premature separation of the placenta from the uterus.

Absolute contraindication A situation that makes a particular treatment or procedure absolutely inadvisable.

Absorption The uptake of nutrients across a tissue or membrane by the gastrointestinal tract.

Acetyl-CoA An important molecule in metabolism, used in many biochemical reactions. Its main use is to convey the carbon atoms within the acetyl group to the citric acid cycle to be oxidized for energy production.

Achilles tendinitis A painful and often debilitating inflammation of the Achilles tendon.

Achilles tendinopathy A term used to describe two characteristics of Achilles tendon injury—inflammation and tendinosis (microtears in the tissue and around the tendon caused by overuse).

Actin Thin contractile protein in a myofibril.

Action The stage of the transtheoretical model during which the individual started a new behavior less than six months ago.

Active transport The energy-requiring transfer of a nutrient across a membrane.

Activities of daily living (ADL) Activities normally performed for hygiene, bathing, household chores, walking, shopping, and similar activities.

Acute coronary syndrome A sudden, severe coronary event that mimics a heart attack, such as unstable angina.

Adduction Movement toward the midline of the body.

Adenosine diphosphate (ADP) One of the chemical by-products of the breakdown of adenosine triphosphate (ATP) during muscle contraction.

Adenosine trisphosphate (ATP) A high-energy phosphate molecule required to provide energy for cellular function. Produced both aerobically and anaerobically and stored in the body.

Adequate Intake (AI) A recommended nutrient intake level that, based on research, appears to be sufficient for good health.

Adherence The extent to which people stick to their plans or treatment recommendations. Exercise adherence is the extent to which people follow, or stick to, an exercise program.

Adipocyte A fat cell.

Adiponectin A hormone related to energy metabolism regulation that facilitates the action of insulin by sending blood glucose into the body's cells for storage or use as fuel, thus increasing the cells' insulin sensitivity or glucose metabolism.

Adipose tissue Fatty tissue; connective tissue made up of fat cells.

Adrenaline An exercise hormone; also called epinephrine.

Aerobic capacity *See* $\dot{V}O_2$max.

Aerobic glycolysis A metabolic pathway that requires oxygen to facilitate the use of glycogen for energy (ATP).

Afferent nervous system The portion of the somatic nervous system that carries impulses from receptors to the central nervous system.

Agonist The muscle directly responsible for observed movement; also called the prime mover.

Allergen A substance that can cause an allergic reaction by stimulating type-1 hypersensitivity in atopic individuals.

Allograft A transplant in which transplanted tissue is sourced from a genetically non-identical member of the same species.

Alpha-glucosidase inhibitors Oral hypoglycemic agents that decrease the carbohydrate absorption rate and slow the increase in postprandial blood glucose level.

Alveoli Spherical extensions of the respiratory bronchioles and the primary sites of gas exchange with the blood.

Alzheimer's disease An age-related disorder of loss of

mental functions resulting from brain tissue changes of cause that is yet to be identified.

Amenorrhea The absence of menstruation.

Amino acids Nitrogen-containing compounds that are the building blocks of protein.

Anabolic Muscle-building effects.

Anaerobic glycolysis The metabolic pathway that uses glucose for energy production without requiring oxygen. Sometimes referred to as the lactic acid system or anaerobic glucose system, it produces lactic acid as a by-product.

Android Pertaining to something that is typically masculine.

Anemia A reduction in the number of red blood cells and/or quantity of hemoglobin per volume of blood below normal values.

Aneurysm A localized abnormal dilation of a blood vessel; associated with a stroke when the aneurysm bursts.

Angina *See* angina pectoris.

Angina pectoris Chest pain caused by an inadequate supply of oxygen and decreased blood flow to the heart muscle; an early sign of coronary artery disease. Symptoms may include pain or discomfort, heaviness, tightness, pressure or burning, numbness, aching, and tingling in the chest, back, neck, throat, jaw, or arms; also called angina.

Anginal threshold The point at which angina symptoms occur.

Annulus fibrosus The outer ring of intervertebral discs.

Anorexia nervosa An eating disorder characterized by refusal to maintain body weight of at least 85% of expected weight; intense fear of gaining weight or becoming fat; body-image disturbances, including a disproportionate influence of body weight on self evaluation; and, in women, the absence of at least three consecutive menstrual periods.

Antagonist The muscle that acts in opposition to the contraction produced by an agonist (prime mover) muscle.

Antecedents Variables or factors that precede and influence a client's exercise participation, including the decision to not exercise as planned.

Antioxidant A substance that prevents or repairs oxidative damage; includes vitamins C and E, some carotenoids, selenium, ubiquinones, and bioflavonoids.

Anxiety A state of uneasiness and apprehension; occurs in some mental disorders.

Aortic aneurysm A general term for any swelling of the aorta, usually representing an underlying weakness in the wall of the aorta at that location.

Apoprotein The protein components of a number of complexes, such as enzymes (apoenzymes), ferritin (apoferritins), or lipoproteins (apolipoproteins).

Apoptosis The programmed cell death or the deliberate suicide of a cell in a multicellular organism for the greater good of the whole individual.

Arrhythmia A disturbance in the rate or rhythm of the heartbeat. Some can be symptoms of serious heart disease; may not be of medical significance until symptoms appear.

Artery A blood vessel that carries oxygenated blood away from the heart to vital organs and the extremities.

Arthritis Inflammation of a joint; a state characterized by the inflammation of joints.

Arthroplasty A surgery to repair, reposition, replace, or remove parts in an arthritic joint.

Arthroscopy A minimally invasive surgical procedure in which an examination and sometimes treatment of damage of the interior of a joint is performed using an arthroscope, a type of endoscope that is inserted into the joint through a small incision.

Arthrosis A degenerative disease of a joint.

Articular cartilage Cartilage covering the ends of the bones inside diarthroidial joints; allows the ends of the bones to glide without friction.

Articulation A joint.

Asthma A chronic inflammatory disorder of the airways that affects genetically susceptible individuals in response to various environmental triggers such as allergens, viral infection, exercise, cold, and stress.

Asthma exacerbation An episode of

progressively worsening shortness of breath, cough, wheezing, and/or chest tightness that results in decreases in expiratory airflow; also called "asthma attack."

Atherogenesis Formation of atheromatous deposits, especially on the innermost layer of arterial walls.

Atherogenic dyslipidemia Formation of atheromatous deposits, especially on the innermost layer of arterial walls due to an abnormal concentration of lipids or lipoproteins in the blood.

Atheroma A deposit or degenerative accumulation of lipid-containing plaques on the innermost layer of the wall of an artery.

Atherosclerosis A specific form of arteriosclerosis characterized by the accumulation of fatty material on the inner walls of the arteries, causing them to harden, thicken, and lose elasticity.

Atopy Allergic hypersensitivity.

Atrophy A reduction in muscle size (muscle wasting) due to inactivity or immobilization.

Autogenic inhibition An automatic reflex relaxation caused by stimulation of the Golgi tendon organ (GTO).

Automated external defibrillator (AED) A portable electronic device used to restore normal heart rhythms in victims of sudden cardiac arrest.

Autonomic nervous system The part of the nervous system that regulates involuntary body functions, including the activity of the cardiac muscle, smooth muscles, and glands. It has two divisions: the sympathetic nervous system and the parasympathetic nervous system.

Autonomic neuropathy A disease of the non-voluntary, non-sensory nervous system (i.e., the autonomic nervous system) affecting mostly the internal organs such as the bladder muscles, the cardiovascular system, the digestive tract, and the genital organs.

Avascular necrosis A disease resulting from the temporary or permanent loss of the blood supply to the bones.

Axon A nerve fiber that conducts a nerve impulse away from the neuron cell body; efferent nerve fiber.

Balance The ability to maintain the body's position over its base of support within stability limits, both statically and dynamically.

Bariatrics The branch of medicine that deals with the causes, prevention, and treatment of obesity.

Baroreceptors A sensory nerve ending that is stimulated by changes in pressure, as those in the walls of blood vessels.

Basal metabolic rate (BMR) The energy required to complete the sum total of life-sustaining processes, including ion transport (40% BMR), protein synthesis (20% BMR), and daily functioning such as breathing, circulation, and nutrient processing (40% BMR).

Base of support (BOS) The areas of contact between the feet and their supporting surface and the area between the feet.

Behavior chain A sequence of events in which variables both preceding and following a target behavior help to explain and reinforce the target behavior, such as participation in an exercise session.

Beta cell Endocrine cells in the islets of Langerhans of the pancreas responsible for synthesizing and secreting the hormone insulin, which lowers the glucose levels in the blood.

Beta receptors Receptors believed to exist on nerve cell membranes of the sympathetic nervous system in order to explain the specificity of certain agents that affect only some sympathetic activities (such as vasodilation and increased heart beat).

Bicipital tendinitis An inflammation of one of the tendons that attach the muscle (biceps) on the front of the upper arm bone (humerus) to the shoulder joint.

Binge eating disorder (BED) An eating disorder characterized by frequent binge eating (without purging) and feelings of being out of control when eating.

Bioavailability The degree to which a substance can be absorbed and efficiently utilized by the body.

Bioelectrical impedance analysis (BIA) A

body-composition assessment technique that measures the amount of impedance, or resistance, to electric current flow as it passes through the body. Impedance is greatest in fat tissue, while fat-free mass, which contains 70–75% water, allows the electrical current to pass much more easily.

Biological value (BV) An estimate of protein quality determined by dividing the nitrogen used for tissue formation by the nitrogen absorbed from food and then multiplying by 100.

Blood pressure (BP) The pressure exerted by the blood on the walls of the arteries; measured in millimeters of mercury (mmHg) with a sphygmomanometer.

Body composition The makeup of the body in terms of the relative percentage of fat-free mass and body fat.

Body mass index (BMI) A relative measure of body height to body weight used to determine levels of weight, from underweight to extreme obesity.

Bolus A food and saliva digestive mix that is swallowed and then moved through the digestive tract.

Bone mineral density (BMD) A measure of the amount of minerals (mainly calcium) contained in a certain volume of bone.

Bone modeling An overall gain in bone mineral that occurs when the rate of bone formation is faster than the rate of bone resorption.

Bone remodeling A locally coordinated activity of osteoclasts and osteoblasts whereby bone can both prevent and repair damage caused by everyday loading. A key feature of remodeling is that it replaces damaged tissue with an equal amount of new bone tissue.

Bradycardia Slowness of the heartbeat, as evidenced by a pulse rate of less than 60 beats per minute.

Bronchiole The smallest tubes that supply air to the alveoli (air sacs) of the lungs.

Bronchitis Acute or chronic inflammation of the bronchial tubes. *See* Chronic obstructive pulmonary disease (COPD).

Bronchospasm Abnormal contraction of the smooth muscle of the bronchi, resulting in an acute narrowing and obstruction of the respiratory airway.

Brush border The site of nutrient absorption in the small intestines.

Bulimia nervosa (BN) An eating disorder characterized by recurrent episodes of uncontrolled binge eating; recurrent inappropriate compensatory behavior such as self-induced vomiting, laxative misuse, diuretics, or enemas (purging type), or fasting and/or excessive exercise (non-purging type); episodes of binge eating and compensatory behaviors occur at least twice per week for three months; self-evaluation is heavily influenced by body shape and weight; and the episodes do not occur exclusively with episodes of anorexia.

Bursa A sac of fluid that is present in areas of the body that are potential sites of friction.

Bursitis Swelling and inflammation in the bursa that results from overuse.

Calcitonin A hormone that acts to reduce blood calcium (Ca++), opposing the effects of parathyroid hormone (PTH).

Calorie A measurement of the amount of energy in a food available after digestion. The amount of energy needed to increase 1 kilogram of water by 1 degree Celsius. Also called a kilocalorie.

Capsule An anatomical term that refers to a cover or envelope partly or wholly surrounding a structure.

Carbohydrate The body's preferred energy source. Dietary sources include sugars (simple) and grains, rice, potatoes, and beans (complex). Carbohydrate is stored as glycogen in the muscles and liver and is transported in the blood as glucose.

Cardiac autonomic neuropathy A disease of the non-voluntary, non-sensory cardiovascular system commonly seen in persons with long-standing diabetes mellitus type 1 and 2.

Cardiac output The amount of blood pumped by the heart per minute; usually expressed in liters of blood per minute.

Cardiac sphincter Sits at the upper portion

of the stomach; prevents food and stomach acid from splashing back into the esophagus from the stomach; also called the esophageal sphincter.

Cardiometabolic risk The identification of factors that increase the likelihood of CVD onset. Managing these risk factors can help a person avoid diabetes and heart disease.

Cardiopulmonary resuscitation (CPR) A procedure to support and maintain breathing and circulation for a person who has stopped breathing (respiratory arrest) and/or whose heart has stopped (cardiac arrest).

Cardiorespiratory endurance The capacity of the heart, blood vessels, and lungs to deliver oxygen and nutrients to the working muscles and tissues during sustained exercise and to remove metabolic waste products that would result in fatigue.

Cardiovascular disease (CVD) A general term for any disease of the heart, blood vessels, or circulation.

Carotenoids Any of a group of red, yellow, or orange highly unsaturated pigments that are found in certain foods (e.g., carrots and sweet potatoes).

Carpal tunnel syndrome A pathology of the wrist and hand that occurs when the median nerve, which extends from the forearm into the hand, becomes compressed at the wrist.

Catabolism Metabolic pathways that break down molecules into smaller units and release energy.

Catecholamine Hormone (e.g., epinephrine and norepinephrine) released as part of the sympathetic response to exercise.

Cell body The portion of a nerve cell that contains the nucleus but does not incorporate the dendrites or axon.

Cellulose An indigestible carbohydrate that comprises much of plants.

Center of gravity (COG) *See* Center of mass (COM).

Center of mass (COM) The point around which all weight is evenly distributed; also called center of gravity.

Central nervous system (CNS) The brain and spinal cord.

Cerebral palsy An umbrella term encompassing a group of non-progressive, non-contagious conditions that cause physical disability in human development.

Cerebral vascular disease A group of brain dysfunctions related to disease of blood vessels supplying the brain.

Chemoprophylaxis The use of drugs, nutritional supplements, or other natural substances to prevent future disease.

Chemical digestion A form of digestion that involves the addition of enzymes that break down nutrients.

Cholelithiasis The presence of stones in the gallbladder.

Cholesterol A fatlike substance found in the blood and body tissues and in certain foods. Can accumulate in the arteries and lead to a narrowing of the vessels (atherosclerosis).

Chronic disease Any disease state that persists over an extended period of time.

Chronic obstructive pulmonary disease (COPD) A condition, such as asthma, bronchitis, or emphysema, in which there is chronic obstruction of air flow. *See* Asthma, Bronchitis, *and* Emphysema.

Chronological age The length of time—in years or months since birth—a person has lived.

Chronotropic incompetence An inability to appropriately increase heart rate. Can be genetically acquired or pathologic.

Chylomicron A large lipoprotein particle that transfers fat from food from the small intestines to the liver and adipose tissue.

Chyme The semiliquid mass of partly digested food expelled by the stomach into the duodenum.

Cirrhosis A consequence of chronic liver disease characterized by replacement of liver tissue by fibrous scar tissue (most commonly caused by alcoholism and hepatitis C).

Claudication Cramplike pains in the calves caused by poor circulation of blood to the leg muscles; frequently associated with peripheral vascular disease.

Coefficient of friction The ratio of the force that maintains contact between an object and a surface and the frictional force that resists the motion of the object.

Cofactor A substance that needs to be present along with an enzyme for a chemical reaction to occur.

Cognitive Pertaining to, or characterized by, that operation of the mind by which people become aware of objects of thought or perception; includes all aspects of perceiving, thinking, and remembering.

Cognitive restructuring Intentionally changing the way one perceives or thinks about something.

Collagen The main constituent of connective tissue, such as ligaments, tendons, and muscles.

Comorbidities Disorders (or diseases) in addition to a primary disease or disorder.

Complete protein A food that contains all of the essential amino acids. Eggs, soy, and most meats and dairy products are considered complete proteins.

Complex carbohydrate A long chain of sugar that takes more time to digest than a simple carbohydrate.

Compression fracture A collapse of a vertebra due to trauma or due to a weakened vertebra in a person with osteoporosis.

Compressive force A force squashing, squeezing, or pressing down on an object.

Computed tomography (CT) A development of x-ray technology to examine the soft tissues of the body. Involves recording "slices" of the body with a CT scanner. A cross-sectional image is then formed by computer integration.

Concentric A type of isotonic muscle contraction in which the muscle develops tension and shortens when stimulated.

Congestive heart failure (CHF) Inability of the heart to pump blood at a sufficient rate to meet the metabolic demand or the ability to do so only when the cardiac filling pressures are abnormally high, frequently resulting in lung congestion.

Consequences Variables that occur following a target behavior, such as exercise, that influence a person's future behavior-change decisions and efforts.

Contemplation The stage of the transtheoretical model during which the individual is weighing the pros and cons of behavior change.

Contractility The ability of muscle tissue (cardiac or skeletal) to contract when stimulated.

Contralateral The opposite side of the body; the other limb.

Coronary angiography A medical imaging technique in which an x-ray picture is taken to visualize the inner opening of the coronary arteries.

Coronary artery bypass surgery (CABG) A procedure in which veins are harvested from a patient's leg and sewn from the aorta to the coronary artery past the blockage.

Coronary artery disease (CAD) *See* Coronary heart disease (CHD).

Coronary heart disease (CHD) The major form of cardiovascular disease; results when the coronary arteries are narrowed or occluded, most commonly by atherosclerotic deposits of fibrous and fatty tissue; also called coronary artery disease (CAD).

Corporation A legal entity, independent of its owners and regulated by state laws; any number of people may own a corporation through shares issued by the business.

Cortical bone Compact, dense bone that is found in the shafts of long bones and the vertebral endplates.

Corticosteroid One of two main hormones released by the adrenal cortex; plays a major role in maintaining blood glucose during prolonged exercise by promoting protein and triglyceride breakdown.

Cortisol A hormone that is often referred to as the "stress hormone" as it is involved in the response to stress. It increases blood pressure and blood glucose levels and has an immunosuppressive action.

Creatine A non-prescription dietary supplement that is being promoted for its ability to enhance muscle strength and physical endurance.

Creatine kinase An enzyme present in muscle, brain, and other tissues that catalyzes the reversible conversion of ADP and phosphocreatine into ATP and creatine.

Creatine phosphate (CP) A storage form of high-energy phosphate in muscle cells that can be used to immediately resynthesize adenosine triphosphate (ATP).

Crepitation *See* Crepitus.

Crepitus A crackling sound produced by air moving in the joint space; also called crepitation.

Crescendo angina Angina pectoris that occurs with increasing frequency, intensity, or duration.

Cross-training A method of physical training in which a variety of exercises and changes in body positions or modes of exercise are utilized to positively affect compliance and motivation, and also stimulate additional strength gains or reduce injury risk.

Cryotherapy Treatment of a disorder with ice or by freezing.

Cytokines Hormone-like low molecular weight proteins, secreted by many different cell types, which regulate the intensity and duration of immune responses and are involved in cell-to-cell communication.

De Quervain's syndrome A pathology of the hand that affects the two tendons that move the thumb away from the hand.

Deconditioning Loss of fitness due to inactivity or inadequate training.

Deep vein thrombosis A blood clot in a major vein, usually in the legs and/or pelvis.

Degenerative joint disease (DJD) A non-infectious, progressive disorder of the weightbearing joints. The majority of degenerative joint disease is the result of mechanical instabilities or aging-related changes within the joint.

Dehydration The process of losing body water; when severe can cause serious, life-threatening consequences.

Delayed onset muscle soreness (DOMS) Soreness that occurs 24 to 48 hours after strenuous exercise, the exact cause of which is unknown.

Dendrite The portion of a nerve fiber that transmits impulses toward a nerve cell body; receptive portion of a nerve cell.

Depression 1. The action of lowering a muscle or bone. 2. A condition of general emotional dejection and withdrawal; sadness greater and more prolonged than that warranted by any objective reason.

DEXA scan *See* Dual-energy x-ray absorptiometry (DEXA).

Diabetes *See* Diabetes mellitus.

Diabetes ketoacidosis (DKA) A feature of uncontrolled diabetes mellitus characterized by a combination of ketosis (the accumulation of substances called ketone bodies in the blood) and acidosis (increased acidity of the blood). Symptoms include slow, deep breathing with a fruity odor to the breath; confusion; frequent urination; poor appetite; and eventually loss of consciousness.

Diabetes mellitus A disease of carbohydrate metabolism in which an absolute or relative deficiency of insulin results in an inability to metabolize carbohydrates normally.

Diastasis recti A separation of the recti abdominal muscles along the midline of the body.

Diastolic blood pressure (DBP) The pressure in the arteries during the relaxation phase (diastole) of the cardiac cycle; indicative of total peripheral resistance.

Dietary Approach to Stop Hypertension (DASH) eating plan An eating plan designed to reduce blood pressure; also serves as an overall healthy way of eating that can be adopted by nearly anyone; may also lower risk of coronary heart disease.

Dietary Reference Intake (DRI) A generic term used to refer to three types of nutrient reference values: Recommended Dietary Allowance (RDA), Estimated Average Requirement (EAR), and Tolerable Upper Intake Level (UL).

Dietary supplement A product (other than tobacco) that functions to supplement the diet and contains one or more of the following ingredients: a vitamin, mineral, herb or other botanical, amino acid, dietary substance that increases total daily intake, metabolite, constituent, extract, or some combination of these ingredients.

Dietary Supplement and Health Education Act (DSHEA) A bill passed by Congress in 1994 that sets forth regulations and guidelines for dietary supplements.

Digestion The process of breaking down food into small enough units for absorption.

Discogenic back pain Dysfunction or degeneration of lumbar intervertebral discs.

Diuretic Medication that produces an increase in urine volume and sodium excretion.

Diverticulosis A condition in which the inner, lining layer of the large intestine (colon) bulges out (herniates) through the outer, muscular layer.

Double product Expressed as a product of heart rate in beats per minute times systolic blood pressure. Bears a close relationship with myocardial work or myocardial VO_2.

Down's syndrome Chromosome abnormality resulting in moderate to severe intellectual disability and characteristic appearance of short trunk and extremities, poor muscle tone, hyperflexibility, and congenital heart defects.

Dual-energy x-ray absorptiometry (DEXA) An imaging technique that uses a very low dose of radiation to measure bone density. Also can be used to measure overall body fat and regional differences in body fat.

Dynamic balance The act of maintaining postural control while moving.

Dyslipidemia A condition characterized by abnormal blood lipid profiles; may include elevated cholesterol, triglyceride, or low-density lipoprotein (LDL) levels and/or low high-density lipoprotein (HDL) levels.

Dyslipoproteinemia Blood lipid disorders.

Dysmorphism An anatomical malformation.

Dyspnea Shortness of breath; a subjective difficulty or distress in breathing.

Dysrhythmia A term for a group of conditions in which there is abnormal electrical activity in the heart.

Eating disorder not otherwise specified (EDNOS) An eating disorder that cannot be classified as either anorexia nervosa or bulimia nervosa.

Eclampsia A serious complication of pregnancy that features coma and convulsions before, during, or shortly after childbirth and is characterized by edema, hypertension, and proteinuria.

Edema Swelling resulting from an excessive accumulation of fluid in the tissues of the body.

Eicosanoids Oxygenated fatty acids that the body uses to signal cellular responses; includes omega-3 and omega-6 fatty acids.

Elastic In muscle physiology, the property of muscle tissue that allows it to change in shape under an applied force (stretch) and then recover or return to its original unloaded state when the force is removed.

Electrical muscle stimulation (EMS) A technique to elicit muscle contraction by delivering electric impulses to the muscles.

Electrocardiogram (ECG) A recording of the electrical activity of the heart.

Electrolyte A mineral that exists as a charged ion in the body and that is extremely important for normal cellular function.

Electron transport chain The chain of reactions in which electron transport generates adenosine triphosphate (ATP).

Elevation The action of raising a muscle or bone.

Embolism An obstruction in a blood vessel due to a blood clot or other foreign matter that gets stuck while traveling through the bloodstream.

Empathy Understanding what another person is experiencing from his or her perspective.

Emphysema An obstructive pulmonary disease characterized by the gradual destruction of lung alveoli and the surrounding connective tissue, in addition to airway inflammation, leading to reduced ability to effectively inhale and exhale.

Employee A person who works for another person in exchange for financial compensation. An employee complies with the instructions and directions of his or her employer and reports to them on a regular basis.

Encephalopathy Brain swelling; can result from hyponatremia.

Endocrine Refers to either the gland that secretes directly into the systemic circulation or the substance secreted.

Endothelium Thin, single-celled layer of epithelial cells that line the circulatory system.

Energy balance The balance between energy taken in, generally as food and drink, and energy expended through normal living and physical activity; when caloric intake equals caloric expenditure resulting in no change in body weight. A positive or negative energy balance will cause weight gain or weight loss, respectively.

Engram A specific, learned, and memorized motor pattern stored in both the sensory and motor portions of the brain, that can be replayed on request.

Enzyme A protein that speeds up a specific chemical reaction.

Ephedra A naturally occurring amphetamine-like compound that can powerfully stimulate the nervous system and heart.

Epiglottis The cartilage in the throat that guards the entrance to the trachea and prevents fluid or food from entering it when an individual swallows.

Epinephrine A hormone released as part of the sympathetic response to exercise; also called adrenaline.

Epiphysis The end of a long bone, usually wider than the shaft (plural: epiphyses).

Esophageal sphincter *See* Cardiac sphincter.

Essential amino acids Eight to 10 of the 23 different amino acids needed to make proteins. Called essential because the body cannot manufacture them; they must be obtained from the diet.

Essential fatty acids Fatty acids that the body needs but cannot synthesize; includes linolenic (omega-3) and linoleic (omega-6) fatty acids.

Essential hypertension Hypertension without an identifiable cause; also called primary hypertension.

Estimated Average Requirement (EAR) An adequate intake in 50% of an age- and gender-specific group.

Estradiol An estrogenic hormone, $C_{18}H_{24}O_2$, produced by the ovaries and used in treating estrogen deficiency.

Estrogen Generic term for estrus-producing steroid compounds produced primarily in the ovaries; the female sex hormones.

Etiology The cause of a medical condition.

Euglycemia A normal glucose response.

Excess post-exercise oxygen consumption (EPOC) A measurably increased rate of oxygen uptake following strenuous activity. The extra oxygen is used in the processes (hormone balancing, replenishment of fuel stores, cellular repair, innervation, and anabolism) that restore the body to a resting state and adapt it to the exercise just performed.

Exercise-induced asthma (EIA) *See* Exercise-induced bronchospasm (EIB).

Exercise-induced bronchospasm (EIB) Transient and reversibly airway narrowing triggered by vigorous exercise; also called exercise-induced asthma (EIA).

Exostosis A benign growth of cartilage or bony material that may occur spontaneously or as a result of the margins of a joint knocking against each other.

Expiratory reserve volume The volume of air that can be forcibly exhaled from the lungs following a normal expiration.

Extension The act of straightening or extending, usually applied to the muscular movement of a limb.

Extrinsic motivation Motivation that comes from external (outside of the self) rewards, such as material or social rewards.

Fascia Strong connective tissues that perform a number of functions, including developing and isolating the muscles of the body and providing structural support and protection.

Fast-twitch muscle fiber One of several types of muscle fibers found in skeletal muscle tissue; also called type II fibers and characterized as having a low oxidative capacity but a high gylcolytic capacity; recruited for rapid, powerful movements such as jumping, throwing, and sprinting.

Fat An essential nutrient that provides energy, energy storage, insulation, and contour to the body. 1 gram of fat equals 9 kcal.

Fat-soluble vitamin Vitamins that, when consumed, are stored in the body (particularly the liver and fat tissues); includes vitamins A, D, E, and K.

Fatty acid oxidation The metabolic pathway that, in the presence of oxygen, breaks down fatty acids to produce energy in the form of adenosine triphosphate (ATP).

Fatty acids Long hydrocarbon chains with an even number of carbons and varying degrees of saturation with hydrogen.

Fatty liver The collection of excessive amounts of triglycerides and other fats inside liver cells.

Female athlete triad A condition consisting of a combination of disordered eating, menstrual irregularities, and decreased bone mass in athletic women.

Fiber Carbohydrate chains the body cannot break down for use and which pass through the body undigested.

Fibrinolysis The breakdown of fibrin, usually by the enzymatic action of plasmin.

Fibrosis Excessive formation of fibrous connective tissue.

Flexibility The ability to move joints through their normal full ranges of motion.

Flexion The act of bending a joint so that the two bones forming it are brought closer together.

Fluoroscopy X-ray guidance used to ensure that a medication reaches its intended destination.

Folate A B vitamin that is essential for cell growth and reproduction.

Foramina Holes or openings in a bone or between body cavities.

Force-couple Muscles working as a group to provide opposing, directional, or contralateral pulls to achieve balanced movement.

Forced expiratory volume in 1 second (FEV_1) The amount of air exhaled in the first one second of maximal exhalation.

Forced vital capacity (FVC) The total amount of air that can be forcibly exhaled after a maximal inhalation.

Free fatty acid (FFA) A fatty acid that is only loosely bound to plasma proteins in the blood. Fatty acids are used by the body as a metabolic fuel.

Free radical A chemical group that has unshared electrons available for a reaction. Free radicals can damage the integrity of DNA and have been implicated as a cause of cancers. Antioxidants, such as vitamin C and vitamin E, neutralize free radicals.

Frontal plane A longitudinal section that runs at a right angle to the sagittal plane, dividing the body into anterior and posterior portions.

Fructooligosaccharide A category of oligosaccharides that are mostly indigestible, may help to relieve constipation, improve triglyceride levels, and decrease production of foul-smelling digestive by-products.

Fructose Fruit sugar; the sweetest of the monosaccharides; found in varying levels in different types of fruits.

Functional age A measure of aging using various indications beyond chronological age; these indices include biological age, social age, and psychological age.

Gait The manner or style of walking.

Gait cycle A single sequence of events between two sequential initial contacts by the same limb.

Galactose A monosaccharide; a component of lactose.

Gastric bypass A surgical procedure that creates a very small stomach; the rest of the stomach is removed. The small intestine is attached to the new stomach, allowing the lower part of the stomach to be bypassed.

Gastric emptying The process by which food is emptied from the stomach into the small intestines.

Gastroesophageal reflux disease A chronic condition in which the lower esophageal sphincter allows gastric acids to reflux into the esophagus, causing heartburn, acid indigestion, and possible injury to the esophageal lining.

Gastrointestinal tract A long hollow tube from mouth to anus where digestion and absorption occur.

General partnership A type of business arrangement in which each partner assumes management responsibility and unlimited liability and must have at least a 1% interest in profit and loss.

Gerontology The study of aging.

Gestational diabetes mellitus (GDM) An inability to maintain normal glucose or any degree of glucose intolerance during pregnancy, despite being treated with either diet or insulin.

Ghrelin A hormone produced in the stomach that is responsible for stimulating appetite.

Glucagon A hormone released from the alpha cells of the pancreas when blood glucose levels are low; stimulates glucose release from the liver to increase blood glucose. Also releases free fatty acids from adipose tissue to be used as fuel.

Glucocorticoid An adrenocortical steroid hormone that increases gluconeogenesis, exerts an anti-inflammatory effect, and influences many bodily functions.

Gluconeogenesis The production of glucose from non-sugar substrates such as pyruvate, lactate, glycerol, and glucogenic amino acids.

Glucose A simple sugar; the form in which all carbohydrates are used as the body's principal energy source.

Glycemic index (GI) A ranking of carbohydrates on a scale from 0 to 100 according to the extent to which they raise blood sugar levels.

Glycemic load (GL) A measure of glycemic response to a food that takes into consideration serving size; GL = GI x grams of carbohydrate.

Glycerol A precursor for synthesis of triacylglycerols and of phospholipids in the liver and adipose tissue.

Glycogen The chief carbohydrate storage material; formed by the liver and stored in the liver and muscle.

Glycogenolysis The breakdown of liver and muscle glycogen to yield blood glucose.

Glycosuria An excretion of glucose in the urine.

Glycosylated hemoglobin (HbA1c) A form of hemoglobin used primarily to identify the plasma glucose concentration over prolonged periods of time.

Golgi tendon organ (GTO) A sensory organ within a tendon that, when stimulated, causes an inhibition of the entire muscle group to protect against too much force.

Gout A disorder of purine metabolism, occurring especially in men, characterized by a raised but variable blood uric acid level and severe recurrent acute arthritis of sudden onset, resulting from deposition of crystals of sodium urate in connective tissues and articular cartilage.

Growth hormone A hormone secreted by the pituitary gland that facilitates protein synthesis in the body.

Gynecomastia Atypical breast tissue development in males.

Gynoid Adipose tissue or body fat distributed on the hips and in the lower body (pear-shaped individuals).

Hand-eye coordination The skillful, integrated use of the eyes, arms, hands, and fingers in fine, precision movement.

Heart rate The number of heart beats per minute.

Heart-rate reserve The reserve capacity of the heart; the difference between maximal heart rate and resting heart rate. It reflects the heart's ability to increase the rate of beating and cardiac output above resting level to maximal intensity.

Hemiarthroplasty Partial hip replacement.

Hemicellulose An indigestible fiber.

Hemodynamic Pertaining to the forces involved in the circulation of blood (e.g., heart rate, stroke volume, cardiac output).

Hemoglobin The protein molecule in red blood cells specifically adapted to carry (by bonding with) oxygen molecules.

Herniated disc Rupture of the outer layers of

fibers that surround the gelatinous portion of the disc.

High-density lipoprotein (HDL) A lipoprotein that carries excess cholesterol from the arteries to the liver.

Histology The anatomical study of the microscopic structure of animal and plant tissues.

Homeostasis An internal state of physiological balance.

Homocysteine A normal by-product of metabolism that can promote development of heart disease.

Hormones A chemical substance produced and released by an endocrine gland and transported through the blood to a target organ.

Hydrostatic weighing Weighing a person fully submerged in water. The difference between the person's mass in air and in water is used to calculate body density, which can be used to estimate the proportion of fat in the body.

Hypercalcemia An abnormally high level of calcium in the blood, usually more than 10.5 milligrams per deciliter of blood.

Hypercapnia A condition marked by an unusually high concentration of carbon dioxide in the blood as a result of hypoventilation.

Hypercholesterolemia An excess of cholesterol in the blood.

Hyperglycemia An abnormally high content of glucose (sugar) in the blood (above 100 mg/dL).

Hyperinsulinemia High blood insulin levels.

Hyperkalemia An increase in serum potassium levels.

Hyperparathyroidism Overactivity of the parathyroid glands resulting in excess production of parathyroid hormone (PTH).

Hyperpnea Abnormally deep or rapid breathing.

Hyperosmolar hyperglycemic nonketotic syndrome (HHNS) An emergency condition in which elevated glucose levels are accompanied by dehydration without ketones in the blood or urine.

Hypertension High blood pressure, or the elevation of resting blood pressure above 140/90 mmHg.

Hyperthermia Abnormally high body temperature.

Hypertonic Having extreme muscular tension.

Hypertriglyceridemia An elevated triglyceride concentration in the blood.

Hypertrophic cardiomyopathy A form of cardiomyopathy in which the walls of the heart's chambers thicken abnormally; a major contributory factor to sudden death in young athletes.

Hypertrophy An increase in the cross-sectional size of a muscle in response to progressive resistance training.

Hyperuricemia An unusually high concentration of uric acid in the blood.

Hypoalphalipoproteinemia A deficiency of high-density (alpha) lipoproteins in the blood.

Hypochondriasis A mental disorder characterized by excessive fear of, or preoccupation with, a serious illness, despite medical testing and reassurance to the contrary.

Hypoglycemia A deficiency of glucose in the blood commonly caused by too much insulin, too little glucose, or too much exercise. Most commonly found in the insulin-dependent diabetic and characterized by symptoms such as fatigue, dizziness, confusion, headache, nausea, or anxiety.

Hypoinsulinemia Waning of the insulin dose.

Hyponatremia Abnormally low levels of sodium ions circulating in the blood; severe hyponatremia can lead to brain swelling and death.

Hypothalamic-pituitary-adrenal axis A complex set of direct influences and feedback interactions among the hypothalamus, the pituitary gland, and the adrenal gland. The fine homeostatic interactions between these three organs constitute a major part of the neuroendocrine system that controls reactions to stress and regulates various body processes including digestion, the immune system, mood, and sexuality, as well as energy usage.

Hypothyroidism Underactivity of the thyroid gland, leading to reduced secretion of thyroid hormones and a reduction in resting metabolic rate.

Hypoxia A condition in which there is an inadequate supply of oxygen to tissues.

Ideal body weight A term used to describe the weight that people are expected to weigh for good health, based on age, sex, and height. Also called ideal weight or desirable body weight.

IgE antibodies Often high in people with allergies, they cause the immune system to react to foreign substances such as pollen, fungus, and animal dander; found in the lungs, skin, and mucous membranes.

Iliotibial band friction syndrome (ITBFS) A repetitive overuse condition that occurs when the distal portion of the iliotibial band rubs against the lateral femoral epicondyle.

Immunocompromised Incapable of developing a normal immune response, usually as a result of disease, malnutrition, or immunosuppressive therapy

Impingement syndrome Reduction of space for the supraspinatus muscle and/or the long head of the biceps tendon to pass under the anterior edge of the acromion and coracoacromial ligament; attributed to muscle hypertrophy and inflammation caused by microtraumas.

Incomplete protein A protein that does not contain all of the essential amino acids.

Independent contractor A person who conducts business on his or her own on a contract basis and is not an employee of an organization.

Inflammation A protective tissue response to injury or destruction of tissues, which serves to destroy, dilute, or wall off both the injurious agent and the injured tissues; classic signs include pain, heat, redness, swelling, and loss of function.

Infrared interactance Body-composition assessment method that involves the use of light absorption and reflection to estimate percent fat and fat-free mass; also called near-infrared interactance (NIR).

Inorganic Non-carbon-containing compounds of mineral, as opposed to biologic, origin.

Insoluble fiber The structural part of the plant that does not form a gel in water; it reduces constipation and lowers risk of hemorrhoids and diverticulosis by adding bulk to the feces and reducing transit time in the colon.

Insulin A hormone released from the pancreas that allows cells to take up glucose.

Insulin resistance An inability of muscle tissue to effectively use insulin, where the action of insulin is "resisted" by insulin-sensitive tissues.

Insulin resistance syndrome *See* Metabolic syndrome (MetS).

Insulin-like growth factor Polypeptides structurally similar to insulin that are secreted either during fetal development or during childhood and that mediate growth hormone activity.

Insulin-like growth factor I (IGF-I) *See* Insulin-like growth factor.

Intake assessment The practice of evaluating a new client based on initial assessment and health-history information.

Intermediate-twitch muscle fiber A muscle fiber that has properties somewhere in between fast-twitch and slow-twitch muscle fibers (i.e., it shares characteristics of both).

Intrinsic factor A glycoprotein—or sugar-protein complex—produced in the stomach that allows vitamin B12 to pass to the portal circulation for absorption.

Intrinsic motivation Motivation that comes from internal states, such as enjoyment or personal satisfaction.

Ipsilateral On the same side of the body or limb.

Ischemia A decrease in the blood supply to a bodily organ, tissue, or part caused by constriction or obstruction of the blood vessels.

Isometric A type of muscular contraction in which the muscle is stimulated to generate tension but little or no joint movement occurs.

Joint mobility The range of uninhibited movement around a joint or body segment.

Joint stability The ability to maintain or control joint movement or position.

Kegel exercise Controlled isometric contraction and relaxation of the muscles surrounding the vagina to strengthen and gain control of the pelvic floor muscles.

Ketoacidosis Occurs when a high level of ketones (beta hydroxybutyrate, acetoacetate) are produced as a by-product of fatty-acid metabolism.

Ketone An organic compound (e.g., acetone) with a carbonyl group attached to two carbon atoms. *See* Ketosis.

Ketosis An abnormal increase of ketone bodies in the body; usually the result of a low-carbohydrate diet, fasting, or starvation.

Kinesthesia Awareness of movement.

Korotkoff sounds Five different sounds created by the pulsing of the blood through the brachial artery; proper distinction of the sounds is necessary to determine blood pressure.

Kreb's cycle A series of chemical reactions that act to break pyruvate down to carbon dioxide, water, and many hydrogen-powered molecules known as NADH and FADH2.

Kyphosis Excessive posterior curvature of the spine, typically seen in the thoracic region.

Labrum Fibrocartilage that helps to increase the stability of the shoulder joint.

Lactase An enzyme that is needed to break the bond between the glucose and galactose molecules in lactose so that they can be digested; a deficiency of this enzyme leads to lactose intolerance.

Lactic acid A metabolic by-product of anaerobic glycolysis; when it accumulates it increases blood pH, which slows down enzyme activity and ultimately causes fatigue.

Lacto-ovo-vegetarian A vegetarian that does not eat meat, fish, or poultry.

Lactose A disaccharide; the principal sugar found in milk.

Lactose intolerance A condition that results from a deficiency in the enzyme lactase, which is required to digest lactose; symptoms include cramps, bloating, diarrhea, and flatulence.

Lacto-vegetarian A vegetarian that does not eat eggs, meat, fish, or poultry.

Laminectomy Surgical removal of the posterior arch of a vertebra.

Lapses The expected slips or mistakes that are usually discreet events and are a normal part of the behavior-change process.

Latent Weak and inactive (e.g., muscles).

Lateral epicondylitis An injury resulting from the repetitive tension overloading of the wrist and finger extensors that originate at the lateral epicondyle; often referred to as "tennis elbow."

Laxity Lacking in strength, firmness, or resilience; joints that have been injured or overstretched may exhibit laxity.

Learned helplessness A psychological state in which people have come to believe that they are helpless in, or have no power or control over, certain situations.

Leptin A hormone released from fat cells that acts on the hypothalamus to regulate energy intake. Low leptin levels stimulate hunger and subsequent fat consumption.

Leukocytes White blood cells.

Liability insurance Insurance for bodily injury or property damage resulting from general negligence.

Life expectancy The average number of years a person can expect to live.

Lifespan The maximum number of years an organism from a given species can live.

Ligand A molecule that binds to another chemical entity to form a larger complex.

Lignin An indigestible fiber.

Limited liability corporation (LLC) A form of business ownership that provides limited liability but is taxed liked a partnership. It is not limited to a certain number of shareholders and owners do not have to be U.S. citizens.

Limited partnerships A hybrid organizational form, with both limited and general partners. A limited partner has no voice in management and is legally liable only for the amount of his or her capital contributions, plus any other debt obligations specifically accepted.

Limits of stability (LOS) The degree of allowable sway from the line of gravity without a need to change the base of support.

Line of gravity A theoretical vertical line passing through the center of gravity, dissecting the body into two hemispheres.

Linoleic acid *See* Omega-6 fatty acid.

Linolenic acid *See* Omega-3 fatty acid.

Lipid The name for fats used in the body and bloodstream.

Lipoprotein An assembly of a lipid and protein that serves as a transport vehicle for fatty acids and cholesterol in the blood and lymph.

Locus of control The degree to which people attribute outcomes to internal factors, such as effort and ability, as opposed to external factors, such as luck or the actions of others. People who tend to attribute events and outcomes to internal factors are said to have an internal locus of control, while those who generally attribute outcomes to external factors are said to have an external locus of control.

Lordosis Excessive anterior curvature of the spine that typically occurs at the low back (may also occur at the neck).

Low-density lipoprotein (LDL) A lipoprotein that transports cholesterol and triglycerides from the liver and small intestine to cells and tissues; high levels may cause atherosclerosis.

Lower cross syndrome A muscle imbalance that positions the pelvis in an anterior or posterior tilt.

Lymphatic system A network of lymphoid organs, lymph nodes, lymph ducts, lymphatic tissues, lymph capillaries, and lymph vessels that produces and transports lymph fluid from tissues to the circulatory system.

Ma huang *See* Ephedra.

Macronutrient A nutrient that is needed in large quantities for normal growth and development.

Macrovascular disease Atherosclerotic processes affecting the large vessels of the body, including coronary, cerebral, and peripheral arteries.

Magnetic resonance imaging (MRI) A diagnostic modality in which the patient is placed within a strong magnetic field and the effect of high-frequency radio waves on water molecules within the tissues is recorded. High-speed computers are used to analyze the absorption of radio waves and create a cross-sectional image based upon the variation in tissue signal.

Maintenance The stage of the transtheoretical model during which the individual is incorporating the new behavior into his or her lifestyle.

Maltose Two glucose molecules bound together; used to make beer.

Maximal aerobic capacity *See* $\dot{V}O_2$max.

Maximal oxygen uptake *See* $\dot{V}O_2$max.

Maximum heart rate (MHR) The highest heart rate a person can attain.

Mechanical digestion The process of chewing, swallowing, and propelling food through the gastrointestinal tract.

Medial epicondylitis An injury that results from an overload of the wrist flexors and forearm pronators.

Melatonin A hormone that plays a role in regulating biological rhythms, including sleep and reproductive cycles.

Menisci The plural form of meniscus; cartilage disks that act as a cushion between the ends of bones that meet in the knee joint.

Meniscectomy The surgical removal of all or part of a torn meniscus.

MET *See* Metabolic equivalents (METs).

Metabolic equivalents (METs) A simplified system for classifying physical activities where one MET is equal to the resting oxygen consumption, which is approximately 3.5 milliliters of oxygen per kilogram of body weight per minute (3.5 mL/kg/min).

Metabolic syndrome (MetS) A cluster of factors associated with increased risk for coronary heart disease and diabetes—abdominal obesity indicated by a waist circumference ≥40 inches (102 cm) in men and ≥35 inches (88 cm) in women; levels of triglyceride ≥150 mg/dL (1.7 mmol/L); HDL levels <40 and 50 mg/dL (1.0 and 1.3 mmol/L) in men and women, respectively; blood-pressure levels ≥130/85 mmHg; and fasting blood glucose levels ≥110 mg/dL (6.1 mmol/L).

Microalbuminuria Small amounts of protein leaking into the urine.

Microdiscectomy The surgical removal of herniated disc material that presses on a nerve root or the spinal cord using a special microscope or magnifying instrument to view the disc and nerves.

Microgonadism Small testicles; associated with long-term use of marijuana.

Micronutrient A nutrient that is needed in small quantities for normal growth and development.

Microvascular disease Atherosclerotic processes affecting small vessels of the body, including retina and renal vessels.

Microvilli Tiny hairlike projections on each cell of every villus that can trap nutrient particles and transport them into the cells for absorption.

Mineral Organic substances needed in the diet in small amounts to help regulate bodily functions.

Minute ventilation A measure of the amount of air that passes through the lungs in one minute; calculated as the tidal volume multiplied by the ventilatory rate.

Mitochondria The "power plant" of the cells where aerobic metabolism occurs.

Monosaccharide The simplest form of sugar; it cannot be broken down any further.

Monounsaturated fat *See* Monounsaturated fatty acid.

Monounsaturated fatty acid A type of unsaturated fat (liquid at room temperature) that has one open spot on the fatty acid for the addition of a hydrogen atom (e.g., oleic acid in olive oil).

Morbid obesity Having a body mass index (BMI) of 40.0 or higher or having a BMI of 35.0 or higher in the presence of at least one other significant comorbidity.

Motivation The psychological drive that gives purpose and direction to behavior.

Motor learning The process of acquiring and improving motor skills.

Multiple sclerosis A common neuromuscular disorder involving the progressive degeneration of muscle function, including increased muscle spasticity.

Muscle dysmorphic disorder An exercise disorder characterized by an obsession to be more lean and muscular, with significant amounts of time devoted to weight lifting and a fixation on one's diet; belief that one's body is small and insufficiently muscular; and two of the following: an uncontrolled focus on a fitness regimen causes the person to miss out on career, social, and other activities; circumstances involving body exposure are avoided; performance at work and in social situations is affected by presumed body deficiencies; potentially detrimental effects of the training program fail to dissuade the individual from pursuing hazardous practices.

Muscle endurance *See* Muscular endurance.

Muscle strength *See* Muscular strength.

Muscular dystrophy A hereditary disease in which the muscles gradually weaken and atrophy.

Muscular endurance The ability of a muscle or muscle group to exert force against a resistance over a sustained period of time.

Muscular strength The maximal force a muscle or muscle group can exert during contraction.

Myalgia Diffuse muscular pain, often accompanied by malaise.

Myocardial infarction (MI) An episode in which some of the heart's blood supply is severely cut off or restricted, causing the heart muscle to suffer and die from lack of oxygen. Commonly known as a heart attack.

Myocardial ischemia The result of an imbalance between myocardial oxygen supply and demand, most often caused by atherosclerotic plaques that narrow and sometimes completely block the blood supply to the heart.

Myocarditis Inflammation of the myocardium, which may lead to acute heart failure.

Myocardium Muscle of the heart.

Myofascial release A general manual massage technique used to eliminate general fascial restrictions; typically performed with a device such as a foam roller.

Myofascial sling A continuous line of action formed by muscles, tendons, ligaments, fascia, joint capsules, and bones that lie in series or in parallel to actively moving joints or muscles.

Myoglobin A compound similar to hemoglobin, which aids in the storage and transport of oxygen in the muscle cells.

Myopathy A neuromuscular disease in which the muscle fibers do not function for any one of many reasons, resulting in muscular weakness.

Myosin Thick contractile protein in a myofibril.

Myotatic stretch reflex Muscular reflex created by excessive muscle spindle stimulation to prevent potential tissue damage.

MyPyramid Food Guidance System An educational tool designed to help consumers make healthier food and physical-activity choices for a healthy lifestyle that are consistent with the 2005 USDA Dietary Guidelines.

Narcolepsy A disorder marked by excessive daytime sleepiness, uncontrollable sleep attacks, and a sudden loss of muscle tone, usually lasting up to 30 minutes.

Negative energy balance A state in which the number of calories expended is greater than what is taken in, thereby contributing to weight loss.

Nephropathy Disease of the kidneys.

Nephrotic syndrome A collection of symptoms that occur because the tiny blood vessels in the kidney become leaky, which allows protein to leave the body in large amounts.

Neurogenic claudication Cramping or pain caused by poor blood circulation, accompanied by pain and paresthesias in the back, buttocks, and legs that is relieved by stooping.

Neuromuscular coordination The ability to activate large and small muscles with the correct amount of force in the most efficient sequence to accomplish a task.

Neuropathy Any disease affecting a peripheral nerve. It may manifest as loss of nerve function, burning pain, or numbness and tingling.

Neurotransmitter A chemical substance such as acetylcholine or dopamine that transmits nerve impulses across synapses.

Nonessential amino acid Amino acids that can be made by the body.

Non-exercise activity thermogenesis (NEAT) Physiological processes that produce heat; a relative newly discovered component of energy expenditure.

Nonsteroidal anti-inflammatory drug (NSAID) A drug with analgesic, antipyretic and anti-inflammatory effects. The term "nonsteroidal" is used to distinguish these drugs from steroids, which have similar actions.

Norepinephrine A hormone released as part of the sympathetic response to exercise.

Normoglycemia *See* Euglycemia.

Nuclear magnetic resonance (NMR) A spectroscopy technique that exploits the magnetic properties of certain nuclei that can provide detailed information on the topology, dynamics, and three-dimensional structure of molecules.

Nucleus pulposus The inner gel of intervertebral discs.

Obesity An excessive accumulation of body fat. Usually defined as more than 20% above ideal weight, or over 25% body fat for men and over 32% body fat for women; also can be defined as a body mass index of >30 kg/m^2 or a waist girth of $\geq$40 inches (102 cm) in men and $\geq$35 inches (89 cm) in women.

Obstructive sleep apnea A condition in which breathing stops for more than 10 seconds during sleep due to part of the airway being closed off while a person is trying to inhale during sleep.

Oligosaccharide A chain of about three to 10 or fewer simple sugars.

Omega-3 fatty acid An essential fatty acid that promotes a healthy immune system and helps protect against heart disease and other diseases; found in egg yolk and cold water fish like tuna, salmon, mackerel, cod, crab, shrimp, and oyster. Also known as linolenic acid.

Omega-6 fatty acid An essential fatty acid found in flaxseed, canola, and soybean oils and green leaves. Also known as linoleic acid.

One-repetition maximum (1 RM) The amount of resistance that can be moved through the range of motion one time before the muscle is temporarily fatigued.

Operant conditioning A learning approach that considers the manner in which behaviors are influenced by their consequences.

Organic A compound that contains carbon.

Orthostatic hypotension A drop in blood pressure associated with rising to an upright position.

Osteoarthritis A degenerative disease involving a wearing away of joint cartilage. This degenerative joint disease occurs chiefly in older persons.

Osteoblast The bone-forming cells.

Osteochondritis A degenerative condition that results in a narrowing of the anterior vertebral body at three or more levels secondary to axial and flexion overload.

Osteoclast The cells that reabsorb or erode bone mineral.

Osteonecrosis The destruction and death of bone tissue, which may stem from ischemia, infection, malignant neoplastic disease, or trauma.

Osteopenia Bone density that is below average, classified as 1.5 to 2.5 standard deviations below peak bone density.

Osteoporosis A disorder, primarily affecting postmenopausal women, in which bone density decreases and susceptibility to fractures increases.

Overload The principle that a physiological system subjected to above-normal stress will respond by increasing in strength or function accordingly.

Overtraining Constant intense training that does not provide adequate time for recovery; symptoms include increased resting heart rate, impaired physical performance, reduced enthusiasm and desire for training, increased incidence of injuries and illness, altered appetite, disturbed sleep patterns, and irritability.

Overweight A term to describe an excessive amount of weight for a given height, using height-to-weight ratios.

Oxidant A chemical compound that readily transfers oxygen atoms or a substance that gains electrons in an oxidation-reduction (redox) reaction.

Oxidative phosphorylation The process by which energy from electrons passed through the electron transport chain is captured and stored to produce adenosine triphosphate (ATP).

Oxygen deficit The energy supplied to muscles through anaerobic mechanisms at the start of exercise, before a steady state of oxygen uptake is reached.

Oxygen uptake reserve The difference between maximal oxygen uptake and resting oxygen uptake.

Pancreatitis An inflammation of the pancreas.

Parasthesia An abnormal sensation such as numbness, prickling, or tingling.

Parasympathetic nervous system A division of the autonomic nervous system that governs the resting functions (i.e., the repair and repose response).

Parathryoid hormone (PTH) A chemical substance produced by the parathyroid glands that is a major element in regulating calcium in the body.

Parkinson's disease (PD) A degenerative disorder of the central nervous system that often impairs the sufferer's motor skills and speech; characterized by muscle rigidity, tremor, a slowing of physical movement and, in extreme cases, a loss of physical movement.

Partnership A business entity in which two or more people agree to operate a business and share profits and losses.

Pars intrarticularis The posterior aspect of the spine, where the vertebral body and posterior elements join together.

Patellofemoral pain syndrome (PFPS) A degenerative condition of the posterior surface of the patella, which may result from acute injury to the patella or from chronic friction between the patella and the groove in the femur through which it passes during motion of the knee.

Pathomechanics Mechanical forces that are applied to a living organism and adversely change the body's structure and function.

Pathogenesis The pathologic, physiologic, or biochemical mechanism resulting in the development of a disease.

Pathophysiology The functional changes associated with, or resulting from, disease or injury.

Peak expiratory flow (PEF) A test used to monitor asthma in which the maximal flow of exhaled air following a complete inspiration is recorded.

Pectin An indigestible fiber.

Peptide bond The chemical bond formed between neighboring amino acids, constituting the primary linkage of all protein structures.

Peptide YY A satiety hormone that is released from the intestines.

Percutaneous transluminal coronary angioplasty (PTCA) A procedure that uses a small balloon at the tip of a heart catheter to push open plaques; usually followed by the insertion of a stent.

Periodization The systematic application of overload through the pre-planned variation of program components to optimize gains in strength (or any specific component of fitness), while preventing overuse, staleness, overtraining, and plateaus.

Periostitis Inflammation of the periosteum (connective tissue covering) of the bone.

Peripheral arterial disease All diseases caused by the obstruction of large peripheral arteries, which can result from atherosclerosis, inflammatory processes leading to stenosis, an embolism, or thrombus formation.

Peripheral nervous system The parts of the nervous system that are outside the brain and spinal cord (central nervous system).

Peripheral neuropathy Damage to nerves of the peripheral nervous system, which may be caused either by diseases of the nerve or from the side effects of systemic illness.

Peripheral vascular disease A painful and often debilitating condition, characterized by muscular pain caused by ischemia to the working muscles. The ischemic pain is usually due to atherosclerotic blockages or arterial spasms, referred to as claudication. Also called peripheral vascular occlusive disease (PVOD).

Peristalsis The process by which muscles in the esophagus and intestines push food through the gastrointestinal tract in a wave-like motion.

Pes cavus High arches of the feet.

Pes planus Flat feet.

Pharmacokinetics The absorption, distribution, metabolism, and excretion of drugs.

Phase III clinical trial Trials performed after preliminary evidence suggesting effectiveness of the drug has been obtained in Phase II; are intended to gather the additional information about effectiveness and safety that is needed to evaluate the overall benefit-risk relationship of the drug; provide an adequate basis for extrapolating the results to the general population and transmitting that information in the physician labeling; usually include several hundred to several thousand people.

Pheochromocytoma An epinephrine-secreting tumor on the adrenal gland.

Phosphagen system A system of transfer of chemical energy from the breakdown of creatine phosphate to regenerate adenosine triphosphate (ATP).

Photokeratitis A burn of the cornea by ultraviolet B rays (UVB).

Physical Activity Readiness Medical Exam Form (PARmed-X) A screening tool used with special populations in conjunction with a physician.

Physical Activity Readiness Questionnaire (PAR-Q) A brief, self-administered medical questionnaire recognized as a safe pre-exercise screening measure for low-to-moderate (but not vigorous) exercise training.

Phytochemical A biologically active, non-nutrient component found in plants; includes antioxidants.

Placenta The vascular organ in mammals that unites the fetus to the maternal uterus and mediates its metabolic exchanges.

Plasma The liquid portion of the blood.

Plastic In muscle physiology, the property of muscle tissue that allows a permanent change in length after an elongation force (stretch) is applied.

Platelet One of the disc-shaped components of the blood involved in clotting.

Plyometrics High-intensity movements, such as jumping, involving high-force loading of body weight during the landing phase of the movement.

Points of contact (POC) The points where the body makes contact with the ground or surface; an aspect of the body's base of support.

Polydipsia Excessive thirst.

Polypeptide A linear chain of amino acids.

Polyphagia Constant hunger.

Polysaccharide A long chain of sugar molecules.

Polyunsaturated fat *See* Polyunsaturated fatty acid.

Polyunsaturated fatty acid A type of unsaturated fat (liquid at room temperature) that has two or more spots on the fatty acid available for hydrogen (e.g., corn, safflower, soybean oils).

Polyuria Frequent urination.

Portal circulation A circulatory system that takes nutrients directly from the stomach, small intestines, colon, and spleen to the liver.

Positive energy balance A situation when the storage of energy exceeds the amount expended. This state may be achieved by either consuming too many calories or by not using enough.

Post-exercise hypotension (PEH) Acute post-exercise reduction in both systolic and diastolic blood pressure.

Postprandial glycemia The concentration of glucose in the blood after eating.

Postprandial lipemia The transient excess of lipids in the blood occurring after the ingestion of foods with a large content of fat; hyperlipemia.

Precontemplation The stage of the transtheoretical model during which the individual is not yet thinking about changing.

Preeclampsia A serious maternal-fetal disease that is diagnosed after 20 weeks of gestation and characterized by persistent hypertension (>140/90 mm/Hg) and proteinuria (24-hour urinary protein level ≥0.3 g).

Prehypertension A blood pressure equal to or greater than 120/80 mmHg.

Premature atrial contraction (PAC) An abnormal heartbeat that originates in the atria and precedes a typical atrial contraction.

Premature ventricular contraction (PVC) A form of irregular heartbeat in which the ventricle contracts prematurely, resulting in a "skipped beat" followed by a stronger beat; also called heart palpitations.

Preparation The stage of the transtheoretical model during which the individual is getting ready to make a change.

Pressor response A disproportionate rise in heart rate during resistance training resulting from autonomic nervous system reflex activity.

Primary hypertension *See* Essential hypertension.

Primary prevention Measures provided to individuals to prevent the onset of a targeted condition.

Process goal A goal a person achieves by doing something, such as completing an exercise session or attending a talk on stress management.

Product goal A goal that represents change in a measurable variable, such as increases in strength scores, reductions in resting heart rate, or weight loss.

Progesterone Hormone produced by the corpus luteum, adrenal cortex, and placenta, the function of which is to facilitate growth of the embryo.

Progressive resistive exercise (PRE) A resistance-training exercise program that employs a systematic increase in repetitions and weight to gradually stress the muscles involved, leading to increased strength.

Proprioception Sensation and awareness of body position and movements.

Proprioceptive neuromuscular facilitation

(PNF) A method of promoting the response of neuromuscular mechanisms through the stimulation of proprioceptors in an attempt to gain more stretch in a muscle; often referred to as a contract/relax method of stretching.

Proprioceptors Somatic sensory receptors in muscles, tendons, ligaments, joint capsules, and skin that gather information about body position and the direction and velocity of movement.

Prostatitis An inflammation of the prostate.

Protection motivation theory A health-risk-reduction theory that emphasizes action based on the severity of a threatened event.

Protein A compound composed of a combination 20 amino acids that is the major structural component of all body tissue.

Protein complementarity Combinations of incomplete plant proteins that together provide all of the essential amino acids.

Protein digestibility corrected amino acid score (PDCAAS) Estimates protein quality by multiplying a particular food protein's chemical score (essential amino acid content in a protein food divided by the amino acid content in a reference protein food) by its digestibility.

Protein efficiency ratio (PER) A measure of protein quality based on experiments with lab animals.

Proteinuria The presence of an excess of serum proteins in the urine.

Protraction Scapular abduction.

Provitamin Inactive vitamins; the human body contains enzymes to convert them into active vitamins.

Pseudoclaudication Pain in the buttock, thigh, or leg that occurs with standing or walking and is relieved by rest in a lying or sitting position, or by flexing forward at the waist.

Pseudotumor cerebri Rare condition in which cerebrospinal fluid outflow is partially obstructed.

Pulmonary function tests (PFTs) A group of tests that measure how well the lungs take in and release air and how well they move oxygen into the blood; includes spirometry, lung volume measures, and diffusion capacity.

Pulmonary hypertension An increase in blood pressure in the pulmonary artery or lung vasculature, leading to shortness of breath, dizziness, fainting, and other symptoms, all of which are exacerbated by exertion.

Pyloric sphincter Separates the stomach from the small intestines.

Pyruvate A biochemical involved in the Kreb's cycle that facilitates adenosine triphosphate production.

Q-angle The angle formed by lines drawn from the anterior superior iliac spine (ASIS) to the central patella and from the central patella to the tibial tubercle; an estimate of the effective angle at which the quadriceps group pulls on the patella.

Quadriplegia Partial or complete paralysis of all four extremities and trunk, including the respiratory muscles from lesions of the cervical cord.

Quantitative computed tomography (QCT) A computerized x-ray technique that uses electronic systems to measure volumetric bone mineral density, plus other measures such as the stress-strain index (SSI) and the geometry of the bone.

Quantitative ultrasound (QUS) A bone density test using sound waves.

Radionuclide stress testing A diagnostic test for coronary artery disease that involves injecting a radioactive isotope (typically thallium or cardiolyte) into the person's vein, after which an image of the heart becomes visible with a special camera.

Range of motion (ROM) The number of degrees that an articulation will allow one of its segments to move.

Rapport A relationship marked by mutual understanding and trust.

Rate-pressure product *See* Double product.

Ratings of perceived exertion (RPE) A scale, originally developed by noted Swedish psychologist Gunnar Borg, that provides a standard means for evaluating a participant's perception of exercise effort. The original scale ranged from 6 to 20; a revised category-ratio scale ranges from 0 to 10.

Recommended Dietary Allowance (RDA) The levels of intake of essential nutrients that, on the basis of scientific knowledge, are judged by the Food and Nutrition Board to be adequate to meet the known needs of practically all healthy persons.

Reduce To restore to the normal place or relation of parts, as to reduce a fracture.

Relapses In behavior change, the return of an original problem after many lapses (slips, mistakes) have occurred.

Relative contraindication A condition that makes a particular treatment or procedure somewhat inadvisable but does not completely rule it out.

Relaxin A hormone of pregnancy that relaxes the pelvic ligaments and other connective tissue in the body.

Renal failure The inability of the kidneys to excrete wastes and to help maintain the electrolyte balance; loss of kidney function.

Renin An enzyme of high specificity that is released by the kidneys and acts to raise blood pressure by activating angiotensin.

Renin-angiotensin-aldosterone system (RAAS) A hormone system that helps regulate long-term blood pressure and extracellular volume in the body.

Residual volume The volume of air remaining in the lungs following a maximal expiration.

Respiratory acidosis A condition in which a build-up of carbon dioxide in the blood produces a shift in the body's pH balance and causes the body's system to become more acidic, resulting in slowed or difficult breathing.

Respiratory synctial virus (RSV) A virus that causes cold-like symptoms but can cause breathing difficulties if the lower respiratory tract (i.e., the lungs) becomes involved.

Resorption The removal stage of the bone remodeling cycle.

Restenosis Recurrent stenosis, or narrowing, of a blood vessel or tubular organ after a surgical correction such as angioplasty.

Resting metabolic rate (RMR) The number of calories expended per unit time at rest; measured early in the morning after an overnight fast and at least eight hours of sleep; approximated with various formulas.

Retinopathy Any non-inflammatory disease of the retina.

Retraction Scapular adduction.

Reversibility The principle of exercise training that suggests that any improvement in physical fitness due to physical activity is entirely reversible with the discontinuation of the training program.

Rheumatoid arthritis An autoimmune disease that causes inflammation of connective tissues and joints.

Risk management Minimizing the risks of potential legal liability.

Rotation Movement in the transverse plane about a longitudinal axis; can be "internal" or "external."

Sagittal plane The longitudinal plane that divides the body into right and left portions.

Saliva Water, salt, and enzyme secretion from the salivary glands that begins digestion.

Sarcomere The basic functional unit of the myofibril containing the contractile proteins that generate skeletal muscle movements.

Sarcopenia Decreased muscle mass; often used to refer specifically to an age-related decline in muscle mass or lean-body tissue.

Satiety A feeling of fullness.

Saturated fat *See* Saturated fatty acid.

Saturated fatty acid A fatty acid that contains no double bonds between carbon atoms; typically solid at room temperature and very stable.

Scaphoid Concave.

Scheuermann's disease A growth disorder characterized by inflammation and osteochondritis of the thoracic vertebrae. This degenerative condition narrows the anterior vertebral body at three or more levels secondary to axial and flexion overload.

Sciatica Pain radiating down the leg caused by compression of the sciatic nerve; frequently the result of lumbar disk herniation.

Scoliosis Excessive lateral curvature of the spine.

Scope of practice The range and limit of responsibilities normally associated with a specific job or profession.

S-Corp A form of business ownership taxed as though it were a partnership. It provides limited liability and is restricted to 75 shareholders and one class of stock. All shareholders must be U.S. citizens and cannot be corporations or partnerships.

Secondary hypertension Hypertension without an identifiable cause.

Secondary prevention The identification and treatment of asymptomatic persons who have already developed risk factors or preclinical disease but in whom the condition is not clinically apparent.

Sedentary Doing or requiring much sitting; minimal activity.

Self–blood glucose monitoring The process of collecting detailed information about blood glucose levels at many time points to enable maintenance of a more constant glucose level.

Self-determination theory A psychological theory suggesting that people need to feel competent, autonomous, and connected to others in the many domains of life.

Self-efficacy One's perception of his or her ability to change or perform specific behaviors (e.g., exercise).

Senescence The process or condition of growing old.

Sensory integration dysfunction A neurological disorder characterized by disruption in the processing and organization of sensory information by the central nervous system; characterized by impaired sensitivity to sensory input, motor control problems, unusually high or low activity levels, and emotional instability.

Sequelae Morbid conditions following or occurring as a consequence of another condition or event.

Serape effect A myofascial sling that facilitates rotational movements of the torso.

Serum cholesterol The level of total cholesterol in the bloodstream.

Shaping Designing a new behavior chain, including antecedents and rewards, to encourage a certain behavior, such as regular physical activity.

Shear force Any force that causes slippage between a pair of contiguous joints or tissues in a direction that parallels the plane in which they contact.

Simple carbohydrate Short chains of sugar that are rapidly digested.

Simple diffusion A process by which molecules diffuse across a membrane based on a concentration gradient without the assistance of a protein carrier.

Sleep apnea The general condition in which breathing stops for more than 10 seconds during sleep.

Slow-twitch muscle fiber A muscle fiber type designed for use of aerobic glycolysis and fatty acid oxidation, recruited for low-intensity, longer-duration activities such as walking and swimming.

SMART goals A properly designed goal; SMART stands for specific, measurable, attainable, relevant, and time-bound.

SOAP note A communication tool used among healthcare professionals; SOAP stands for subjective, objective, assessment, plan.

Sole proprietorship A business owned and operated by one person.

Soluble fiber A type of fiber that forms gels in water; may help prevent heart disease and stroke by binding bile and cholesterol; diabetes by slowing glucose absorption; and constipation by holding moisture in stools and softening them.

Somatosensory system The physiological system relating to the perception of sensory stimuli from the skin and internal organs.

Somnolence A state of drowsiness; sleepiness.

Specificity Exercise training principle explaining that specific exercise demands made on the body produce specific responses by the body; also called exercise specificity.

Spina bifida occulta A serious birth abnormality

in which the spinal cord is malformed and lacks its usual protective skeletal and soft tissue coverings, but is covered by a layer of skin. This form of spina bifida rarely causes disability or symptoms.

Spinal stenosis A medical condition in which the spinal canal narrows and compresses the spinal cord and nerves.

Spirometry Pulmonary function testing that measures lung function by assessing the amount (volume) and/or speed (flow) of air that can be maximally inhaled and exhaled; used in the diagnosis and management of asthma.

Spondylolithesis Forward displacement of one vertebra over another; usually occurs at the 4th or 5th lumbar vertebrae.

Spondylolysis A stress fracture in the posterior aspect of the spine.

Sprain A traumatic joint twist that results in stretching or tearing of the stabilizing connective tissues; mainly involves ligaments or joint capsules, and causes discoloration, swelling, and pain.

Stable angina Typical set of symptoms (discomfort in chest, a heavy, viselike, and/or squeezing pain that often radiates to the shoulders, jaw or neck) that usually occurs at predictable times, such as during stress or exercise; once activity ceases, the pain usually goes away.

Standard of care Appropriateness of an exercise professional's actions in light of current professional standards and based on the age, condition, and knowledge of the participant.

Starch A plant carbohydrate found in grains and vegetables.

Static balance The ability to maintain the body's center of mass (COM) within its base of support (BOS).

Stenosis The narrowing of any tube-like structure within the body (e.g., coronary artery stenosis, spinal stenosis).

Stimulant A substance that activates the central nervous system and sympathetic nervous system.

Stimulus control A means to break the connection between events or other stimuli and a behavior; in behavioral science, sometimes called "cue extinction."

Strain A stretch, tear, or rip in the muscle or adjacent tissue such as the fascia or tendon.

Stress echocardiography Cardiac ultrasound; the sound waves of an ultrasound are used to produce images of the heart at rest and at the peak of exercise.

Stress urinary incontinence The involuntary loss of urine that occurs with physical exertion and a rise in abdominal pressure.

Stroke A sudden and often severe attack due to blockage of an artery into the brain.

Stroke volume The amount of blood pumped from the left ventricle of the heart with each beat.

Subacute The characteristic of a condition intermediate between chronic and acute inflammation, exhibiting some of the characteristics of each.

Subluxation An incomplete dislocation; though relationship is altered, contact between joint surfaces remains.

Sucrose Table sugar; a disaccharide formed by glucose and fructose linked together.

Supraventricular dysrhythmia Any abnormal cardiac rhythm originating above the ventricles.

Sympathetic nervous system A division of the autonomic nervous system that activates the body to cope with some stressor (i.e., the fight or flight response).

Sympathomimetic A characteristic of medications that mimic the effects of the sympathetic nervous system.

Symphysitis Irritation of the pubic symphysis caused by increased motion at the joint.

Synapse The region of communication between neurons.

Syncope A transient state of unconsciousness during which a person collapses to the floor as a result of lack of oxygen to the brain; commonly known as fainting.

Syndrome X *See* Metabolic syndrome (MetS).

Synergistic dominance A condition in which the synergists carry out the primary function of a weakened or inhibited prime mover.

Synovial cell Fibroblasts lying between the

cartilaginous fibers in the synovial membrane of a joint.

Synovial fluid Transparent, viscous lubricating fluid found in joint cavities, bursae, and tendon sheaths.

Synovial membrane The connective-tissue membrane that lines the cavity of a synovial joint and produces the synovial fluid; also called synovium.

Synovium *See* Synovial membrane.

Systolic blood pressure (SBP) The pressure exerted by the blood on the vessel walls during ventricular contraction.

Tachycardia Elevated heart rate over 100 beats per minute.

Tendinitis Inflammation of a tendon.

Tendonosis A condition that involves microscopic tears of the tendon caused by repeated trauma.

Tenosynovitis An inflammation of the synovial sheath that surrounds a tendon.

Teratogenic Nongenetic factors that can cause birth defects in the fetus.

Tertiary prevention The care of established disease, with attempts made to minimize the negative effects of disease, restore optimal function, and prevent disease-related complications.

Testosterone The steroid hormone produced in the testes; involved in growth and development of reproductive tissues, sperm, and secondary male sex characteristics.

Thermic effect of food An increase in energy expenditure due to digestive processes (digestion, absorption, metabolism of food). Also called thermic effect of feeding.

Thermoregulation Regulation of the body's temperature.

Thrombophlebitis Inflammation of a vein.

Thyroid hormone Hormones secreted by the thyroid gland and responsible for controlling the metabolic rate.

Tidal volume The volume of air inspired per breath.

Tolerable Upper Intake Level (UL) The maximum intake of a nutrient that is unlikely to pose risk of adverse health effects to almost all individuals in an age- and gender-specific group.

Total peripheral resistance (TPR) The resistance to the passage of blood through the small blood vessels, especially arterioles.

Trabecular bone Spongy or cancellous bone composed of thin plates that form a honeycomb pattern; predominantly found in the ends of long bones and the vertebral bodies.

Trace element An element essential to nutrition or physiologic processes, found in such minute quantities that analysis yields a presence of virtually none.

Trans fats *See* Trans fatty acid.

Trans fatty acid An unsaturated fatty acid that is converted into a saturated fat to increase the shelf life of some products.

Transcient ischemia Momentary dizziness, loss of consciousness, or forgetfulness caused by a short-lived lack of oxygen (blood) to the brain; usually due to a partial blockage of an artery, it is a warning sign for stroke.

Transcutaneous electrical nerve stimulation (TENS) A technique used for pain relief in which nerves are electronically stimulated to block the transmission of pain information to the brain.

Transferrin A protein in blood plasma that carries iron derived from food intake to the liver, spleen, and bone marrow.

Transitional vertebra A malformation of the spine where one vertebra has the characteristics of two types of vertebrae typically occurring at the cervicothoracic, thoracolumbar, or lumbosacral junction.

Translate The act of moving a rigid body in which all parts move in the same direction at the same speed.

Transtheoretical model of behavior change (TTM) A theory of behavior that examines one's readiness to change and identifies five stages: precontemplation, contemplation, preparation, action, and maintenance.

Transtheoretical stages of change *See* Transtheoretical model of behavior change (TTM).

Transverse plane Anatomical term for the imaginary line that divides the body, or any of its parts, into upper (superior) and lower (inferior) parts. Also called horizontal plane.

Trendelenburg gait A drop of the pelvis on the side opposite of the stance leg, indicating weakness on the side of the stance leg.

Triacylglycerol Stored triglycerides.

Trigger *See* Antecedent.

Triglyceride Three fatty acids joined to a glycerol (carbon and hydrogen structure) backbone; how fat is stored in the body.

Trochanteric bursitis The painful inflammation of the bursa surrounding the greater trochanter of the femur.

Type 1 diabetes *See* Type 1 diabetes mellitus (T1DM).

Type 1 diabetes mellitus (T1DM) Form of diabetes caused by the destruction of the insulin-producing beta cells in the pancreas, which leads to little or no insulin secretion; generally develops in childhood and requires regular insulin injections; formerly known as insulin-dependent diabetes mellitus (IDDM) and childhood-onset diabetes.

Type 2 diabetes *See* Type 2 diabetes mellitus (T2DM).

Type 2 diabetes mellitus (T2DM) Most common form of diabetes; typically develops in adulthood and is characterized by a reduced sensitivity of the insulin target cells to available insulin; usually associated with obesity; formerly known as non-insulin-dependent diabetes mellitus (NIDDM) and adult-onset diabetes.

Unsaturated fatty acids Fatty acids that contain one or more double bonds between carbon atoms; typically liquid at room temperature and fairly unstable, making them susceptible to oxidative damage and a shortened shelf life.

Unstable angina In contrast to stable angina, unstable angina occurs in individuals at unpredictable times, or even at rest; unstable angina may progress to a myocardial infarction.

Valsalva maneuver A strong exhaling effort against a closed glottis, which builds pressure in the chest cavity that interferes with the return of the blood to the heart; may deprive the brain of blood and cause lightheadedness or fainting.

Valgus Characterized by an abnormal outward turning of a bone, especially of the hip, knee, or foot.

Varus Characterized by an abnormal inward turning of a bone, especially of the hip, knee, or foot.

Vasoconstriction Narrowing of the opening of blood vessels (notably the smaller arterioles) caused by contraction of the smooth muscle lining the vessels.

Vasodilation Increase in diameter of the blood vessels, especially dilation of arterioles leading to increased blood flow to a part of the body.

Vasopressin Hormone released by the posterior pituitary gland during exercise; reduces urinary excretion of water and prevents dehydration.

Vegan A vegetarian that does not consume any animal products, including dairy products such as milk and cheese.

Vegetarian A person who does not eat meat, fish, poultry, or products containing these foods.

Ventilatory rate The number of breaths per minute.

Ventricular function Function of heart muscle's (myocardium) contraction mechanics. For example, ventricular ejection fraction is a measure of ventricular contractility (rate and force with which the myocardium contracts).

Ventricular tachycardia A rapid heart beat (usually at least 100 beats per minute) that originates in one of the ventricles of the heart.

Vertical banded gastroplasty A gastroplasty for the treatment of morbid obesity in which an upper gastric pouch is formed by a vertical staple line, with a cloth band applied to prevent dilation at the outlet into the main pouch.

Vestibular system Part of the central nervous system that coordinates reflexes of the eyes, neck, and body to maintain equilibrium in accordance with posture and movement of the head.

Villi Finger-like projections from the folds of the small intestines.

Visceral Pertaining to the internal organs.

Visceral adiposity *See* Visceral obesity.

Visceral obesity Excess fat located deep in the abdomen that surrounds the vital organs; closely related to abdominal girth. Its accumulation is associated with insulin resistance, glucose intolerance, dyslipidemia, hypertension, and coronary artery disease. Abdominal girth measured at the level of the umbilicus with values ≥40 inches (102 cm) in men and ≥35 inches (89 cm) in women are strong indicators of visceral obesity.

Visual system The series of structures by which visual sensations are received from the environment and conveyed as signals to the central nervous system.

Vital capacity The volume of air that can be maximally inhaled and exhaled in one breath.

Vitamin An organic micronutrient that is essential for normal physiologic function.

$\dot{V}O_2$max Considered the best indicator of cardiovascular endurance, it is the maximum amount of oxygen (mL) that a person can use in one minute per kilogram of body weight. Also called maximal oxygen uptake and maximal aerobic capacity.

Waist circumference Abdominal girth measured at the level of the umbilicus; values ≥40 inches (102 cm) in men and ≥35 inches (89 cm) in women are strong indicators of abdominal obesity and associated with an increased health risk.

Waist-to-hip ratio A useful measure for determining health risk due to the site of fat storage. Calculated by dividing the ratio of abdominal girth (waist measurement) by the hip measurement.

Water-soluble vitamins Vitamins that require adequate daily intake since the body excretes excesses in the urine; dissolvable in water.

Xanthine A chemical compound that is a precursor of uric acid and is found in blood, urine, and muscle tissue.

Yogic breathing A pattern or breathing technique based on the principles of yoga. Also referred to as pranayama, the science of breath control. There are many styles of yogic breathing.

INDEX

A

B

C

D

E

F

G

H

I

J

K

M

N

O

P

Q

R

S

T

U

V

W

X

Y

Z